HANDBOOK OF
EXPERIMENTAL IMMUNOLOGY

Handbook of
Experimental Immunology

EDITED BY

D.M.WEIR

M.D.(Edin.)

Immunology Unit, Bacteriology Department
University of Edinburgh Medical School

BLACKWELL SCIENTIFIC PUBLICATIONS
OXFORD AND EDINBURGH

© Blackwell Scientific Publications 1967

This book is copyright. It may not be
reproduced by any means in whole or
in part without permission. Application
with regard to copyright should be
addressed to the publisher.

SBN: 632 04330 X

First Published 1967

Printed in Great Britain in the City of Oxford at
THE ALDEN PRESS
and bound at
THE KEMP HALL BINDERY, OXFORD

Contents

v

Section 2 · Antigens

Section 3 · Methods for the Study and Demonstration of Antigen-Antibody Interaction

PART A · METHODS UTILIZING PRIMARY INTERACTION

Contents

Contributors

APPLEYARD, G. *Microbiological Research Establishment, Porton, Salisbury, Wiltshire*

ANDRES, GIUSEPPE A. *Instituto di Patologia Medica, Università di Roma, Rome*

AUGUSTIN, ROSA *Immunochemistry Unit (Cancer Research), University of Liverpool*

BATCHELOR J.R. *Department of Pathology, Guy's Hospital, Medical School, London, SE*1

BITENSKY, LUCILLE *The Mathilda and Terence Kennedy Institute of Rheumatology, Hammersmith, London, W*6

BROCKLEHURST W.E. *Pharmacology Department, University of Edinburgh*

DAVIES D.A.L. *Searle & Co. Ltd, Lane End Road, High Wycombe, Bucks.*

DRESSER D.W. *National Institute for Medical Research, Mill Hill, London, NW*7

FAHEY J.L. *Immunology Branch, National Cancer Institute, National Institutes of Health, Bethesda, Md.*

FARR, RICHARD S. *Division of Allergy, Immunology and Rheumatology, Scripps Clinic and Research Foundation, La Jolla, California*

FREEMAN, TRISTRAM *Medical Research Council, National Institute for Medical Research, Mill Hill, London*

FURTH R. VAN *Department of Microbial Diseases, University Hospital, Leiden, The Netherlands*

GESNER B.M. *Department of Medicine, New York University*

HERBERT W.J. *Trypanosomiasis Research Unit, Royal (Dick) School of Veterinary Studies, University of Edinburgh*

HOLBOROW E.J. *Medical Research Council, Rheumatism Research Unit, Taplow, Maidenhead, Berks.*

HOWARD J.G. *Cellular Immunology Unit, Zoology Department, University of Edinburgh*

HSU, KONRAD C. *Department of Microbiology, Columbia University, New York*

A*   ix

HUNTER W.M. *Medical Research Council, Clinical Endocrinology Research Unit, Edinburgh*

JOHNSON G.D. *Medical Research Council, Rheumatism Research Unit, Taplow, Maidenhead, Berks.*

LAWLER, SYLVIA D. *Department of Clinical Research, Royal Marsden Hospital, London SW3*

LEVINE, LAWRENCE *Graduate Department of Biochemistry, Brandeis University, Waltham, Massachusetts*

LONGBOTTOM, JOAN L. *Medical Research Council, Clinical Immunology Research Group, Department of Medicine, Institute of Diseases of the Chest, London SW3*

LUMSDEN W.H.R. *Trypanosomiasis Research Unit, Royal (Dick) School of Veterinary Studies, University of Edinburgh*

LUTZ W. *Department of Social Medicine, University of Edinburgh*

MICHIE D. *Department of Machine Intelligence and Perception, University of Edinburgh*

MINDEN, PERCY *Division of Allergy, Immunology and Rheumatology, Scripps Clinic and Research Foundation, La Jolla, California*

ÖUCHTERLONY O. *Department of Bacteriology, University of Göteborg*

PARDOE, GRACE I. *Department of Experimental Pathology, University of Birmingham, England*

PARKER, CHARLES W. *Division of Allergy and Immunology, Department of Medicine, Washington University School of Medicine, St. Louis, Missouri*

PEPYS J. *Medical Research Council, Clinical Immunology Research Group, Department of Medicine, Institute of Diseases of the Chest, London SW3*

PINCKARD R.N. *Immunology Unit, Department of Bacteriology, University of Edinburgh*

SEEGAL, BEATRICE C. *Department of Microbiology, Columbia University, New York*

SOULSBY E.J.L. *Department of Parasitology, University of Pennsylvania, Philadelphia*

STANWORTH D.R. *Department of Experimental Pathology, University of Birmingham, England*

STELOS, PETER *Hahnemann Medical College and Hospital, Philadelphia*

STUART A.E. *Immunopathology Research Unit, Pathology Department, University of Edinburgh*

SUTHERLAND I.W. *Sub-Department of General Microbiology, University of Edinburgh*

TERRY, ELIZABETH W. *Immunology Branch, National Cancer Institute, National Institutes of Health, Bethesda, Md.*

TYRRELL D.A.J. *Medical Research Council and Ministry of Health, National*

Institute for Medical Research, Common Cold Research Unit, Salisbury, Wiltshire

WEIR D.M. *Immunology Unit, Department of Bacteriology, University of Edinburgh*

WORTIS H.H. *National Institute for Medical Research, Mill Hill, London NW7*

ZWARTOUW H.T. *Microbiological Research Establishment, Porton, Salisbury, Wiltshire*

Preface

The aim of this volume is to bring together discussion of the underlying principles, practical details and applications of some widely used procedures in experimental and applied immunology and to include other less well-known methods such as fluorescence polarization and radioimmunoassay techniques which may have potential applications. Many of the methods dealt with here have been described in journals and other publications often in the materials and methods section of a paper when the underlying principles, limitations and applications of the procedure have necessarily received scant attention.

The book is primarily intended for the experimental immunologist with some background laboratory knowledge; however, it is hoped that some of the descriptions and discussion will be of interest to workers in applied immunological fields.

The scope of the volume is not exhaustive and it is hoped in future editions to widen the field covered and perhaps alter the balance as trends demand. The subjects have been grouped so as to deal with some of the experimental procedures used in the study of immunoglobulins, their isolation and properties and the preparation of antigens from bacteria, viruses and tissues. These sections are followed by discussion of methods involving antigen-antibody reactions including their application, in the later chapters of this section, to the study of fungi, viruses, protozoa and helminths. Methods for the study of 'cellular' immune reactions are grouped in section 4. This division is convenient but admittedly arbitrary as the mechanisms do not depend only on cellular reactions and may in fact involve locally acting immunoglobulins produced by sensitized cells, e.g. Chapter 33, 'Localized Haemolysis in Gel', or circulating immunoglobulins acting as opsonins. After a description of some methods used in the study of allergic reactions, a section on statistical methods is appended with particular application to immunological data.

I would like to thank the many contributors for their hard work and co-operation in the production of this volume, Dr W.J.Herbert and Dr H.K. Ghosh for kindly providing much of the immunological data used in the statistical appendix, my colleague Dr. R.N.Pinckard for helpful discussion, and Professor Robert Cruickshank for support and encouragement throughout. Miss S.McDiarmid kindly helped with the large correspondence involved in the planning and allocation of the chapters and Mrs D.E.J.Suckling prepared the index. Finally, I should particularly like to acknowledge the continued guidance and encouragement of Mr Per Saugman of Blackwell Scientific Publications and his colleague Mr J.L.Robson for his help in the production of the volume.

D.M.WEIR

SECTION 1
Antibodies

PART A

ISOLATION OF
IMMUNOGLOBULIN

CHAPTER 1

Salt Fractionation

PETER STELOS

Introduction

The isolation of proteins by precipitating them out of solution with high concentrations of neutral salts has been in use for about a century. Salt fractionation procedures have been replaced in part by newer methods such as electrophoresis, chromatography and gel filtration (see Chapters 2 and 3). It is still a useful procedure, particularly when dealing with large volumes of protein solutions. In practice, it is often found that several methods are needed to obtain a protein preparation having a reasonable degree of purity. For example, the γM and γG globulin fractions would be bound in the precipitate obtained by adding a solution of saturated ammonium sulphate to a serum sample to give a concentration of 50 per cent in ammonium sulphate. The γM fractions could then be separated from the γG fraction by chromatography on DEAE-cellulose, by zone electrophoresis, by gel filtration on Sephadex G-200, or by density gradient centrifugation. On the other hand, one could easily obtain the γG fraction in relatively pure state by adding to the serum sample a solution of saturated ammonium sulphate to give a final concentration of 33 per cent in ammonium sulphate.

There have been a number of reviews on the salt fractionation of serum proteins in recent years. Attention is called to the reviews by Fuller [1], Keller & Block [2] and Pennell [3]. This section deals with fractionation methods involving ammonium sulphate and sodium sulphate since these are by far the two most widely used by immunologists.

General considerations

The solubility of a protein depends on the number and arrangement of its

3

polar and nonpolar groups and the dipole nature of these groups. These groups interact with one another in the same molecule and with neighbouring protein molecules. In the presence of pure water, interactions between charged polar groups are diminished owing to the high dielectric constant of water. Some proteins, however, may still be soluble in water as a result of interactions between their charged polar groups and the surrounding water molecules. Thus serum albumins, for example, are found to be soluble in pure water, presumably because the interaction between protein and water is more favourable than that between neighbouring protein molecules. On the other hand, the euglobulins are generally insoluble in water because the interaction between neighbouring protein molecules is more favourable than that of protein and water molecules. Euglobulins may be made soluble by the addition of small amounts of neutral salt. Within limits, it is found that increasing the salt concentration will increase the solubility of most proteins. This phenomenon is known as the 'salting-in effect' and results from the energetically favourable interaction of the charged groups on the protein with those of the ions of neutral salts.

At high concentrations of neutral salts most proteins will be precipitated out of aqueous solutions. This phenomenon is known as the 'salting-out effect' and was one of the first used in the isolation of proteins. The addition of high concentrations of salt lowers the activity of water molecules and hinders their interaction with the charged polar groups of protein molecules, thus favouring the interaction between neighbouring protein molecules. In such an event, the insolubility of the protein would be increased and would result in the precipitation of the protein from solution. For a quantitative account of the subject, the books by Cohn & Edsall [4] and Edsall & Wyman [5] should be consulted.

Fractionation with ammonium sulphate

The γ globulins of many mammalian sera may be precipitated out of solution by adding saturated ammonium sulphate (SAS) to the serum to give a final concentration of one-third saturation in ammonium sulphate. This method has been widely used and requires no special skill or equipment.

The SAS solution is prepared by dissolving enough ammonium sulphate in distilled water to give a saturated solution. Table 1.1 presents the properties of SAS solutions at various temperatures. For example, at 20° C, 536·3 g of ammonium sulphate dissolved in 1 litre of distilled water will give a saturated solution. This solution will be 4·06 M in ammonium sulphate. It should also be noted that the solubility of ammonium sulphate in saturated solutions at temperatures ranging from 0 to 30° C is not as extreme as that of sodium sulphate solutions.

To prepare saturated solutions of ammonium sulphate that can be used at temperatures between 0 to 30° C, the following procedure is recommended. For every litre of SAS needed, weigh out about 550 g of ammonium sulphate. Place the weighed salt in a 1 litre beaker (or larger if more than 1 litre is to be prepared) and add about 600 ml of distilled water. Heat the mixture slowly until all of the salt is dissolved. While the solution is still hot, filter it through coarse filter paper to remove any insoluble impurities. (Ammonium sulphate of technical grade usually contains material which is insoluble in hot or cold water.) When the clarified solution reaches room temperature, bring the volume to about 990 ml, and add enough concentrated ammonium hydroxide to bring the pH to about 6·5 (this pH is near the isolectric point of many of the γ globulins). Finally the volume is made up to the 1 litre mark. At this

TABLE 1.1

Saturated solutions of ammonium sulphate (AS) and of sodium sulphate (SS) in water at various temperatures#

Temperature C	0°	10°	20°	25°	30°
Per cent AS by weight	41·42	42·22	43·09	43·47	43·85
Grammes AS per 1000 ml solution	514·7	525·0	536·3	541·2	545·9
Moles AS per 1000 ml solution	3·90	3·97	4·06	4·10	4·13
Grammes AS to add to 1000 ml water	706·9	730·5	755·8	766·8	777·6
Per cent SS by weight	4·47	8·25	16·04	21·81	29·14
Grammes SS per 1000 ml solution	46·2	89·1	184·9	264·0	374·0
Moles SS per 1000 ml solution	0·325	0·628	1·30	1·95	2·65
Grammes SS to add to 1000 ml water	46·8	90·2	191·0	279·0	411·0

Compiled from International Critical Tables.

stage the solution should contain a small amount of undissolved salt, indicating that a saturated solution has been achieved. Prior to use the solution should be thoroughly shaken, and when allowed to settle it should contain some undissolved salt.

To precipitate out the γ globulins, one volume of SAS is added to every 2 volumes of serum. For example, 50 ml of SAS is added for every 100 ml of serum. The SAS is added dropwise to the serum with constant stirring. The mixture is allowed to stand for 15 minutes or longer and centrifuged. The sediment is washed twice with 100 ml of 40 per cent SAS, centrifuging, and discarding the supernatant each time. The sediment is dissolved in about 100 ml of 0·9 per cent NaCl, and the globulin fraction is again precipitated with 50 ml of SAS. After washing the precipitate two times with 100 ml 40 per cent SAS each time and discarding the supernatants, it is again dissolved in

100 ml of 0·9 per cent NaCl. The precipitation step at 33 per cent SAS, washing with 40 per cent SAS is repeated for a third time.

For convenience, the γ globulin fraction can be stored in the 40 per cent SAS suspension at refrigerator temperatures for an indefinite period of time, apparently with no deleterious effect. The high concentration of ammonium sulphate prevents most forms of microbial growth and has not been shown to cause any measurable changes in chemical or biological properties.

For further experimentation, the γ globulin suspended in 40 per cent SAS may be centrifuged, and the sediment dissolved in a small volume of any desired solvent. The solution may then be dialysed against the solvent with several changes of the dialysate to remove ammonium sulphate. Alternatively the solution may be placed on a Sephadex G25 column previously equilibrated with the desired solvent to remove the ammonium sulphate and to equilibrate the γ globulin fraction with this solvent.

Rabbit γ globulin fractions prepared by this method will usually consist of about 95 per cent γ globulin as judged by Tiselius electrophoresis, with the remainder consisting mainly of β globulin and some α globulin.

Another method commonly used to precipitate out the globulin fractions is that of dialysing the serum against known concentrations of ammonium sulphate solutions. In this method, the serum is placed in a dialysis bag and allowed to dialyse against the ammonium sulphate solution. It is thought that the protein is subjected to milder treatment than that obtained by adding SAS directly to the serum. The dialysis method, however, requires that the solution be constantly stirred and a sufficiently long time be allowed for the attainment of dialysis equilibrium. Moreover, the precipitate would still have to be washed to remove occluded protein. These considerations would indicate that no real advantage is to be gained by this method.

Some workers prefer to express the concentration of ammonium sulphate in terms of molarity rather than per cent saturation. Table 1.1 shows the molarity of saturated solutions of ammonium sulphate. At 25° C, for example, a saturated solution has a molarity of 4·10; and the molarity of a 33 per cent SAS would be 1·37. The molarity of saturated solution at temperatures between 0° and 30° C can be easily interpolated from the data given in Table 1.1.

Ammonium sulphate precipitation of urinary proteins
It may be convenient sometimes to precipitate out proteins from large volumes of solution by adding the salt directly to the solution. Bence-Jones proteins may be prepared from the urine of myeloma patients by adding ammonium sulphate to a concentration of 75 per cent saturation [6]. The amount of salt to be added can be calculated by measuring the volume of the sample, and by referring to Table 1.1, noting how much salt is needed to bring the

solution to 75 per cent in SAS. For example, for every 1000 ml of urine at 25° C, 0·75 × 766·8 = 575 g of ammonium sulphate is added.

For isolating proteins from urine the following procedure is recommended. The urine is first dialysed against running tap water (cold). About 24 hours is sufficient if the dialysis bag is agitated during the dialysis. Any insoluble material is removed by filtration through a coarse filter paper. The clarified urine is brought to pH 5·5 (near the isoelectric point of many Bence-Jones proteins) by the drop-wise addition of 6 N acetic acid, and the volume measured in a graduated cylinder. The sample is placed in a suitable beaker, e.g. for a 1 litre sample a 2 litre beaker is used. While the solution is stirred either magnetically or mechanically, 575 g of ammonium sulphate is slowly added in small portions. The salt should not be added rapidly because it will form lumps. After the salt has been added, the suspension is centrifuged, and the supernatant is discarded. The sediment is dissolved in a small volume of the desired solvent and is dialysed against this solvent to remove ammonium sulphate. The solution may then be used for further experimentation. If the urinary proteins are to be lyophillized, the sediment is taken up in a small volume of distilled water, and is dialysed extensively against distilled water prior to lyophillization.

The major advantage of this method is that it allows a concentration of urinary proteins from a large volume of sample, since proteins of immunological interest may be present in rather low concentrations. Since many mammals may excrete urinary proteins resembling Bence-Jones protein, a similar fractionation procedure could be used to isolate them. These proteins appear to have properties in common with the light chains of γ globulin and are useful in structural and biosynthetic studies of γG antibodies [7].

Fractionation with sodium sulphate
The major advantage of sodium sulphate over ammonium sulphate in protein fractionation is that it contains no nitrogen. A major disadvantage is the insolubility of sodium sulphate as compared to ammonium sulphate. Further, the solubility of saturated solutions of sodium sulphate is markedly temperature dependent. The solubility of saturated solutions of this salt increases from 4·47 per cent at 0° C to 21·81 per cent at 25° C (Table 1.1), whereas the solubility of saturated solutions of ammonium sulphate show but a relatively small change, i.e. 51·5 per cent at 0° C and 54·1 per cent at 25° C. In order to control the solubility of sodium sulphate solutions, it is therefore necessary to maintain the temperature of the solution rather closely, and preferably at close to 25° C or higher where the solubility is sufficiently high to allow precipitation of the globulin fractions.

The method most widely used by immunologists is the one devised by Kekwick [8]. In this procedure, which is slightly modified, 18 g of sodium sulphate is added per 100 ml of serum (at room temperature, about 25° C). The precipitate is washed with 100 ml of 18 per cent sodium sulphate, centrifuged and the supernatant discarded. (The supernatant may contain other immunoglobulins, but the procedure outlined here is for the preparation of γ globulin fractions.) The sediment is washed again with 100 ml of 18 per cent sodium sulphate, centrifuged and the sediment is dissolved in 40 ml of pH 8 borate-buffered saline. To prepare this buffer, 8 g of sodium chloride and 12·4 g of boric acid are weighed and dissolved in about 950 ml of distilled water; after adjusting the pH to 8 with 15 N sodium hydroxide, the volume is brought to the 1 litre mark. The globulin solution (40 ml) is again precipitated by adding sodium sulphate to a concentration of 12 g per 100 ml, or, in this case, 4·8 g per 40 ml. The precipitate is washed twice with 100 ml of 12 per cent sodium sulphate, centrifuging and discarding the supernatant each time. The precipitate is dissolved in 20 ml of pH 8 borate buffered saline and the globulin reprecipitated by adding sodium sulphate to a concentration of 12 g per 100 ml, e.g. 2·4 g per 20 ml.

The precipitated globulins may finally be dissolved in a small volume of any desired solvent and dialysed against this solvent to remove the sodium sulphate prior to further experimentation. The globulin fraction prepared by this method has been shown to be better than 98 per cent γ globulin as judged by Tiselius electrophoresis, and the yield amounted to about 7 per cent of the total serum protein [8].

For small serum samples, a dialysis method described by Marrack and co-workers [9] may be convenient. The serum sample was dialysed against several changes of 18 per cent sodium sulphate. After washing the precipitate several times with 18 per cent sodium sulphate, it was dissolved in buffer and redialysed against several changes of 15 per cent sodium sulphate. The precipitate was washed several times with 15 per cent sodium sulphate, redissolved in a small volume of buffer, and again precipitated by dialysis against 15 per cent sodium sulphate. Rabbit globulin fractions prepared by this method were found to contain better than 95 per cent of the protein migrating as γ globulin [9]. The use of 15 per cent sodium sulphate as against 12 per cent in the Kekwick procedure may account for the lower purity of the γ globulin preparation.

References

[1] FULLER J.F. (1953) The isolation of proteins. In *The Proteins*, Vol. 1, pp. 1–85, ed. NEURATH H. & BAILEY K. New York: Academic Press
[2] KELLER S. & BLOCK R.J. (1960) Separation of proteins. In *Analytical Methods of Protein Chemistry*, Vol. 1, pp. 2–30, ed. ALEXANDER P. & BLOCK R.J. New York: Pergamon Press

[3] PENNELL R.B. (1960) Fractionation and isolation of purified components by precipitation methods. In *The Plasma Proteins*, Vol. I, pp. 9–50, ed. PUTNAM F.W. New York: Academic Press

[4] COHN E.J. & EDSALL J.T. (1943) *Proteins, Amino Acids and Peptides*. New York: Reinhold Publishing Corp

[5] EDSALL J.T. & WYMAN J. (1958) *Biophysical Chemistry*, pp. 263–282. New York; Academic Press

[6] PUTNAM F.W. & STELOS P. (1953) Proteins in multiple myeloma II. Bence–Jones proteins, *J. biol. Chem.* **203,** 347

[7] PUTNAM F.W., MIGITA S. & EASLEY C.W. (1962) Structural and immunochemical relationships among Bence–Jones proteins. In *Protides of the Biological Fluids*, Vol. 10, pp. 93–107, ed. PEETERS H. Amsterdam: Elsevier Publishing Company

[8] KEKWICK R.A. (1940) The serum proteins in multiple myelomatosis. *Biochem. J.* **34,** 1248

[9] MARRACK J.R., HOCH H. & JOHNS R.G.S. (1951) The valency of antibodies. *Brit. J. exp. Path.* **32,** 212

CHAPTER 2

Preparative Electrophoresis

PETER STELOS

Introduction

Preparative electrophoresis may be used for the separation of proteins that are sufficiently different from one another in net electric charge under appropriate conditions of pH and ionic strength. Until the advent of ion-exchange columns suitable for the chromatography of proteins [1], electrophoresis was a widely used tool in the separation and analysis of serum proteins. Ion-exchange columns, composed of diethylaminoethyl- or carboxymethyl-cellulose, have a high capacity and are extremely useful for fractionating large volumes of serum. However, the fractions obtained are usually diluted, and the process involves the use of many buffers or a suitable gradient device as well as a long period of time for the elution of all serum proteins. In some instances, the fractions obtained as single chromatographic peaks may show two or more components when analysed by electrophoresis (for details of these methods see Fahey & Terry Chapter 3). The choice of procedure should obviously be made with an eye to the type of information that is desired.

This section deals with preparative electrophoresis on a moderate scale. It deals specifically with zone electrophoresis in a starch-supported medium or in polyacrylamide gels. Pevikon, which is a co-polymer of polyvinyl chloride and polyvinyl acetate, has been used in recent years as a replacement for potato starch [2]. Much of what will be described for starch holds also for Pevikon. The procedures described below are designed for use with apparatus that can be readily built in the laboratory. No attempt will be made to cover the modifications of this basic technique for use with the more elaborate preparative electrophoresis models that are commercially available since the procedures involved are fully described in company manuals. Attention is also called to recent publications dealing with various aspects of preparative electrophoresis [3, 4, 5, 6, 7, 8, 9].

General considerations

Electrophoresis refers to the migration of charged particles in solution under the influence of an electric field. Although most preparative electrophoresis methods make use of some supporting medium, such as starch or Pevikon,

10

it should be remembered that the actual environment through which the charged proteins migrate is composed of about 50 per cent buffer solution. The supporting medium serves as a matrix in which the electrolyte is embedded and is usually not involved to a great extent in the electrophoretic process. The term zone electrophoresis [10] has been applied when electrophoresis is carried out in a supporting medium to distinguish it from moving-boundary electrophoresis which is carried out entirely in a liquid phase. Ideally, a supporting medium should be completely insoluble in aqueous buffers, exhibit no electro-osmotic effect, and should not have any adsorptive capacity for proteins. Although most substances used as supporting media have one or two of these properties, electro-osmotic flow to a varying degree is common to all of them. Electro-osmosis or electro-endosmosis results whenever an electromotive force is applied to a solid phase suspended in a liquid phase. Such an effect is manifested by a backward flow of electrolyte so that at pH 8·6 the serum proteins may move to the cathode as well as to the anode. The γ globulins are actually observed to migrate to the cathode with most supporting media, even though they are negatively charged at pH 8·6. This effect is quite noticeable with potato starch as a supporting medium and is rather small with Pevikon.

It has become customary to carry out electrophoresis of serum proteins at pH 8·6 since at this pH all of the proteins are negatively charged and will migrate to the anode. Barbital buffer of 0·1 ionic strength and pH 8·6 has been most frequently used. The major disadvantage of this buffer is that protein content cannot be measured by Kjeldahl analysis or absorbancy at 280 mμ unless the protein fractions are dialysed to remove barbital. Protein content may be measured, however, by the phenol reagent in the presence of barbital buffer.

Another preparative method that is described in some detail is an adaption to a larger scale of the one described by Ornstein & Davis [7]. In this method the supporting medium is polyacrylamide gel. The major advantage of this method over that of zone electrophoresis in a starch block is that it separates proteins according to size and shape as well as electric charge. It can therefore be used to achieve a separation of molecules that have the same charge but have appreciably different molecular weights. The reader should consult the article by Ornstein & Davis [7] for the principles involved in this method.

Briefly, the gel is prepared in glass cylinders in three successive stages. The first stage consists of forming the lower gel, which contains 7·5 per cent acrylamide. After this has polymerized, the spacer gel is added, which contains 5 per cent acrylamide, and is therefore more porous than the lower gel. The third stage consists of the sample which can be mixed with acrylamide solution in order to gel, or may be mixed with 10 per cent sucrose and layered over the spacer gel. The unique feature of this method is the sharp concentration of protein that is achieved as the protein migrates from the sample layer into the spacer gel and towards the lower gel. This concentration effect results from the fact that the larger porosity of the spacer gel permits a rapid migration of protein. At the interphase of spacer and lower gels, proteins of different mobility appear as fine sharp zones (or disks) stacked one on top of the other according to their relative mobility. As the different proteins migrate into the lower gel which is less porous, they encounter an increased resistance. Their movement through this gel will then be inversely proportional to their size and shape and directly proportional to their net charge. Presumably, those proteins of greater molecular weight will be impeded more than those of smaller molecular weight.

It is possible to vary the concentration of acrylamide in order to have gels of different porosity. Gels of smaller pore size, for example, may be used to allow passage of low molecular weight proteins while excluding larger proteins. Urea may also be incorporated into the gels, and such gels would be useful in studies concerned with the sub-unit structure of the immunoglobulins or of other proteins.

Apparatus for zone electrophoresis in a horizontal direction

There are many commercially available models that can be used for zone electrophoresis. All of them have in common (*a*) a tray to hold the supporting medium, (*b*) two buffer vessels which make contact with each end of the tray and in which electrodes are immersed, and (*c*) a regulated DC voltage power supply. The following is a description of an apparatus that can be constructed at little expense (see Fig. 2.1.). It consists of two identical rectangular plates made of Plexiglass, 46 cm long, 12 cm wide and 0·5 cm thick, separated by thin plastic strips, 0·5 cm thick, placed at each side of the bottom plate. The plates can be held together during electrophoresis by brass pins which are inserted in holes drilled at 10 cm intervals along the side edges of the plates and plastic strips. The buffer vessels can be made of glass or plastic; they should be rectangular in shape and have a 1 litre capacity. Salt bridges, made from glass tubing of 1 cm diameter and filled with KCl-agar (90 ml KCl, 10 ml H_2O and 3 g agar), serve to connect the buffer vessels to the glass beakers (600 ml) in which the electrodes are immersed. The electrodes are the same as those used in Tiselius electrophoresis and are made of silver. They are placed in 50-ml beakers on the bottom of the 600-ml beakers. The electrodes are prepared by filling the beakers with 400 ml of buffer after which 25 ml of saturated potassium chloride are injected into the 50-ml beakers (which contain the silver wire) by means of a syringe and needle, care being taken not to inject air that would disturb the dense KCl layer covering the electrodes. The advantage of using this electrode arrangement over others is that no changes in pH will occur during electrophoresis. The electrode assemblies should be interchanged after each experiment to insure proper functioning of the reversible Ag-AgCl electrode reactions. Contact between the tray and the buffer vessels is made by thick filter papers which should be first wetted with buffer. The regulated DC power supply need not be expensive. A unit having an output of 500 volts is satisfactory.

This apparatus has been used in starch block experiments involving up to 6 ml of serum. Assuming a protein content of 60 mg per ml, 360 mg of protein would appear to be the capacity of this system. The block could be made wider and thicker to accommodate more protein. Making the block much thicker would present difficulties caused by the gravitational tendency of the

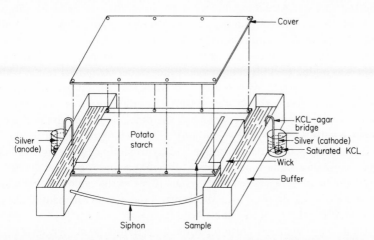

FIG. 2.1. Schematic drawing of an apparatus suitable for zone electrophoresis in a horizontal direction using starch, Pevikon or any other material as supporting medium.

buffer to settle to the bottom. This would result in a buffer gradient in the block and would be manifested by an uneven migration of protein as viewed from top to bottom. Making the block too wide would present problems of maintaining a uniform potential gradient across the width of the block. It should be borne in mind, however, that the dimensions given here are in no sense the maximum limits permissible; considerable latitude for improvisation exists. It should also be remembered that the block can be made smaller if less amounts of protein are to be used.

Experimental procedure
In a typical experiment involving the apparatus just described the following procedure was used. A thick slurry was made by thoroughly mixing in an 800-ml beaker about 300 ml of pH 8·6 barbital buffer and an equal volume of

purified potato starch (*not* the hydrolysed starch that is used in starch gel electrophoresis). The potato starch was purchased from J.T. Baker Chemical Co., Phillipsburg, N.J. and could be used without prior washing. The slurry should not be lumpy. The bottom plate of the block was prepared by covering it with wax paper or Parafilm and with the plastic strips in place along the sides. Removable plastic strips were also placed at the front and back ends so that the bottom plate now formed a tray. The slurry was poured to completely fill the tray and allowed to settle for 10 minutes. Excess buffer was removed by blotting with paper towels or filter paper, and the surface was made flush with the plastic strips by sliding a sharp-edged spatula transversely along the surface. A rectangular slit 1 cm in width was cut 9 cm from one end of the block. About 3 ml of undiluted rabbit serum was mixed with an equal volume of dry starch and the slurry was poured into the slit. Usually, this sufficed to cover the slit; if not, some of the starch removed in forming the slit was added to fill it completely. Filter paper strips, cut to the width of the block, were wetted with buffer and placed at the ends of the block to provide contact with the buffer vessels. Another sheet of wax paper (or Parafilm) was placed over the surface of the block, and the top plate fastened into place with the brass screws and nuts. The rectangular buffer vessels were each filled with 800 ml of the buffer and hydrostatic equilibrium was established by use of a syphon or a rubber tube connecting the buffer vessels. The ends of the block now rested on the inner edges of the buffer vessels with the filter paper wicks dipping into the buffer, and the experimental set-up as shown in Fig. 2.1 was thus established.

After a 15 minute equilibration period, a current of 30 ma (about 300 volts) was passed through the apparatus for 24 to 30 hours. Progress of the albumin front could be followed by adding a few crystals of bromphenol blue to the serum in the slit. The entire apparatus could be fitted into a refrigerator, but a cold room would also be suitable. It is mandatory to use low temperatures to inhibit the growth of micro-organisms.

After electrophoresis, the block was removed from the refrigerator, allowed to dry partially, and was cut in 1 cm segments. Each segment was placed in a 15 ml centrifuge tube to which 3 ml of buffer were added, and the mixture was thoroughly stirred. The tubes were centrifuged, and the supernatant solutions were assayed for protein content. Protein was measured by the Lowry *et al* method [11].

An example of the use of this procedure in comparing the distribution of antibody activity in antiserums obtained in the early and late stages of the immune response is given in Figs. 2.2 and 2.3. In the early response, the antibody activity is shown to be in the fast migrating γ globulin fraction whereas in the late response, the antibody activity is found in both the fast and slow migrating γ globulins. In conjunction with sedimentation analysis, it was further shown that the fast migrating antibody had an S_{20} of 18S and the slow migrating antibody had an S_{20} of 6S [12, 13].

The use of Pevikon as a supporting medium involves the same procedure as that described for potato starch. Pevikon, or Pevikon C-870, can be purchased from Stockholm's Superfosfat Fabriks A.-B., Stockholm, Sweden. Details of this method are described by Tomasi & Kunkel [2].

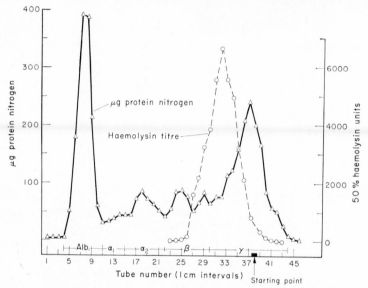

FIG. 2.2. Zone electrophoresis in a starch-supporting medium of a rabbit anti-serum against sheep red cells obtained during the early stage of immunization. The antibody activity is represented by a single peak which is centred between the β and γ globulin fractions.

—△—△ μg Protein nitrogen   ○ - - ○ Haemolysin titre

Zone electrophoresis in polyacrylamide gels

An apparatus suitable for the separation of 30 mg of protein is shown schematically in Fig. 2.4. The solutions used in making the lower and spacer gels were those described by Ornstein & Davis for their standard system [7]. The sample, 30 mg of rabbit γ globulin, was mixed with 2 ml of the standard buffer and 200 mg of sucrose. It was layered on top of the spacer gel after the upper vessel was filled with buffer. A current of 10 ma (about 170 volts) was passed through the apparatus for 10 hours in the cold room. At the end of the experiment, the marker dye (bromphenol blue) had migrated about 7 cm into the lower gel. A longitudinal slice which removed about one-eighth of the gel was made and stained with Buffalo Black. The rest of the gel was frozen with solid carbon dioxide. The stained slice was then used to locate the protein zones in the unstained gel, and the latter gel was sliced by a razor blade to isolate the corresponding protein zones. After cutting the gel segments into smaller pieces, they were placed in a Potter-Elvehjem glass homogenizer fitted with a Teflon pestle, and were thoroughly ground with about 2 volumes of buffer. Gel particles were removed by centrifugation and the supernatants

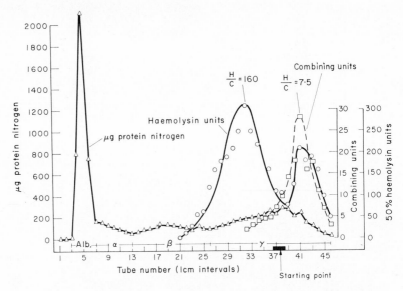

Fig. 2.3. Zone electrophoresis in a starch-supporting medium of a rabbit anti-serum against sheep red cells obtained during the late *stage* of immunization. The antibody activity is represented by two peaks. The curve marked combining units parallels the distribution of the second hemolytic curve. The ratio of hemolysin units to combining units (H/C) is a measure of the hemolytic efficiency and the faster migrating fraction (18S antibody) is seen to be more efficient than the slower migrating fraction (6S antibody).

△—△ μg Protein nitrogen   ○—○ Haemolysin titre   □ - - □ Combining units

analysed for protein content. It was found that about 70 per cent of the protein was recovered.

Although the amount of protein used was quite small, it may be possible to use larger amounts. In other experiments, 50 mg of protein were used in columns of the same design but of a diameter of 3 cm instead of 2·5. How large the diameter can be made is not known, but it would appear that heat gradients, extending laterally from the centre of the gel, might impose some limit. This limitation could be removed if the gel column were cooled efficiently during electrophoresis.

Experiments were also tried with polyacrylamide gels in rectangular vessels. These experiments were inconclusive, and the cylindrical gels were thought preferable because they were easier to work with and no major departure from the system devised by Ornstein & Davis [7] was involved.

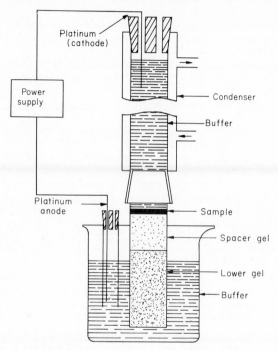

FIG. 2.4. Schematic drawing of an apparatus for zone electrophoresis in polyacryl amide gel. The lower glass cylinder is 2·5 cm in diameter and 15 cm in height. The condenser is connected to the lower glass cylinder by a ground glass joint (24/40) and is 30 cm in height.

It should be noted that urea can be incorporated in the gels. Such urea-polyacrylamide gels should be helpful in isolating polypeptide chains for further study. Experiments with small gels indicated that reduced and alkylated antibodies could be separated into many bands. Some of these bands appeared to be common for antibodies of different specificities while others appeared to be unique for a given antibody specificity [14, 15].

References

[1] SOBER H.A. & PETERSON E.A. (1958) Protein chromatography on ion exchange cellulose. *Fed. Proc.* **17,** 1116

[2] TOMASI T. & KUNKEL H.G. (1964) Isolation of 7S and 19S gamma globulins. In *Methods in Medical Research*, pp. 80–86, ed. EISEN H.F. Chicago: Year Book Medical Publishers, Inc.

[3] KUNKEL H.G. & TRAUTMAN R. (1959) Zone electrophoresis in various types of supporting media. In *Electrophoresis*, pp. 226–262, ed. BIER M. New York: Academic Press, Inc.

[4] BODMAN J. (1960) Agar gel, starch block, starch gel and sponge rubber electrophoresis. In *Chromatographic and Electrophoretic Techniques*, Vol. II, pp. 91–157, ed. SMITH I. London: William Heinemann Medical Books Ltd.

[5] SVENSSON H. (1960) Zonal density gradient electrophoresis. In *Analytical Methods of Protein Chemistry*, Vol. 1, pp. 195–244, ed. ALEXANDER P. & BLOCK, R.J. New York: Pergamon Press

[6] RAYMOND S. (1962) A convenient apparatus for gel electrophoresis. *Clin. Chem.* **8,** 455

[7] ORNSTEIN L. & DAVIS B.J. (1962) *Disc Electrophoresis* preprinted by Distillation Products Industries. Rochester: New York

[8] HJERTEN S. (1963) 'Molecular-sieve' electrophoresis in cross-linked polyacrylamide gels. *J. Chrom.* **11,** 66

[9] LEWIS U.J. & CLARK M.O. (1963) Preparative methods for disk electrophoresis with special reference to the isolation of pituitary hormones. *Anal. Biochem.* **6,** 303

[10] TISELIUS A. & FLODIN P. (1953) Zone electrophoresis. *Adv. in Prot. Chem.* **8,** 461

[11] LOWRY O.H., ROSEBROUGH N.J., FARR A.L. & RANDALL R.J. (1951) Protein measurement with the phenol reagent. *J. Biol. Chem.* **193,** 265

[12] STELOS P. (1956) Electrophoretic and ultracentrifugal studies of rabbit hemolysins. *J. Immunol.* **77,** 396

[13] STELOS P. & TALMAGE D.W. (1957) The separation by starch electrophoresis of two antibodies to sheep red cells differing in hemolytic efficiency. *J. Infect. Dis.* **100,** 126

[14] STELOS P., GROSSBERG A.L., ROHOLT O.A. & PRESSMAN D. (1964) Electrophoretic properties of reduced rabbit antibodies. *Fed. Proc.* **23,** 2115

[15] STELOS P., GROSSBERG A.L. & PRESSMAN D. (1964) Discrete molecular forms of rabbit 6S anti-hapten antibodies. *Abstracts* II–186, VI Int. Cong. of Biochem., New York

CHAPTER 3

Ion Exchange Chromatography and Gel Filtration

J.L.FAHEY & ELIZABETH W.TERRY

1. Column chromatography

Introduction

Chromatographic techniques for protein fractionation have had profound effects in immunology. Substituted cellulose chromatography was introduced 10 years ago by Peterson & Sober [1, 2] and gel-filtration (exclusion) chromatography more recently by Porath & Flodin [3]. The former technique has been particularly advantageous in the preparation of pure IgG ($7S\gamma_2$ globulin) from whole serum and made it possible for Porter [4] to separate the two types of immunoglobulin fragments (Fab and Fc) produced by papain digestion. Gel filtration has been widely used to isolate antibodies of different molecular weights and to separate the heavy and light polypeptide chains of the immunoglobulin molecule [5].

Substituted cellulose chromatography and gel-filtration chromatography, together with other methods such as zone electrophoresis (see Stelos, Chapter 2), form basic tools in laboratories concerned with the preparation of immunoglobulins. For example DEAE-cellulose chromatography has been exceedingly valuable as a simple one-step procedure for preparing purified serum IgG. DEAE-cellulose has the additional advantage of high capacity for adsorption of protein so that large amounts of serum can be fractionated readily. DEAE-cellulose chromatography also has been useful for preparation of myeloma proteins, but has not been useful in the preparation of normal immunoglobulin components other than IgG, because of the large number of additional serum proteins that are eluted in most DEAE-cellulose chromatogram fractions. Some of these fractions can be further separated by gel filtration or by zone electrophoresis.

Gel filtration has the advantage of separating the IgM from the IgG molecules on the basis of size. The intermediate size IgA molecules can also be purified by recycling chromatography. The major limitation of this powerful tool is a low capacity in terms of millilitres of serum or milligrammes of protein mixture that can be applied to the column to achieve good resolution.

B

19

Thus, prior fractionation by some other technique is often useful as a preliminary step before preparation of proteins on a gel-filtration column.

Zone electrophoresis (see Chapter 2) is useful for immunoglobulin characterization and as a preliminary step in purification of many proteins of the immunoglobulin family. The slowest migrating IgG molecules can be prepared in purified form by zone electrophoresis alone, but electrophoretic fractions containing the rest of the immunoglobulin family are contaminated by other serum proteins. Most readily available zone electrophoresis equipment is limited to a top capacity of 10 to 15 ml serum.

Much of the equipment required for the two chromatographic procedures is interchangeable. The common facilities are listed in Table 3.1.

TABLE 3.1.

Column chromatography equipment

Columns and connecting tubing
Fraction collector
Ultraviolet spectrophotometer
pH meter
Dialysis tubing
Ultrafiltration or other equipment
  for concentrating fractions

Columns

Chromatography columns of glass or plastic, suitable either for substituted cellulose chromatography or for gel filtration, are commercially available.*
Two general types of column are used and both are illustrated in Fig. 3.1.
The plastic columns with removable top and bottom pieces usually permit entry and egress of fluid through small holes in the centre of the top and bottom plates. Glass columns generally have a fixed filter near the bottom. The top may be closed with a one-hole stopper or with a socket-type joint which can be fused onto the top of the commercially available glass columns. The use of ball and socket joint connections is described by Peterson & Sober [6]. A packing reservoir (shown above the empty glass column in Fig. 3.1) is prepared by fusing ball and socket joints onto the top and bottom of a 1 litre thick-walled suction flask [6] and sealing the side arm opening.

One important consideration in selecting and using chromatography columns is the amount of 'dead' space in which eluate can collect and mix between the bottom of the gel or resin and the actual site of entry of the

* In U.K., Wright Scientific Ltd, London, N.W.6, manufacture a wide range of plastic columns with minimal dead space.

eluate into the collection tube. In general, columns are designed either with a flat bottom and an outflow tube projecting directly from the centre of the bottom disc, or with a bowl-shaped bottom which tapers below the filter into an outflow tube. Columns with bowl-shaped bottoms are satisfactory if the design of the outlet tube prevents back-up of eluate into the bowl. Mixing problems encountered with this type of column may be eliminated by placing

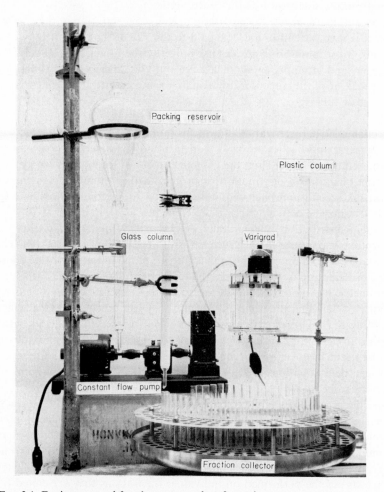

FIG. 3.1. Equipment used for chromatography of proteins.
    On the left is a glass column fitted with a ball and socket joint at the top. Above it is a reservoir suitable for packing a DEAE-cellulose column. In the centre is an operating column connected to a variable gradient device by tubing passing through a pump which delivers buffer from the varigrad to the substituted cellulose column. On the right is a plastic column with removable end pieces.

a partially straightened paper clip or other 'drip stick' into the outflow tube, or minimized by filling the bowl below the filter with glass beads. Flat bottoms for columns eliminate the mixing problem, but unless carefully designed may create uneven flow through the column, the buffer in the centre being more readily able to pass out of the column than buffer travelling down the sides. The flat bottom may be altered for optimal operation so that there is a slight taper from the sides towards the centre outlet.

If an automatic device for recording protein concentration in the emerging effluent is used, attention must be paid to the size of the outflow tube of the column. Most monitoring devices use polyethylene tubing of relatively small diameter, and attempts to adapt a large outflow tube to small tubing may cause back-up of the effluent in any available space between the resin or gel and the narrow tubing.

Detection and characterization of proteins in the effluent

Two general approaches are used to detect and characterize the proteins in column effluents. In the first, the protein content of fractions is measured so that the quantitative distribution of protein in the column effluent may be known. A second approach requires detection of specific components (e.g. antibody, enzyme activity, etc.) in the effluent.

Protein distribution is commonly determined by quantitative ultraviolet absorption measurements at wavelengths of about 280 mμ or 260 mμ. These techniques depend upon the phenylalanine, tryptophane and tyrosine content of the proteins and do not measure the total quantity of protein. The spectrophotometric techniques, however, are particularly useful because of ease and rapidity of handling the samples, because they can be coupled to automatic recording devices for continuous measurement of the effluent, and because little or no sample is consumed in the test. Folin-Ciocaulteau techniques may also be used. Biuret methods are generally less sensitive to protein content. Nitrogen determinations are not usually practical because of the number of fractions to be assayed.

Specific protein characterization is commonly carried out by zone electrophoresis, starch gel electrophoresis, immunoelectrophoresis, by immunochemical techniques such as Ouchterlony analysis, antibody-in-agar (immunoplate) quantitative measurements, antibody assay, by enzymatic assay, by binding of isotopically labelled substances, or by other specific tests. Such tests may be performed on individual fractions as they are eluted from the column or on pooled and concentrated fractions from selected regions of the total effluent.

Concentration of fractions

Proteins are eluted from columns in relatively large volumes of buffer. The fractions may be concentrated by ultrafiltration, by lyophilization or by use of an absorbent such as carbowax or polyglucose granules outside a dialysis bag. A convenient procedure for negative pressure ultrafiltration has been described by Peterson & Sober [2,6].

Identification and quantification of specific immunoglobulins

Specific forms of immunoglobulin are usually identified on the basis of unique antigenic properties of the heavy or light polypeptide chains. The immunoglobulins IgG, IgA, IgM and IgD are distinguished by antiserums specific for the γ, α, μ or δ chains respectively. The Type K (I) or Type L (II) immunoglobulins are recognized on the basis of unique antigenic properties of kappa (Type I) and lambda (Type II) light polypeptide chains.

Qualitative techniques such as immunoelectrophoresis or gel diffusion (Ouchterlony) analysis are useful for identification of immunoglobulins and for testing the purity of chromatographic fractions. Quantitative techniques such as precipitation methods, antibody-in-agar plates (immunoplate), immune inhibition or other methods, however, provide greater information about the chromatographic distribution of immunoglobulin components.

The preparation of polyvalent antiserum and of specific antiserum for use in qualitative and quantitative tests for immunoglobulins is beyond the scope of this report. Proper analytic reagents, however, are as important as proper chromatographic techniques for successful fractionation of complex mixtures of protein such as serum.

2. Ion-exchange chromatography

Introduction

Ion-exchange chromatography involves the electrostatic binding of proteins onto a cellulose resin suspended in buffer and packed into a column. Elution may be effected either by changing the pH of buffer passing through the column, thus affecting the charge on the protein molecules, or by increasing the molarity of the buffer, thus providing more salt ions to compete with the proteins for charged groups on the resin. Conditions for chromatography are selected to take advantage of net charge differences between serum proteins and to assure a net charge on the resin opposite that of the proteins. By a gradual increase in salt concentration (with or without a fall in pH), proteins are eluted in order of increasing numbers of charged groups bound to the resin. Additional information on theory and practice of substituted cellulose chromatography is included in a review by Peterson & Sober [6].

Both anion and cation exchange resins are available. Diethylaminoethyl (DEAE) cellulose is a frequently used anion exchanger. Carboxymethyl (CM) cellulose is often utilized as a cation exchanger. Either of these resins may be used for the fractionation of serum proteins and preparation of immunoglobulins. Because DEAE-cellulose has been used most extensively, the discussion below is concerned with use of this adsorbent. The cation exchange resins are considered separately (see p. 36).

When serum is added to a DEAE-cellulose column under suitable conditions, most of the serum proteins will adsorb onto the resin. When buffers of low molarity and pH greater than 6·5 are used, much of the IgG of human serum (and the corresponding immunoglobulins of many other species) is not adsorbed and passes through with the first buffer volume.

The adsorbed serum proteins can be eluted by increasing the salt concentration either by use of a gradient or by stepwise increments. Net charge is one of the factors determining the elution of serum protein molecules from a DEAE-cellulose column. As shown in Fig. 3.2, the electrophoretically slower migrating proteins tend to be eluted earlier than rapidly migrating proteins. Size of the charged surface may also be a factor. Molecules of larger size tend to be eluted later than smaller molecules with the same net charge density per unit surface area, e.g. IgM molecules are eluted later than IgA.

Procedure for DEAE-cellulose column chromatography

Solutions and equipment

In addition to the items noted in Table 3.1 DEAE-cellulose chromatography requires:

Diethylaminoethyl-cellulose
Constant flow pump
Variable gradient devices (Varigrad)
Columns with sintered glass filter at bottom and socket joint at top*
Funnel with ball and socket joints*
Ball and socket glass adaptors for connecting tubing in certain systems*
Air pressure source and pressure gauge (at least 0–10 lb)*

Solutions for cleaning and washing DEAE-cellulose:

0·3 M KH_2PO_4; 0·5 N NaOH; and 95 per cent ethanol
Initial buffer: 0·005 or 0·01 M phosphate buffer, pH 8·0
Limit buffer: 0·3 M phosphate buffer, pH 8·0
Tris or potassium phosphate buffers are usually satisfactory.

Preparation of adsorbent

DEAE-cellulose may be obtained in floc or powder form. Floc cellulose generally gives better flow rates than DEAE powder. Both forms seem to have similar protein-binding capacities.

* Needed for packing glass columns similar to those shown in Fig. 3.1.

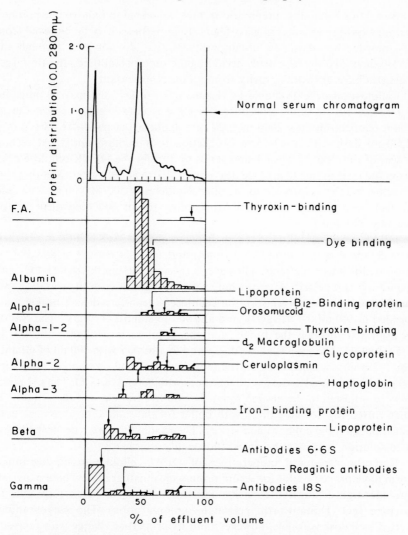

FIG. 3.2. Two dimensional analyses of serum proteins by DEAE-cellulose chromatography and electrophoresis.

Three millilitres of serum were fractionated on 3 g of DEAE-cellulose packed in a glass column. A total of 300 ml buffer was used in a gradient elution system with an initial buffer 0·015 M, pH 8 tris phosphate and a final buffer of 0·30 M, pH 4 tris phosphate. The gradient was produced with a two-chamber system [8] similar to that shown in Fig. 3.3 except that a 250 ml round flask replaced the beaker as a mixing chamber and a 125 ml Erlenmeyer flask was used as a reservoir. The pH gradient change is shown in Fig. 3.4. The buffer flow rate was 20 ml per hour, and 100 fractions of 3 ml each were collected. The protein content as determined by the optical density at 280 mμ is shown at the top of the figure. The effluent fractions were then divided into sixteen pools, concentrated and analysed by paper electrophoresis [8]. Individual serum components were identified by specific tests.

New DEAE-cellulose preparations must be treated to remove fine particles before exposure to sintered glass filters. Fine particles may be removed from the powder by sieving to obtain particles that do not pass through the #230 sieve [6] or by repeatedly decanting the supernatant fluid after the larger particles have settled by gravity from a dilute suspension.

Cellulose adsorbents should be cleaned prior to use, and may be prepared for re-use by the same procedure. Washing is conveniently carried out at room temperature in a 2000 ml (120 mm diameter) coarse filter on top of a 2000 ml flask with a side arm connection to a vacuum outlet. At certain stages of the cleaning it is advantageous to transfer the DEAE-cellulose cake from the filter funnel to a 1 litre beaker in order to add the next solution prior to returning the suspension to the filter. Volumes of 500–800 ml may be used at each step if 50 g of dry DEAE-cellulose (or its wet equivalent) is the starting material.

DEAE-cellulose is allowed to remain overnight in 0·3 M KH_2PO_4 in a beaker. The cellulose is transferred to a funnel and most of the 0·3 M KH_2PO_4 is aspirated through the filter. The cake is re-suspended in 0·3 M KH_2PO_4 and aspiration is repeated. After washing with distilled water until aspiration rate has slowed (about five rinses), the cellulose is transferred to a beaker, suspended in 500 ml 0·5 N NaOH, and allowed to stand 1–4 hours. The NaOH is aspirated through the funnel and the cellulose is washed with 500 ml 0·5 N NaOH. The resin is allowed to stand in a beaker with 500 ml of ethanol for 1–2 hours, washed once on the funnel with 500 ml of ethanol, once with 800 ml 0·05 N NaOH, and five to ten times with 800 ml of H_2O. The pH range may be adjusted to the desired range by careful titration, and the cellulose is then rinsed two to three times with buffer (of the same type as will be used when packing the column) and stored. The funnel filter may be cleaned with acid solution, and must be rinsed thoroughly afterwards.

Recently introduced preparations of DEAE-cellulose in microgranular form have proved useful for serum protein chromatography. These materials provide high adsorption capacity and can be used in batch technique to prepare IgG (D.Stanworth, personal communication). The microgranular DEAE-cellulose is fragile, however; and its properties change with repeated handling.

Packing the DEAE-cellulose column
The glass column and reservoir shown at the left of Fig. 3.1 are clamped together. A rubber tube attached to the bottom of the column is clamped and the column is filled with the initial phosphate buffer. Sufficient initial buffer is thoroughly mixed with clean, buffered DEAE-cellulose to prepare a *thin* suspension (dilution about 1:10) which is poured into the funnel on top of the column. An air line with attached pressure gauge is connected to

the top of the funnel by means of ball and socket joints secured with a clamp (not shown in Fig. 3.1). The clamp at the bottom of the column is then removed allowing the buffer to flow through the column. The pressure gauge is adjusted to 2 lb initially and the pressure increased at intervals as the cellulose packs and flow rate decreases until a pressure of 10 p.s.i. is reached and the packed resin approaches the top of the column. (Some lots of DEAE-cellulose pack too tightly at 10 p.s.i. and lower pressure is sufficient for column packing and rinsing.) During packing the funnel must be swirled frequently to maintain an evenly divided suspension of DEAE-cellulose. Care must be taken to replace the apparatus in a strictly vertical position. Columns may be packed with cellulose to within $1\frac{1}{2}$ to 2 inches of the top. Excess resin may be carefully taken off after removal of the pressure line and a flat resin top prepared. Packing should be done at room temperature whether or not the column is to be run in the cold. The column is then washed with approximately 200 ml of initial buffer. The pH of the column eluate should be stabilized at pH 8·0.

TABLE 3.2.

Glass column dimensions	Approximate amount of DEAE-cellulose	Serum sample	Effluent volume
1 cm × 25 cm	2 g	1–2 ml	100–150 ml
2 cm × 12 cm	5 g	5 ml	200–300 ml
2 cm × 20 cm	10 g	10 ml	300–400 ml
2 cm × 37 cm	20 g	20 ml	400–800 ml

Preparation and application of sample
Samples to be placed on the ion-exchange cellulose column should be equilibrated with the starting buffer, usually by dialysis. Dialysed serum should be centrifuged to remove insoluble material.

Buffer remaining above the surface of the cellulose is allowed to sink into the adsorbent. The serum sample is layered over the resin with a pipette. Care should be taken to avoid creating unevenness on the top of the adsorbent. (The volume of serum that may be applied to various columns is given in Table 3.2.) Immediately after the sample has passed into the cellulose, the sides of the column above the resin are rinsed twice with several ml of starting buffer. These are separately allowed to pass into the resin. Following the second rinse, a few millilitres of buffer are placed above the cellulose. The top of the column is sealed by a stopper or ball joint through which tubing from the pump enters the column. The tubing should reach to the buffer above the

B*

cellulose. The tubing passing through the pump has been previously primed with starting buffer.

Control of elution
Elution of adsorbed proteins often is best accomplished by a gradient of gradually increasing salt concentration. Various devices have been designed to produce a concentration of pH gradient in the buffer flowing into a cellulose column. One of these, the varigrad [7] has nine chambers, connected sequentially, into which buffer can be placed. As buffer is pulled from

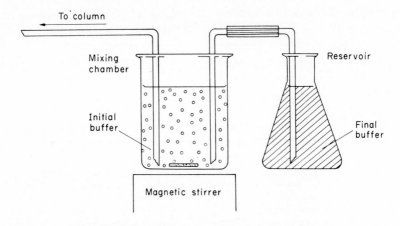

FIG. 3.3. Simple arrangement for producing an elution gradient.
    The mixing chamber (250 ml beaker) contains the initial or starting buffer. The reservoir (125 ml Erlenmeyer flask) contains the final or limit buffer. Prior to starting the elution gradient, the fluid levels in the two vessels should be approximately even. The tubing to the column and the tubing connecting the two vessels are filled with initial buffer and are clamped until the elution is to begin.

Chamber 1 by the pump, the level of fluid in all chambers re-equilibrates. The buffer in each chamber is stirred continuously to ensure thorough mixing.
    The varigrad chambers can be filled with buffers of different molarity to regulate the gradient and to achieve different protein elution patterns [7]. Frequently used is a gradient produced by filling cylinders 1, 2, 3, 5 and 7 of the varigrad with initial buffer, cylinders 6, 8 and 9 with the final buffer, and cylinder 4 with a mixture of 90 per cent starting buffer and 10 per cent of the final buffer. For small columns a roughly similar gradient can be obtained by filling chambers 1 and 2 with starting buffer and chamber 3 with final buffer, and not using the remaining six chambers. The same volume of buffer is placed in each chamber of the varigrad, the total volume being determined

by the total effluent volume necessary to remove the protein from the column. The flow rate can be adjusted with the pump. Rates of 0·5 to 1 ml per minute have proved convenient.

Elution gradients can be created by using two or three interconnected vessels, initially containing buffers of different pH or molarity. A simple and useful system created from a beaker and Erlenmeyer flask is illustrated in Fig. 3.3. The gradient change in pH with two buffer systems is shown in Fig. 3.4. This gradient is similar to that produced in the varigrad systems

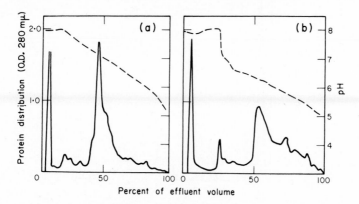

FIG. 3.4. Comparison of buffers (by DEAE-cellulose chromatography of normal serum) in gradient elution systems with progressive increase in hydrogen ion concentration (fall in pH) and progressive increase in molarity (0·015 to 0·30 M phosphate). The chromatographic system is the same as that represented in Fig. 3.2. [(a) Tris PO$_4$ buffers, (b) potassium PO$_4$ buffers]. The better buffering capacity of tris phosphate is readily apparent. - - - - - pH, ——— protein.

described above. By changing the relative shape and volume of the two flasks, the gradient may be changed.

A 0·005 M, 0·01 M or 0·015 M phosphate buffer is generally used as the initial buffer. A 0·3 M phosphate is used as final buffer. Chromatograms produced by elution gradients with increasing salt concentration and falling pH formed by tris phosphate buffers are shown in Figs. 3.2, 3.4–3.7. Chromatograms produced by buffers with constant pH (pH8) are shown in Figs. 3.8 and 3.9.

Distribution of immunoglobulins and other serum proteins
The serum proteins are separated by DEAE-cellulose chromatography into a series of fractions as shown in Fig. 3.2. The first peak of protein elution contains only IgG (6·6S γ globulin) but all of the remaining chromatogram peaks contain mixtures of proteins [2, 8]. The distribution of normal serum protein components is described by Goodman *et al* [9] and Tombs *et al* [10].

The locations of many normal serum protein components are indicated in Fig. 3.2.

Serum components, such as enzymes, may be associated with several molecular forms and chromatography can be useful in separating these forms. Lactic dehydrogenase is identified in three distinct chromatogram components (Fig. 3.5). These are found to represent electrophoretically different classes of

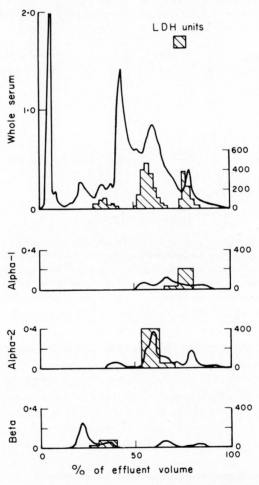

FIG. 3.5. Chromatographic distribution of the lactic dehydrogenases.

Serum from a patient with malignant melanoma and metastases to the liver had a serum level of 502 u/0·1 ml. Chromatography was carried out on a DEAE-cellulose column as illustrated in Fig. 3.2. Serum α_1, α_2 and β globulin fractions were prepared by zone (block) electrophoresis and subjected to chromatography under similar conditions.

enzyme, but the distinction is more clearly seen on DEAE-cellulose chromatography than on zone electrophoresis.

Serum protein chromatograms may reflect the serum protein changes of

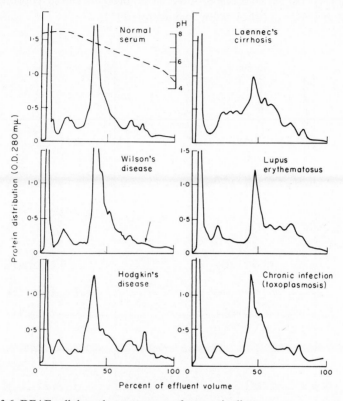

FIG. 3.6. DEAE-cellulose chromatograms of serums in disease.

In each case, the disease was in an active and advanced state. In the Wilson's Disease
serum the absence of a ceruloplasmin peak is indicated by the arrow. In the other
diseases the low peak at about 40 per cent of the elution volume represents low
serum albumin levels. The increased components seen in the other disease serums
represent increase of some α and β globulin components. Some of the changes in
chronic infection are shown in Fig. 3.7, and the changes in Hodgkin's Disease are
described in detail elsewhere [11]. Chromatography was carried out as described in
Fig. 3.2. The change in pH in the effluent during DEAE-cellulose chromatography
with tris phosphate buffers is shown with the normal serum chromatogram.

disease (Fig. 3.6). The distortions caused by disease, however, are better
seen by combining DEAE-cellulose chromatography with zone electrophoresis.
In Fig. 3.7, the protein distribution in serum from a patient with chronic
infection is compared with that of a normal serum. Striking change in serum

proteins and glycoproteins can be detected in a number of diseases by combining DEAE-cellulose chromatography with other analytic techniques. Combined procedures for example, proved valuable in a study of Hodgkin's Disease [11]. Decreased levels of some serum proteins and glycoproteins and marked increases of others were demonstrated [11].

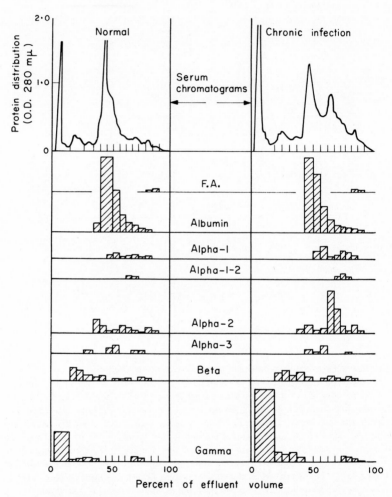

FIG. 3.7. Two dimensional analysis of serum protein changes in disease (DEAE-cellulose chromatography + zone electrophoresis).

Three millilitres of normal serum and 3 ml of serum from a patient with active pulmonary tuberculosis were fractionated on DEAE-cellulose columns as described in Fig. 3.2. The effluent from each column was divided into sixteen pools, concentrated and analysed by paper electrophoresis.

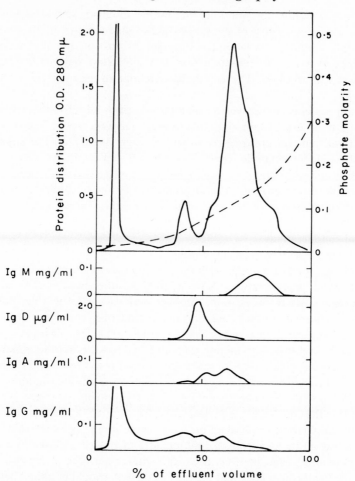

FIG. 3.8. Immunoglobulin distribution on DEAE-cellulose chromatography.

Five millilitres of normal human serum were dialysed against 0·015 M, pH 8 potassium phosphate buffer and applied to a 2 × 22 cm column containing 8 g of DEAE-cellulose equilibrated with the same buffer. Elution was performed with 500 ml of buffer in a gradient from 0·015 to 0·30 M phosphate at pH 8. The change in phosphate concentration is shown by the dashed line. Immunoglobulin distribution was determined with the quantitative assay of each component using the antibody-in-agar plate technique [12] except for IgM where the estimate was made from Ouchterlony tests. The serum donor had a low level of IgA and a high level of IgD, but the chromatographic distribution of these two proteins was similar to that in other serums [31].

The gradient elution (increasing molarity) at a constant pH used here (and in all subsequent figures) differs from the chromatographic procedure used in the previously illustrated chromatograms where progressive lowering of pH was also produced, as in Fig. 3.4.

Immunoglobulin distribution on DEAE-cellulose chromatography is shown in Fig. 3.8. Most of the serum IgG is eluted in the first fraction, but some IgG continues to be eluted throughout most of the effluent volume. IgD appears in a fairly discrete region. IgA is eluted more broadly and overlaps with IgD and IgM. The last immunoglobulin to emerge from the column is IgM.

Serum proteins are recovered quantitatively from DEAE-cellulose columns [2], but it is less certain that quantitative recovery always occurs if the substituted anionic groups are present in high density on the supporting material. Under suitable conditions recovery of antibody activity from DEAE-cellulose columns has been good as would be expected because of the mild conditions employed for adsorption and elution. In specific experiments, it is advisable to use quantitative methods to determine recovery.

Special considerations

Evaluating DEAE-cellulose preparations

Marked variations are observed in the performance of commercially available DEAE-cellulose preparations. Not only are there differences between suppliers, but separate lots from the same supplier may vary considerably. Some are useless for immunoglobulin preparation. The nitrogen content of the DEAE-cellulose preparations has not proved to be a good guide to their performance. One test is useful in determining the value of DEAE-cellulose preparations. (I) A standard column 1×25 cm is packed with the test DEAE-cellulose. Two millilitres of normal human serum is added and chromatography carried out in the usual way. The resolution of serum proteins is determined (*a*) by measuring the OD at 280 mμ of the elution fractions, (*b*) by locating the elution site of transferrin (iron-binding protein)—none should be in the first protein peak—and (*c*) by localizing the elution sites of IgA (β_{2A} globulin) and IgM (γ_{1M} globulin) by Ouchterlony tests with specific antiserums. Neither should be in the first protein peak and the bulk of the IgA should be eluted before the bulk of the IgM globulins. (II) One millilitre of macroglobulinaemic serum (containing 50 mg IgM per ml) is chromatographed to determine whether or not the DEAE-cellulose has the capacity to adsorb this load of IgM. The test behaviour of adequate and inadequate preparations of DEAE-cellulose is compared in Fig. 3.9. This test may have to be carried out at several initial buffer salt concentrations such as 0·02 M, 0·01 M or 0·005 M phosphate (pH 8 potassium phosphate) to ascertain the conditions under which useful fractionation can be achieved.

Sample size, column dimensions, elution volumes

Serum proteins can generally be separated adequately on the basis of 1 ml of whole serum per g of dry DEAE-cellulose. The maximal amount of serum that can be used, however, will vary with the properties of the adsorbent as noted above. Column dimensions, sample size and effluent volume relationships which we have found useful for routine work are listed in Table 3.2. The relative amount of serum can be increased if the DEAE-cellulose is a good adsorbent and a low ionic strength initial buffer is used.

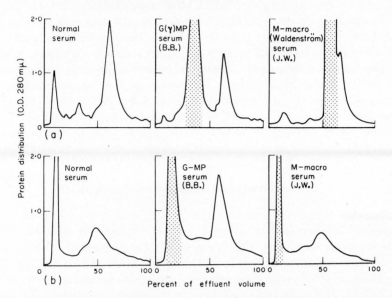

FIG. 3.9. Comparison of adequate (*a*) and inadequate (b) DEAE-cellulose preparations.

One millilitre of serum was applied to a column containing 2 g of prepared DEAE-cellulose and protein was eluted in 150 ml of buffer with a gradient of 0·01 M to 0·30 M phosphate (potassium) pH 8 buffer. Serum BB contains a G-myeloma protein and serum JW has large amounts of Waldenström macroglobulin. The shaded area indicates the location of the anomalous protein after chromatography of myeloma or macroglobulinemic serums. Both of the anomalous proteins are adsorbed to the good DEAE-cellulose preparation under the initial conditions for chromatography, and are eluted later in an appropriate fraction of the effluent. With the poor DEAE-cellulose preparation little of the anomalous proteins are adsorbed and both proteins appear in the first effluent fraction. As a result, no distinction is made between these proteins (although they have different properties on suitable adsorbents) and they are not separated from the normal IgG fraction of serum.

Stepwise elution

Stepwise changes (in contrast to a gradient) in elution buffers may be advantageous for purification of specific proteins. Proper use of stepwise elution techniques usually requires preliminary explorations to establish the best conditions for separating specific components. Stepwise techniques have been used to separate $7S\gamma_2$ and $7S\gamma_1$ globulins of guinea-pigs [13] and to separate blood group antibodies in human serum [14, 15].

Carboxymethyl (CM)-cellulose chromatography

CM-cellulose is a cation exchanger and is used with buffer systems below pH 7. Serum proteins are eluted from CM-cellulose in reverse order relative to DEAE-cellulose chromatography. The most cathodal migrating proteins are eluted last rather than first from the columns. Immunoglobulins adsorb to CM-cellulose in acetate buffer at pH 5·5. Either acetate or phosphate buffers may be employed successfully. Elution of proteins is achieved by increasing pH and by raising ionic strength. Conditions must be chosen carefully to obtain good recovery of immunoglobulins. Sober & Peterson [16] have reported fractionation of IgG on CM-cellulose columns. Porter [4] found CM-cellulose to be of value in separating the papain produced fragments of rabbit IgG.

3. Gel filtration (exclusion) chromatography

Introduction

Exclusion chromatography utilizing gels of cross-linked dextran, agar, agarose or polyacrylamide beads is a method for the separation of substances of different molecular dimensions. This method has proved valuable for fractionation of serum proteins, enzymes, hormones, nucleic acids and other substances; as a method for desalting or removing excess dyes, etc., from solutions of macromolecules; and has been utilized for estimation of molecular weights of proteins. The gel filtration technique has been reviewed by Porath [17], Tiselius *et al* [18] and by Laurent & Killander [19] and is also described in literature provided by suppliers of the gel beads.

Gel-forming beads are allowed to swell in buffer, water or other solution, and are packed in a column. The column volume is occupied by the bead material, the solution within the beads, and the solution between the beads. Protein molecules larger than the bead pores will pass unhindered through the column and emerge with the void volume (Fig. 3.10). Smaller molecules will enter the beads.

The number of beads entered by a particular molecular group determines its rate of passage through the column. Solute molecules within the gel beads maintain a concentration equilibrium with solute in the liquid phase outside the gel. Thus, a particular molecular species moves as a band through the column. Molecular weight plus molecular shape and hydration affect the behaviour of molecules during exclusion chromatography. In general, however, protein molecules appear in the column eluent in order of decreasing size.

A number of gels of different molecular exclusion limits have been prepared and these separate molecules in various size ranges. Sephadex G-200* (exclusion limit—molecular weight about 200,000) has been used extensively for separation and purification of the serum proteins, and the immunoglobulins in particular. Techniques for separation of serum proteins on Sephadex

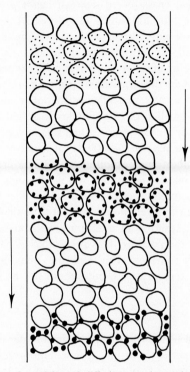

FIG. 3.10. Separation of particles of different size by exclusion chromatography (gel filtration).

Three sizes of molecules are shown being separated by the gel beads. The largest molecules are excluded from the bead pores and emerge with the void volume (adapted from Tiselius, Porath & Albertsson, 1963). The intermediate size particles are excluded from some of the bead pores. The smallest particles pass freely into the gel beads.

G-200 are described below. Similar techniques are used with acrylamide and methylenebis-acrylamide copolymer bead (Bio-Gel P300)† filtration.

Procedure for Sephadex G-200 chromatography
Reagents and equipment
Sephadex G-200, Sephadex G-25 (coarse). Tubing and glassware for column

* Pharmacia Fine Chemicals, New York, N.Y., London and Uppsala, Sweden.
† BioRad Laboratories, Richmond, California.

operation. Stock solutions of: (*a*) Tris-HCl, 1·0 M, pH 8·0 and (*b*) NaCl, 1·0 M for preparation of buffer that is 0·2 M NaCl and 0·1 M tris-HCl.

Preparation of gel column

Commercially obtained cross-linked dextran beads are sieved using a U.S. Standard Sieve Series No. 200 which has pores 74 μ in diameter. Smaller Sephadex beads which pass through the sieve are discarded, and, those remaining are retained. This fraction is allowed to swell for 1 week in an excess of buffer consisting of 0·1 M Tris-HCl and 0·2 M NaCl. Any fine particles discernable by opacity of the supernatant fluid are removed by decantation.

The column (4 × 55 cm) is half-filled with buffer and the outflow tap is clamped. A slurry of swollen G-25 Sephadex is added to form a 1 cm layer over the outlet filter (or cotton plug). When this has settled, a thick slurry of G-200 is added. When a layer of G-200 has formed at the bottom, the outflow tap is opened and additional amounts of G-200 are added at frequent intervals until the Sephadex column is 45-50 cm high. Buffer is allowed to flow overnight to permit the gel beads to settle. The surface can be made smooth by stirring the top layer and allowing it to settle while buffer is flowing through the column. Addition of a 25-cm extension tube to the top of the column will facilitate the pouring. It is preferable to pack the column at the temperature at which it will be run. Columns may be moved from room temperature to lower temperatures, but should not be moved from lower to higher temperatures.

Column operation

The sample is applied to the top of the column under the buffer solution by introduction of a pipette to within a few millimetres of the gel surface. Sample should be expressed smoothly and steadily. This may be facilitated by using a syringe driven by a synchronous motor. The density of the sample may be increased by addition of sucrose—to a 3 per cent sucrose concentration in serum with the buffers described above. If a 1 molar NaCl buffer is used, addition of sucrose to a 10 per cent concentration may be necessary.

The column is connected by an airtight system to a buffer reservoir. A hydrostatic head of pressure of 6–12 cm has proved generally useful. Higher pressure tends to pack the column and decreases flow rate. Flow rates of about 1–2 ml/cm^2/hour are usual with this technique.

Flodin & Killander [20] have recommended using a hydrostatic head of 100–200 cm. This is possible if relatively small beads of Sephadex G-200 are used to prepare the column. Flow rates may be slow under these conditions.

The protein distribution in the eluate may be determined by measuring the optical density at 280 mμ through a system for continuous monitoring of the effluent or by examination of individual effluent fractions.

Reverse flow chromatography is a process in which the sample and buffer enter the column at the bottom and emerge at the top. This technique is advantageous for maintaining good buffer flow rate and avoiding gel packing. Plastic columns (Fig. 3.1) are packed with Sephadex beads in the standard way. Long thin plastic tubing is attached to inflow and outflow taps on the column and tube openings are adjusted to appropriate heights for desired buffer flow rates—the outflow tube over a fraction collector and the inflow tubing in a buffer reservoir. Serum is added by placing the free end of the inflow tubing into the sample (the other end of the tubing is attached to the bottom of the column) and allowing the serum to be drawn into the tubing.

Recycling chromatography

Proteins differing only slightly in size may be incompletely separated by passage through a standard gel filtration column. Resolution can be improved by use of very long columns (usually not technically feasible) or recycling chromatography [21]. By this modification [21], selected column fractions are passed through the column several times to amplify small differences in filtration rate. Recycling chromatography can be performed as a continuous process [21] with the aid of equipment for monitoring protein content of the effluent. Recycling chromatography is usually performed as a reverse flow process.

Exclusion chromatography with boiled gels

Columns prepared from larger beads of G-200 which have been treated by boiling have been introduced recently by Rapp & Borsos [22]. These may be run under a low buffer head, and have the advantage of fast flow rates (0·75 1 ml/min).

Sephadex G-200 is sieved on U.S. series 200 mesh, beads between 74 and 120 μ being retained [22]. Thirty grammes of the sieved material are placed in 1–1·2 litres of buffer (0·1 M tris–0·2 M NaCl), covered and boiled on a heating stirplate for 5–10 minutes. The slurry is then cooled to room temperature and poured into a 4×55 cm column without further addition of buffer to column or gel. The slurry is poured into the column as the gel packs until it reaches approximately 3(2–5)cm from the top of the column.

After packing, the column is washed overnight with buffer to stabilize the gel. Samples are applied with a disposable pipette, generally without addition of sucrose, and the buffer level on top of the gel brought up to approximately 1 cm from the rubber stopper on the top of the column. It is necessary to leave an air space between the buffer and the top of the column to absorb the changes in pressure within the column when the stopper is removed.

Buffer in a reservoir is maintained at a constant level approximately 4–10 cm from the bottom of the gel in the column to assure that buffer flow is not too rapid.

Distribution of immunoglobulins

Whole serum, when applied to a G-200 column, yields three major peaks of protein in the effluent (Fig. 3.11). IgM is present in the first peak in addition to α_2 macroglobulin, both having molecular weights of approximately

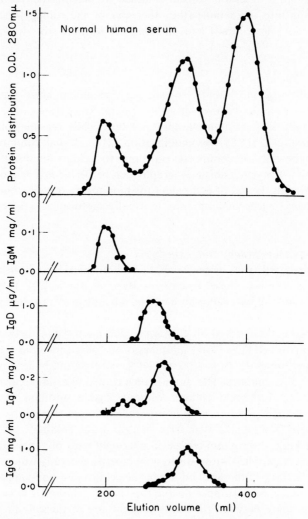

FIG. 3.11. Immunoglobulin distribution following G-200 Sephadex gel filtration of normal human serum.

900,000. Large lipoproteins and, in some serums, haemoglobin–haptoglobin complexes, which can be detected by characteristic colour, also appear in the first peak.

The second peak consists largely of IgG. The effluent fractions of the leading side of this peak are contaminated with IgA and IgD and those on the back side of the peak may contain non-immune globulins and albumin. The third peak contains albumin and globulins with molecular weights under 100,000. The distribution of individual serum components has been described by Flodin & Killander [20] and Fireman et al [23].

Serum IgA is eluted before the peak of IgG (Fig. 3.11). Serum IgA is heterogeneous in size, however, and also appears in the first protein peak and in the region between the first two peaks. IgD is eluted just before the major IgA peak (Fig. 3.11).

The use of gel filtration techniques for the estimation of protein molecular weight is described by Whitaker [24] and Andrews [25].

Separation of polypeptide chains

The polypeptide chains of immunoglobulins were shown by Edelman & Poulik [26] and by Porter [27] to be dissociated by reduction, alkylation and acidification. The heavy and light polypeptide chains may be separated by gel filtration using Sephadex G-75 as described by Fleischman, Pain & Porter [5]. Subsequently, Sephadex G-100, G-200, or intermediate size became available and have been used to separate polypeptide chains. The G-200 columns have the advantage of separating partly aggregated (or incompletely dissociated) material into several fractions.

Sephadex G-200 columns for separating polypeptide chains may be prepared with 1 N acetic acid, 8 M urea, or 5 M guanidine. If guanidine is to be used in a column of boiled Sephadex, the Sephadex must be boiled in 5 M NaCl, because guanidine cannot be heated to high temperatures. The gel bed can be equilibrated with 5 M guanidine after the column is packed.

4. Preparation of purified immunoglobulins

IgG may be purified by DEAE-cellulose chromatography of serum from man, rabbit and many other species. IgG is not readily obtained by this method, however, from some species such as the mouse [28]. In addition to the technique for chromatography described above, Levy & Sober [29] used a buffer of lower pH and an excellent DEAE-cellulose adsorbent to obtain human serum IgG. This material (in pH 6·3 buffer) could be applied directly to CM-cellulose columns for further fractionation.

IgM can be prepared by a combination of zone electrophoresis (selecting the slower migrating fractions to reduce contamination with IgA, β lipoprotein and α_2 macroglobulin) and Sephadex G-200 gel filtration (taking the ascending half of the first elution peak) to obtain the larger immunoglobulin molecules.

IgA may be partly purified from normal serum by combining zone electrophoresis to obtain the β globulin region with Sephadex G-200 chromatography, to collect the fractions eluted after IgM and before IgG. DEAE-cellulose chromatography may be helpful for preparing A-myeloma proteins from ammonium sulphate or electrophoretic fractions of whole serum.

IgD is normally present in small amounts and is similar to several other immunoglobulin groups in physical properties [31]. IgD has been purified from serums with D-myeloma proteins or from serums with abundant IgD but little IgG or IgA, obtained from patients with selective immunoglobulin deficiency syndromes.

References

[1] PETERSON E.A. & SOBER H.A. (1956) Chromatography of proteins. I. Cellulose ion-exchange adsorbants. *J. Am. Chem. Soc.* **78,** 751

[2] SOBER H.A., GUTTER F.J., WYCKOFF M.M. & PETERSON E.A. (1956) Chromatography of proteins. II. Fractionation of serum protein on anion-exchange cellulose. *J. Am. Chem. Soc.* **78,** 756

[3] PORATH J. & FLODIN P. (1959) Gel filtration: A method for desalting and group separation. *Nature, Lond.* **183,** 1657

[4] PORTER R.R. (1959) The hydrolysis of rabbit γ-globulin and antibodies with crystalline papain. *Biochem. J.* **73,** 119

[5] FLEISCHMAN J.B., PAIN R.H. & PORTER R.R. (1962) Reduction of γ-globulins. *Arch. biochem. Biophys.* **Suppl. 1** 174

[6] PETERSON E.A. & SOBER H.A. (1962) Column chromatography of proteins: Substituted cellulose. In *Methods in Enzymology*, eds. COLOWICK S.P. & KAPLAN N.O. Vol. V, pp. 3–27. Academic Press: New York

[7] PETERSON E.A. & SOBER H.A. (1959) Variable gradient device for chromatography. *Anal. Chem.* **31,** 857

[8] FAHEY J.L., McCOY P.F. & GOULIAN M. (1958) Chromatography of serum proteins in normal and pathological sera: The distribution of protein-bound carbohydrate and cholesterol, siderophilin, thyroxin-binding protein, B12-binding protein, alkaline and acid phosphatases, radioiodinated albumin and myeloma proteins. *J. Clin. Invest.* **37,** 272

[9] GOODMAN H.C., DEVAUX ST. CYR. C., CLEVE H. & GRABAR P. (1961) Immuno-electrophoretic studies of normal human serum fractionated by anion exchange cellulose column chromatography in Protides of the Biological Fluids. In *Proc. of 8th Colloquim*, ed. PEETERS H. Elsevier: Amsterdam

[10] TOMBS M.P., COOKE K.B., BURSTON D. & MACLAGEN N.F. (1961) The chromatography of normal serum proteins. *Biochem. J.* **80,** 284

[11] GOULIAN M. & FAHEY J.L. (1961) Abnormalities in serum proteins and protein-bound hexose in Hodgkin's disease. *J. Lab. Clin. Invest.* **57,** 408

[12] FAHEY J.L. & McKELVEY E. (1965) Quantitative determination of serum immuno-globulins in antibody-agar plates. *J. Immunol.* **94,** 84

[13] YAGI Y., MAIER P. & PRESSMAN D. (1962) Two different anti-insulin antibodies in guinea pig antiserum. *J. Immunol.* **89,** 442

[14] ABELSON N.M. & RAWSON A.J. (1959) Studies of blood group antibodies. I Fractiona-tion of anti-A and anti-B isohemagglutinins by anion-cation cellulose chromato-graphy *J. Immunol.* **82,** 435

[15] ABELSON N.M. & RAWSON A.J. (1961) Studies of blood group antibodies. V. Fractiona-tion of examples of anti-B, anti-A, B, anti-M, anti-P, anti-Jk, anti-Le, anti-D, anti-CD, anti-K, anti-Fy, anti-s and anti-Good. *Transfusion* **1,** 116

[16] SOBER H.A. & PETERSON E.A. (1958) Protein chromatography on ion exchange cellu-lose. *Fed. Proc.* **17,** 1116

[17] PORATH J. (1960) Gel filtration of proteins, peptides and amino acids. *Biochim. biophys. Acta* **39,** 193

[18] TISELIUS A., PORATH J. & ALBERTSSON P.A. (1963) Separation and fractionation of macromolecules and particles. *Science* **141,** 13

[19] LAURENT T.C. & KILLANDER J. (1964) A theory of gel filtration and its experimental verification. *J. Chromatog.* **14,** 317

[20] FLODIN P. & KILLANDER J. (1962) Fractionation of human serum proteins by gel filtration. *Biochim. biophys. Acta* **63,** 403

[21] PORATH J. & BENNICH H. (1962) Recycling chromatography. *Arch biochem. Biophys.* **Suppl. 1,** 152

[22] BORSOS T. & RAPP H.J. (1965) Estimation of molecular size of complement components by sephadex chromatography. *J. Immunol.* **94,** 510

[23] FIREMAN P., VANNIER W.E. & GOODMAN H. (1964) Immunochemical studies of human serum fractionated by gel filtration with Sephadex G-200. *Proc. Soc. exp. Biol. Med.* **115,** 845

[24] WHITAKER J.R. (1963) Determination of molecular weights of proteins by gel filtration on sephadex. *Anal. Chem.* **35,** 1950

[25] ANDREWS P. (1964) Estimation of the molecular weights of proteins by sephadex gel filtration. *Biochem. J.* **91,** 222

[26] EDELMAN G.M. & POULIK M.D. (1961) Studies on structural units of the γ-globulins. *J. exp. Med.* **113,** 861

[27] PORTER R.R. (1962) The structure of gamma-globulin and antibodies. In *Basic Problems in Neoplastic Disease*, eds. GELHORN A. & HERSCHBERG, E. pp. 177–194. Columbia University Press: New York

[28] FAHEY J.L. (1966) Chromatographic Separation of Immunoglobulins. In *Methods of Immunology*, eds. CHASE M. & WILLIAMS, C.A. in press

[29] LEVY H.B. & SOBER H.A. (1960) A simple chromatographic method for preparation of gamma globulin. *Proc. Soc. exp. Biol. Med.* **103,** 250

[30] STRAUSS A.J.L., KEMP P.G., JR., VANNIER W.E. & GOODMAN H.C. (1964) Purification of human serum γ-globulin for immunologic studies: γ-globulin fragmentation after sulfate precipitation and prolonged dialysis. *J. Immunol.* **93,** 24

[31] ROWE D.S. & FAHEY J.L. (1965) A new class of human immunoglobulins. II. Normal serum IgD. *J. exp. Med.* **121,** 185

CHAPTER 4

Ultracentrifugation of Immunoglobulins

D.R.STANWORTH

Introduction

Ultracentrifugation has, of course, played a leading role in the characterization of immunoglobulins. Indeed, it was the first technique to demonstrate convincingly the existence of more than one class of γ globulin in animal sera.

Early studies [1] employing the high speed ultracentrifuges developed by the Svedberg group in Uppsala, revealed the presence of 5–10 per cent of a high molecular weight component (18–19S) in horse and human serum globulin fractions, in addition to the major 7S component. The subsequent demonstration that isoagglutinin activity was associated with the macroglobulin component [2] moreover, dispelled speculation that possibly some animal species (e.g. human) produced 7S antibodies, whilst others (e.g. horse) produced the 19S type. Purified antibodies of both sedimentation classes, isolated from antisera raised in many different animal species, have since been characterized by ultracentrifugation [3].

The type of antibody produced in response to a particular antigen (e.g. pneumococcal polysaccharide) would seem to depend on the species of animal immunized. As is now well known, however, other factors are involved and different types of antibody are produced at different stages following immunization. In this connection, it is interesting to note, in retrospect, that a secondary immunization process (e.g. in horses) was observed to lead to the appearance of 'ultracentrifugally inhomogeneous components' (e.g. 17S, 12S and 7S) [3], in addition to the 19S antibody component detected in a first-bleeding of the animals.

The use of highly specific immuno-diffusion techniques has led to the further characterization of the different sedimenting classes of immunoglobulin, revealing structural relationships in that all contain one type of polypeptide chain—the 'light' chain—in common,* as well as the existence of new classes of immunoglobulin (e.g. γD [4]); nevertheless, as will be indicated, ultracentrifugation (in its many different forms) still has an important function to fulfil,

---

* The immunoglobulin nomenclature recently compiled by WHO will be used throughout the rest of the article, where necessary, i.e. 19S γ globulin will be referred to as γM; 7S γ globulin as γG, etc.

44

at a time when the study of immunoglobulins is beginning to attract the attention of molecular biologists as well as immunologists.

The characterization of immunoglobulins (in serum or in isolated form) by moving boundary procedures carried out in analytical rotors, is dealt with in section A. Besides providing an outline of the various methods used in the determination of the molecular size of native immunoglobulins, this section indicates how analytical ultracentrifugation is being applied to the study of their association and dissociation products (which are not readily defined by other techniques).

As has happened, however, in the field of electrophoresis, the classical moving boundary procedures are being replaced by more practicable and flexible zone-separation techniques. Hence, zone-centrifugation is described in some detail in section B, together with various forms of boundary analysis performed in preparative ultracentrifuge tubes. As will be illustrated, these techniques, which are both analytical and preparative, are of particular application to the characterization of antibodies present in serum in only trace amounts and not readily isolated in pure form.

A short final section (C) considers recent development in ultra-centrifugation techniques, which could prove pertinent to the future study of immunoglobulins.

Section A

Boundary ultracentrifugation in analytical rotors

No attempt will be made to provide a detailed theoretical background to the methods in use within this field. Such a need is adequately fulfilled by general books and review articles [1, 5, 6, 7, 8, 9]. Nevertheless, before describing procedures which have been developed for the *isolation* of immuno-globulins, an outline will be given of the principal techniques employed in the characterization of these proteins in the analytical ultracentrifuge.

1. *Determination of relative composition*
To many investigators, the conventional schlieren pattern (refined by the introduction of a phase-plate into the optical system of the Spinco Model E ultracentrifuge) still provides the most useful guide to the ultracentrifugal composition of protein mixtures. By this procedure, for example, it is possible to differentiate the serum immunoglobulin pattern observed in Waldenström macroglobulinaemia from that observed in myelomatosis (as shown in Fig. 4.1). Furthermore, human myeloma sera can be subdivided into a γG group and the less common γA groups, according to whether an increase solely

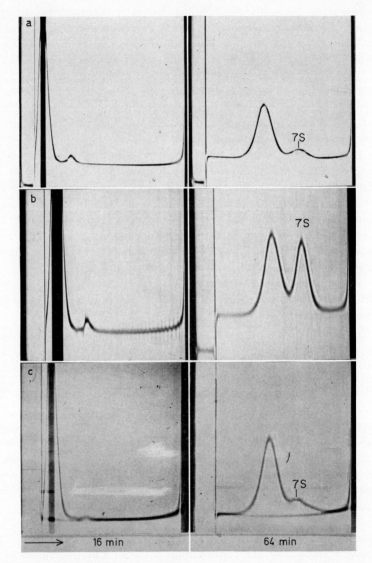

Fɪɢ. 4.1. Analytical ultracentrifugation patterns of human hyperglobulinaemic sera (59,780 rev/min, 20° C, solvents: barbitone pH 8·6, I=0·05 containing 0·2 ᴍ NaCl, or phosphate, pH 7·5, 0·01 ᴍ containing 0·15 ᴍ NaCl). Photographs taken at 16 and 64 min (except where otherwise stated).

(a) Normal human serum (dil 1/5).

(b) γG myeloma serum (dil 1/5) (showing marked elevation of 7S component).

(c) γD myeloma serum (dil 1/5) (showing increase in 7S component concentration).

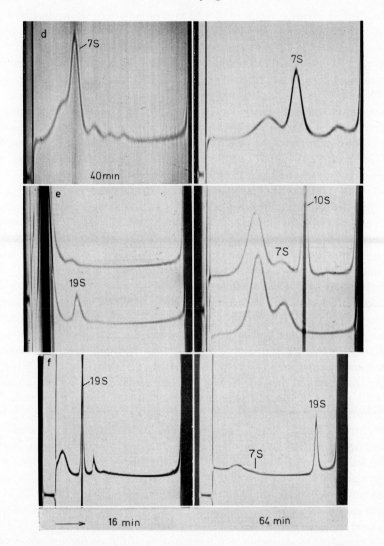

(d) γA myeloma serum (dil 1/5) (showing marked elevation of 7S component and additional abnormal components sedimenting between 7S and 19S).

(e) Top (wedge-window cell): γA myeloma serum (dil 1/5) (showing excessive amounts of abnormal 10S component). Bottom (standard cell): γA myeloma serum (dil 1/5) (showing increases in both 7S and 19S peaks, but no abnormal intermediate-sedimenting components).

(f) Waldenström macroglobulinaemic serum (dil 1/20) (showing gross elevation of 19S component and small amounts of faster sedimenting abnormal components).

in the 7S peak is observed (as in the γG myeloma pattern shown in Fig. 4.1b) or additional abnormal components sedimenting between the 7S and 19S peak are detected (as in the various forms of γA myeloma, now referred to as 'atypical γA myeloma' rather than 'atypical macroglobulinaemia' as was the practice). The much rarer γD myeloma [10], also shows an increase in the 7S peak of its serum ultracentrifugal pattern (see Fig. 4.1c).

In γA myeloma sera, an abnormal increase in the 7S peak is also frequently observed (Fig. 4.1d), but this is accompanied by the appearance of the faster sedimenting minor components (sometimes referred to as 'Z' components) not seen in the γG and γD myeloma patterns. Occasionally, however, the predominant increase in γ globulin concentration is associated with an abnormal 8–12S peak [11] (as shown in Fig. 4.1e). A protein responsible for this effect, isolated in pure form from a hyperglobulinaemic serum (but not identified as a γA globulin by antigenic analysis) [12], was shown to have a sedimentation coefficient (S_0) of 9·70S (molecular weight around 400,000) and to be split into half-molecules (6·25S) on reduction by 2-mercaptoethanol. Yet another type of γA myeloma serum pattern, recently described [13], and also illustrated in Fig. 4.1e., showed a marked increase in both the 7S and 19S peak areas (together with trace amounts of two abnormal components sedimenting between the 7S and 19S peaks). The serum concerned was shown to possess two distinct paraproteins (of β and γ_1 electrophoretic mobility), both of γA antigenic type (as revealed by gel-diffusion precipitin analysis with specific rabbit anti-γA globulin serum).

The discovery of this last-named type of γA myeloma serum immuno-globulin pattern emphasizes the importance of not basing a diagnosis of Waldenström macroglobulinaemia solely on the observed increase in the ultracentrifugal peak, which (as in this case) could represent the presence of polymerized 7S γA globulin. There are, however, other ultracentrifugal indications which help to avoid confusing this type of myeloma serum ultra-centrifugal pattern with that of a macroglobulinaemic serum. For instance, in the author's experience, an increase in the concentration of the 7S component rarely accompanies the marked increase in macroglobulin (19S γM, etc.) level found in the sera of cases with macroglobulinaemia. This observation is supported by the results of quantitative gel-diffusion precipitin analyses, carried out in parallel with ultracentrifugal analyses, on a group of fourteen macroglobulinaemic sera [14] in only one of which was the 7S component concentration abnormally raised (i.e. above 1200 mg/100 ml). In contrast however, Filliti-Wurmser *et al* [15] have produced *statistical* evidence of an increase in the 7S peak in the ultracentrifugal patterns of 57 Waldenström macroglobulinaemic sera (of which only three contained macroglobulin levels below 1·0 g/100 ml). This study revealed also a bimodal distribution of the predominant macroglobulin components, at 17·0S and 18·3S.

Another distinctive characteristic of macroglobulinaemic sera patterns is the presence of varying amounts of faster sedimenting 29S and 38S components* (seen in the pattern in Fig. 4.1f), in addition to the excessive level of the principal macroglobulin (19S) component. Moreover, it has been

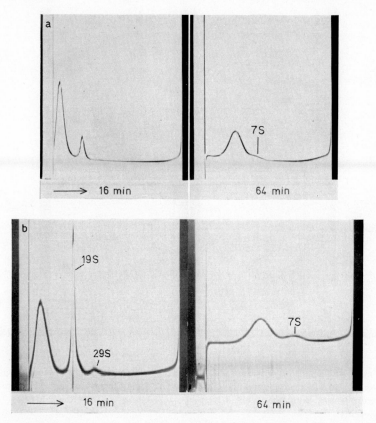

FIG. 4.2. Analytical ultracentrifugation patterns of serum (diluted 1/5) of supposed early case of Waldenström macroglobulinaemia (a), and the pattern of a sample of serum taken from the same patient, $6\frac{1}{2}$ years later (b). (59,780 rev/min, 20° C, photographs taken at 16 and 64 min).

shown [14] that the appearance of such components—assumed to be *in vivo* polymerization products of the 19S macroglobulin molecule—is dependent upon the serum level of the 19S component. Thus, it has been calculated that the 29S component should be detectable when the 19S component concentration level has reached 600 mg/100 ml, whilst the 38S component should appear

* Assigned different S_0 values by various investigators.

in the ultracentrifugal pattern of macroglobulinaemic sera if the 19S component level is higher than 1000 mg/100 ml.*

Like the major 19S γM components of macroglobulinaemic sera [16], the faster sedimenting components (i.e. 29S and 38S) are dissociated (to 7S

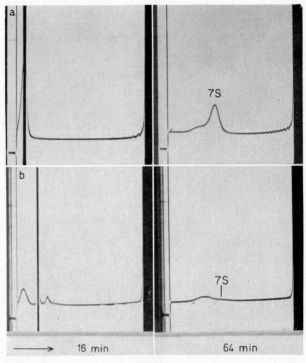

FIG. 4.3. Effect of: (a) reduction (0·1 M 2-mercaptoethanol) and (b) lowering of pH (to 4·2) on the macroglobulin components of a Waldenström macroglobulinaemic serum (shown untreated in Fig. 4.1f).
Solvents:
(a) 0·1 M 2-mercaptoethanol in barbitone buffer (pH 8·6, I = 0·05) containing 0·2 M NaCl.
(b) Acetate buffer (pH 4·2, I = 0·1).
Serum samples diluted 1/20.
(Conditions of ultracentrifugation as in Fig. 4.1).

* This point is also indicated by Fig. 4.2, which compares the ultracentrifuge patterns of samples of serum taken over a 6½ year period, from a steatorrhea patient who was found initially to have also a mild degree of macroglobulinaemia, manifested by a raised 19S component level of 465 mg/100 ml (i.e. 9 per cent total protein) as shown in patterns a. Ultracentrifugation of the second serum sample (pattern b)—6½ years later—shows that the 19S component level has increased to 26 per cent total protein; in addition, 29S component (4 per cent) and a trace of 38S component are now detectable.

sub-units) by reducing agents such as 2-mercaptoethanol (as shown in Fig. 4.3). In contrast, lowering of pH (e.g. to 4·2) fails to dissociate the macro-globulin components. This provides another example of the application of analytical ultracentrifugation to the characterization of the abnormal sedimenting γ globulin constituents found in certain hyperglobulinaemic sera. If, for example, the 29S and 38S macroglobulin peaks had comprised a γM antibody-antigen complex, they would have been disrupted by the acid pH, in a similar manner to the dissociation of the 22S complex (comprising γM rheumatoid factor and γG globulin) observed sedimenting ahead of the 19S

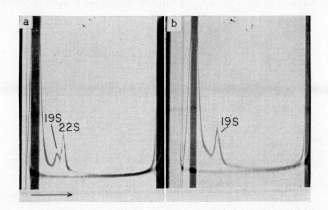

FIG. 4.4. Analytical ultracentrifugation patterns of rheumatoid arthritic serum (dil 1/2) in phosphate-citrate buffer, pH 7·0, 0·05 M, containing 0·15 M NaCl at (a) pH 7·0 (b) pH 4·6.

Photographs taken at 59,780 rev/min, 20° C, in double-sector cell containing solvent in the other compartment.

Note that the 22S complex (comprising rheumatoid factor and 7S γG globulin) is completely dissociated at the acid pH.

peak in the ultracentrifugal patterns of rheumatoid arthritic sera (as is shown in Fig. 4.4).

This effect should be differentiated, however, from the acid-dissociation ($<$pH 4·0) of *in vivo* aggregated γG globulin (e.g. of So = 14·6S) observed recently in the serum of a patient with multiple myeloma associated with hyperviscosity syndrome [105], and of a patient classified as suffering from a typical macroglobulinaemia, who revealed autopsy changes of polyarteritis nodosa [106].

Similarly, ultracentrifugal analysis (and starch-gel electrophoresis) have been employed to demonstrate that the components sedimenting faster than the 7S peak in γA myeloma sera are probably polymeric forms of 7S monomers [13]. For instance, neither concentrated urea solution (30 per cent

C

w/v) nor acid pH (3–4) showed any 'depolymerizing' effect, whereas 0·1 M 2-mercaptoethanol reduced the intermediate sedimenting components to 7S sub-units [17]. On the other hand, conclusive evidence is not yet available to support the contention that the high molecular weight components (i.e. >7S) observed in the ultracentrifugal patterns of purified preparations of normal serum γA globulin (to the extent of 19 per cent of the total protein) [18] are naturally occurring polymeric forms of this class of immunoglobulin. It has not proved easy, for instance, to demonstrate intermediate sedimenting (between 7S and 19S) γA globulin components at this concentration level in zone-centrifugal fractions of normal human serum (as is seen from Fig. 4.27).

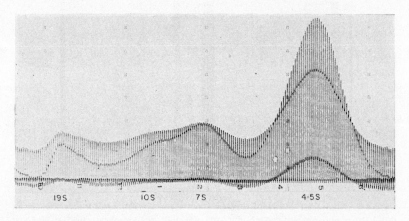

FIG. 4.5. Gel-filtration (Sephadex G. 200) pattern of normal human serum deprived of a major portion of the γG globulin component (by preliminary batch DEAE-cellulose chromatography). Gilford plots shown (monitoring at 280 mμ through 2 mm, 5 mm and 10 mm cells, full-scale deflection = 3·00 optical density units, 3 min readings).

Gel-filtration (Sephadex G. 200) of human serum, on the other hand, reveals a γA globulin distribution maximum slightly ahead of the γG globulin (i.e. peaking in a fast shoulder on the γG peak) [19, 20] (see Fahey and Terry Chapter 3). Moreover, a preliminary removal of the bulk of the γG globulin constituent (by batch DEAE-cellulose chromatography) leads to a serum gel-filtration pattern in which a separate elution peak ahead of the 7S peak is becoming apparent (as shown in Fig. 4.5, where the automatic monitoring technique referred to in section B3 was employed).

Obviously, it is always essential to employ more than one type of fractionation procedure if the serum immunoglobulins are to be estimated precisely. Analytical ultracentrifugation offers, however, the most reliable 'one-stage' method of quantitating the amounts of the abnormally sedimenting γ globulin components in γA myeloma and macroglobulinaemic sera. It is, of course, also applied to the estimation of the gross increase in the 7S and 19S fractions in myeloma and macroglobulinaemic sera respectively, although here it must be recognized that other serum proteins which sediment in these regions will not be differentiated. These include α_2 and β globulins (forming 32 per cent of the total) in the 7S peak, and α_2 macroglobulin in the 19S peak (forming about 67 per cent of the total in normal serum) [35].

It has been customary, therefore, to perform specific quantitative gel-diffusion precipitin estimations on the whole serum, in order to avoid estimating these non-γ globulin components separating in the 7S and 19S ultracentrifugal peaks. Similar immunological assays are employed in the sera of hypogammaglobulinaemic patients [21], where (in the case of untreated individuals) the γ globulin level is often below the limits of detection of the schlieren optical system of the analytical ultracentrifuge (i.e. below 50 mg/100 ml). Nevertheless, there are potential limitations of quantitative gel-diffusion precipitin estimations which must be guarded against. For instance, it is most important that the antiserum employed should be directed against all types of antigenic determinants likely to be encountered in any paraprotein falling within the particular class under estimation. It is also possible that errors in quantitation will be caused by the presence of polymerized forms of an immunoglobulin (e.g. γA), which will interfere with the accurate estimation of the level of the monomeric protein in hyperglobulinaemic sera. Finally, it should be realized that the results of quantitative precipitin analysis are expressed in terms of a reference standard (usually an arbitrarily selected normal human serum.)

A comparison of the results obtained by parallel ultracentrifugal and quantitative precipitin analyses of the γM globulin levels in a group of thirteen macroglobulinaemic sera is shown in Fig. 4.6. The ultracentrifugal values (which include the three forms of macroglobulin, where present) were obtained by determination of the areas under the peaks of enlarged ($\times 10$) tracings of the schlieren patterns (by the method of 'counting squares') and then relating these to the total serum protein determined independently by a biuret method. The gel-diffusion precipitin values are expressed as percentages of the γG globulin level in a standard human serum (from a healthy adult, assumed to have a normal serum γM globulin level of 50 mg/100 ml). As will be noticed, the immunological assay appears to be underestimating the total macroglobulins measured by ultracentrifugation, in the excessively high macroglobulin concentration range (even after allowing for the normal level of α_2 macroglobulin in the 19S peaks). This effect can possibly be attributed to the slower gel-diffusion rate of the polymeric forms of 19S macroglobulin also present.

A technical point worth mentioning is the necessity of diluting (usually at least ten times) macroglobulinaemic sera prior to ultracentrifugation, in order to eliminate the 'concentration bar' (due to self-sharpening of the 19S boundary) and thus permit the accurate determination of the area under the schlieren peak. It should be added, too, that the accuracy of concentration

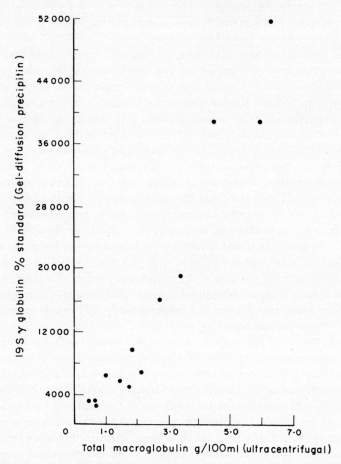

FIG. 4.6. Comparison of γM globulin contents of thirteen macroglobulinaemic sera, estimated by both analytical ultracentrifugation and quantitative gel-diffusion precipitin analysis (reproduced from *Clinica Chimica Acta* (1963), **8**, 91, by permission of the Elsevier Publishing Company).

estimations in general can be improved by the automatic fitting of a baseline to the serum schlieren pattern, by the use of a double-sector cell (as illustrated in Fig. 4.4), or by including in the rotor an extra cell containing the solvent. The latter arrangement also allows the direct comparison of two protein mixtures (as indicated by Fig. 4.1e), if one of the cells contains a wedge-window and providing the menisci are aligned by careful addition (with an accurate microsyringe) of the same volume of liquid into each cell.

Ultracentrifugal analysis has also been applied widely, of course, to an analysis of the composition of immunoglobulins isolated (by various fractionation procedures) from serum, urine and other body fluids. As already mentioned, for example, it has been employed to establish the purity of γA

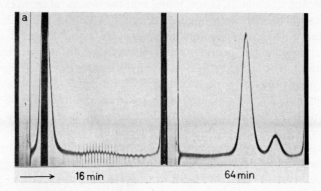

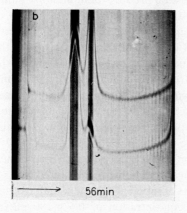

Fig. 4.7. Analytical ultracentrifugation patterns of (a) low-temperature ethanol preparation (Squibb) of human γG globulin (showing 20–40S aggregates, responsible for the convective disturbance spikes, and 15 per cent 10S dimer) and (b) fractions obtained by Sephadex G. 200 fractionation (top pattern, fraction enriched in 10S component; and bottom pattern, fraction enriched in 7S γG component).

Ultracentrifugation conditions: 59,780 rev/min, 20° C, solvent, phosphate buffer (pH 7·5, 0·01 M) containing 0·15 M NaCl.

globulin preparations isolated from normal human serum, and has revealed the presence of polymerized material (possibly formed as a result of the isolation procedure). Similarly, it has revealed association products in human γG globulin preparations isolated from normal human serum by low temperature ethanol (or ether) fractionation. For example, analytical ultracentrifugation of a Squibb preparation of human γG globulin* (used for poliomyelitis prophylaxis) revealed aggregated (20–40S) γ globulin and 15 per cent of dimer (10S), in addition to the native 7S form (as shown in Fig. 4.7a).

* Obtained through the courtesy of the American Red Cross Blood Program.

Gel filtration (on Sephadex G. 200) revealed a comparable size distribution, whilst recycling of the 10S fraction provided material enriched in dimer to the extent of 50 per cent total γG globulin (see Fig. 4.7b).

Ultracentrifugation has also thrown light on the mechanism of the structural alterations occurring in solutions of purified preparations of γG globulin (containing of the order of 1·0 g per cent protein) during storage [22], which are characterized by a 'splitting' of the immunoelectrophoresis precipitin line (as indicated in Chapter 7). It was found that the structural changes occurred in two stages. The first, involving formation of 10S dimer (up to 20 per cent of the total protein), was accompanied by a substantial degree of unfolding of the γG globulin polypeptide chains (as revealed by marked increase in laevorotation). The second stage involved the appearance of 5S component in the ultracentrifugal pattern, accompanied by a decrease in the level of 10S component, but only slight (if any) increase in laevorotation. The 5S degradation product was further degraded to 3·5S material, both of these sub-units showing properties similar to those of products of proteolytic enzyme digestion of γG globulin, and being responsible for the 'split-line' effect observed on immunoelectrophoresis of the stored human γG globulin. (The implications of these observations are considered in Chapter 7.)

The approximate sizes of enzymatic digestion products of immunoglobulins are usually determined by analytical ultracentrifugation, as are those of native immunoglobulin fragments (for example the Bence-Jones proteins, comprising monomeric or dimeric forms of light chains) isolated from the urine of patients with hyperglobulinaemia. The schlieren peaks shown by the latter proteins are difficult to resolve from each other, and from contaminating low molecular weight serum proteins e.g. albumin (due to boundary spreading occurring at the relatively long times of ultracentrifugation necessary at 59,780 rev/min). Recent investigations have indicated, however, that this problem will possibly be solved by the use of the high speed (max. 67,770 rev/min) titanium rotors now available for use in Spinco Model E machines. For instance [23], analytical ultracentrifugation at this higher speed has revealed a new intermediate in papain digests of rabbit γG globulin, sedimenting with an $S_{20,w}$ rate of $5·25 \pm 0·05S$ at a concentration of 0·6 g/100 ml (in 0·05 M acetate buffer, pH 5·5). This papain cleavage fragment was resolved from a faster moving 5·9S peak (assumed to represent structurally altered intact rabbit γG globulin) and from a slower moving 3·5S peak (assumed to be a mixture of Fab and Fc pieces).

Another important application of boundary ultracentrifugation in analytical rotors (in parallel with free-solution electrophoretic analysis) has been in the investigation of antibody-antigen reactions, where quantitative analysis of schlieren patterns has provided information about the size and composition of the soluble complexes formed at varying antigen-antibody ratios [24]. Recently, Gilbert [25] has indicated how his general mathematical treatment of reversibly reacting systems can be applied to the numerical analysis of the schlieren patterns obtained by sedimentation (and electrophoresis) of antigen-antibody systems. The model system chosen comprised a univalent antigen (molecular weight 70,000) and a bivalent antibody (molecular weight 150,000).

Analytical ultracentrifugation at varying pH has been employed [26] to determine the avidity of a γM antibody (rheumatoid factor) for antigen (γG globulin) preparations of different origins (isologous and autologous). In this

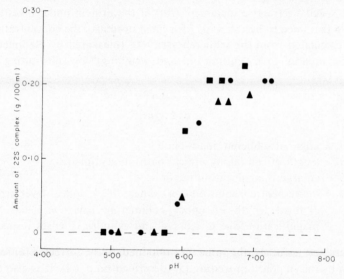

FIG. 4.8. Relationship between amount of artificially-formed 22S complex detectable and pH of reaction mixture. ■ rheumatoid factor and isologous normal human γG globulin; ● rheumatoid factor and autologous γG globulin; ▲ rheumatoid factor and isologous rheumatoid γG globulin.

investigation, constant amounts of human γG globulin and rheumatoid factor were mixed and dialysed against buffers of varying pH, the resultant mixture being examined in the ultracentrifuge for the presence of undissociated 22S complex (as indicated by Fig. 4.4a). The amount of dissociation occurring at each pH was determined by measurement of reduction of the area of the 22S peak as well as by the proportionate increase in area of the 7S peak. The plotting of degree of dissociation against pH (Fig. 4.8) failed to reveal any difference in the avidity of normal human γG globulin, isologous rheumatoid γG globulin or autologous rheumatoid γG globulin for rheumatoid factor. Such sedimentation data can also be used to confirm that the γM rheumatoid factor antibody molecule combines with approximately 6 molecules of antigen (γG globulin) [27], thus substantiating one of the few pieces of evidence yet available of the existence of multiple combining sites on γM antibody molecules.

The main drawback of the application of analytical ultracentrifugation for such purposes is the relative insensitivity of the schlieren optical system. Nevertheless, changes in protein concentration were calculated from the schlieren areas (by substitution in the equation shown below) with an error not exceeding 0·01 g/100 ml (providing that the protein concentration exceeded about 0·05 g/100 ml).

If the specific refractive increment (Δn) of the protein under investigation is known (assumed to be 186×10^{-5} for most proteins), the concentration (C) can be calculated from the schlieren area (A), (measured by planimetry, by 'counting squares' or by cutting out and weighing)* by substituting in the equation [28]:

$$C = \frac{A \tan \theta}{a \cdot I \cdot \Delta n E^2}$$

where θ = angle of schlieren phase-plate
a = length of cell (along optical path) in centimetres
E = enlarger magnification factor
I = instrument constant $b.m_x.m_c$, where 'b' = optical lever arm (cm)
= focal length of upper collimating lens; 'm_x' and 'm_c' = magnification due to camera and cylindrical lenses respectively.

For greatest accuracy, the value thus obtained can be corrected for sectorial dilution by the standard procedure [5] (described on p. 64). It is also important, when dealing with multicomponent systems, to correct for the Johnston–Ogston [29] effect for superimposed gradients of slow components on faster boundaries, if necessary [5, 6].

Finally, it is possibly worth mentioning the role of analytical ultracentrifugation in establishing the homogeneity of protein preparations. When a single schlieren peak has been observed, it is important to ascertain whether polydispersity is contributing to boundary spreading (by establishing whether the apparent diffusion constant, obtained from the ultracentrifuge pattern, is larger than the measured diffusion coefficient [5]). Even if this criterion of homogeneity is satisfied, however, it is possible that a minor contaminant is present in an amount below the limits of detection of the schlieren optical system.

It is customary, therefore, to confirm the purity of immunoglobulin (and

---

* Alternatively, areas can be determined by summation of ordinates under the curve, measured by means of a micro-comparator or plate assessor (as described in section A3).

other protein) preparations by performing gel-diffusion precipitin tests with antisera directed against all possible contaminants, whilst immunogenicity testing constitutes an even stricter criterion of purity. On the other hand, size heterogeneity (comprising polymeric forms of the immunoglobulins, already mentioned) is only readily demonstrable by ultracentrifugation (or gel filtration).

2. Determination of sedimentation coefficient

The other main application of boundary ultracentrifugation in analytical rotors is, of course, in the determination of sedimentation rate, from which the molecular weight can be determined (if the preparation is homogeneous) by substituting in the classical Svedberg equation:

$$M = \frac{RTS}{D(1-\bar{v}\rho)} \text{ at infinite dilution,}$$

where M = molecular weight
R = gas constant $(8\cdot314 \times 10^7 \text{ ergs}/°\text{C/mole})$
T = absolute temperature
S = sedimentation coefficient (S_0) in Svedberg units
D = diffusion coefficient (D_0)
$\bar{v}$ = partial specific volume of solute
ρ = density of solution at 20° C

As will be noted, the use of this equation in calculating molecular weight requires a separate determination of diffusion coefficient (D_0) either by a direct method (employing a Gouy diffusiometer or Tiselius cell) or indirectly by a comparative technique (as referred to in section B3). The accuracy of the latter procedures, however, is dependent upon the use of an appropriate range of reference proteins. Alternatively, the diffusion coefficient can be determined by measuring the broadening of an ultracentrifuge schlieren peak after sedimentation for varying times (and constant concentration) at very low speeds in a synthetic boundary cell [30]. As when determining sedimentation coefficients, it is necessary to correct for concentration dependence and for the Johnston–Ogston effect. Recently developed equilibrium techniques, however, avoid the necessity of determining sedimentation or diffusion coefficients in calculating molecular weight (as will be outlined in section A3).

As defined by Svedberg [1], the apparent sedimentation coefficient (S_{app}) is the sedimentation velocity (dx/dt) in a standard centrifugal field $(\omega^2 x)$,

i.e. $$S_{app} = \frac{dx/dt}{\omega^2 x}$$

c*

where $x =$ distance between the midpoint of the peak and the axis of rotation

$t =$ time (sec.)

$$\omega = \text{angular velocity} = 2\pi\,\frac{\text{rev/min}}{60}\;(\text{sec}^{-1}).$$

The most exact value of S is obtained by using the above in the integral form:

$$S_{\text{app}} = \frac{ln.x_2 - ln.x_1}{\omega^2(t_2 - t_1)}$$

where x_2 and x_1 are the distances (cm) between the peak maxima (P) and the axis of rotation at times t_2 and t_1 (in seconds)

or
$$S_{\text{app}} = \frac{2\cdot303}{\omega^2\,60}\,\frac{\log x_2 - \log x_1}{t_2 - t_1}$$

where t_2 and t_1 are in minutes.

The tabulation of data obtained by measurement of schlieren plates is illustrated in Table 4.1, where it will be noted that the distance of the peak (P_1) from the axis of rotation (i.e. x) at photo time (t) has been determined by subtraction of the distance between peak and outer reference line (i.e. $RL_2 - P_1$) from the known distance between the reference line and axis of rotation (i.e. 7·33 cm at maximum speed). The distance between peak and reference line (i.e. $RL_2 - P_1$) is measured (three times) with a microcomparator reading to 0·01 mm. A correction for acceleration time (during linear acceleration) is made by switching on the ultracentrifuge automatic camera at 4 min (i.e. when $\frac{2}{3}$ operating speed is reached) after starting the rotor (which took 6 min to reach the operating speed of 59,780 rev/min).

The apparent sedimentation coefficient can be readily obtained from such data (shown in Table 4.1), by plotting $\log x$ against t. The slope of the resulting curve gives $S_{\text{app}}.60\,\omega^2/2\cdot303$, from which the apparent sedimentation coefficient (S_{app}) can be calculated.

Computational methods [31] have been developed to determine apparent sedimentation coefficients by the graphical procedure just outlined. Any deviation from a linear $\log x$ against t relationship (which could be due either to heterogeneity of the schlieren peak under observation or to non-ideal sedimentation) is readily detected. Moreover, if a linear relationship obtains, the computer fits the best straight line to the points (by least squares analysis) and then calculates the slope.

In taking advantage of such a facility, it is of course necessary to obtain data from sedimentation analysis in a form which can be handled by a digital computer. This is being achieved in the author's laboratory by the use of an

TABLE 4.1

Specimen data obtained by micro-comparator measurement of schlieren plate in the determination of sedimentation coefficient

Run No. 2064. Rheumatoid factor preparation in phosphate buffer
(pH 6·9, 0·06 M) cont. 0·15 M NaCl
59,780 rev/min at 20° C, 60° phase-plate angle

Frame no.	Time (t) min	1st reading			2nd reading			3rd reading			Mean (RL_2-P_1) (on plate) cm	RL_2-P_1 /Magn. factors cm	Distance of peak from axis of rotation (x) cm
		Peak position (P_1)	Ref. line position (RL_2)	Difference (RL_2-P_1) cm	Peak position (P_1)	Ref. line position (RL_2)	Difference (RL_2-P_1) cm	Peak position (P_1)	Ref. line position (RL_2)	Difference (RL_2-P_1) cm			
1	4	18·675	15·878	2·797	18·521	15·723	2·798	18·650	15·855	2·795	2·797	1·308	6·022
2	8	14·533	11·935	2·598	14·378	11·789	2·589	14·324	11·735	2·589	2·592	1·212	6·118
3	12	10·342	7·967	2·375	16·374	13·998	2·376	10·139	7·754	2·385	2·379	1·112	6·208
4	16	6·115	3·942	2·173	12·139	9·964	2·175	5·897	3·726	2·171	2·173	1·016	6·314
5	20	2·928	0·964	1·964	7·947	5·983	1·964	6·195	4·231	1·964	1·964	0·918	6·412
6	24	3·763	2·015	1·748	3·762	2·007	1·755	4·804	3·053	1·752	1·752	0·819	6·511

electronic plate assessor* (as illustrated in Fig. 4.9). The results of measurements carried out by manual movement over cross-wires of a magnified ($\times 10$) image of a schlieren pattern are obtained rapidly (to an accuracy of 0·01 mm) in digital form and in typed form (on an IBM Type B typewriter), besides being punched directly on to paper tape.

This procedure leads to much greater speed in plate measurement (about ten times the speed of measurement by means of a travelling microscope), as well as reducing operator errors. Furthermore, the assessor has a valuable facility for editing data tape merely by the selection of push-button controls

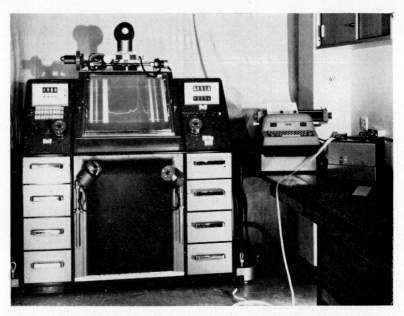

Fig. 4.9. The AGI plate assessor and ancillary IBM typewriter and tape-punch.

sited on the main console. The tape is then fed into the computer, together with a programme suitable for the calculation of sedimentation coefficients (as already described).

The simultaneous type-out of the plate measurements (a specimen of which is shown in Table 4.2, for direct comparison with the data obtained by micro comparator shown in Table 4.1) provides a valuable check on the data on the tape, besides affording a means of manual calculations of S_{app} (if required).

In other methods of obtaining sedimentation data, the need for a photographic record has been eliminated by employment of u.v. optical systems and automated recording techniques. For instance, Lamers *et al.* [32] have devised

* Manufactured by Aeronautical and General Instruments Co Ltd, Croydon, London.

a 'split-beam' recording system in which the centrifuge cell is scanned by a masked photomultiplier*, whilst Spragg *et al.* [33] have employed an oscillating mirror system for recording optical densities. Both systems have depended on the installation of a monochromator (in place of previously supplied filters) into the u.v. optical system of the Model E ultracentrifuge, and also the

TABLE 4.2

Data typed out directly, following measurement of the schlieren plate by means of the plate assessor (cf. the measurements from the same plate listed in Table 4.1, obtained by the conventional microcomparator technique).

The run number and 'position measured' number ('000' refers to meniscus, '001' to the peak and '099' to reference line RL_2) are typed in by operating buttons on the main console of the assessor. The last two columns (providing the distance, RL_2-P_1, between peak and reference line; and the meniscus position) are typed in manually. The y ordinate readings are irrelevant.

```
, 2064 004
,       000.  00000 00057.0 00001 00057.0 00001 00057   00001
,       001.  00190 00057.0 00192 00057.0 00191 00057   00191
,       099.  02982 00057.0 02982 00057.0 02984 00057   02982 02981
, 2064 008                                              2.790
,       000.  00000 00057.0 00001 00057.0 00001 00057   00001
,       001.  00392 00057.0 00396 00057.0 00394 00057   00394
,       099.  02983 00057.0 02984 00057.0 02986 00057   02984 02983
, 2064 012                                              2.590
,       000.  00000 00057.0 00001 00057.0 00001 00057   00000
,       001.  00598 00057.0 00599 00057.0 00598 00057   00598
,       099.  02985 00057.0 02985 00057.0 02987 00057   02985 02985
, 2064 016                                              2.387
,       000.  00000 00057.0 99998 00057.0 00001 00057   00000
,       001.  00807 00057.0 00806 00057.0 00810 00057   00808
,       099.  02982 00057.0 02984 00057.0 02979 00057   02981 02981
, 2064 020                                              2.173
,       000.  00000 00057.0 00001 00057.0 00002 00057   00001
,       001.  01017 00057.0 01017 00057.0 01017 00057   01017
,       099.  02983 00057.0 02981 00057.0 02981 00057   02981 02980
, 2064 024                                              1.964
,       000.  00000 00057.0 00000 00057.0 00001 00057   00000
,       001.  01228 00057.0 01229 00057.0 01230 00057   01229
,       099.  02984 00057.0 02982 00057.0 02984 00057   02984 02984
                                                        1.755
```

replacement of the standard mercury lamp by a reliable light source (e.g. stable xenon arc lamp) having a uniform spectral coverage in the visible and u.v. range. Measurements can also be taken from these systems in forms suitable for processing in a digital computer (besides monitoring by means of pen tracings).

It is of course necessary to correct the apparent sedimentation coefficients obtained by the methods outlined, to standard conditions (i.e. water at 20° C) by substituting in the equation:

$$S_{20,\,\mathrm{w}} = S_{\mathrm{app.}\,t^\circ,\,\mathrm{solv.}} \cdot \frac{\eta_{t^\circ,\mathrm{w}}}{\eta_{20^\circ,\mathrm{w}}} \cdot \frac{\eta_{t^\circ,\,\mathrm{solv.}}}{\eta_{t^\circ,\mathrm{w}}} \left(\frac{1 - \bar{v}_{20^\circ,\mathrm{w}} \cdot \rho_{20^\circ,\mathrm{w}}}{1 - \bar{v}_{t^\circ,\,\mathrm{solv.}} \cdot \rho_{t^\circ,\,\mathrm{solv.}}} \right)$$

* Now commercially available for installation in Spinco Model E machines.

where η, ρ and $\bar{v}$ are the viscosity, density and partial specific volume terms respectively for water (w) or solvent, at 20° C or at the temperature of centrifugation ($t°$). The first correction term is avoided by setting the RTIC system of the Model E machine to control the rotor temperature at 20° C. This leaves the need to correct for the density and viscosity of the chosen solvent system (which should contain at least 0·2 M neutral salt, in order to eliminate primary and secondary charge effects).

Finally, it is essential to ascertain the dependence of sedimentation coefficient ($S_{20,w}$) on concentration (C), by determining the sedimentation rate at varying finite concentrations (up to about 1 g protein/100 ml). The concentration values plotted (determined from the areas under the schlieren peaks, as already described on p. 58) should be first corrected for the decrease in concentration of the sedimenting component with increasing time and with increasing distance from the axis of rotation. This can be accomplished (to a good approximation) for a two-component system, by substituting in the square law equation [1]:

$$C_0 = C_t \left(\frac{x_t}{x_m} \right)^2$$

where C_0 and C_t are the concentrations at the start, and after time t respectively

x_m and x_t are the distances from the axis of rotation to the meniscus and peak respectively.

Extrapolation of the $S_{20,w}$ against C_0 plots to zero concentration then provides the value of the sedimentation coefficient at infinite dilution (i.e. S_0), from which the molecular weight can be calculated (by substitution in the Svedberg equation, on p. 59).

The plots obtained from ultracentrifugal analysis of isolated immunoglobulin preparations are shown in Fig. 4.10. These comprise total γG globulin fractions isolated from individual human* sera by batch DEAE-cellulose ion-exchange chromatography [34]; a '10S' γA globulin preparation isolated by Deutsch [12] from a human myeloma serum (as indicated in section A1) and a γM globulin isolated by Miller & Metzger [59] from the serum of a patient with Waldenström macroglobulinaemia.

The marked concentration dependence exhibited by these immunoglobulins (particularly the γM and γA globulins) emphasizes the futility of reporting a sedimentation coefficient of an isolated preparation without expressing the concentration of the solution analysed. If, however, it is possible to deter-

---

* The sedimentation coefficients of γG globulins isolated from the sera of other species show a similar concentration dependence [3].

mine the sedimentation coefficient of an immunoglobulin at only one concentration, some idea of the S_0 value can be obtained from the appropriate $S_{20,w}$ against C plot shown in Fig. 4.10. Alternatively, an approximate correction for concentration dependence can be made by substituting in the expression:

$$S_0 = S^{obs}(1 - k \cdot C)$$

assuming the reported slope of the $S_{20,w}$ against C plot for the immunoglobulin in question (e.g. $k = 0·005$ ml/mg for γG globulin [35]). If other components are present, it is necessary to correct for the concentration effect of these on the sedimentation rate of the observed peak, by substituting in the equation [35]:

$$S_i^0 = S_i^{obs}/(1 - \Sigma_1^i k_i c_i)$$

where S_i represents the sedimentation rate which would have been observed if the ith component were the only component present. Wallenius *et al* [35] have applied this procedure to the determination of the sedimentation coefficients of the principal components observed in schlieren patterns of electrophoretic fractions of human serum. They also found it necessary to make Johnston–Ogston corrections in analyses of solutions containing more than 6 mg/ml of 19S component.

3. Sedimentation equilibrium methods for the determination of molecular weight
Technical developments in this field of ultracentrifugation have obviated the necessity for separate determination of sedimentation (and diffusion) coefficients in order to obtain molecular weight values (as just described).

A major advance has been the avoidance of prolonged sedimentation equilibrium analyses by the exploitation (by Archibald [36]) of the conditions obtaining during the approach to equilibrium. Archibald realized that there was no net flow of solute through the surface at the meniscus or bottom of the ultracentrifuge cell. Hence, the conditions for equilibrium are satisfied in these regions (at any time) and molecular weight can be determined by substituting values of the concentration (c) and concentration gradient (dc/dx)—at the meniscus or at the bottom of the cell—in a thermodynamic form [5] of the Svedberg equation (for an ideal two-component system), viz:

$$M = \frac{RT}{(1 - \bar{v}\rho)\,\omega^2} \cdot \frac{dc/dx}{x.}$$

A discrepancy between the molecular weight values thus obtained from measurement at the top and bottom of the cell indicates heterogeneity, possibly due to the formation of aggregates in a solution containing a single

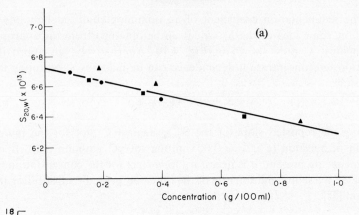

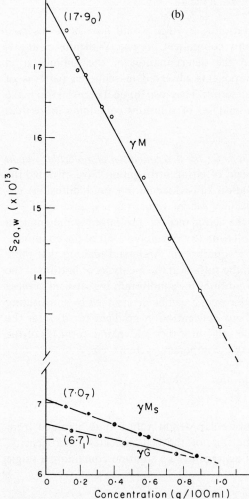

FIG. 4.10. $S_{20,w}$ against concentration (C) plots of the principal immunoglobulins.

(a) Various human γG globulin preparations, isolated from individual normal sera by batch DEAE-cellulose chromatography (shown by courtesy of Dr D.E. Normansell).

(b) γM globulin and its subunits (γMs) isolated from a Waldenström macroglobulinaemic serum (reproduced from *J. biol. Chem.*, (1965) **240**, 3325 by courtesy of Drs F.Miller and H.Metzger and the publishers, The American Soc. of Biological Chemists Inc., Baltimore.

(c) 10S γA globulin, isolated from a myeloma serum, and its 7S reduction fragment (reproduced from the *Journal of Molecular Biology*, (1963) **7**, 662 by courtesy of Dr H.F. Deutsch and the publishers, Academic Press Inc, New York).

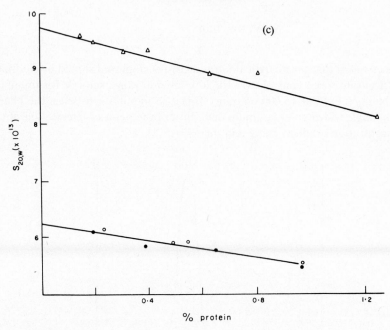

molecular species. When looking for such effects, it is important to ensure that the bottom of the cell forms the shape of a true sector from the axis of rotation, if necessary by including a drop of silicone oil (e.g. Dow Corning No. 555 Silicone fluid or Kel-F Polymer Oil No. 1) in the bottom of the cell in order to combat convective disturbances. Use of an immiscible liquid of this type aids the detection of aggregated material, the accumulation of which at the bottom of the cell leads to a thickening of the sharp interface between aqueous and non-aqueous liquids [37].

One of the main advantages of the Archibald method is that it provides a means of obtaining the weight average molecular weight, even of polydisperse systems in non-ideal solution. Moreover, by employing relatively high centrifugal fields in the study of such systems, it is possible to remove higher molecular weight aggregates or impurities before obtaining measurements solely on the principal component (an advantage not shared by other methods of determining molecular weight, such as light-scattering).

The selection of appropriate experimental conditions for determination of the molecular weight of proteins by this procedure has been discussed by Schachman [5], Elias [7] and others. The speed necessary to obtain measurable concentration gradients at the top and bottom of the cell (as shown in the tracing of the schlieren pattern in Fig. 4.11) can be calculated approximately from the following equation [28]:

$$\text{Speed (rev/min)} = \sqrt{\frac{5 \cdot 10^{11}}{M(1-\bar{v}\rho)}}$$

It is essential that the analytical ultracentrifuge employed should be equipped for accurate speed control over the low rev/min range suitable for immunoglobulins (i.e. 8000–15,000 rev/min). It is also important to select the phaseplate angle which gives optimum definition of the point of intersection of the concentration gradient curve and meniscus.

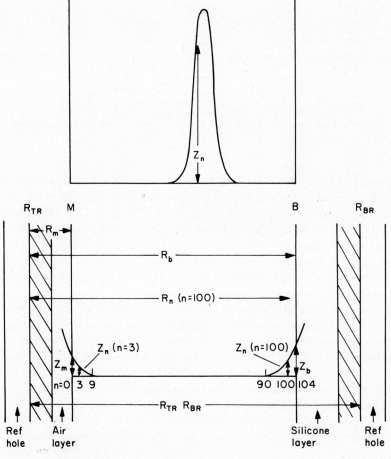

Fig. 4.11. Schematic diagram, illustrating the measurement of concentration gradient curves obtained in Archibald analyses (reproduced from *Methods in Enzymology* (1957), **4**, 57, by courtesy of Dr H.K.Schachman and the publishers Academic Press Inc, New York).

The determination of the values of C (at the top and bottom of the cell) and dc/dx, for substitution in the modified form of the Svedberg equation shown on p. 65, presents a daunting prospect to some potential users of the Archibald procedure for determining molecular weight. Simplified methods of obtaining these values have, however, been devised (as will be outlined).

It is customary to determine the initial concentration (C_0) by performing an additional ultracentrifugal analysis on the protein solution under investigation, using a synthetic boundary cell as a refractometer [38]. Providing identical experimental conditions to those obtaining in the main ultracentrifugal analysis are adopted, a direct measure of the initial concentration which includes all the relevant optical parameters is obtained in terms of the area under the schlieren peak on the photographic plate (measured by one of the methods referred to in Section A1, or by summation of ordinates, as will be described). This avoids the need to determine absolute solute concentration or the optical constants of the ultracentrifuge, because values of dc/dx, usually referred to as 'z' values, are obtained in the same form.

If the available ultracentrifuge is equipped with Rayleigh interference optics, greater accuracy in the determination of the initial concentration (from a synthetic boundary run) can be achieved, merely by counting the number of fringes from one side of the boundary to the other [5]. Recently [39], moreover, the measurement of displacement of a single Rayleigh fringe as a function of radial distance (x) has been used to obtain dc/dx (by fitting a second degree polynomial in x, extrapolating and differentiating). Good agreement with the published molecular weight values were obtained for solutions of ribonuclease and bovine serum albumin. In an alternative, graphical, method dc/dx was obtained from the tangent to the fringe drawn after photographic enlargement.

Both graphical and numerical methods have been employed to obtain values of dc/dx from schlieren patterns (e.g. as in Fig. 4.11), obtained from the main Archibald run, involving centrifugation for short periods of time at relatively low speeds. Details of these evaluation procedures can be found elsewhere [28]. Briefly, starting from the meniscus ($n = O$), the ordinates of the concentration gradient curves (at the top of the cell) are measured at regular intervals (e.g. 1 mm) on a tracing of an enlarged pattern (taking as base-line an extrapolation, to the meniscus, of the straight plateau region of the curve). The distances (Zn) thus obtained represent dc/dx values and incorporate the optical constants of the ultracentrifuge, the solute concentration, the refractive index increment of the solute and the enlarger magnification factor (none of which needs to be evaluated when a separate synthetic boundary cell run is undertaken).

These distances can be measured by a graphical procedure, involving the superimposition of transparent graph paper upon a tracing of the enlarged

Archibald pattern. They are, however, more readily obtained by the use of a two-dimensional comparator. Furthermore, this approach is now facilitated by the use of plate assessors (referred to in section A2), which provide the distances measured rapidly and in a form which can be handled directly by digital computers. The AGI assessor, in use in the author's laboratory, is particularly useful in this respect in that it possesses an incrementing device which ensures movement by constant distances (e.g. 0·2 mm on the plate) along the x axis, prior to location of the cross-wires on an enlargement ($\times 10$) of the gradient curve by movement along the y axis. The error incurred by this incrementing procedure is as little as 0·01 mm (on the plate), irrespective of the increment selected. The distances (x) of the ordinates from the axis of rotation are, of course, provided in similar form to the ordinate values (Z).

A similar procedure can be employed to determine dc/dx values from the concentration gradient curve at the bottom of the cell (taking the solution-silicone oil interface as reference).

The values of dc/dx and x thus obtained are substituted in the following equation [38], to correct for the change in concentration at the meniscus and bottom of the cell.

Concentration at meniscus:

$$C_m = C_0 - \frac{1}{x_m^2} \int_{x_m}^{x} x^2 \, (dc/dx) \, dx.$$

Concentration at bottom of cell:

$$C_b = C_0 + \frac{1}{x_b^2} \int_{x}^{x_b} x^2 \, (dc/dx) \, dx$$

where x refers to a position in the plateau region (where $dc/dx = 0$). If the material under investigation is known to be homogeneous, these equations can be combined, thus avoiding the need to determine C_0 by a separate synthetic boundary run. Substitution of the above concentration values (C_m or C_b) and the dc/dx values (at the meniscus or cell bottom) in the modified Svedberg equation given on p. 65 provides an estimate of the molecular weight at the two cell positions.

If the Archibald run is not performed in a double sector cell which contains solvent in the other compartment, it is sometimes necessary to correct the ordinate values (Zn) measured as outlined, to allow for base-line curvature caused by sedimentation of low molecular weight molecules in the solvent (when speeds greater than about 10,000 rev/min are used). The greatest error, however, is caused by imprecise location of the meniscus, on which depends the accuracy of the dc/dx values (at meniscus or cell bottom) and the accurate summation of the ordinates under the concentration gradient curves. Traut-man [40] has pointed out that an error of 0·1 mm in fixing the position of the meniscus (x_m) can lead to an error of 10 per cent in dc/dx, and consequently in the molecular weight. He has overcome this problem by incorporating a double-slit device in the ultracentrifuge optical system, which produces interference fringes flanking the central shadow area of the meniscus; this enables its precise location (to within 0·005 mm). Alternatively [41], the position of the meniscus can be determined from the intersection of Archibald plots

i.e.
$$\frac{RT}{\omega^2} \cdot \frac{dc/dx}{x, C} \text{ versus } x$$

obtained from schlieren patterns photographed at different times and rotor speeds. Pain [58] has located the meniscus accurately in sedimentation equilibrium experiments by taking photographs at a bar angle of 90° as soon as the rotor attained running speed.

Greater accuracy in summation of the ordinates under the concentration gradient curve at the top of the cell can be achieved by including an extra ordinate at a distance of half an increment (i.e. at $n = 0.5$) from the apparent meniscus position (by use of the Newton-Cotes integration formula) [42].

When dealing with non-ideal solutions, Archibald determinations should be performed at several different concentrations (below 1 g/100 ml) and the $M_{app} (1 - \bar{v})$ concentration plot extrapolated to zero concentration.

The procedure has been applied to the determination of the molecular weights of various immunoglobulins and their sub-units. For example Charlwood [43] applied it to the analysis of rabbit γG globulin (isolated by sodium sulphate precipitation) and its papain digestion fragments. Ultra-centrifugal speeds of 8,210 and 12,590 rev/min were adopted, measurements being made from five photographic exposures at 8 or 16 minute intervals and protein concentrations being determined by separate differential refractometer measurements. The molecular weight of whole γG globulin thus obtained (namely 187,000 ± 1,400), from measurement at a single protein concentration (assuming $\bar{v} = 0.735$), was in fair agreement with the mean value (172,700) [44] obtained by Archibald analysis of a solution (0·96 per cent) of rabbit γG globulin comprising about 40 per cent anti-ovalbumin antibody (isolated by low temperature ethanol precipitation, sodium sulphate precipitation or by DEAE-cellulose chromatography). An appreciably lower molecular weight value (137,000) for the rabbit γG globulin was obtained, however, from S_0 and D_0 values (by the method outlined in section A2), thus emphasizing the importance of correcting for concentration dependence in Archibald determinations too.

It is conceivable, also, that the relatively high values reported in the literature for rabbit γG globulin (150,000–188,000) [45] could be attributed to impurities in the preparations examined or, more likely, to the presence of small amounts of aggregates (such as the 10S dimeric form, referred to in section A1). In this connection, it should be noted that where it is necessary to prevent aggregation (e.g. of γ globulin fragments) by the use of 6 M urea (or some similar type of reagent) a synthetic boundary run (to determine the initial solute concentration, for Archibald analysis) is not easily performed. Trautman & Crompton [41], however, have indicated how this problem can be overcome by employing a method of calculating molecular weights from data obtained at different exposures during the Archibald approach to sedimentation equilibrium, without having to determine the initial concentration. A least squares slope obtained by plotting data from runs carried out at different speeds provides a single Z-average molecular weight value in the form: $M_{app}(1-\bar{v})$, as well as giving an indication of heterogeneity. Correction for concentration dependence is then achieved by extrapolation of the $M_{app}(1-\bar{v})$ against ρ plot to zero concentration.

By this method, ribonuclease was found to possess a molecular weight of 14,000 in the absence of urea and 12,500 in the presence of 6 M urea. A similar procedure has been applied to the determination of the mol. wts. of heavy and light polypeptide chains of horse γG globulin [46], which were found to be 105,000 and 40,000 respectively (assuming $\bar{v} = 0.74$) in 8 M urea: 0.2 M KCl: 0.1 M formic acid (pH 3.5). In contrast, values of M_{app} for light chain determined at three different concentrations in KCl-phosphate buffer (pH 7.7), gave a molecular weight of 50,000 (with little concentration dependence).

Edelman and Poulik [47] have used the same technique to ascertain the effect of various dissociating reagents (including urea, 2-mercaptoethanol, etc.) on the $M_{app}(1-\bar{v})$ values of human as well as rabbit γG globulin; the former preparation being a Cohn fraction II (containing a trace of 19S component) and the latter isolated as a pseudo-globulin.

An alternative to the Archibald procedure, which has been applied successfully to the determination of the molecular weight of immunoglobulin fragments, relies on achieving sedimentation equilibrium in relatively short times (e.g. 14 hours for ribonuclease) by the use of short columns (1–3 mm) of solution [48]. Both schlieren and interference optics have been employed in the application of this technique (devised by Van Holde and Baldwin [48]) to the determination of the molecular weight of γG globulin sub-units. The apparent molecular weight (M_{app}) can be calculated from the following equation, defining the conditions obtaining at the mid-point of short columns in equilibrium:

$$M_{app} = \frac{1}{\bar{r}} \cdot \frac{dc}{C \, dr} \cdot \frac{R.T}{\omega^2(1-\bar{v}\rho)}$$

$\bar{r}$ = distance from centre of column to axis of rotation, dc/dr = concentration gradient at the mid-point, and C = protein concentration at mid-point (within 1 per cent of the initial concentration, if sufficiently short columns are employed). The change in protein concentration across the cell is determined by numerical integration of the schlieren curve, as described earlier for the Archibald procedure. Determination of the initial concentration (e.g. by a separate synthetic boundary cell run) is not necessary.

It is convenient to obtain the apparent molecular weight from the slope of the plot*:

$$\frac{1}{r}\left(\frac{dn_c}{dr}\right) \text{ versus } n_c \text{ where } n_c \text{ represents the refractive increment.}$$

An upward curvature of this plot suggests the presence of aggregates, which are confirmed if there are discrepancies between the weight average molecular weight (M_w) and Z-average molecular weight (M_z)—both of which are obtained from the Van Holde and Baldwin procedure.

Molecular weights can also be calculated directly from interference patterns [49], the dc/dr value being obtained from measurement of the fringe difference between two points equidistant from the centre of the column. A recent report [103] describes the combined use of schlieren and interference optics in the determination of molecular weights of chymotrypsinogen A and ribonuclease A by the Van Holde and Baldwin procedure. At sedimentation equilibrium, concentration gradients in the cell were recorded by both optical systems.

Owing to the appreciable non-ideality of the solvents employed in the examination of γG globulin sub-units (e.g. 6 M urea, 6 M guanidine solution, etc.), it is essential to obtain the true molecular weight by extrapolation of apparent values (M_{app}) to zero protein concentration.

Sedimentation equilibrium analysis in short columns has provided convincing evidence in support of the model of the rabbit γG globulin molecule postulated by Porter [50]. For example, Small *et al.* [51] have determined the molecular weights of the 'heavy' and 'light' polypeptide chains in 5 M guanidine hydrochloride, using 3 mm columns and interference optics. They found good agreement between the weight average and Z-average molecular weights of the two types of chains, and of whole γG globulin. In a more exhaustive study, Marler *et al.* [52] have employed both schlieren and interference optics to obtain accurate molecular weights of papain-cleavage fragments as well as polypeptide chains (in 6 M guanidine

---

* This relationship is also used in the form $\frac{1}{r} \cdot \frac{(dz)}{(dr)}$ against Zn, where z represents the ordinates under the schlieren curve (as in the Archibald measurement procedure outlined on p. 68).

hydrochloride). Their data indicate that papain splits the two heavier (γ) polypeptide chains of the rabbit γG globulin molecule into approximately equal halves.

Similar types of investigation have been carried out, by other workers, on the polypeptide chains of rabbit γG globulin [53] and on peptic-digestion fragments [54]. In the latter study, involving the sedimentation of a 3S fragment in 1·7 mm columns in a double sector cell at 11,272 rev/min, over a protein concentration range of 0·3—0·5 per cent, the Z-average molecular weight was found to be 81,500, whereas the weight-average value was 55,000 (in good agreement with the molecular weight determined from S_0 and D_0 values). As already mentioned, such a discrepancy suggests the presence of aggregates, which are also indicated from the curvature of the plot referred to above. When, therefore, greater care was taken in the isolation of the γG globulin fragment in question, apparent M_z and M_w values of 91,300 and 91,900 respectively were obtained (assuming $\bar{v} = 0·730$) and there was no indication of aggregation from the

$$\frac{1}{r}\left(\frac{dn_c}{dr}\right) \text{ versus } n_c \text{ plot.}$$

Yphantis [55] has reduced the time taken to reach equilibrium in the Van Holde and Baldwin technique, by employing even shorter columns (around 0·7 mm). For example, in analyses on bovine ribonuclease (run at 0·5 per cent and 1·0 per cent protein concentrations and 12,590 and 15,220 rev/min respectively), equilibrium was established in about 40 minutes. This technique permits the use of higher running speeds (and therefore lower protein concentrations), whilst maintaining the mid-point concentration close to the original concentration, but at the cost of some precision in the molecular weight value obtained. A further development by Yphantis [55] has been the construction of multichannel cell-centre pieces, comprising 6 or 8* observation channels, which are filled from side-pocket reservoirs (by the method used to fill the Kegeles [56] type synthetic boundary cell). Thus, three or four solvent-sample (of different concentration) pairs can be analysed simultaneously, the reference base-lines being provided in each case.

Yphantis [57] has also indicated how molecular weights can be determined by equilibrium ultracentrifugation of relatively dilute protein solutions (e.g. 0·003–0·2 per cent) at faster ($\times 3$) than usual operating speeds. Under such conditions, it is possible to study polydisperse solutions, and to estimate the size of the slowest sedimenting component.

Pain [58] has used a multichannel cell to determine the weight-average molecular weights of the polypeptide chains of rabbit and horse γG globulins

* Obtainable from Beckman Instruments.

in urea buffers. He measured the refractive increment for the solute in each solution by separate synthetic boundary cell runs. Other investigators, however, have avoided separate concentration determinations by applying interference optics to the analysis of the boundaries formed in multichannel cells.

A major drawback in using this type of cell has been the changes in protein concentration caused by adsorption of protein from the short liquid columns analysed. Pain [58] appears to have overcome this problem, even when using concentrated urea solutions as solvents, judging by the reproducibility and linearity of the $1/M_{app}$ versus C plots he obtained from separate runs in a multichannel cell. He also obtained an extrapolated value of 151,000 for the molecular weight of whole horse γG globulin (from separately determined values of S_0, D_0, and $\bar{v}$) which was in reasonable agreement with the sum of the weights of the constituent polypeptide chains, assuming that the Porter structure also obtains for the γG globulin of this species.

Molecular weight determinations on immunoglobulins have so far been confined largely to γG globulins and their sub-units, owing to the ease of isolation of this protein in pure form and its ready dissociation into polypeptide chains or enzyme-digestion fragments. As indicated, sedimentation equilibrium methods have proved useful in studying the sub-units, whilst the molecular weight of the whole γG globulin has usually been deduced from separate determinations of sedimentation and diffusion coefficients (as outlined in section A2). These data have also been used to calculate frictional coefficients (as indicated by Svedberg & Pedersen [1]).

On the other hand, the sedimentation equilibrium techniques are not easily applied to the study of γM and γA globulins, owing to their larger molecular sizes and to the difficulties experienced in the isolation of their sub-units. Hence, here too, molecular weights have been determined from S_0 and D_0 values. For example, this method has been used to demonstrate that a human macroglobulin isolated from the serum of a patient with Waldenström macroglobulinaemia is comprised of 5 sub-units, possessing a molecular weight (185,000) which is 16 per cent higher than the molecular weight of homologous γG globulin examined in parallel [59]. More recent studies [60], on the distribution of the disulphide links in the γM molecule, have provided evidence that each of these sub-units comprises four polypeptide chains.

The molecular weights of a 9·7S γA globulin (myeloma) and its sub-units obtained by reduction [12] (referred to in Section A1) have been determined in a similar manner and found to be 424,000 and 190,000 respectively. It is also interesting to note that this whole γA molecule was found to have an axial ratio (a/b) of 20, whilst the axial ratio of its sub-units ($a/b = 6$) was similar to that of human γG globulin.

Section B

Preparative ultracentrifugation

The methods outlined in the previous section are applicable to the characterization of the immunoglobulins present in high proportions in hyperglobulinaemic sera or in the form of purified preparations, isolated by various physico-chemical fractionation procedures or by dissociation of specific antigen-antibody precipitates. In every case, separation was accomplished in analytical cells, and followed by one or other of the various types of optical systems available. In no case, however, was it possible to recover any of the sedimented fractions on completion of ultracentrifugation.

Preparative ultracentrifugation, on the other hand, offers a means of achieving this objective, in addition to providing information about sedimentation behaviour. Moreover, providing that a sufficiently sensitive assay system is available, it is possible to ascertain the sedimentation characteristics of an antibody without having to isolate it from the complex mixture of proteins within the antiserum.

Such advances have resulted from the development of density gradient centrifugation techniques (for a concise review see Charlwood [104]). Before dealing with these, however, it is worth mentioning other types of investigation of immunoglobulins which can be undertaken with a preparative ultracentrifuge.

1. *Moving boundary separations*

Trautman [6], for example, has described methods of determining sedimentation coefficients by ultracentrifugation in swinging-bucket or angle rotors. A rough procedure involves the determination of the time taken to sediment a biologically active substance from the meniscus to a pellet (under well-defined conditions), and merely requires the biological assay of two fractions. This is a technique which can be carried out in any type of preparative rotor and at the same time—where a faster sedimenting active component is being separated from slower moving material—a partial purification is being effected, although many recycles are necessary to achieve a high degree of purification (with a proportionate sacrifice of yield).

γM antibodies have been isolated in this manner [2], but the method is handicapped by the high losses in activity resulting from the denaturation occurring during pellet formation. Müller-Eberhard and his associates [61] have attempted to overcome this problem by the addition of a much slower sedimentating protein, to stabilize the high molecular weight immunoglobulins. Thus, these workers added albumin at the beginning of the fifth cycle of an eight-cycle process designed to isolate γM globulin from normal human serum. It was afterwards necessary to isolate the albumin from the γM globulin fraction by a zone-electrophoresis step.

Obviously, the other classes of immunoglobulins (i.e. γG, γA and γD), which all possess sedimentation coefficients in the region of 7S, would not be readily separable by this approach.

A more precise measurement of sedimentation rate can be obtained by treating the tube in a swing-out rotor as if it were an analytical ultracentrifuge cell. In this 'boundary locator' technique (as Trautman [6] terms it), the centrifuge is stopped before the boundary reaches the bottom of the tube, and several fractions from different levels down the tube are taken for assay. This provides a means of establishing that a plateau region still exists in the tube, whereupon the boundary position is located (as illustrated in Fig. 4.12) by plotting a boundary location function u^* (i.e. average concentration times

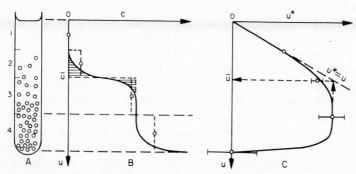

FIG. 4.12. Schematic illustration of measurement procedure used in the 'boundary location' technique (reproduced from *Instrumental Methods of Experimental Biology* (1964), by courtesy of Dr R.Trautman and the publishers, Macmillan Co, New York).

volume) against volume (u), and its displacement converted into a sedimentation rate by substitution in the expression:

$$S_{obs} = F_s(\log \bar{r} - \log r_a)/t'$$
$$\text{(in Svedbergs)}$$

where F_s is a speed factor (i.e. $10^{13} \, ln.10/(60 \, \omega^2)$),

r_a and $\bar{r}$ are the radii corresponding to the starting level and the boundary location (determined as shown in Fig. 4.12) respectively, and t' is the time in min (after correction for acceleration and deceleration time).

The S-rate thus obtained is converted to an $S_{20,w}$ value in the usual manner. Greatest accuracy will be achieved if the temperature of centrifugation is controlled, as can be accomplished by the use of a swing-out rotor fitted with a thermistor device, in a Spinco Model E ultracentrifuge. If this facility is not available, it is necessary to check the temperature immediately before and after centrifugation, preferably in a "dummy" solvent tube which has been centrifuged simultaneously with the test samples.

As in moving boundary analyses in the analytical ultracentrifuge, careful speed control is essential when using preparative machines for the determination of sedimentation behaviour. Slow acceleration (approx. 2000 rev/min) and deceleration (without braking) minimize convective disturbances. This is particularly necessary when density-gradient stabilization is not operative, whereupon very slow deceleration times (e.g. 15–20 min) between 5,000 rev/min and rest have been employed [62]. The time consumed in acceleration and deceleration can be estimated graphically, and added to the total time at maximum speed (calculated from the odometer readings of the ultracentrifuge).

When relatively pure substances are being examined by this technique, there is often inadequate boundary stabilization (in contrast to that provided by contaminating boundaries in crude mixtures such as serum). It then becomes necessary to create a density gradient by means of sucrose or some other appropriate solute, in order to prevent the occurrence of radial convection. When preparing such density gradients (e.g. from 2·5 and 5·0 per cent sucrose solutions), the sample is dissolved in the two sucrose solutions forming the bottom two layers, and sample solution alone forms the top layer. In correcting the observed sedimentation rate (as already described above), it is customary to employ a value for the sucrose density obtained by averaging the density over the whole tube.

Hogeboom & Kuff [62] have adopted this procedure in determining the sedimentation coefficients of proteins (over a range of 4–2000S) in dilute solution ($<0·1$ per cent). The sampling technique employed (for 5 ml tubes from a SW-39 rotor) is illustrated in Fig. 4.13. Injection of 50 per cent sucrose solution (at a constant flow-rate of 0·09 ml/min) through a hypodermic needle (25 gauge) piercing the bottom of the tube (about 5 mm above its base) gently forces the tube contents into the collecting chamber, which has a perforated base. Removal of samples (by means of a silicone-coated pipette) at 3 minute intervals yields aliquots (0·27 ml) which are weighed in order to obtain accurate volume determinations. Protein concentrations are determined by dividing the concentration of sedimenting material in each sample by the original concentration, and then plotting the resultant fractional concentration against the distance from the meniscus to the mid-point of each sample. Measurements [62] carried out on a concentrated (0·83 per cent) solution of human immune serum globulin, comprising 6·17S component (74 per cent) and 8·8S component (22 per cent) assigned a sedimentation coefficient ($S_{20,w}$) of 6·34S to the main component.

The method is not readily applicable to determining sedimentation co-efficients in multi-component systems, although this difficulty has been partially overcome by plotting concentration *increment* (occurring over successive 1 mm. intervals) against distance, and thereby producing sedimentation patterns analogous to those obtained by schlieren optics from analysis in the Model E machine. This problem does not arise, of course,

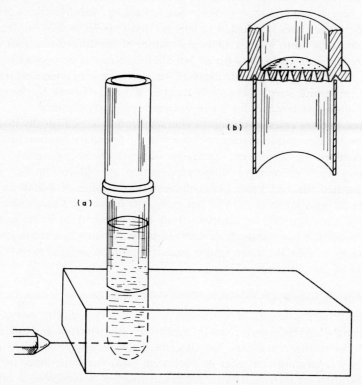

FIG. 4.13. A sampling device involving elution from the top of a density gradient tube (reproduced from the *Journal of Biological Chemistry*, (1954) **210**, 733 by permission of Drs G.H.Hogeboom and E.L.Kuff and the publishers, the American Society of Biological Chemists, Baltimore).

if one is dealing with a biologically active substance. For instance, the sedimentation coefficient of an enzyme present in a complex protein mixture has been determined [63].

Trautman *et al* [64] have applied the boundary locator technique to the determination of the S-rate of a complement-fixing virus particle, and obtained a value of 13·2S (compared with a value of 14S obtained by analytical ultracentrifugation) on the basis of the complement fixation titration (assay error $\pm$ 25 per cent) of just four fractions (withdrawn in a pipette) from triplicate analyses in 5 ml lusteroid tubes in a SW-39 rotor. In other studies [65], bovine plasma albumin-γG globulin mixtures and hemocyanin have been employed in systems designed to simulate situations where numerous samples cannot be taken (e.g. when examining certain biological systems). Samples were withdrawn, after centrifugation, by means of a Pasteur pipette (1 mm bore at tip) and their volumes determined by measurement in graduated centrifuge tubes (graduated in 0·01 ml divisions up to 0·04 ml, then in wider divisions up to 6·5 ml). Optical densities of the diluted fractions were measured as usual at 280 mμ (or at 346 mμ in the case of hemocyanin solutions). Alternatively, ultracentrifugation was carried out in quartz centrifuge tubes (2 ml) which were subsequently scanned at 1 mm intervals by the use of a special adaptor (Spinco) for a conventional spectrophotometer.

Hence, in these cases involving the characterization of biologically inactive proteins, the concentration term to be used in the boundary location function is determined by a physical technique instead of by biological assay. By using such preparative ultracentrifugation procedures, it has been demonstrated that sedimentation coefficients in the range of 4–100S can be determined with an error of $\pm$10 per cent. It is important to note that this order of accuracy can be achieved from measurements of a biologically active substance (e.g. antibody) present in trace amounts in a crude protein mixture *even when the assay system available provides only an approximate measure of concentration.*

2. *Use of separation cells*

Ultracentrifugal analyses of antibodies and other biologically active substances have also been performed in separation cells, which fit into analytical rotors. As in the procedures just described, this technique is based on a boundary separation and relies on biological assay (or some other form of concentration measurement) after ultracentrifugation is complete. It affords an advantage, however, in that use of the schlieren optical system of the analytical ultracentrifuge provides an indication of the progress of separation of a particular component (e.g. the 7S component of serum), which can be used as an internal reference against which to compare the rate of sedimentation of antibody activity.

Two types of separation cell have been employed. In the fixed partition type [66] (suitable only for use with high molecular weight solutes) a piece of filter paper placed on top of a perforated plate, sited two-thirds of the way down the cell, serves as a barrier which prevents remixing at the end of the run of the material situated in the two compartments. A cell of different design [67] incorporates a movable partition, which takes up position on deceleration of the cell at the end of the run. This type can be used with both low and high molecular weight solutes.

There are, however, disadvantages in using both types of cell [5]. Consequently, their application to the characterization of antibodies has been restricted. Where such an investigation has been attempted, it has been the practice either to compare the titres of antibody in the top and bottom compartments (in a simplified treatment) [68] or to measure the relative depletion of antibody in the top compartment after centrifugation [68, 69]. In the former method, the ratio of antibody activity in the bottom and top compartments at the end of a run is divided by the ratio of the 7S component concentration in the two compartments, determined from measurements involving graphical integration of the schlieren pattern, to obtain a specific activity (which should be unity if the antibody assayed is of the 7S class). This approach demonstrated that the haemagglutinating antibody in the serum of a non-allergic individual immunized with ragweed pollen extract was of the order of 7S, whereas the skin-sensitizing antibodies present in the sera of ragweed-sensitive individuals ranged from 3–25S. The other method, based on measurement of solute transport, revealed a similar difference in behaviour of the two types of antibody. Moreover, results obtained by application of this method [69] showed a similar large variation (ranging over several Svedberg units) for the sedimentation coefficient of reagin to ragweed, separated in a moving partition cell (in contrast to the appreciably less variable values obtained by zone-centrifugation, which will be discussed later).

Some of this variability can obviously be attributed to the difficulty in obtaining accurate end-point P-K titration (as this antibody assay method was employed on both occasions). This is suggested by the much more reliable results from measurements performed on a reference human γG globulin preparation (1 per cent solution), based on protein concentrations determined by nitrogen estimation [69]. The S-rate of 7·4S obtained was close to the value given by conventional analytical ultracentrifugation.

It is possible, too, that denaturation of the labile reagin molecule contributed to the variable S-rate values obtained for this antibody, although it would be expected that separation cells would share the advantages of other boundary separation procedures in ensuring that the active molecules are maintained in their native environment (in contrast to the artificial solvent medium into which zone separations proceed). Separation cells also provide an alternative means of isolating a slow-moving component in a relatively homogeneous state (in the top compartment).

There are, however, many advantages in using instead a pre-formed density gradient in a swing-out rotor. In fact, the system employed in the rough method of determining sedimentation rate referred to earlier (in section B

p. 76), which relies on the assay of biological activity in just two fractions from a density gradient separation in a 5 ml tube in a SW-39 rotor (e.g. the top 4 ml and the bottom 1 ml), can be considered as 'a separation cell without a partition'. Taking this idea a stage further, Yyphantis [70] has likened the conditions obtaining in boundary ultracentrifugation in a mild preformed sucrose density gradient to a multicomponent separation cell. Moreover, use of a density gradient overcomes the problem of stabilizing dilute boundaries (e.g. at concentrations below 0·01 g per cent).

3. *Zone-centrifugation*

The preparative procedures described so far have all involved boundary separations, such as occur in the analytical ultracentrifuge cell (referred to in section A), and are therefore not readily applicable to the study of *mixtures* containing antibodies falling into the different classes of immunoglobulin. Zone-centrifugation in relatively steep density gradients (e.g. 10–30 per cent sucrose), on the other hand, provides a means of determining the sedimentation characteristics of more than one type of immunoglobulin (e.g. γG and γM globulins) simultaneously in a single run. A large number of small volume fractions are obtained for biological assay, thus providing a precise indication of the sedimentation distribution of a biologically active substance (or substances). Moreover, as with other types of zone separation procedures, it is possible (at least theoretically) to obtain absolute resolution (see Fig. 4.14) of the multiple components within a mixture (providing there is sufficient difference in their sedimentation rates) in contrast to the *relative* separations achieved by the boundary procedures already outlined.

As in zone-electrophoresis in slabs of solid supporting medium, it is possible to make direct comparative analyses by centrifuging the test sample simultaneously with reference substances (e.g. purified immunoglobulin preparations) in a swing-out rotor. In this event, it is of course essential to ensure that the same volumes of solvent and sample are used in each tube, and that tube distortion is minimized. This problem is now simplified by the availability of polypropylene tubes, and, more recently, of the much less expensive polyallomer (copolymer of ethylene and propylene) tubes, which are considerably more uniform than the previously used lusteroid tubes. Another approach (as will be described) is the use of isotopically labelled internal standards, which are added to the test sample in trace amounts.

Zone-centrifugation possesses most of the advantages already attributed to boundary ultracentrifugation in density gradients, besides permitting the recovery of the sedimented fractions for further study. It is much cheaper to perform than analytical ultracentrifugation (e.g. in a Spinco Model E machine). Moreover, the technique of automatic monitoring of the contents of the zone-centrifuge tubes, which is being developed in the author's laboratory, provides a composite sedimentation pattern which could ultimately replace the need for the conventional schlieren patterns obtained by boundary separation in analytical machines (as outlined in section A).

For these reasons, zone-centrifugation is the technique of most value to the experimental immunologist. The remainder of this article will be devoted, therefore, to detailed technical aspects and to examples of application of this method to the study of immunoglobulins.

As in systems which have been employed in the zone separation of virus particles [71] and subcellular particles [72], a density gradient is used merely

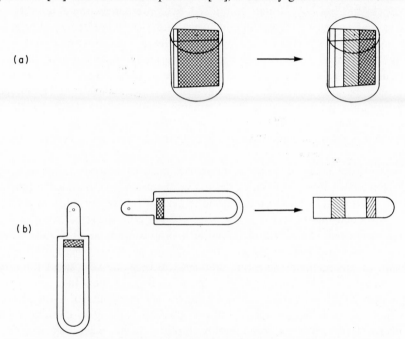

FIG. 4.14. Schematic illustration of difference between (a) moving boundary ultracentrifugation and (b) zone-centrifugation in a density gradient.

to prevent radial convection which would lead to serious disturbances of the moving zones (as the separations are made in non-sector shaped tubes). A slight density gradient of solvent has the effect of directing convection across the centrifugal field, thus producing eddy-type currents [6]. Apparently there have been numerous unsuccessful attempts to stabilize ultracentrifugal zones by means of the porous types of solid media used in zone-electrophoresis, which on theoretical grounds would not be expected to work.

Preformed gradients have also been used in isodensity ultracentrifugal techniques, to separate serum lipoproteins [73] for example. This method

D

would appear to have little application to the isolation of immunoglobulins however, owing to insufficient difference between their partial specific volumes.

Preparation of the density gradient prior to zone-centrifugation can be achieved merely by gently layering the less dense solution on top of the denser solution and leaving the two layers to mix, by standing the tube overnight at 4° C; alternatively the speed of mixing of the two layers can be enhanced by rotating the tubes at an angle of 30° or by stirring with a saw-toothed wire. More reproducible gradients are obtained, however, by the use of a gradient-forming device. Most of the apparatus currently in use is based on a design of Bock & Ling [74], which comprised two interconnecting reservoirs, a stirrer and valves to regulate the delivery rate. The more dense solution is intimately mixed with the less dense one, and the resulting mixture is delivered to the bottom of the centrifuge tube as a perfectly linear density gradient. This device has since been modified and refined by several workers. For example, an apparatus has recently been described [75] which has the advantage of being able to form reproducible gradients rapidly in three tubes (small or large) simultaneously. The simple gradient-forming device (based on the Bock & Ling design) employed in the author's laboratory is shown in Fig. 4.15.

Apart from sucrose, many other solutes such as dextran and inorganic salts have been used for forming density gradients. A medium used recently, in the separation of guinea-pig antibodies against foot-and-mouth virus [76], is of particular interest because, by using a 65 per cent saturated $NaNO_3(v/v)$ solution above a 75 per cent saturated KBr (v/v) solution at 20° C, a positive density (from 1·25–1·29 g/ml) but a negative viscosity (1·6–1·0 cp) gradient is set up. In this manner, the S-rate gradient can be made very slight (nominally reducing the S-rate to about 1/7 of its $S_{20,w}$ value). In contrast, in zone-centrifugation carried out at a temperature of about 10° C (at 35,000 rev/min for 18 hours), where a sucrose gradient ranging in concentration from 10–40 per cent (w/v) is commonly employed, it has been calculated that the S-value at the top of the tube would be one-half of the $S_{20,w}$ value, and would decrease to as low as 1/11 of the $S_{20,w}$ value at the bottom of the tube. This results in a progressive retardation of the faster 19S zone, relative to the 7S zone, besides causing a dilution of both moving zones.

The choice of medium will naturally be influenced by the properties of the immunoglobulin(s) to be ultracentrifuged. For instance, sucrose has been found to have a stabilizing effect on the activity of labile skin-sensitizing antibody during the zone-centrifugation of allergic sera at 4° C [77].

The protein concentration and manner of application of the test sample above the preformed gradient are other important factors to be considered, if high resolution of zones is to be obtained. A raining down of visible droplets follows the layering on of the sample. This effect can be minimized by using a very dilute starting sample, and by blurring the lower boundary as it is applied [6]. The author has found it necessary to dilute normal serum to at least three times its volume if this effect is to be reduced sufficiently, when using sucrose density gradients. Undiluted serum (1 ml in a 6·5 ml tube) has been used, at room temperature; stabilization against droplet formation being achieved by a massive 'density shelf' formed by a high density salt solution [76].

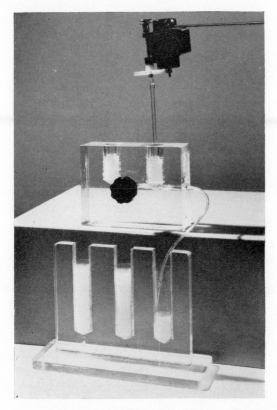

Fig. 4.15. Illustrating the use of a simple gradient-forming device.

Varying volumes of test sample have been used as starting band in zone-centrifugation, ranging from 1 ml down to 0·1 ml (in a 5 ml tube). Obviously, in selecting a suitable starting volume, it is necessary to compromise between the demands of yield and purity. When determining the sedimentation characteristics of antibodies and enzymes, a small volume (i.e. 0·1–0·2 ml) is chosen in order to achieve maximum resolution, providing that the assay technique is sufficiently sensitive.

Antibodies

Zone-centrifugation of immunoglobulins has usually been performed in sucrose density gradients. For example, Kunkel and his associates [78, 79] have separated mixtures of 7S and 19Sγ globulins in 10–40 per cent sucrose

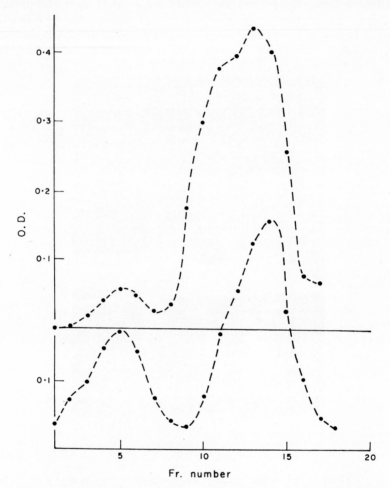

FIG. 4.16. Density-gradient centrifugation patterns of normal and pathological human sera (reproduced from *The Plasma Proteins* (1960), Vol. 1, 279, by permission of Dr H.G.Kunkel and the publishers, Academic Press Inc, New York).

gradients, the 19S zone moving to the bottom of the tube (5 ml) after 18 hour centrifugation in a SW-39 rotor at 35,000 rev/min, whilst the 7S zone remained above the mid-portion of the tube. In fractionations of whole serum (diluted 1:1 with isotonic saline), bromophenol blue was added to mark the albumin, whilst (after centrifugation) the position of the 19S zone was revealed by its scattering of a narrow beam of light. Sampling of the fractions was achieved either by withdrawal through a Pasteur pipette, or by piercing a hole in the bottom of the tube and collecting the drops (under the control of negative pressure) into a fraction collector. Kunkel [78] has pointed out that, although the latter sampling technique provides pure bottom fractions, it has a disadvantage in that the top fractions may be contaminated slightly by heavier material. Optical density measurement (at 280 mμ) of the fractions provides a protein distribution curve (as illustrated in Fig. 4.16).

This approach demonstrated that the 19S component could be resolved from the slower moving components in normal and macroglobulinaemic

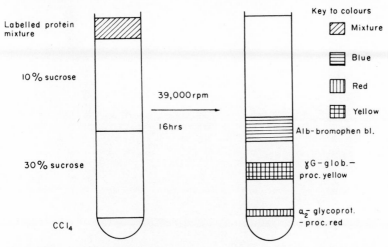

FIG. 4.17. Use of external dye-labelled reference proteins: albumin, γG globulin and α_2 macroglobulin (reproduced from *Analytical Biochemistry* (1961), **2**, 324, by courtesy of the publishers, Academic Press Inc, New York).

sera (Fig. 4.16). A high degree of separation between a 19S antibody (anti-A) and a 7S antibody (anti-Rh$_0$) was also accomplished [78].

A similar technique has been applied to the classification of the size distribution of the saline anti-A and anti-B isoagglutinins in a large number of human sera [80]. Agglutination titrations carried out on five broad fractions from various corresponding levels in the density gradient tube after centrifugation revealed, in addition to '19S' and '7S' patterns, a third 'mixed' size pattern. It now seems probable that this group contained intermediate sedimenting antibodies (8–11S), of the type since revealed by Rockey & Kunkel [78] on zone-centrifugation of certain human sera. It remains to be demonstrated whether the isoagglutinating activity found in this sedimentation region of human serum is caused by the presence of polymerized forms of γA antibody (or even γG antibody), or whether it represents yet another class of antibody analagous to the $10S\gamma_1$ antibody [82] identified in a fraction of purified horse antihapten antibody.

The density gradient system used in the author's laboratory [83] is similar to that of the Kunkel group, but with certain modifications. Narrower starting sample bands (0·25 ml and 0·5 ml) have been employed, in an attempt

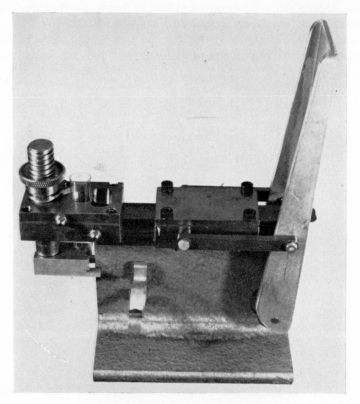

Fig. 4.18. Mechanical tube slicer.

to improve resolution. This practice, in effect, extends the length of medium in which the moving zones can separate. The time available for separation of zones in the 4·5S–7S region of serum has also been increased on occasions by placing a small volume (0·3 ml) of a dense immiscible liquid (e.g. carbon tetrachloride) at the bottom of the 5 ml tubes in a SW-39 rotor, in order to prevent loss of the 19S proteins as a result of pellet formation.

Dye-labelled reference proteins, representative of the three main sedimenting classes of serum proteins (i.e. 4·5S, 7S and 19S) have been used as external

markers, in the location of zones separated in tubes centrifuged simultaneously in a SW-39 rotor [83]. Cellulose-reactive Procion dyes, which have also
been used for coupling to antigens [84], have proved suitable labels, which

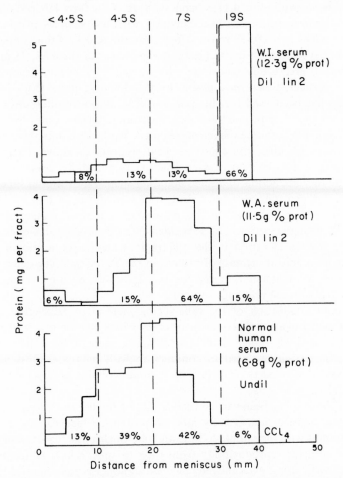

FIG. 4.19. Zone-centrifugation patterns of normal human, γG myeloma (WA) and
Waldenström macroglobulinaemic (WI) sera (reproduced from *Analytical Bio-
chemistry* (1961), **2**, 324, by courtesy of the publishers, Academic Press Inc, New
York).

cause no alteration in the sedimentation characteristics of the reference
proteins. Thus 19S α_2 glycoprotein was labelled with Procion Brilliant Red,
whilst 7S γG globulin was labelled with Procion Brilliant Yellow (by mixing
the protein with a solution of the dye at pH 7·4, allowing to stand at room
temperature for 30–60 minutes, and dialysing away the unbound dye). The

4·5S albumin reference protein was labelled with Evans Blue or with bromo-phenol blue.

Complete separation of the three coloured zones (blue, yellow and red) is observed as shown in Fig. 4.17, when a mixture of the three labelled reference proteins is ultracentrifuged simultaneously with test samples placed in the other two tubes in a SW-39 rotor. Afterwards, alignment of the sample tubes alongside the reference tube indicates the positions of the 4·5S, 7S and 19S zones, which are readily recoverable by using a tube slicing procedure. A mechanical slicer, based on a design by Randolph & Ryan [83] (shown in Fig. 4.18) has been used for this purpose. This offers an alternative to the decantation and drip-out methods of harvesting separated zones (referred to earlier). As many as thirteen segments (3 mm in depth) were thus obtained from a 5 ml lusteroid tube, with an 80 per cent recovery of liquid. The plotting of the total protein content of each fraction (obtained by measurement of optical density at 280 mμ of diluted aliquots) against the mean distance from the meniscus provides a characteristic zone-centrifugation pattern. This is illustrated in Fig. 4.19, where the pattern of a normal human serum is compared with the patterns of a Waldenström macroglobulinaemic serum (showing a gross elevation in the 19S region) and a γG myeloma serum (showing a significant increase of protein in the 7S region). The demarcation of the various sedimentation regions was indicated by direct comparison with the dye-labelled reference proteins.

The main application of the tube-slicing method of recovering density gradient centrifugation fractions is in cases where one or two well-defined zones are required, rather than in a complete scan of the tube contents. Hence, this technique—used in conjunction with reference substances—is recommended if a particular class of immunoglobulin (e.g. γG or γM) is required.

This approach has been carried further [86] by the use of internal reference substances, namely radioactively labelled proteins, which can be mixed in trace amounts with the sample to be examined. Such a practice overcomes the need for accurate reproducibility from tube to tube, which is an absolute requisite when using external reference substances (as just described). It is also possible to use two different markers in the same tube. For example (as shown in Fig. 4.20), Charlwood [86] has employed ^{125}I-labelled γM globulin and ^{131}I-labelled γG globulin simultaneously in a comparative study of the sedimentation rates of anti-insulin antibodies. A similar technique has also been used in the characterization of anti-nuclear antibodies (and their anti-gens) and in controlling the isolation of normal and pathological macro-globulins, where trace-labelled normal γG globulin was employed to decide which fractions could be pooled to give maximum yield for any specific level of contamination. Moreover, it has been possible to locate antibodies by means of a simplified procedure, employing 7S and 19S reference globulins labelled with the *same* isotope.

It should be noted that all these separations were performed in a fixed angle rotor (usually Spinco No. 40) which, despite its failure to achieve as high a degree of zone sharpness as that obtained using a swing-out rotor, has an advantage in that considerably more material can be handled (e.g. twelve antisera could be screened simultaneously).

The use of isotopically labelled proteins as internal reference substances offers a valuable alternative to employing well-characterized enzymes [87],

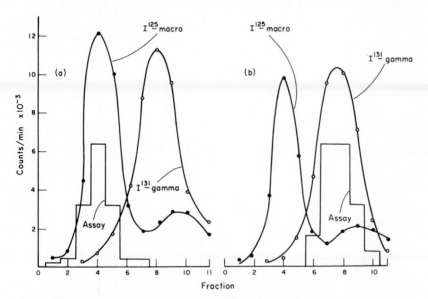

FIG. 4.20. Use of ^{125}I-γM and ^{131}I-γG globulins as trace internal reference proteins in the characterization of anti-insulin antibodies: (*a*) human serum 287, (*b*) human serum 496 (reproduced from *Analytical Biochemistry* (1963), **5**, 226, by courtesy of Dr P.A.Charlwood and the publishers, Academic Press Inc, New York).

as the sensitivity of radioactivity measurements is comparable to that of enzyme assay and, therefore, permits the addition of a minimum amount of foreign material (the sedimentation coefficient of which can be assumed to be equal to its S_0 value).

Both types of marker have been employed in the determination of comparative sedimentation rate by zone-centrifugation, in a similar manner to the use of reference substances in moving boundary analysis carried out in separation cells (as described in section 4B2, p. 80). Martin & Ames [87], for example, have applied sucrose density gradient centrifugation (in a SW-39

D*

rotor) to the determination of the sedimentation coefficients of several enzymes in crude protein mixtures, employing three well-characterized enzymes (of approx. molecular weight: 68,000; 75,000 and 170,000) as reference substances.

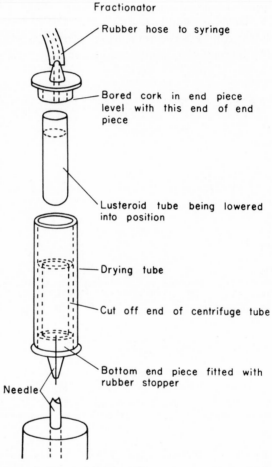

FIG. 4.21. A simple device for sampling zone-centrifuge tubes (reproduced from the *Journal of Biological Chemistry* (1961), **236,** 1372, by courtesy of Drs R.G.Martin and B.N.Ames, and of the publishers, the American Society of Biological Chemists, Baltimore).

In this technique, 0·1 ml of sample (containing not more than 2 per cent protein) is layered over 4·55 ml of buffered sucrose gradient. After zone-centrifugation, a constant number (308 ± 5) of drops—divided into as many as forty-four fractions—is collected by means of a simple fractionator* (illustrated in Fig. 4.21), the rate of flow being controlled at approximately one drop per second by a syringe connected to the top of the tube. By the use of this recovery procedure, volume differences of less than 3 per cent between the first and last fractions were recorded.

An important advantage of this technique is the use of preformed *linear* gradients—formed from 20 per cent w/v (0·584 M) and 5 per cent w/v (0·146 M) sucrose, each in 0·05 M tris-HCl buffer at pH 7·5—in which the viscosity and density of the sucrose gradient (over a temperature range of 3–15° C) are such that essentially linear migration of most biological substances occurs. Under such conditions of sedimentation, the ratio of the distances travelled from the meniscus by any two substances will remain constant. This means that there is no need for careful control of temperature, time and speed of centrifugation, etc., when comparing the behaviour of an unknown substance with that of a standard. The relative sedimentation rate (R) can be determined after any time of centrifugation by substitution in the expression:

$$R = \frac{\text{distance travelled from meniscus by unknown}}{\text{distance travelled from meniscus by standard}}$$

and because of the nearly constant rate of sedimentation,

$$R = \frac{S_{20,w} \text{ of unknown}}{S_{20,w} \text{ of standard}}$$

(assuming both macromolecules possess the same partial specific volume).

Martin & Ames [87] have pointed out that, as most proteins have partial specific volumes between 0·700 and 0·750 ml per g, the assumption of a partial specific volume of 0·725 ml per g, will result in less than 3 per cent error in the estimation of $S_{20,w}$ for most proteins. (This applies to γG, γM and γA globulins, on the basis of partial specific volume values so far reported in the literature.)

Approximate molecular weights have also been obtained from zone-centrifugation determinations, by substituting in the equation [5]:

$$\frac{S_1}{S_2} = \left(\frac{MW_1}{MW_2}\right)^{2/3}$$

as the ratio S_1/S_2 is equal to R (defined above) for most proteins (assuming both unknown and standard to be spherical molecules). The same type of calculation could be made, of course, from data obtained by the moving boundary procedures described earlier (in section B1, p. 76).

* A more elaborate fractionator has been described by Szybalski [88], whilst a simple tube puncturing device has been described recently by Salo [89].

(a)

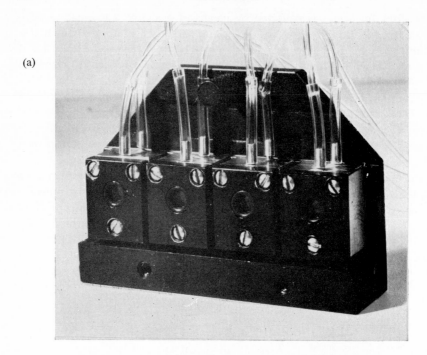

(b)

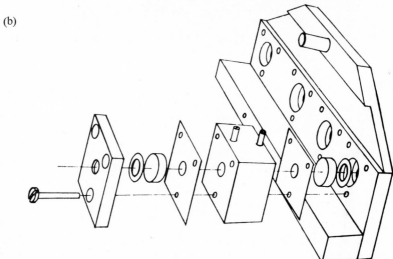

FIG. 4.22. Gilford flow-through assembly. (a) 10 mm cells (0·10 ml capacity) on carrier, (b) schematic diagram of assembly of component parts (reproduced by courtesy of Gilford Instruments, Oberlin, Ohio).

The shape factor can be taken into account by using a diffusion constant (D_0) value, determined directly by classical procedures (dependent on schlieren or interference optics) or comparatively by gel filtration [90] (where the biological assay of column fractions can reveal the elution volume of an active component in a crude protein mixture) or by a gel-diffusion precipitin technique [91] (dependent upon the availability of an antiserum directed against the protein in question). Only an *approximate* molecular weight is obtained, however, from D_0 values determined by the latter comparative methods, by substitution in the Svedberg equation (shown on p. 59 of section A).

Anderson & Vannier [69] have applied the comparative zone-centrifugation technique of Martin & Ames [87] to the determination of the sedimentation coefficients of human skin-sensitizing antibodies to ragweed, employing human γG globulin ($S_0 = 6\cdot8S$) as reference standard. Diluted samples of allergic sera (comprising 0·1 ml serum: 0·1 ml buffered saline) were

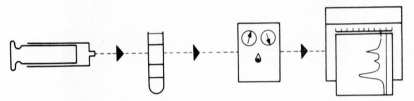

FIG. 4.23. Schematic illustration of the automatic monitoring of zone-centrifugation tubes.

separated in a buffered sucrose (5–20 per cent) gradient at temperatures between 0–5° C, in 5 ml tubes in a SW-rotor at 35,000 rev/min, for varying lengths of time. As mentioned earlier, the sedimentation coefficients thus obtained (viz. 7·4–7·9S) were much more reliable than the values (ranging from 2·9–10·2S) obtained by parallel determinations in a moving partition cell.

The whole process of zone-centrifugation has been simplified and refined by the development of automatic zone sampling and zone analysis techniques, to replace the various procedures already described. In the author's laboratory [91], these improvements have been achieved by the use of a Gilford 2000 Multiple Sample Absorbance Recorder* which possesses important features not found in similar types of instrument. For instance, the provision of micro-flow-through cells (an example is shown in Fig. 4.22) of 0·03, 0·06 and 0·1 ml capacity (and 2, 5 and 10 mm depth respectively)—controlled by an automatic cuvette positioner—facilitates simultaneous monitoring of three sample tubes in addition to a solvent blank. Moreover, the recording

* Manufactured by Gilford Instruments Inc, Oberlin, Ohio, U.S.A.

system permits the selection of any value between 0·1 and 3·0 optical density units as full-scale deflection, over which range a linear optical density— concentration relationship obtains. This extends considerably the limits of detection of protein zones. For example, assuming the extinction coefficient (E $^{1\ cm}_{1\ per\ cent}$) of immunoglobulins at 280 mμ is of the order of 14 optical

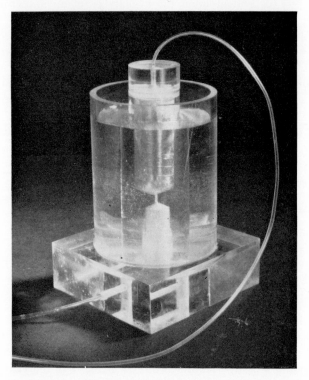

FIG. 4.24. Zone-centrifuge tube holder (constructed by Mr M.Doughty). The base of the tube is pierced by a No. 19 gauge syringe needle set into the base of the holder, whereupon the separated zones are gently forced out through the tapered perspex cap which fits tightly on to the top of the tube.

density units, a protein level of 7 mg/100 ml would be readily detectable (i.e. at least ten times lower than the limit of detection of the schlieren optical system).

A schematic illustration of the sampling and recording system is shown in Fig. 4.23. A monochromator (Unicam S.P. 500) permits monitoring at any selected wave-length in the visible or u.v. region*. The separated zones are

* An automatic dual-wavelength selecting device is also available, which permits simultaneous monitoring at any two wavelengths in the visible or u.v. region.

gently forced out of the centrifuge tubes (5 ml polyallomer) by pumping dense (60 per cent w/v) sucrose solution into the bottom through a hypodermic needle (No. 19 gauge) set into the base of the tube-holder (shown in detail in Fig. 4.24). A modified (slowed-down) Gilford constant-flow system (Model 105S) has been mainly used for this purpose (pumping 60 per cent sucrose through a 10 ml syringe at a rate of 0·11 ml/m) but recent investigations have shown a peristaltic pump to be superior. It also has the advantage of permitting the simultaneous sampling of three centrifuge tubes. The contents of the tubes are then led out from the top through a tapered perspex cap connected by fine-bore (1 mm) PVC tubing to the flow-through cell (which, like the analytical ultracentrifuge cells, comprises a central corrosion-resistant compartment bounded by quartz windows). The effluent is finally collected in

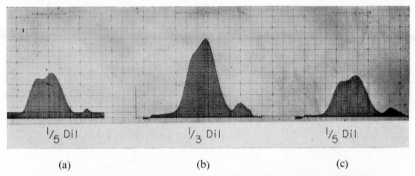

(a)   (b)   (c)

FIG. 4.25. Gilford zone-centrifugation patterns of samples (0·25 ml) of normal human serum diluted (a) 1/5, (b) 1/3 and (c) 1/5, obtained by successive monitoring through a 5 mm cell. Full-scale deflection 3·0 optical density, 5 sec readings; conditions of zone-centrifugation: 18 hours, 39,000 rev/min in SW-39 rotor at 12° C in 10–30 per cent buffered sucrose gradient.

a fraction collector, controlled by a drop-counter, and equipped with an event-marker which indicates position of tube change on the recorder chart.

In this manner, a virtually continuous plot of the distribution of the sedimented zones is obtained (as indicated in Fig. 4.25). The design of the flow-through cells, which provides a minimum cell-volume with maximum light-path and which ensures a minimum mixing within the cell, is a critical factor in achieving precisely separated zones. In the sampling techniques described earlier, the degree of definition revealed was limited by the volume of the sample required for protein assay (by separate u.v. absorption or colorimetric measurement). Other limitations of indirect sample analysis were the necessity to dilute the samples, to transfer these to and from micro-silica cells (prior to analysis at 280 mμ), and the sacrifice of material if a colorimetric analytical technique were used.

When employing a 5 mm flow-through cell (0·06 ml capacity) in the automatic sampling procedure, it is customary to recover thirty-three fractions (each comprising eleven drops of approximate volume 0·015 ml) from a polyallomer tube ($2 \times \frac{1}{2}$ in.) containing 0·25 ml sample and 5·0 ml sucrose

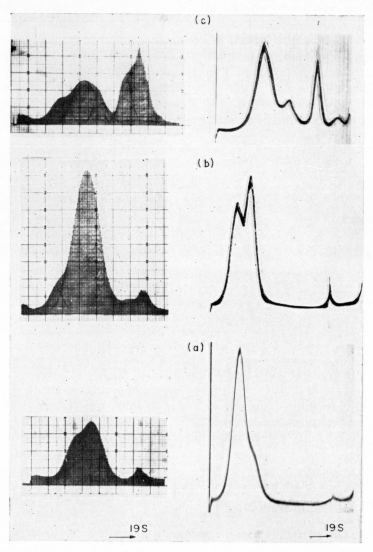

Fɪɢ. 4.26. Zone-centrifugation and schlieren patterns of (a) normal human serum, (b) γG-myeloma serum, (c) Waldenström macroglobulinaemic serum (conditions of moving boundary ultracentrifugation as in Fig. 4.1 and of zone-centrifugation as in Fig. 4.25).

gradient. The 19S peak of human serum patterns sometimes shows a spurious shape, owing to the turbulence created when the dense eluting sucrose solution (60 per cent w/v) enters the flow-through cell behind the macroglobulin zone. Nevertheless, this effect does not prevent the accurate location of the 19S zone; furthermore, it is reduced appreciably by keeping the tube cool (at centrifugation temperature) and by precooling the eluting sucrose solution. It could be avoided by withdrawing the sample through tubing connected to a needle, piercing the bottom of the centrifuge tube, by applying a gentle air pressure to the top of the tube. This sampling procedure suffers from a disadvantage, however, in that the density of the tube effluent passing through the flow-through cell continuously decreases. In contrast, the continuous

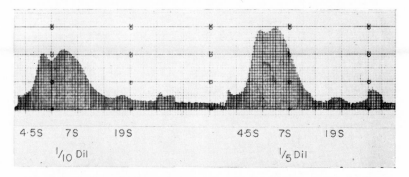

Fig. 4.27. Zone-centrifugation pattern of the most common type of γA myeloma serum. Conditions of ultracentrifugation and monitoring as in Fig. 4.25. (Also depicted, in schlieren form, in Fig. 4.1d.)

increase in density occurring during sampling from the top of the tube encourages the rapid voiding of the cell and, hence, maximum definition of the zone-centrifugation pattern.

The reproducibility of the monitoring technique is indicated by a comparison of the normal serum patterns shown in Fig. 4.25 which were obtained by successive analysis of the contents of three tubes (5 ml) centrifuged simultaneously in a SW-39 rotor. As was found with other sampling methods (described earlier), only a partial resolution of the 4·5S and 7S serum components was achieved under conditions optimal for the separation of the 7S and 19S components. This was also indicated by gel-diffusion precipitin analysis, employing specific antisera, where considerable overlap of the major components (e.g. albumin and γG globulin) comprising these serum sedimentation classes was observed.

Despite this limitation, however, zone-centrifugation followed by automatic monitoring of the separated zones offers a valuable alternative to moving

boundary ultracentrifugation in analytical rotors, particularly as far as the
study of the immunoglobulins is concerned. For example, in Fig. 4.26, the
zone-centrifugation patterns of normal, Waldenström macroglobulinaemic and γG myeloma sera are compared with the corresponding schlieren

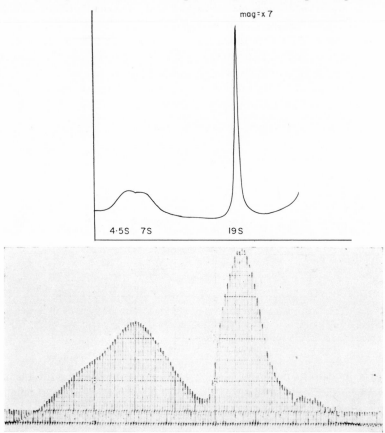

FIG. 4.28. Comparison of zone-centrifugation (below) and schlieren patterns (above)
of a partially purified preparation of horse serum α_2 macroglobulin (approx. 1·5 g per
cent). Schlieren photograph taken after 17 min centrifugation at 59,780 rev/min and
20° C (conditions of zone-centrifugation and tube monitoring as in Fig. 4.25).

patterns (photographed at a time before the separation of the 4·5S and 7S
components was complete). A pronounced increase in the level of γM or γG
globulin is apparent in the zone-centrifugation patterns of the macroglobulinaemic and myeloma sera respectively, indicating there is no need for
schlieren analytical patterns in order to differentiate between the two types of
hyperglobulinaemia. On the other hand, γA myeloma serum patterns (see

Fig. 4.27) containing an increase in 7S component concentration and small amounts of intermediate sedimenting (between 7S and 19S) components, are not readily differentiated from γG myeloma patterns.

As already mentioned, however, it is possible to recover the separated zones (which can then be analysed by specific gel-diffusion precipitin techniques) after these have passed through the autoanalyser cell. The

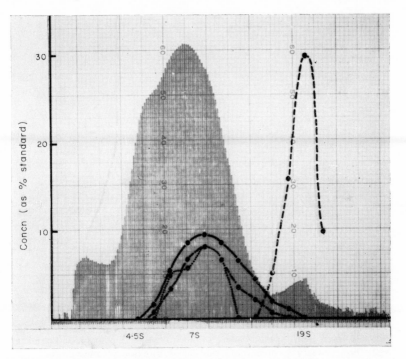

FIG. 4.29. Distribution of γG (●– · –●), γM (●– – –●), γA (●—●) and γD (●· ·●) immunoglobulins in zone-centrifugation fractions of normal human serum. Immunoglobulins estimated (by Dr D.S.Rowe) by quantitative gel-diffusion precipitin analysis. (Conditions of zone-centrifugation and tube monitoring as in Fig. 4.25.)

macroglobulin zone is, of course, the most readily recovered with minimal contamination from slower sedimenting material. For instance, a highly pure specimen of horse serum α_2-macroglobulin was obtained from a horse serum protein preparation which had been deprived of the γM globulin constituent by prior ammonium sulphate precipitation. Automatic sampling permitted precise delineation of the optimum point of separation between the 7S and 19S zones (as shown in Fig. 4.28, where the zone-centrifugation and schlieren patterns are compared). The fractions comprising the 19S zone can then be combined, dialysed to remove the sucrose and concentrated by ultrafiltration through Visking tubing.

The distribution of the four classes of immunoglobulins (i.e. γG, γM, γA and γD) within the zone-centrifugation patterns of normal human serum has been determined by quantitative gel-diffusion precipitin analysis by means of the radial immunodiffusion technique [93] (performed directly on the zone-

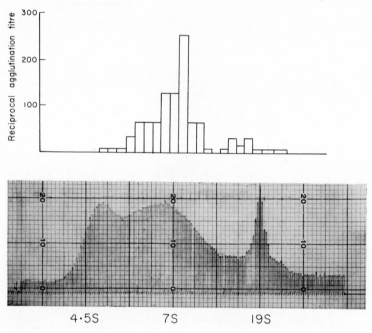

FIG. 4.30. Zone-centrifugation pattern of human anti-tetanus toxoid serum taken 7 weeks post primary immunization, showing distribution of antibody activity as determined directly by passive hemagglutination of sheep cells coated with toxoid. 0·25 ml serum (diluted 1/2 after reconstitution from freeze-dried solid) was centrifuged in a SW-39 rotor for 18 hours at 39,000 rev/min, 4° C, in a 10–30 per cent buffered sucrose gradient. The fractions were recovered and monitored (at 5 second intervals by passage through 5 mm cells), as described in the text.

centrifugation fractions). As might be expected (see Fig. 4.29) there was no evidence of any separation between the three low molecular weight immunoglobulins (i.e. γG, γA and γD), nor was any of the polymeric form of γA globulin apparent (although this would not be readily detected by the gel-diffusion technique employed). The γM globulin, on the other hand, was well separated from the others, although it would of course be mixed with α_2-macroglobulin. Hence, none of the immunoglobulins can be isolated from whole serum simply by means of zone-centrifugation. A complementary fractionation procedure such as zone-electrophoresis (see Chapter 2) or ion-exchange chromatography (see Chapter 3) is necessary before or after the ultracentrifugation step.

On the other hand, as already indicated, the sedimentation characteristics of an antibody γ globulin can be determined from a single zone-centrifugation run, providing a sufficiently sensitive assay system is available. Moreover, agglutination titrations can be made directly on the sedimentation fractions after auto-analysis without the necessity of first removing the sucrose. Similarly, the distribution of anti-tetanus toxoid antibodies in the sera of humans at varying stages following immunization with the toxoid has been followed (in collaboration with Dr M.W.Turner), by agglutination titration, using toxoid-coated tanned red cells (Fig. 4.30). Other types of antibody activity recovered in zone-centrifugation fractions following auto-analysis have included skin-sensitizing activity (in human allergic sera fractions) and lymphocyte transformation activity (in rabbit anti-human leucocyte sera). The method has also proved useful in establishing the size character-istics of anti-Rh antibodies.

The automatic sampling technique described has yet to be applied to the determination of sedimentation coefficients, a field in which its precision and reproducibility should prove important factors. It has been applied already to comparative analyses, in which purified immunoglobulins (run simultan-eously in separate tubes) are employed as reference substances, in ascertaining the sedimentation class to which a particular antibody belongs. When using a constant-flow syringe, however, it has been possible to monitor only one tube at a time. Consequently, in spite of the high degree of reproducibility achieved between tubes centrifuged simultaneously, slight differences in spread of the sample and reference patterns have been observed. In such cases, it has been the custom to align patterns by the matching of an easily recognized feature common to all patterns, such as the point of maximum upward sweep of the base-line caused by the entrance of the 60 per cent sucrose solution into the auto-analyser cell. This problem has since been overcome, however, by synchronized monitoring of sample and reference tubes, employing a four-channel peristaltic pump.

Section C

Future Developments

The constant refinement of commercially available ultracentrifuges and the development of faster machines and rotors is leading inevitably to more precise analysis of the immunoglobulins (as well as the other serum proteins).

For example, the use of high speed titanium rotors to improve the resolution of protein digestion fragments of γG globulin has already been cited (in section A p. 56). In the field of preparative ultracentrifugation, too, the use of much faster swing-out rotors (providing a gravitational field of 410,000 g at the maximum speed of 65,000 rev/min*) will result in substantial increase in the degree of resolution of serum protein achieved by zone-centrifugation techniques. By using such speeds (together with maximum rotor stabilization, temperature control, etc.) followed by the automatic monitoring of the centrifuge tube contents (as described in section B p. 95) it should be possible to obtain zone-centrifugation patterns showing a degree of resolution comparable to that observed in schlieren patterns (obtained from conventional boundary analysis in analytical rotors). It is conceivable, therefore, that the analytical ultracentrifuge will be displaced ultimately by a preparative ultracentrifuge-auto-analyser combination.

It seems likely that such technical advances will also lead to the further application of zone-centrifugation to the determination of sedimentation coefficients of antibodies and their sub-units. The newly developed technique of density gradient centrifugation in analytical rotors [94] should find a similar use (providing the antibody can be obtained in pure form). This technique, in which relatively shallow sucrose gradients (e.g. 1·1–3 per cent; 2–7 per cent) have been employed [95] in a 30 mm Kegeles type synthetic boundary cell, and which requires one-tenth of the volume of sample needed for conventional ultracentrifugal analysis, would appear, however, to have the greatest application as a direct method for the examination of reversibly interacting systems (e.g. antibody-antigen interactions and γ globulin aggregation phenomena).

There are already many signs that the use of digital computers will greatly facilitate the interpretation of ultracentrifugation data. Methods of collecting this data in suitable form, involving the use of plate assessors, and the automatic monitoring of the rotating ultracentrifuge cell, have been mentioned in section A p. 62. It is conceivable that further developments will involve the replacement of the ultracentrifuge recording system by a television camera on line to a computer. Various investigators [96, 97] have discussed the compilation of digital computer programmes for evaluating ultracentrifugal data, and programmes are now available for the calculation of sedimentation velocity and molecular weight (from Archibald data†). It seems likely, too,

* A new type of preparative ultracentrifuge (Model L2 65), now being produced by Beckman Instruments Co Ltd, will reach these speeds as will the M.S.E. "Super-speed" 65 machine. A comparable machine (Model B. 60) manufactured by International Equipment Co, takes a 6-place (5 ml) swing-out rotor at a maximum speed of 60,000 rev/min ($\equiv 405,900$ g).

† For other details, see the Beckman publications 'Fractions' (1965), No. 1, p. 10 and (1966), No. 1, p. 2.

that computers will facilitate the complete evaluation of the massive amount of data obtained from the use of Rayleigh interference optics in the determination of molecular weight by sedimentation equilibrium analysis [98].

Interference optics should also prove useful in differential sedimentation analysis, where it is possible to measure—with high precision—small changes in sedimentation rate (such as might occur as a result of antibody-antigen interaction, or following limited degradation or association of the γ globulin molecule).

The equipping of analytical ultracentrifuges with monochromators and scanning devices will no doubt encourage the study of antigen (or hapten) —antibody interactions, in a similar manner to the recent use of this recording system in a study of the rôle of sub-units in the regulation and catalytic activity of an enzyme (aspartate transcarbamylase [99]).

In the isolation of immunoglobulins, there is every indication that the problem of overcoming the capacity restrictions encountered in the use of swing-out rotors (in preparative zone-centrifugation) will be solved by using zonal ultracentrifuges [100], which permit the introduction of the gradient and sample layer into the rotor during rotation, and the subsequent recovery of the separated zones without having to bring the rotor to rest. Fisher & Canning [101] have applied this technique (using a B IV rotor) to the isolation of 19S serum macroglobulins, which they separated cleanly from the slower sedimenting serum proteins in one step. The lower practical limit of separation with this rotor appeared to be of the order of 10S, however, hence it would obviously be unsuitable for the isolation of other types of immunoglobulin.

The separation of other protein components along with the immunoglobulins in the major sedimenting fractions of serum complicates any attempt at a single-stage fractionation. Nevertheless, zone-centrifugation has been employed to advantage in conjunction with other types of isolation procedure (as indicated in section B p. 103). In this connection, a recent report of the combination of zone-centrifugation and gel-diffusion precipitin analysis [102] is of particular interest, as such an 'immunocentrifugation' technique could provide a valuable adjunct to immunoelectrophoresis (in the qualitative analysis of immunoglobulins).

Finally, it is predicted that ultracentrifugation will find increasing application in the elucidation of the *conformation* of the immunoglobulin molecules. Already, sedimentation equilibrium methods have provided valuable information about the size of the γG and γM globulin sub-units (whilst in dissociated form) and recombination and hybridization experiments are in progress to establish how these fit together to form the parent molecule. Ultracentrifugation should also prove a valuable tool in ascertaining the significance of conformational changes in relation to the varied biological activities of immunoglobulin molecules. In this connection, the study of reversible-reacting systems, in both analytical cells and preparative ultracentrifuge tubes, should throw further light on the mechanism of antibody-antigen interaction, on γ globulin polymerization and on the combination of antibody γ globulin with other key substances, such as cell surface constituents and lymphocyte ribonucleic acid (RNA).

Acknowledgements

The author is grateful to Drs D.E.Normansell and S.P.Spragg for their comments on this article, and to Mr M.Doughty for his technical assistance in developing the automated zone monitoring procedure described in section B p. 95. He is also indebted to Dr Grace Pardoe, and to Messrs M.Doughty and R.Stuckey, for much help in preparing the manuscript and illustrations.

References

[1] SVEDBERG T. & PEDERSEN K.O. (1940) *The Ultracentrifuge*. London: Oxford University Press; New York: Johnson Reprint Corporation

[2] PEDERSEN K.O. (1945) *Ultracentrifugal Studies on Serum and Serum Fractions*. Uppsala: Almquist & Wiksell

[3] KABAT E.A. & MAYER M.M. (1961) *Experimental Immunochemistry*, 2nd ed. Springfield, Illinois: Charles C. Thomas

[4] ROWE D.S. & FAHEY J.L. (1965) A new class of human immunoglobulins II. Normal serum IgD. *J. exp. Med.* **121**, 185

[5] SCHACHMAN H.K. (1959) *Ultracentrifugation in Biochemistry*. New York: Academic Press

[6] TRAUTMAN R. (1964) Ultracentrifugation. In *Instrumental Methods of Experimental Biology*, chapter 7, ed. NEWMAN D.W. New York: Macmillan Co; London: Collier-Macmillan

[7] ELIAS H.S. *Theory and Application of Ultracentrifugal Techniques*. Munich: Beckman Instruments G.m.B.H.

[8] WILLIAMS J.W. (1963) Ed. *Ultracentrifugation in Theory and Experiments*. New York: Academic Press

[9] CLAESSON S. & MORING-CLAESSON I. (1961) Ultracentrifugation. In *Laboratory Manual Methods in Protein Chemistry* **3**, 119

[10] ROWE D.S. & FAHEY J.L. (1965) A new class of human immunoglobulins I. A unique myeloma protein. *J. exp. Med.* **121**, 171

[11] IMHOF J.W. & BALLIEUX R.E. (1961) Atypical β2A-myeloma. A clinical study of ten patients with fast sedimenting (S_{20} 8–12S) serum proteins and an immunochemical analysis of these pathological protein components. *Acta med. Scand.* **170**, 449

[12] DEUTSCH H.F. (1963) Molecular transformations of a γ_1-globulin of human serum. *J. molec. Biol.* **7**, 662

[13] VAERMAN J.P., FUDENBERG H.H., VAERMAN C. & MANDY W.J. (1965) The significance of the heterogeneity in molecular size of human serum γA-globulins. *Immunochemistry* **2**, 263

[14] RATCLIFF P., SOOTHILL J.F. & STANWORTH D.R. (1963) Physicochemical and immunological studies of pathological serum macroglobulins. *Clin. chim. Acta,* **8,** 91

[15] FILLITI-WURMSER S., GENTOU C. & HARTMANN L. (1964) Existence de deux variétés 17S ou 18·3S de γM et d'une augmentation de globulines 6·6S sériques dans la maladie de Waldenström. *Revue fr. d'Études. clin. biol.* **9,** 398

[16] DEUTSCH H.F. & MORTON J.I. (1958) Human serum macroglobulins and dissociation units. I. Physico-chemical properties. *J. biol. Chem.* **231,** 1107

[17] FRANKLIN E.C. (1962) Two types of γ_1A-globulin in sera from normals and patients with multiple myeloma. *Nature, Lond.* **195,** 393

[18] HEREMANS J. (1960) *Les Globulines Sériques du Système Gamma; Leur Nature et Leur Pathologie.* Paris: Masson

[19] FIREMAN P., VANNIER W.E. & GOODMAN H.C. (1963) The association of skin-sensitizing antibody with the β_2A globulin in sera of ragweed-sensitive patients. *J. exp. Med.* **117,** 603

[20] TERR A.I. & BENZ J.D. (1964) Gel filtration of human skin-sensitizing antibody and β_2A globulin. *J. Allergy* **35,** 206

[21] SOOTHILL J.F., KEKWICK R.A., VALLET L., CUTBUSH M., THOMAS A.R., MOLLISON P.L. & GELL P.G.H. (1961) Estimation of γ-globulin in the serum of patients with hypo-gamma globulinaemia. *J. clin. Path.* **14,** 470

[22] JAMES K., HENNEY C.S. & STANWORTH D.R. (1964) Structural changes occurring in 7S γ-globulins. *Nature, Lond.* **202,** 563

[23] NELSON C.A. (1964) Isolation of a new intermediate in the papain cleavage of rabbit γ-globulin. *J. biol. Chem.* **239,** 3727

[24] SINGER S.J. & CAMPBELL D.H. (1952) Physical chemical studies of soluble antigen-antibody complexes. 1. The valence of precipitating rabbit antibody, *J. Am. chem. Soc.* **74,** 1794

[25] GILBERT L.M. & GILBERT G.A. (1965) Generalized treatment of reversibly reacting systems in transport experiments, illustrated by an antigen-antibody reaction. *Biochen. J.* **97,** 7c

[26] NORMANSELL D.E. & STANWORTH D.R. (1966) Ultracentrifuge studies of the reactions of rheumatoid factor with native human γG-globulin. *Immunology* **10,** 527

[27] FRANKLIN E.C., EDELMAN G.M. & KUNKEL H.G. (1959) In *Immunity and Virus Infections,* ed. NAJJAR V.A., New York: John Wiley

[28] SCHACHMAN H.K. (1957) In *Methods in Enzymology* **4,** 57, ed. COLOWICK S.P. & KAPLAN N.O. New York: Academic Press

[29] JOHNSTON J.P. & OGSTON A.G. (1946) A boundary anomaly found in the ultracentrifugal sedimentation of mixtures. *Trans. Faraday Soc.* **42,** 789

[30] EHRENBERG A. (1957) Determination of molecular weights and diffusion coefficients in the ultracentrifuge. *Acta chem. Scand.* **11,** 1257

[31] BILLICK I.W. (1962) Velocity sedimentation studies on pressure and concentration-dependent systems. *J. phys. Chem.* **66,** 1941

[32] LAMERS K., PUTNEY F., STEINBERG I.Z. & SCHACHMAN H.K. (1963) Ultracentrifuge studies with absorption optics. 3. A split-beam photoelectric scanning absorption system. *Arch. biochem. biophys* **103,** 379

[33] SPRAGG S.P., TRAVERS S., & SAXTON T. (1965) Oscillating mirror system for recording optical densities from the Spinco model E analytical ultracentrifuge. *Analyt. Biochem.* **12,** 259

[34] STANWORTH D.R. (1960) A rapid method of preparing pure serum gamma-globulin. *Nature, Lond.* **188,** 156

[35] WALLENIUS G., TRAUTMAN R., KUNKEL H.G. & FRANKLIN E.C. (1957) Ultracentri-

fugal studies of major non-lipid electrophoretic components of normal human serum, *J. biol. Chem.* **225**, 253

[36] ARCHIBALD W.J. (1947) A demonstration of some new methods of determining molecular weights from the data of the ultracentrifuge. *J. phys. Colloid Chem.* **51**, 1204

[37] COHEN S.S. & SCHACHMAN H.K. (1957) Physical studies on the RNA of turnip yellow mosaic virus. *Virology*, **3**, 575

[38] KLAINER S.M. & KEGELES G. (1955) Simultaneous determination of molecular weights and sedimentation constants. *J. phys. Chem.* **59**, 952

[39] ROBERTS J.L. & CONWAY G.F. (1964) An application of the Rayleigh optics of the ultracentrifuge to molecular weight determinations by the Archibald method. *Biochim. biophys. Acta*, **88**, 201

[40] TRAUTMAN R. (1958) Optical fine-structure of a meniscus in analytical ultracentrifugation in relation to molecular weight determinations using the Archibald principle. *Biochim. biophys. Acta* **28**, 417

[41] TRAUTMAN R. & CRAMPTON C.F. (1959) Application of the Archibald principle for the ultracentrifugal determination of the molecular weight in urea solutions of histone fractions from calf thymus. *J. Am. chem. Soc.* **81**, 4036

[42] MELLOR J. W. (1955) *Higher Mathematics for Students of Chemistry and Physics*. New York: Dover Publications Inc.

[43] CHARLWOOD P.A. (1959) Ultracentrifugal examination of digestion products from rabbit γ-globulin. *Biochem. J.* **73**, 126

[44] CAMMACK K.A. (1962) Molecular weight of rabbit gamma-globulin. *Nature, Lond.* **194**, 745

[45] PORTER R.R. (1960) γ-globulin and antibodies In *The Plasma Proteins* **1**, 246, ed. PUTNAM F.W. New York: Academic Press

[46] FLEISCHMAN J.B., PAIN R.H. & PORTER R.R. (1962) Reduction of γ-globulins, *Arch. biochem. Biophys.* Supplement **1**, 174

[47] EDELMAN G.M. & POULIK M.D. (1961) Studies on structural units of the γ-globulins. *J. exp. Med.* **113**, 861

[48] VAN HOLDE K.E. & BALDWIN R.L. (1958) Rapid attainment of sedimentation equilibrium. *J. phys. Chem.* **62**, 734

[49] WOODS E.F., HIMMELFARB S. & HARRINGTON W.F. (1963) Studies on the structure of myosin in solution. *J. biol. Chem.* **238**, 2374

[50] PORTER R.R. (1962) In *Symposium on Basic Problems in Neoplastic Disease*, p. 177, ed. GELLHORN A. & HIRSCHBERG E. Columbia University Press. New York

[51] SMALL P.A., KEHN J.E. & LAMM M.E. (1963) Polypeptide chains of rabbit gamma-globulin. *Science, N.Y.* **142**, 393

[52] MARLER E., NELSON C.A. & TANFORD C. (1964) The polypeptide chains of rabbit γ-globulin and its papain-cleaved fragments. *Biochemistry* **3**, 279

[53] PALMER J.L., NISONOFF A. & VAN HOLDE K.E. (1963) Dissociation of rabbit gamma-globulin into sub-units by reduction and acidification. *Proc. nat. Acad. Sci., (Wash.)* **502**, 314

[54] UTSUMI S. & KARUSH F. (1965) Peptic fragmentation of rabbit γG-immunoglobulin. *Biochemistry* **4**, 1766

[55] YPHANTIS D.A. (1960) Rapid determination of molecular weights of peptides and proteins. *Ann. N.Y. Acad. Sci.* **88**, 586

[56] KEGELES G. (1952) A boundary-forming technique for the ultracentrifuge. *J. Am. chem. Soc.* **74**, 5532

[57] YPHANTIS D.A. (1964) Equilibrium ultracentrifugation of dilute solutions. *Biochemistry* **3**, 297

[58] PAIN R.H. (1963) The molecular weight of the peptide chains of γ-globulin. *Biochem. J.* **88**, 234

[59] MILLER F. & METZGER H. (1965) Characterization of a human macroglobulin I. The molecular weight of the sub-unit, *J. biol. Chem.* **240**, 3325

[60] MILLER F. & METZGER H. (1965) Characterization of a human macroglobulin II. Distribution of the disulphide bonds. *J. biol. Chem.* **240**, 4740

[61] MÜLLER-EBERHARD H.J., KUNKEL H.G. & FRANKLIN E.C. (1956) Two types of γ-globulin differing in carbohydrate content. *Proc. Soc. exp. Biol. Med.* **93**, 146

[62] HOGEBOOM G.H. & KUFF E.L. (1954) Sedimentation behaviour of proteins and other materials in a horizontal preparative rotor. *J. biol. Chem.* **210**, 733

[63] LEVINTOE L., MEISTER, A., HOGEBOOM G.H. & KUFF E.L. (1955) Studies on the relationship between the enzymatic synthesis of glutamine and the glutamyl transfer reaction. *J. Am. chem. Soc.* **77**, 5304

[64] TRAUTMAN R., SAVAN, M. & BREESE S.S. (1959) Partition by zone ultracentrifugation of the two complement-fixing particles in the foot-and-mouth disease virus system. *J. Am. chem. Soc.* **81**, 4040

[65] TRAUTMAN R. & BREESE S.S. (1959) Moving boundary theory applied to preparative ultracentrifugation. *J. phys. Chem.* **63**, 1592

[66] TISELIUS A., PEDERSEN K.O. & SVEDBERG T. (1937) Analytical measurements of ultracentrifugal sedimentation. *Nature, Lond.* **140**, 848

[67] YPHANTIS D.A. & WAUGH D.F. (1956) Ultracentrifugal characterization by direct measurement of activity: II Experimental. *J. phys. Chem.* **60**, 630

[68] GYENES L., GORDON J. & SEHON A.H. (1961) Ultracentrifugal characterization of antibodies in sera of ragweed-sensitive individuals. *Immunology*, **4**, 177

[69] ANDERSEN B.R. & VANNIER W.E. (1964) The sedimentation properties of the skin-sensitizing antibodies of ragweed-sensitive patients. *J. exp. Med.* **120**, 31

[70] YPHANTIS D.A. (1963) In *Ultracentrifugal Analysis in Theory and Experiment*, p. 227, ed. WILLIAMS J.W. New York: Academic Press

[71] BRAKKE M.K. (1953) Zonal separations by density-gradient centrifugation. *Arch. biochem. Biophys.* **45**, 275

[72] DE DUVE C., BERTHET J. & BEAUFAY H. (1959) Gradient centrifugation of cell particles. Theory and applications. In *Progress in Biophysics and Biophysical Chemistry*, **9**, 325, ed. BUTLER J.A.V. & KATZ B. New York: Pergamon Press

[73] DE LALLA O.F. & GOFMAN J.W. (1954) Ultracentrifugal analysis of serum lipoproteins. *Meth. biochem. Analysis* **1**, 459

[74] BOCK R.M. & LING N.S. (1954) Devices for gradient elution in chromatography. *Analyt. Chem.* **26**, 1543

[75] SAMUELS S. (1964) A continuous density gradient apparatus for use in zonal ultracentrifugation. *Analyt. Biochem.* **7**, 164

[76] COWAN K.M. & TRAUTMAN R. (1965) Antibodies produced by guinea-pigs infected with foot-and-mouth disease virus. *J. Immunol.* **94**, 858

[77] STANWORTH D.R. (1959) Studies on the physico-chemical properties of reagin to horse dandruff. *Immunology* **2**, 384

[78] KUNKEL H.G. (1960) Macroglobulins and high molecular weight antibodies. In *The Plasma Proteins*, **1**, 279, ed. PUTNAM F.W. New York: Academic Press

[79] EDELMAN G.M., KUNKEL H.G. & FRANKLIN E.G. (1958) Interaction of the rheumatoid factor with antigen-antibody complexes and aggregated gammaglobulins. *J. exp. Med.* **108**, 105

[80] FUDENBERG H.H. & KUNKEL H.G. (1958) In *Proc. Seventh Congr. of the International Soc. of Blood Transfusion*, Rome (1959) Basel: S. Karger.

[81] ROCKEY J.H. & KUNKEL H.G. (1962) Unusual sedimentation and sulfhydryl sensitivity of certain isohemagglutinins and skin-sensitizing antibody. *Proc. Soc. exp. Biol. Med.* **110,** 101

[82] ROCKEY J.H., KLINMAN N.R. & KARUSH F. (1964) Equine antihapten antibody. I. 7S β_2A and 10S γ_1-globulin components of purified anti-β-lactoside antibody. *J. exp. Med.* **120,** 589

[83] STANWORTH D.R., JAMES K., & SQUIRE J.R. (1961) Application of zone centrifugation to the study of normal and pathological human sera. *Analyt. Biochem.* **2,** 324

[84] HESS R. & PEARSE A.G.E. (1959) Labelling of proteins with cellulose-reactive dyes. *Nature, Lond.* **183,** 260

[85] RANDOLPH M.L. & RYAN R.R. (1950) A slicer for sampling liquids. *Science, N.Y.* **112,** 528

[86] CHARLWOOD P.A. (1963) Application of radioactively-labelled marker proteins in density gradient ultracentrifugation. *Analyt. Biochem.* **5,** 226

[87] MARTIN R.G. & AMES B.N. (1961) A method for determining the sedimentation behaviour of enzymes. Application to protein mixtures. *J. biol. Chem.* **236,** 1372

[88] SZYBALSKI W. (1960) Sampling of virus particles and macromolecules sedimented in an equilibrium density gradient. *Experientia,* **16,** 164

[89] SALO T. (1965) A simple tube-puncturing device for use with density-gradient centrifugation. *Analyt. Biochem.* **10,** 344

[90] ANDREWS P. (1965) The gel-filtration behaviour of proteins related to their molecular weights over a wide range. *Biochem. J.* **96,** 595

[91] ALLISON A.C. & HUMPHREY J.H. (1960) A theoretical and experimental analysis of double diffusion precipitin reactions in gels, and its application to the characterization of antigens. *Immunology* **3,** 95

[92] STANWORTH D.R. (1964) Zone centrifugation. In *Proc. Tenth Congress of the International Society of Blood Transfusion,* p. 1181. Stockholm 1966, Basel: S. Karger

[93] MANCINI G., VAERMAN J.P., CARBONARA A.O. & HEREMANS J.F. (1964) In *Proc. XIth. Colloquium Protides of the Biological Fluids,* Bruges (1963), p. 370, ed. PEETERS H. Amsterdam: Elsevier

[94] ROSENBLOOM J. & SCHUMAKER V.N. (1963) Analytical ultracentrifugation of T4 bacteriophage DNA in preformed sucrose density gradients. *Biochemistry* **2,** 1206

[95] HESS E.L., OBERHAUSER D.F. & HORN R. (1965) Density gradient centrifugation in the analytical ultracentrifuge. *Fedn Proc. Am. Socs exp. Biol.* **24,** Part 1., 289

[96] SPRAGG S.P. (1963) Use of a digital computer for evaluating ultracentrifuge data. *Nature, Lond.* **200,** 1200

[97] TRAUTMAN R. (1963) In *Ultracentrifugal Analysis in Theory and Experiment,* p. 203, ed. WILLIAMS J.W. New York: Academic Press

[98] SCHACHMAN H.K. (1963) The ultracentrifuge: problems and prospects. *Biochemistry,* **2,** 887

[99] GERHART J.C. & SCHACHMAN H.K. (1965) Distinct sub-units for the regulation and catalytic activity of aspartate transcarbamylase. *Biochemistry,* **4,** 1054

[100] ANDERSON N.G., BARRINGER H.P., BATELAY E.F. & FISHER W.D. (1964) The B-IV zonal centrifuge. *Life Sci.* **3,** 667

[101] FISHER W.D. & CANNING R.E. (1964) Isolation of macroglobulin by rate zonal centrifugation. *Am. Zool.* **4,** 310

[102] PRINS H.K. & SMINK D.A. (1964) Zone ultracentrifugation. In *Proc. Xth Congr. Int. Society of Blood Transfusion,* pp. 1186. Stockholm, 1966. Basel: S. Karger

[103] CHERVENKA C.H. (1966) Use of combined schlieren and interference optics for

determination of molecular weights from sedimentation equilibrium data. *Analyt. Chem.* **38,** 356

[104] CHARLWOOD P.A. (1966) Density gradient separations in the ultracentrifuge. *Brit. Med. Bull.* **22,** 121

[105] KOCHWA S., SMITH E., BROWNELL M. & WASSERMAN L.R. (1966) Aggregation of IgG globulin *in vivo*. II. Physicochemical properties of the isolated protein. *Biochem.* **5,** 277

[106] STANWORTH D.R. (1966) Unpublished observation.

CHAPTER 5

Isolation of Specific Antibody from Complexes of Antigen and Antibody

PETER STELOS

Introduction

The isolation of antibodies in as pure a state as possible is obviously one of the goals of immunology. Ideally, what is desired is the isolation and character-ization of antibodies; all having the same specificity, and all being identical in physical and chemical properties. It would then be possible to apply the methods of protein chemistry to such a preparation and thereby learn what rôle chemical composition has to play in antibody specificity. Indeed, the chemical basis for biological specificity constitutes one of the major aims of biology.

During the past 50 years, there have been many ingenious attempts to prepare antibodies in a relatively pure state. It is not the purpose here to describe all of these attempts nor to merely catalogue all of the methods now in use. Rather, the intention is to point out some of the major problems encountered in the isolation of antibodies and to describe some of the solutions that appear to be feasible.

General considerations

The central fact about antibodies is that they will combine only with the antigen that induced their formation or with substances closely related chemically to the inducing antigen. All purification methods, therefore, must start with the reaction of a particular antiserum with its specific antigen, or antigen, if modified, with all of its specific combining sites intact. It is obvious that if antigen is modified, for example, to make it more insoluble, this may alter some of its antigenic determinant groups so that they are incapable of reacting with their specific antibodies. It would appear then that all antigens that have been chemically treated for whatever reason may be different from the antigen originally used for inducing antibody formation. This is not to say that the antigen used for immunization has not undergone some change before it can act as an inducer for antibody synthesis. The

112

mechanism of the antigen stimulus in antibody synthesis is completely unknown.

Another problem to be considered is the fact that antibodies of a given specificity may have different association constants (for further details see Pinckard and Weir, Chapter 14). That is, a given antigen will not induce the formation of antibodies all of which will react to the same degree with the inducing antigen. Apart from the heterogeneity due to different classes of antibody, e.g. γM, γG and γA, there is evidence that even within a particular class differences in reactivity to a given antigen are present. All purification procedures, therefore, may be considered to be selective procedures in the sense that only those antibody molecules which are capable of forming antigen-antibody complexes of a minimum bond energy will be removed from a particular antiserum.

The nature of the immune response is another factor to be considered. It is known that the antibody response is conditioned by the immunization schedule, route of administration, nature of the antigen and other factors. To obtain a predominance of γM antibodies, early collection of antiserum might be indicated whereas, if γG antibodies are wanted, one would use hyperimmune antiserum. In any event, the two classes of antibodies can be easily separated by chromatography, electrophoresis or gel-filtration methods.

Antibody purification may be viewed as generally involving four steps: (1) the reaction of antiserum with its specific antigen or modified antigen; (2) the removal of non-antibody protein by thorough-washing of the insoluble antigen-antibody complex; (3) the dissociation of the antigen-antibody complex; and (4), the physical separation of antibody from antigen. Table 5.1 is but a partial list of various methods which have been used in antibody purification.

Preparation of bovine serum albumin (BSA) coupled to diazotized poly-aminopolystyrene (PAS)

The PAS was a commercial product from Norsk-Hydro-Elektrisk-Kvaelslofak tieselskab, Oslo, Norway. Methods for preparing PAS have been described [6, 7]. About 50 g of the material was suspended in 800 ml distilled water in a 1 litre beaker. After standing for 20 minutes, the supernatant containing many fine particles was decanted and discarded. This operation was repeated three or more times and the last supernatant contained very few fine particles. The suspension was poured onto a Buchner funnel and air was allowed to pass through until the precipitate was a fairly dry cake. The cake was then scraped from the filter paper and allowed to dry at room temperature overnight.

Into a 400 ml beaker immersed in an ice bath, 10 g of the dry PAS was

TABLE 5.1

Some Methods Used for Isolating Specifically Purified Antibodies

Antigen	Modification of antigen	Separation of antibody from antigen	Refs.
Protein	Thiolation of protein	Reaction with mercurials; dissociation at acid pH	1, 2, 3
Protein or protein-hapten	Coupling of protein by diazotized p-amino-benzyl-cellulose	Dissociation at acid pH	4, 5
Protein or protein-hapten	Coupling of protein by diazotized polyamino-polystyrene	Dissociation at acid pH	6, 7, 8
Protein or protein-hapten	Thiolation and polymerization of protein to form insoluble matrix	Dissociation at acid pH	9
Hapten	Hapten coupled by diazo reaction to fibrinogen	Dissociation by excess hapten	10
Hapten	Multivalent (precipitating) hapten	Precipitate dissolved in excess hapten and multivalent hapten precipitated at acid pH	11
Hapten	Hapten coupled by diazo reaction to protein	Precipitate dissolved in excess hapten and antibody separated on DEAE-cellulose	12, 13
Hapten	Hapten coupled by diazo reaction to protein	Precipitate dissolved in excess hapten; protein-hapten precipitated by Streptomycin	14
Hapten	Hapten coupled by diazo reaction to tyramine-cellulose	Dissociation at acid pH	15
Polysaccharide	None	Dissociation at high salt concentration (polysaccharide is insoluble)	16
Polysaccharide	None	Digestion of precipitate with specific carbohydrase	17
Polysaccharide	None	Dissociation at acid pH (polysaccharide is insoluble)	18

suspended in 150 ml of 2 N HCl. To the suspension, stirred by magnetic agitation, 50 ml of 1 M NaNO$_2$ was added dropwise. This amount of NaNO$_2$ was sufficient to give a positive test when the reaction mixture was tested with starch-KI paper.

The suspension was poured onto a Buchner funnel and the precipitate washed with 2 litres of cold distilled water and with 800 ml of cold borate-buffered saline at pH 8. (To make a 1 litre solution, 8 g of NaCl and 12·4 g of boric acid are added to about 900 ml of distilled water. The solution is adjusted to pH 8 with 15 N NaOH and distilled water is added to bring the volume to 1 litre.) The precipitate on the filter paper was allowed to dry partially, after which it was scraped from the filter paper and transferred to a 400 ml beaker. To this was added 2 g of BSA (Armour) which had been dissolved in 100 ml of pH 9 borate buffer. (The buffer was made by adding enough 2 N NaOH to the pH 8 borate-saline buffer to bring the pH to 9.) The mixture was placed in a cold room, and was stirred gently by magnetic agitation overnight.

The suspension was next filtered through a Buchner funnel, and the filtrate was saved in order to determine how much BSA had reacted with the diazo-tized PAS. A portion of the filtrate was dialyzed against pH 9 borate buffer with several changes, and the protein content measured by differential refractometry or absorbancy at 280 mμ.

After the precipitate on the Buchner funnel had dried partially, it was scraped from the filter paper. Excess diazo groups were quenched by reacting them with β-naphthol at pH 8 to 9. The β-naphthol was prepared by pulverizing 5 g of it with a mortar and pestle. The fine powder was then dissolved in 2 ml of 2 N NaOH in a 50 ml beaker. (Heating the mixture in a hot-water bath facilitated solution.) The solution was then diluted to 2 litres with distilled water, and the pH was adjusted to 8 to 9 by dropwise addition of dilute acetic acid. Any resulting precipitate was removed by filtration. The β-naphthol solution was then placed in a cold room, and again, any resulting precipitate was removed by filtration. To this clear solution was added the partially dried precipitate of BSA–PAS, and the suspension was stirred by magnetic agitation overnight in the cold room.

The suspension was again poured onto a Buchner funnel, and the precipitate in the funnel was washed with 2 litres of cold distilled water, followed by 1 litre of cold 0·9 per cent NaCl, then by 100 ml of cold 0·1 M glycine-HCl buffer at pH 2·3, and finally by 200 ml of cold pH 8 borate buffer. After allow-ing the precipitate to dry in the funnel by passing air through it, it was scraped from the filter paper into a 400 ml beaker.

The immunoadsorbent thus prepared was stored in the refrigerator until needed. Some preparations have been stored for as long as 6 months without any loss of adsorbing capacity.

E

Usually, about 0·7 g of BSA were found to have reacted with 10 g of diazotized PAS under the conditions described here. Attempts to increase the amount of BSA coupling to the PAS by increasing the concentration of BSA in the reaction mixture have been unsuccessful.

The same procedure described above was used to react 1 g of ovalbumin with 10 g of diazotized PAS. About 0·37 g of ovalbumin were coupled to 10 g of PAS in one experiment.

Procedure for the isolation of rabbit anti-protein antibodies by a batch method

To remove complement, it is necessary to add a heterologous antigen-antibody system to the antiserum. It has been found that adding 32 μg of ovalbumin and 288 μg of anti-ovalbumin to 1 ml of rabbit anti-BSA serum will remove the complement [19]. After establishing the equivalence point of an anti-ovalbumin serum, the necessary amounts of reagents may be added to a given volume of anti-BSA serum. In a typical experiment, it was found that the rabbit anti-ovalbumin serum contained 4·5 mg of antibody per ml. To 315 ml of anti-BSA serum were added 10 mg (315 ml × 32μg) of ovalbumin and 20 ml (= 90 mg of anti-ovalbumin) of anti-ovalbumin serum. The mixture was allowed to stand overnight in the refrigerator, after which the suspension was centrifuged and the sediment discarded.

The decomplemented serum was then added to the immunoadsorbent, prepared as above, in a 400 ml beaker, and the suspension stirred by magnetic agitation for about 4 hours in the cold. The suspension was poured onto a Buchner funnel, and the filtrate was saved. The precipitate in the funnel was washed with 3 litres of cold 0·9 per cent NaCl. At this time, the filtrate had a reading of 0·024 optical density units at 280 mμ, indicating that most of the inert proteins had been removed from the adsorbent. The filter cake was allowed to partially dry, and was scraped from the filter paper into a 250 ml beaker. About 75 ml of cold glycine-HCl buffer at pH 2·3 were added to this, and the beaker was placed in an ice bath. The suspension was stirred rather vigorously by magnetic agitation for 20 minutes, after which it was poured onto a Buchner funnel. After collecting the filtrate, an additional 10 ml of the pH 2·3 glycine-HCl buffer were added to the filter cake to remove occluded protein. The combined filtrates were neutralized by adding dropwise 1 N NaOH while the solution was stirred. The small amount of pink precipitate was removed by high-speed centrifugation. The supernatant had an optical density of 1·22 at 280 mμ and a volume of 115 ml. Assuming that 1 mg per ml of γ globulin has an optical density of 1·5, then the filtrate contained 115 ml × 1·22/1·5 = 94 mg of antibody. A second treatment of the immunoadsorbent with 75 ml of pH 2·3 glycine-HCl buffer yielded another 27 mg of antibody.

The original antiserum contained 1·4 mg of antibody per ml, or a total of 490 mg. Therefore, the efficiency was $121/490 \times 100 = 24\cdot8$ per cent.

For further use, the adsorbent was washed with 200 ml of pH 8 borate buffer while still in the Buchner funnel, allowed to dry partially, and scraped from the paper into a 400 ml beaker. It was then stored in the refrigerator.

Reabsorption of the filtrate with the same adsorbent and repetition of the procedure just described yielded 92 mg of antibody. A third cycle yielded 71 mg and a fourth, 52 mg. The four absorptions thus accounted for 336 mg out of a total of 490 mg originally present.

In terms of precipitability, 90 to 95 per cent of the protein in all four preparations were precipitated by adding an equivalent amount of antigen. In the ultracentrifuge, 95 per cent of the protein had a sedimentation co-efficient of 6S and 5 per cent, of 9S.

TABLE 5.2

Properties of immunoadsorbents prepared by reacting 2 g of BSA or 1 g of ovalbumin with 10 g of diazotized PAS

Protein	g protein g PAS	ml antiserum adsorbed	mg total antibody	mg antibody recovered after cycle			
				1	2	3	4
BSA	0·07	315	490	121	92	71	52
Ovalbumin	0·04	188	380	97	46	50	—

The same procedure described here was used to prepare rabbit anti-ovalbumin antibodies. Table 5.2 summarizes and compares the results obtained with the two immunoadsorbents. Generally, the efficiency of the two adsorbents in removing antibody from specific antisera was about the same.

Procedure for the isolation of rabbit anti-protein antibodies by a column method

The BSA-PAS immunoadsorbent prepared as described above was used [8]. The preparation, 10 g, was mixed with 10 g of Solka-Floc (Brown Co, Berlin, N.H.), suspended in 400 ml of 0·9 per cent NaCl, and packed into a column (1·7 cm × 25 cm). The bottom of the column was first packed to a height of 2 cm with a slurry of Solka-Floc suspended in 0·9 per cent NaCl. Solka-Floc is a cellulose product derived from wood pulp which acts as a 'filler' and permits a more rapid flow of liquid through the column. About 35 ml of rabbit anti-BSA serum, decomplemented as above, were placed on the column, and 0·9 per cent NaCl was passed through continuously until the effluent was free of protein (OD at 280 mμ was less than 0·020). The adsorbed antibodies were eluted by passing through 20 ml of pH 3 citrate-phosphate buffer (158 ml of 0·1 M citric acid, 41·1 ml of 0·2 M Na_2HPO_4 and enough distilled water to make 1 litre). Effluent fractions containing protein, as measured by absorbancy at 280 mμ, were combined and neutralized by dropwise addition of 1 N NaOH. The small amount of pink precipitate was removed by centrifugation or filtration. The clarified supernatant was precipitated by addition of an equal volume of saturated ammonium sulphate and stored in this state until needed.

All procedures were done in a cold room (5° C) and the antibodies were in acid pH for not more than 2 to 3 hours. Between 80 and 90 per cent of the eluted proteins were precipitable by an equivalent amount of antigen. The recovery of anti-BSA antibody, in the above experiment, accounted for 50 per cent of the total present in the original serum. After washing the column with 50 ml of pH 8 borate buffer, it could be used for additional adsorptions.

The method just described was also used for the isolation of anti-ovalbumin antibodies. However, only 10 per cent of the antibody was removed from the antiserum after one passage through the column.

Comparison of the batch method with the column method indicates that the latter is probably more efficient, especially with anti-BSA serum. The batch method, however, can handle larger amounts of antiserum, and the process requires much less time than the column method.

References

[1] SINGER S.J., FOTHERGILL J.E. & SHAINOFF J.R. (1960) General method for isolation of antibodies. *J. Am. chem. Soc.* **82**, 565

[2] SINGER S.J. (1964) Purification of antiprotein antibodies by thiolated antigen procedure. In *Methods in Medical Research*, Vol. 10, pp. 87–90, ed. EISEN H.N. Chicago: Year Book Medical Publishers

[3] EISEN H.N., ARONSON N. & SIMMS, E.S. (1964) Preparation of purified anti-gamma-globulin antibodies. In *Methods in Medical Research*, Vol. 10, pp. 91–93, ed. EISEN H.N. Chicago: Year Book Medical Publishers

[4] MALLEY A. & CAMPBELL D.H. (1963) Isolation of antibody by means of an immunological specific adsorbent. *J. Amer. chem.* **85**, 487

[5] MOUDGAL N.R. & PORTER R.R. (1963) The use of antigen-cellulose suspensions for the isolation of specific antibodies. *Biochem. biophys. Acta* **71**, 185

[6] GYENES L. & SEHON A.H. (1960) Preparation and evaluation of polystyrene-antigen conjugates for the isolation of antibodies. *Can. J. biochem. Physiol.* **38**, 1235

[7] YAGI Y., ENGEL K. & PRESSMAN D. (1960) Quantitative determination of small amounts of antibody by use of solid adsorbents. *J. Immunol.* **85**, 375

[8] STELOS P. & PRESSMAN D. (1962) Papain digestion of antigen-antibody precipitates. *J. biol. Chem.* **237**, 3679

[9] ONOUE K., YAGI Y. & PRESSMAN D. (1965) Immunoadsorbents of high capacity. *Immunochemistry* 2, 181

[10] KARUSH F. & MARK R. (1957) The preparation and properties of purified anti-hapten antibodies. *J. Immunol.* 78, 296

[11] EPSTEIN S.I., DOTY P. & BOYD W.C. (1956) A thermodynamic study of hapten-antibody dissociation. *J. Am. chem. Soc.* 78, 3306

[12] KOSHLAND M.E., ENGLEBERGER F. & KOSHLAND D.E. JR. (1959) General methods for labeling of active site of antibodies and enzymes. *Proc. Nat. Acad. Sci. (Wash.)* 45, 1470

[13] GROSSBERG A.L. & PRESSMAN D. (1964) Purification of anti-p-azobenzoate antibodies. In *Methods in Medical Research*, Vol. 10, pp. 103–105, ed. EISEN H.N. Chicago: Year Book Medical Publishers

[14] EISEN H.N. (1964) Preparation of purified anti-2, 4-dinitrophenyl antibodies. In *Methods in Medical Research*, Vol. 10, pp. 94–102, ed. EISEN H.N. Chicago: Year Book Medical Publishers

[15] VANNIER W.E., BRYAN W.P. & CAMPBELL D.H. (1965) The preparation and properties of a hapten-cellulose antibody adsorbent. *Immunochemistry* 2, 1

[16] HEIDELBERGER M. & KABAT E.A. (1938) The dissociation of antibody from pneumococcus specific precipitates and specifically agglutinated pneumococci. *J. exp. Med.* 67, 181

[17] KABAT E.A. (1954) Purification of human antidextrans. *Science* 120, 782

[18] HILL W.C. & CEBRA J.J. (1965) Horse anti-SI immunoglobulins 1. Properties of γM-antibody. *Biochemistry* 4, 2574

[19] TALIAFERRO, W.H. & TALMAGE D.W. (1955) Absence of amino acid incorporation into antibody during the induction period. *J. Inf. Dis.* 97, 88

PART B

STUDIES ON THE SYNTHESIS AND PROPERTIES OF THE IMMUNOGLOBULINS

CHAPTER 6

In vitro Technique for Immunoglobulin Synthesis

R.VAN FURTH

Introduction

In studies on the site of antibody or immunoglobulin formation, tissue culture has been widely employed [1, 2, 3]. In early experiments, *in vitro* synthesis was established by the increase of the antibody titre or immunoglobulin content in the culture fluid in comparison to that in the extract of a non-cultured sample [4, 5, 6, 7, 8, 9]. Subsequently, isotopic assay was used [10, 11, 12, 13, 14, 15, 16, 17]. This method requires that the synthesized antibodies or immunoglobulins in the culture fluid are isolated by specific precipitation and then measured by the incorporation of radioactive amino acids into these proteins. The method is very sensitive, but the different types (IgG and IgM) of the synthesized proteins can be distinguished only if the culture fluid is fractionated.

With the technique for the synthesis of serum proteins *in vitro* described by Hochwald, Thorbecke & Asofsky [18], the different classes of immunoglobulins can be determined directly, but this method has limitations for the assay of antibody formation. In the present chapter this technique will be described in detail.

Methods

Principle

The outline of the method is shown in Fig. 6.1. Tissue fragments or cell

120

suspensions are incubated in the presence of radioactive amino acids. The *de novo* synthesized immunoglobulins are detected and identified by auto-radiography of the immunoelectrophoretic pattern.

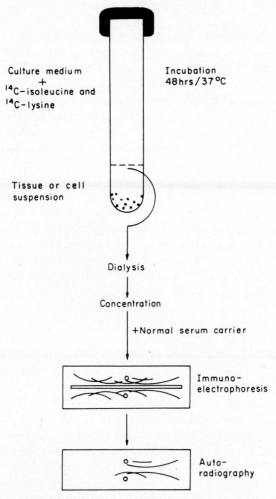

Culture medium
+
^{14}C−isoleucine and
^{14}C−lysine

Incubation
48hrs/37°C

Tissue or cell
suspension

Dialysis

Concentration

+Normal serum carrier

Immuno−
electrophoresis

Auto−
radiography

FIG. 6.1. Outline of the technique for examining immunoglobulin synthesis *in vitro*.

Tissues

Tissue samples are minced with surgical blades in a petri dish containing Hank's balanced salt solution. Discrete tissue fragments are then placed with a capillary pipette against the wall of a roller tube. The fluid which drains to the bottom of the tube is removed. The optimal wet weight of the cultured tissue ranges from 50 to 150 mg, depending on the nature of the tissue.

Bone-marrow samples, collected in 0·1 per cent heparin without preservative, are suspended in Hank's solution and further prepared in the same way as the tissue fragments.

Lymphocyte suspensions from peripheral blood are prepared from samples collected in siliconized bottles, which contain 4 mg heparin per 100 ml blood. The erythrocytes of these samples are sedimented with a 5 per cent solution of dextran (molecular weight 200,000, 30 ml solution to 100 ml blood) for 30 minutes at 37° C. The supernatant fraction, rich in leucocytes is centrifuged at 650 g for 7 minutes at 20° C. The leucocytes are resuspended in a few drops of Hank's solution and transferred to the roller tube. The minimum number of lymphoid cells for detecting immunoglobulin synthesis *in vitro* is 0·1 to 0.5×10^8 cells for normal peripheral blood. After antigen stimulation a smaller number of cells may be sufficient. If the granulocyte count in the peripheral blood is high, as in normal peripheral blood samples, the granulocytes are first removed by filtering the leucocyte-rich supernatant fraction through a nylon fibre column at room temperature [19]. The granulocytes of a 100 ml blood sample are separated by 4 g nylon fibres (3 denier, 1˙5 inch, type 200, Du Pont De Nemours & Co, treated with Duponal-R.A. as described by the manufacturer) which are packed in a glass column (12 mm diameter) to a height of 12 cm. The commercially available leucocyte filter (Leuko-Pak ™, Fenwal Laboratories, Morton Grove, Ill.) can also be used.

Culture medium
The culture medium, which contains no serum is prepared with 100 ml Hank's balanced salt solution (Oxoid, London) to which 2 ml of an amino acid stock solution (fifty times as concentrated as shown in Table 6.1), 0·5 per cent (w/v) ovalbumin, glucose to a final concentration of 0·5 per cent (w/v), 1 per cent (v/v) BME vitamin mixture (Microbiological Associates Inc, Bethesda, Md.) and 100 U/ml penicillin is added. The pH is adjusted to 7·4 with an isotonic solution of 1·4 per cent sodium bicarbonate solution.

The medium is sterilized by passage through a Millipore filter. The radioactive amino acids are then added: 1 μc/ml ^{14}C L Lysine (uniformly labelled 124 μc/mmole, Schwarz Bio Research, Orangeburg, N.Y.) and 1 μc/ml ^{14}C L Isoleucine (uniformly labelled, 110 μc/mmole, Schwarz Bio Research, Orangeburg, N.Y.).

Cultures
For each culture 1 ml of medium containing 2 μc is used. The tubes can be gassed with 5 per cent CO_2 in air. The cultures are incubated for 48 hours at 37° C under continuous rotation (10 rotations per hour) and then frozen at

$-20°$ C. After being thawed the culture fluid is centrifuged at 18,000 g for 20 minutes at $4°$ C. To remove the excess of radioactive amino acids the cell-free supernatant solution is dialysed against 0·015 M phosphate buffer (pH 7·6) for 72 hours at $4°$ C. Thereafter the culture fluid is concentrated by lyophilization and dissolved in 0·1 ml twice-distilled water.

TABLE 6.1

Constituents of amino acid mixture in the culture medium*

Amino acids	Concentration† mM
L—Arginine · HCl	0·2
L—Histidine	0·1
Glycine	0·3
L—Alanine	0·3
L—Serine	0·5
L—Threonine	0·3
L—Valine	0·3
L—Leucine	0·3
L—Aspartic acid	0·15
L—Glutamic acid	0·15
L—Asparagine · H_2O	0·3
L—Glutamine	1·5
DL—Phenylalanine	0·2
L—Tyrosine	0·1
L—Tryptophan	0·03
L—Proline	0·15
Hydroxy—L—proline	0·15
L—Cysteine · HCl · H_2O	0·2
L—Methionine	0·2

* After Neumann & McCoy [55].
† Concentration in final culture medium.

Immunoelectrophoresis

To ensure comparable results, immunoelectrophoretic analysis of the concentrated culture fluid is carried out under strict standard conditions [20, 21]. Microscope slides are coated with 2·5 ml 1·3 per cent agar gel (Noble, Difco) in 0·05 M Veronal buffer (pH 8·6). Because the concentrated culture fluid often contains too little protein to provide a well-defined reproducible precipitation line, a carrier serum is added. The antigen well (about 1 μl) is first filled with serum. After the serum has been absorbed into the agar (3–4 minutes) the concentrated culture fluid is added three times to the antigen well.

E*

Electrophoresis (3·5 V/cm) is carried out at room temperature. The immuno-electrophoretic pattern is developed with an antihuman serum or with an antiserum specific for one immunoglobulin or Bence-Jones protein. The unprecipitated radioactive proteins on the slides are removed by washing in phosphate buffered saline, for 72 hours, with three changes. Next the slides are dried and stained with amido black.

Agarelectrophoresis
The culture fluid is analysed by electrophoresis on agar gel according to Wieme [22]. Slides are prepared with 0·9 per cent agar gel (Noble, Difco)

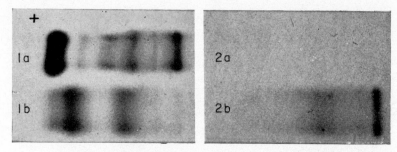

FIG. 6.2. Autoradiography of cellulose acetate electrophoresis.

1. *Cellulose acetate membrane*
(a) Serum with homogeneous band in γ globulin region, from patient with mono-clonal IgG in serum, but without signs of multiple myeloma in the bone marrow.
(b) Culture fluid of bone-marrow sample; no homogeneous band in gammaglobulin region visible on membrane stained with amido black.

2. *Autoradiograph of cellulose acetate membrane*
(a) Nothing visible.
(b) Homogeneous band with same electrophoretic mobility as monoclonal IgG in serum.

in 0·05 M Veronal buffer (pH 8·6). A 5 mm long slit is filled once with the concentrated culture fluid and the electrophoretic separation (30 V/cm) is done under cooling with petroleum ether. No carrier serum is added. The slides are fixed in 5 per cent acetic acid in 70 per cent ethanol and then washed, dried and stained with amido black.

The electrophoresis of the culture fluid is also carried out on a cellulose acetate membrane [23, 24]. With a sample applicator (Beckman) 0·25 μl of the culture fluid is applied to the membrane. Electrophoresis is done for 20 minutes, 25 V/cm, in a Microzone Cell (Beckman), which contains 0·075 M Veronal buffer (pH 8·6). No carrier serum is used. After the membrane is fixed, stained and dried at 70° C a strip of it is cut off. This strip, which contains the electropherograph of the culture fluid and of the serum of the same individual, is mounted on a microscope slide and exposed for auto-radiography (Fig. 6.2) [45].

Autoradiography
Sheet film (Kodak RS Pan, 650 ASA) is cut into strips to fit the microscope slides. A strip is placed between the electrophoretic slide and a blank slide; these slides are clamped together with a clothes-pin. The optimal exposure time is 21 days for the immunoelectrophoresis and 7 days for the agar electrophoresis slides, with the quoted amino acids and the degree of labelling given. The films are developed with 10 per cent Rodinal solution (Agfa) for 10 minutes at 20° C.

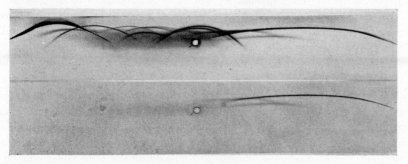

FIG. 6.3. Spleen.

Above: Immunoelectrophoretic pattern of carrier serum and culture fluid of an adult spleen developed with horse anti-human serum.
Below: Autoradiograph with labelled IgG, IgA and IgM lines (from reference 37).

Indication of *in vitro* synthesis
The labelled proteins of the culture fluid and the proteins of the carrier serum precipitate together on the immunoelectrophoresis slide. The autoradio-graphic lines on the film strip can therefore be identified by the comparison of these lines with the lines on the immunoelectrophoresis slide (Figs. 6.1 and 6.3). A labelled immunoglobulin line indicates the synthesis of this protein *in vitro*.

The intensity of the autoradiographic lines is graded thus: − = negative; (+) = just visible; + = clearly visible; + + + + = very dark (see Table 6.2).

Quantitative studies

The following is an example of the kind of study that can be made of the amount of immunoglobulins synthesized under the experimental conditions described.

A suspension of spleen cells was cultured for 6, 12, 24 and 48 hours in a medium containing only ^{14}C lysine. After incubation the culture fluid was treated with a diphtheria toxoid-antitoxin precipitate to correct for non-specific adsorption of radioactive substances. After the addition of a small amount of purified IgG, the labelled IgG was precipitated with specific anti-IgG serum in slight excess. The amount of radioactive amino acid incorporated into the precipitated IgG was measured and also the lysine pool of the spleen cells was determined. From these data it has been calculated that the total amount of IgG synthesized during the initial 6 hours of incubation was about 1·25 μg per 10^8 lymphoid cells [26, 27]. This value agrees well with the results obtained for unstimulated rabbit spleens [17], whereas after antigen stimulation the immunoglobulin or antibody production was at least tenfold higher [28, 17, 14, 16, 29]. The initial rate of synthesis was not maintained during the 48 hours of incubation, but decreased markedly after 12 hours [26, 27]. The addition of 20 per cent foetal calf serum to the medium caused no distinct increase of the immunoglobulin production, as judged from the autoradiographic assay [30].

The amount of radioactive immunoglobulin in the precipitation line on the immunoelectrophoresis slide was determined and the result was compared with the intensity of this line on the autoradiograph. The concentrated culture fluid was diluted serially in saline and the diluted solutions were subjected to immunoelectrophoresis in duplicate on the same slide; anti-IgG serum was used. One precipitation line of the slide was cut out, the proteins were extracted from the agar and the amount of radioactive protein was quantitatively determined. The duplicate precipitation line on the slide wax exposed for autoradiography during 3 weeks and the intensity of the line graded. The results of this study show that the score of + + + corresponds to about 0·0125 μg radioactive IgG. The limit of visibility (+) is reached at approximately 0·0002 μg labelled immunoglobulin in the precipitation line, under the given experimental conditions [26, 27].

Specificity of the method

The possibility has to be considered that the immunoglobulins become radioactive by non-specific adsorption of labelled amino acids during incubation or by precipitation of labelled proteins on the antigen-antibody precipitate during immunoelectrophoresis. Therefore different control experiments had to be performed.

The incubation of dead tissues or serum with the radioactive medium gives no labelled immunoglobulin lines. When puromycin was added to the culture, the *in vitro* formation of immunoglobulins was inhibited. The intensity of the IgG line on the autoradiograph and the amount of IgG synthesized per culture tube showed good correlation with the concentration of puromycin. The autoradiograph of a peptide map, prepared from IgG synthesized *in vitro*, showed the labelling of different peptide spots in a pattern comparable with the 'fingerprint' of serum IgG. From these experiments it may be concluded that the labelling of the immunoglobulin lines, visible on the autoradiographs, results from the *in vitro* incorporation of ^{14}C amino acids into the immunoglobulin molecule [26, 25].

The use of a hydrolysate of labelled algal or yeast proteins is not recommended. This mixture of radioactive amino acids may give a non-specific

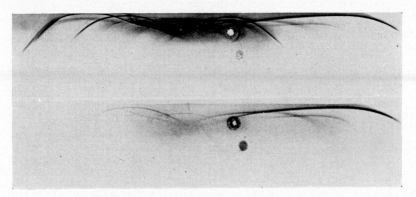

FIG. 6.4. Peripheral blood lymphocytes—infectious mononucleosis.

Above: Immunoelectrophoretic pattern of carrier serum and culture fluid prepared with $1·3 \times 10^8$ mononuclear cells (horse anti-human serum).
Below: Autoradiograph showing the synthesis of IgG, IgA and IgM. Note also the labelling of α_2 macroglobulin, α_1A globulin and part of the albumin line (from reference 42).

labelling of serum proteins, probably due to the binding of amino acids such as cysteine [18].

For the autoradiographic assay it is essential to use amino acids with a high specific activity. Instead of ^{14}C lysine and ^{14}C isoleucine, other labelled amino acids such as valine or leucine may also be used. These amino acids may be preferable to isoleucine, because the γ globulin molecule contains three times as many valine and leucine molecules as of isoleucine [31]. However, appropriate control experiments must be included, if a different medium is used.

The double diffusion test in agar gel [32] cannot be applied for the detection of immunoglobulin or antibody synthesis because other labelled proteins of the culture fluid adsorb non-specifically onto the immune precipitate [33]. However, if the labelled immunoglobulins are isolated first, this technique may well be used. In this way the antigenic type of the L chain of labelled IgM was determined [34].

Frequently other lines are found to be labelled. The haptoglobin line is seen in cultures from tissues with an active erythropoiesis, such as bone marrow and the foetal liver. This labelling is due to the binding of ^{14}C haemoglobin to haptoglobin of the carrier serum [35, 26, 36, 37]. However, the labelling of the haptoglobin line in liver cultures may depend on the synthesis of this protein [38]. In a large variety of tissue cultures the α_2-macroglobulin line is labelled (Fig. 6.4.) This labelling may be considered to be non-specific. It might be that α_2 macroglobulin is a carrier of labelled tissue products such as enzymes, or that this protein is ubiquitously synthesized *in vitro* [35, 39]. In a number of autoradiographs the albumin line and some α globulin lines, often only the part near the electrophoresis axis, are weakly

TABLE 6.2

Combined autoradiography results of the synthesis of immunoglobulins by normal human tissues *in vitro*

Organs	Autoradiography*		
	IgG	IgA	IgM
Spleen	+ +	+ +	+
Lymph node	+ +	+	+
Bone marrow	+ + +	+ +	+
Thymus	+ +	(+)	—
Thoracic duct lymphocytes	+ +	+ +	+ +
Peripheral blood lymphocytes	+	+	(+)

* The intensity of the autoradiographic image is graded from: — = negative; (+) = just visible; + = clearly visible; to + + + + = very dark.

labelled (Fig. 6.4). This labelling is probably due to coprecipitation of radio-active tissue products onto the precipitation line. Whether some of these proteins are synthesized *in vitro* has not been checked. In cultures of the adult and foetal liver, however, a distinct labelling of albumin, α and β globulin lines are found [40, 38, 36, 37].

Discussion

The method described here is a simple and sensitive technique to study the site of formation of serum proteins. Although the autoradiographic assay gives only semi-quantitative data on protein production, the results obtained under standard conditions can be well compared. Different applications will now be discussed.

The site of immunoglobulin formation has been extensively studied with this method in man and animals [18, 40, 26, 41]. In man the spleen, lymph nodes, bone marrow and thymus synthesize different patterns of immunoglobulins (Fig. 6.3; Table 6.2) [37]. Also circulating lymphocytes, obtained from normal subjects and from patients with abnormalities of the lymphocytes, incubated without specific antigens or phytohaemagglutinin, show the formation of immunoglobulins *in vitro* (Fig. 6.4; Table 6.2) [42]. This technique has also been applied to study immunoglobulin formation during foetal life [43, 56]. In the human foetus, the spleen showed the synthesis of IgG and IgM after the twentieth week of gestation (Fig. 6.5) [26, 36].

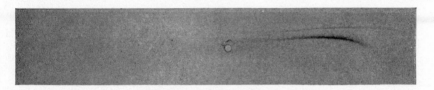

FIG. 6.5. Foetal spleen.

Autoradiograph of a spleen culture from a 22 week old foetus showing labelling of IgG and IgM. Note the absence of IgA. Immunoelectrophoresis developed with horse anti-human serum (from reference 36).

Cultures of plasma cell tumours in mice and pathological bone-marrow samples in man demonstrated the formation of abnormal immunoglobulins with the same characteristics as the paraproteins in the serum [35, 44].

In these studies, the autoradiography of the electrophoresis pattern, on agar or on cellulose acetate, is more sensitive for the detection of a homogeneous band in the immunoglobulins than the stained slide (Fig. 6.2) [44, 45].

Antibody formation *in vitro* can also be detected by autoradiography. The culture fluid and a carrier serum with specific antibody activity is separated electrophoretically; the precipitation line is developed with the antigen [43]. To distinguish between the formation of IgG and IgM antibodies, the culture fluids have to be fractionated first.

The formation of auto-antibodies *in vitro* has been accomplished so far only for cold auto-haemagglutinins [34]. Attempts to demonstrate the *in vitro* synthesis of rheumatoid factor and antinuclear antibodies failed, probably because these antibodies interacted with antigens in the culture [46, 47].

The sites of formation of other serum proteins have also been extensively studied by the technique described. These studies showed that complement is labelled in cultures of various organs [40, 48, 57] and C-reactive protein is synthesized exclusively by the liver [49]. The autoradiographic assay of the immunoelectrophoresis pattern is also used to detect the synthesis of albumin and other serum proteins by a cell-free system from the liver [50, 51].

A disadvantage of the described method is the lack of information about the cellular localization of the immunoglobulin production. By immuno-fluorescent staining of the cell suspensions the morphology of the cells containing immunoglobulins can clearly be observed [26, 52, 53, 54]. When both techniques are applied to the same sample, the immunofluorescent staining performed before incubation may indicate which cells are involved in the synthesis *in vitro* [36, 37, 42, 44, 45].

References

[1] STAVITSKY A.B. (1961) *In vitro* studies of the antibody response. In *Advanc. Immunol.* **1**, 211, ed. TALIAFERRO W.H. & HUMPHREY J.H. New York/London: Academic Press

[2] THORBECKE G.J. & BENACERRAF B. (1962) The reticulo-endothelial system and immunological phenomena. In *Progress in Allergy*, **6**, 559, ed. KALLÓS P. & WAKSMAN B.H. Basel/New York: S. Karger

[3] GOWANS J.L. & McGREGOR D.D. (1965) The immunological activities of lymphocytes. In *Progress in Allergy*, **9**, 1, ed. KALLÓS P. & WAKSMAN B.H. Basel/New York: S. Karger

[4] FAGRAEUS A. (1948) Antibody production in relation to the development of plasma cells. *In vivo* and *in vitro* experiments. *Acta med. Scand.* **Suppl. 204**

[5] FAGRAEUS A. (1948) The plasma cellular reaction and its relation to the formation of antibodies *in vitro*. *J. Immunol.* **58**, 1

[6] KEUNING F.J. & VAN DER SLIKKE L.B. (1950) The role of immature plasma cells, lymphoblasts and lymphocytes in the formation of antibodies, as established in tissue culture experiments. *J. Lab. clin. Med.* **36**, 167

[7] THORBECKE G.J. & KEUNING F.J. (1953) Antibody formation *in vitro* by haemopoietic organs after subcutaneous and intravenous immunization. *J. Immunol.* **70**, 129

[8] THORBECKE G.J. & KEUNING F.J. (1956) Antibody and gamma-globulin formation *in vitro* in haemopoietic organs. *J. inf. Diseases* **63**, 157

[9] ROBERTS S., ADAMS E. & WHITE A. (1949) Influence of mode of immunization on the relationship between the development of tissue titres and the release *in vitro*. *J. Immunol.* **62**, 155

[10] RANNEY H.M. & LONDON I.M. (1951) Antibody formation in surviving cells. *Fed. Proc.* **10**, 562

[11] KESTON A.S. & KATCHEN B. (1956) Incorporation of glycine-2 C^{14} into homologous antibody by rabbit tissue slices. *J. Immunol.* **76**, 253

[12] STEINER D.F. & ANKER H.S. (1956) On the synthesis of antibody protein *in vitro*. *Proc. nat. Acad. Sci. U.S.* **42**, 580

[13] ASKONAS B.A. & WHITE R.G. (1956) Sites of antibody production in the guinea-pig. The relation between *in vitro* synthesis of anti-ovalbumin and γ-globulin and distribution of antibody-containing plasma cells. *Brit. J. exp. Path.* **37**, 61

[14] ASKONAS B.A. & HUMPHREY J.H. (1958) Formation of specific antibodies and gamma-globulin *in vitro*. A study of the synthetic ability of various tissues from rabbits immunized by different methods. *Biochem. J.* **68,** 252

[15] STAVITSKY A.B. (1958) *In vitro* production of diphtheria antitoxin by tissues of immunized animals. III. Incorporation of amino acids into antibody; relationship to antibody synthesis and sensitivity relative to other methods. *Brit. J. exp. Path.* **39,** 661

[16] STAVITSKY A.B. & WOLF B. (1958) Mechanisms of antibody globulin synthesis by lymphoid tissue *in vitro*. *Biochem. biophys. Acta* **27,** 4

[17] THORBECKE G.J. (1960) Gamma globulin and antibody formation *in vitro*. I. Gamma-globulin formation in tissues from immature and normal adult rabbits. *J. exp. Med.* **112,** 279

[18] HOCHWALD G.M., THORBECKE G.J. & ASOFSKY R. (1961) A new technique for the demonstration of the synthesis of individual serum proteins by tissues *in vitro*. *J. exp. Med.* **114,** 459

[19] GREENWALT T.J., GAJENOSKI M. & MCKENNA J. (1963). A new method for preparing buffy coat-poor blood. *Transfusion* **2,** 221

[20] GRABAR, P. & WILLIAMS C.A. (1953) Méthode permettant l'étude conjuguée des propriétés électrophorétiques et immunochimiques d'un mélange de protéines. Application au sérum sanguin. *Biochem. biophys. Acta* **10,** 193

[21] SCHEIDEGGER A. (1955) Une microméthode de l'immuno-électrophorese. *Int. Arch. Allergy* **7,** 103

[22] WIEME R.J. (1959) Studies on agar gel electrophoresis. *Editions Arscia*, Bruxelles

[23] GRUNBAUM B.W., KIRK P.P.L. & ATCHLEY W.A. (1960) Microelectrophoresis on cellulose acetate membranes. *Anal. Chem.* **32,** 1361

[24] GRUNBAUM B.W., ZEC J. & DURRUM E.L. (1963) Application of an improved micro-electrophoresis technique and immunoelectrophoresis of the serum proteins on cellulose acetate. *Microchem. J.* **7,** 41

[25] VAN FURTH R., SCHUIT H.R.E. & HIJMANS W. (1966) The formation of immuno-globulins by human tissues *in vitro*. I. Methods and their specificity. *Immunology* **11,** 1

[26] VAN FURTH R. (1964) The formation of immunoglobulins by human tissues *in vitro*. Doctorate thesis, Leiden

[27] VAN FURTH R. (1966) The formation of immunoglobulins by human tissues *in vitro*. II. Quantitative studies. *Immunology* **11,** 13

[28] VAUGHAN J.H., DUTTON A.H., DUTTON R.W., GEORGE M. & MARSTON R.Q. (1960) A study of antibody production *in vitro*. *J. Immunol.* **84,** 258

[29] HELMREICH E., KERN M. & EISEN H.N. (1961) The secretion of antibody by isolated lymph node cells. *J. biol. Chem.* **236,** 464

[30] VAN FURTH, R. (1965) Unpublished observations

[31] CRUMPTON M.J. & WILKINSON J.M. (1963) Amino acid compositions of human and rabbit gammaglobulins and of the fragments produced by reduction. *Biochem. J.* **88,** 228

[32] OUCHTERLONY Ö. (1962) Diffusion-in gel methods for immunological analysis II. In *Progress in Allergy*, **6,** 30, (ed. KALLÓS P. & WAKSMAN B.H. Basel/New York: S. Karger

[33] THORBECKE G J. & VAN FURTH R. (1963) Unpublished observations

[34] VAN FURTH R. & DIESSELHOFF-DEN DULK M. (1966) The formation of cold auto-haemagglutinins with anti-I specificity *in vitro J. Immunol.* **96,** 920

[35] THORBECKE G.J., HOCHWALD G.M. & JACOBSON E.B. (1962) Autoradiography of immunoelectrophoresis in the study of serum protein formation by mouse plasma cell tumors and a few other transplantable tumors. *Ann. N.Y. Acad. Sci.* **101,** 255

[36] VAN FURTH R., HIJMANS W. & SCHUIT H.R.E. (1965) The immunological development of the human fetus. *J. exp. Med.*, **122**, 1173

[37] VAN FURTH R., SCHUIT H.R.E. & HIJMANS W. (1966) The formation of immuno-globulins by human tissues *in vitro*. III. Spleen, bone marrow, lymph nodes and thymus. *Immunology* **11**, 19

[38] WILLIAMS C.A., ASOFSKY R. & THORBECKE G.J. (1963) Plasma protein formation *in vitro* by tissues from mice infected with staphylococci. *J. exp. Med.* **118**, 315

[39] PHILLIPS M.E. & THORBECKE G.J. (1965) Serum protein formation of donor type in rat-into-mouse chimaeras. *Nature, London*, **207**, 376

[40] ASOFSKY R. & THORBECKE G.J. (1961) Sites of formation of immunoglobulins and of a component of C'_3. II. Production of immunoelectrophoretically identified serum proteins by human and monkey tissues *in vitro*. *J. exp. Med.* **114**, 471

[41] THORBECKE G.J., ASOFSKY R., HOCHWALD G.M. & JACOBSON E.B. (1964) Auto-radiography of immunoelectrophoresis in the study of ^{14}C-amino acid incorporation into serum proteins by tissues *in vitro* and *in vivo*. In *Protides of the Biological Fluids*, **11**, 125, ed. PEETERS H. Amsterdam/London/New York: Elseviers Publ. Cy.

[42] VAN FURTH, R., SCHUIT, H.R.E. and HIJMANS, W. (1966). The formation of immuno-globulins by human tissues *in vitro*. IV. Circulating lymphocytes in normal and pathological conditions. *Immunology* **11**, 29

[43] SILVERSTEIN A.M., THORBECKE G.J., KRANER K.L. & LUKES R.J. (1963) Fetal response to antigenic stimulus. III. Gamma-globulin production in normal and stimulated fetal lambs. *J. Immunol.* **91**, 384

[44] VAN FURTH R., SCHUIT H.R.E. & HIJMANS W. (1966) The formation *in vitro* of para-proteins in multiple myeloma and Waldenström's macroglobulinaemia. *Brit. J. Haemat.* **12**, 202

[45] VAN FURTH R., SCHUIT H.R.E., HIJMANS W. & HUIBRECHTSE L. (1966) *In vitro* formation of monoclonal IgG by non-myeloma bone marrow. *Fed. Proc.* **25**, 309

[46] LEVENE H.I., FRANKLIN E.C. & THORBECKE G.J. (1961) *In vitro* formation of 7S and 19S γ-globulins by tissues from normal subjects and patients with rheumatoid arthritis. *J. Immunol.* **86**, 440

[47] VAN FURTH R. & HIJMANS W. (1963) Unpublished observations

[48] THORBECKE G.J., HOCHWALD G.M., VAN FURTH R., MÜLLER-EBERHARD H.J. & JACOBSON E.B. (1965) Problems in determining the sites of synthesis of complement components. In *Ciba Foundation Symposium on Complement*, ed. WOLSTENHOLME G.E.W. & KNIGHT J. J.&A.Churchill Ltd, London

[49] HURLIMANN J., THORBECKE G.J. & HOCHWALD J. (1966) The liver as site of C reactive protein formation. *J. exp. Med.* **123**, 365

[50] DECKEN A. VON DER (1963) Labelling of immunologically specific proteins by ribo-nucleoprotein particles from rat-liver and chick-liver cell sap. *Biochem. J.* **88**, 385

[51] GANOZA M.C., WILLIAMS C.A. & LIPMANN F. (1965) Synthesis of serum proteins by a cell-free system from rat liver. *Proc. nat. Acad. Sci. U.S.* **53**, 619

[52] VAZQUEZ J.J. (1961) Antibody- or gamma globulin-forming cells, as observed by the fluorescent antibody technique. *Lab. Invest.* **10**, 1110

[53] VAZQUEZ J.J. (1964) Kinetics of proliferation of antibody forming cells. In *The Thymus in Immunobiology*, ed. GOOD R.A. & GABRIELSON A.E. New York/Avanston/London: Harper & Row

[54] BALFOUR B.M., COOPER E.H. & ALPEN E.L. (1965) Morphological and kinetic studies on antibody-producing cells in rat lymph nodes. *Immunology* **8**, 230

[55] NEUMAN R.E. & McCOY Th.A. (1965). Growth-promoting properties of pyruvate,

oxalate and α-ketoglutarate for isolated Walker carcinosarcoma 256 cells. *Proc. Soc. exp. Biol. Med.* **98,** 303

[56] THORBECKE G.J. & VAN FURTH R. (1966) Ontogeny of immunoglobulin synthesis in various mammalian species. In *Ontogenetic Approaches to Immunity*, ed. SMITH R.T., MIESCHER P.A. & GOOD R.A. Gainesville, University of Florida Press (in press)

[57] PHILLIPS M.E. & THORBECKE G.J. (1966) Studies on the serum proteins of chimeras. I. Identification and study of the site of origin of donor type serum proteins in adult rat-into-mouse chimeras. *Int. Orch. Allergy* **29,** 553

CHAPTER 7

Structural and Biological Characteristics
of the Immunoglobulins

D.R.STANWORTH & GRACE I.PARDOE

Introduction

This chapter has been written with the experimental immunologist in mind. An exhaustive theoretical coverage of the subject has not been attempted, as several excellent review articles published recently fulfil this purpose [1, 2, 3, 4, 5, 6].

The aim has been to provide an outline of the principal techniques employed in the investigation of the structural and biological characteristics of the immunoglobulins. Examples have been selected to illustrate how the application of such techniques is furthering knowledge of the chemistry of these proteins, and how, in turn, this is leading to a better understanding of the mechanism of their varied biological activities.

Inevitably, the main emphasis has been placed on the most abundant and most easily isolated γG globulin type. Nevertheless, many of the techniques (sometimes with suitable modifications) used in the study of these immunoglobulins are applicable to the other immunoglobulin classes.

Section A provides a background to the subject, indicating the structural relationships obtaining between the different classes of immunoglobulins within the same species, and between the corresponding class in different species. Section B deals with the isolation and characterization of immunoglobulin sub-units. Finally, the conformation of immunoglobulins is considered in section C, which also provides examples of how structural changes influence the biological properties of the molecules.

134

SECTION A. STRUCTURAL RELATIONSHIPS BETWEEN THE IMMUNOGLOBULINS

1. Human immunoglobulin classes

Comparative gel-diffusion precipitin analyses, performed on both normal and pathological immunoglobulins and their sub-units, have led to the elucidation of the antigenic relationships obtaining between the four main classes of human immunoglobulins. The structural basis of this relationship is illustrated diagrammatically in Fig. 7.1, which is based on the Porter model [7] of the rabbit γG globulin molecule (see also Fig. 7.6), comprising two 'heavy' (H) polypeptide chains (of about 50,000 mol. wt.) and two 'light' (L) chains (of about 20,000 mol. wt.). Recent evidence that the γM globulin molecule (at least in one Waldenström macroglobulinaemic serum) probably comprises five 7S sub-units [8, 9] (see also section C1b), and that the 7S monomeric form of γA globulin tends to polymerize [10], is also taken into account.

The nomenclature for human immunoglobulins proposed by a committee set up by the World Health Organization [11] has been adopted, although the previously used symbols have been included for comparison. The recently discovered γD class [12] of immunoglobulins is also included, designated according to the new system of nomenclature. (The four classes of immunoglobulin can also be differentiated by immunoelectrophoretic analysis, as shown in Fig. 7.2.)

As indicated in Fig. 7.1, the antigenic relationships observed between the various immunoglobulin classes can be attributed to the possession of common 'light' polypeptide chains. In each immunoglobulin class, however, molecules can be recognized [13] with two different antigenic forms (κ or λ) of light chain, which have been shown recently to possess quite distinct primary structures (referred to in section B2).

A γG globulin fraction of normal human serum was found to comprise about 60 per cent of type I (now termed K) material (with κ light chain) and about 30 per cent type II (now termed L) material (with λ light chain) [14]. A similar relative distribution of types K and L molecules is assumed to obtain amongst the other normal immunoglobulin classes (i.e. γA, γM and γD) [2]. In contrast, the pathological immunoglobulins (paraproteins) found in myeloma and Waldenström macroglobulinaemia comprise molecules with only one or other of the two 'light' chain types. This applies also to the Bence-Jones proteins, which usually occur as light chain dimers (of about 40,000 mol. wt.), but which are occasionally found in the monomeric (single chain) form [15].

Certain human antibody fractions have also been found to comprise molecules of only one light chain type. For instance, every one of the Coombs-positive cold isoagglutinins isolated from the sera of six cases of haemolytic

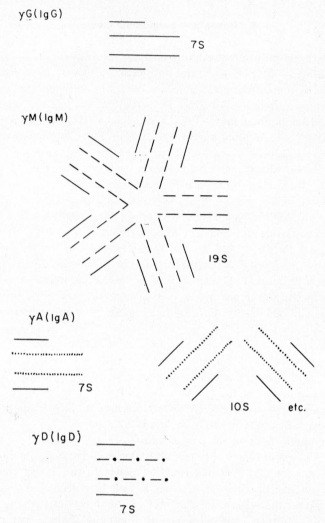

Fig. 7.1. Schematic illustration of structural relationships between the four major classes of human immunoglobulins (based on the Porter model of the γG globulin molecule). Key to heavy polypeptide chain antigenic types:

——γ; — — —μ; - - - - - - -α; ·—·—·— δ.

The light chains of each class of immunoglobulin exist in two distinctive antigenic forms, κ and λ.

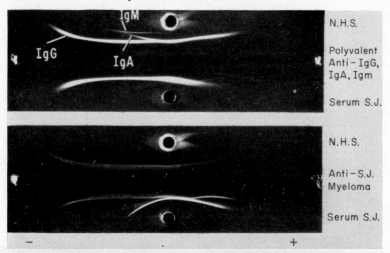

FIG. 7.2. Immunoelectrophoretic comparison of γD (IgD) myeloma protein (in serum of patient S.J.) with principal immunoglobulins (IgG, IgM and IgA) of normal human serum (NHS). (Reproduced by permission of Drs D.S.Rowe and J.L.Fahey from *J. exp. Med.* (1965), **121**, 171.)

anaemia were found to be of type K [16]. Individual 19S anti-γG globulin factors isolated from the sera of rheumatoid arthritic patients, and 7S γ globulin Rh antibodies, on the other hand, have been found to comprise both type K and type L molecules [17]. Moreover, antibody activity to thyroglobulin has been demonstrated (by radioimmunoelectrophoresis) in both

TABLE 7.1

Heavy chain sub-types of human γG globulin (abridged from Fudenberg [2])

Indicator system: primate antiserum to myeloma proteins [19]	Indicator system: rabbit antiserum to myeloma proteins [20]	Indicator system: rabbit antiserum to 'H chain' disease proteins [22]	Location of antigenic determinants on heavy chain
γ2a (11 per cent)*	Ne (heterologous)		Fc
γ2b (77 per cent)	We		Fc
γ2c (9 per cent)	Vi	Zu (20 per cent)‡	Fd
γ2d (3 per cent)	Ge†	Cr (80 per cent)‡	

* Per cent incidence of 274 γG myeloma proteins investigated by Terry and Fahey.
† There is only indirect evidence of correlation of this group with γ2d.
‡ Per cent incidence of 5 'H chain' disease paraproteins studied.

light chain types (i.e. κ and λ) of each of the three main cases of human immunoglobulins, in the sera of seven patients with chronic thyroiditis [18].

Antigenic differences in the *heavy* polypeptide chains of human γG globulins have also been detected, by means of monkey antisera raised against normal human γG globulin [19] and rabbit antisera raised against individual myeloma proteins [20] (as illustrated in Fig. 7.3). It has been shown that the γG globulin fraction of a normal individual's serum contains

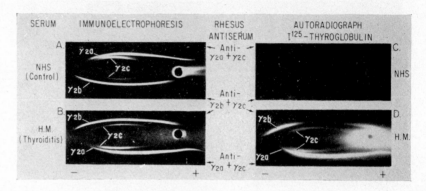

FIG. 7.3. Immunoelectrophoretic characteristics of human γ_{2a}, γ_{2b} and γ_{2c} globulin antibodies against thyroglobulin. Plates developed with rhesus monkey antiserum raised against pooled normal human γ_2G globulin.

A. Immunoelectrophoretic pattern of normal human serum (NHS).

B. Immunoelectrophoretic pattern of serum from patient with chronic thyroiditis and circulating antibodies to thyroglobulin.

C. Autoradiograph showing no non-specific binding of ^{125}I-thyroglobulin by NHS precipitin arcs.

D. Autoradiograph showing ^{125}I-thyroglobulin specifically bound by γ_{2a}, γ_{2b} and γ_{2c} globulin in thyroiditis serum.

(Reproduced by courtesy of Drs W.D.Terry & J.L.Fahey from *Science* (1964), **146**, 400.)

molecules with four different types of heavy chains (listed in Table 7.1). On the other hand, γG globulin preparations isolated from myeloma sera contain only one of the four types of heavy chain.

Human antibodies (e.g. to thyroglobulin [19, 21]) have been shown to occur in three of the different heavy chain forms (i.e. γ_{2a}, γ_{2b}, γ_{2c}) of γG globulin. As in the case of serum paraproteins, however, the urinary paraproteins (γG globulin Fc pieces) found in the urine of five cases of Franklin's ('heavy chain') disease comprise molecules of a single heavy chain type (four being of γ_{2d} type, and one of γ_{2c} type) [22].

Finer, genetically determined, antigenic differences have been revealed within both the heavy and light polypeptide chains of the various classes

TABLE 7.2

Classification of the principal immunoglobulins in various mammalian species

Species	Class of Immunoglobulin					References
	γG (7S)	γM (19S, 29S, 38S)	γA (7S, 10S, etc.)	γD (7S)	γE (γX) (8S)	
Human	γ₁ (? reagin) γ₂ (γ2a, γ2b, γ2c, γ2d)	γM	γA			18, 19, 20, 21
Mouse	γ₁ (γF)* γ2a, γ2b (γG-Be₁) (γG-Be₂)*	γM	γA			26, 27, 28, 29
Guinea pig	γ₁ γ₂	γM	γA			37, 38, 39, 40, 41
Rat	γ₁ (? mast cell sensitizing antibody) γ₂ γ2a, γ2b	γM	?γA			46, 47, 48, 452
Horse	γ₁ (10S) γ₂ γa, γb, γc	γM	γA			31, 60, 61, 62
Rabbit	γ₁ (? isologous skin-sensitizing antibody) γ₂	γM	γA (6S, 9S)			6, 32, 455

* Alternative nomenclature.

of human immunoglobulins and their sub-units (isolated from certain patho-logical urines). For instance, the Gm allotypic determinants have been located on the heavy chains within the Fc part of the human γG globulin molecule, whilst the InV determinants have been shown to be associated with the light chains (of normal and pathological human γG globulin molecules), and, presumably with the light chains of γA and γM globulin molecules showing InV activity [23, 24]. The genetic control of these allotypic specificities is considered by Dr S. Lawler in the next chapter (8). Peptide mapping of tryptic digests of γG globulins of known Gm type [25, 421, 422] has suggested that the antigenic determinants involved are probably associated with a small number of side chains on the γG globulin molecule.

2. Characteristics of the immunoglobulin classes identified in other animal species

The characterization of the human immunoglobulins, referred to in the previous section (A1), has been greatly facilitated by the ready availability of large amounts of paraproteins in myeloma and macroglobulinaemic sera. As might be expected, therefore, the lack of similar naturally occurring sources of materials in the sera of other species has impeded the characterization of their various immunoglobulin constituents. In Table 7.2, an attempt has been made to classify the immunoglobulins of those animal species, in addition to human, which have been studied in any detail (i.e. mouse, horse, rabbit, rat, guinea-pig). Their immunoelectrophoretic characteristics are shown in Fig. 7.4.

Myeloma proteins have been found in sera of mice (C3H or BALB/c) transplanted with plasma-cell tumours [26]. As in the case of paraproteins isolated from the sera of patients with multiple myeloma, the mouse myeloma proteins can be divided into two distinctive antigenic groups (of β and γ electrophoretic mobilities). Moreover, the mouse myeloma proteins in the γ group resemble human γG myeloma protein in comprising only 7S sedimenting material, whereas the β group shows multiple sedimenting components (e.g. 7S, 9S, 11S and 13S) [27], as do the serum globulins comprising the most common sedimenting class of *human* γA myeloma proteins (shown in Fig. 4.1d). Subsequent, more extensive, studies [28] have led to the detection of four major classes of mouse immunoglobulins, namely γ_2 and γ_1 (7S) globulins, γA globulin and γM globulin (differentiated by their distinctive electrophoretic mobilities and by their specific antigenic determinants, as illustrated by the immunoelectrophoresis pattern in Fig. 7.4a). Radioimmunoelectrophoretic analysis of mouse antiserum raised against haemocyanin indicated that all four immunoglobulin classes possess antibody activity.

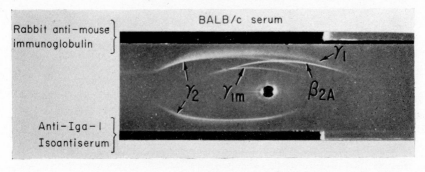

(a)

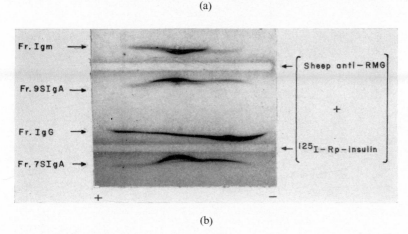

(b)

Fig. 7.4. Immunoelectrophoretic characteristics of the principal immunoglobulins of various mammalian species.

(a) Immunoelectrophoresis of serum from hyperimmunized BALB/c mice. A 'polyvalent' rabbit anti-mouse immunoglobulin antiserum (in top trough) revealed four mouse immunoglobulin classes: γ_1 (i.e. γ_1G), γ_2 (i.e. γ_2G), γ_1M (i.e. γM) and β_2A (i.e. γA). Iso-antiserum anti-Iga-1 (in the bottom trough) identified the Iga-isoantigen on γ_2 (i.e. γ_2G) globulin.

(Reproduced by courtesy of Drs J.L.Fahey, J.Wunderlich and R.Mishell from *J. exp. Med.* (1964), **120**, 223.)

(b) Rabbit immunoglobulins IgM (i.e. γM), 9S and 7S IgA (i.e. γA) and IgG (i.e. γG) demonstrated in Sephadex G200 fractions of purified antibody against the p-azo-phenylarsonate group (Rp) demonstrated by radioimmunoelectrophoresis. After electrophoresis of each fraction in agar on a slide, a mixture of sheep antiserum against whole macroglobulin fraction of normal rabbit serum (labelled sheep anti-RMG) and ^{125}I-Rp-insulin (2 μg/ml sheep antiserum) was diffused overnight. Protein concentrations of the antibody fractions applied in the wells were: IgM fraction, 4·7 mg/ml. IgA fractions: 9S, 4·3 mg/ml; 7S, 3·4 mg/ml. IgG fraction, 5·0 mg/ml.

(Reproduced by courtesy of Drs K.Onoue, Y.Yagi and D.Pressman from *J. exp. Med.* (1966), **123**, 123.)

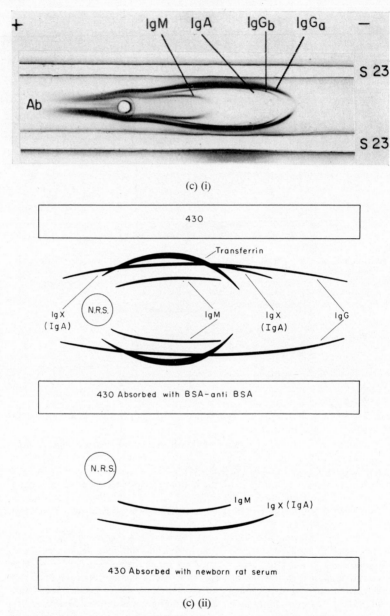

(c) (i)

(c) (ii)

Fig. 7.4. (c) (i) Immunoelectrophoretic pattern of whole purified rat anti-DNP antibody ('Ab') developed with rabbit antiserum ('S23').

(Reproduced by courtesy of Drs R. A. Binaghi and E.S.de Merle from *Int. Arch. All.* (1966), **30,** 589.)

Fig. 7.4. (c) (ii) Immunoelectrophoretic analysis of normal rat serum (NRS) against rabbit–anti-rat serum ('430'). Recent investigations [452] suggest that the IgX component is analogous to the IgA component of human serum.

(Reproduced by courtesy of Drs B.G.Arnason, C.de Vaux St. Cyr and P.Grabar from *Nature, Lond.* (1963), **199,** 1199.)

As with human γG globulins, heavy chain sub-classes (γ_{2a} and γ_{2b}) of the mouse 7S γ_2 component have been identified by means of appropriate heterologous antisera [29]. Furthermore, both of these γ globulins, which are of similar electrophoretic mobility, have been shown to possess antibody activity

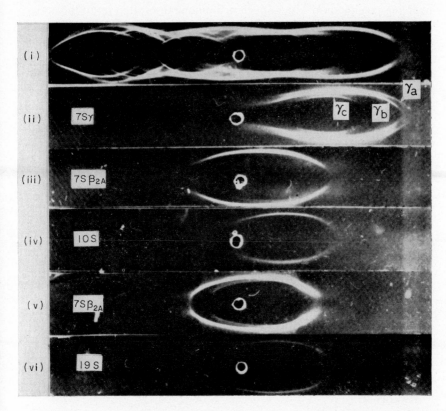

FIG. 7.4. (d) Immunoelectrophoresis of equine serum and purified anti-β lactoside (Lac) antibody, developed with rabbit antiserum against normal equine serum. Samples analysed: (i) normal equine serum; (ii) γG globulin anti-Lac antibodies; (iii) 7S γA globulin anti-Lac antibody; (iv) isolated 10S γ_1 globulin anti-Lac antibody; (v) anti-Lac antibody preparation; (vi) 19S component isolated from purified equine anti-Lac antibody.

(Reproduced by permission of Drs J.H.Rockey, N.R.Klinman and F.Karush from *J. exp. Med.* (1964), **120**, 589.)

(in an antiserum raised against haemocyanin), whereas a genetically controlled isoantigenic determinant (Iga-1) was found to be confined to the γ_{2a} subgroup, and absent from γ_{2b} molecules (in a study of the corresponding mouse myeloma proteins).

Most of the studies on the immunoglobulins of other species have been carried out on *antibody* γ globulin, isolated from sera in which the antibody level has been enhanced by deliberate antigenic stimulation. In this approach, it is usual to obtain an antibody-rich fraction by an initial isolation step involving precipitation with antigen or immunoabsorption on to the antigen coupled (specifically or non-specifically) to a suitable carrier (as described in Chapter 5). Final purification of the recovered antibody (and subfractionation into the different immunoglobulin classes) is then achieved by various physico-chemical procedures such as gel filtration, ion-exchange chromatography or zone-centrifugation. Some antibody γ globulin fractions such as the

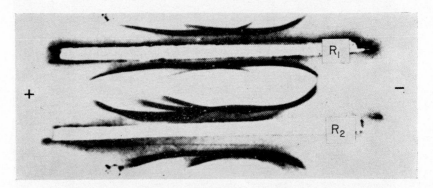

Fig. 7.4. (e) Immunoelectrophoretic patterns of guinea-pig anti-2,4-dinitrophenyl bovine γ globulin antibody (top and bottom) and of guinea-pig anti-pipsyl guinea-pig albumin (centre), developed with rabbit antisera ('R₁' and 'R₂') raised against pooled guinea-pig serum. Both antisera reveal two main precipitin arcs in the guinea-pig antibody preparations with different electrophoretic mobilities corresponding to the γ_1 and γ_2 forms. (In addition, rabbit antiserum R_2 reveals, in the pipsyl antibody preparation only, an additional precipitin line, not clearly demonstrated by rabbit antiserum R_1.)

(Reproduced by courtesy of Drs G.J.Thorbecke, B.Benacerraf and Z.Ovary from *J. Immunol.* (1963), **91**, 670.)

high molecular weight (γM) globulin antibodies produced in horses, cows and pigs in response to immunization with pneumococcal organisms (or their capsular polysaccharides [30]) are readily obtained in high yield by this procedure. In a recent investigation [31], for example, the bulk (82 per cent) of a composite horse antibody fraction (against pneumococcus type I organisms) isolated in this way, comprised γM antibodies, while the remainder contained γG and γA antibodies (which were subfractionated by gel filtration followed by DEAE cellulose chromatography). Similarly, γG globulin antibodies are readily obtained when rabbits are immunized by a whole range of commonly used antigens. On the other hand, the isolation of other classes of immunoglobulin antibodies, produced at appreciably lower serum levels following immunization, presents a much greater technical challenge. For instance, the isolation of the γM globulin components from rabbit and rat antisera involves the use of multi-stage fractionation procedures, resulting in low yields of purified immunoglobulins. Similar difficulties hamper the isolation of rabbit γA globulin, which is found at extremely low serum levels (e.g. 13 μg/ml of pooled antiserum [32]), even after prolonged immunization. Onoue *et al* [32] estimated that their yield of 7S γA antibody from 3 litres of starting rabbit antiserum (raised against the p-azophenyl arsonate group) amounted to only about 15 mg.

Until the problem of isolation of the relatively minor immunoglobulin components from the various animal species has been resolved, it is not possible to obtain unequivocal evidence about their structural relationships (by application of similar procedures to those outlined in section B, which have revealed the relationships between the human immunoglobulins illustrated in Fig. 7.1). Present knowledge about the properties of the immunoglobulins of other species is therefore based largely on comparative gel-diffusion precipitin analyses or immunoelectrophoresis (in which the precipitin arcs are revealed either by means of an antiserum raised in a different species, or by the use of radioisotopically labelled antigen [33]). The immunoelectrophoretic characteristics of species which have already been studied in some detail, shown in Fig. 7.4, should be compared with the immunoelectrophoretic patterns of the principal human immunoglobulins (γG, γM, γA, γD) shown in Fig. 7.2.

As already mentioned, an attempt has been made (in Table 7.2) to classify the immunoglobulins so far identified in the various species according to their distinctive antigenic, electrophoretic and biological (e.g. skin-sensitizing activity) properties. As will be seen, a consistent immunoglobulin pattern is beginning to emerge, and it seems possible that, as in the case of the human immunoglobulins, the antigenic relationships between the main immunoglobulin classes (i.e. γG, γA, γM, etc.) of other animal species will be attributable, at least in part, to the possession of common antigenic determinants within their Fab portions.

In contrast, however, to the main classes of *human* immunoglobulin, where structural relationships have been shown to be confined to the light polypeptide chains, evidence has been obtained (from allotype studies [34]) to indicate that *rabbit* γG and γM globulins possess common determinants on the Fd portion of their *heavy* polypeptide chains (see Fig. 7.6 for an explanation of the nomenclature). Furthermore, similarities in certain biological activities (e.g. placental transmission [35, 305], skin reactivity [36]) shown by rabbit γG and γM globulins suggest structural similarities within the *Fc* regions of their heavy chains too (as will be further described in section B).

Finer antigenic differences have been detected in the heavy chains of the γG globulin molecules of species other than human and mouse. These γG globulin sub-groups (listed in Table 7.2), which are distinct from the other major classes of γ globulin (γM, γA, etc.) and from the light chain sub-groups (types K and L), have similar or closely related immunoelectrophoretic mobilities (as indicated in Figs. 7.2 and 7.4). It is of interest that such heavy chain sub-classes appear to be associated with the electrophoretically 'slower' ('γ_2') of the two main distinguishable forms of non-human γG globulin. Nevertheless, as already mentioned with reference to mouse γ globulins [28], a faster migrating form ('γ_1') of γG globulin has been detected in several species. In the mouse, this γ_1 form has been shown to possess specific antigenic determinants which distinguish it from the two sub-classes [29] (γ_{2a}, γ_{2b}) of the electrophoretically slower (γ_2) form. Similarly, two antigenically and electrophoretically distinguishable forms (γ_1 and γ_2) of γG globulin have been identified [37] in guinea-pig antibody fractions from antisera raised against protein antigens (e.g. ovalbumin [38], insulin [39]) or hapten groups [40] (e.g. 2,4-dinitrophenyl). These two forms of specifically purified antibodies showed a double arc on immunoelectrophoresis, not observed with the whole γG globulin. This effect has been explained by the findings from papain digestion studies [41] (see section B), which indicated that the two antibody γG globulin forms possess common antigenic determinants in their Fab portions, but distinctive determinants in their Fc portions. Such structural differences are responsible for the quite distinctive biological properties shown by the two forms (γ_1 and γ_2) of guinea-pig γG globulin (and by the corresponding forms found within the γG globulins of other species such as mouse). Thus, the γ_1 form of guinea-pig γG globulin elicits skin reactions (of the P-K type) in other animals of the same species, and sensitizes chopped guinea-pig lung for antigen-induced histamine release [40], whereas the γ_2 form is only capable of evoking skin reactions (of the PCA type) in *heterologous* skin [42]. This latter (i.e. γ_2) form inhibits skin reactions produced by the γ_1 form (in homologous animals) [40]. Moreover, of the two forms, the γ_2 is unique in fixing complement, participating in immune lytic reactions [40], mediating Arthus reactions [43] and selectively binding to macrophages [43] (to which, as in heterologous skin sensitization, it becomes attached through its Fc portion).

γG antibodies of other mammalian species (e.g. man, rhesus monkey, dog and mouse) [44] which have the ability to evoke PCA reactions in guinea-pigs have also proved to be of the electrophoretically slower (γ_2) class, none of them being able to elicit homologous skin reactions. γ_2G antibodies of other species (e.g. cow, horse, sheep [45]) lack the structure (presumably within the Fc portions) necessary for binding to guinea-pig tissues.

It is tempting to generalize, and to speculate that the homologous skin-sensitizing antibodies found in the antisera of other species will also prove to be a γ_1 form of γG globulin. In addition to the naturally occurring skin-sensitizing antibodies (reagins) found in the sera of hypersensitive humans, similar types of (isologous) tissue-sensitizing antibodies have been detected in the sera of rats [46, 47, 48] (immunized with a variety of antigens injected together with *Bordetella pertussis* organisms or complete Freund's adjuvant) and of dogs [49, 50] which have acquired a spontaneous hypersensitivity to ragweed pollen. The activity of these antibodies is found in the fast γ globulin region on electrophoresis of the sera from hypersensitized animals. Moreover, the rat and dog antibodies possess the characteristics of human reagins, for instance, heat lability (when subjected to 56° C for 30 minutes), persistence at the site of passive transfer for relatively long periods (e.g. 18hr) and sedimentation in the ultracentrifuge at a rate of about 8S.

The difficulty in isolating sufficient amounts of such antibodies for direct characterization (by the procedures outlined in section B) has led to the application of correlative procedures (where the distribution of reaginic activity is compared with that of readily characterized immunoglobulins) and indirect procedures (such as the study of the effect of removing selected immunoglobulins from hypersensitive sera by absorption with specific antisera). As a result of the application of such methods, some investigators [51, 52, 53] claimed that human reagin was an immunoglobulin of the γA class, but the lack of correlation between P-K activity and γA globulin distribution in human allergic serum [54] suggested otherwise (see also Chapter 35). Ishizaka [55] has recently obtained data to suggest that reagin is not a γA type of globulin. Instead, he has postulated (possibly prematurely) that it represents a new class of immunoglobulin (which he has designated 'E').* Further evidence is required, however, to exclude the possibility that, as in the other animal species mentioned, human isologous skin-sensitizing antibodies are an electrophoretically fast (γ_1) sub-class of γG globulins. Such an analogy with guinea-pig γ_1G globulins would imply that human reagins become attached to passively sensitized human skin through their Fc portions, a fundamental question which has yet to be answered by more direct experimentation.

In this connection, the biological properties and antigenic relationships recently attributed to various rabbit immunoglobulins [32, 56] are of possible relevance. As in the case of mice and guinea-pigs, the production of isologous skin-sensitizing antibodies (in P-K type tests) has been demonstrated in the sera of a small proportion of rabbits, following immunization with the hapten group, p-azo-phenyl arsonate, coupled to bovine γ globulin. It has been claimed [32], however, that such activity is associated with a minor, 7S γA, immunoglobulin antibody component (found at levels of about 13 μg antibody/ml of selected pooled serum), but not with a 9S form of γA globulin present in the antiserum at comparable concentration levels. The γG globulin component of the rabbit antisera, on the other hand, was shown to

---

* Bennick & Johansson (*Immunology*. In Press) have recently discovered a myeloma counterpart of this immunoglobulin (designated, initially, "IgX").

F

mediate PCA reactions in heterologous (guinea-pig) skin (in keeping with the behaviour of the γ_2 sub-type of the γG globulin of other species such as mouse and guinea-pig). As, however, the identification of the supposed γA globulin component in the rabbit antisera (of which only a few contained significant amounts of this antibody) was not altogether convincing, it is still possible that the P-K type activity (observed in passively sensitized rabbits) is associated with an antigenically and electrophoretically distinctive γ_1 sub-type of rabbit γG globulin (by analogy with the known behaviour of the γ_1 sub-types of the γG antibodies produced in guinea-pig and mice sera).* Hence, further investigations of the rabbit immunoglobulin system will be awaited with much interest, as these can be expected to throw further light on the relationship between the structure and function of the various immunoglobulin classes in general.

Sela & Mozes [57] have separated electrophoretically fast ('γ_1') and slow ('γ_2') forms of γG globulin from rabbit antisera (raised against synthetic polypeptides and native protein antigens) by chromatography on DEAE-Sephadex A50 (using 0·02 M potassium phosphate buffer, pH 8·0, with a salt gradient up to 0·3 M phosphate). The difference in behaviour of the two forms is attributed to their possession of distinctive Fab fragments combined with a common Fc fragment (i.e. designated by the older terminology as 'I III I' and 'II III II'). Antibodies directed against acidic determinants were found predominantly in the first (electrophoretically slow) chromatographic fraction, whereas those directed against basic determinants were eluted mainly in the second (electrophoretically fast) fraction. Evidence has been obtained [58] for the existence of corresponding types of γG globulin in fractions isolated from *human* sera, showing interesting conformational differences (as will be described in section B). Neither the rabbit nor the human forms has been differentiated antigenically, however. For instance, testing with horse anti-rabbit γG globulin serum has failed to distinguish antigenic differences between γ_1 and γ_2 forms of rabbit γG globulin, separated by ion-exchange chromatography [59]. Similarly prepared fractions of human serum were indistinguishable on gel-diffusion testing with rabbit or monkey anti-human γG globulin antisera [58].

Other recently discovered types of immunoglobulin include the human 7S γD globulin [12] (illustrated in Fig. 7.1) and the horse 10S γ_1 globulin [60]. Antibody activity has yet to be shown associated with the former, but the latter was demonstrated (by equilibrium dialysis) to possess specific hapten-binding activity. The horse 10S γ_1 globulin was identified, together with five other antigenically distinct immunoglobulins (γA, γM and three antigenically distinct γG globulins) in horse antiserum directed against p-azo-phenyl-β-lactoside (lac.). These were separated from antigen by DEAE-cellulose

* This is suggested by recent findings of Zvaifler & Becker [455].

chromatography and zone electrophoresis (in solvents containing lactose), following specific precipitation with lac-human serum albumin and lac-haemocyanin complexes. The three horse γG globulins have been classified as γ_2 globulins in Table 7.2, on the basis of their relatively slow electrophoretic mobility (as shown in Fig. 7.4). A highly purified preparation of the horse antibody γ globulin (isolated by a combined rivanol, ammonium sulphate precipitation and zone-electrophoresis separation procedure), often referred to as 'T component', has been shown [61] (by amino-acid analysis) to be more closely related to horse γG globulin than to γA globulin. In other studies [62] on horses immunized with diphtheria toxin or with human γ_2 globulin, antibodies of the T component (or γ_1) type were found to be produced at a later stage in the immune response than antibodies of the γ_2 globulin type. Moreover, the former gave a flocculation curve on optimal proportion titration, whereas the latter showed a typical precipitin curve.

It can be expected that many of the gaps in the immunoglobulin classification shown in Table 7.2 will be filled from the results of future investigations with refined techniques. In this connection, it is interesting to note that *mouse* γA globulin has been observed to produce dual precipitin arcs on immunoelectrophoresis [28, 63], possibly reflecting the existence of γA heavy chain (i.e. α chain) sub-groups* analogous to the $\gamma_2 G$ heavy chain (i.e. γ chain) sub-groups already identified in this (and other) species. It is possible that similar dual precipitin arcs associated with human γM globulins represent a subdivision of the γM heavy chain (i.e. μ chain), but a simpler explanation attributes such effects to the existence of polymeric forms of human γM globulin (i.e. 29S and 38S) in the preparations tested [64].

As in the study of human immunoglobulins mentioned in the previous section (A1), the delineation of allotypic specificities by use of *iso-antisera* is clarifying fine structural relationships between the polypeptide chains of several other species (notably rabbit and mouse). The results of such investigations point to a different form of heavy and light chain structure in rabbit γG globulin, from that assigned to the corresponding class of human immunoglobulin (depicted in Fig. 7.1). In fact, this type of immunogenetic approach has led to the suggestion that the rabbit γG globulin molecule might be composed of three (instead of two) pairs of polypeptide chains (i.e. two pairs of heavy chains and one pair of light chains) [1].

Similarities in structure between the corresponding immunoglobulin classes of the species represented in Table 7.2 have been inferred by their vertical alignment in the construction of the table. Apart from the γG globulins, however, there is no direct evidence of such interspecies relationships (owing to the problems of isolation of sufficient of the other classes of

* Evidence for the existence of two such human γA globulin subclasses has been reported recently from several laboratories [444, 445, 446].

immunoglobulins from species other than human and mouse, as already discussed). Investigations of the cross-reactivity between the γG globulins (total) of a range of species (human, rhesus monkey, baboon, ox, horse, sheep, rat and chicken) have provided evidence that the species specific antigenic determinants of the γG globulin homologues are mainly located on the Fc portions of their molecules. This finding is based on quantitative precipitin estimations [65], using rabbit anti-human γG globulin (and anti-Fab and anti-Fc antisera), and also rheumatoid arthritic sera (containing rheumatoid factor, i.e. human anti-human γG globulin). In cross-reactivity studies employing the latter 'antiserum', the various γG globulin homologues were tested in soluble heat-aggregated form [65], or in the form of insoluble bis-diazotized benzidine-linked γG globulin complexes coated on to human erythrocytes [66]. As will be indicated in section C, conformational studies suggest that such treatments expose antigenic determinants which are normally masked by the folding of the polypeptide chains in the native molecules.

It will be interesting to establish whether the other classes of immunoglobulin (e.g. γM and γA globulin) show similar interspecies cross-reactivities. The results of such investigations should help to elucidate the role of antibodies of these types in immune responses. Furthermore, it will be important to establish whether the physico-chemical properties (e.g. electrical charge) of such antibodies are influenced by the characteristics of the antigen, as appears to be the case in the production of antibodies of the γG type (in rabbits) [57]. Recent data of the Sela group [67] indicate a similar correlation between the electrophoretic mobility of purified antibodies of the γM globulin class and the net electrical charge of the antigen.

SECTION B. CHARACTERIZATION OF IMMUNOGLOBULIN SUB-UNITS

1. Methods of production and isolation

(a) Proteolytic cleavage
The now classical experiments of Porter [68] involving the papain digestion of rabbit γG globulin have provided a basis for subsequent work on the isolation and characterization of immunoglobulin sub-units.

In his initial digestion studies, Porter incubated rabbit γG globulin (150 mg) (isolated by diethylamino-ethyl-(DEAE-) cellulose chromatography, or sodium sulphate precipitation) with mercuripapain (1·5 mg) in 0·1 M phosphate buffer pH 7·0, containing 0·01 M cysteine and 0·002 M ethylene-diamine-tetra-acetate disodium salt (EDTA) to activate the enzyme. After incubation at 37° C for 16 hours, the solution was dialysed against several changes of water, with vigorous stirring, over a period of 48 hours (to remove the cysteine and EDTA, and thereby facilitate oxidation and inactivation of the enzyme).

The non-dialysable digestion products were either lyophilized or fractionated directly by ion-exchange chromatography after dialysis against acetate buffer, pH 5·5. Column fractionation on carboxymethyl- (CM-) cellulose (as shown in Fig. 7.5) separated the digest into three major peaks (I, II and III),

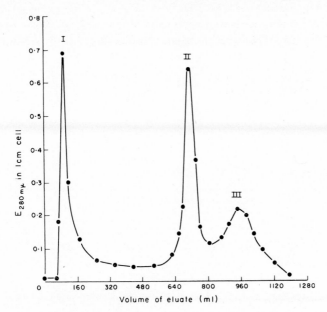

Fig. 7.5. Chromatography of papain-digest of rabbit γG globulin on carboxy-methylcellulose. Weight of digest 150 mg. Column $20 \times 2 \cdot 4$ cm. Volume of mixing chamber 1200 ml. Gradient from 0·1 M sodium acetate, pH 5·5 to 0·9 M sodium acetate, pH 5·5, commencing at 200 ml eluate volume.
(Reproduced by courtesy of Prof R.R.Porter, f.r.s., from *Biochem. J.* (1959), **73**, 119.)

comprising fragments which together constituted 90 per cent of the total original γG globulin molecule. Fragments I and II (now termed Fab fragments) proved to be of extremely similar chemical composition and molecular weight (50,000–55,000), and each retained the power to combine (but not form precipitate) with antigen when the digested γG globulin contained antibodies. The third fragment, III (now termed Fc) had a larger molecular weight (about 80,000), crystallized readily (hence the use of the postscript 'c' in the terminology) and possessed much of the antigenicity of the original molecule. As will be indicated in section B3b, subsequent studies have demonstrated that many different biological activities are associated with this portion of the molecule.

On the basis of these findings, Porter [68] concluded that the rabbit γG globulin molecule is comprised of two pieces (Fab) with very similar structure, containing the antibody receptor sites, joined to a third piece (Fc) of quite different character. This supposition has since been fully substantiated, whilst reductive cleavage studies (by the methods outlined later in this section) have led to the formulation of the now familiar polypeptide chain structure for rabbit (and human) γG globulin depicted in diagrammatic form in Fig. 7.6, which shows the W.H.O. recommended terminology for the sub-units [11].

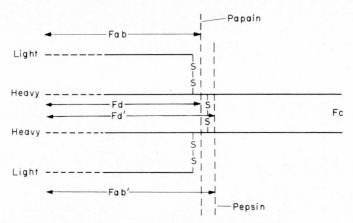

Fig. 7.6. Schematic representation of γG globulin structure (based on the original Porter model) showing the supposed sites of papain and pepsin cleavage. (The broken lines indicate regions of marked variability in primary amino acid sequence.)

The γG globulins of other species, such as human and mouse, have been similarly split by papain digestion into pieces of approximately one-third the size of the original molecules. As in the case of the rabbit γG globulin digestion products, antigen-binding activity was found to be associated with the type of fragment (electrophoretically 'slow') isolated in greater yield (i.e. twice the amount of the other, electrophoretically 'fast', fragment [69]).

Edelman *et al* [70] used immunoelectrophoresis to demonstrate antigenic differences between the electrophoretically slow and fast fragments obtained by papain digestion of human γG globulin (Cohn fraction II) preparations. As will be indicated later (see Fig. 7.15b, for example), this technique has proved invaluable in following the course of γ globulin proteolysis. The papain digestion fragments of *human* γG globulin were found to possess different chromatographic properties from those shown by rabbit γG globulin fragments, and hence were not similarly separable by a single-stage fractionation on carboxymethyl-cellulose [71]. Franklin [72], however, succeeded in obtaining relatively pure preparations of human γG globulin fragments by a two-stage chromatographic procedure involving sub-fractionation of the carboxymethyl-cellulose chromatographic fractions on diethylaminoethyl-cellulose (as shown in Fig. 7.7). Two of the three major 3·5S fragments

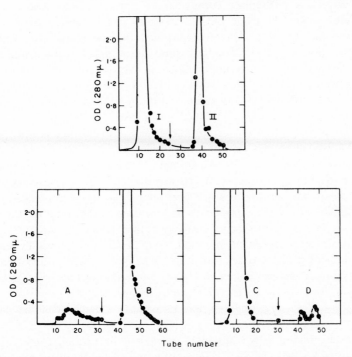

FIG. 7.7 Chromatographic patterns of papain digest of human γG globulin. Top: first step on CM-cellulose (0·01 M phosphate buffer, pH 7·6). The arrow indicates the start of NaCl gradient (up to 0·4 M). Bottom: rechromatography of peak I (left) and peak II (right) on DEAE-cellulose (0·01 M phosphate buffer, pH 8·0). The arrow indicates the start of NaCl gradient (up to 0·3 M). Fraction B is equivalent to Fc, and fractions A and C to Fab.

(Reproduced by permission of Dr E.C.Franklin from *J. Clin. Invest.* (1960), **39**, 1933.)

(originally termed 'A' and 'C') thus separated were shown to be closely related antigenically, although differing in electrophoretic mobility, whilst the third fragment (originally termed 'B') possessed distinctive antigenic properties. As indicated by Fig. 7.6, the former (electrophoretically slow) A and C fragments are now referred to as Fab, and the latter (electrophoretically fast) B fragment as Fc. The antigenic relationship between these fragments of human γG globulin and other human immunoglobulins (γM and γA) were determined by gel-diffusion precipitin analysis [73]. Rowe [442, 450] used ammonium sulphate at 60 per cent saturation to isolate the slow (Fab) component from a papain digest of pooled human γG globulin.

An alternative method of separating the fragments has involved zone-electrophoresis of papain digests of γG globulin in slabs of potato starch [74]. Alternatively, a particulate copolymer of polyvinyl acetate and chloride (marketed under the trade name 'Pevikon') can be employed as electrophoresis medium [75]. This material has the advantage that separated fractions may also be analysed for carbohydrate content without interference by contamination with the support medium. Moreover, it does not cause the electro-osmotic cathodal flow which limits the use of other polyvinyl resins such as polyvinyl chloride. Measurement of the protein eluted from segments (e.g. 1 cm), by means of a modified Folin assay [76], provides the type of electrophoretic pattern of normal human γG globulin digests illustrated in Fig. 7.8. As might be expected from the immunoelectrophoresis pattern shown by papain digests of γG globulin, a certain degree of overlapping of the Fab and Fc zones occurs. Consequently, it has been customary to carry out a preliminary testing of small portions of the electrophoretic fractions, using antiserum directed specifically against each type of fragment, to ensure that only homologous fractions are combined (prior to concentration by ultrafiltration). A convenient and rapid sampling can be achieved by removing serial sections from the edge of the starch block by means of a cork borer [77]. These samples are then eluted with a drop of saline and tested by micro-gel-diffusion precipitin analysis. Having thus mapped out the extent of overlap, the regions of starch containing pure Fab and Fc fragments can be eluted *en bloc*.

A faster-moving 2·1S component, related antigenically to the Fc piece, and termed F'c [98] or Fc' [271] has also been isolated by this procedure [85]. This fragment, which has also been identified in concentrated normal urine [271], occurs only at low concentrations in cysteine-activated papain digests of human γG globulins (comprising about 10 per cent of the intact molecules) and needs special antisera for its detection (by immunoelectrophoresis, as in Fig. 7.14). It can also be separated [85] from the fast-migrating sub-components of the Fc fragment (shown in Fig. 7.24), and from undigested γG globulin, by a combined chromatographic procedure involving elution from CM-cellulose by acetate buffer (0·01 M, pH 5·4) followed by re-chromatography on DEAE-cellulose in phosphate buffer (0·05 M, pH 7·8). The Fc' fragment is eluted in the 'tail portion' of the three peaks thus obtained. Alternatively, it has been separated from Fab and Fc fragments by gel filtration on Sephadex G150, but the product thus obtained is contaminated by free light chains [261]. Zone-electrophoresis (in starch or 'Pevikon') blocks would seem therefore to offer the best method of obtaining a pure preparation of the Fc′ fragment.

Greater resolution of the Fab and Fc pieces has been achieved by selecting myeloma γG globulins of slow electrophoretic mobility for papain digestion [74] (see Fig. 7.8). As will be described later, it has also proved advantageous

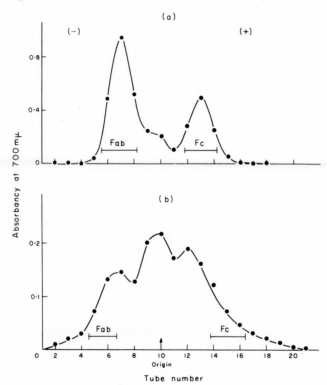

FIG. 7.8. Separation of Fab and Fc fragments from papain digests of human γG globulin by zone electrophoresis in starch.

(a) Digest (1 hour) of γG myeloma protein.

(b) Digest (5 minutes) of normal γG globulin.

Absorbancy at 700 mμ determined by Folin reaction.

(Reproduced by courtesy of Drs M.Fougereau and G.M.Edelman from *J. exp. Med.* (1965), **121**, 373.)

first to remove the undigested γG globulin and low molecular weight peptides by gel filtration on Sephadex G100 [58].

Further light has been thrown on the mechanism of papain hydrolysis of rabbit γG globulin by digestion studies using pepsin at pH 4·5 [78]. Proteolysis is achieved by incubation (at 37° C for 18 hours) of the protein (in

F*

0·07 M acetate buffer, pH 4·5–5·0, containing 0·05 M NaCl) with crystalline enzyme (at an enzyme–substrate ratio of 1/100). After digestion, the enzyme is inactivated by adjusting the pH of the reaction mixture to 8·0 and dialysing against cold borate-buffered saline (pH 8·0, I = 0·16). In addition to small peptides, this treatment produced a 5·25S fragment (of 106,000 mol. wt.), now termed F(ab')$_2$, which retains antigen-precipitating activity (when antibody, such as rabbit antiovalbumin, is used as starting γG globulin). Subsequent reduction of this material with cysteine (0·01 M) or 2-mercaptoethylamine (0·01 M) at pH 8·0, produces non-precipitating ('univalent') 3·5S antibody fragments (Fab') possessing very similar properties to the Fab fragments obtained by *papain* digestion in the presence of cysteine [79, 80]. As a result of further investigations [81], it was inferred that the two 3·5S Fab fragments of rabbit antibody γG globulin (each containing an antigen-combining site) are linked by a single labile disulphide bond (as shown in Fig. 7.6), which is ruptured by the cysteine employed to activate the proteolytic enzyme. Pepsin digestion in the absence of reducing agent, on the other hand, leaves this disulphide bond intact, but appears to degrade that part of the molecule corresponding to the Fc piece.

Further evidence suggesting that the two Fab portions of the rabbit γG globulin molecule are linked by a disulphide bond has been obtained by employing a two-stage cleavage process, in which hydrolysis by *water-insoluble* papain (papain coupled to a copolymer of p-amino-phenylalanine and leucine) which has been washed free from thiol, was followed by reduction with cysteine (0·01 M) [82]. The limited cleavage of 3–5 peptide bonds per molecule (achieved after 5 minutes' enzymatic digestion) proved sufficient to render the γG globulin molecule susceptible to subsequent reduction by cysteine, to give three pieces having properties similar to those obtained by digestion with cysteine-activated soluble papain in the usual way.

Jaquet & Cebra [83] have isolated a pure preparation of fragment I dimer (i.e. the Fab dimer, F(ab)$_2$ by the consecutive action of insoluble papain and dodecyl sulphate (0·5 per cent) on rabbit γG globulin (isolated from rabbit antiovalbumin antiserum by ammonium sulphate precipitation, followed by DEAE-cellulose chromatography). As in the case of the 5S fragment obtained by pepsin digestion [78], the insoluble-papain digestion product (now termed Fab dimer) precipitated with specific antigen, but lacked antigenic determinants characteristic of the Fc pieces. The Fab dimer was, however, found to have a smaller molecular weight (84,000) than the highly purified pepsin fragment (of 90,000 mol. wt.). This suggests that the sites of cleavage by papain and pepsin are different, as is indicated by the results of other recent investigations by Utsumi & Karush [84] (and as is illustrated diagrammatically in Figs. 7.6 and 7.10). Such a difference is further manifested by the contrasting ease of reoxidation of the two enzymatic digestion products following reduction [83]. Thus, the 5S pepsin fragment is readily reoxidized, whereas there is almost no tendency for the "univalent" 3·5S moieties of the papain Fab dimer to recombine.

In their more detailed study, Utsumi & Karush [84] employed gel filtration (Sephadex G75) to separate the fragments produced by peptic digestion of rabbit γG globulin. Solutions of the protein (1–2 per cent w/v) in 0·2 M acetate

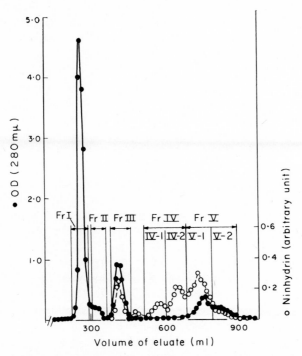

FIG. 7.9. Gel filtration (on Sephadex G75) of peptic digest of γG globulin. A sample (150 mg) of a 20 hour digest was passed through two columns (54 × 3 cm) in tandem at room temperature. Solvent: 0·2 M NaCl–0·01 M sodium phosphate buffer (pH 8·2) containing 0·002 M EDTA.

(Reproduced by courtesy of Drs S.Utsumi and F.Karush from *Biochemistry* (1965), **4**, 1766.)

buffer (pH 4·5) were incubated at 37° C for varying times (4–96 hours) with twice-crystallized pepsin (enzyme/substrate concentration 1/100 to 2/100). The type of pattern obtained by filtration of a 20 hour digest is shown in Fig. 7.9. Ninhydrin scanning revealed peptides (e.g. fraction IV) deficient in aromatic amino acids, and so not detected by scanning the eluates for absorbance at 280 mμ. The fractions isolated from the peptic digests possessed the following characteristics. Fraction I comprised only the fragment designated

'Pep-I' (60±2 per cent of the total protein), which was shown to be anti-genically identical to papain fragment I (Fab piece), but of slightly higher molecular weight 92,000/2 (compared with 40,700 for the Fab piece) and richer in carbohydrate. Fraction II (obtained in 2 per cent yield) was eluted from the column in the same position as pepsin, and contained mainly 3S fragments of similar antigenicity to papain fragments I (Fab) and III (Fc). (The amount of this fraction recovered varied considerably, depending on the time of digestion.) Fraction III comprised a fragment designated 'Pep-III''. This migrated as a single 2·4S peak in the ultracentrifuge and could be crystallized from dilute neutral buffer at 4° C (even at protein concentrations of 0·5 per cent), to give quadrilateral-shaped crystals closely resembling those shown by papain fragment III (Fc). (Goodman [284] obtained a fragment of similar properties by peptic digestion of papain fragment III of rabbit γG globulin.) The Pep-III' fragment was shown, however, to be of 27,000 mol. wt. (compared with Fc piece, 50,000 mol. wt.), to lack interchain disulphide bonds, to lack the carbohydrate found in the papain digestion Fc fragment, and to possess some *but not all* of its antigenic determinants. Fraction IV, comprising a third fragment ('Pep-IV') peculiar to peptic digestion of rabbit γG globulin, was recognizable only by the ninhydrin reaction. It contained a second carbohydrate moiety (comprising all of the fucose, and 70 per cent of the hexose and hexosamine, of the total γG globulin), which appeared to be identical with that found in papain fragment III (Fc). It seems probable that its immunogenic inactivity, as revealed by its failure to react with antiserum against rabbit γG globulin heavy chain, is connected with its lack of tyrosine (see section B3a). The final fraction ('V') eluted from the Sephadex G75 column was shown to comprise peptides (<5000 mol. wt.) which were shown to be antigenically active by their capacity to inhibit the precipitation of papain fragment III (Fc) by goat entiserum directed against rabbit γG globulin heavy chain, which had been absorbed with the peptic digestion fragment Pep-III'.

From such observations, and the results of other studies employing varying digestion times, it was concluded that pepsin initially splits rabbit γG globulin into two major fragments, Pep-I (i.e. the 5S F(ab')$_2$ referred to earlier) and a 3·5S fragment designated Pep-III, which is antigenically indistinguishable from papain fragment III (Fc). Further action of pepsin results in the degradation of Pep-III (i.e. Fc) fragment into the Pep-III' fragment and the smaller peptides Pep-IV and Pep-V. The Pep-I and Pep-III' fragments do not seem to be further broken down by prolonged incubation with pepsin at pH 4·5. The Pep-III' fragment would appear to resemble the 2·1S Fc' fragment isolated from *papain* digestion of *human* γG globulin in the presence of cysteine (by the method outlined on page 154). This fragment, which constitutes about 10 per cent of the intact molecule, was found to be immuno-

TABLE 7.3

Comparison of peptic and papain digestion products of rabbit γG globulin

	Pep-I (5S)	Pep-II* (3·3S)	Pep-III (3·3S)	2 hour digestion pH 4·5 → Pep-III' (2·4S)	+ Pep-IV (carbohydrate-rich, devoid of aromatic residues, antigenically inactive)	+ Pep-V
Peptic fragment (separated on G75 Sephadex) [84]	Pep-I (5S)	Pep-II* (3·3S)	Pep-III (3·3S)	Pep-III' (2·4S)	Pep-IV (carbohydrate-rich, devoid of aromatic residues, antigenically inactive)	Pep-V
Corresponding papain fragment	F(ab)$_2$ (produced by insol. papain) [82]	Fab, Fc	Fc	? F'c [98] (2·1S)		Low mol. wt. peptides (<5000) [71]

* Produced in negligible yield (2 per cent) by 18–24 hours' peptic digestion (pH 4·5).

logically active even after reductive cleavage in the presence of urea. It carries at least one antigenic determinant in common with the Fc fragment, but lacks its hexose (see also pages 225–239) [85].

The properties of the various peptic digestion fragments are summarized in Table 7.3, in which they are compared with fragments obtained by papain digestion. A schematic illustration of the tentative disposition of the peptic fragments within the rabbit γG globulin molecule (as proposed by Utsumi and Karush) is shown in Fig. 7.10. This model also incorporates two asymmetric inter-heavy chain disulphide bonds, in an attempt to explain the conflicting evidence concerning the number and stability of such bonds (outlined

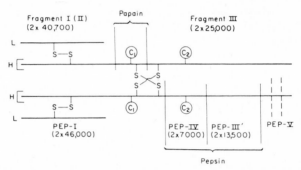

FIG. 7.10. Diagram depicting relationship of peptic fragments (Pep-I, Pep-IV, Pep-III′ and Pep-V) to the papain fragments I and III and to the heavy (H) and light (L) chains, showing the positions of the carbohydrate moieties (C_1 and C_2) and the inferred location of the points of papain and peptic cleavage. Each inter-heavy chain disulphide bond is asymmetric with respect to its half-cystine groups. Measured molecular weights are given in parentheses. The value for Pep-IV is approximate and based on the mass recovery from a known quantity of rabbit γG globulin, ignoring the carbohydrate.

(Reproduced by courtesy of Drs S.Utsumi and F.Karush from *Biochemistry* (1965), **4**, 1766.)

later in section B1b). The observed difference in the size of the F(ab)$_2$ and F(ab′)$_2$ fragments obtained by digestion with insoluble papain and pepsin respectively, is attributed to the location of different sites of cleavage by the two enzymes (owing to their different specificities). Moreover, the F(ab′)$_2$ fragment includes the carbohydrate moiety (of rabbit γG globulin), supposedly removed in the form of low molecular weight peptides by papain digestion.

According to this structural model, the Fd fragment (i.e. the N-terminal end of the heavy chain located in the Fab portion of the molecule) should prove to be of lower molecular weight than the corresponding fragment (designated Fd′) comprising the portion of the heavy chain in the Fab′ pieces in the 5S peptic fragment (Pep-I) of rabbit γG globulin (see also Fig.

7.6). Attempts by Heimer [86] to demonstrate such size differences between the Fd and Fd' fragments of *human* γG globulin were complicated, however, by the technical difficulties commonly encountered in the study of these *human* fragments, namely, their tendency to aggregate even in the presence of 1 N propionic acid. Recently, however, Press *et al* [209] have succeeded in isolating Fd fragment from a *human myeloma* γG globulin, by utilizing the observation that dissociation occurred in weak acid (0·2 N acetic acid containing 0·015 M NaCl) conditions, presumably because the light chains were of type L (which are more readily dissociated than type K [285]) and because the Fd fragment behaves as a dimer in the weaker acid. Press *et al* [209] are of the opinion, however, that it is unlikely that this method can be applied generally, and suggest that, for chemical studies, cleavage of the heavy chain by cyanogen bromide is probably preferable (although in this method all biological activity so far investigated has been lost).

The relative positions of the three peptic digestion fragments constituting the Fc portion (i.e. Pep-III, Pep-IV and Pep-V fragments) shown in the diagram of Utsumi & Karush [84] (see Fig. 7.10) is arbitrary; it now seems probable [87] that the reverse arrangement obtains in the rabbit γG globulin molecule. Nevertheless, it can be inferred that fragments Pep-IV and Pep-III' are contiguous, because the peptic degradation of papain fragment III (Fc) results in the loss of the antigenic determinants associated with Pep-V, without loss of the carbohydrate (associated with fragment Pep-IV). (This provides an example of the use of a carbohydrate prosthetic group as a marker in the location of overlapping γG globulin fragments obtained by different degradative procedures.)

Inman & Nisonoff [258] have shown that the crystallized Fc fragment of rabbit γG globulin (prepared by digestion with papain in the presence of a relatively high (0·05 M) concentration of cysteine) dissociated into 1·8S half-fragments (of 24,000 mol. wt. at pH 2·4) in 0·05 M NaCl at pH 2·7. These were isolated by gel filtraton of this preparation (18 mg) through a column (2·5 × 125 cm) of a mixed bed of cross-linked polyacrylamide Biogels P60 and P100, equilibrated with 0·05 M NaCl at pH 2·4. Under these conditions, the dissociated Fc fragment was resolved from both smaller molecules (^{131}I-labelled ribonuclease) and larger molecules (^{125}I-labelled rabbit γG globulin) as is shown in Fig. 7.11. The conditions employed are similar to those required for the dissociation of rabbit γG globulin into half molecules (as outlined later in section B2b).

Other proteolytic enzymes [88] such as trypsin and various sulphydryl-activated plant proteases resembling papain (for example bromelain and ficin) have been used to cleave γG globulins. For example, Hanson & Johansson [89] have isolated several tryptic degradation products from human γG globulin (DEAE-Sephadex A50 sub-fraction of Cohn fraction II) by gel filtration on Sephadex G75. The two major fractions (5S and 3·5S) thus obtained resembled the two fractions separated in a similar manner from insoluble papain-hydrolysed human γG globulin [90], whilst immunoelectrophoretic analysis also pointed to similarities between the two types of proteolytic digestion fragments.

Asahi *et al* [351] have recently reported the isolation of univalent antibody fragments from tryptic digestion (in the presence of cysteine) of rabbit γG globulin from antisera against bacterial α-amylase (purified by ether precipi-

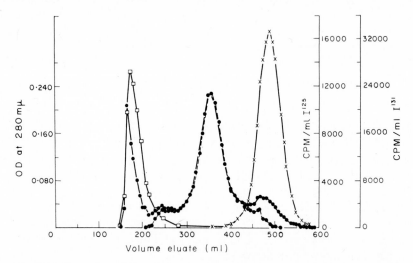

Fig. 7.11. Separation of dissociation products of Fc fragment of rabbit γG globulin by gel filtration on a mixed bed of Biogels P60 and P100; eluent 0·05 M NaCl (pH 2·4). Mixture contained 18 mg of purified Fc (prepared by papain digestion in the presence of 0·05 M L-cysteine), ^{125}I-labelled γG globulin (4 mg) and ^{131}I-labelled ribonuclease (4 mg). ●, optical density at 280 mμ, corrected for contribution of γG globulin or ribonuclease, as estimated from the radioactivity measurements; □, counts per minute of ^{125}I; ×, counts per minute of ^{131}I.

(Reproduced by courtesy of Drs F.P.Inman and A.Nisonoff from *J. biol. Chem.* (1966), **241**, 322.)

tation, followed by DEAE-cellulose chromatography). For digestion, rabbit γG globulin (40 mg) and crystalline trypsin (1·4 mg), dissolved in 0·1 M tris-HCl buffer (pH 7·5, containing 0·01 M cysteine and 0·005 M calcium acetate) (4 ml) were incubated at 37° C for 24 hours; the mixture was dialysed against 0·01 M acetate buffer, pH 5·4. After separating the small amount of precipitate by centrifugation, the supernatant was fractionated on DEAE-cellulose (according to the method of Porter [68]).

Skvaril [91] has demonstrated that the 'split line' effect observed in stored

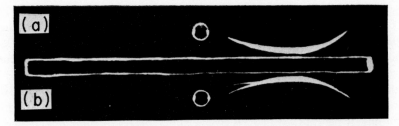

FIG. 7.12. Immunoelectrophoretic patterns of human γG globulin: (a) normal; (b) heated at 37° C (showing a typical 'split-line' effect). Antiserum: rabbit anti-whole human serum.
(Reproduced from *Nature, Lond.* (1964), **202**, 563.)

preparations of human γG globulin (see Fig. 7.12) could be reproduced by tryptic digestion of freshly prepared material (which initially produced only a single precipitin line). Substantial evidence has since been obtained (from ultracentrifugal and starch-gel electrophoretic analyses and optical rotation measurements) by James *et al* [92], indicating that the structural changes occurring in human γG globulins during storage, and at an enhanced rate when incubated at 37° C (outlined diagrammatically in Fig. 7.13) involve a dimerization process, during which a proportion (up to 20 per cent) of the γG globulin molecules become unfolded, followed by proteolytic degradation

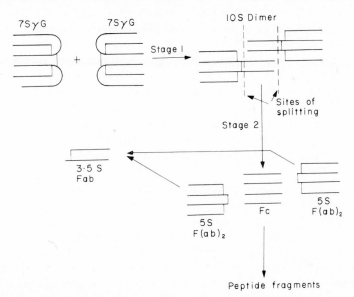

FIG. 7.13. Schematic illustration of structural alterations occurring in human γG globulin during ageing.

similar to that achieved by the papain (or peptic) digestion of native (7S) γG globulin (in the absence of reducing agent). Fab dimers, and at a later stage Fab monomeric (3·5S) fragments, are obtained by gel filtration on Sephadex G200, whereas the Fc piece is degraded to small peptides (as occurs during the peptic digestion of rabbit γG globulin, referred to earlier). This finding has been substantiated by the studies of Connell & Painter [93], who have employed amino-acid analysis to show that the fragments appearing in solutions (16 per cent w/v in 0·3 M glycine buffer, pH 6·7) of human γG globulin (Cohn fraction II, prepared from out-dated plasma) during storage at 2° C were identical to similar fragments isolated from *plasmin* digests of human γG globulin. Plasmin digestion was achieved by incubating at 37° C, a solution (10 per cent w/v) of human γG globulin in 0·3 M glycine—0·05 M tris (hydroxymethyl) aminomethane buffer (pH 7·5) (10 ml) with plasmin solution (0·75 ml, containing 15 mg protein/ml of a potency of 140 units) for varying times up to 24 hours.

The similarity of the multi-banded patterns (in the anode region) shown by natural (storage) and plasmin-produced Fc fragments, when subjected to starch-gel electrophoresis in borate buffer, provided further evidence that the changes occurring naturally in human γG globulin during storage result from the presence of traces of contaminating plasmin. Like plasmin-induced and papain-induced Fab fragments, the Fab fragments from aged immune human sera were shown to possess antibody activity [93] (as measured by toxin neutralization tests in guinea-pigs or rabbits, and virus neutralization tests in tissue culture). In other studies [94], however, the efficacy of aged, fragmented preparations of immune human serum γG globulins were shown to be impaired when compared with fresh (unfragmented) material, when tested for their ability to induce passive immunization of guinea-pigs against tetanus toxin, and monkeys against poliomyelitis virus type I. It is probable that the loss of the Fc fragment, due to the structural changes occurring on ageing, results in the rapid excretion of the antibody fragments by the passively immunized animals (as the catabolic studies outlined in section B3b suggest).

Rabbit γG globulin has been shown to behave differently from human γG globulin after trypsin treatment, in that 3·5S fragments were not produced in the absence of a reducing agent [95, 96]. The amount of *human* γG globulin fraction susceptible to tryptic degradation at pH 7·5 is increased by the presence of cysteine (0·01 M), which results in the production of slightly increased yields of 3·5S fragment (e.g. 60 per cent, compared with the 50 per cent produced in the absence of cysteine [95, 96]). Approximately 45 per cent of rabbit γG globulin (Cohn fraction II) was degraded by trypsin in the *presence* of cysteine (0·01 M), i.e. a little less than the amount of 3·5S product obtained by tryptic digestion of human γG globulin in the *absence* of reducing agent. Hence, it appears that the peptide bonds of the rabbit γG globulin are less accessible to the enzyme than are the bonds in human γG globulin. (The γG globulins of different species vary also in their susceptibility to papain cleavage [88].)

This raises the interesting question of the mechanism of the degradation of γG globulin by proteolytic enzymes (see also section C, dealing with the conformation of immunoglobulins). Studies involving a comparison of the products of digestion in the presence of N-ethylmaleimide (0·05 M) or iodo-acetate (0·1 M) [96] have provided evidence that the *free sulphydryl groups* of human γG globulin are involved in the cleavage of disulphide bonds during the fragmentation of this immunoglobulin by trypsin (at pH 8·0). The interpretation of such findings is complicated, however, by the probable heterogeneity of the γG globulin preparations studied. Indeed, an appreciable array of evidence is accumulating to suggest that *human γG globulin fractions, at least, comprise molecules of different conformation, which differ in their*

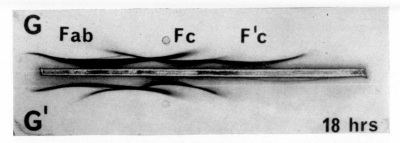

FIG. 7.14. Immunoelectrophoretic patterns of human γG globulin (Cohn fraction II) after digestion in the presence (G) and absence (G′) of cysteine.
(Reproduced by courtesy of Dr M.D.Poulik from *Nature, Lond.* (1966), **210**, 133.)

susceptibility to proteolytic degradation (as the incomplete conversion of this protein to 3·5S fragments by trypsin and other proteolytic enzymes suggests). For instance, human myeloma γG globulins have been differentiated according to their behaviour when digested with cysteine-activated papain (by the classical Porter [68] procedure). Of a group of twenty immunoglobulins of this class [22], 90 per cent (termed 'C' or 'papain-insensitive') produced not only Fab and Fc fragments, but also an immunoelectrophoretically distinct F′c precipitin arc (shown in Fig. 7.14) after digestion at 37° C for 18 hours. No Fc (or F′c) fragments were detected, however, in papain digests (18 hours) of the remaining 10 per cent of the myeloma γG globulins (termed 'type Z' or 'papain-sensitive'); i.e. all their Fc portions had been destroyed by this time. Other investigators [97, 98] have made similar observations, employing starch-gel electrophoresis and analytical ultracentrifugation, in addition to immunoelectrophoresis, to identify the papain digestion products.

These observations of the variability in behaviour of myeloma γG globulins to proteolytic digestion are not too surprising, in view of the readily demonstrable antigenic differences between immunoglobulins of this class. Of greater interest, however, is the finding that γG globulin molecules representative of both structural forms (i.e. 'papain-resistant' and 'papain-sensitive', depicted diagrammatically in Fig. 7.38) appear to be present in preparations (e.g. Cohn II fractions) of *normal* human γG globulin, although these have yet to be distinguished antigenically.

The study of these two structural forms of human γG globulin has been facilitated by the use of gel filtration on Sephadex G100, combined with automatic effluent monitoring (in a Gilford Multiple Sample Absorbance Recorder), used both as an analytical and preparative tool [58]. Thus, papain digestion (at pH 7) of human γG globulin (e.g. Cohn fraction II, 1, 2) for 4 hours at 37° C in the *absence* of cysteine (followed by inactivation of the enzyme with 0·01 M N-ethylmaleimide) resulted in the isolation (in the first peak of the Sephadex G100 elution pattern, as shown in Fig. 7.15) of 'papain-resistant' γG globulin. This material, which comprised about 30–35 per cent of the total γG globulin (depending on its method of preparation), was found to be digested completely, however, when reincubated with papain in the *presence* of cysteine (0·01 M). The products of digestion (Fab, Fc) of that part of the γG globulin (65–70 per cent) which was degraded initially by papain in the *absence* of cysteine, were isolated in the second peak from the Sephadex G100 separation of the digest (indicated by immunoelectrophoretic analysis, as in Fig. 7.15b), and the low molecular weight peptides (showing absorbance at 280 mμ) were eluted at a much later stage as the third peak (indicated by the wide separation between the third peak and the previous first and second peaks, shown in Fig. 7.15a). It seems possible that these fragments (of which the one-dimensional high-voltage electrophoretograms are shown in Fig. 7.26) are similar to the low molecular weight (<5000) peptides separated in low yields (2–3 per cent) by ion-exchange chromatography after papain digestion of human γG globulin in the presence [71] or absence [99] of cysteine.

Hence, the two structural forms of human γG globulin can be readily distinguished by the character of the Sephadex G100 elution patterns of their papain digests (for 4 hours at 37° C) performed in the absence of cysteine. This approach offers important advantages over the practice employed in the differentiation of the two forms of myeloma (and normal) γG globulins (mentioned earlier), depending on the appearance of the immunoelectrophoretic pattern of the products after extensive papain digestion (18 hours at 37° C) in the presence of cysteine [22] or of differences in the complex patterns (see Fig. 7.24) obtained after starch-gel electrophoresis of the digests obtained using papain in the absence of cysteine [98]. Thus, two myeloma

(a)

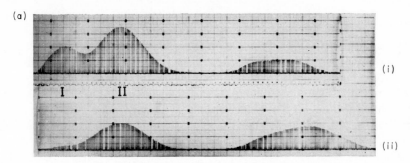

(i)

I   II

(ii)

(b)

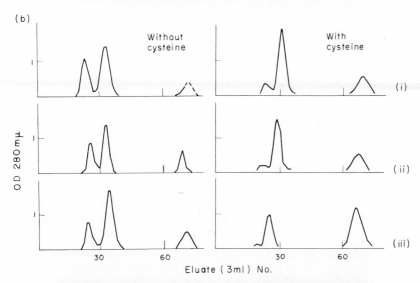

Without cysteine

With cysteine

(i)

(ii)

(iii)

OD 280mμ

30   60   30   60

Eluate (3ml) No.

(c)

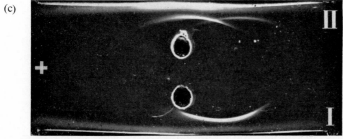

Fig. 7.15

(a) Sephadex G100 gel-filtration patterns (automated plots) of papain digests (4 hours) of human γG globulin (Cohn fraction II 1,2) in the (i) absence and (ii) presence of cysteine (0·01 M).

(b) Tracings of gel-filtration patterns shown by (i) 2 hours', (ii) 4 hours', and (iii) 18 hours' digestion in the absence and presence of cysteine.

(c) Immunoelectrophoretic patterns of Sephadex G100 fractions I and II isolated from the papain digest (4 hours) in the absence of cysteine.

Antiserum: rabbit anti-human γG globulin.

γG globulins, which would be classified as 'papain-sensitive' on the basis of their immunoelectrophoretic patterns after prolonged (18 hours) digestion with cysteine-activated papain, were recognized by the almost complete absence of a first peak (of undigested protein) when papain digests (2 hours) in the *absence* of cysteine were analysed by gel filtration on Sephadex G100. In contrast, a third myeloma γG globulin preparation (which showed cryoglobulin properties) was digested to a limited extent only by papain (in the *absence* of cysteine), with the result that most of the material was eluted unchanged in the first peak of a Sephadex G100 separation of the digest.

Rabbit γG globulin [71, 100] (and the γG globulins of other mammalian species [71]) have also been found to be heterogeneous with respect to susceptibility to papain proteolysis. This has been demonstrated by Sephadex G200 gel filtration of digests after limited proteolysis (e.g. 10 minutes) by mercuripapain in the presence of cysteine (0·01 M) and EDTA (0·002 M), followed by inhibition of the enzyme with a 1·5 M excess of iodoacetamide [100]. The gel-filtration pattern (reproduced in Fig. 7.16) showed three peaks, comprising fractions with sedimentation coefficents (S_{20} values) of 6·9S, 5·0S and 3·6S. The residual undigested rabbit γG globulin, isolated in the first fraction (comprising 5–10 per cent of the total γG globulin after digestion with 1 per cent papain for 10 minutes), was more resistant to the action of papain (when redigested) than was the starting γG globulin preparation. This resistance did not appear to be related to the composition of the Fab component of the molecule (being independent of the presence of fragments I or II), but the papain-resistant fraction was found to possess more hexose (almost double) than the whole rabbit γG globulin preparation. The 5S fraction appears to be an *intermediate* in the enzymatic degradation of rabbit γG globulin, comprising one Fab and one Fc fragment (due to fracture of one heavy polypeptide chain before the other, with the release of a single Fab sub-unit).

Technical difficulties, caused by the lability of their heavy polypeptide chains, have hampered similar proteolysis studies of the other main classes of immunoglobulins (γM, γA). Consequently, most investigations of the subunits of these immunoglobulins have been made on the products of reductive cleavage (obtained by similar methods to those outlined below; see also section C1, b and c). Miller & Metzger [447] have, however, employed trypsin for the cleavage of a γM globulin and its sub-units (γMs), as is outlined in section C.

(b) Chemical dissociation

(i) *Reductive cleavage*

The first method, applied by Edelman & Poulik [101] to the reductive cleavage of human and rabbit γG globulin involved extensive reduction (with

0·1M 2-mercaptoethylamine or 2-mercaptoethanol) in the presence of a potent denaturing agent (6 M urea). Although this approach demonstrated that the γG globulin molecule possessed more than one kind of polypeptide chain, it has several disadvantages. These include difficulties of fractionation in the presence of urea, resulting in poor recoveries, insolubility of the products in the usual aqueous solvents and loss of biological activity.

These problems are avoided to a large extent by adopting mild reducing conditions at near neutral pH as described by Fleischman *et al* [102]. It is thus possible to obtain dissociation products which are soluble in ordinary

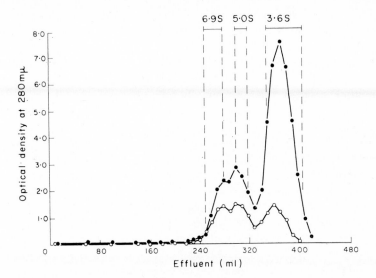

FIG. 7.16. Sephadex G200 gel-filtration patterns of papain digest (10 minutes) of rabbit γG globulin. ●, pool of γG globulin without prior digestion; ○, 6·9S fraction from pool of γG globulin previously digested (10 minutes) with 1 per cent papain. (Reproduced by courtesy of Dr J.W.Goodman from *Biochemistry* (1965), **4**, 2350.)

solvents at neutral pH, and which retain their biological activity (presumably because under these conditions, the rupture of intra-chain disulphide bonds, with resultant molecular rearrangements leading to aggregation, does not occur). The reductive cleavage procedure adopted by these investigators is as follows: after degassing by suction on a water-pump, nitrogen is bubbled slowly through a 2 per cent (w/v) solution of the γG globulin (DEAE-cellulose fraction from human, rabbit or horse serum), dissolved in 0·55 M tris-HCl buffer, pH 8·2. (Tris = tris-(hydroxymethyl)-amino-methane.) 2-Mercapto-ethanol is added, to a final concentration of 0·75 M, and the mixture kept at room temperature for 1 hour. It is then cooled in ice-water, and an equal volume of 0·75 M iodoacetamide (previously degassed and cooled to 0° C) is added. Trimethylamine is cautiously added to maintain the pH at about 8, and, after 1 hour, the solution is dialysed overnight against 100 vol. cold saline, any slight precipitate being removed by centrifugation.

The ten sulphydryl groups liberated from the interchain disulphide bonds ruptured by this reductive treatment are alkylated by the iodoacetamide. Subsequent fractionation of the reduction mixture by gel filtration in acid (N) solution, or in detergent such as sodium dodecyl sulphate [103], leads to the separation of the heavy and light polypeptide chains. This can be accomplished by dialysing the reduced protein (100–200 mg) against cold 1 N acetic or 1 N propionic acid overnight, and then fractionating on a column (3 × 65 cm) of Sephadex G75 (pre-equilibrated with the acid) in the cold-room.

A typical gel-filtration pattern obtained by this procedure is shown in Fig. 7.17, which was obtained by the fractionation of reduced rabbit γG globulin. The larger fraction (initially referred to as 'A' [7] or 'H' [105]) obtained in 70–75 per cent yield, was found to comprise *heavy* polypeptide chains whilst the smaller fraction (initially referred to as 'B' [7] or 'L' [105]), obtained in 25–30 per cent yield, comprises *light* polypeptide chains. This evidence, together with the finding that the amino acids, carbohydrate, and N-terminal amino acids of rabbit γG globulin can be accounted for in terms of the chains [106] provides support for the now familiar four-chain structure for the γG globulin molecule (postulated by Porter [68]). As shown in Fig. 7.6, this comprises two polypeptide chains of 50,000 mol. wt., and two of 20,000 mol. wt., linked by inter-chain disulphide bonds.

In other investigations, the reduction of rabbit γG globulin in 6 M guanidine hydrochloride, followed by fractionation of the polypeptide chains in the same solvent, has provided a slightly higher yield of light chain (about 33 per cent), and therefore a revised estimate of its molecular weight as 25,000 [107, 108, 449]. It is significant that reduction under these conditions produced no further diminution in molecular weight, presumably because only intra-chain disulphide bonds were newly exposed by the denaturing agent.

Cohen [109] has adopted similar methods to those developed by Fleischman *et al* [102] to show that the *human* γG globulins molecule also conforms to the Porter four-chain polypeptide structure. Moreover, by reduction and gel filtration through Sephadex G75 in 1 N acetic acid, he demonstrated that the heavy and light polypeptide chains are present in equal proportions in the human γM and γA globulin molecules, as well as in the γG globulin molecule. The structural similarities of the light chains from the main immuno-globulin classes and the distinctive nature of their heavy chains have been demonstrated by studies of their serological cross-reactivity, by starch-gel electrophoresis and by peptide-mapping techniques (as outlined in section B2).

The polypeptide chain composition of the papain digestion fragments of human and rabbit γG globulins has also been ascertained by peptide mapping of tryptic hydrolysates [74], by analysis of molecules reconstituted from chains labelled with different radioactive iodine isotopes [74] and by gel-diffusion precipitin analysis using rabbit [109, 74, 111] or goat antisera [106], directed specifically against the different polypeptide chains or papain digestion

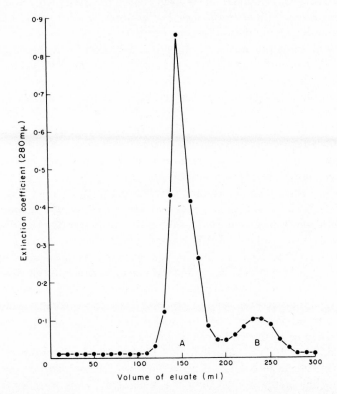

Fig. 7.17. Fractionation of reduced rabbit γG globulin on Sephadex G75 in 1 N acetic acid.
(Reproduced by courtesy of Drs J.B.Fleischman, R.H.Pain and R.R.Porter, F.R.S., from *Arch. biochem. Biophys.* (1962), **Sup. 1**, 174.)

fragments. Thus, Fc piece has been shown to contain only heavy chain, whereas light chain has been located in the Fab pieces. Moreover, the N-terminal section of the heavy chain (originally named 'A piece' and now referred to as Fd piece) has been isolated (in stable dimeric form) from Fab pieces of rabbit γG globulin following reduction and alkylation, by gel filtration on Sephadex G75 in 1 N propionic acid [106]. It has not, however, proved possible to obtain a reaction between the Fd part of normal human γG globulin Fab piece and specific rabbit anti-heavy chain antiserum [111] (possibly because of its weak antigenicity, or because its antigenicity is destroyed during the separation of parent Fab piece by papain digestion).

A single fractionation of reduced γG globulin on Sephadex G75 in acid fails to provide a clear-cut separation of the heavy and light chains, as might be expected. The contamination of each chain preparation by the other can be established by various techniques. For example, where there is a clear-cut electrophoretic differentiation between the two types of chain (as in the case of chains from human or horse γG globulin), starch-gel electrophoresis in 8 M urea in 0·2 M formate buffer, pH 8·4, can be employed [102]. Alternatively, where the electrophoretic patterns of the heavy and light chains overlap (as in the case of rabbit γG globulin chains), cross-contamination has been detected by the assay of N-terminal amino acids [102]. The purity of polypeptide chain preparations has also been determined, of course, by gel-diffusion precipitin analysis. Isotopically labelled chain preparations have been employed as markers in chain fractionation procedures, and as antigens in specific precipitation tests for purity [112].

Refractionation of combined (and ultrafiltered) eluates, comprising selected areas of the initial gel-filtration peaks, provides relatively pure chain preparations (with, inevitably, some sacrifice in yield). For example, a recycled heavy chain preparation isolated by Fleischman *et al* [102] was shown to contain not more than 3 per cent of light chain (according to N-terminal amino-acid assay). Even after recycling heavy and light chain fractions of guinea-pig γ_2G globulin in 4 M guanidine hydrochloride on Sephadex G200, however, Lamm *et al* [112] found it necessary to combine only those eluates which were proved to be immunochemically pure (as shown in Fig. 7.18), if preparations of a high degree of purity were to be obtained.

Koshland *et al* [113] have investigated the effects of various reduction procedures on the recoveries of heavy and light chains of three specifically purified rabbit antibody γG globulins, separated by gel filtration through Sephadex G200 equilibrated with 0·01 M tris buffer (pH 8·0) containing detergent (0·01 M sodium dodecyl sulphate) to solubilize and dissociate the chains [103]. The range of reducing conditions employed involved the use of 2-mercaptoethanol concentrations varying from 0·05–1·0 M, and urea concentrations from 0 to 12 M. When 2-mercaptoethanol alone was used, it was added to a solution of the antibody (0·5–1·0 per cent w/v in 0·1 M tris buffer, pH 8·0). The reduction was allowed to proceed under nitrogen for 1 hour, prior to the addition of dry iodoacetamide or iodoacetic acid in 10 per cent molar excess of the concentration of 2-mercaptoethanol used. The alkylating solution was maintained for 0·5 hour at pH 7·5–8·0 with 5 N NaOH. When reduction was carried out in the presence of urea, the reaction time was extended to 24 hours at room temperature (in order that maximum randomization of the protein structure would be achieved). The alkylated proteins were freed from the other products of the reaction by dialysis for 48 hours against changes (4 litres) of distilled water, and concentrated to

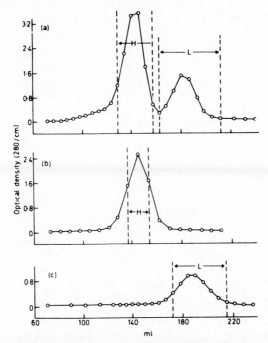

FIG. 7.18. Non-specific guinea-pig γ_2G globulin after mild reduction and alkylation.

(a) Separation in 4 M guanidine on Sephadex G200.

(b) A second filtration of the indicated portion of the heavy (H) chain peak, comprising eluates that were pure by immunochemical criteria. (About 1 per cent of the optical density, eluted where the light (L) chains would be expected. is not evident because of the reduction in scale.)

(c) A second filtration of the indicated portion of the light (L) chain peak, comprising eluates containing pure light (L) chains. (About 1·5 per cent of the optical density, eluted where heavy (H) chains would be expected, is not evident because of the reduction in scale.)

(Reproduced by courtesy of Drs M.E.Lamm, V.Nussenzweig and B. Benacerraf from *Immunology* (1966), **10**, 309.)

dryness by rotary flash evaporation. The dried alkylated preparations were taken up in the tris-detergent buffer to a concentration of 10–20 mg/ml, allowed to stand (4 hours at room temperature, or overnight in the cold), and any insoluble material removed by centrifugation. The clear supernatant (containing at least 95 per cent of the initial protein) was filtered through Sephadex G200, using a column (1·4 × 100 cm) and a flow-rate of 12–15 ml hour for samples of less than 25 mg, while for samples of 25–125 mg, a

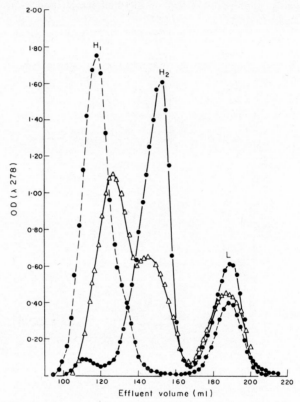

Fig. 7.19. Sephadex G200 fraction of reduced and alkylated antibody directed against the p-phenylarsonic acid group (from a¹a¹b⁴b⁴ doubly homozygous rabbit). ●- - -●- - -●, separation after mild reduction (with 0·05 M 2-mercaptoethanol); —△—△—△—, separation after more extensive reduction (with 0·1 M 2-mercapto-ethanol and 10 M urea); ●—●—●, separation after complete reduction (with 0·5 M 2-mercaptoethanol and 12 M urea). Eluant: 0·01 M sodium dodecyl sulphate in 0·01 M tris buffer, pH 8·0.

(Reproduced by courtesy of Drs M.E.Koshland, F.M. Englberger and R.Shapanka from *Biochemistry* (1966), **5**, 641.)

column (2·2 × 100 cm) and a flow-rate of 6–7 ml/hour were used. The absorbance of the eluates (2–2·5 ml fractions) was read at 278 mμ. Representative gel-filtration curves thus obtained are shown in Fig. 7.19. After 'mild reduction' (with 0·05 M 2-mercaptoethanol), all the heavy chain was recovered in the fastest moving (H_1) fraction, with only a shoulder on the descending limb to indicate the presence of small amounts of slower-moving material. After 'intermediate reducing conditions' (using 0·1 M 2-mercaptoethanol and 10 M urea), the heavy chain was distributed between the H_1 fraction and the second, slower-moving, H_2 fraction. After 'complete reduction' (by 0·5 M 2-mercaptoethanol and 12 M urea), the heavy chain was eluted almost exclusively in the H_2 fraction. In contrast, the rate of filtration of the third component (i.e. light chain) was independent of disulphide bond cleavage. As only trace amounts of light chain were found in the H_1 fraction, the *two* heavy chain fractions (i.e. H_1 and H_2) could not be attributed simply to a

TABLE 7.4

Effect of the extent of reduction on the separation of rabbit antibody sub-units by gel filtration (reproduced by courtesy of Drs M.E. Koshland, F.M. Englberger and R. Shapanka from *Biochem.* (1966) **5**, 641)

Antibody preparation	No. of expts	Recovered (per cent)		Total
		Heavy chain $(H_1 + H_2)$	Light chain	
After mild reduction				
Arsonic	5	74·5 ± 4·4	18·9 ± 1·7	93·4 ± 4·3
Ammonium	3	74·3 ± 3·7	18·5 ± 2·1	92·8 ± 2·9
After intermediate reduction				
Arsonic	2	72·2 ± 8·5	22·6 ± 1·1	94·7 ± 9·5
Lac	3	71·2 ± 2·1	22·4 ± 2·3	93·6 ± 5·4
After complete reduction				
Arsonic	6	68·3 ± 2·7	24·1 ± 1·2	92·4 ± 3·1
Ammonium	5	70·7 ± 1·1	25·2 ± 0·9	95·9 ± 1·5
Lac	3	65·7 ± 0·2	24·5 ± 0·3	90·2 ± 0·1

complex of light and heavy chains (in H_1), as compared with pure heavy chains (in H_2). Instead, the differences in rate of filtration were considered to reflect other properties, such as the aggregation or swelling of the partially reduced chain. The yields of heavy and light chains obtained following the various reducing conditions employed are given in Table 7.4.

Attempts to separate the κ and λ light chains from normal human γG globulin by electrophoresis, chromatography, gel filtration and salt precipitation have proved unsuccessful. Cohen [114] has, however, isolated partially purified preparations (each showing ten electrophoretic fractions when analysed in urea-glycine starch gels). These were obtained by exploiting the fact that λ chains (for the most part) dissociate from reduced alkylated γG globulin at a *higher pH* than κ chains. Thus, a preparation constituting about 15 per cent of the total light chain and comprising over 80 per cent λ chains, was obtained by dissociation of reduced human γG globulin in 0·1 M acetate buffer (pH 3·6). Subsequent fractionation by gel filtration in 1 N acetic acid of the residual undissociated (at pH 3·3) γG globulin, led to the recovery of 60 per cent of the total light chain, comprising about 90 per cent of κ chain.

Reductive cleavage of rabbit γG globulin (DEAE-cellulose sub-fraction of sodium sulphate precipitated material) under somewhat different conditions from those used in the isolation of the polypeptide chains (as just described) has led to the dissociation of the molecule into two sub-units of approximately equal size, i.e. into *half-molecules* [115]. This was achieved by reduction with 0·1 M 2-mercaptoethylamine, addition of excess p-chloromercuribenzoate (to prevent reoxidation) and acidification to pH 2·5 in aqueous salt solution. A close similarity between the amino-acid compositions of the sub-units and whole γG globulin, together with other evidence, points to each sub-unit comprising a heavy and light chain. Furthermore, it has been shown that in one-half to two-thirds of the rabbit γG globulin molecules, the two halves are linked together by a *single labile disulphide bond* [116]. It is probable that papain and pepsin cleave such molecules on *opposite 'sides'* of this bond [117] (as is indicated in Fig. 7.6).

The location of this disulphide bond, bridging the heavy chains in the two halves of the rabbit γG globulin molecule, was deduced by estimation of the amount of S-carboxymethyl-L-cysteine derivative recovered after hydrolysis and alkylation with iodoacetamide [116]. A similar technique has been employed to demonstrate that single disulphide bonds link the heavy and light chains in each half of the rabbit γG globulin molecule [117]. Moreover, studies [104, 118] on Bence-Jones proteins have indicated that cysteine residues in the C-terminal positions of the κ type of light chains, and in the penultimate position in the C-terminal residue in λ type of light chains, are involved in such inter-chain bridging within human γG globulin molecules.

It seems likely that the ingenious diagonal electrophoresis technique [119], which has been used to locate the disulphide bridges in chymotrypsinogen-A, will prove of great value in the precise location of the disulphide bonds in immunoglobulin molecules (once the problem of molecular heterogeneity has been overcome, and it can be certain that peptides derived from a homogeneous population of γG globulin are being examined). Application of some such technique will be necessary to resolve the apparent discrepancies [1] in the number of interchain disulphide bonds being assigned by different workers to the γG globulin molecule. It is important to carry out reductive cleavage studies on highly purified preparations under rigidly controlled conditions, in the presence and absence of denaturing agents, in order to differentiate between inter- and intra-chain bonds. Cecil & Stevenson [120] are making investigations of this type, using *sulphite* as cleaving agent. The reactivity of the protein with this reagent at pH 7·0 offers a means of *estimating the disulphide bonds*, the extent of reaction being determined by estimating the amount of thiol formed. Inter-chain disulphide bonds normally interact with sulphite alone. Such reactions are performed at 25° C with 0·5 M sodium sulphite, adjusted to pH 7·0 with dilute nitric acid, and stopped by the addition of aliquots (1 ml) to 8 M urea-0·3 N HNO_3 (4 ml) to give a final pH of 2·5, the presence of the urea preventing precipitation of the γG globulin. The *total* content of disulphide (intra- as well as inter-chain) bonds on the other hand is determined by carrying out the reaction in the presence of urea or guanidine hydrochloride, using a slight excess of phenyl-mercuriacetate to prevent oxidation of the thiol groups formed.

The relative labilities of the two types of inter-chain disulphide bonds (i.e. H—H and H—L) in rabbit γG globulin have been compared by reduction with increasing concentrations of 2-mercaptoethanol at pH 8·2, or with 2-mercaptoethylamine at pH 5·0 [121].

Thiol groups can be measured by amperometric titration with phenyl-mercuriacetate (at $-0·3$ volts). Alternatively, the colorimetric procedure of Jocelyn [122], employing di-(5-carboxy-4-nitrophenyl)disulphide, provides a rapid and reliable procedure. For example, this method has been applied to the estimation of thiol groups revealed on denaturation of human γG globulin, in studies [123] of its reactivity with rheumatoid factor. Karush *et al* [124] have recently developed an assay for disulphide groups based on the measurement of the quenching of fluorescence of fluorescein mercuric acetate by disulphide-containing materials in alkaline solution. This highly sensitive and specific procedure, which can be used for the detection of disulphide groups either on paper or in solution, should find wide application in the study of immunoglobulins. When used as a freshly prepared spray solution (2×10^{-4} M fluorescein mercuric acetate in 1·5 N NaOH) as little as 10^{-10} mole of disulphide can be detected on paper.

The studies of Cecil & Stevenson [120] have shown that urea is less effective than guanidine hydrochloride in unfolding human and rabbit γG globulins (DEAE-cellulose chromatography fractions). A similar effect has been reported from investigations on pig γG globulin [125]. The number of disulphide bonds reacting with sulphite alone (i.e. probably all the inter-chain disulphide bonds) was found to be six bonds per molecule of human, and 6·5 bonds per molecule of rabbit, γG globulin. These numbers are about one bond per molecule less than were found to react with 2-mercaptoethanol (0·2 M) in the absence of reducing agent [187].

A mild reducing agent, 1,4-dithiothreitol, has been employed as a cleaving agent in the degradation of relatively concentrated (>2 per cent w/v) solutions of human γG globulin [126]. Careful addition of the reagent to a solution (2 g/100 ml) of human γG globulin in 0·55 M tris buffer (pH 8·1) achieved almost complete reduction within 30 minutes (as revealed by electrophoresis in 8 M urea- formic acid-starch gel), no further degradation being observed when the reaction time was increased to 2 hours and the concentration of 1,4-dithiothreitol to 0·3 M. Marked reduction occurred with protein concentrations up to 10 per cent (w/v), but it was then necessary to increase the concentrations of the 1,4-dithiothreitol and alkylating agent (iodoacetamide). Much of the degraded protein was in the form of half-molecules, rather than light and heavy chains, when γG globulin concentrations greater than 6g per cent were employed.

(ii) *Other methods of chemical cleavage*
Although chemical reagents such as cyanogen bromide [127, 128, 138] have been used for the selective cleavage of peptide bonds in the polypeptide chains of a number of enzymes and their precursors (e.g. ribonuclease, trypsinogen), this method has until recently found little application to the isolation of fragments of immunoglobulins. Cahnmann *et al* [129] claim to be the first to apply the technique to the isolation of biologically active fragments of γG globulins; they used a DEAE-cellulose sub-fraction of rabbit γG globulin, isolated from an antiserum against bovine serum albumin. The cleaving agent employed was cyanogen bromide, which specifically breaks the methionyl bonds, and has the advantage that it causes practically no side-reactions [127].

A typical cleavage technique is as follows: A solution of the γG globulin (50 mg/ml) in phosphate buffer (0·0175 M, pH 6·3) is mixed with an equal volume of cyanogen bromide (15 mg/ml) in 0·6 M HCl. After being kept in a tightly closed vessel at room temperature for 4 hours, the reaction mixture is dialysed at 4° C for 1 hour against phosphate buffer (0·02 M, pH 7·8, containing 0·15 M NaCl). It is, of course, important to carry out a parallel control experiment (omitting cyanogen bromide), against which any apparent cleavage by the chemical reagent can be assessed.

It was shown that such treatment led to the cleavage of about half of the methionine residues in the original γG globulin, namely, those in the Fc portion, with the concomitant release of a 5·3S fragment, possessing properties similar to those of the 5S peptic digestion products (i.e. F(ab')$_2$, together with lower molecular weight fragments (resulting from the disruption of the Fc portion of the molecule). Reduction of the 5·3S cyanogen bromide cleavage fragment with cysteine (0·01 M, pH 8·0) at 37° C for 8 hours produced a 3·5S fraction, which gave a similar starch-gel (in 8 M urea-formic acid) pattern to that shown by papain Fab piece, and which lacked the antigen (BSA) precipitating ability of the parent 5·3S fragment.

Cyanogen bromide has also been used to cleave the heavy chains of rabbit γG globulin [130] in sequential studies on the C-terminal peptide. Incubation of heavy material (500 mg) with cyanogen bromide (1 g) in 70 per cent formic acid (25 ml) for 24 hours at 25° C, and at 4° C, converted 95 per cent and 92 per cent respectively of the methionine to homoserine and produced six components, revealed by starch-gel electrophoresis (in urea-formate), which were partially separable by gel filtration through Sephadex G100 in N acetic acid. Similar conditions have been employed to cleave the heavy chains of a human myeloma γG globulin into five fragments [209], which were partially separable by gel filtration through Sephadex G100 in N acetic acid or, more readily, in urea-formate buffer (pH 3·3) [211] and identified by starch-gel electrophoresis.

It seems probable that other methods of chemical cleavage will be developed to provide fragments of different characteristics from those readily obtainable by the commonly used enzymatic degradation procedures. In this connection, a combination of chemical and enzymatic treatments might prove useful. For instance, blockage of a particular type of amino-acid side-chain could prevent specific proteolytic cleavage at these positions along the polypeptide chain. This has been demonstrated following the blockage of the ε-amino groups of lysine residues of proteins (such as ribonuclease and lysozyme) by treatment with ethyl-thiol-trifluoracetate [131] or carbon disulphide [132], whereupon subsequent tryptic digestion cleaved the peptide chain only at the sites of its arginine residues. These forms of substitution yield water-soluble peptides, in contrast to the tryptic digestion products obtained following substitution by other reagents (discussed in a recent review article by Hill [133]). Moreover, the trifluoracetyl and dithiocarbamyl groups are easily removed under mild conditions.

2. Methods of analysis of sub-units

Many of the methods employed in the characterization of immunoglobulin sub-units have been mentioned already in the previous section (B1). Of these, immunodiffusion and immunoelectrophoresis (which rely, of course, on the presence of reactive antigenic determinants in the sub-unit) are described in detail in Chapter 19, and ultra-centrifugation has been discussed in Chapter 4, where the problems presented by the use of solvents (e.g. 6 M urea solution), needed to prevent aggregation of the sub-units, are considered. Of the other main physico-chemical procedures, zone-electrophoresis (see Chapter 2) and gel filtration (see Chapter 3) have proved particularly useful in the isolation as well as the characterization of the products of immunoglobulin dissociation. The supporting media employed in the former method range from paper to starch gel, depending on the size of the fragments being examined. In gel

G

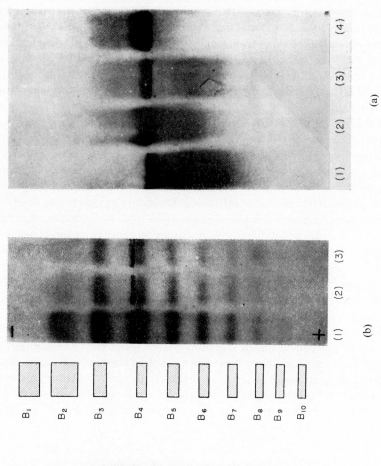

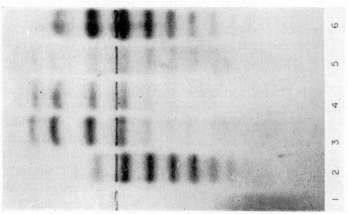

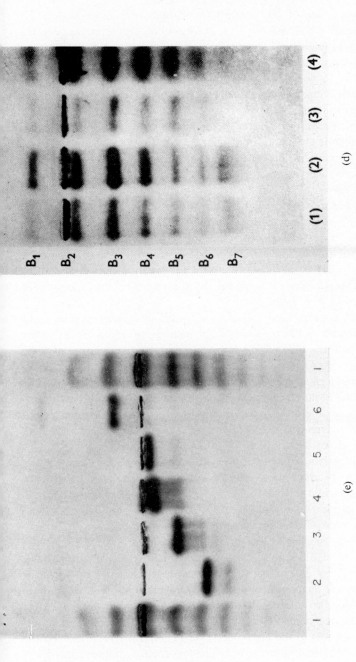

FIG. 7.20. Electrophoresis in 8 M urea-glycine starch gels. (a) $\gamma_1(1)$ and $\gamma_2(2)$ subfractions of normal human γG globulin and of heavy chains of these $\gamma_1(3)$ and $\gamma_2(4)$ subfractions.
(b) Light chains from $\gamma_1(1)$ and $\gamma_2(2)$ subfractions of normal human γG globulin and from normal human γM globulin (3). A diagrammatic representation of the ten components of human light chains is shown on the left.
(c) Light chains from γG globulins: (1) rabbit; (2) guinea-pig; (3) bovine; (4) horse; (5) baboon; (6) human.
(d) Light chains from guinea-pig γG globulins: (1) and (2) two different preparations of anti-(ovalbumin)γG globulin; (3) anti-(bovine serum albumin) γG globulin; (4) guinea-pig γG globulin.
(e) Light chains of human γG globulins: (1) and (7) normal γG globulin; (2–6) five pathological γG globulins.
(Patterns reproduced by permission of Professor S.Cohen and Professor R.R. Porter, F.R.S., from *Biochem. J.* (1964) **90**, 278.)

filtration, the pore size of the dextran (Sephadex) or polyacrylamide gel employed is varied when dealing with sub-units of different size. Peptide fragments thus isolated and identified are ultimately characterized by chemical analysis (as outlined in sub-section B2b).

(a) Physico-chemical analysis of sub-units
Starch-gel electrophoresis

Starch-gel electrophoresis procedures, based on the method devised originally by Smithies [134] for the analysis of genetic variations in serum proteins, have provided valuable means of analysing immunoglobulin sub-units. The inclusion of 8 M urea or some other suitable denaturing agent in the buffer prevents reaggregation of the sub-units during electrophoresis at alkaline or acid pH. Electrophoresis is carried out in horizontal [135] or vertical [134] trays of starch (or in narrow columns of polyacrylamide [136]) gel, using a discontinuous buffer system (i.e. buffers of different compositions in bridging and electrolyte solutions). The vertical procedure (in which the gel is covered with petroleum jelly) is particularly useful for simultaneous comparative analysis of several samples (as indicated by the results of immunoglobulin sub-units, shown in Fig. 7.20).

Samples (approximately 0·05 ml) at concentrations of the order of 3–12 mg/ml are subjected to electrophoresis for periods of 15–24 hours under voltage gradients of the order of 5 V/cm at an ambient temperature of 4° C. After removing the petroleum jelly, the gel is sliced in a horizontal plane along its length (using a dermatome knife blade or some other slicing device). The cut gel surfaces are stained, for example, with Amido Black 10B [134].

Poulik [137] has developed a two-dimensional procedure involving conventional vertical starch-gel electrophoresis in a large tray ($22 \times 28 \times 0.6$ cm), accommodating about 500 ml of gel. In this method, the use of buffer containing 2-mercaptoethanol for electrophoresis in the second dimension permits sub-fractionation of the sub-units separated by electrophoresis (in the absence of reducing agent) in the first dimension (e.g. a complex electrophoretic pattern of the papain digestion products of rabbit γG globulin has been obtained in this manner, as shown in Fig. 7.21).

Vertical starch-gel electrophoresis of the light chains of human γG globulin (at concentrations of 3–12 mg/ml) in formate buffer (0·05 M formic acid/ 0·01 N NaOH, pH 2·9–3·0) in 8 M urea (at a voltage gradient of 6 V/cm for 16–18 hours at room temperature) using 0·2 M formic acid—0·08 N NaOH in the electrode vessels, produced a diffuse band [101]. A similar analysis, using 8 M urea and 0·035 M glycine buffer (pH 8·8) for the gels and 0·3 M boric acid— 0·06 N NaOH (pH 8·2) in the electrode vessels [139], however, resolved the pooled human γG globulin light chains into ten distinct components (designated B1–B10 by Cohen and Porter, and now presumably L1–L10), three of which moved toward the cathode and seven towards the anode.* Such patterns were obtained by analysis of the light chains from both electrophoretically 'fast' and 'slow' human γG globulin and from other immunoglobulins (e.g. γM) as shown in Fig. 7.20. Individual bands, eluted from the starch-gel and re-run under similar conditions, moved as individual components with the same mobility as shown originally, whereas in urea-formic

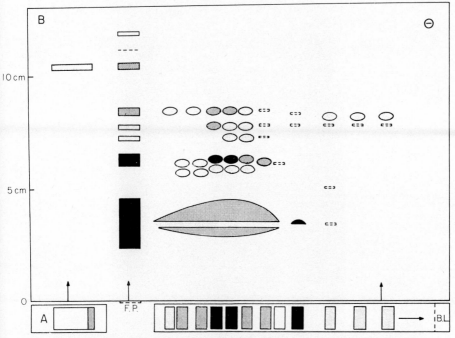

FIG. 7.21. Electrophoretic map of papain-digested rabbit γG globulin. (A) Drawing of the separated intermediates. (B) Drawing of the micro-subunits of the intermediates after electrophoresis in urea-2-mercaptoethanol starch gel. F.P. = filter-paper application spot control. B.L. = brown line.
(Reproduced by courtesy of Dr M.D. Poulik from Protides of Biological Fluids, Bruges (1264), p. 400. Ed. Peeters, H., Elsevier (Amsterdam).)

acid gels their mobility fell within the range of that of whole light chains. Light chains isolated from γG globulins of other species showed a similar heterogeneity (but variable band number and mobility) when analysed in urea-glycine gel (as shown in Fig. 7.20). Moreover, light chains separated from two different preparations of guinea-pig antibody against bovine serum

---

* Light (and heavy) polypeptide chains from specific anti-hapten antibodies and from γG globulins of normal rabbit serum have also been resolved into distinct multiple components by disc electrophoresis on polyacrylamide gels in the presence of urea [438].

albumin (isolated from different antisera) were found (in urea-glycine gel) to contain all the bands of normal guinea-pig γG globulin light chains, but in different relative intensity (as also shown in Fig. 7.20). In contrast,

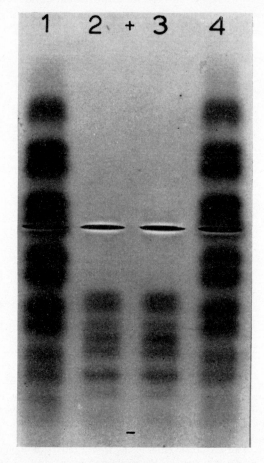

FIG. 7.22. Electrophoresis in alkaline-urea starch gels of purified light chains of partially reduced proteins. 1, 4. Normal human γG globulin light chains. 2. Human 7S γA myeloma globulin light chains. 3. Human 17S γA myeloma globulin light chains.

(Reproduced by courtesy of Drs J.P.Vaerman, H.H.Fudenberg, C.Vaerman and W.J.Mandy from *Immunochemistry* (1965), **2**, 263.)

the light chains of human myeloma γG globulins were found to be homogeneous in urea starch gels at alkaline pH (7–8), as well as at acid pH. The mobilities of the bands shown by such light chains (and by the light chains from γA myeloma and γM globulins) were unrelated to those of the parent proteins, but appeared to correspond to one or other of the components (B1–B10) of normal γG globulin light chains (as indicated by Fig. 7.20). No consistent correlation was found between the antigenic type (K or L) of the light chains and their electrophoretic mobility, despite the differences in amino-acid compositions (after 24 hours acid hydrolysis) of the myeloma light chains of different mobility.

In contrast to the findings of Cohen & Porter [139], Vaerman *et al* [140] have observed sharp bands in the urea starch-gel (pH 7 or 8) patterns of the light chains of partially reduced γA myeloma proteins (as shown in Fig. 7.22). Moreover, the mobility of these bands appeared to be unrelated to those of normal human γG globulin light chains. These investigators have obtained evidence from starch-gel electrophoresis in support of the hypothesis that the heterogeneity shown by preparations of normal and pathological γA globulins is due to polymerization of the 7S form.

The heavy chains of normal human γG globulin migrate as diffuse bands in urea-glycine starch gels (at pH 7–8), showing approximately the same spread as the parent γG globulin. The heavy chains from electrophoretically fast ($γ_1$) and slow ($γ_2$) sub-fractions of normal human γG globulin are, however, somewhat less heterogeneous and have the same relative mobilities as the parent molecules (see Fig. 7.20) as do heavy chains from myeloma γG globulins (when analysed on polyacrylamide gels in 8 M urea-0·05 M tris buffer, pH 8·8).

Many attempts have been made to explain the reason for the multiple banding observed in the urea-glycine starch-gel patterns of normal γG globulin light chains. Cohen & Porter [139] have carried out experiments which indicate that the effect was not an artefact. Furthermore, the same workers have obtained evidence against the effect being due to unequal reduction of light chains, variable hydrolysis of amide groups during fractionation of the chains in 1 N acetic acid, or to reaction of the amino groups with cyanate which is in equilibrium with urea at neutral and alkaline pH. Consequently, they [139] have suggested on the basis of their urea starch-gel analyses of the light chains isolated from γG myeloma globulins, and from the serum γG globulin of a colostrum-deprived calf, that the complexity of the light chain pattern possibly reflects cellular differentiation. Feinstein [141], however, has recently offered an interesting explanation for the origin of the banding patterns of the immuno-globulin light chains, as a result of observations using charged thiol reagents. He has demonstrated (as shown in Fig. 7.23) that the addition of a single carboxyl group to one light chain of a Bence–Jones protein (which usually gives one band on electrophoresis) alters its pattern by a single band spacing, as would be expected if light chains in the electrophoretic medium were of almost identical size and shape. Chains with identical net charge travel as a single band, even where they differ in amino-acid composition (such as is now known to occur within the N-terminal portion of different Bence-Jones proteins, as is shown in Fig. 7.33). Electrophoresis was performed in starch gel containing glycine buffer (0·05 M, pH 8·5) with 8 M urea. The charge increment was added to several Bence–Jones proteins by carboxymethylation of a cysteine residue with iodoacetate

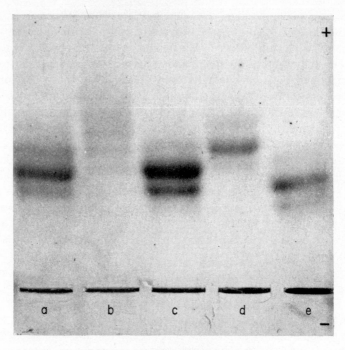

FIG. 7.23. Urea starch-gel electrophoretic patterns.

(i) Effect of carboxymethylation of a cysteine residue on the electrophoretic pattern of a Bence-Jones protein (type L): (a) iodoacetamide treated, reduced and iodacetate treated; (b) randomly carboxymethylated; (c) iodoacetate treated, reduced and iodoacetamide treated; (d) reduced and iodoacetate treated; (e) reduced and iodacetamide treated.

(0·3 M), following reduction with 2-mercaptoethanol (0·15 M) for 1 hour in tris buffer, pH 8·2; alkylation with uncharged iodoacetamide (0·25 M) served as a control [141]. Quantitative estimation of the amount of carboxymethyl-cysteine liberated after hydrolysis *in vacuo* with 6 N HCl at 106° C for 24 hours, confirmed that a single charge had been introduced into a peptide light chain. Furthermore, the banded patterns of normal light chains were simulated (see Fig. 7.23) by random introduction of carboxyl groups into

Bence-Jones protein, after reduction, by prolonged treatment with iodoacetate at pH 10. Similar studies have been carried out using heavy chains from pathological γG, γA and γM globulins. It is also interesting to note that *rabbit* Fab fragments yield urea starch-gel electrophoresis band patterns [142] of similar

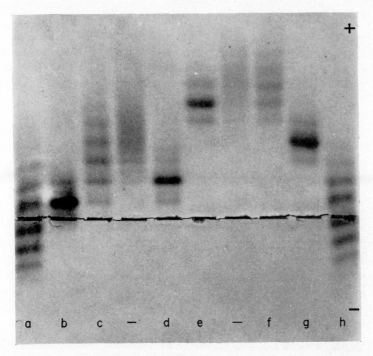

FIG. 7.23

(ii) Electrophoretic patterns: (a) and (h), light chains isolated from normal human γG globulin; (b) Bence-Jones protein (type K) reduced and iodoacetamide treated; (c) Bence-Jones protein (type K) randomly carboxymethylated; (d) Bence-Jones protein (type K) reduced and iodoacetate treated; (e) Bence-Jones protein (type L) reduced and iodoacetate treated; (f) Bence-Jones protein (type L) randomly carboxymethylated; (g) Bence-Jones protein (type L) reduced and iodoacetamide treated. Electrophoresis in starch gel containing glycine buffer (pH 8·5; 0·05 M) and 8 M urea.

(Reproduced by courtesy of Dr A.Feinstein from *Nature, Lond.* (1966), **210**, 135.)

spacing to that shown by the light chains and Fd portions (of heavy chains) within such fragments.

The use of radioactive isotopically labelled iodoacetate as carboxymethylating agent in this procedure offers a valuable method for locating and estimating sulphydryl groups in heterogeneous systems, as these can be titrated separately after resolving the various components by urea starch-gel electro-

G*

phoresis. In this connection, it is worth noting that Feinstein [141] has successfully used electrophoresis in agar gel cooled with petroleum ether [143] to measure mobility changes in light chains following reduction and carboxymethylation. This technique has the advantage of requiring very little material (e.g. 10 μl of a 1 per cent w/v protein solution), and it provides results in an hour.

Substitution of thiol groups by charged alkylating reagents also influences the ion-exchange chromatographic properties of immunoglobulin sub-units, as might be expected. For instance, Franklin & Stanworth [144] have shown that reductive cleavage products of γM globulins which have been alkylated by iodoacetate are eluted from DEAE-cellulose columns (using the Sober–Peterson [110] stepwise procedure) in the same buffer (0·05 M sodium dihydrogen phosphate) as that removing any unchanged parent γM globulin. In contrast, sub-units alkylated by iodoacetamide are eluted in the first solvent (phosphate buffer, 0·01 M, pH 7·5), well clear of contamination by intact γM globulin. Obviously, therefore, the latter reagent should be chosen for alkylation of γM globulin sub-units, where their subsequent isolation by DEAE-cellulose chromatography is intended.

Starch gel electrophoresis has been used in the characterization of the products of proteolytic cleavage of immunoglobulins. For example [97, 98], it has been applied to the analysis of papain digests (in the presence and absence of cysteine) of human γG globulins from normal (Cohn fraction II) and pathological myeloma proteins. As indicated in Fig. 7.24, the Fc fragments of both normal and myeloma γG globulins (after digestion with papain for 18 hours at 37° C) resolve into a series of bands (nine to eleven in number), the mobility and intensity of which depend on the inclusion or omission of cysteine in the digestion mixtures. The three faster-moving bands (and a fourth, demonstrable at high sample concentrations, i.e. containing 4–5 per cent sub-component) were only observed in papain digests in the presence of cysteine and were associated with the Fc′ fragment referred to earlier (in section B1). (Details of the various methods employed in the isolation of this 2·1S fragment, which is antigenically related to the 3·5S Fc piece of human γG globulin, are given on page 154, section B1).

Starch-gel electrophoresis has also been employed for the *preparation* of immunoglobulin sub-units. For example, Goodman [147] used this method to recover immunologically active non-dialysable fragments (2·3–3·2S) from peptic digests of the papain Fc fragment of rabbit γG globulin. After starchgel electrophoresis in 0·2 M sodium borate buffer (pH 8·4), at a potential difference of 250 V for 15 hours at room temperature, the separated bands were located by staining a thin slice of the gel. Sections of the gel corresponding to the positions of the bands were then excised and minced, and the protein eluted from them by electrodialysis [148]. Gel filtration (or ion-exchange chromatography), however, offers a more practicable method of isolating immunoglobulin sub-units, whether these be polypeptide chains (as outlined in section B1) or low molecular weight peptides (as will be described later).

Gel filtration

The use of gel filtration on columns of Sephadex G100, followed by automatic effluent monitoring, as a means of assessing the extent of proteolysis of γG globulins, has already been indicated [58] (see Fig. 7.15). Fragments devoid

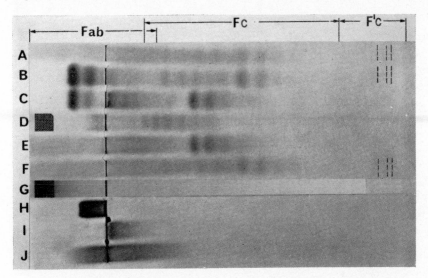

FIG. 7.24. Comparative starch-gel electrophoresis of human γG globulin (Cohn fraction II) and γG myeloma proteins ('T' and 'N') after digestion with papain in presence and absence of cysteine.

Human γG globulin: A, F, papain digest in presence of cysteine; E, papain digest in absence of cysteine; J. native protein.

Myeloma γG globulins: B, papain digest of protein T in presence of cysteine; C, papain digest of protein T in absence of cysteine; I, native protein T; G, papain digest of protein N in presence of cysteine; D, papain digest of protein N in absence of cysteine; H, native protein N.

(Reproduced by courtesy of Drs M.D.Poulik and J.Shuster from *Nature, Lond.* (1965), **207**, 1092.)

of aromatic amino acids can be located by measuring UV absorption at 230 mμ instead of the customary 280 mμ, or by the ninhydrin reaction [263] (the intensity of which varies directly as the concentration of $-NH_2$ groups and hence inversely as the size of the peptide, and so is useful only for peptides of low molecular weight). Carbohydrate distribution may be assessed by scanning for hexoses using the orcinol method [150]; where the column support is itself carbohydrate in nature (e.g. Sephadex gel, cellulose, substituted

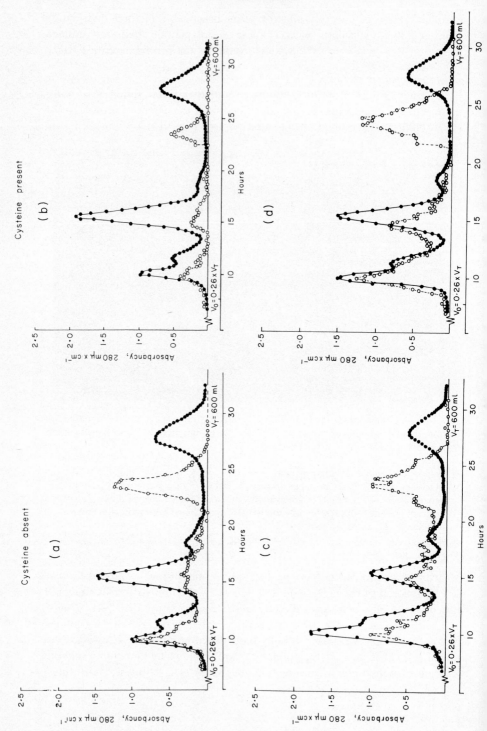

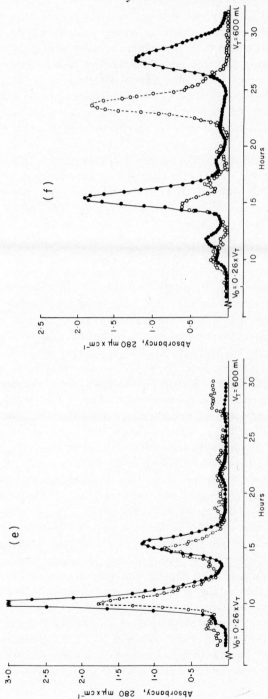

Fig. 7.25. Gel-filtration (Sephadex G150) patterns of proteolytic enzyme digests of human γG globulin (Cohn fraction II) in the presence and absence respectively of cysteine. ●, optical density at 280 mμ; ○, hexoses (orcinol reactivity). Digestion conditions: enzyme:substrate ratio 1:100. Incubation, 37° C, 30 hours in phosphate buffer (I = 0·1, pH 6·8) containing 0·002 M disodium salt of EDTA. In (b), (d) and (f), 0·01 M cysteine was also present.

Gel filtration: column (75 × 3·2 cm) eluted with 0·5 M tris-HCl buffer, pH 8·2, containing 0·002 M disodium salt of EDTA; flow-rate 2·5 cm/hour.

(a), (c) and (e) digestions in the absence of cysteine.

(Reproduced by kind permission of Dr H.Bennich.)

celluloses), it is essential to carry out assays of column eluates known to be free from any protein or peptide components in order to obtain a correction for traces of carbohydrate eluted from the column support medium. This is especially so when working with the carbohydrate-poor immunoglobulins (e.g. γG). For fragments, a preferred scanning method is the sensitive L-fucose assay procedure [151], which gives virtually nil readings for hexoses. As a class, immunoglobulins have a higher ratio of fucose to sialic acid [152] than most other serum proteins, and there are sensitive specific assay systems for both of these carbohydrates.

Typical results of chemical analyses of various enzymatic digests of human γG globulin are shown in Fig. 7.25. Other examples of the application of gel filtration, through Sephadex G75 and G100 in 1 N acetic or propionic acid, to the analysis of the products of proteolytic and reductive cleavage of γG globulins are presented in Figs. 7.9 and 7.17. This technique has also been applied to hapten interaction studies [153], in order to establish the location of the antigen-combining sites on the heavy or light chains of rabbit antibody (as will be considered further in section B3). In a similar type of application [154], synthetic polyacrylamide gel (Biogel P10) has been used in the characterization of the tryptic peptides from the active sites of rabbit antibody γG globulin molecules (identified by affinity labelling [250]).

Smaller peptide fragments of immunoglobulins are more readily separated by gel filtration on columns of Sephadex G25 or G10 or by ion-exchange chromatography (e.g. on Dowex 50 or Dowex 1, as described later). For instance, the low molecular weight (probably 2000–5000) fraction separated after the Fab and Fc fragments (and the undigested protein) from Sephadex G100 filtration of papain digests of human γG globulin (i.e. the material comprising the third peak of the patterns shown in Fig. 7.15) can be subfractionated by filtration through Sephadex G10 (as shown in Fig. 7.26a). As will be seen, the profile of the pattern thus obtained (by automatic effluent monitoring) was different when cysteine was included in the papain digestion. This can be attributed to the presence of peptides liberated when the papain-resistant form (see page 166) of human γG globulin is unfolded by the reductive treatment. Peptide differences can also be demonstrated by one-dimensional high-voltage electrophoresis at pH 3·5 (as shown in Fig. 7.26b), whereupon additional acidic spots are observed in digests incorporating cysteine.

Combination of gel filtration and peptide mapping techniques offers a useful means of reducing the complexity of the mixtures of peptides obtained by proteolysis of immunoglobulins (or their sub-units). For example, gel filtration of tryptic digests of oxidized samples of human γG globulin on Sephadex G25 provides the type of profile shown in Fig. 7.27a. Subsequent peptide-mapping (by paper-partition chromatography and high-voltage electrophoresis in directions at right-angles to each other [433]) provides in effect a

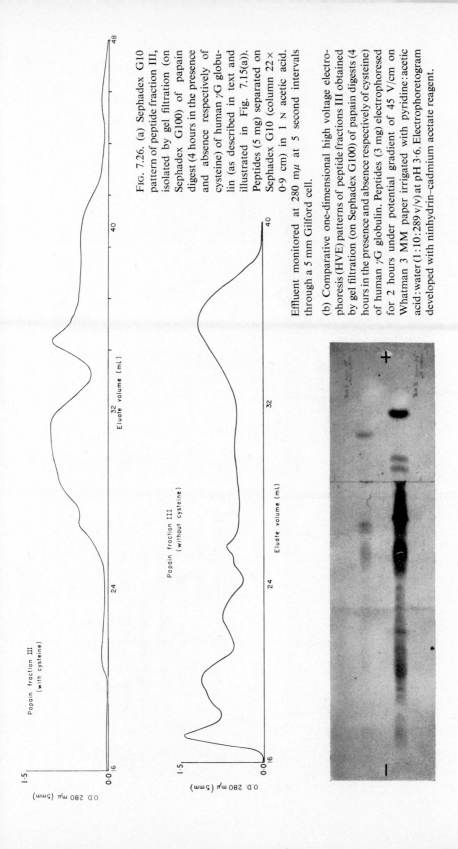

Fig. 7.26. (a) Sephadex G10 pattern of peptide fraction III, isolated by gel filtration (on Sephadex G100) of papain digest (4 hours in the presence and absence respectively of cysteine) of human γG globulin (as described in text and illustrated in Fig. 7.15(a)). Peptides (5 mg) separated on Sephadex G10 (column 22 × 0·9 cm) in 1 N acetic acid. Effluent monitored at 280 mμ at 5 second intervals through a 5 mm Gilford cell.

(b) Comparative one-dimensional high voltage electro-phoresis (HVE) patterns of peptide fractions III obtained by gel filtration (on Sephadex G100) of papain digests (4 hours in the presence and absence respectively of cysteine) of human γG globulin. Peptides (3 mg) electrophoresed for 2 hours under potential gradient of 45 V/cm on Whatman 3 MM paper irrigated with pyridine:acetic acid:water (1:10:289 v/v) at pH 3·6. Electrophoretogram developed with ninhydrin–cadmium acetate reagent.

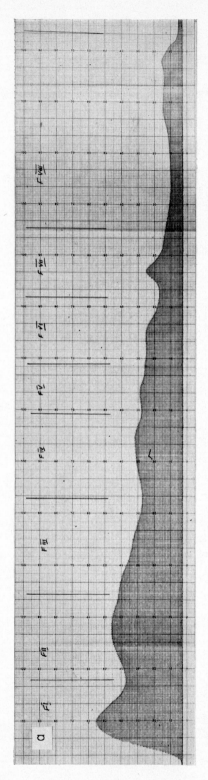

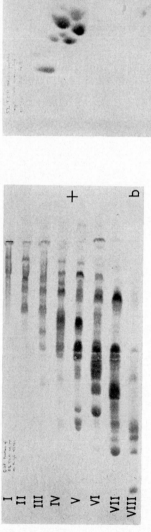

FIG. 7.27

(a) Sephadex G25 profile of tryptic peptides (soluble in 5 per cent trichloracetic acid) of human γG globulin (produced as described in text). Peptides (100 mg) separated on column (80 × 2 cm) in 0·2 M ammonia at flow-rate of 12 ml/hour. Effluent monitored at 280 mμ every 5 seconds through Gilford cell.

(b) One-dimensional HVE patterns of Sephadex G25 fractions concentrated (rotary evaporation), desalted and lyophilized. Portions (3 mg) analysed under conditions described in caption to Fig. 7.26 (b).

(c) Two-dimensional map of peptides recovered from Sephadex G25 fraction VIII using conditions described in caption to Fig. 7.30.

'three-dimensional' fingerprinting technique [155], in which the peptides are separated according to their size, partition coefficient and charge. That the preliminary separation on Sephadex reduces the complexity of the γG globulin digest is illustrated in Fig. 7.27b, which shows the one-dimensional high-voltage electrophoresis patterns of the various size-groups of peptides analysed after concentration of the combined column effluents by rotary evaporation at 37° C and subsequent deionization by passage through columns of ion-exchange resin (Dowex 50 × 2). A two-dimensional map of one of the fractions ('number VIII') is shown in Fig. 7.27c.

It is possible to discern differences in the peptide compositions of tryptic digests of oxidized γG globulins, even by one-dimensional high-voltage electro-

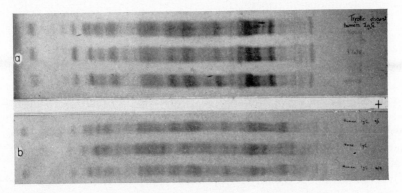

FIG. 7.28. Demonstration of isospecific (a) and heterospecific (b) differences in one-dimensional HVE patterns of tryptic peptides of oxidized γG globulins.
(a) Comparison of peptides of human γG globulins from three normal subjects.
(b) Comparison of peptides of human and horse γG globulins. Portions (2 mg) of peptides (soluble in 5 per cent trichloracetic acid) analysed under conditions similar to those employed in Fig. 7.26 (b).

phoresis. This is illustrated in Fig. 7.28, which demonstrates the detection of isospecific differences (Fig. 7.28a) between the γG globulins of three human subjects and species differences (Fig. 7.28b) between human and horse γG globulins.

Another combined gel-filtration and peptide-mapping technique, which has been applied to the peptides in a tryptic digest of the α chain of haemoglobin [156], involves the direct transfer of extruded zones (2 cm) from a narrow (3 mm internal bore) column of Sephadex G25 in phenol:acetic acid:water (1 : 1 : 1 w/v/v) to Whatman No. 3 MM paper, followed by paper-partition chromatography or two-dimensional mapping (i.e. paper chromatography followed by high-voltage electrophoresis). The use of the phenol:acetic acid: water system as displacing solvent in gel filtration of peptides has been shown [157] to counteract the retardation of aromatic peptides through adsorption on to the gel, thereby permitting an estimation of molecular size by this method. A newly developed lyophilic cross-linked dextran derivative (Sephadex LH-20, now available from Pharmacia AB) should also prove useful in avoiding this retardation.

The development of thin-layer chromatography on Sephadex (and other supporting media) for the separation of peptides should find application in the analysis of enzymatic digests of immunoglobulins. Ballieux [158] has successfully combined thin-layer chromatography and high-voltage electrophoresis at pH 3·5 in layers (0·2 mm thick) of Kieselgel G (Merck), to obtain well-defined peptide maps of tryptic digests of human γG globulin. A smaller number of spots was observed, however, than with the conventional 'fingerprinting' technique on paper.

To prepare samples for peptide mapping by the technique developed by Ingram [159], it is essential to ensure maximum and reproducible digestion of the protein, if representative fingerprints are to be obtained. This is accomplished by enzymatic digestion of protein molecules which have been unfolded by some form of denaturation treatment. Although some proteins (e.g. haemoglobins) may be sufficiently denatured by heating a solution (in a narrow tube) at pH 8·0 for 4 minutes at 90° C, followed by rapid cooling, this treatment is less satisfactory for immunoglobulins. These proteins have many disulphide bonds maintaining their tertiary structure (discussed in section C) and these bonds must be ruptured by oxidation or reduction.

It is not possible to identify glycopeptides in peptide analyses of proteolytic digests of oxidized proteins, since the methods presently available for identifying non-reducing carbohydrates on chromatograms all depend on oxidation (periodate-Schiff [160], periodate-silver oxide [161], periodate-benzidine [162] reagents) of a cis-glycol structure within the hexose molecule; which is destroyed equally well by the performic acid oxidation procedure. In such cases, it is necessary to denature the protein by the method of Ingram [159], and to subject it to extensive proteolytic digestion, by adding further amounts of enzyme after intervals of 4–5 hours. In the author's laboratory, improved degradation has been achieved by proteolytic digestion with trypsin or pronase (the proteolytic enzyme of *Streptomyces griseus*), under conditions of continual dialysis against a volatile buffer, e.g. ammonium acetate or carbonate. The dialysable peptides are recovered from the dialysable material by rotary evaporation, repeated twice to remove as much ammonium salt as possible. Peptides are recovered from the non-dialysable material by precipitation of undigested protein (and enzyme) with 5 per cent trichloracetic acid, and removal of the latter with ether, as described elsewhere.

Maximal enzymatic digestion of pituitary thyrotropin glycoprotein was achieved [163] by cleaving the disulphide bonds with sodium borohydride [164]. In a typical experiment, thyrotropin preparation (60 mg), dissolved in

6 M urea containing 0·02 per cent EDTA (15 ml) was reduced by the careful addition of sodium borohydride (60 mg) to the reaction mixture, which was gently stirred, and kept at 41° C under a stream of nitrogen for $1\frac{1}{2}$ hours; the temperature was rapidly reduced to 25° C and iodoacetic acid (45 mg) added; the solution was adjusted to pH 8·5 with 6 N HCl and alkylated for 20 minutes. The entire reaction mixture was then applied to a column (3·4 × 40 cm) of Sephadex G25 equilibrated with water. The reduced alkylated glycoprotein emerged unretarded, having been separated completely from urea and salts. Anfinsen & Haber [165] used a similar procedure to remove urea and salts, thus avoiding dialysis losses. It is probable that this would prove a satisfactory alternative method for treating immunoglobulins (or their major sub-units) prior to enzymatic digestion, particularly where studies of the glycopeptides are envisaged, since non-reducing carbohydrate terminal units are resistant to sodium borohydride under the conditions used.

A convenient oxidative procedure for denaturing immunoglobulins prior to tryptic digestion for peptide mapping, devised by Hirs [166], uses performic acid. The protein (40 mg), dissolved in formic acid (1 ml) is treated with performic acid solution (1·2 ml) in an ice-bath for 2·5 hr. The performic acid solution is prepared by oxidizing formic acid (9·5 ml) with hydrogen peroxide (100 vol., 30 per cent solution, 0·5 ml) at room temperature for 2·5 hr. The excess reagents may be removed from the oxidized protein by dialysis against distilled water, or by lyophilization. Kimmel *et al* [167] recommend an alternative procedure for treatment of oxidized protein (e.g. papain) prior to proteolytic digestion for peptide sequence studies. The oxidized protein (in a total volume of 30 ml) is precipitated by the addition of 25 per cent trichloracetic acid solution (20 ml); the precipitate is collected by centrifugation and washed (× 5) with portions (10 ml) of 10 per cent trichloracetic acid, or until the washings give a negative test for peroxide with starch-potassium iodide test paper. The precipitate is then washed with portions (50 ml) of absolute ethanol (× 3) followed by ether (× 3) and air-dried at room temperature for several days. It has been shown by Smith *et al* [168] that if lyophilized directly after oxidation, the oxidized protein contained enough residual peroxide to interfere seriously with the subsequent enzymic proteolysis.

After equilibrating with 0·2 M ammonium acetate or carbonate buffer (pH 8·6–8·8) (2 ml), the oxidized protein is incubated with trypsin (at a 1/100 enzyme/substrate ratio) at 37° C for 16 hours. The volatile buffer is removed by rotary evaporation, and the residue (dissolved if necessary in the minimum volume of distilled water) extracted with an equal volume of 10 per cent trichloracetic acid (TCA) solution. The precipitate is collected by centrifugation, re-extracted (× 2) with an equal volume of 5 per cent TCA solution, and the combined aqueous extracts are washed (at least × 3) with an equal volume of ether (to remove TCA), and concentrated by rotary evaporation or partial freeze-drying.

For desalting prior to chromatography, the peptide solution (adjusted to pH 3·3 with dilute acetic acid) is applied to a column of ion-exchange resin (e.g. Dowex 50×2 in the ammonium cycle) and subsequently eluted at alkaline pH with 0·5 N ammonium hydroxide. (After use, the column may be regenerated by irrigating with 1 N NH_4OH.)

Peptides may be separated by two-dimensional chromatography-electrophoresis, or by two-dimensional electrophoresis, on Whatman No. 3 MM filter-paper (57×46 cm). In the former technique, the sample (3 mg), dissolved in pyridine : acetic acid : water (1 : 10 : 289, pH 3·5, 0·03 ml) is applied as a band (1 cm long) on the base-line. Separation is achieved by descending chromatography in the first direction for 18 hours, using 1-butanol : acetic acid : water (12 : 3 : 5), and in the second direction (at right-angles to the first) by electrophoresis (e.g. 2000–4000 V and ca. 100 mA for 1–2 hr) in pyridine : acetic acid : water (1 : 10 : 289, pH 3·5). It is preferable to carry out partition chromatography *prior to* electrophoresis, as residual traces of salts are removed by this procedure. An alternative electrophoresis step may be made in pyridine : acetic acid : water (10 : 0·4 : 90, pH 6·5). Two-dimensional electrophoresis may be carried out in, for example [179], pyridine : acetic acid : water (25 : 25 : 950, pH 4·7), followed in the second direction (at right-angles to the first) in acetic acid : 88 per cent formic acid : water (87 : 25 : 888, pH 1·9).

After drying, the chromatogram is revealed by reaction with ninhydrin [149]. The colour of the transient purple ninhydrin chromophore may be stabilized by incorporating cadmium acetate into the spray reagent. A convenient reagent [170] is prepared *immediately before use* by mixing freshly prepared ninhydrin (1 per cent w/v in acetone) solution (100 ml) with cadmium acetate (0·5 per cent w/v in water, 75 ml, and glacial acetic acid, 25 ml) solution (15 ml). The cadmium acetate stock solution may be stored, but the ninhydrin solution is unstable and is prepared as required. The ninhydrin chromophore is developed at 80° C for about 20 minutes. The maps may be preserved by wrapping in polythene sheeting, and stored at 4° C. Colour photography (on Kodak Ektachrome type B film) provides a valuable additional record of the peptide maps.

It is sometimes useful to employ stains for specific amino acids in peptide mapping. Baglioni [171] describes the use of a sequence of sprays on the same chromatogram. A convenient spray sequence is (i) isatin, revealing proline and hydroxy-proline; (ii) ninhydrin, reacting with N-terminal amino acids and ε-amino groups of lysine; the ninhydrin colour being bleached by treatment with acetone; (iii) *p*-dimethylaminobenzaldehyde, which gives the pink colour due to tryptophane; (iv) Sakaguchi reagent (consisting of α-naphthol followed by sodium hypochlorite or hypobromite), giving the deep red colour due to arginine and (v) Pauly reagent, for histidine. A similar sequential identification procedure for amino-acid location in peptides has been described by Easley [172].

The presence of glycopeptides in peptide maps (and other chromatograms) may be established by the use of specific spray reagents. One of the most

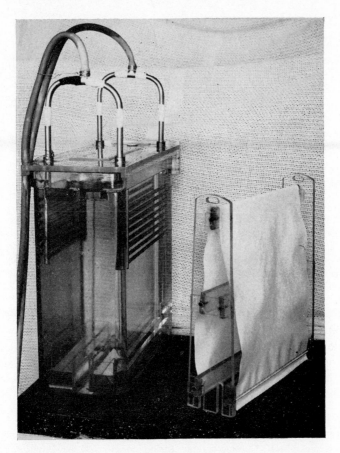

FIG. 7.29. Vertical peptide mapping apparatus adapted from standard glass chromatography tanks (supplied by Shandon Scientific Co. Ltd., London).

satisfactory is the periodate-benzidine reagent of Mowery [162]. The periodate reagent is prepared by dissolving sodium metaperiodate, $NaIO_4$ (0·645 g) in distilled water (75 ml) and adding tertiary-butanol (25 ml) to the solution. The benzidine reagent comprises benzidine (3 millimoles) dissolved in tertiary-butanol (50 ml), mixed as required with ammonium nitrate (60 millimoles) in

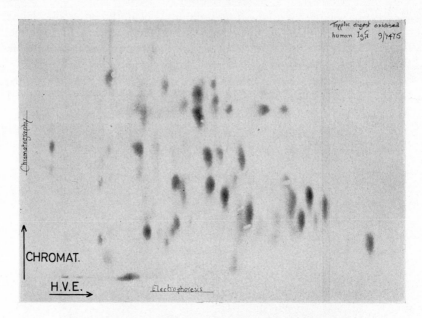

Fig. 7.30. Typical two-dimensional fingerprint of peptides (soluble in 5 per cent tri-chloracetic acid) derived from tryptic digestion of oxidized human γG globulin. Sample (3 mg) applied to Whatman 3 MM paper. Descending chromatography in n-butanol:acetic acid:water (120:30:50) for 18 hours at 20° C, followed by high-voltage electrophoresis for 1·5 hours, potential gradient 45 V/cm, in pyridine:acetic acid:water (1:10:289), pH 3·5. Map developed with ninhydrin–cadmium acetate spray.

water (50 ml). In practice, the chromatogram is sprayed on *both sides* with the periodate reagent and allowed to oxidize at room temperature for 30 minutes. The chromatogram is then heavily sprayed on both sides of the paper with the benzidine reagent, when glycopeptides are revealed as white spots on a blue background.

Fig. 7.31. Comparative tryptic peptide maps of immunoglobulins.
(a) (i) Tryptic peptide maps of four Bence-Jones proteins ('Ag', 'Lo', 'Mo' and 'Ln') of antigenic type K. Chromatography (in n-butanol:acetic acid:water 4:1:5) in vertical direction; high-voltage electrophoresis (for 1 hour at 2000 V in pyridine:acetic acid:water 1:10:289, pH 3·7) in horizontal direction, cathode to right. Circled 'x' on vertical axis marks position of phenol red indicator after chromato-graphy. Chromatograms developed with ninhydrin.
(a) (ii) Tryptic peptide maps of four Bence-Jones proteins ('Sh', 'Ol', 'Ha' and 'Bo') of antigenic type L. Conditions as described above. Circled peptides gave positive arginine test.
(Reproduced by permission of Drs F.W.Putnam and C.W.Easley from *J. biol. Chem.* (1965), **240**, 1626.)

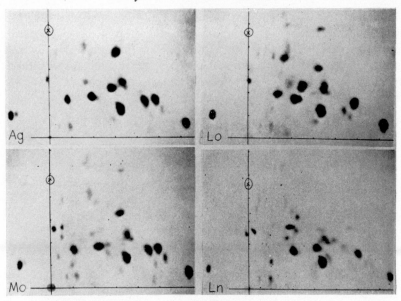

FIG. 7.31 (a) (i)

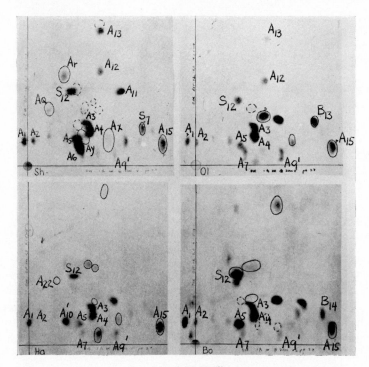

FIG. 7.31 (a) (ii)

Equipment for electrophoresis is commercially available, and may be of vertical or horizontal design. In the former, the sheet of paper is cooled by immersion in a solvent such as the light petroleum fraction, 'Varsol', which is immiscible with both sample and buffer used. In the horizontal apparatus, the paper is cooled between water-cooled metal plates. In the author's laboratory,

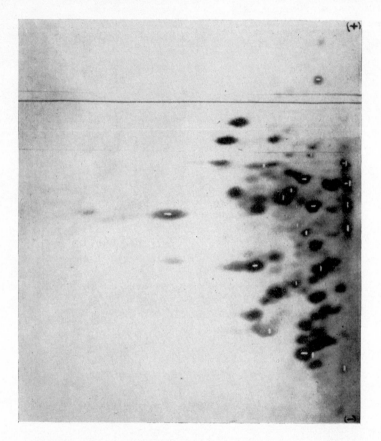

FIG. 7.31 (b) (ii) Peptide map of heavy chains of a γA myeloma globulin (key as above).

equipment of vertical design has been made by adapting standard glass chromatography tanks. Extension pieces of Whatman 3 MM paper are sewn to the chromatogram, which is draped over a Perspex frame (as shown in Fig. 7.29). In Fig. 7.30 are shown typical 'fingerprints' of tryptic digests of human and horse γG globulins, obtained by using this equipment for the separation in the second direction, following descending partition chromatography in the first direction. (The patterns shown in Fig. 7.26, 7.27 and 7.28 were also obtained using the apparatus shown in Fig. 7.29.)

Peptide mapping of the immunoglobulins is, of course, simplified by the examination of digests of their proteolytic or reductive cleavage fragments.

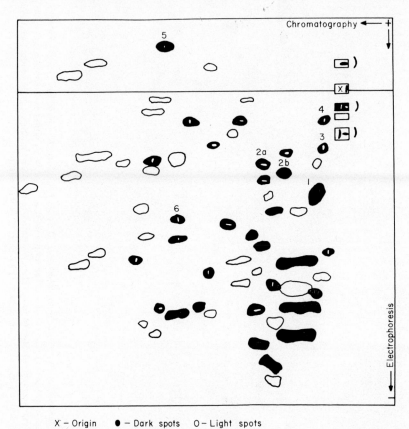

X — Origin   ● — Dark spots   O — Light spots

FIG. 7.31

(b) (iii) Drawing of composite peptide map of heavy chains of γM globulin (key as above).

(Reproduced by courtesy of Drs B.Frangione and E.C.Franklin from *Arch. biochem. Biophys.* (1965), **111**, 603.)

The oxidized Fab fragments of rabbit and human γG globulin are less readily digested by trypsin or chymotrypsin, however, than are the Fc fragments. Pepsin and pronase, on the other hand, effect extensive digestion of rabbit Fab pieces, and trypsin and chymotrypsin readily degrade the oxidized polypeptide *chains* of immunoglobulins.

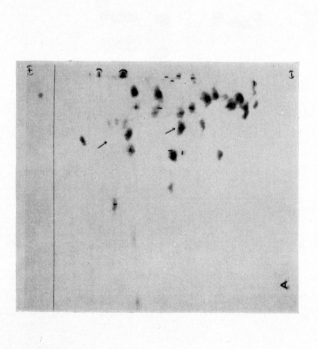

Fɪɢ. 7.31

(b) (i) Representative tryptic peptide maps of (A) heavy chains from normal human γG globulin which was Gm(a + b + f +); (B) heavy chains from γG myeloma globulin, which was Gm(a + b − f −). Technique of Katz *et al* [433] employed; chromatographic separation being carried out prior to high-voltage electrophoresis. Map developed with ninhydrin, Sakaguchi arginine reagent and Pauly reagent (for histidine). Key for specifically stained spots: —, arginine; /, histidine;), carbohydrate.

Peptide mapping has provided confirmatory evidence of the structural similarities between the light chains [174] of the various immunoglobulin classes (γG, γM, γA, etc.), whilst demonstrating marked differences in their heavy chains [175] (as is illustrated schematically in Fig. 7.1). Similarly, it has also been used to substantiate the composition of the polypeptide chains of the Fab and Fc fragments of human γG globulins [74]; and the antigenic similarities between the Bence–Jones proteins and the light chains of the corresponding serum myeloma γG [176] or γA [177] globulins. It has also revealed marked structural differences between Bence–Jones proteins or myeloma γG globulin light chains [178, 179] of the κ and λ types, only a few spots being observed as common to the tryptic digest patterns of both types of light chain. (These differences have since been confirmed by sequential amino-acid analysis, as will be outlined in the next sub-section.) As mentioned previously, the 'finger-printing' technique has also been employed to demonstrate fine structural differences between the heavy chains and Fc fragments of Gm(a+) and Gm(a−), and of Gm(b+) and Gm(b−) γG globulins [25, 421, 422]; and recently, between γG globulins of different InV type [181, 427].

Inevitably, too, peptide mapping has found wide application in attempts to define antibody specificity in primary structural terms. Initial investigations [182] failed to distinguish differences between rabbit antibodies of different specificities. More recent studies have, however, demonstrated differences in amino-acid composition between rabbit antibodies directed against haptenic groups of different charge [183]. Moreover, similar differences have been demonstrated by quantitative amino-acid analysis [184]. Nevertheless, it will be necessary to carry out sequential analysis in order to obtain unequivocal evidence of a relationship between antibody activity and primary structure.

Representative peptide maps of tryptic digests of immunoglobulin subunits are shown in Figs. 7.31 and 7.32. Figure 7.31 includes maps obtained by the chromatography/high voltage electrophoresis technique, whilst the patterns shown in Fig. 7.32 were obtained by two-dimensional high-voltage electrophoresis [74] (in pyridine : acetic acid : water 25 : 25 : 950, pH 4·7, in the first dimension, and in acetic acid : 88 per cent formic acid : water 87 : 25 : 888, pH 1·9, in the second dimension). The presence of spots appearing in the same places in peptide maps of both heavy and light chains [74] in a given solvent sequence raises the possibility that the chains have certain amino-acid sequences in common. Moreover, comparison of the map of peptides from whole heavy chains with those from the corresponding Fc fragments permits examination of the peptides of the Fd fragments (see Fig. 7.6 for nomenclature) without the problem of isolating this part of the molecule. For example, Frangione & Franklin [185] have adopted this

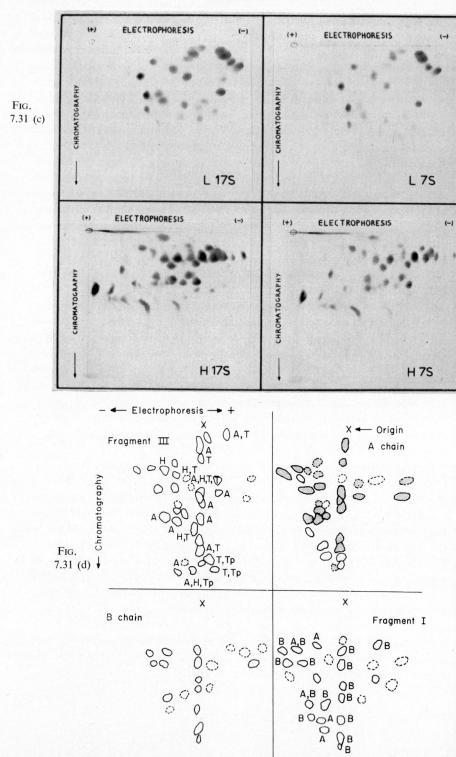

FIG.
7.31 (c)

FIG.
7.31 (d)

approach to demonstrate that much of the variability of different myeloma γG globulins resides in the Fd parts of the molecules.

(b) Chemical analysis of immunoglobulin sub-units

Chemical analysis of *whole* immunoglobulin molecules provides information of limited value, because of the great complexity of these glycoproteins. Thus, although qualitatively the same amino acids and carbohydrate constituents are present in the three principal groups (γG, γM and γA) of immuno- globulins of human and other mammalian species so far analysed, the relative proportions of these constituents vary considerably among the classes. For example, the human γG globulins are relatively poorer in carbohydrates, but richer in lysine than the γM or γA globulins. For meaningful structural studies, well-characterized polypeptide fragments and sub-units must be isolated in a high state of purity. Two main approaches have been adopted: (i) analysis of low molecular weight fragments of particular interest (e.g. portions of the molecule showing specific biological activities) which have been isolated and partially characterized by the methods already indicated in this section; (ii) systematic sequential analysis of well-defined sub-units (e.g. the composite polypeptide chains). Each of these approaches relies on qualita- tive and quantitative amino-acid estimations, terminal amino-acid assay (as will be outlined) and the determination of the location, composition and sequence of the carbohydrate prosthetic groups.

FIG. 31(c) Tryptic peptide maps of isolated light and heavy polypeptide chains of γA myeloma globulins (17S and 7S). Chromatography in n-butanol:acetic acid:water (120: 30:50) for 24 hours at 4° C, followed by high-voltage electrophoresis for 100 minutes under voltage gradient of 35 V/cm, in pyridine:acetic acid:water (1:10:289), pH 3·7, using the method of Katz *et al* [433]. Chromatograms developed (by dipping) in 0·25 per cent ninhydrin in dry acetone or by spraying with ninhydrin. (Reproduced by courtesy of Drs J.P.Vaerman, H.H.Fudenberg, C.Vaerman and W.J. Mandy for *Immunochemistry* (1965), **2**, 263.)

(d) Tracings of tryptic peptide maps of S-carboxymethylated chains and fragments of rabbit γG globulin. High-voltage electrophoresis at pH 6·5 in 0·2 M pyridine acetate for 3 hours at a potential gradient of 10 V/cm, followed by chromatography for 14 hours in pyridine:n-butanol:acetic acid:water (50:75:15:60). Chromatograms developed by spraying with ninhydrin or specific sprays. Peptides present in all patterns traced with smooth line. Peptides observed only occasionally indicated by dashed line. Peptides in maps of fragment III (i.e. Fc) containing specific amino acids indicated by capital letters: A, arginine; H, histidine; T, tyrosine; TP, tryptophane. Peptides in maps of 'A' (i.e. heavy) chain found also in maps of 'frag- ment III' (i.e. Fc) are shaded. Peptides in 'Fragment I' (i.e. Fab) which are derived from 'B' (i.e. light) chains are indicated by letter B; peptides from 'A' (i.e. heavy) chains are indicated by letter A. Other even fainter areas were observed with greater sample loads in maps of 'B' (light) and 'A' (heavy) chains of fragment I(Fab). (Reproduced by courtesy of Dr C.A.Nelson, M.E.Noelken, C.E.Buckley, C.Tanford and R.L.Hill from *Biochemistry* (1965), **4**, 1418.)

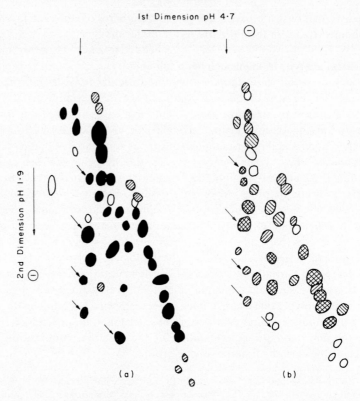

FIG. 7.32. Composite drawings of tryptic peptide maps obtained by two-dimensional high-voltage electrophoresis (as described in text).

(a) Light (L) chain patterns (i.e. composite drawings of maps of human γG globulin light (L) chains Fab(ii) fractions).

▨ Peptides present in patterns of heavy (H) chains and Fab(ii) fractions.

☐ Peptides present in light chains but not found in Fab(ii) fractions.

■ Peptides present in both light chains and in Fab(ii) fractions.

(b) Heavy (H) chain patterns (i.e. composite drawings of maps of human γG globulin heavy (H) chains, Fab(i) fraction and Fc fragment).

▨ Peptides of heavy chains present in Fc fragment but not found in Fab(i) fragment.

▨ Peptides of heavy chains present in Fab(i) fragment but not found in Fc fragment.

☐ Peptides present in hydrolysates of heavy chains, but not found in Fab(i) nor in Fc fragments.

▩ Peptides of heavy (H) chains present in both Fab(i) and Fc fragments.

Diagonal arrows indicate ninhydrin-positive spots which were common to patterns of both light and heavy chains. Vertical arrows indicate positions of origins.

(Reproduced by courtesy of Drs M. Fougereau and G. M. Edelman from *J. exp. Med.* (1965), **121**, 373.)

The analytical data appertaining to whole immunoglobulins which have been characterized in any detail [1, 186, 187, 188, 189, 213] are presented in Tables 7.5, 7.6 and 7.7. The amino-acid compositions of the heavy and light chains of various immunoglobulins are given in Tables 7.8 and 7.9 (whilst

TABLE 7.5

Amino-acid compositions of the main classes of human immunoglobulins (reproduced from data in *Clin. Chim. Acta* (1964) **10**, 293, by permission of Drs N.Heimberger, K.Heide, H.Haupt and H.E.Schultze)

	γG globulin (mol. wt. 160×10^3)		γM globulin (mol. wt. 10^7)		γA globulin (mol. wt. 160×10^3)	
	% w/w	moles/mole	% w/w	moles/mole	% w/w	moles/mole
Lysine	6·96	87	4·88	381	4·57	57
Histidine	2·28	27	1·83	133	1·93	23
Ammonia	1·46	146	1·23	768	2·02	202
Arginine	4·02	41	5·05	324	4·55	47
Aspartic	7·69	107	7·12	619	6·15	86
Threonine	7·18	114	7·23	716	7·65	121
Serine	9·69	178	6·45	799	7·93	146
Glutamic acid	11·26	140	10·62	825	10·52	130
Proline	6·05	100	5·27	544	6·26	104
Glycine	3·35	84	3·06	528	3·22	90
Alanine	3·18	72	3·51	493	3·87	87
½ (Cystine)	2·20	34	1·58	155	2·10	33
Valine	8·10	131	6·49	655	6·00	97
Methionine	0·85	10	1·16	89	0·80	10
Isoleucine	2·14	30	2·70	239	1·74	25
Leucine	7·21	102	6·33	560	7·76	110
Tyrosine	5·97	62	4·21	258	4·38	43
Phenylalanine	4·29	47	3·96	269	3·66	40
Tryptophane	3·83	33	2·86	152	3·30	28
Total	97·71	1552	85·98	8507	88·41	1479
Hexoses	1·10	10	5·40	300	3·20	28
Acetyl hexosamine	1·30	9	4·40	199	2·90	21
N-acetyl neuraminic acid	0·30	1–2	1·30	42	1·80	9
Fucose	0·20	2	0·70	42	0·22	2
Total	100·61		97·78		96·53	

TABLE 7.6

Carbohydrate compositions of the main classes of human immunoglobulins (moles/mole)

Constituent	γG (160,000)					γA (160,000)	γM (960,000)
Mannose	5·07	*7·25	†9·25	5·75	10·67	14·2	174
Galactose	3·02	3·62	4·62	3·45		14·2	87
Fucose	2·1	2·04	1·95	2·6	2·92	2·1	40
N-acetyl glucosamine	8·43	9·65	9·65	10·1	10·77	21·0	144
N-acetyl neuraminic acid	1·03	0·93	2·43	0·89	0·95	9·3	41·3
Reference	8	437	437	217	436	186	8

* Electrophoretically slower fraction ⎱ Electrophoresis in polyvinyl
† Electrophoretically faster fraction ⎰ chloride, pH 8·6

TABLE 7.7

Amino-acid analysis of immunoglobulins

(reproduced by courtesy of Professors S. Cohen & R.R. Porter
from *Adv. Immunol.* (1964) **4**, 287)

Amino acid	Amino-acid residue (g/100 g protein)				
	Rabbit IgG	Human IgG	Human IgM	Horse IgG	Horse IgA (T)*
Lysine	5·76	7·06	4·91	6·77	6·50
Histidine	1·73	2·44	1·98	2·58	2·57
Arginine	4·42	4·02	4·75	3·34	3·02
Aspartic acid	8·08	7·77	6·95	7·25	7·31
Threonine	10·37	7·04	6·17	8·31	7·13
Serine	8·32	9·13	6·58	9·68	9·29
Glutamic acid	11·05	11·18	9·92	10·27	9·36
Proline	6·79	6·40	4·95	6·02	6·52
Glycine	3·98	3·37	2·91	3·68	3·53
Alanine	3·71	3·29	3·12	3·60	3·28
Valine	8·36	7·92	5·77	8·14	7·74
Methionine	1·13	0·93	1·02	0·78	0·59
Isoleucine	3·49	2·16	2·83	3·14	2·70
Leucine	6·73	7·40	6·09	6·63	6·51
Tyrosine	6·17	5·76	5·44	5·55	4·93
Phenylalanine	4·15	4·07	3·85	3·79	3·47
Cystine	2·63	2·07	2·30	2·08	1·90
Tryptophan	2·90	2·63	2·47	2·57	2·47
Carbohydrate	2·40	2·80	12·30	2·40	4·90
	101·6	97·4	95·70	97·80	94·80

*Now referred to as IgG(T) [189].

data from analyses of purified antibodies are given later in Tables 7.17 and 7.18 in section B3a). As will be noted from Table 7.9, there is a close similarity between the compositions of the light chains of human γG and γM globulins, in contrast to the obvious differences between the heavy chains. This provides evidence in support of the findings of comparative antigenic analyses (illustrated schematically in Fig. 7.1), as well as of those obtained by peptide mapping and urea-starch-gel electrophoresis (discussed earlier in this section).

TABLE 7.8

Comparison of the amino-acid composition of the polypeptide chains of the immunoglobulins of various species (reproduced by courtesy of Professors S. Cohen and R.R. Porter from *Adv. Immunol.* (1964) **4**, 287)

(a) Amino-acid composition of heavy chains

| | Residues/50,000 g | | | | |
	Rabbit IgG	Human IgG	Human IgM	Horse IgG	Horse IgA (T)*
Lysine	23	29	20	26	27
Histidine	7	10	7	10	12
Arginine	16	12	18	10	10
Aspartic acid	33	33	34	30	34
Threonine	49	34	38	37	33
Serine	49	50	42	45	46
Glutamic acid	40	39	40	38	38
Proline	36	33	29	31	38
Glycine	33	28	28	28	28
Alanine	24	19	26	22	22
Valine	41	41	36	46	45
Methionine	5	4	5	4	3
Isoleucine	15	8	13	13	11
Leucine	30	31	30	28	31
Tyrosine	17	17	12	16	16
Phenylalanine	14	13	16	13	12
Half-cystine	10	7	7	3	6
S-carboxymethyl-cysteine	4	4	3 (?4)	3 (?4)	4
Tryptophan	8	8	7	8	7
Hexose	4·5	4	20	5	10
Hexosamine	4	4·5	12	4	7

* Now referred to as IgG(T) [189].

Quantitative amino-acid analysis

In common with N- and C-terminal group assays, quantitative amino-acid analysis is an essential tool for primary structural studies. The application of this technique has been widely extended as a result of the automation [145] of the classical procedure of Stein & Moore [195], involving the quantitative

H

chromatographic separation of acid (6 N HCl) hydrolysates of the protein on columns of ion-exchange resins (Amberlite IR 120 or Dowex 50 cation-exchange, and Dowex 1 anion-exchange types). The effluents are monitored by reacting with ninhydrin in the presence of a reducing agent (necessary to prevent formation of aldehydes by a combined decarboxylation and oxidation of the amino acids, with lower yields of chromophore). The ninhydrin chromo-phore is specific for amino ($-NH_2$) groups, so that the colour yield/mole of

TABLE 7.8 (b) Amino-acid composition of light chains

| | Residues/20,000 g | | | | |
	Rabbit IgG	Human IgG	Human IgM	Horse IgG	Horse IgA (T)*
Lysine	8	10	10	10	10
Histidine	2	3	2	2	2
Arginine	3	6	5	4	4
Aspartic acid	16	13	13	12	13
Threonine	25	15	15	17	19
Serine	19	24	24	28	32
Glutamic acid	18	20	19	16	16
Proline	10	11	11	11	12
Glycine	15	11	12	16	18
Alanine	13	12	12	12	13
Valine	18	13	13	14	14
Methionine	0·9	0·6	0·7	0·8	0·4
Isoleucine	6	5	5	10	7
Leucine	11	13	13	11	12
Tyrosine	10	8	8	6	6
Phenylalanine	5	6	5	4	4
Half-cystine	6	3	3	3	3
S-carboxymethyl-cysteine	1	1	1	1	1
Tryptophan	4	2	3	3	3
Hexose	0·3	0·25	0	0·4	0·6
Hexosamine	0·2	0·2	0·3	0·1	0·1

* Now referred to as IgG(T) [189].

individual amino acids is measured in calibration of the system. The amino acids are eluted from the ion-exchange resins successively, their concentration being a function of the peak area from which the molar ratios of the consti-tuent amino acids may be calculated.

Obviously, many factors can influence the accuracy of quantitative amino-acid analysis, despite the now ready availability of automated techniques. Foremost among these is the heterogeneity encountered in immunoglobulin preparations. This problem has been circumvented in the analysis of human immunoglobulins by employing the relatively homogeneous and abundant preparations isolated from sera of patients with myelomatosis or macro-

TABLE 7.9

Comparison of the amino-acid compositions of various
immunoglobulins and their sub-units
(a) Amino-acid composition of human γG globulin and of
the heavy and light chains
(This table, and Table 7.9(c), are reproduced by courtesy
of Drs M.J.Crumpton and J.M.Wilkinson from *Biochem.
J.* (1963) **88**, 228)

Amino acid	Human γG globulin	Heavy chain	Light chain
Lys	7·06	7·35	6·23
His*	2·44	2·62	1·75
Arg	4·02	3·81	4·57
Asp	7·77	7·64	7·33
Thr†	7·04	6·83	7·42
Ser†	9·13	8·60	10·28
Glu	11·18	10·05	13·04
Pro	6·40	6·41	5·10
Gly	3·37	3·23	3·33
Ala	3·29	2·73	4·19
Val*	7·92	8·15	6·27
Met	0·93	1·02	0·42
Ileu	2·16	1·86	2·74
Leu	7·40	7·11	7·29
Tyr†	5·76	5·52	6·16
Phe	4·07	3·77	4·31
CyS‡	2·07	1·41	1·51
CyS·CH$_2$·CO$_2$H	0	1·15	0·69
Try	2·63	2·79	2·15
Total	94·6	92·1	94·8

* Amounts determined after 72 hours of hydrolysis only.

† Corrected to zero time for decomposition during hydrolysis.

‡ Calculated as cysteic acid after oxidation and hydrolysis of the protein.

globulinaemia. Nevertheless, the complete separation of such immunoglobulins (particularly the γM globulins) from other serum proteins often presents a difficult task. In isolating normal human serum γM globulin for amino-acid analysis [188], this drawback has been met by the use of West African sera as starting material, as these are almost free from haptoglobin, and contain relatively low concentrations of β-lipoprotein. Antibody γ globulin can be separated from other serum proteins by precipitation with specific antigen (as was the practice used in isolating the antibodies whose amino-acid composition is given in Table 7.17). This still leaves the possibility of antibody heterogeneity,

TABLE 7.9 (b) Amino-acid compositions of heavy and light chains of human immunoglobulins IgG and IgM. (Reproduced by courtesy of Professor S.Cohen, and Drs H.Chaplin and E.M. Press from *Biochem. J.* (1965) **95**, 259)

	Heavy chain 50,000			Light chain 20,000		
Assumed mol. wt.	IgG	IgM[(1)]	IgM[(2)]	IgG	IgM[(1)]	IgM[(2)]
Lys	29	20	21	9·7	9·6	9·5
His	9·6	7·6	8·3	2·5	2·4	2·7
Arg	12	17	18	5·8	5·3	4·6
Asp	33	33	35	13	13	14
Thr	34	38	38	15	15	15
Ser	50	42	39	24	24	24
Glu	39	40	41	20	19	19
Pro	33	29	28	11	11	12
Gly	28	28	29	11	12	13
Ala	19	26	28	12	12	12
Val	41	36	38	13	13	13
Met	3·9	5·3	5·0	0·6	0·7	0·6
Ileu	8·2	13	13	4·9	4·7	4·6
Leu	31	30	32	13	13	12
Tyr	17	12	12	7·6	8·0	6·1
Phe	13	15	16	6·0	5·3	5·3
Cys (half)	6·9	7·4	5·7	2·9	3·3	
CyS·CH$_2$·CO$_2$H	3·6	3·2	4·5	0·9	1·1	1·3
Try	7·5	7·6	7·8	2·3	2·7	2·8

IgM[(1)] was prepared from defibrinated plasma of U.K. blood donor; IgM[(2)] was prepared from West African serum.

however, which must be eliminated when looking for small differences in the composition of different antibodies of the same immunoglobulin class, raised in the same species. A high degree of accuracy has been achieved in such studies of specifically purified rabbit γG globulin antibodies (as will be outlined in section B3a) by using automated techniques of improved precision and by analysing hydrolysates of Fab *sub-units*, rather than the much larger whole antibody molecules.

Several automatic analysers are commercially available which will perform a complete analysis of the amino acids in protein hydrolysates in 21 hours. Recent technical refinements involving the use of columns of highly homogeneous micro-bead resins under high pressure (about 100–200 lb/sq. in.) have dramatically reduced these times (to 3–5 hours), besides permitting analyses of very small samples (<0·1 ml). Moreover, the introduction of

7.9 (c) Amino-acid composition of rabbit γG globulin, the heavy and light chains and the A piece (Fd) and B piece (light chain)

Amino acid	Rabbit γG globulin	Heavy chain	Light chain	A piece (Fd)	B piece (light chain)
Lys	5·76	5·79	4·99	4·22	4·78
His*	1·73	1·79	0·89	1·06	0·98
Arg	4·42	4·90	2·04	3·85	2·13
Asp	8·08	7·53	8·91	6·18	9·18
Thr†	10·37	9·79	12·20	11·98	12·24
Ser†	8·32	8·52	8·36	9·93	8·08
Glu	11·05	10·39	11·80	7·35	11·31
Pro	6·79	7·03	4·85	6·47	4·83
Gly	3·98	3·71	4·47	4·76	4·40
Ala	3·71	3·37	4·75	3·87	4·51
Val*	8·36	8·07	8·69	8·68	9·02
Met	1·13	1·21	0·33	0·77	0·57
Ileu	3·49	3·39	3·49	2·36	3·30
Leu	6·73	6·79	5·56	7·21	6·07
Tyr†	6·17	5·52	7·79	5·68	7·66
Phe	4·15	4·07	3·88	3·56	3·92
CyS‡	2·63	1·91	2·68	2·00	—
CyS·CH$_2$·CO$_2$H	0	1·17	0·80	1·54	0·73
Try	2·90	2·91	1·71	2·98	—
Total	99·2	97·9	98·2	94·5	—

* Amounts determined after 72 hours of hydrolysis only.

† Corrected to zero time for decomposition during hydrolysis.

‡ Calculated as cysteic acid after oxidation and hydrolysis of the protein.

automatic interpretive procedures increases the speed and accuracy of measurement of the chromatographic patterns obtained by simultaneous monitoring of column effluents at 570 mμ and 440 mμ (for proline and hydroxyproline determination).

When analysing protein hydrolysates, it is customary to add an internal standard (e.g. nor-leucine), and this is also included in the standard calibration mixture of amino acids, measurements of which are interspersed between estimations of components of protein hydrolysates. For accurate determination of amino-acid composition, it is necessary to carry out analyses (in duplicate) on hydrolysates (after 24, 48 and 72 hours) and to extrapolate the values thus obtained to zero time. Of the amino acids destroyed by prolonged acid hydrolysis, threonine, serine, tyrosine, cysteine and cystine are estimated by

7.9 (d) Amino-acid composition of type L γA myeloma globulin (Ha), the autologous Bence-Jones protein and related products. (Reproduced by courtesy of Drs G.M.Bernier, K.Tominga, C.W.Easley and F.W.Putnam from *Biochemistry* (1965) **4**, 2072)

Amino acid	γA globulin	Papain digest	Bence-Jones protein	Reduced alkylated Bence-Jones protein	Light chain (acetic acid)	Light chain (SDS)	Heavy chain (SDS)
			(g amino-acid residues/100 g protein)*				
Lysine	5·44	5·37	6·27	6·28	6·22	5·81	5·27
Histidine	2·53	2·05	2·37	2·18	2·27	2·36	2·67
Arginine	5·40	5·60	5·42	5·26	5·32	5·76	5·55
Aspartic acid	7·87	7·92	6·77	6·86	7·01	7·43	8·26
Threonine	8·99	8·47	8·32	8·49	8·48	8·51	8·38
Serine	9·54	9·80	11·06	11·45	10·83	9·77	8·13
Glutamic acid	11·00	10·49	11·52	11·57	11·41	11·12	11·24
Proline	8·04	8·31	6·77	7·23	7·22	7·63	8·93
Glycine	4·25	4·31	4·04	4·00	4·17	4·31	4·49
Alanine	4·86	4·57	5·80	5·69	5·69	5·24	4·95
Valine	6·85	7·51	7·22	7·07	7·36	6·91	6·36
Methionine	0·66	0·46	0	0·03	0·12	0·26	1·00
Isoleucine	1·44	1·72	1·96	1·96	1·87	1·75	1·90
Leucine	9·45	8·07	7·57	7·66	7·58	8·92	10·02
Tyrosine	4·35	5·33	6·99	6·79	(6·10)†	5·10	2·96
Phenylalanine	4·23	4·48	2·79	2·66	(3·50)†	4·19	4·71
CM-cysteine	0	0	0	2·17	0·44	1·94	1·14
Half-cystine	2·44	2·64	2·14	0	1·43	Trace	1·06

* Expressed as the percentage of the total recovered amino acids. Tryptophan was not determined but was assumed to be 3 per cent for calculation purposes. Correction factors were not applied for partial destruction of amino acids during hydrolysis.

† Parentheses signify poor resolution of phenylalanine and tyrosine.

S.D.S. refers to sodium dodecyl sulphate.

extrapolation to zero time. Tryptophane is assayed on the original protein by the method of Spies & Chambers [190], and cystine may be conveniently determined after oxidation to cysteic acid and isolation by ion-exchange chromatography on Amberlite IR 120 or Dowex 1 × 8, as described by Moore [191]. Ammonia (amide nitrogen) is also calculated by extrapolation to zero time. Reliable results can be obtained with as little as 0·1 μmole of solute.

Hence, the technique is particularly valuable for determining the amino-acid composition of peptides or glycopeptides, separated as described later. As mentioned earlier (in section B1), it has also found useful application in the quantitative determination of the amount of carboxymethylcysteine produced on reduction and alkylation of γG globulin (from which the number of interchain disulphide bonds can be deduced).

Qualitative, as well as quantitative, amino-acid (and sugar) estimation plays an important role in the elucidation of polypeptide structure (particularly in sequential analysis). Technical details can be obtained from other sources [192, 428, 429].

Besides forming the basis of quantitative amino-acid analysis, ion-exchange chromatography has also been used to separate peptides from proteolytic digests of whole proteins. For example, Hirs *et al* [193] have separated peptides, containing 20–25 amino-acid residues from tryptic hydrolysates of oxidized ribonuclease, using Dowex 50×2. Guidotti *et al* [194] fractionated the tryptic peptides of human haemoglobin on Dowex 50×2 (H^+), eluting with a pyridine acetate buffer, and scanning the eluates by the ninhydrin procedure of Moore & Stein [195], using 0·2 ml aliquots. Kimmel *et al* [167] effected an initial separation of peptides from a tryptic digestion of oxidized papain on Dowex 50×2. Bulked fractions were then chromatographed on Dowex 1×2 in acetate form, and the degree of separation achieved assessed by two-dimensional paper chromatography and ionophoresis as already described. When using Dowex 50 or similar strongly acidic cation-exchange resins in the H^+ cycle, however, the emergent anions (present as the free acids) may be labile, and must be neutralized as soon as possible. Terminal non-reducing residues may be hydrolysed from glycopeptides by the strongly acidic resin. Moreover, such procedures give imperfect separation of peptides, hampered by the difficulty of detection, since the colour yield obtained by reaction with ninhydrin decreases with increasing peptide size. This is demonstrated by the attempts of Nelson *et al* [401] to differentiate the column (Dowex 50×8) chromatographic patterns of tryptic digests of the heavy and light chains of antibody and normal rabbit γG globulins (revealed by monitoring with ninhydrin in the automatic amino-acid analyser). The problem has been partially resolved in the automatic continuous method developed by Catravas [196] (and now commercially available from Technicon Instruments Co Ltd). This provides an estimate of the size and distribution of the ninhydrin peaks before and after *alkaline* hydrolysis (using a sample volume less than one-fifth of that required by other ion-exchange resin chromatographic separation techniques).

Despite technical advances incorporated in this procedure, however, it has little direct application to the analysis of the complex peptide mixtures obtained by enzymatic digestion of oxidized immunoglobulins. A preliminary separation of such mixtures into groups of various sizes by sucessive gel filtration through Sephadex G25 and G10 (as mentioned in section B1), followed by further fractionation by ion-exchange chromatography or two-dimensional paper chromatography/ionophoresis separation procedures, affords a better means of resolving their complexity. Alternatively, a combination of column chromatographic techniques (on Dowex 1 × 2) followed by gel filtration (through Sephadex G25) might prove a more useful separation procedure; this approach has been adopted in the separation of the tryptic peptides of Knoxville No. 1 haemoglobin [197].

Terminal amino-acid residue analysis

N-terminal and C-terminal amino-acid assays are the other major techniques employed in the chemical analysis of polypeptides and their digestion fragments. Apart from their essential role in the determination of amino-acid sequence in peptides and glycopeptides, these procedures are also used to demonstrate polypeptide chain heterogeneity and to ascertain the number of different chains present in protein cleavage mixtures. The Sanger [180] and Edman [198] techniques have been most widely used for determining N-terminal amino acids. In the Sanger technique, interaction with 1-fluoro-2,4-dinitrobenzene converts the free amino groups to the corresponding 2,4-dinitrophenyl compounds, which are readily identified by paper chromatography after acid hydrolysis. In the Edman method, the protein is treated with phenylisothiocyanate to form a phenylthiocarbamyl (PTC) peptide which is then cleaved by anhydrous HCl in nitromethane to give the phenylthiohydantoin of the N-terminal amino acid. This derivative is soluble in the organic solvent, and is identified by chromatography, whilst the remainder of the protein (or peptide) is insoluble, and may be recovered for further reaction. Hence, an important advantage of the Edman technique is that it permits stepwise cleavage of single amino-acid residues (starting from the N-terminal end of the polypeptide chain) for several cycles (e.g. 5–7 have been frequently achieved). A difficulty often encountered in the application of this technique, however, is the insolubility of phenylthiocarbamyl protein derivatives and large phenylthiocarbamyl peptides in the anhydrous acid medium used for cyclization. Fraenkel–Conrat *et al* [199] have devised a means of overcoming this problem by performing all operations on a layer of the protein adsorbed on Whatman No. 1 filter paper.

An alternative N-terminal assay procedure, devised by Gray & Hartley [200], should find wide application in structural determinations of immunoglobulins, because of its high sensitivity (about 100 times more sensitive than the fluordinitrobenzene method of Sanger [180]). This employs a fluorescent reagent (1-dimethylaminonapthalene-5-sulphonyl chloride, known as dansyl chloride) which reacts with amino-acid phenolic groups, yielding derivatives which are highly resistant to acid hydrolysis and which exhibit intense yellow fluorescence under ultraviolet (u.v.) light. The method is applicable to as little as 10^{-4}–10^{-3} μmole of peptide. For example, in applying it to the determination of the N-terminal residues in peptides of the heavy chains of human γG globulin, Press *et al* [209] used 0·005 μmole of peptide, dissolved in 0·1 M NaHCO$_3$ (15 μl). To this was added a solution of dansyl chloride in acetone (1 mg/ml, 15 μl) and the reaction allowed to proceed for 3 hours at room temperature [200], whereupon the product was dried *in vacuo*, 6 N HCl (20 μl) added, the tube sealed, and hydrolysis continued for 6–12 hours at 105° C. After removing the acid *in vacuo*, the hydrolysate was extracted into acetone and separated by thin-layer chromatography on silica gel-G, developed initially with chloroform–acetic acid (7 : 3) and scanned under a u.v. lamp; after drying, the chromatogram was developed with ethanol–aq. ammonia (S.G.: 0·880) (9 : 1, v/v) and again viewed under a u.v. lamp.

The sequential degradation of N-terminal amino acids may also be achieved by the use of leucine amino peptidase, which requires the presence of a free α amino group, and acts not only on N-terminal leucine residues, but also on peptides having an N-terminal amino acid with an aliphatic side chain. The efficiency of the enzyme increases with the size of the side chain. Margoliash [202] defines the conditions for the use of this peptidase for sequential degradation of peptides.

An interesting outcome of N-terminal assays on the polypeptide chains of rabbit γG globulin was the finding that these amino acids (alanine, aspartic acid) were almost entirely confined to the light chains, in contrast to normal human γG in which N-terminal amino acids have been found in both chains [1]. This observation has since been attributed to the termination of the heavy chains of rabbit γG globulin by pyrrolidone carboxylic acid residues, as also were the heavy chains of a human myeloma γG globulin [201]. The recent observations [209] that both the heavy chain of a human myeloma γG globulin and also its isolated Fd portion were terminated by pyrrolid-2-one-5-carbonylvalyl-threonine provides support for the Porter structural model of γG globulin (shown in Fig. 7.6), as does the finding that both the heavy chain and the Fc fragment have the same C-terminal residue, glycine.

Both enzymatic and chemical methods have been employed in the characterization of C-terminal residues. For instance, carboxypeptidase-A selectively removes neutral amino acids, whilst carboxypeptidase-B hydrolyses C-terminal arginine, lysine and acyl derivatives. (Details of the use of these enzymes are given by Margoliash [202].) The alternative hydrazinolysis [203] method has serious disadvantages, such as low recoveries and the complete loss of C-terminal cystine, cysteine, asparagine and glutamine residues [204]. Nevertheless, it sometimes proves superior to the enzymatic procedures as, for example, in the determination of the terminal residues in the C-terminal

H*

peptides of the heavy chains of a human myeloma γG globulin [209]. In this case, digestion of the heavy chain with carboxypeptidase-A before or after oxidation with performic acid released only traces of amino acid. Hydrazinolysis, however, gave yields (after correction for losses) of 0·9 mole of glycine and 0·1 mole of serine per mole of heavy chain, whilst the Fc fragment gave 1·1 moles of glycine/mole.

Primary structural analysis

The characterization of the *primary structure* of a protein involves the following steps: (a) isolation of a highly purified sample; (b) chemical and physico-chemical characterization to determine molecular weight, nitrogen content, number and nature of prosthetic groups (such as carbohydrate); (c) isolation of pure preparations of constituent polypeptide chains; (d) accurate determination of their amino-acid compositions; (e) production of overlapping peptides by proteolytic procedures of differing specificity; (f) elucidation of the amino-acid sequences by serial identification of the terminal residues after sequential degradation. (Technical details for these procedures are described by Leggett Bailey [192] and Morris [428].)

Thus, the task is of immense magnitude, despite such technical developments as improved fractionation procedures (e.g. gel filtration) for peptides, and the standardization of the Edman N-terminal amino-acid degradation [205]. Moreover, it is not greatly facilitated by adopting as a guide the analytical procedures which were applied to the now well-characterized proteins such as haemoglobin, since each protein has distinctive structural features. The characterization of immunoglobulins is further complicated by marked heterogeneity within a particular class (e.g. γG). Hence, initial primary structural analyses have been performed on the much more homogeneous and more readily available paraproteins such as urinary Bence–Jones proteins and serum myeloma γG globulins.

Already, sequential analysis has provided important information about the structures of Bence-Jones proteins (which are the free light chains of the patients' myeloma γG globulins, and are closely related to normal human γG globulin light chains). As mentioned previously, peptide mapping (as well as terminal amino-group assay and determination of amino-acid composition of isolated peptides) has demonstrated gross primary structural differences between light chains of the two antigenic types, K and L [178]. As shown by Fig. 7.33, based on the investigations of the Putnam group [206, 426], Hilschman *et al* [207] and Baglioni *et al* [427, 443], sequential analysis of the amino-acid sequence of three Bence-Jones proteins has now revealed fascinating structural differences between light polypeptide chains of the same antigenic type (namely K). In contrast to the many structural differences revealed between the N-terminal halves of the three polypeptide chains, only one

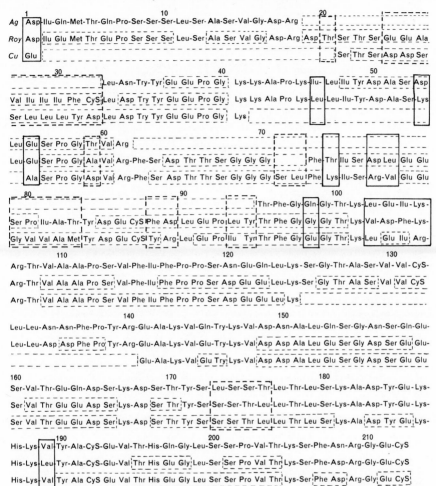

Fig. 7.33. Comparison of known partial amino-acid sequence of three Bence-Jones proteins ('Ag', 'Roy' and 'Cu') of antigenic type K. Known sequences are indicated by joining together the abbreviations for the amino acids by dashes (e.g. Asp—Ilu—Glu). Areas of undetermined sequence are enclosed by a horizontal dashed line. In cases of known composition, the amino-acid residues are placed in order of their elution from ion-exchange column of the analyser if the sequence is unknown for any protein. If, however, the sequence is known for one protein, the residues enclosed by a dashed line (undetermined sequence) are ordered to correspond with the known sequence. Regions of probable homologous and non-homologous interchanges are emphasized by enclosure in a box with a solid line. Regions of possible interchange are enclosed with a vertical dashed line. Data for specimens 'Roy' and 'Cu' are derived from report by Hilschman and Craig [207] (which did not report which glutamic and aspartic acid residues are present as amides).

(Reproduced by courtesy of Drs K.Titani, F,Whitley, L.Avogadro and F,W, Putnam from *Science* (1965), **149,** 1090.)

7.34(a)

Type I
Stable monomer —Lys.Ser.Phe.AspNH₂.Arg.Gly.Glu.Cys

Stable dimer —Lys.Ser.Phe.AspNH₂.Arg.Gly.Glu.Cys
                                                                        |
                                                                       Cys

γ globulin —Lys.Ser.Phe.AspNH₂.Arg.Gly.Glu.Cys
            —Lys.Ser.Phe.AspNH₂.Arg.Gly.Glu.Cys
                                                                        |
                                                                   A chains

Type II
Stable monomer —Lys.Thr.Val.Ala.Pro.Thr.Glu.Cys.Ser.

Stable dimer —Lys.Thr.Val.Ala.Pro.Thr.Glu.Cys.Ser
                                                                     |
                                                                    Cys

γ globulin —Lys.Thr.Val.Ala.Pro.Thr.Glu.Cys.Ser
            —   Thr.Val.Ala.Pro.Thr.Glu.Cys.Ser
                                                                     |
                                                                A chains

7.34(b)

Protein		Ref.
B.J.	Leu.Tyr.Ala.Cys.Glu(Val,Thr,His,Gln,Gly,Leu)(Ser,Ser,Pro,Val,Thr)Lys. Ser.Phe. Asn.Arg. Gly.Glu.Cys	
	190 200 210	
Roy	Leu.Tyr.Ala.Cys.Glx.Val(Thr,His,Glx,Gly)Leu.Ser(Ser,Pro,Val,Thr)Lys. Ser.Phe. Asx.Arg. Gly.Glx Cys	207
Cum	Val(Tyr,Ala,Cys,Glx,Val,Thr,His,Glx,Gly,Leu,Ser,Ser,Pro,Val,Thr)Lys. Ser.Phe. Asx. Arg. Gly(Glx. Cys)	207
Ag	Val.Tyr.Ala.Cys.Glu.Val.Thr.His.Gln.Gly.Leu.Ser.Ser.Pro.Val.Thr.Lys. Ser.Phe. Asn.Arg. Gly.Glu.Cys	207
Rad	Val.Tyr.Ala.Cys.Glu(Val,Thr,His,Gln,Gly,Leu)(Ser,Ser,Pro,Val,Thr,Lys)(Ser,Phe)(Asn,Arg) Gly.Glu.Cys	
Day	(Val,Tyr,Ala,Cys,Glx,Val,Thr,His,Glx,Gly,Leu,Ser,Ser,Pro,Val,Thr,Lys)(Ser,Phe, Asn,Arg)(Gly,Glu,Cys)	
Man	(Val,Tyr,Ala,Cys,Glx,Val,Thr,His,Glx,Gly,Leu,Ser,Ser,Pro,Val,Thr,Lys)(Ser,Phe, Asn,Arg)(Gly,Glu,Cys)	
Ker	Leu.Tyr.Ala.Cys.Glu(Val,Thr,His,Gln,Gly,Leu)(Ser,Ser,Pro,Val,Thr)Lys. Ser(Phe, Asn,Arg)(Gly,Glu,Cys)	

Protein		Ref.
Ag	Ile.Phe.Pro.Pro.Ser.Asn. Glu.Gln.Leu.Lys.Ser.Gly.Thr.Ala.Ser.Val.Val.Cys.Leu	207
Rad	Ile(Phe,Pro,Pro,Ser)Asp. Glx Glx Leu(Lys,Ser,Gly,Thr,Ala,Ser)Val.Val.Cys.Leu	
B.J.	(Ile,Phe,Pro,Pro,Ser,Asx)(Glx,Glx,Leu)Lys(Ser,Gly,Thr,Ala,Ser)Val.Val.Cys.Leu	
Ker	(Lys,Ser,Gly,Thr,Ala,Ser)Val(Val,Cys,Leu)	
	120 130	
Roy	Ile(Phe,Pro,Pro,Ser, Asx,Glx,Glx)Leu.Lys.Ser(Gly,Thr,Ala,Ser)Val(Val,Cys)Leu	207

7.34(c)

Protein		Ref.
B.J.	————Tyr.Tyr.Cys.Gln.Gln.Tyr.Glu.Asn.Leu(Pro,Tyr) ————	
Ker	————Tyr.Tyr.Cys.Gln.Gln.Tyr.Asp.Asp.Leu.Pro.Pro.Thr.Phe.Gly.Pro.Gly.Thr.Lys. ————	
Rad	———— Tyr.Cys.Gln.Gln.Tyr.Glu.Thr.Ser. Pro.Thr.Thr.Phe. ————	
	90 100	
Roy	.........Tyr(Tyr,Cys,Glx,Glx,<u>Phe</u>,Asx,Asx,Leu,Pro,<u>Leu</u>,Thr,Phe)Gly(Gly,Gly,Thr)Lys.	207
Cu	(....Tyr,Tyr,Cys,Glx,Glx)Arg.Leu(<u>Glx,Ile</u>,Pro,Tyr,Thr,Phe,Gly,Glx,Gly,Thr)Lys.	207
Ag	————Thr.Phe.Gly.Gln.Gly.Thr.Lys	207

Protein	23	Ref.
B.J.	Arg.Val.Thr.Ile. Thr.Cys.Gln.Ala.Ser.Gln.Asp.Ile.Asn.Lys.	
Ker	Asp.Arg.Ile.Thr.Ile. Thr.Cys.Gln.Ala(Ser.Gln.Asp,Ile,Lys)	
Day	Val(Thr,Ile, Thr.Cys.Gln.Ala,Ser,Gln,Asp,Ile.<u>Ser,Asx,Phe</u>,Leu,Asx,Try,Tyr)	
Roy	Asx.Arg(Val/Iso ,Thr,Ile, Thr.Cys.Glx,Ala,Ser,Glx,Asx,Ile,<u>Ser, Iso/Val</u>.<u>Phe</u>)Leu(Asx.Try.Tyr)	207
Ag	Leu.Asn.Try.Tyr.	207
Rad	Ala.Thr.Leu.Ser.Cys.Arg.Ala.Ser.Gln	

structural difference was detected between the C-terminal portions of the chains. It has been concluded that such multiple structural differences are incompatible with the concept of the single point mutations sometimes postulated for the abnormal haemoglobins. Instead, it is proposed that chromosomal rearrangements are responsible for these (and probably, also, for variability in antibody structure). Sub-units corresponding to the variable N-terminal half of whole Bence-Jones proteins have been separated by gel filtration on Sephadex G75 and identified by peptide mapping [214].

Milstein [104, 118] has obtained further evidence of structural similarities between the C-terminal portions of the light chains of γG globulins. As shown in Fig. 7.34, the same C-terminal amino-acid sequence is postulated for the region in the vicinity of the disulphide bridges linking the light to the heavy chain in γG globulin molecules, and the light chains together in the stable dimeric form of Bence-Jones proteins. Other sequential studies carried out by the Porter group [208] have demonstrated close similarities between the arrangement of amino acids in a C-terminal octa-decapeptide isolated from a heavy chain of rabbit γG globulin and from a human myeloma γG globulin. These studies have now been extended [209], as the result of the isolation in high yield of a nineteen-residue peptide from the C-terminal end of the heavy chain of human γG globulin, following splitting at its four methionine residues by the action of cyanogen bromide (using the technique described already on page 179). The amino-acid sequence of this C-terminal peptide is:

$$
\begin{array}{ccc}
\text{NH}_2 & & \text{NH}_2 \\
| & & | \\
\end{array}
$$

His—Glu—Ala—Leu—His—Asp—His—Tyr—Thr—

$$
\begin{array}{c}
\text{NH}_2 \\
| \\
\end{array}
$$

—Glu—Lys—Ser—Leu—Ser—Leu—Ser—Pro—Gly—COOH

As a result of this work, in which both the N- and C-terminal amino-acid sequences in the heavy chain of the human γG globulin molecule have been

---

Fig. 7.34.

(a) Suggested structure around the interchain disulphide bridge in human Bence-Jones proteins and in γG globulins.
(Reproduced by courtesy of Dr C.Milstein from *Nature, Lond.* (1965), **205**, 1171.)

(b) Comparison of the peptides containing cysteine residues 192 and 132, and C-terminus, of several Bence-Jones proteins (type K).

(c) Comparison of the peptides containing cysteine residues 86 and 23 respectively of several Bence-Jones proteins (type K).
(Reproduced by courtesy of Dr C.Milstein from *Nature, Lond.* (1966), **209**, 370.)
Glx and Asx mean that no distinction between glutamine and glutamic acid and between aspuragine and aspartic acid is available. Proteins Rad, Day and Man: InV(b+); Ker and Roy: InV(a+).

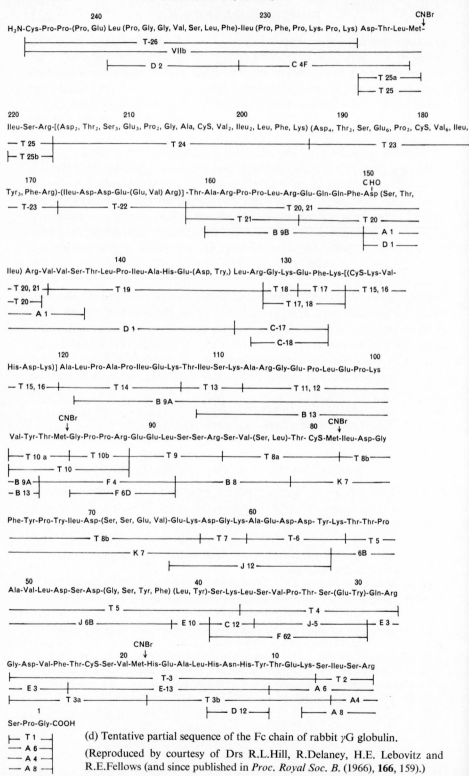

7.34 (d)   *Tentative partial sequence of F$_c$ chain of IgG*

(d) Tentative partial sequence of the Fc chain of rabbit γG globulin.

(Reproduced by courtesy of Drs R.L.Hill, R.Delaney, H.E. Lebovitz and R.E.Fellows (and since published in *Proc. Royal Soc. B.* (1966), **166**, 159).)

elucidated, and in which it has been shown that only one of each is present per mole of chain, it is concluded that the heavy chain is most probably a single polypeptide chain (and not two chains [1], as considered possible by some investigators).

The nineteen amino-acid residues at the C-terminal end of the myeloma γG globulin heavy chain show only two replacements when compared with the corresponding section of the C-terminal end of the heavy chain of normal rabbit γG globulin. Consequently, Press *et al* [209] have suggested that the Fc fragment of immunoglobulins from mammalian species may have a unique sequence showing relatively little variation from one species to another, the greater variability being confined to the Fd fragment of the chain. In other words, it is suggested that the heavy chains might resemble the light chains which have been shown (by the studies on Bence-Jones proteins referred to already) to possess a variable half (at the N-terminal end) and a stable half (at the C-terminal end). The cross-reactivity studies described in Section A2 would seem to suggest, however, that the heavy chains of all mammalian γG globulins are not alike in this respect, for it was found that rabbit anti-human γG globulin and human anti-human γG globulin (i.e. rheumatoid factor) formed appreciably more precipitate when reacted with the aggregated Fc fragment of human γG globulin than with the corresponding aggregated fragment of some other species such as horse. This finding could be due to structural dissimilarity within that part of the heavy chain in the Fc fragment remote from the C-terminal end, which is exposed as a result of the aggregation process. This implies that, like the light chains, the heavy chains *within the Fc portion* of the molecule possess a stable structure at the C-terminal end and a variable structure at the N-terminal end. It is in the latter part of the Fc heavy chain that new determinants might be expected to become exposed as a result of the conformational changes outlined in section C (resulting in the induction of the biological activities associated with aggregated γG globulins). In view of the observations of Naunton & Dintzis [210] that polypeptide chains are synthesized from the N-terminal amino acid to the C-terminal, it would appear that the variable portions of both the light and heavy chains of γG globulins are synthesized in response to a specific inductive stimulus (the antigen), in a manner reminiscent of the synthesis of induced enzymes in response to the presence of a specific inducer.

The elucidation of the amino-acid sequence of the heavy and light polypeptide chains of the immunoglobulins is proceeding at a rapid pace. For instance, Press *et al* [211, 454] have obtained improved separation of the fragments cleaved from heavy chains by cyanogen bromide, by performing Sephadex G100 filtration in urea-formate (pH 3·3). In a comparison of the eleven C-terminal residues in the heavy chains of human, rabbit and horse γG globulins, replacements were observed only in the 2 and 4 positions.

Moreover, Hill *et al* [212, 417] have determined the partial sequence of the whole Fc region of the heavy chain of *rabbit* γG globulin, from the analysis of tryptic and chymotryptic peptides (as reproduced in Fig. 7.34(d)).

Carbohydrate analysis

As already mentioned, all the immunoglobulins contain small amounts of *carbohydrate*, and so are glycoproteins. Since in many serum proteins, notably follicular stimulating hormone (FSH), transferrin and fibrinogen, biological activity is intimately connected with the carbohydrate moieties, the nature and distribution of the carbohydrate components is of potential interest. It is necessary initially to establish the number and molecular sizes of the carbohydrate units. In the case of the 'carbohydrate-poor' γG globulins, examination of the molar ratios (see Table 7.6) indicates that the five constituent sugars (N-acetyl-*D*-glucosamine, N-acetyl-neuraminic acid, *L*-fucose, *D*-galactose and *D*-mannose) are present in molar ratios of 8 : 1 : 2 : 3 : 5. Experience with other serum glycoproteins (e.g. orosomucoid, transferrin, fibrinogen) suggests that all these five sugars are present in complex chains, rather than attached individually as *single* non-reducing end-groups to amino acids. Other studies with mammalian serum glycoproteins (orosomucoid, transferrin, FSH, fetuin), submaxillary (ovine, bovine, porcine) and pleural (human and bovine pleuromucoid) glycoproteins indicate that the carbohydrate is glycosidically linked to the protein chain; essentially similar conclusions have been reached from studies of avian (ovalbumin, ovomucoid) glycoproteins. In any glyco-protein, the oligosaccharide prosthetic groups may be similar or quite different. Studies on the intact glycoprotein afford only an average picture from which it is not possible to deduce the unique fine structure for each oligosaccharide unit. It is therefore important to find conditions of proteolytic degradation which leave part of the peptide chain attached to the carbohydrate units; moreover, in the case of γG globulin, because of the low carbohydrate content of the native protein, the isolation of intact glycopeptide units is an essential prelude to the determination of fine structure. Studies of the carbohydrate group, with reference solely to its immediate vicinal amino acids, have usually been made after somewhat drastic proteolytic procedures, involving successive proteolysis with enzymes of different specificity, e.g. trypsin, pepsin, pronase.

Extensive studies on the nature of the carbohydrate of human γG globulin (Cohn II 1, 2 fraction) have been carried out by the Smith group [215, 216, 217]. These have indicated that the polysaccharide is uniquely attached to the protein through an aspartyl residue. Details of the technical procedures employed are as follows: glycopeptides were prepared by hydrolysing a salt-free suspension of heat-denatured human γG globulin (Cohn II 1, 2) (50 g) in water (250 ml) at 60° C with recrystallized mercuripapain (175 mg), dimercaptopropanol (0·25 ml) and EDTA (4·7 g). The progress of the reaction was followed by the increase of colour developed when an aliquot was reacted with ninhydrin reagent. In the first experiment, similar additions of mercuri-papain and dimercaptopropanol were made at 2, 8, 23, 43 and 70 hours, and the reaction proceeded for 98 hours, pH being maintained near 6·5 by the addition as required of 1 N LiOH. It was subsequently found that hydrolysis (as revealed by increased ninhydrin colour) was virtually complete in 4–6 hours, although a slight increase in ninhydrin yield continued up to 48 hours. The final ninhydrin colour indicated a cleavage of about half of the total

TABLE 7.10

Yields of glycopeptides recovered from a papain digest of heat-denatured human γG globulin (Cohn II 1, 2) by the combined fractionation procedure indicated in the text (estimated from the recovery of hexose determined by the orcinol/sulphuric acid method, no correction being made for loss of material removed in samples). This table and Tables 7.11–7.13 are reproduced by courtesy of Drs J.W. Rosevear and E.L. Smith from *J. biol. Chem.* (1961) **236,** 425

Step	Procedure	Yield for each step (per cent)	Cumulative yield (per cent)
1	Papain digestion	98	98
2	Resin treatment	72	71
3	Ethanol precipitation	84	60
4	Zone electrophoresis	90*	54†

* Material recovered in the three major glycopep-tides.

† In making cuts to obtain each glycopeptide free of the others, approximately half of the material was excluded; however, such material could be recovered in large part by pooling and resubmitting to the column electrophoretic procedure.

peptide bonds of human γG globulin. The glycopeptides were recovered from the supernatant after proteolysis by centrifugation, and treatment with Dowex 50×8 (20–50 mesh, H^+ cycle), the eluate (pH 2) being immediately neutralized with LiOH. Approximately 72 per cent of the hexoses but only 1·6 per cent of the amino acids applied to the resin were recovered in the eluate, which was poured into nine volumes of cold ethanol containing a little lithium chloride (to aid flocculation). The precipitated glycopeptides were recovered by centrifugation and drying *in vacuo* (over phosphorus pentoxide and NaOH

TABLE 7.11

Composition of glycopeptides isolated from a papain digest of heat-denatured γG globulin

Analytical figures given are uncorrected for possible hydrolytic destruction and are given for the anhydrous material. Values for glucosamine are calculated for the N-acetylated derivative.

Residue	Glycopeptide 1			Glycopeptide 2			Glycopeptide 3		
	mmole residue per g	g residue per 100 g	Residues per 4800 g*	mmole residue per g	g residue per 100 g	Residues per 4200 g*	mmole residue per g	g residue per 100 g	Residues per 2800 g*
Hexose	1·50	24·3	7·3	1·81	29·3	7·6	2·80	45·3	7·8
Glucosamine	1·24	25·1	6·0	1·43	29·1	6·0	1·11	22·5	3·1
Fucose	1·41	6·0	2·0	0·50	7·4	2·1	0·71	10·4	2·0
Sialic acid	0·21	7·0	1·0	0·14	4·5	0·6	0·071	2·4	0·2
Aspartic acid	0·44	5·1	2·1	0·43	5·0	1·8	0·65	7·5	1·8
Glutamic acid	0·69	8·9	3·3	0·56	7·3	2·4	0·32	4·1	0·9
Tyrosine	0·19	3·1	0·91	0·23	3·7	0·95	0·39	6·4	1·1
Phenylalanine	0·097	1·4	0·47	0·09	1·3	0·38	0·12	1·7	0·3
Threonine	0·056	0·6	0·27	0·018	0·2	0·08	0·04	0·4	0·1
Serine	0·093	0·8	0·45	0·051	0·4	0·22	0·07	0·6	0·2
Valine	0·050	0·5	0·24	0·072	0·7	0·30			
Alanine	0·029	0·2	0·14	0·022	0·1	0·09			
Lysine							0·14	1·8	0·4
Total		83·0			89·0			103·1	

* Estimated molecular weights were obtained by averaging the calculated values for best fit of whole numbers of residues. Those figures which gave calculated molecular weights in excess of 10,000, 11,000 and 7000 for glyco-peptides 1, 2, and 3, respectively, were excluded from the calculation.

pellets). Paper electrophoresis of the dried material revealed three well-defined hexose-contaning fractions; a larger sample was fractionated by preparative starch-column electrophoresis based on the data from the pilot paper ionophoresis. The sample (in veronal buffer, pH 8·5, I = 0·05) was applied to the starch column (48 × 3 cm) [267] arranged so that the positive power lead was connected to the lower electrode, ensuring migration of the negatively charged glycopeptides into the starch, when electrophoresed at 5° C and 450 V for 48 hours. Fractions were recovered from the column by elution with the same buffer. Scanning by photometric orcinol and nin-hydrin reactions, revealed three glycopeptide peaks, designated 'I', 'II'

TABLE 7.12

Probable molar composition of glycopeptides from papain digestion of heat-denatured human γG globulin, calculated from the data given in Table 7.11 (after correction for a loss of glucosamine of the order of 20 per cent during acid hydrolysis)

Constituent	Glycopeptide 1	Glycopeptide 2	Glycopeptide 3
Glutamic acid	3	2	1
Aspartic acid	2	2	2
Tyrosine	1	1	1
N-acetylglucosamine	8	8	4
Galactose	3	3	3
Mannose	5	5	5
Fucose	2	2	2
Sialic acid	1	1	0
Molecular weight	4430*	4300*	3010

* These values have been computed on the basis of the above composition with the assumption that one acetyl is present on the sialic acid residue. It has also been assumed that all of the glucosamine is N-acetylated.

and 'III', recovered by pooling and ethanol precipitation as described above. The yields of glycopeptides by this fractionation procedure are shown in Table 7.10.

The glycopeptides were analysed for amino acids (as described already), for free amino groups [218], hexoses, using a modified orcinol–sulphuric acid procedure [217], hexosamine [219], *L*-fucose [220], sialic acid [221] and uronic acids [222]. The data thus obtained are presented in Tables 7.11 and 7.12. The hexosamine was identified as glucosamine and the sialic acid as N-acetylneuraminic acid by paper chromatography using appropriate standard sugars and specific spray reagents [173, 227]. The amino-acid sequences of the glycopeptides were determined by the methods already outlined. Using the Sanger technique [180], the dinitrophenyl derivatives (N-terminal amino acids) obtained are indicated in Table 7.13. The glycopeptides resisted further degradation by pepsin, papain, trypsin or chymotrypsin; carboxypeptidase was also without effect, suggesting the absence of a free C-terminal amino acid. Leucine amino peptidase, however, cleaved successive N-terminal amino acids. For this procedure, carried out in 0·06 M tris buffer containing 0·002 M magnesium chloride, pH 8·5, glycopeptide (4 mg) in buffer (1 ml) was incubated with aminopeptidase (1·8 mg) in buffer (1 ml) at 40° C for 24 hours. The cleaved amino acids, separated from the glycopeptide by dialysis, were identified by column chromatography; the residual glycopeptide was analysed for amino-acid content after hydrolysis with 6 N HCl (as previously described). The sum of the calculated molar ratios of the dialysed amino acids and of the amino acids of the residual glycopeptide corresponded to the composition of the original glycopeptide. Exhaustive treatment of the glycopeptides with leucine amino peptidase, controlled by rigorous analysis

TABLE 7.13

Dinitrophenyl (DNP) derivatives obtained from glycopeptides of human γG globulin

Sample	Ether phase	Aqueous phase
Glycopeptide 1	DNP-glutamic acid	O-DNP-tyrosine, aspartic acid, glutamic acid, glucosamine
Glycopeptide 2	DNP-glutamic acid	O-DNP-tyrosine, aspartic acid, glutamic acid, glucosamine
Glycopeptide 3	DNP-aspartic acid	O-DNP-tyrosine, aspartic acid, glutamic acid, glucosamine

of the residues, indicated that the largest glycopeptide isolated in this very detailed study contained the sequence:

Glu—Glu—Asp(NH_2)—Tyr—Glu—Asp—(carbohydrate)

In a further study of the nature of the carbohydrate prosthetic groups of this large glycopeptide, Rothfus & Smith [223] carried out a Smith periodate oxidation [239]. Periodate oxidation has been applied extensively to the elucidation of carbohydrate structure, based upon the quantitative measurement of the consumption of the oxidant, the concomitant formation of formic acid and formaldehyde and the properties of the oxidized carbohydrate after its subsequent reduction to a polyalcohol. The information, however, is difficult to interpret in the case of glycoproteins since certain amino acids (e.g. cystine, cysteine, N-terminal tyrosine, N-terminal threonine and N-terminal serine) are also readily oxidized; furthermore, titrimetric measurement of the evolved formic acid is confused by the changed pK_a

values of the oxidized protein. Information can, however, be obtained as to the nature of the linkage between carbohydrate and protein [224], but there exist severe limitations to the use of this general procedure, especially where the overall carbohydrate content is as low as in the case of the γG globulins. The technique will possibly prove of more value in the study of the relatively carbohydrate rich γA and γM globulins.

More meaningful results were obtained [223] by applying the Smith degradation procedure to the glycopeptide I isolated from human γG globulin by Rosevear & Smith [217]. After controlled periodate oxidation, the product is reduced by sodium borohydride, when very mild acid hydrolysis preferentially cleaves the sensitive acetal bonds. The residual resistant oligo-saccharide may be recovered and subjected to further oxidation. Using this procedure, it was found [217] that, as in the other serum glycoproteins, N-acetyl-neuraminic acid and *L*-fucose probably occupied positions near the non-reducing terminal of the carbohydrate chain, and that all the sugars were in the pyranose form. Much of the mannose and N-acetyl-*D*-glucosamine resisted oxidation, whereas the galactose as well as the fucose and N-acetyl-neuraminic acid were oxidized completely. The pyranose structure of the readily oxidizable components was inferred from the recovery and positive identification of polyols (glycerol, derived from hexoses, and 1,2-propylene glycol, derived from methyl pentoses, i.e. fucose), implying a substituent on C_2 of galactose. In the oxidation procedure used, glycopeptide (0·5 per cent w/v) was oxidized in aqueous sodium periodate (0·06 M) at 28° C in the dark. Aliquots (1 ml) were withdrawn at intervals and the amount of periodate reduced was determined by arsenite titration. The increase in acidity was followed by potentiometric titration of aliquots (1 ml), after stopping the oxidation by the addition of ethylene glycol (0·05 ml). The accuracy of this method was followed by a parallel oxidation of erythritol. After stopping oxidation (after 7 hours) by the addition of ethylene glycol, concentrating by lyophilization and partially desalting by gel filtration (Sephadex G25 column, 0·9 × 150 cm), the ninhydrin- and orcinol-positive components (all in the excluded fraction) were pooled and concentrated to approximately 50 ml, and reduced with sodium borohydride (200 mg) for 4 hours at room temperature, when the final pH was 10·1. After neutralizing (with dilute HCl), and concentrating by partial lyophilization, the reduction product was desalted as before. Glycopeptide fractions (in a total volume of 50 ml) were analysed by paper chromatography, after hydrolysis of aliquots with 2 N HCl for varying times up to 12 hours, revealing the presence of mannose and glucosamine (deacetylated by the acid hydroly-sis) which had resisted oxidation, and glycerol and 1,2-propylene glycol (derived from the oxidation of galactose and fucose respectively).

The glycosidic bonds involving oxidized hexose residues are more acid-labile than those between unoxidized residues. The products of very mild acid-hydrolysis (0·1 N HCl at room temperature for 24 hours) of the residual oxidized/reduced glycopeptide, analysed by paper chromatography, revealed only oligosaccharides containing glucosamine. Glyceraldehyde and glycol-aldehyde were determined in the hydrolysates by the acid/diphenylamine reaction of Dische & Borenfreund [226] by dichromatic readings at 660 mμ (for glycolaldehyde) and 520 mμ (for glyceraldehyde). The glycolaldehyde could have arisen from hexoses linked through C_4 or C_6, or from non-reducing end-groups such as *L*-fucose, while the glyceraldehyde must have arisen from oxidized hexoses bearing a substituent on C_2 (probably galactose). Infra-red spectroscopy of the glycopeptide indicated a complete absence of ester linkages, from which it was deduced that the mode of linkage of the carbohydrate to the protein is probably through a *stable glycosylamine bond through the amide group of asparagine.*

Further work has been carried out by Clamp & Putnam [161], on a glyco-peptide derived by sequential proteolysis with pepsin and pronase of human γG globulin (Cohn II 1, 2). For the proteolysis, γG globulin (20 g) in 0·1 M sodium chloride adjusted to pH 2 (550 ml) was incubated with pepsin (0·25 g) for 48 hours at 37° C, pH being maintained at 2 throughout the incubation. After neutralizing with 1 N NaOH and concentrating to small volume (*in vacuo*), the digest was dried over phosphorus pentoxide. The product was triturated with ethanol, water (300 ml) was added, and the filtrate adjusted to pH 8·5 with 1 N NaOH. It was then made 0·02 M with respect to calcium chloride, incubated with pronase (0·4 g) at 37° C for 48 hours, neutralized and dried as before. The glycopeptides were extracted from the pronase digestion with 90 per cent (w/v) phenol-water, and precipitated by the addition of ethanol; the precipitate was then washed serially with a mixture of ethanol and phenol-water, acetone, ether and dried. The product (1·53 g.) had a hexose content of 3·2 per cent. A portion of this material (1·4 g), dissolved in water, was filtered through Sephadex G25 (150 × 2·25 cm), the hexose fractions being pooled and concentrated (rotary evaporation) to dryness, yielding crude glycopeptide material (0·11 g, hexose content 40·1 per cent). Final purification was achieved by preparative paper chromatography on Whatman 3 MM paper, irrigated with the organic phase of a solvent mixture comprising 1-butanol:acetic acid:water (4:1:5) in which glycopeptides are immobile. Elution of the base-line residual material with water resulted in the recovery (after evaporation to dryness) of material (20 mg) containing 43·6 per cent hexose. Chemical analyses indicated the molar ratios of the constituents of this glycopeptide material, given in Table 7.14. It is noted that, apart from the aspartic acid, the amino-acid components of the glycopeptide isolated from peptic and pronase degradation of human γG globulin (chiefly serine and threonine) differ from those located as vicinal to the aspartic-acid residue carrying the carbohydrate chain in the papain glycopeptides isolated by Rosevear & Smith [217], namely:

Asp—Tyr—Glu—Asp
| |
NH$_2$ Carbohydrate

It is thus possible that in the pepsin-pronase glycopeptides, the aspartic acid

TABLE 7.14

Amino-acid and amino-sugar analysis of purified glycopeptides* recovered from human γG globulin (Cohn fraction II) after sequential pepsin and pronase proteolysis (as described in the text) (reproduced by courtesy of Drs J.R.Clamp and F.W.Putnam from *J. Biol. Chem.* (1964) **239**, 3233)

| Amino acid | HCl hydrolysis | | Molar ratio† |
	2 N at 98° C for 6 hours	6 N at 105° C for 22 hours	
	μmole‡		
Lysine	Trace	0·04	0·17
Ammonia	0·85	0·95	
Amino sugar	0·98	0·48	4·08
Aspartic acid	0·18	0·24	1·00
Threonine	0·13	0·17	0·71
Serine	0·13	0·18	0·75
Glutamic acid	Trace	0·03	0·12
Proline	Trace	0·05	0·21
Glycine	Trace	0·03	0·12
Alanine	Trace	0·02	0·08
Peptides	Present	Absent	

* Amino acids present at 0·01 μmole or less are not included.

† The molar ratios are calculated relative to aspartic acid (1·0). The amino-sugar value is taken from the 2 N HCl hydrolysis, and the other values from the 6 N HCl hydrolysis.

‡ Glycopeptide hydrolysate, 0·54 mg, applied to column.

carrying the carbohydrate chain is N-terminal rather than C-terminal as observed in the papain glycopeptides (as also suggested for rabbit γG globulin by Press [435]).

Further light has been shed on the sequence and nature of the anomeric linkages of the carbohydrate chains by work carried out by Pardoe [228]. Glycopeptides were isolated by proteolysis of heat-denatured pooled human γG globulin (Cohn fraction II 1, 2) using trypsin and pronase respectively under conditions of continual dialysis at optimum pH (as already mentioned). The glycopeptides were recovered from the digest (after holding at 100° C for 1 minute to inactivate and coagulate the enzyme) in the supernatant after centrifugation, by concentration (rotary evaporation) and extraction of the residue with trichloracetic acid (as previously described). Fractionation on Sephadex G25 monitored with orcinol and ninhydrin indicated that whereas there was a considerable ninhydrin-positive peak in the included moiety, substantially all the carbohydrate was present in the ninhydrin-positive material of the excluded fraction. High-voltage electrophoresis in one dimension (on Whatman 3 MM paper) resulted in the separation of ten ninhydrin spots, of which only two were positive to the periodate-benzidine spray [162] reagents (mentioned earlier), in the case of the pronase digestion; the tryptic glycopeptide fraction, also recovered from Sephadex G25 fractionation of the digest, showed a similar paper electrophoretic pattern, but a single carbohydrate-positive spot was obtained. Paper chromatography of both pronase and tryptic digests, irrigated with n-butanol:acetic acid:water (12 : 3 : 5 v/v) yielded in each case a single large spot on the origin, whereas mobile carbohydrate-negative peptides were separated; preparative paper chromatography in this solvent system resulted in the recovery of carbohydrate-containing peptide material. High-voltage electrophoresis of these products yielded a single carbohydrate-positive spot from the tryptic digest, but two spots of rather similar electrophoretic mobility were located in the pronase digestion fraction.

Induced glycosidic enzymes of known and defined specificity were isolated and partially purified from cell-free culture filtrates of *Klebsiella aerogenes* NCIB 9479 [229, 230]. By this means, specific α-L-neuraminidase, α-L-fucosidase, β-D-galactosidase, N-acetyl-β-D-glucosaminidase were isolated and their strict specificity determined by incubating with various substrates [230, 272]. Incubation of tryptic glycopeptide with neuraminidase, followed by subsequent gel filtration (through Sephadex G25) resulted in the recovery of all the neuraminic acid in the included moiety, the residual (excluded) glycopeptide containing no bound sialic acid; all the remaining carbohydrate components were, however, still present. The residual glycopeptide, when incubated with either α-L-fucosidase or β-D-galactosidase, lost L-fucose or D-galactose respectively, these sugars being recovered from the Sephadex G25 included moiety, and determined (by Dische & Shettles assay [220]; orcinol assay [150] and specific galactose oxidase colorimetric reaction [273] respectively). The original glycopeptide was degraded by α-L-fucosidase, but not by β-D-galactosidase. Glycopeptide, from which either L-fucose or D-galactose had been removed enzymatically, was susceptible to cleavage by β-D-glucosaminidase, some material being recovered in the

Sephadex G25 included fraction which, after acid hydrolysis (3 N HCl for 2 hours at 100° C), contained components giving a positive reaction with the Elson-Morgan reagents [274] indicative of hexosamine. These experiments have shown that the sialic acid and fucose are α-glycosidically linked, whereas the galactose and N-acetyl-*D*-glucosamine are β linked. Moreover, the terminal sequence shows sialic acid and *L*-fucose on different chain ends, probably linked to galactose. Since previous work [230, 272] has shown that N-acetyl-β-*D*-glucosaminidase from this source tends to cleave oligosaccharides, the sequence next to galactose awaits further elucidation. The anomeric linkage of mannose has not yet been ascertained, but Li [419] has shown the presence of α-linked *D*-mannose residues in the glycoproteins orosomucoid (α_1-acid glycoprotein), ovalbumin and ovomucoid; the presence of a similar mannose linkage in other glycoproteins, including immunoglobulins, seems highly probable.

From these structural studies [161, 217, 223, 228], it is concluded that carbohydrate is attached as a single polysaccharide chain to the heavy chain of human γG globulin. Attachment is by a glycosyl linkage to the amide group of asparagine. The carbohydrate linked to the amino acid is N-acetyl-*D*-glucosamine, and the resistance of this sugar to periodate oxidation indicates that it carries a substituent on the C_3 or C_4 positions. The ease with which galactose is oxidized by periodate, and removed (after prior removal of neuraminic acid or fucose) by the action of β-*D*-galactosidase, implies that this sugar is near the non-reducing terminal of the chain, while the resistance of the mannose residues to acid hydrolysis would suggest their position to be near to the reducing N-acetyl-*D*-glucosamine residues attached to the protein. The arrangement of the carbohydrate in the chains is thus similar to that deduced for orosomucoid [230].

Structural studies have also been carried out by Nolan & Smith on glycopeptides isolated by a similar proteolytic degradation of rabbit [275] and bovine [276] γG globulins. For example [275], they used a rabbit γG globulin preparation isolated from pooled sera of rabbits hyperimmunized with *Pneumococcal* polysaccharide SVII (Squibb), which contained γ_2G globulin (93 per cent), γ_1G globulin (1 per cent) and approximately 3 per cent each of α_1 and α_2 globulins. This preparation (40 g) was incubated at 60° C for 29 hours with mercuripapain activated by dimercaptopropanol, by a similar procedure to that used by Rosevear & Smith [217] for the degradation of human γG globulin (already discussed), pH being maintained between 6·3 and 6·8 by the addition of 1 N NaOH, and the course of proteolysis being followed by the increased reactivity with ninhydrin. The insoluble residue, removed by centrifugation, contained only about 0·4 per cent of the total hexoses. A multi-stage purification procedure, monitored by ninhydrin and orcinol reactions, was adopted for the recovery of glycopeptides. The first step involved treatment with Dowex 50 × 8, yielding hexose-containing material

(8·5 g), which was subjected (in 500 mg portions) to gel filtration on Sephadex G25 (column size $122 \times 2·8$ cm), when the glycopeptides were eluted as a single peak in the excluded moiety. A sample of the glycopeptides (500 mg) was fractionated by gradient elution from a column ($85 \times 2·8$ cm) of DEAE-cellulose in veronal buffer (pH 8·4, $I = 0·005$ to $0·5$), a total of 3 litres of effluent being collected in the recovery of five glycopeptide fractions, which were shown to be homogeneous when examined by two-dimensional chromatography and electrophoresis on paper (as previously described). Recoveries of hexose obtained by this multi-step purification procedure are

TABLE 7.15

Recovery of glycopeptides from a papain digest of heat denatured γG globulin, after isolation by the multistep fractionation procedure described in the text. (This Table and Tables 7.16a and 7.16b are reproduced by courtesy of Drs. C.Nolan and E.L.Smith from *J. Biol. Chem.* (1962) **237,** 446)

Step	Preparation	Yield (as per cent of total hexose)	
		Each step (per cent)	Over-all (per cent)
1	Papain digestion	99	99
2	Dowex 50 treatment	97	96
3	Gel filtration	96	92
4	DEAE-column chromatography	95	88
5	Gel filtration	95*	83

* This value represents the minimal recovery of each of the individual glycopeptide fractions obtained from step 4. The over-all recovery from step 4 (88 per cent) is a better representation of the total recovery.

given in Table 7.15. Chemical analysis revealed the molar ratios and estimated residues shown in Table 7.16. The amino-acid sequence of 'glycopeptide IV', investigated by Edman [198, 205] degradation and leucine aminopeptidase (as already indicated), was:

$$
\begin{array}{ccccc}
\text{Glu} & \text{Glu} & \text{Glu} & \text{Phe} & \text{Asp} \\
| & | & & & | \\
\text{NH}_2 & \text{NH}_2 & & & \text{Carbohydrate}
\end{array}
$$

The sequence of amino acids in a glycopeptide fraction isolated by similar proteolytic degradation of bovine γG globulin [276] was found to be:

TABLE 7.16

(a) Composition of glycopeptides isolated from rabbit γG globulin

The values listed have not been corrected for destruction except in the case of glucosamine, as noted. In calculating the number of residues of each component, the weighted average of the concentrations of the amino-acid components in the stock solution of the glyco-peptide was taken as the concentration of the glycopeptide. The aspartic-acid value was excluded from the average in the case of glycopeptide 4. Sialic acid was calculated as N-acetylneuraminic acid.

Residue*	Glycopeptide 2		Glycopeptide 3		Glycopeptide 4	
	Molar ratio	Estimated residues	Molar ratio	Estimated residues	Molar ratio	Estimated residues
Hexose	2·9	3	2·7	3	3·7	4
Glucosamine†	4·0	4	3·3	4	3·9	4
	(4·6)		(4·3)		(4·5)	
Fucose	1·0	1	0·8	1	0·9	1
Sialic acid	None	0	None	0	0·26	0
Aspartic acid	1·03	1	1·00	1	1·28	1
Glutamic acid	1·94	2	1·05	1	2·97	3
Phenylalanine	0·97	1	0·91	1	1·01	1

 * In addition to the amino acids listed, glycopeptide 4 contained threonine, serine and glycine in amounts equivalent to 0·17, 0·19 and 0·21 residues, respectively. Other amino acids were absent from the glycopeptide preparations or present in amounts equivalent to less than 0·1 of a residue.

 † The glucosamine values in parentheses were obtained in conjunction with the amino-acid analyses with an automatic amino-acid analyser and are corrected for an estimated 47 per cent destruction. The other values were obtained by a p-dimethylaminobenzaldehyde method.

(b) Amino-acid sequence of peptides separated from glycopeptide 4 by leucine amino-peptidase and papain hydrolysis

Enzyme	Substrate	Products
Leucine amino-peptidase	Glycopeptide 4	(Glu, 1·00; Glu-NH₂, 0·77; Phe, 0·36; Asp, 0·16)*
Papain	Glycopeptide 4	Peptide P1 (Glu, Glu-NH₂)
		Peptide P2 (Glu, Glu-NH₂ Glu-NH₂)
		Peptide P3 (Glu-NH₂, Phe, Asp.(CHO))
Leucine amino-peptidase	Peptide P3	(Glu-NH₂, Phe, Asp.(CHO))
Sequence		Glu. Glu-NH₂.Glu-NH₂.Phe.Asp.(CHO)

 * The values represent the molar ratios of the amino acids released by leucine amino-peptidase. CHO represents carbohydrate.

Lys—Pro—Arg—Glu—Glu—Glu—Phe—Asp

| |

NH$_2$ Carbohydrate

As is shown in Table 7.6, the carbohydrate compositions of the γG globulins of human and various animal species are very similar. The carbohydrate content of the γM and γA immunoglobulins is higher than that of the γG globulins; no information is at present available of the carbohydrate content of the γD immunoglobulins. The carbohydrate prosthetic groups seem to be confined to the heavy chains of the various classes of human, rabbit, and horse immunoglobulins examined, although trace amounts found in light chain preparations cannot be unequivocally attributed to contamination by heavy chains. Chemical analyses of papain digestion fragments appeared to indicate that the carbohydrate groups are located at two distinct sites on the heavy chain in rabbit and horse γG globulins [1, 106]. As already mentioned in section B1, two carbohydrate-containing fragments were isolated from peptic digests (at pH 4·5) of rabbit γG globulin by gel filtration on Sephadex G75 [84, 435, 453]. One appeared to be located in a region of the molecule close to the C-terminal end of the papain Fab fragment (as shown in Fig. 7.10), whilst the other (which contained all the fucose of the rabbit γG globulin) was isolated in an immunogenically inactive fragment (of 14,000 mol. wt.) derived from the heavy chains comprising the Fc region.

In recent studies, Bolton *et al* [402] have used the method of gas-liquid chromatography to identify carbohydrate components in hydrolysates of glycopeptides and glycoproteins. This sensitive procedure permits a complete quantitative analysis to be performed on micro-amounts of biological materials (containing about 0·25 mg total carbohydrate) by a single simple step, thus having considerable advantages over classical methods of carbohydrate analysis. After methanolysis, the trimethylsilyl ethers of the constituent sugars can be obtained quantitatively and rapidly (1–3 minutes). The method has been used for quantitative determination of neutral and amino sugars including N-acetyl-neuraminic acid.

A major problem in chemical analysis of glycopeptides has been the quantitation of the ratios of the two hexoses usually encountered, galactose and mannose. A separation was achieved by Eylar & Jeanloz [225], by using Dowex 1 × 8 initially in the carbonate form, and subsequently preferentially eluting the mannose as borate complex. The galactose was later eluted at greatly increased ionic strength. A recent variation of this technique [403] uses the strongly basic anion-exchange resin in the sulphate cycle, the adsorbed sugars being eluted sequentially with 86 per cent ethanol. The separations depend on the partition of the sugars between the water-rich resin phase and the less polar external solution of the ethanol. The method has been automated [405, 416]. Details of methods for the qualitative and quantitative analysis of the component sugars of glycopeptides derived from glyco-proteins are discussed by Northcote [430] and by Neuberger & Marshall [431].

3. Biological activities associated with sub-units

(a) Activities located in Fab fragments

Massive efforts are being made to identify and characterize the antigen-combining sides of antibody molecules. As already mentioned (in section B1), studies with papain and pepsin digestion fragments from 'bivalent' rabbit γG globulin molecules have shown that one antigen receptor site is located in each of the two Fab portions of the molecule, thus accounting for the failure of the 3·5S Fab fragments to form precipitin lattices whilst retaining their capacity to combine with antigen. Subsequent studies have been directed towards establishing the role in antigen combination of the light chains and of those portions of the heavy chains within the Fab fragments of the antibody molecule (i.e. the Fd piece); and to the identification of the key amino acids within the active sites.

As mentioned earlier (in section B2), Edelman *et al* [231] concluded that the light chains (but not the heavy chains) of reduced and alkylated guinea-pig anti-hapten (2,4-dinitrophenyl-polylysine) antibody were probably associated with antibody activity on the grounds that their starch-gel electro-phoresis patterns (in 8 M urea at pH 3·5) showed a discrete banding, which appeared to correlate with the specificity of the parent antibody. It was not possible, however, to carry out direct hapten-binding tests on the separated heavy and light chains, as their activity was destroyed by the conditions employed in their isolation (involving reduction with 0·1 M 2-mercaptoethanol in 8 M urea for 2 hours at room temperature, followed by alkylation with iodoacetamide). A similar limitation restricted the approach of Franek & Nezlin [232], wherein very high losses (98 per cent) of antibody activity were incurred by using an equally drastic procedure for the separation of the heavy and light chains of horse antibody (against diphtheria and tetanus toxoid), involving the cleavage of disulphide bonds with sodium sulphite and cupric nitrate (yielding S-sulpho derivatives), followed by fractionation on Sephadex G100 in 0·05 M formic acid–6 M urea.

The problem of isolating heavy and light chains in active form was partially resolved by applying the relatively mild isolation procedures devised by Fleischman *et al* [102] (outlined in section B2), which permitted the retention of a substantial amount of the original antibody activity. Although, as might be expected, neither the heavy nor light chain preparations prepared in this manner (from horse or rabbit γG globulin fractions containing antibodies against various protein antigens) retained the ability to precipitate with its specific antigen, the heavy chain, but not the light chain, caused a marked delay in the time of precipitation if added to antiserum before the addition of antigen. Furthermore, only the heavy chain was co-precipitated with the specific antigen–antibody precipitate. There are, however, several disadvantages to exploiting the latter property as a test system, which cause difficulties in quantitation of antibody activity.

In consequence, most of the other studies on the nature of the active sites of antibodies have relied on the use of highly purified anti-hapten antibodies, the specific activity of which can be readily measured by various methods. In preparing such antibodies (e.g. anti-DNP-bovine γG globulin), use is made of their excessive affinity for the homologous hapten (ε-N-2,4-dinitrophenyl-*L*-lysine, or briefly, ε-N-DNP-lysine) [233]. Because of this strong affinity, however, subsequent dissociation of the antibody from specific precipitate is difficult, and is more readily achieved by the use of 2,4-dinitrophenol, which has a relatively low affinity for the anti-DNP antibody, but which can be employed at high concentration (0·1 M). Approximately 50–60 per cent of the anti-hapten antibody can be thus extracted from the specific precipitate in the form of the DNP-antibody complex (provided that a sufficient volume of 0·1 M 2,4-dinitrophenol is used). Inclusion of streptomycin in the hapten solution prevents the antigen from simultaneously dissolving, because of the ability of this antibiotic to form highly insoluble salt-like complexes with extensively substituted dinitrophenyl proteins (which are polyanionic at pH > 4). Subsequent passage of the soluble DNP–antibody complex through Dowex 1 removes the dissociable hapten, leaving purified anti-hapten antibody which can be concentrated by ammonium sulphate precipitation, and dialysed exhaustively to remove any residual free hapten. An outline of such a purification scheme, which provides antibody of which approximately 85–90 per cent precipitates with DNP-bovine γG globulin, is given in Fig. 7.35. In an alternative procedure, the yield of anti-hapten antibody is increased by extracting the initial specific precipitate with ε-N-DNP-*lysine*, which is bound much more strongly by the antibody than is 2,4-dinitrophenol itself, and therefore competes more effectively with the precipitated antigen (DNP-bovine γG globulin) for antibody-binding sites. The difficult task of removing the ε-N-DNP-lysine from its soluble complex with the anti-hapten antibody is accomplished by passing the ε-N-DNP-lysine-antibody complexes through large columns (4·5 × 31 cm) of Sephadex G25 (using 1 g Sephadex per 1 mg antibody protein) saturated with 0·1 M 2,4-dinitro-phenol. In this way, the ε-N-DNP-lysine can be displaced from antibody by the dinitrophenol, which is subsequently removed by dissociation on Dowex 1, as described in the previous method. Eisen [234] gives full experimental details for both methods.

In another method of purifying anti-DNP-hapten antibodies [112] (referred to in more detail later), the initial specific precipitate is formed by interacting the antiserum with antigen incorporating hapten linked to a heterologous protein 'carrier'. Similarly, the initial step in the purification of anti-p-azo-benzoate antibodies [235] produced by immunization with γ globulin azo-benzoate, involved precipitation with antigen incorporating a heterologous 'carrier' (namely, ovalbumin-azo-benzoate). In this case, use is made of ion-exchange chromatography on DEAE-cellulose to separate the antihapten

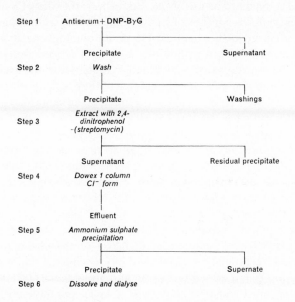

Fig. 7.35. Outline of the scheme employed in the purification of anti-2,4-dinitrophenyl-bovine γG globulin antibody.

(Reproduced by courtesy of Drs F.S.Farah, M.Kern and H.N.Eisen from *J. exp. Med.* (1960), **112**, 1195.)

antibody from the antigen, which remains bound to the column after dissociation of the specific precipitate by 0·1 M p-nitrobenzoate at pH 7·0.

Various methods have been employed in the measurement of antibody–hapten affinity. Of these, *equilibrium dialysis* has found widest application in the determination of the hapten-binding capacity of antibody sub-units. After attaining equilibrium, the concentration of hapten on each side of the membrane is determined by measurement of some distinctive property such as absorbance, fluorescence or radioactivity. Moreover, since the formation of hapten–antibody complex is reversible, it is immaterial whether antibody and hapten are placed in separate compartments or in the same compartment [236].

(Full details of the equilibrium dialysis technique and methods of hapten-conjugation are given in Chapter 14.) Utsumi & Karush [237] used equilibrium dialysis at neutral pH to measure the number of intact combining sites, and the average dissociation constants, of the heavy and light chains of a specifically purified rabbit anti-hapten (anti-p-azo-phenyl-β-lactoside) antibody. The heavy and light chain preparations were obtained by mild reduction (with 2-mercaptoethanol) and alkylation under anaerobic conditions, followed by gel filtration through Sephadex G200 in M tris buffer, pH 8·0 (containing 0·03 M sodium decyl sulphate). The use of the detergent (rather than 1 N acetic or 1 N propionic acid) affords a means of studying the activity of the chain preparations in unaggregated form at neutral pH; specific binding capacity is, however, lost by its removal. By this method, the *heavy* chains were found to contain nearly all of the original hapten-combining sites, although the average association constant was somewhat lower than that of the original antibody preparation [238]. Again, however, no activity was found in the light chain preparation.

In a similar approach, Metzger & Singer [153] used purified rabbit antibodies directed against the 2,4-dinitrophenyl determinant (anti-DNP) which, as already mentioned, have the advantage of an unusually high affinity for the homologous hapten (ε-N-2,4-dinitrophenyl-lysine) [240], resulting in the retention of antibody activity under adverse conditions (e.g. even at the pH of 1 N propionic acid). A typical experimental procedure is as follows: After reduction of the interchain disulphide bridges of rabbit anti-DNP antibody (and normal rabbit γG globulin control) with 2-mercaptoethanol in 0·55 M tris buffer, pH 8·2, and subsequent alkylation of the liberated sulphydryl groups with iodoacetamide (by the method of Fleischman *et al* [102] described earlier in section B1), followed by overnight dialysis against 0·16 M NaCl, the dialysis sac is opened and ε-N-DNP-lysine (2 moles per mole protein) added. Dialysis is continued against 1 N propionic acid containing ε-N-DNP-lysine (6×10^{-6} M). By thus adding the specific hapten to the reduced anti-DNP *before* exposing the protein to 1 N propionic acid, appreciable binding capacity can be retained in the subsequent presence of the acid. This capacity ('r'), usually expressed as the number of moles of hapten bound per mole of antibody protein, is calculated from absorbance measurements made at 280 mμ (for protein) and at 360 mμ (for the ε-N-DNP-lysine hapten), using the dialysate as blank, assuming

$$E \frac{1 \text{ per cent}}{1 \text{ cm}} = 14\cdot6 \text{ at } 280 \text{ m}\mu \text{ for the protein,}$$

$$E \frac{1 \text{ per cent}}{1 \text{ cm}} = 0\cdot89 \times 10^4 \text{ at } 360 \text{ m}\mu \text{ for the antibody-bound } \varepsilon\text{-N-DNP-lysine.}$$

The number of moles of ε-N-DNP-lysine bound per mole of antibody protein was thus calculated to be 1·65 at a protein concentration of 0·95 mg/ml in 1 N propionic acid (containing ε-N-DNP-lysine 6×10^{-6} M). In contrast, the control normal rabbit γG globulin had the same absorbance as the dialysate at 360 mμ (after correcting for the small intrinsic absorbance at this wavelength by the protein), indicating that it had failed to bind any of the hapten.

In subsequent separations of the heavy and light chains of the reduced and alkylated antibody (and normal) γ globulins containing excess hapten, samples (50 mg) of protein were applied successively to a column ($75 \times 2·8$ cm) of Sephadex G75 equilibrated with 1 N propionic acid containing 6×10^{-6} M ε-N-DNP-lysine. Elution patterns obtained by absorbance measurements at 280 mμ and 360 mμ (using equilibrating mixture as control) are compared in Fig. 7.36, which also includes the patterns given by reduced and alkylated anti-DNP (and normal) rabbit γG globulin in the absence of hapten. This revealed that the ε-N-DNP-lysine was eluted with the *heavy* chain in the first peak of the reduced and alkylated anti-DNP antibody, but not with the light chain peak, under conditions where essentially no association of ε-N-DNP-lysine with either heavy or light chain peaks of *normal* γG globulin occurred. In addition, however, a third of the theoretical yield of light chains was eluted with the heavy chains, instead of in the customary second peak (i.e. the heavy : light chain distribution in the first and second peaks changed to 21 : 4 instead of the normal distribution of 19 : 6 observed in the fractionation of normal rabbit γG globulin equilibrated with 6×10^{-6} M ε-N-DNP-lysine and 1 N propionic acid). These findings suggest that the light chains may play a direct role in the combination of hapten with heavy chains. Alternatively, however, they might merely reflect the influence of the hapten in maintaining the conformation of the heavy chains necessary for combination with light chains.

Similarly, studies with highly purified polypeptide chains of guinea-pig γ_2G globulin antibody, directed against the DNP-haptenic group [112], suggested that *light* chains were also involved in the binding of hapten by the heavy chains. Anti-DNP antibodies were isolated from sera of guinea-pigs immunized with DNP-bovine γG globulin by precipitation at equivalence with DNP-bovine fibrinogen in the presence of 0·01 M disodium ethylene diamine tetra-acetate, and subsequent elution of the washed precipitate with 0·1 M 2,4-dinitrophenol in the presence of streptomycin. The antibody was then freed of the dissociable hapten by passing the soluble antibody–dinitrophenol complex through a column of Dowex 1 ×8 (200–400 mesh) equilibrated with 0·01 M phosphate buffer (containing 0·15 M NaCl) at pH 7·4. The heavy and light chains were separated by mild reduction of the antibody by dithioerythritol and alkylation by iodoacetamide, followed by gel filtration on Sephadex G200 in the presence of 4 M guanidine-hydrochloride (as described in detail in section B2, and illustrated in Fig. 7.18). Hapten-binding activity was determined by equilibrium dialysis at room temperature, using (^{3}H)-DNP

I

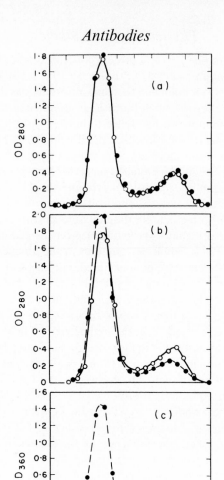

Fig. 7.36.(a) Sephadex G75 elution patterns of reduced, alkylated normal rabbit γG globulin (open circles) and anti-DNP antibodies (closed circles) from the same column equilibrated with 1 M propionic acid. (b) Protein elution patterns, and (c) DNP-lysine elution patterns of reduced, alkylated rabbit γG globulin (open circles, solid line) and anti-DNP antibodies (closed circles, dashed line) containing excess DNP-lysine from a Sephadex G75 column equilibrated with 1 M propionic acid containing 6×10^{-6} M ε-DNP-lysine.

(Reproduced by courtesy of Drs H.Metzger and S.J. Singer from *Science* (1963), **142**, 674.)

coupled to ε-amino-caproic acid (with a specific activity of 19·5 mc/1 mM) as hapten. Initial volumes of 0·8 ml were employed inside and ouside the sac, and the hapten concentration (2·6–3·0 × 10⁻¹⁰ moles) resulted in about 6000 counts/min/10⁻⁹ moles of hapten (when hapten (0·45 ml) was added to phosphor (15 ml) and counted in a Packard Tris-Carb Liquid Scintillation Counter). The amounts of protein used ranged from 84 to 600 μg, and mixtures of heavy and light chains were made in molar ratios of 1:1 or 1:2. Protein concentrations were determined from absorbance measurements, assuming that $E_{1\,cm}^{1\%} = 13\cdot3$ at 280 mμ and the moles of antibody-combining sites equal the moles of heavy chain (assuming a molecular weight of 5×10^4). When only light chains were employed (for purposes of comparison), the moles of protein were calculated assuming a molecular weight of 2×10^4. The change in volume during dialysis was determined by weighing the dialysis sac and its contents before and after dialysis. About 2 per cent of the hapten was found bound to the dialysis sac. Significant hapten binding was thus observed only when specific *heavy* chains were present with *light* chains. Moreover, *specific* light chains were more effective in this respect than non-specific light chains (from non-antibody guinea-pig γ_2 G-globulin). After recombination of specific heavy and specific light chains, about 9 per cent of the potential binding sites were occupied by hapten (representing a maximum of about 29 per cent of recovery of the activity of native antibody at a similar hapten:binding site ratio).

In another approach [241], attempts have been made to locate the active site of an antibody by precipitin formation with antigen incorporating a radio-active isotopically labelled hapten (¹⁴C-polytyrosyl-gelatin), followed by removal of the hapten carrier (gelatin) by specific enzymatic digestion (with collagenase). This leaves ¹⁴C-polytyrosyl groups firmly bound to the antibody. As these could only be fully dissociated at pH 1·8, the heavy and light chains of the reduced and alkylated antibody, labelled in this manner, were separated on Sephadex G75 in 1 N propionic acid. Unequivocal conclusions could not be drawn from the distribution of radioactivity within the fractions isolated, owing to appreciable (80 per cent) dissociation of the hapten from reduced and unreduced antibody in 1 N propionic acid, although the detection of radioactivity in a peak eluted ahead of the heavy chain peak suggested that the polytyrosyl group might be bound to heavy chain dimer (or possibly to undissociated antibody).

More precise location of the active sites of anti-hapten antibody molecules has been obtained by techniques involving specific or differential hapten labelling. The specific methods have developed out of the extensive studies carried out mainly by the Pressman group, involving the general blocking of different polar groups and side chains within the antibody molecule by chemical substitution. In these earlier investigations, for example [242], the effect of acetylation of anti-hapten (specifically purified rabbit anti-p-azobenzoate antibody) on its reaction with hapten (p-azobenzoate) was determined. It was found (from equilibrium dialysis studies) that there was little loss in binding capacity (even when over 90 per cent of the amino groups of the rabbit antibody were acetylated), although the treatment resulted in loss of precipitating power. In other experiments [243], acetylation (of 96 per cent of rabbit anti-BSA amino groups) was shown to destroy antigen-precipitating ability without preventing the combination of antibody with antigen, to form soluble complexes detectable by electrophoresis and ultra-centrifugation. Evidence, thus obtained and substantiated by studies of the effect of iodination [244, 245, 246] and of variation of pH [247] on hapten binding, all points to *tyrosine* residues playing an important role in the active sites of rabbit antibodies. The effect of iodination with ^{131}I on antibody activity has been studied [244] in systems involving specific precipitation of rabbit anti-ovalbumin and anti-BSA antibodies, tissue localization of rabbit anti-kidney antibody and cell binding of rabbit anti-human erythrocyte antibody. In each system, the antibody activity was found to decrease rapidly with iodination, thirty iodine atoms per antibody molecule essentially destroying activity. The effect of iodination (on the binding capacity of rabbit anti-phenyl-arsonic acid antibody) has been determined [245] by the equilibrium dialysis technique, which revealed a direct correlation between the uptake of iodine and the decrease in hapten-binding capacity; there was also evidence that only one iodine-reactive group is present at each binding site. In a comparison of the effect of iodination on the active sites of four anti-hapten antibodies [248], the order of increasing sensitivity to iodination was found to be:

anti-p-azophenyl-trimethylammonium $\leqslant$ anti-p-azobenzoate $<$
anti-3-azopyridine $<$ anti-p-azophenylarsonate.

The ability of hapten (when present during iodination) to protect antibody against loss of activity, was interpreted as further evidence that the iodine-reactive group was within the active site. Moreover, this reactive group, which appeared to be a tyrosyl residue, was present in the active site of each anti-hapten antibody, although the extent to which it was involved in hapten binding appeared to differ for each antibody studied. In later studies [249], incorporating quantitative amino-acid analysis, the iodine-reactive group was firmly identified as a *tyrosyl* residue, by the combined use of catalytic photo-oxidation (which selectively alters the iodine-reactive histidine residue) and iodination (which effected a significant decrease in binding capacity by *tyrosyl* residues only).

The specific labelling techniques to be outlined depend on the ready availability of this type of amino-acid residue within the region of the hapten-binding site of the antibody. For instance, in 'affinity labelling' (similar to that employed in the identification of the active sites of enzymes), use is made of a bifunctional specific hapten, i.e. a hapten carrying a reactive substituent such as a diazonium radical, which is capable of forming a covalent link preferentially with a protein side chain (i.e. tyrosyl) at the anti-hapten antibody active site, to which the hapten is drawn by electrostatic attraction as a result of the affinity of its specific antigenic determinant (e.g. phenylarsonate). Thus, rabbit anti-p-phenylarsonic acid antibody was reacted with p-phenylarsonic acid diazonium fluoborate under the described conditions [250]. Reagent stock solutions were prepared (in water at 0° C) immediately prior to use. A solution of diazonium reagent, $3 \cdot 03 \times 10^{-4}$ M ($0 \cdot 1$ ml) was added with stirring to an ice-cold protein solution containing 6 mg anti-hapten antibody (rabbit anti-phenylarsonic acid) or normal rabbit γG globulin in $2 \cdot 9$ ml $0 \cdot 17$ M borate buffer, pH $8 \cdot 0$, containing $0 \cdot 12$ M NaCl. Thus, the initial molarities of the components of the reaction mixture were protein: $1 \cdot 25 \times 10^{-5}$ and diazonium radical: $1 \cdot 01 \times 10^{-5}$; the rabbit γG globulin (molecular weight taken as 160,000) had an extinction coefficient (1 per cent, 1 cm) = $14 \cdot 6$ at 280 mμ. Reactions were terminated after varying times (1 minute to 24 hours) by the addition of freshly prepared ice-cold tyramine solution ($0 \cdot 32$ M, adjusted to pH $8 \cdot 0$, $0 \cdot 2$ ml), whereby any unreacted diazonium reagent was rapidly removed. After denaturing the azo-protein (precipitated by adding ethanol to a concentration of 75 per cent) and exhaustive washing (to remove residual reagents), the nature and distribution of azo-derivative covalently bound to protein was assessed spectrophotometrically. The washing procedure involved successive centrifugation and decantation of the precipitated protein with ethanol (5 ml), ether (2×5 ml), ethanol (5 ml) and 1 per cent sodium chloride (1 ml) and, finally, 1 per cent sodium chloride (5 ml). The penultimate washing (ethanol containing a little NaCl) prevented turbidity in the supernatant. The washed azo-protein precipitate was dissolved (at 37° C) in a solution of sodium lauryl sulphate ($0 \cdot 5$ per cent) in phosphate buffer ($0 \cdot 02$ M, pH $6 \cdot 2$) ($1 \cdot 5$ ml) and clarified by centrifugation (10,000 rev/min, 10 minutes). The ultraviolet absorption spectrum of the protein solution was recorded automatically over the range 310–600 mμ, initially at pH $6 \cdot 2$ and then after the addition of $0 \cdot 5$ N NaOH to give a final molarity of $0 \cdot 15$ M.

The effect on the coupling reaction of prior blocking of the antibody active sites by specific hapten has been investigated by including the hapten (sodium p-nitrophenylarsonate) in the antibody solution (prior to addition of the diazonium reagent) in 500-fold molar excess over the protein (i.e. at $6 \cdot 25 \times 10^{-3}$ M). Applying this inhibition technique [250], it was shown that two moles of bifunctional hapten were taken up per mole of antibody; the initial rate of formation of azo-tyrosyl derivative was about 400 times greater than the (non-specific) uptake by normal rabbit γG globulin. In contrast, the rate of reaction of bifunctional hapten (e.g. p-phenylarsonic acid diazonium fluoborate) with anti-hapten antibody which had been protected by (reversible) blockage of its active site with hapten (p-nitrophenylarsonate) was as slow as the uptake by normal rabbit γG globulin. Other evidence of labelling of tyrosyl residues at the active site of the antibody molecule was provided by comparison of the UV absorption spectra of the reaction products [250].

Other reagents used as bifunctional haptens include p-carboxyphenyl-diazonium fluobenzoate [250]; p-nitrophenyl-diazonium fluoborate and 2,4-dinitrophenyl-diazonium fluoborate [251]. Other potential reagents which have been used to locate the active sites of enzymes include 4-(iodoacetamido)-salicylic acid [252] and p-nitrophenyl-bromoacetyl-α-amino-isobutyrate [253] (shown to modify a methionine residue near the active site of trypsin). Even at low concentrations (10^{-6} M), some of these reagents (e.g. p-nitrophenyl-diazonium fluoborate) react extremely rapidly with the anti-hapten antibody (at relatively low pH, e.g. 5·0), and in consequence the coupling technique, outlined above, must be modified [251].

In another, 'paired' or '*differential*', labelling procedure [254] a radioactive label is incorporated into the active sites of anti-hapten molecules by covalent linkage to the tyrosyl residues, in the presence and absence of specific hapten. Subsequent proteolytic digestion of the labelled antibody yields peptides which are compared (by the peptide mapping technique previously described in section B2) with peptides obtained by similar proteolysis of unlabelled antibody, whereby evidence of preferential labelling is obtained. In applying this technique, one sample of specifically purified anti-hapten antibody is iodinated with ^{131}I-labelled iodine in the presence of hapten and another portion is iodinated to the same extent with ^{125}I-labelled iodine in the absence of hapten. The preparations are then mixed and subjected to pepsin proteolysis. The resultant peptides are isolated by paper chromatography and high-voltage electrophoresis and counted. It is concluded that any peptide, for which the ratio of the two isotopes differs from that in the original mixture, is derived from a portion of the molecule in which the antibody-hapten complex has affected iodination. Moreover, this region can be localized within a specific polypeptide chain by fractionating the mixture of labelled antibody samples into heavy and light chains prior to peptic digestion and peptide mapping.

In a typical experiment [255], specifically purified rabbit anti-p-azophenyl-arsonate antibody (30·1 mg) dissolved in borate buffer, pH 8·0 (1·9 ml) was added to 1 M glycine buffer, pH 9·0 (1·5 ml) and iodinated (at 0° C) by the dropwise addition of ^{125}I-labelled hypo-iodite ($1·4 \times 10^8$ counts/min) (6·5 μmoles) in 1 M glycine buffer (2·8 ml). Another portion of the same antibody solution containing, in addition, sodium-phenyl-arsonate (60 μmoles) was similarly treated, except that the hypo-iodite was labelled with ^{131}I ($4·9 \times 10^8$ counts/min). After 2 hours at 0° C, both preparations were individually transferred to dialysis sacs and dialysed against borate buffer containing

0·15 M NaCl (2 litres), the dialysate being changed twice daily for 3 days. During the second dialysis, potassium iodide (0·25 g) was added to the outer solution. The iodine uptake per molecule of protein was 25·9 atoms (for the ^{125}I-labelled preparation) and 26·1 atoms (in the case of the ^{131}I-labelled preparation). In order to study the isolated polypeptide chains, portions (equivalent to 19 mg protein) of each solution were mixed, concentrated by pervaporation and then dialysed against 0·55 M tris-HCl buffer, pH 8·2. After adjusting the protein concentration to 20 mg/ml, the heavy and light chains were isolated by the method of Fleischman *et al* [102] (described previously), i.e. after reduction with 0·75 M 2-mercaptoethanol and alkylation, followed by gel filtration through Sephadex G75 (column size 51 × 2·8 cm) in 1 N propionic acid. The radioactivity of the eluates (expressed as ^{131}I counts/min/tube), plotted against the eluate number, revealed a gel-filtration pattern typical for reduced γG globulin (similar to that shown in Fig. 7.17). Thus, 74 per cent of the ^{131}I activity was located in the first (heavy chain) fraction and 26 per cent in the second (light chain) fraction. The former (heavy chain) fraction, subdivided into two fractions, and the light chain fraction were dialysed against distilled water (9 volumes). For peptide analysis, the solutions were lyophilized and the residues were taken up in 0·5 M formic acid containing pepsin (0·33 mg/ml), resulting in a concentration of iodinated protein of 10 mg/ml in each case, and incubated at 37° C for 16 hours. Dialysed lyophilized portions of the protein before and after reduction and alkylation were also digested. The digests were lyophilized and the peptides separated by two-dimensional paper chromatography and electrophoresis as described (in section B2b). Radio-autographs (on Kodak industrial X-ray film, type XX) were prepared and areas on the paper corresponding to spots on the radio-autographs were excised. The concentrations of ^{125}I/^{131}I (in counts/min) on each piece of paper were determined, and the ^{125}I : ^{131}I ratio calculated for each spot.

The patterns of the digest of (i) the mixture of the two iodinated proteins, or (ii) the reduced and alkylated (but unfractionated) mixture were found to be essentially similar. The ratio ^{125}I : ^{131}I was essentially unity for most spots (i.e. it was the same as in the original mixture). It was, however, high for three spots, indicating that more of the iodinated peptides, represented by these spots, came from the antibody iodinated (^{125}I) in the absence of hapten than from antibody combined with hapten during iodination (^{131}I). Moreover, these same three high ratio spots were observed in peptide maps of peptic digests of the light chain fraction, but not in those of peptic digests of the heavy chain subfractions. Thus, it was shown that the binding of hapten affects primarily the iodination of the *light* chains of the antibody. Before concluding unequivocally from this evidence that the high-ratio peptides originated from the hapten-binding site located in the light chains, it will be necessary to establish that the observed effect is not due to a *conformational change* occurring during hapten–antibody combination, leading to an altered rate of iodination at locations other than at the active site.

The paired-label technique has also been used [256] to demonstrate chemical differences between the Fab fragments of types I and II (separated by carboxy-methyl cellulose chromatography) from whole-rabbit γG globulin and from specifically purified rabbit anti-p-azobenzoate antibody.

In other chemical substitution studies [257], specific amidation (by reaction with ethyl acetimidate hydrochloride) of the ε-amino groups (of lysine) of a series of rabbit antibodies has indicated that lysine side chains are not normally present in the active sites. Esterification of carboxyl groups, however, has been shown to influence hapten binding. Furthermore, the interesting observation [259] has been made that when the carboxyl groups of a rabbit antibody directed against a positively charged hapten (phenyltrimethylammonium) are blocked by esterification with diazoacetamide, its binding activity is destroyed. On the other hand, the hapten-binding ability of antibody directed against a negatively charged hapten (e.g. p-(p-azobenzene)-azobenzoate) was un-affected by such treatment. The latter type of antibody did, however, show decreased hapten-binding power in the presence of various anions [260], the effect decreasing in the order $CNS^- > NO_3^- > I^- = Br^- > Cl^-$, sug-gesting the presence of a positively charged group in the active site. Results consistent with these findings have been reported recently by Sela & Mozes [57], who have demonstrated a dependence of the chemical nature of the active sites of rabbit antibodies on the net electrical charge of the antigen (various synthetic polypeptides) Thus, antibodies directed against acidic antigens were eluted predominantly in the first peak on chromatography on DEAE-Sephadex A50 (in 0·02 M potassium phosphate buffer, pH 8·0), whereas antibodies against basic antigens were found mainly in a second peak (observed by subsequent gradient elution using 0·3 M phosphate buffer at pH 8·0).

The antibodies thus separated differ in the composition of their Fab fragments, but possess a common Fc portion (demonstrated by peptide mapping [262]), i.e. in the older terminology, antibody eluted in the first peak from DEAE-Sephadex comprises portions (I III I), whilst the composition of the second peak can be represented as (II III II). Moreover, it has been shown that antibodies with specificities directed towards the same determinant (the 2,4-dinitrophenyl group) belong exclusively to one or other of these two immunoglobulin fractions, depending upon the electrical charge of the macro-molecular carrier (e.g. synthetic acidic and basic polypeptides, polylysyl-rabbit serum albumin) to which the determinant was attached. Consequently, it is concluded that 'the antigen is not just a macromolecular carrier to which specific determinants are attached, but rather that the biosynthesis of the antibody is controlled both by the specificity determinants (in the formation of the specific combining sites) and by other parts of the antigenic molecule (in defining areas of the antibody which do not include the antigen combining sites)' [57].

The experimental approaches outlined above have narrowed down the location of these regions to the Fab portion of the antibody molecule, but (as the findings have indicated) the relative roles of the light chains and Fd portions (of the heavy chains within the Fab fragment) are still far from clear. Evidence is being obtained, however, to suggest that the specific antigen-binding groups are located in the Fd portion of the molecule, their configuration being influenced by the conformation of the neighbouring light chains. A similar effect has been observed in studies of the structural basis of Gm(f) specificity, the folding of the heavy polypeptide chains (within the Fd portion) containing the allotypic specificity being influenced by the neighbouring light chains [420, 439]. Conformational investigations of the type outlined in section C should throw further light on the relative contributions of the heavy and light polypeptide chains to antibody activity. It will be necessary, however, to elucidate the amino-acid sequences within the chains in order to establish the precise role played by primary structure.

Peptide mapping (described in section B2b) has been used in attempts to demonstrate structural differences amongst rabbit γG globulins, which are related to antibody specificity. The maps of peptides from tryptic digests of oxidized fragments Fab (I), Fab (II) (separated on CM-cellulose) and Fc, from papain digests of normal γG globulin, were shown to be identical to patterns obtained for corresponding γG globulin fragments isolated from specific rabbit antisera directed against *Salmonella* H antigen and horse γ globulin (containing at least 20–25 per cent antibody) [264]. There were, however, slight differences discernible between the patterns of the Fab (I) and Fab (II) fragments (revealed by ninhydrin or specific arginine [332] reagents). Gitlin & Merler [182] obtained essentially similar results, although they reported minor differences between the patterns of peptide maps obtained from enzymatic digests of rabbit antibodies directed against *Pneumococcus* types II, III, VI, VII, and XII capsular polysaccharides. Similarly, early determinations of amino-acid composition [265] failed to reveal any significant differences between rabbit γG globulin antibodies of differing specificity.

Significant differences in the amino-acid composition of rabbit antibodies have been demonstrated from analyses of highly purified specific antibodies, however, by using automatic amino-acid analytical techniques of improved precision, and expressing the results as molar ratios (thus obviating the necessity for an accurate preliminary determination of the amount of protein hydrolysed) and by studying sub-units (e.g. papain digestion fragments) rather than whole γG globulin molecules (thereby reducing the standard error, in terms of residues per mole, by a factor of 3). Incorporation of these refinements in amino-acid analyses of univalent fragments of rabbit antibody [266] (isolated by DEAE-cellulose fractionation of a sodium sulphate precipitate) ensured that the standard deviations of nearly all replicate measurements were less than *one residue per fragment*. There are disadvantages, however, in this approach, which must be considered when interpreting data obtained by quantitative amino-acid analytical techniques, particularly when measuring only slight differences in composition. Reservations should similarly be made when interpreting (qualitative) peptide maps. These include (i) the possibility of introducing artefacts by enzymatic digestion, (ii) contamination of one antibody fragment by another, and (iii) incomplete enzymatic digestion. Despite such potential limitations, the application of this procedure to Fab fragments [266] has revealed consistent differences of three to four amino acid residues (other than glutamic) with charged side chains, corresponding to the different relative binding strength to CM-cellulose (and different electrophoretic mobilities) of the various antibody fragments studied.

In other studies, by the Koshland group [183, 184], comparative quantitative amino-acid analyses have been made of three specifically purified anti-hapten antibodies directed against (i) the negatively charged phenylarsonic group [183], (ii) the positively charged phenyltrimethylammonium group [183], (iii) the uncharged phenyl-β-lactoside (lac) group [184]. Samples of antibodies or their sub-units were prepared for analysis in the following way [113]: precipitated protein, obtained by the addition of 50 per cent trichloracetic acid to a final concentration of 7–8 per cent, and separated by centrifuging, was washed with cold absolute ethanol (3 ml) and air-dried in the reaction tube. Constant boiling-point HCl (0·4 ml/mg protein) was added and the contents of the tube subjected to repeated freezing and thawing under reduced pressure, to remove any dissolved oxygen. The sample was hydrolysed at $110° \pm 1°$ C (using a boiling toluene bath) for 20 hours and analysed (in a Beckman autoanalyser). Using the same pipette, aliquots (containing 1·0–1·3 mg) of each sample were applied to the short and long columns of the analyser. A standard mixture of amino acids, and hydrolysed antibody, were analysed alternately, and samples to be compared (e.g. light chains from two antibodies isolated from the same rabbit) were analysed using the same batch of ninhydrin reagent. Amino-acid recoveries from intact antibody were normalized to a leucine content of 89, 91 and 89 per cent for the (i) arsonic, (ii) phenyltrimethylammonium and (iii) lac antibodies respectively. These values represent the average recovery of moles leucine/mole antibody applied for nine preparations of each antibody. The moles of antibody applied were calculated from micro-Kjeldahl (total nitrogen) analyses of aliquots of the hydrolysates, assuming a total nitrogen content of 16 per cent and a molecular weight of 160,000 for the proteins. (The standard error of the mean in these

values ranged from 0·7 to 1·1.) In similar experiments, an average of 11·2±
0·07 moles leucine/23,000 g light chain was found for five preparations of
antibody directed against substituted ammonium haptens, while for two anti-
lac preparations, 11·4±0·39 moles leucine/23,000 g light chain were recovered.
The amino-acid data for all three light chains were therefore normalized to 11
moles leucine, whilst the leucine standards used for the heavy chains were
derived from the leucine recoveries from the whole molecules and their light
chains.

The results of amino-acid analyses of hydrolysates of the whole anti-
hapten molecules indicated that rabbit antibody directed against the negatively
charged p-phenylarsonic acid group possessed a higher content of arginine
and iso-leucine in comparison with the antibody directed against the
positively charged p-amino-phenyl-trimethyl ammonium ion, which had a
higher content of aspartic acid and leucine. The third antibody, directed
against the neutral phenyl-β-lactoside group, on the other hand, was characterized by a higher aspartic acid and a lower serine and threonine content. The
probability that each of the three antibodies was isolated reproducibly from
a separate pool of differently charged rabbit γG globulin molecules was found
to be negligible. Moreover, the findings could not be attributed to the concentration of the antibodies into known genetic types of rabbit γG globulin,
since the amino-acid differences outlined were also observed when antibodies
were prepared in rabbits, homozygous for $(a^1a^1b^4b^4)$ γG globulin production.
Hence, these data have been interpreted as evidence that antibodies possess
differences in primary structure, which are associated with their immunological specificities. Moreover, a recent extension of these investigations [113],
involving the determination of the amino-acid compositions of the heavy and
light chains isolated from the same three anti-hapten antibodies, has permitted
the location of amino-acid differences within the two types of sub-unit.
Heavy and light chains were isolated using a range of reducing conditions
(given in Table 7.4), with varying concentrations of 2-mercaptoethanol
(0·05–1·0 M) and urea (0–12 M) as described on page 172, followed by gel
filtration through Sephadex G200 (equilibrated with 0·01 M tris buffer, pH 8·0
containing 0·001 M EDTA and either 0·01 M sodium dodecyl sulphate or 0·05 M
sodium sulphate, to solubilize and dissociate the chains, as described by
Utsumi & Karush [103]). The amino-acid compositions of the polypeptide
chains, determined as previously described, are shown in Table 7.17.

The characteristic differences in amino-acid composition, observed in the
previous studies, were found to be distributed in *both* the heavy and light
chains. For instance, statistical analysis (at the 99·9 per cent confidence level)
showed that the differences in contents of serine, and part of the tyrosine,
were located in the respective heavy chains, whereas differences in the aspartic
acid and balance of the tyrosine contents were located in the light chains.

The consistent fractional recoveries of many of the amino acids in the three antibody light chains were interpreted as evidence that each antibody consisted of at least two types of light chains (in agreement with the heterogeneity revealed by urea–starch-gel electrophoresis, mentioned earlier). New differences were also revealed, in the content of proline, valine and alanine

TABLE 7.17 (a) (Reproduced by courtesy of Drs M.E. Koshland, F.M.Englberger and R.Shapanka from *Biochem.* (1966) **5**, 641)

Average amino-acid recoveries* from the heavy chains of three antibodies isolated from $a^1a^1b^4b^4$ rabbits

| Amino acid | Residues per 53,000 g | | |
	Arsonic antibody	Ammonium antibody	Lac antibody
Lys	25.3 ± 0.12†	25.4 ± 0.17†	25.5 ± 0.098*
His	6.73 ± 0.039	6.87 ± 0.13	7.17 ± 0.11
Arg	19.7 ± 0.089	19.5 ± 0.16	19.6 ± 0.058
Asp	33.1 ± 0.25	34.5 ± 0.19	33.5 ± 0.30
Thr	50.4 ± 0.31	50.7 ± 0.28	49.9 ± 0.098
Ser	53.1 ± 0.25	52.4 ± 0.27	50.3 ± 0.36
Glu	39.3 ± 0.12	40.0 ± 0.13	39.2 ± 0.32
Pro	42.9 ± 0.25	43.1 ± 0.29	41.9 ± 0.26
Gly	34.6 ± 0.18	34.9 ± 0.049	34.5 ± 0.36
Ala	23.0 ± 0.29	23.1 ± 0.13	22.7 ± 0.36
Val	42.4 ± 0.24	42.5 ± 0.20	42.0 ± 0.31
Met	5.97 ± 0.078	5.93 ± 0.16	6.11 ± 0.081
Ileu	16.4 ± 0.078	16.3 ± 0.065	16.2 ± 0.13
Leu	33	34	33
Tyr	17.1 ± 0.13	17.0 ± 0.12	14.9 ± 0.042
Phe	15.3 ± 0.057	15.3 ± 0.053	15.1 ± 0.12
CM-Cys	13.7 ± 0.058	13.8 ± 0.18	13.2 ± 0.13

* Hydrolysis time, 20 hours.
† Standard error of the mean.

in the sub-units, which were not observed in the analyses on the whole antibody molecules (because, it was suggested, the preparations of whole antibody assayed were of mixed allotype, or because a difference in an amino-acid yield in one chain was obscured by a compensating change in another chain). Finally, the close agreement between the composition of the intact antibodies and their compositions calculated by summation of the amino acids present in their respective heavy and light chains (assuming two pairs of each chain per antibody molecule) is interpreted as substantiation of the Porter four-chain structure of γG globulin, besides providing additional evidence of the homogeneity of the chain preparations used in the quantitative amino-acid analysis.

These findings indicate how the determination of the amino-acid composition of polypeptide chain sub-units of rabbit anti-hapten antibodies can be employed in the characterization of the active sites of antibody molecules.

TABLE 7.17 (b)

Average amino-acid recoveries* from the light chains of three antibodies isolated from $a^1a^1b^4b^4$ rabbits

Amino acid	Arsonic antibody	Residues per 23,000 g Ammonium antibody	Lac antibody
Lys	9.27 ± 0.081†	9.20 ± 0.036*	9.81 ± 0.037*
His	1.27 ± 0.028	1.27 ± 0.014	1.40 ± 0.022
Arg	3.05 ± 0.035	2.61 ± 0.060	3.20 ± 0.056
Asp	19.1 ± 0.12	20.2 ± 0.058	21.8 ± 0.17
Thr	30.5 ± 0.11	30.2 ± 0.043	31.0 ± 0.16
Ser	21.6 ± 0.12	21.4 ± 0.085	21.5 ± 0.12
Glu	21.2 ± 0.12	20.8 ± 0.063	20.7 ± 0.18
Pro	11.9 ± 0.046	12.1 ± 0.043	12.7 ± 0.07
Gly	19.9 ± 0.078	19.9 ± 0.098	19.9 ± 0.10
Ala	16.5 ± 0.10	15.5 ± 0.014	15.8 ± 0.22
Val	20.8 ± 0.14	21.7 ± 0.15	22.5 ± 0.12
Met	0.87 ± 0.011	0.41 ± 0.020	0.86 ± 0.046
Ileu	7.47 ± 0.029	6.79 ± 0.030	7.31 ± 0.080
Leu	11	11	11
Tyr	10.8 ± 0.11	10.9 ± 0.067	10.1 ± 0.14
Phe	6.57 ± 0.024	6.77 ± 0.030	7.06 ± 0.060
CM-Cys‡	7.26 ± 0.021	7.08 ± 0.054	7.03 ± 0.25

* Hydrolysis time, 20 hours.
† Standard error of the mean.
‡ Average of three different determinations.

They support the evidence obtained from the hapten-binding studies referred to earlier, which indicate that both heavy and light chains are involved in antibody specificity. Furthermore, the observation that the average amino-acid composition of the light chain preparation from each antibody is specific for that antibody, despite the multiplicity of side chains involved, has prompted the hypothesis that light chain contains two regions identified with specificity, one of *invariant* amino-acid composition and sequence (in all light chains for a given antibody, providing the major light-chain contribution to antibody specificity) and the other of *variable* amino-acid composition and sequence (serving to modify the quantitative effect of the 'invariant' region). This suggestion is consistent with the presence of two regions (of constant and variable amino-acid compositions respectively) revealed in human Bence–Jones proteins by sequential analyses (as indicated in Fig. 7.33, section B2b). It is also pertinent to the conclusion of Sela & Mozes [57] (cited earlier) that antibody biosynthesis is controlled both by specific determinants on the antigen molecule, and by other parts which define areas of the antibody molecule which do not include the antigen-combining site.

Comparative amino-acid analyses have also been made of four different *human* antibodies [268], isolated from the serum of the same individual, following immunization with the minimal dose of each non-protein antigen (dextran, levan, teichoic acid and purified blood-group substance A). Specific precipitates were isolated by sequential absorption with each antigen. These were washed ($\times 6$) in the cold with 0·15 M NaCl and hydrolysed directly; except in the case of three of the four anti-A substance precipitates examined, which were extracted ($\times 2$) with trichloracetic acid (to ensure removal of the antigen present), followed by ether (to remove residual trichloracetic acid). Samples of γG globulin from the serum of the antibody donor (isolated by DEAE-cellulose chromatography), of pooled γG globulin and of pooled γM globulin (at least 90 per cent pure) from other human sera were also examined. Samples were hydrolysed by the procedure described in section B2b and the amino acids determined in a Technicon autoanalyser. Elution from the ion-exchange column was accomplished by the buffer gradient system introduced by Piez & Morris [269], the amino-acid contents of the effluents being monitored by reaction with ninhydrin (as previously mentioned [145]). The autoanalyser was calibrated by carrying out twenty analyses of a standard amino-acid mixture (supplied by Beckman Instruments Inc., Palo Alto, California), to which had been added 0·1 μmoles each of L-cysteic acid, D,L-hydroxylysine and methionine sulphoxide. This standard mixture was used to check each new batch of buffer or ninhydrin reagent. Hydroxylysine enantiomorphs appeared as twin peaks at 501 ml and 504 ml of column effluent, relative to the lysine peak at 552 ml, both in standard mixtures and in the antibody hydrolysates which contained this residue.

The amino-acid compositions thus determined are presented in Table 7.18, which includes the values reported by other investigators for pooled human γG globulins [71] and pooled human γM globulins [270]. The values given were obtained after hydrolysis for 22 hours/110° C, and have not been extrapolated to zero time, so are uncorrected for destruction of labile hydroxy amino acids. The results are expressed as moles of amino-acid residue/mole (160,000 g in the case of γG globulins), assuming that the samples examined

TABLE 7.18

Amino-acid composition of antibodies and normal γG globulin from one individual.

(Reproduced by courtesy of Drs E.W.Bassett, S.W.Tanenbaum, K.Pryzwansky, S.M.Beiser and E.A.Kabat from *J. exp. Med.* (1965) **122**, 251)

Designation	Antilevan					Antidextran		Antiteichoic acid		Anti 'A'				γG-globulin			Pooled γG		Pooled γG[71]	Pooled γM		*Pooled γM[270]
	II_1	I_2	II	II	II	I_1	II_3	I_3	II_3	205	206	II_4	I_4	146	147	148	140	141		187	188	
Hours hydrolysed	22	22	22	48	72	22	22	22	22	22	22	22	22	22	48	72	22	22	22	22	22	20
Aspartic acid	122	123	123	122	—	119	118	122	125	122	121	122	120	123	123	120	118	117	117	111	112	127
Threonine	113	113	114	106	—	108	110	109	111	126	128	120	124	111	105	99	113	113	115	116	116	140
Serine	146	144	146	124	151	148	147	150	151	156	155	153	150	146	126	106	156	153	171	141	141	173
Glutamic acid	152	155	152	152	151	149	149	149	150	148	150	147	145	146	143	143	145	142	143	139	136	151
Proline	103	99·2	99·5	102	102	102	99·4	108	108	109	112	104	108	107	108	108	115	115	112	97·1	97·1	106
Glycine	102	102	100	102	101	100	99·2	119	121	108	109	108	110	107	104	108	106	107	98·9	105	105	112
Alanine	86·2	84·7	84·5	85·7	85·4	79·2	79·0	82·4	84·0	84·4	81·5	83·0	84·2	81·4	79·9	79·9	81·2	80·8	75·4	85·4	82·6	97·9
Valine	131	132	132	131	131	133	135	102	102	116	114	116	113	139	136	139	127	129	129	106	104	124
Half-cystine†	37·1	34·9	39·9	32·2	31·9	39·1	37·2	34·0	34·5	31·2	30·4	30·4	32·0	35·1	35·5	35·9	33·6	35·2	30·4	35·1	36·4	29·3
Methionine†	14·4	13·7	14·6	14·3	13·3	14·8	16·5	16·4	16·7	13·4	13·7	14·0	14·9	13·7	13·1	13·9	12·0	12·2	7·5	13·3	12·7	17·8
Isoleucine	33·8	32·0	34·9	32·2	31·9	31·0	31·0	33·6	34·4	33·4	34·0	33·2	34·1	34·4	33·7	34·6	26·6	28·7	33·7	42·9	42·3	38·7
Leucine	116	115	116	118	116	108	110	109	111	116	114	113	110	116	116	115	113	113	108	98·0	98·0	114
Tyrosine	45·3	44·7	46·5	45·6	45·8	55·9	56·9	53·6	53·0	52·4	54·1	(9)	(15)	55·9	57·0	57·0	58·2	57·9	61·2	40·5	41·6	43·4
Phenylalanine	54·9	52·8	54·3	54·3	53·7	54·1	56·3	54·5	54·7	48·4	47·4	48·8	49·0	52·0	52·1	50·7	47·2	46·6	46·7	47·8	46·4	52·8
Lysine	93·4	94·0	93·0	93·9	91·8	87·0	88·0	80·8	83·0	80·1	81·2	78·6	76·5	93·3	92·9	93·2	89·9	89·5	90·9	64·7	63·4	78·0
Histidine	28·6	27·2	27·4	27·8	28·5	25·9	26·3	29·1	28·3	28·3	29·0	26·2	26·9	30·1	30·6	29·6	26·9	27·2	27·1	26·0	25·3	27·0
Arginine	46·5	46·1	46·5	47·1	46·5	46·5	48·6	58·1	59·1	56·2	56·0	53·8	55·0	47·8	49·5	47·5	45·1	45·2	42·5	55·0	56·1	62·2
Hydroxylysine	‡	‡	‡	‡	‡	3·2	3·2	3·7	3·6	‡	‡	‡	‡	‡	‡	‡	‡	‡	—	4·3	3·6	—
Glucosamine	5·0	6·1	7·2	5·0	§	6·4	5·5	5·5	6·2	(17·8)	(14·7)	6·4	5·8	2·4	§	§	7·5	8·7	—	12·9	12·3	—

* The data of Heimer et al [270] were converted into residues per 160,000 g of γM, based upon the premise that the original percentages were given as g anhydroamino acid per 100 g of protein. With the exception of isoleucine and half-cystine, these amino-acid residue values are consistently higher than found here for γM. On the other hand, the data of Chaplin et al, [188], when calculated into residues as above, provide for a lower residual amino-acid composition of γM, except for tyrosine.

† Sum includes oxidation products.
‡ None detected in the protein hydrolysate.
§ Trace quantity (less than 0·1 residue) found.

contained 2·6 per cent tryptophane [187], and a non-nitrogenous carbohydrate content of 2 per cent in γG and 10 per cent in γM globulins respectively [30]. Estimations of half-cystine and methionine include the sum of their respective oxidation products. The compositions of the anti-A substance and anti-teichoic acid antibody preparations were less reliable than those of the anti-levan and anti-dextran preparations, owing to contamination by about 10–20 per cent γM globulin. Nevertheless, the values for a number of amino acids (e.g. methionine, aspartic and glutamic acids) are very uniform throughout all the antibodies tested, despite their production by hydrolysis of antigen-antibody complexes. In contrast, differences ranging from seven to thirty-two residues were found in the contents of glycine, valine, leucine, tyrosine, arginine, lysine and threonine of the various antibodies. Furthermore, these differences were not correlated with the Gm types of the antibodies (which were as follows: anti-levans, a − b − ; anti–dextrans, a − b − ; anti-teichoic acid, a − b − ; anti-'A', a + b − ; normal γG globulin being a + b +). Hydroxylysine was found in two of the four antibodies (anti-dextran and anti-teichoic acid) and in pooled γM globulin, but not in pooled γG globulin (which was also shown to be deficient in this amino acid by Crumpton & Wilkinson [187]).

Thus, human antibodies of different specificity, isolated from the *same* individual, have been shown to possess more striking differences in amino-acid composition than were shown by the various rabbit anti-hapten antibodies studied by the Koshland group [113] (referred to earlier).

(b) Activities associated with the Fc fragments

The many and varied biological activities found to be associated with the Fc fragments of γG globulin molecules are listed in Table 7.19, together with their principal modes of assay. Obviously, any attempt to associate certain of these activities (e.g. control of placental transmission, or rate of catabolism) with well-defined sites within the structure of the Fc fragment is restricted by the extent of the animal experimentation required for their assay. This situation contrasts, for instance, with the relative ease with which the antigen-combining sites (within the Fab fragments) can be delineated by equilibrium dialysis measurements on sub-units of highly pure anti-hapten antibodies (as described in the previous section, B3a). Nevertheless, inhibition techniques are beginning to aid in the precise location of certain activities (e.g. skin attachment, rheumatoid-factor reactivity) associated with the Fc fragments of γG globulin molecules.

A certain degree of caution must be exercised in interpreting results obtained by some of the assay systems listed in Table 7.19, because of the possibility that the configuration of the γG globulin sub-units may have been altered during manipulation prior to testing. Thus, as Brambell *et al* [277] have pointed out, for instance, it is possible that the relative rates of transmission of papain digestion fragments (Fab and Fc) of rabbit γG globulin across the foetal yolk-sac membrane might have been influenced by slight conformational changes occurring during their preparation and (trace) iodination. Similar artefacts could, of course, influence other properties, such as the rate of catabolism of γG globulin sub-units. Nevertheless, a substantial amount of indirect evidence, obtained by comparative testing of the different classes of immunoglobulins (i.e. γG, γM, γA, etc.) supports findings from direct studies on the enzyme digestion fragments of γG globulin, which point to the Fc portion being closely involved in the activities listed in Table 7.19. Thus, for example, homologous γG globulins are transmitted across foetal membranes more readily than heterologous γG globulins [278]; moreover, within the human species, the γG globulin is transmitted whereas the γM [279] and γA [280] globulins (which, as indicated in Fig. 7.1, possess distinctive Fc portions) are not transmitted. Similarly, of these three classes of human immunoglobulin, only the γG globulin is capable of passively sensitizing guinea-pig tissue [281, 282] or of reacting with rheumatoid factor [283] in the *in vitro* systems indicated in Table 7.19.

That such activities are intimately dependent upon the heavy chain structure within the Fc portion of the γG globulin molecules is also suggested indirectly by comparing the activities of the various immunoglobulin types isolated from the sera of other mammalian species. In this connection, it is interesting to find that, unlike the case of the corresponding human γ globulins, *rabbit γG* and γM globulins both reach the rabbit foetus [35, 305]; furthermore, rabbit antibodies of *both classes* are capable of producing reverse Arthus reaction [36] in guinea-pigs. It is possible that the difference in transmission across the foetal membranes shown by homologous human and rabbit γM globulins reflects a difference in the mode of transfer in the two species, because in humans transfer of globulins is believed to occur across the placenta (as in rhesus monkeys), whereas in rabbits transfer is effected *via* the uterine cavity and the vascular, foetal, yolk-sac splanchnopleura [169]. Nevertheless, it seems likely that the 'Fc portions' of human and rabbit γM globulins play an important role in their differing behaviour during membrane transmission and in guinea-pig skin sensitization. This is suggested by evidence from studies on rabbit allotypes, which have shown that the a locus phenotypes are present on both rabbit γM and γG globulin molecules [286] (and probably on γA globulin molecules [287]). This could mean that part of the heavy chain (within the Fd piece) is common to these three immunoglobulins, although (as Cohen & Porter [1] have suggested) this observation could also represent the manifestation of a six-chain polypeptide structure in the case of *rabbit γG* globulin. Obviously, if such a structure existed (in contrast to the commonly accepted four-chain structure of *human γG* globulin, shown in Fig. 7.6), it could be expected to have a profound

TABLE 7.19

Biological activities associated with the Fc region of γG globulin molecules

Activity	Assay system	Type of γ globulin (or sub-units) examined	References
Complement fixation	Determination of (1) complement-fixing activity, (2) inhibition of immune haemolysis (e.g. using sheep erythrocytes and fresh guinea-pig serum)	Rabbit antibody γG globulin sub-units (alone and combined with antigen) Normal γG globulin (in non-aggregated and aggregated form)	288, 290, 310
	Enhancement of opsonization of erythrocytes and bacteria	Mouse antibodies	311
Skin fixation	Direct (and inhibition) PCA reactivity in guinea-pigs	γG globulin antibodies (human, rabbit, etc.)	281
	Reverse PCA reactivity in guinea-pigs; inhibition of Schultz-Dale reaction (using guinea-pig tissue)	Normal (and antibody) rabbit γG globulin and sub-units; normal human γG globulin	312, 313, 282
Membrane transmission	Injection of antibody or isotopically labelled normal γ globulin into uterine lumen of rabbit at 24th day of pregnancy followed by examination of foetal serum, etc.	^{131}I-labelled normal rabbit γG globulin (or sub-units) Guinea-pig antitoxin, rabbit antitoxin, etc.	277
	Measurement of interference of uptake of guinea-pig agglutinins by suckling (11 day) mice	Normal rabbit γG globulin (and sub-units)	321

Method	Procedure	Material	References
Macrophage fixation	Determination of extent of rosette formation following incubation (1 hour at room temperature) of passively sensitized homologous macrophages with sheep erythrocytes (heterologous macrophages are less suitable)	Guinea-pig γ_2G antibodies against sheep erythrocytes	43
Microsome fixation	Displacement of synthesized γ globulin from microsome	γG globulin and sub-units	328
Elimination and catabolism	Determination of half-lives of ^{131}I-labelled homologous or heterologous γ globulin, by serum and urine measurement	Rabbit, guinea-pig, mouse, human γG globulins	314
	Effect of administration of heterologous γ globulin (or sub-units) on γ globulin turnover in mice	Wide range of γG globulins	315, 316, 404
Specific antigenicity (reactivity with rheumatoid factor and other anti-γG globulin antisera)	Haemagglutination (or inhibition of agglutination) of antibody-coated erythrocytes	Human, rabbit, etc., γG globulin (normal and antibody) and sub-units	320, 304 317 66, 451
	Agglutination of particles of polystyrene latex pretreated with γG globulin		
	Quantitation of precipitation reaction, using aggregated γG globulins		65, 318
	Ultracentrifugal determination of amount of RF–γG globulin complex formed		456

influence on the biological activities associated with the Fc portion of the γG globulin molecule.

Other interesting observations of possible relevance in this context are the findings that parts of the rabbit γG globulin molecule, other than the Fc portion, are involved in complement fixation (to specific precipitates). Taranta & Franklin [288] found that neither 5S peptic digestion fragments (F(ab')$_2$) nor 3·5S papain digestion fragments (Fab) of rabbit anti-ovalbumin, anti-bovine serum albumin and anti-pneumococcal polysaccharide SVI fixed guinea-pig complement (when incubated for 18 hours at 4° C in the presence of fresh guinea-pig serum). Other investigators, however, have demonstrated substantial fixation of guinea-pig complement by peptic digests of rabbit anti-sheep erythrocyte γG globulin antibody [289] (in the presence of sheep erythrocytes), and of rabbit and sheep anti-human serum albumin and anti-ovalbumin antibodies [290] (present as *washed* specific precipitate with antigen). Peptic digestion fragments of rabbit anti-sheep erythrocyte antibodies were found, however, to fix insufficient complement for lysis of the sheep erythrocytes (in contrast to the lytic activity of intact antibodies). Further evidence, suggesting that Fab fragments are also involved in complement fixation, has been obtained from application of procedures [291, 292] involving the dissociation of specific antigen-antibody precipitates following complement fixation. The complexity of the systems employed, however, and the wide scope for conformational rearrangements during manipulation, cause inevitable reservations about the results obtained.

The finding that human γM as well as γG globulin antibodies of the same species fix complement provides indirect evidence that the molecular configuration outside the Fc region is involved in some way, whilst the demonstration [293] of activity in guinea-pig γ_2 but not γ_1 globulin molecules, implicates the Fc portion (at least of the γG globulin molecules of this species). This last observation is of some relevance when interpreting the results of investigations with antibodies of species such as human and rabbit, which are also now known to comprise γG globulin sub-fractions. Terry has reported [308] that of the four heavy chain sub-classes of human γG globulin, only the γ_{2d} type fails to fix complement (although it has the capacity to evoke PCA reactions, as mentioned later).

As in the determination of some of the other activities (e.g. skin fixation) listed in Table 7.19, the use of an inhibition system permits the study of *non-antibody* sub-units of γG globulin. Thus, for example [289], it was shown that the Fc (papain digestion) fragments of normal rabbit γG globulin (DEAE-cellulose sub-fraction of sodium sulphate precipitated fraction), as well as of antibody γG globulin, inhibited immune haemolysis of sheep erythrocytes by rabbit antibody (primarily owing to its ability to interact with guinea-pig complement, but also to some extent by interacting with the sheep erythrocytes). In this procedure, varying amounts of Fc fragment (or its parent normal rabbit γG globulin) were pre-incubated with either sheep erythrocyte suspension or pooled guinea-pig sera for 30 minutes at $0°$ C. The remaining reactants (guinea-pig complement or sheep erythrocytes, and γ_2G haemolytic antibody) were added and the tubes incubated at $37°$ C. (Full details of the quantitation of complement fixation are given in Chapter 20.)

It seems probable that the interaction of guinea-pig complement with rabbit γG globulin Fc piece thus observed was due to the latter being in *aggregated* form, since pronounced complement-binding activity is shown by Fc fragments which have been aggregated by heat-treatment or by coupling with bis-diazotized benzidine [294]. In contrast, both aggregated Fab pieces I and II failed to fix complement (as did complexes of these papain digestion fragments with antigen). Furthermore, as the studies of Ishizaka's group [294] have shown, the structure responsible for complement fixation by aggregated whole γG globulins, and by soluble complexes of antibody γG globulin and homologous antigen (in certain proportions, e.g. Ag_3Ab_2), appears to reside in the Fc portion of the γG globulin molecule. It seems likely (on the basis of optical rotation measurements, as outlined in section C), that tertiary structural alterations within the Fc portions of antibody γG globulin molecules, brought into close proximity by interaction with homologous antigen (or by non-specific aggregation processes), result in complement fixation (and guinea-pig skin reactivity, as will be discussed later). Moreover, it is possible that a similar interaction occurs between the Fc portions of adjacent haemolytic γG globulin antibody molecules *on the erythrocyte surface*. In support of this, it has been concluded from electron-microscopy studies [295], and by the use of new complement-fixation tests [296] based on the fixation and transfer of the activated first complement component (C'_{1a}), that at least two γG globulin molecules are required in close proximity to fix one molecule of complement and to initiate lytic action. This observation is supported by other recent findings that aggregates of human [297] and rabbit [298] (non-antibody) γG globulin molecules, as small as dimers (10S) are capable of fixing complement, as well as forming precipitate with rheumatoid factor [297], as is indicated in Table 7.20. The suceptibility to proteolysis, of such human γG globulin association products resulting in the break-down of their (presumably combined) Fc portions (as illustrated in Fig. 7.13), suggests that here, too, tertiary structural changes within this part of the molecule result in the formation of a configuration responsible for complement fixation (and the induction of other activities such as guinea-pig skin fixation and rheumatoid-factor reactivity). In contrast to the requirement of two adjacent γG globulin antibody molecules to initiate haemolysis, it was found that a single γM antibody molecule, bound to the erythrocyte surface, was sufficient to fix complement [295, 296]. Even here, however, it is possible that the unfolding of this relatively large antibody molecule, which occurs as a result of its combination with the cell surface, results in an intra-molecular interaction between the '*Fc portions*' of its five (or six) 7S sub-units subsequent complement fixation.

It is worth mentioning a practical outcome of studies on complement binding. The uptake of complement by aggregated molecules provides a valuable guide to the extent of denaturation induced in a γG globulin preparation during its isolation (as is shown by the data in Table 7.21). It is important to carry out such a screening on γG globulin preparations intended for intravenous injection, to avoid the administration of the toxic aggregates. These have been removed by ultracentrifugation (7 hours at 40,000 g, to remove 30–100S aggregates; and 7 hours at 100,000 g to remove 8–9S

TABLE 7.20

Ability of human γG globulin fractions containing varying amounts of the 10S form and larger aggregates to react with rheumatoid factor and to fix complement [297]

	Per cent composition			Rheumatoid factor precipitation		Complement fixation
				μg N pptd. from rheumatoid	μg N pptd. from 0·3 ml rheumatoid	
			> 10S	factor prepn./mg	arthritic serum/mg	Per cent complement fixed by 0·1 mg
Sample	7S	10S	(20–40S)	sample	sample	sample
a	70	15	15	15·6	3·1	20
b	100	—	—	0·3	0·2	3·0
c	90	10	—	0·4	0·3	6·4
d	50	50	—	3·3	1·5	10
e	40	60	—	6·1	2·6	16·5
f	(38)	(12)	(50)	63·3	11·2	52

components) or by limited proteolysis (e.g. by peptic digestion) [316]. A major disadvantage of the latter procedure, however, is that the fragments (2·4S, 5S) so produced are rapidly eliminated from the circulation [314]. Other attempts to remove anti-complementary activity have involved digestion with pepsin at extremely low enzyme:globulin ratios (1:100,000), incubation at 37° C at pH 4·0 for 6 hours, or reduction (e.g. with mercaptoethylamine) followed by alkylation (with iodoacetamide). Such measures often lead, however, to the production of unstable γG globulin preparations. A much milder procedure [297] relies on the separation of large aggregates (20–40S) and 10S dimer by gel filtration on Sephadex G200, preferably employing automatic effluent monitoring (to minimize handling), although this leads inevitably to some sacrifice of yield owing to overlapping of the 10S and 7S elution fractions (even where re-cycling is preformed).

Although human antibody γG globulin, after reduction with 0·1 M 2-mercaptoethanol and dialysis against iodoacetamide [300], failed to fix complement, its ability to combine with antigen (measured by the anti-globulin consumption test) was unimpaired, a finding of both academic and practical importance. As pointed out by Wiedermann and his co-workers [300], this precludes the use of the effect of 2-mercaptoethanol on complement fixation as an indirect method of distinguishing between γG and γM type antibodies. The findings of these investigators further emphasize the important role played by interchain disulphide bridges (particularly within

TABLE 7.21

Physico-chemical and biological properties of γG globulin preparations incubated at various temperatures (Reproduced by courtesy of Dr C.S.Henney from [385])

Incubation temperature* (° C)	Per cent aggregated material formed on incubation of 1 per cent solution λ_c	Free SH groups/ mol.	Minimum skin reactive dose (μg N)	Per cent human complement fixed by 50 μg protein	μg N pptd. by 5 mg protein from 0·3 ml RA serum
Room temp. (18–20)	0·2	202	None detectable	> 64	0	0·8
37	0·8	202	None detectable	64	0	3·0
45	1·0	204	0·1	—	4	4·8
50	1·8	213	0·15 (52° C)	16	—	12·0
55	2·3	216	—	—	10	18·0
60	9·3	220	0·30	5	58	28·0
63	12·9	224	0·50	< 5	84	38·0

* Incubation for 10 minutes in all cases.

the Fc portion) in maintaining the conformation of the γG globulin molecule essential for complement fixation. Although reduced and alkylated whole human γG globulin antibodies failed to fix complement after non-specific (heat at 60° C for 5–25 minutes) aggregation, the aggregate retained its capacity to precipitate rheumatoid factor. This suggests that the same reactive site (presumably within the Fc portion of the molecule) is not involved in the two activities (complement fixation, rheumatoid-factor reactivity). Attempts have been made to provide direct evidence of this, and it has been found that isolated rheumatoid factor does not appear to inhibit complement-fixation activity in haemolytic systems using sheep erythrocytes sensitized with dilute glycerinated rabbit haemolysin [301].

Recently, Ishizaka *et al* [302] have shown that specific precipitate formed between antigen and rabbit anti-BSA antibody, which had been reduced by 0·1 M 2-mercaptoethylamine (pH 5·0) followed by alkylation with iodoacetate, fixed complement to the extent of 62 per cent (on a weight basis) of that fixed by untreated antibody-antigen precipitate. Moreover, the complement-fixing capacity of the specific precipitates did not change on exposure to pH 2·5 in 0·1 M NaCl. It has been deduced from these findings that antibody reconstructed from half-molecules (see section B1b) is capable of fixing complement (when combined with antigen), and that the inter-heavy chain disulphide bridges of intact antibody molecules are not essential for complement fixation. Other comparative studies [303] have been made to establish whether complement fixation and guinea-pig skin attachment are associated with a common γG globulin structure within the Fc portion of the molecule. Relatively drastic reduction of rabbit γG globulin and Fc fragments (0·2–0·3 per cent) by 0·1 M 2-mercaptoethylamine in borate-buffered saline containing 2 M urea (for 24 hours at room temperature), followed by alkylation (with a 10-fold molar excess of iodoacetamide or iodoacetate) resulted in almost complete loss of tissue affinity, but had little effect on complement fixation *in vitro*. As Ishizaka has speculated [303] these findings could be attributed to a difference in steric requirements (within the Fc portion of the molecule) for tissue binding and complement fixation.

Before drawing too firm conclusions from this type of approach, it will be necessary to obtain far greater control over the structural alterations induced by the experimental conditions adopted, and to improve the methods used to characterize the biologically active products. This has been done in the case of induction of reactivity with rheumatoid factor, in preparations of γG globulin (as will be outlined further in section C). Here, optical rotatory dispersion measurements provide a quantitative assessment of the degree of tertiary structural alteration induced by various *in vitro* denaturation treatments. It is interesting to find that the various forms of aggregation process employed (e.g. heat denaturation, bis-diazobenzidine coupling, formation of soluble complex with specific antigen) induce guinea-pig skin reactivity, as well as ability to precipitate with rheumatoid factor. This suggests that, as in the case of guinea-pig skin reactivity, the determinants reactive with rheumatoid factor are located within the Fc portion of the γG globulin molecule. Direct and inhibition tests (indicated in Table 7.19) on γG globulin sub-units have provided substantial evidence in support of this contention. As with the other biological activities already discussed, however, it is becoming obvious that the spatial configuration of the polypeptide chains within the Fc region of the γG globulin molecule plays a critical role in its reactivity with rheumatoid factor [406].

Inhibition of haemagglutination systems (comprising γG globulin-coated tanned erythrocytes and purified rheumatoid factor [304]) are now being used in attempts to characterize further the γG globulin determinants involved in combination with rheumatoid factor. The observation [385] that the γG globulins of some species (such as horse) when denatured to a similar extent to human γG globulin (as revealed by optical rotatory dispersion measurements) are relatively unreactive with rheumatoid factor, suggests that primary structure plays an important role in this particular γG globulin activity. Hence, chemical analysis (by methods outlined in section B2b) is being carried out on peptides cleaved from the rheumatoid-factor-combining sites located within the Fc region of reactive γG globulin molecules. In a somewhat different approach to this problem, Goodman [147] has tested products of pepsin digestion of rabbit γG globulin Fc (papain) piece, by determining their capacity to sensitize sheep erythrocytes for agglutination by rheumatoid serum. Thus, the peptic fractions (3·5 mg), dissolved in buffered saline, pH 8·0 (20 ml), were absorbed overnight at 4° C with washed packed sheep erythrocytes (2 ml) from 2-day-old blood. These absorbed protein solutions were then used to coat tanned sheep erythrocytes, which were subsequently assayed for agglutinability by various rheumatoid sera. Some of the dialysable fractions from peptic digestion of Fc piece, fractionated by preparative starch-gel electrophoresis and gel filtration on Sephadex (G25 and G50) columns (by the procedures outlined in section B2a) were thus shown to have retained reactivity with rheumatoid factor. These fractions also showed an ability to combine with specific antibody (as revealed by the delay they imposed on flocculation of goat antiserum directed against rabbit γG globulin Fc piece with homologous antigen), and skin reactivity (revealed by their ability to elicit reverse PCA reactions in guinea-pigs).

This illustrates the manner in which the problem of delineating the biologically active sites within the Fc portion of the molecule is being tackled. Studies of the isolated peptides from the rheumatoid-reactive and complement-fixation sites are aided by the availability of *in vitro* assay systems. Skin reactivities of non-dialysable (2·5S to 3·6S) peptic digestion fragments of Fc piece of rabbit γG globulin, separated by electrophoresis in polyacrylamide gel, have been assayed by inhibition of direct PCA activity [306]. Although the reverse PCA test is a more sensitive method (see Chapter 22), it has the inherent disadvantage of requiring *reactivity with antibody* in addition to 'fixation' to guinea-pig skin tissue. It is possible, however, that inhibition of the *in vitro* release of histamine from rabbit platelets by antigen–antibody combinations [307] will be developed into a more satisfactory method of determining guinea-pig skin reactivity of low molecular weight peptides.

Another important characteristic associated with the Fc region of the γG globulin molecule is the structure controlling its catabolism. This has been established by the studies of Spiegelberg & Weigle [314] on the catabolism

TABLE 7.22

Per cent radioactivity excreted in urine during the first 3 days following injections of γ globulin and γ globulin fragments. †(This table, and Table 7.23, are reproduced by courtesy of Drs H.C.Spiegelberg and W.O.Weigle from *J. exp. Med.* (1965), **121**, 323)

Animals	Source of γ globulin	7S γ globulin Total I*	7S γ globulin Protein I*	Pepsin 5S i.e. F(ab')₂ Total I*	Pepsin 5S i.e. F(ab')₂ Protein I*	Papain 3·5S I (S) i.e. Fab Total I*	Papain 3·5S I (S) i.e. Fab Protein I*	Papain 3·5S III (F) i.e. FC Total I*	Papain 3·5S III (F) i.e. FC Protein I*	Duration of digestion
Rabbit	Rabbit	43·3	0·6	89·5	25·0	80·4	21·7	68·1	1·9	18 hrs.
						77·3	13·0	52·5	2·1	5 min.
Guinea-pig	Rabbit	31·3	2·3	86·5	35·2	77·5	46·2	74·3	11·9	18 hrs.
						87·8	41·6	56·9	10·7	5 min.
Mouse	Rabbit	26·0	0·7	79·2	15·1	90·8	33·3	57·6	6·2	18 hrs.
						64·0	17·2	58·7	3·8	5 min.
Guinea-pig	Guinea-pig	50·2	2·8	85·7	9·3	91·7	28·0	85·9	14·8	18 hrs.
								61·0	12·0	5 min.
Rabbit	Guinea-pig	47·8	1·8	82·3	4·3	95·0	13·9	84·3	6·7	18 hrs.
								69·9	4·3	5 min.
Mouse	Guinea-pig	37·1	1·1	80·5	4·2	80·9	3·7	79·2	3·6	18 hrs.
								65·1	2·2	5 min.
Mouse	Mouse	45·5	1·9	77·7	2·9	85·6	9·7	67·9	2·2	18 hrs.
Rabbit	Mouse	69·9	1·6	78·5	4·3	72·8	18·2	66·5	3·5	18 hrs.
Guinea-pig	Mouse	66·3	2·0	89·7	3·9	83·2	25·9	81·3	5·5	18 hrs.
Rabbit	Mouse	42·2	0·5	83·9	2·5	96·9	3·6	72·7	8·9	18 hrs.
								66·5	6·6	5 min.
Guinea-pig	Human	29·9	0·8	91·9	5·4	94·9	35·3	96·8	18·8	18 hrs.
								39·7	6·0	5 min.
Mouse	Human	40·9	0·9	97·1	2·8	84·8	6·7	86·5	10·3	18 hrs.
								52·6	9·9	5 min.

Total I*, total recovered I^{131} activity. Protein I*, total TCA precipitable recovered I^{131} activity. † Average of three to six animals.

in rabbits, guinea-pigs, and mice of homologous and heterologous γG globulin fragments obtained by pepsin and papain digestion. The elimination of radioactive-iodine labelled papain Fc fragment into the urine was *slow*, and closely related to the rate of elimination of the intact γG globulin, whereas the pepsin fragment and papain Fab fragments were rapidly catabolized and eliminated in all species examined (as indicated by the data in

TABLE 7.23

Half-lives of different γ globulins and γ globulin fragments*

| | | | γ globulin fragments | | |
| | | | | | Papain 3·5S |
Animal	Source of γ globulin	7S γ globulin average (range)	Pepsin 5S F(ab')₂	I (S) (Fab)	II (F)† average (range) (Fc)
Rabbit	Rabbit	6·0 (4·5–7·5)	<0·5	<0·5	4·7 (4·1–5·6)
Guinea-pig	Rabbit	4·3 (4·0–4·7)	<0·5	<0·5	4·0 (3·9–4·1)
Mouse	Rabbit	5·7 (5·3–6·4)	<0·5	<0·5	4·4 (3·6–5·9)
Guinea-pig	Guinea-pig	4·2 (3·4–5·0)	<0·5	<0·5	2·2 (1·7–2·5)
Rabbit	Guinea-pig	3·3 (2·9–3·7)	<0·5	<0·5	2·1 (1·6–2·5)
Mouse	Guinea-pig	4·9 (4·6–5·2)	<0·5	<0·5	2·2 (2·0–2·4)
Mouse	Mouse	4·0 (3·0–5·2)	<0·5	<0·5	1·0 (0·8–1·1)
Rabbit	Mouse	1·5 (1·2–1·7)	<0·5	<0·5	1·4 (1·3–1·5)
Guinea-pig	Mouse	2·3 (2·2–2·5)	<0·5	<0·5	1·5 (1·4–1·7)
Rabbit	Human	5·0 (3·7–5·8)	<0·5	<0·5	3·8 (2·6–4·9)
Guinea-pig	Human	3·8 (3·7–3·9)	<0·5	<0·5	3·1 (3·0–3·4)
Mouse	Human	4·5 (4·2–4·9)	<0·5	<0·5	2·9 (2·6–3·6)
Rabbit	Horse	1·7 (1·6–1·8)	<0·5	—	—
Rabbit	Bovine	1·6 (1·4–1·8)	<0·5	—	—

* Half-life given in days.
† Half-life of F papain fragment (III), i.e. Fc, obtained after 5 minutes' digestion with papain.

Tables 7.22 and 7.23). Moreover, prolonged incubation (18 hours at 37° C) with cysteine (0·01 M) effected structural alterations in the papain Fc fragment, resulting in a rapid catabolism of a large portion of it within 24 hours of injection. Similar findings have been reported by Fahey & Robinson [315], who showed that the passive administration of homologous γG globulin (chick) or its papain Fc fragment (but not the Fab fragment) resulted in an increased turnover rate of the γG globulin; and by Sell [404] who showed that bovine γG globulin was less effective than the γG globulins of other species (e.g. mouse, guinea-pig, human and rabbit) in increasing the *fractional* catabolic rate of human, mouse, bovine and guinea-pig γG globulins in the mouse. These findings have important practical implications in connection with the use of antibody fragments as prophylactic and therapeutic agents. The rapid catabolism of the pepsin and papain digestion fragments (i.e. F(ab')$_2$ and Fab) suggest that their use for such purpose in man is limited [314]. Thus, although the commonly used practice of administering pepsin-digested horse antitoxin (i.e. F(ab')$_2$) fragment for the prophylactic treatment of tetanus and diphtheria [322] avoids exposing the human recipient to the heterologous (horse) antigenic determinants, which are destroyed by peptic degradation of the Fc portion of the antibody molecule, the removal of that segment also destroys the structure controlling its rate of catabolism. On the other hand, preliminary studies [327] have indicated that the dimerization of human γG globulin (presumably by interaction through its Fc segments) fails to affect its rate of catabolism in rabbits.

In attempting to identify the various biological activities associated with the Fc portion of the γG globulin molecule, it is important to establish whether these are carried on the same molecule, rather than on molecules of different γG globulin sub-classes. This is emphasized by recent observations on the properties of the γ_1 and γ_2 forms of guinea-pig (and mouse) γG globulin (outlined in section A2), which have shown homologous skin-sensitizing activity to be associated with the electrophoretically fast (γ_1) form, whilst complement fixation and heterologous skin-sensitizing activity is associated with the slower (γ_2) form. Furthermore, in this connection, recent observations of Terry [308] on the skin-sensitizing activity of human γG myeloma proteins of different heavy chain sub-classes are of much interest. Proteins of the γ_{2b}, γ_{2c} and γ_{2d} types (see Table 7.1) gave positive reverse PCA reactions, whereas γ_{2a} myeloma proteins were unreactive, irrespective of light chain type (κ or λ). Inhibition testing suggested that the lack of reactivity of the γ_{2a} molecules could be attributed to their failure to combine with a critical tissue receptor site. It will be interesting to ascertain whether both of the conformational forms of *human* γG globulin, referred to earlier (in section B1), possess skin reactivity. Preliminary studies in the authors' laboratory have indicated that the 'papain-resistant' form has a greater tendency to form aggregates following reductive cleavage by cysteine (0·01 M) and dialysis against N-ethyl maleimide (0·01 M).

The possibility that the *carbohydrate* prosthetic groups of γG globulins are essential for the biological activities listed in Table 7.19 has only been investigated to a limited extent. As already mentioned in section B2b, the carbohydrate is covalently linked to the heavy chains within the Fc part of the γG globulin molecule (human, rabbit, horse, etc.). Smiley & Horton [323] isolated glycopeptides by pronase digestion of human γ_2G globulin (obtained by DEAE-cellulose chromatography of Cohn fraction II). Pronase digestion at an enzyme : protein ratio of 1 : 100 proceeded overnight at 60° C, and the entire digest was filtered through a column of Sephadex G25 equilibrated with 0·01 M phosphate buffer, pH 7·0. The excluded fraction shown (by ninhydrin and orcinol monitoring as described in section B2) to contain the glyco-peptides was refractionated on Sephadex G75, when the glycopeptides were recovered as a single peak (identified by the orcinol reaction) in the included moiety, free from residual undigested material and large peptides (containing no carbohydrate). Finally, residual pronase was removed by Dowex 50 × 8 (H^+ form) and the product lyophilized. The molar ratios of the carbohydrate constituents were sialic acid : fucose : galactose : mannose : N-acetylglu-cosamine, 1 : 2 : 3 : 4 : 9, and the principal amino acids were aspartic, glutamic, serine and threonine. This glycopeptide fraction (without further purification) was examined for biological activity.

The addition of the glycopeptide to antibody-sensitized sheep erythrocytes prior to the addition of complement failed to prevent haemolysis, although (in the same experiment) *aggregated* human $\gamma_2 G$ globulin effected complete inhibition. The inhibitory effect of the glycopeptide on skin fixation of rabbit $\gamma_2 G$ antibody globulin (anti-BSA) in the guinea-pig was tested by adding a large excess of the glycopeptide to the antibody solution prior to injection; the control injection was of antibody alone. Intravenous injection of the antigen (bovine serum albumin, 1 mg) and Evans blue dye (3 mg) demon-strated no effect by the presence of the glycopeptide on capillary permeability (i.e. on PCA activity). Nor was an inhibitory effect observed when the glyco-peptides were included in a system comprising aggregated human γG globulin and high-titre rheumatoid-arthritic sera, examined either by the latex or sensitized sheep red-cell agglutination procedures.

In the authors' laboratory, a somewhat different approach (412] was made to assess the influence of the carbohydrate (particularly the terminal non-reducing sugars, N-acetyl-neuraminic acid and *L*-fucose) on the interaction of aggregated human γG globulin with rheumatoid factor. Human γG globu-lin, aggregated (as described in section C2) by heat, dilute HCl or dilute NaOH treatment, was incubated with neuraminidase (induced enzyme isolated from culture filtrates of *Klebsiella aerogenes* NCIB 9479 [229]) under identical conditions of continual dialysis (described earlier in section B2). Suitable con-trols were included. The recovered γG globulins were then examined for quantitative precipitation with rheumatoid factor, and the cleaved neuraminic acid was recovered quantitatively from the dialysates and analysed by the sensitive Warren [413] procedure. Although the total neuraminic (= sialic) acid was recovered in each case from the dialysates, there was no difference in the amount of specific precipitate formed by the aggregated γG globulin before or after its removal. Similar results were obtained when the terminal

L-fucose residues were removed from the aggregated human γG globulin preparations by the action of specific α-*L*-fucosidase (induced in *K. aerogenes* NCIB 9479 [230]), whereupon the whole of the *L*-fucose was removed (and recovered quantitatively in the dialysate) without any effect on the amount of specific precipitate formed.

Possible light is shed on the lack of activity of the carbohydrate moiety in native human γG globulin by its insensitivity to neuraminidase. It was reported by Robert *et al* [325] that only a proportion of the neuraminic acid is cleaved readily from bovine γG globulin by neuraminidase. Similar results have been obtained in the authors' laboratory, and by Labat & Berger [441], with human γG globulin. It is possible that the role of carbohydrate is a structural rather than a functional one, as suggested by Eylar [326]. Moreover, since extracellular proteins (including, of course, immunoglobulins) are glycoproteins, whereas intracellular proteins seldom seem to be, it is possible that the carbohydrate prosthetic group is attached to the protein after synthesis of the polypeptide chains within the cell, as suggested in recent studies by Neutra & Leblond, [390, 440]. The isolation from colostra and milk (of various species) of specific oligosaccharide nucleotides having the general formulae:

$$\alpha N\text{-acyl-NA2} \rightarrow \beta D\text{-Galp } 1 \rightarrow 4\beta D \text{ GpNAc } 1 \rightarrow DPU;$$

$$\alpha N\text{-acyl-NA2} \rightarrow \beta D\text{-Galp } 1 \rightarrow 6\beta D \text{ GpNAc } 1 \rightarrow DPU;$$

$$\alpha L\text{-Fucp } 1 \rightarrow \beta D\text{-Galp } 1 \rightarrow 4\beta D \text{ GpNAc } 1 \rightarrow DPU;$$

$$\beta D\text{-Galp } 1 \rightarrow 4\beta D \text{ GpNAc } 1 \rightarrow DPU^*$$

* Key: DPU = uridine diphospho-
           Galp = galactopyranosyl
     GpNAc = N-acetyl-D-glucosaminyl
         Fucp = Fucopyranosyl
   N-acyl-NA = N-acyl-neuraminic acid; acyl may be acetyl or glycolyl

suggests a possible role of these in glycoprotein biosynthesis, since they transfer the oligosaccharide prosthetic groups to suitable receptor molecules [146].

SECTION C. CONFORMATION OF IMMUNOGLOBULINS

1. Spatial arrangement of sub-units

(a) Sub-units of γG globulin

As indicated in the previous section, antigenic and chemical analysis of the polypeptide chains comprising the molecular fragments obtained by papain digestion has provided strong evidence in support of the Porter structural model of γG globulin (depicted diagrammatically in Fig. 7.6). Nevertheless, the demonstration of the presence in γG globulin preparations of molecules with differing susceptibility to enzyme digestion, and with different numbers of inter-chain disulphide bonds (as already mentioned in section B) has exposed the inadequacy of schematic models. It is important, therefore, to elucidate the *spatial arrangement* of the polypeptide chains within the γG globulin molecule, as such an arrangement can be expected to have a critical influence on the various activities of the molecule (as will be illustrated). This sub-section is devoted to the main experimental techniques which are being applied to the study of such questions, and is succeeded by sub-sections dealing with the conformation of the less well characterized γM and γA globulins.

It is interesting to note that the biological activities associated with the papain digestion fragments (Fab and Fc) of the rabbit γG globulin molecule are unaffected by the cleavage of the molecule (into three pieces of about 50,000 mol. wt.). This has prompted Cohen & Porter [1] to suggest that the γG globulin molecule has a *tripartite structure*, and that papain cleavage of one or two peptide bonds (within the region linking the F(ab)$_2$ and Fc pieces) leaves the configuration of the fragments unaltered (despite the limited production of low molecular weight peptides observed after papain proteolysis). This suggestion is supported by the finding of Goodman & Gross [329] that no new antigenic sites are exposed in the fragments as a result of the papain treatment. The type of structure envisaged has been represented in diagrammatic form by Noelken *et al* [330] (and is shown in Fig. 7.37). In this model, the site of papain cleavage has been depicted as an extended flexible part of the heavy chain, in contrast to the compact globular Fab and Fc regions. Evidence in support of this partially flexible structure is provided by studies of fluorescence depolarization (see Chapter 12 for an account of the method) (which have indicated that the observed rotational relaxation time of a fluorescent dye attached to γG globulin is smaller than would be expected for a compact sphere [407]), and by the observation [88] that a whole range of proteolytic enzymes (of differing specificity) attacks a similar region of the heavy chain (assumed to be the most readily accessible). Further evidence that this region, in the vicinity of the labile inter-heavy chain disulphide bond, is particularly susceptible to attack by proteolytic enzymes, is provided by results of studies on the reversible dissociation of the Fc fragment of rabbit γG globulin. Inman & Nisonoff [408] concluded that the decrease in the S-carboxymethylcysteine content of alkylated Fc fragments after prolonged papain digestion, and the loss of the capacity for re-oxidation if alkylation is omitted, are due to the gradual removal of the region of the Fc fragment which contains the inter-chain disulphide bond.

The findings from studies on the enzymatic digestion of γG globulins in the presence and absence of reducing agent (0·01 M cysteine) cited in section B1 suggest, however, that the folding of the polypeptide chains in some γG globulins masks their sites of proteolysis and that it is necessary to cleave intra-chain disulphide bonds to gain access to these sites. It seems probable that the behaviour of the 'papain-resistant' human γ_1G globulin, separated from papain digests by gel filtration on Sephadex G100 (as mentioned in section B1) can be attributed to such a configurational arrangement. This is illustrated schematically in Fig. 7.38, where cleavage of additional intra-chain disulphide bridges in the heavy chains of the resistant form (e.g. by 0·01 M cysteine) might be expected to lead to an unfolding of the molecule (as was indicated by an

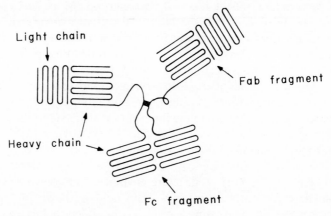

Fig. 7.37. Schematic representation of a possible model for γG globulin. The *short heavy line* represents the single disulphide bond between the two heavy chains. (Reproduced by courtesy of Drs M.E.Noelken, C.A.Nelson, C.E.Buckley and C. Tanford from *J. biol. Chem.* (1965), **240**, 218.)

increase in laevorotation) and the exposure of new side chains (as suggested by an increase in immunoelectrophoretic mobility and the isolation of additional acidic peptides not observed in digestion products of the more common 'papain-sensitive' form of human γG globulin). Such a structure could also possibly explain the apparent masking of the light chains in some γG globulin molecules, as indicated by the demonstration of agglutinating factors directed against buried antigenic determinants [331] (revealed by peptic digestion of human γ_2G globulin) and by the difficulty in eliciting antibodies directed against light chain determinants by immunization with whole γG globulin. Similarly, studies with trypsin [96], in the presence and absence of various alkylating agents (N-ethyl maleimide, iodoacetamide) have indicated that human γG globulin comprises molecules with different conformations (as indicated by the variable lability of their disulphide bonds and differing susceptibility to enzyme digestion).

Cohen & Porter [1] have suggested that the two inter-chain disulphide bonds assigned, in the original Porter model, to the C-terminal end of the heavy chains, might instead be intra-chain bonds. This is consistent with the finding of Palmer & Nisonoff [116], who showed that a large proportion (two-thirds) of rabbit γG globulin molecules dissociate into equivalent halves in dilute salt solution, after rupture of a single labile disulphide bond (by mild reduction and acidification). Moreover, it has since been shown [408] that the crystalline Fc fragment of rabbit γG globulin, prepared by papain digestion in the presence of 0·05 M L-cysteine, dissociates into half-fragments (1·8S, 24,000 mol. wt. at pH 2·4) under similar conditions (i.e. 0·05 M NaCl at pH 2·7). This provides further evidence that the *non-covalent* interactions between the heavy chains

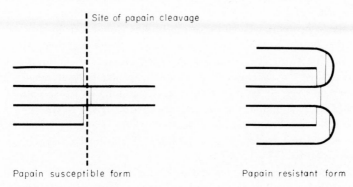

FIG. 7.38. Schematic illustration of possible structural variations differentiating papain-susceptible and papain-resistant forms of γG globulin.

of rabbit γG globulin are largely localized in the Fc region. On the other hand, it was found that the crystalline Fc fragment prepared by proteolysis in the presence of *low concentrations of reducing agent* (e.g. 0·001 M cysteine) is largely undissociable at low pH. Similarly, proteolysis with papain in the presence of 0·05 M cysteine for 1 or 4 hours, followed by dialysis (to remove the cysteine) but omitting an alkylation step, also yielded an undissociable fragment at low pH (owing to reformation of an inter-chain disulphide bond). In both cases, however, dissociation could be achieved by further reduction and alkylation.

Hence, reversible dissociation of the Fc fragment of rabbit γG globulin can be achieved under appropriate conditions. The production of *covalently* linked half Fc fragments under different dissociation conditions (e.g. by the use of insoluble papain, followed by prolonged treatment with detergent [82])

K

is attributed to intra-molecular disulphide bond interchange. The formation of such artefacts will confuse any attempted elucidation of γ globulin structure. It is important, therefore to recognize the existence of such structural heterogeneity when interpreting presently available data on the conformation of γG globulins. Some of these data have been obtained from investigations on what must obviously have been heterogeneous populations of molecules. There is also the problem of the conformational changes induced by isolation procedures. An obvious example of this is the ease of formation of dimer (and sometimes larger polymeric forms) in lyophilized (Cohn fraction) preparations of γG globulins. Obviously any change involving the cleavage of intra- or inter-chain disulphide bonds can be expected to have an important influence on the conformation of immunoglobulin molecules.

Early hydrodynamic measurements (such as viscosity, diffusion) on rabbit antibody γG globulin preparations [30] showed the molecular dimensions to be of the order of 265 Å long and 37 Å wide (when hydrated to the extent of 0·2 g water/g protein). γG globulin antibodies isolated from sera of other species (e.g. man, monkey, horse) were shown to have similar width, and lengths varying from 204 Å to 338 Å [333]. Horse γM globulin antibody (directed against *Pneumococcus* type specific capsular polysaccharide) on the other hand, proved to be about three times as long as horse antitoxin γG globulin [333]. A similar order of size has been assigned to the γG globulin molecule following low angle X-ray scattering measurements, which indicate that the anhydrous molecule is a cylinder of elliptical cross-section with dimensions of $240 \times 57 \times 19$ Å [334].

Electron-microscopy provides the other main procedure for determining the shape of immunoglobulin molecules. Two approaches have been adopted. In the first, direct observations are made on γG globulin preparations, by using shadow-casting or negative contrast techniques. Thus, Hall *et al* [335], for example, obtained evidence of a dimer-like granular structure, with average dimensions close to those provided by hydrodynamic measurements. Recently, however, Höglund & Levin [336] have reported substantially different values for the dimensions of human γG globulin (zone-electrophoresis fraction), namely 150×60 Å, based on the measurement of three hundred and ten particles. The measured lengths of the γG globulin molecules were found to deviate considerably more from the mean value than did the lengths of albumin molecules (examined by a similar technique). γM globulin molecules were also observed and found usually to be ellipsoid (300×200 Å, on the basis of one hundred and ten molecules measured) although irregular forms (double forms or particles with clefts) were occasionally observed. Stroboscopy [337] has revealed some definite chain structure in a few γM globulin molecules (as shown in Fig. 7.39), which are thought to be possibly in an open, swollen form.

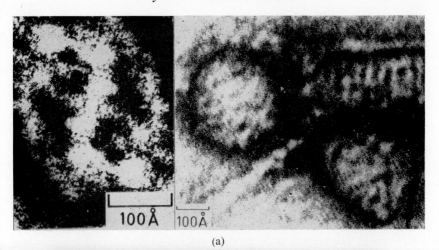

(a)

(b)

FIG. 7.39. (a) Stroboscopy picture of a twofold symmetrical γM globulin molecule appears to have an open, swollen structure with some chain units.
(Reproduced by courtesy of Dr S.Höglund.)
(b) Electron micrograph of normal bovine γM globulin, showing rod-like sub-structure. Negative staining, magnification about 400,000.
(Reproduced by courtesy of Drs E.A.Munn and A.Feinstein.)

In preparation for electron-microscopy, the protein solutions examined by Höglund & Levin [336] were first dialysed against 0·1 M ammonium carbonate buffer (pH 8·8), as it was found that the use of other volatile buffers at lower pH (e.g. ammonium acetate, pH 6·8) caused molecular aggregation. After dialysis, the protein solutions were diluted with the same buffer and fixed for 2 minutes with 5 per cent formalin in 1 per cent buffered osmic acid [338]; formalin alone was used for negative staining. In preparations for shadow casting, solutions containing about 0·05 per cent protein were applied to freshly cleaved mica by a high-pressure spray gun [339], driven by air and supplied with two air filters. This technique was found to give a minimum number of aggregates in the specimens, which were shadowed with platinum in a Siemens evaporating unit (essentially as described by Hall [340]). Afterwards, the specimen was backed with carbon [341], floated on double-distilled water and picked up on platinum discs with 70 mμ holes, or on copper grids. The heights of the protein molecules were inferred by examining shadowed specimens containing a mixture of the proteins and 880 Å-polystryrene latex particles (Dow Chemical Co).

The specimens were examined in the Siemen's Elmiskop 1 instrument, using the double condenser lens at a magnification of 20,000 and 40,000, a 400 μ condenser aperture and a 50 μ objective aperture (at an operating voltage of 60 kV). The sizes of the protein molecules were calculated from prints with an ocular micrometer, graduated to 0·1 mm. Measurements were also made on both shadowed and unshadowed 880 Å-polystyrene latex particles. All widths were corrected for an exaggeration of about 60 Å by the metal cap. Rowe [342] has criticized the molecular dimensions obtained by Höglund & Levin [336] in this manner, on the grounds that the molecular weights calculated from them differ grossly from those generally accepted for the proteins (γG and γM globulins, albumin and α_2 macroglobulin) examined.

In negative staining, performed by Höglund & Levin [336], phosphotungstic acid at pH 7·0 was added to fixed protein solutions (containing about 0·05 per cent protein) to a final concentration of about 1 per cent. One drop of this solution was placed (using a micropipette) on the carbon grid, prepared according to Spencer [343]. After 3 minutes, excess liquid was sucked off with a piece of filter paper.

In an alternative approach, several investigators have examined γ globulin *antibodies* in combination with large antigenic particles or molecules (which can be seen very clearly in negative staining). The complexes examined include rabbit γG globulin antibodies combined with polyoma and verruca vulgaris virus [344], tobacco mosaic virus [346], or influenza virus [347]; bacterial (*Salmonella typhimurium*) flagella [348]; horse spleen ferritin [345, 349]; γM globulin antibodies interacting with the tail of T_2-phage [337]. Measurement of inter-flagellar distances under conditions of negative staining [348] have indicated that the minimum length of rabbit antibody γG globulin molecules is about 180 Å. The individual antibody molecules could not be resolved by this technique, however, and hence no definite conclusions

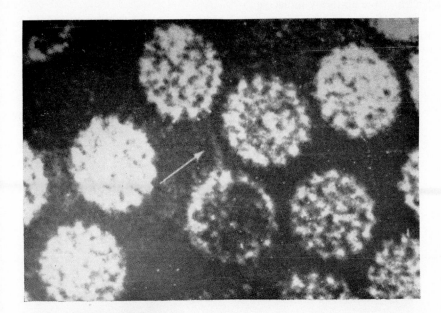

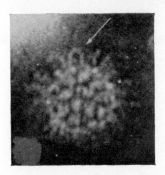

FIG. 7.40

(a) Goat antibody molecule (270 Å) linking two polyoma virus particles (near equivalence, antigen excess). Magnification ×40,000.

(b) Goat antibody molecule with both ends binding same virus particle. Magnification ×40,000.

Negatively stained preparations produced by mixing drop of aqueous suspension of washed pellet of antigen–antibody complex with equal amount of 3 per cent phosphotungstic acid, adjusted to pH 6·0 with KOH, and placing a drop of mixture on 400-mesh carbon-formvarcoated grid.

(Reproduced by courtesy of Drs J.Almeida, B.Cinader and A.Howatson from *J. exp. Med.* (1963), **118**, 327.)

could be reached about their precise shape and thickness. Electron-microscopic examination [344] of negatively stained aggregates of virus antigen (polyoma or verruca vulgaris virus) and rabbit or goat γG globulin antibody, on the other hand, has revealed the antibody molecules as *cylindrical rods* with a long axis of 250–270 Å and a short axis of 35–40 Å. The combining sites were at opposite ends of the antibody molecules (as shown in Fig. 7.40), separated by a distance of 250–270 Å, i.e. the same order of magnitude as the length of the antibody molecule.

The electron-microscopic (negative contrast) observations of Feinstein & Rowe [349] on complexes of horse spleen ferritin and rabbit anti-ferritin

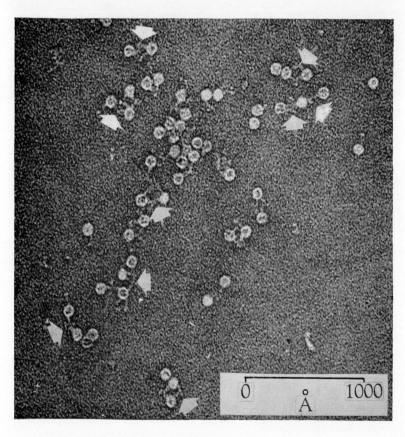

7.41

antibody γG globulin have led to the interesting suggestion that when cross-linking of antigenic particles occurs, the antibody molecule 'clicks open' to varying degrees about a 'hinge-point' located at one end (as illustrated in Fig. 7.41). This permits a linkage twice as long as the original antibody molecule (approximately 100 Å in length), in which the two binding sites are thought to be situated fairly close to each other in a compact structure (which is unaffected when only a single antigen is bound to the antibody). Corroborative evidence in support of this theory has been obtained by examination of ferritin-bound monovalent fragments of antibody, produced by reduction (by 2-mercaptoethanol) of pepsin-treated insoluble complexes of

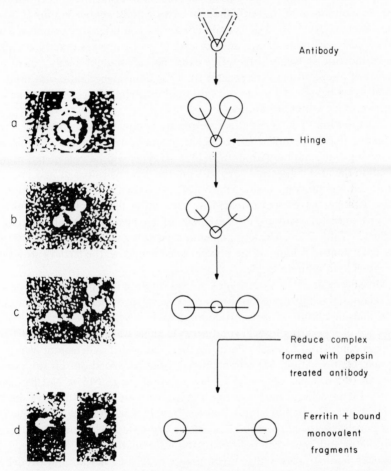

FIG. 7.41. Selected areas (right) from an electron micrograph (left) illustrating the various types of linkage observed in ferritin–anti-ferritin complexes (a–c) and the effect of reduction following papain treatment (d). A diagrammatic representation of the 'click-open' theory of cross-linking, referred to in the text, is also shown. Microscopy details: Antigen–antibody complex in 8 per cent sodium tungstoborate, pH 6·2, dried down over holes in carbon film, photographed at an initial magnification × 40,000 and an accelerating voltage of 80 kV.

(Reproduced by courtesy of Drs A.Feinstein and A.J.Rowe from *Nature, Lond.* (1965), **205**, 147.)

ferritin–anti-ferritin. This revealed rod-like structures, not more than 100 Å in length, with no sign of a kink, suggesting that the hinge-point is associated with a disulphide bond.

Details of preparation of the specimens examined by Feinstein & Rowe [349] (kindly supplied by Dr A.J.Rowe) are as follows: the concentration of the γG globulin used (in both shadow casting and negative staining) was of the order of $10^{-2}–10^{-3}$ g/100 ml. The ferritin–anti-ferritin complexes were prepared by using moderate antigen excess, as complexes exactly at equivalence did not spread satisfactorily over the substrate. Usually, an antigen excess of about 50 per cent greater than the equivalence ratio was used, the exact value being not too critical (although probably varying from one antigen–antibody system to another).

Examination of *soluble* antigen–antibody complexes has provided further evidence that structural changes occur in antibody γG globulin molecules, following combination with antigen [350, 415] (as will be considered in more detail in the next subsection). Apart from the demonstration of new immunogenic determinants by immunization of rabbits with the soluble complexes, these changes have been revealed by estimating the number of sulphydryl groups liberated, and by measurement of changes in optical rotation (as shown in Table 7.26). The latter technique affords a useful means of determining the extent of folding of the polypeptide chains (i.e. the tertiary structures) of the γG globulin molecule.

Measurement of the variation of optical rotation of a protein solution with wavelength (i.e. the 'optical rotatory dispersion') provides a greater amount of information about tertiary structure than is revealed by the more usual practice of measuring optical rotation at a single wavelength (e.g. 589·5 mμ). This is considered to offer one of the best methods for detecting *changes* in protein conformation. Measurements are usually carried out on solutions of protein (0·5–1·0 per cent w/v) in salt solutions (e.g. 0·15 M NaCl or KCl) in 0·5–1·0 dm cells, over a wavelength range of about 200–600 mμ, in a spectropolarimeter. The Bellingham & Stanley 'Pepol 60' instrument,* employed for this purpose in the authors' laboratory, incorporates a Unicam SP 500 monochromator and both xenon (covering the wavelength range 240–600 mμ) and tungsten light sources. Other investigators have used a Rudolph Model 80S spectropolarimeter or a Cary Model 60 instrument. Further details on instrumentation are given by Djerassi [409]. When a high degree of accuracy is required, the temperature of the cell compartment can be kept constant by jacketing with water from a thermostatically controlled water-bath. Protein concentrations are determined by micro-Kjeldahl nitrogen determination, or by a colorimetric procedure such as the Folin assay (modification of Lowry *et al* [76]), standardized by nitrogen estimation.

---

* Supplied by Bellingham & Stanley Ltd, 71 Hornsey Rise, London, N.19.

The specific optical rotation, $[\alpha]_\lambda$ is calculated from the data thus obtained by substitution in the equation:

$$[\alpha]_\lambda = \frac{100}{d.c.} \cdot \alpha_\lambda$$

where α_λ = optical rotation at wavelength λ

d = path-length in decimetres

c = protein concentration in g/100 ml.

The optical dispersion characteristics of *randomly coiled* proteins and polypeptides are defined by the simple Drude equation:

$$[\alpha]_\lambda = \frac{A}{\lambda^2 - \lambda_c^2}$$

where A = a constant (including a refractive index correction term)

λ_c = the optical rotatory dispersion constant.

These constants can be determined (with varying degrees of accuracy) by different graphical procedures. A method proposed by Yang & Doty [410] permits λ_c to be obtained directly, without independent calculation of A, from the slope of the plot of $[\alpha]_\lambda \cdot \lambda^2$ against $[\alpha]_\lambda$.

When an α helical structure is present in the protein conformation, however, anomalous dispersion plots are obtained. In an attempt to allow for such complications, Moffitt & Yang [352] have modified the simple Drude equation, on the assumption that the α-helix structure behaves as a single absorbing system. They have thus derived an empirical relationship for the mean residue relation at wavelength λ,

$$[m']_\lambda = \frac{a_0 \cdot \lambda_0^2}{\lambda^2 - \lambda_0^2} + \frac{b_0 \cdot \lambda_0^4}{(\lambda^2 - \lambda_0^2)^2}.$$

The mean residue rotation, $[m']_\lambda$, is defined as

$$[\alpha]_\lambda^T \left(\frac{\text{m.r.w.}}{100} \right) \left(\frac{3}{n^2 + 2} \right)$$

where $[\alpha]_\lambda^T$ = specific rotation at temperature $T°$ and wavelength λ

m.r.w. = mean residue weight

$\quad = \dfrac{\text{molecular weight of the molecule}}{\text{number of peptide units in the molecule}}$

n = refractive index at wavelength λ

K*

b_0 and λ_0 = constants characteristic of the helix

a_0 = a constant incorporating both helical and intrinsic residue contributions (which can be calculated separately by a modification of the Mofitt-Yang equation).

When calculating the values of a_0 and b_0, the value of λ_0 (i.e. the optical dispersion constant for helices, which gives linear Moffitt plots) is usually assumed to be 212 mμ (a value obtained from observations on a large number of synthetic polypeptides). The slope of the straight line obtained by substitution of this value for λ_0 and plotting $[m']_\lambda$ $(\lambda^2 - \lambda_0^2)$ against $\{1/(\lambda^2 - \lambda_0^2)\}$ provides the value of b_0, whilst its intercept on the ordinate axis determines a_0. The value of b_0 is zero when the configuration is a random coil (e.g in the denatured state).

An assessment of the accuracy and reliability of optical rotatory dispersion measurement can be obtained from the review article by Urnes & Doty [353]. Briefly, this indicates that absolute rotations can be measured with relatively great precision (often with an average error of $\pm 0\cdot002°$), with the result that rotatory data, accurate to within 1 per cent, can be obtained. Values of λ_c and b_0, obtained by graphical assessment, are, however, reproducible only to within several per cent; consequently, the best estimate of helical content by any single parameter can be considered valid only within ± 5 per cent. Another point worth mentioning is the importance of using carefully purified reagent in studies concerned with the solvent effect of 2-chloroethanol.

It is thus evident that four main parameters, $[\alpha]$, λ_c, a_0 and b_0, may be obtained from optical rotation measurements, providing an estimate of the extent of configurational changes occurring in proteins. Studies are often made of the changes in the protein solution following denaturation (e.g. by heat, extremes of pH, urea, guinidine) or 'renaturation' treatment (e.g. by lowering the activity of the solvent, water, by the addition of lithium bromide or 2-chloroethanol). As implied, the denaturation treatments usually decrease the helical content of the protein, whilst renaturation treatments accomplish an apparently reverse effect (by lowering intramolecular bond formation).

Hamaguchi & Migita [354] have made use of the latter effect in devising an optical rotatory technique for differentiating Bence-Jones proteins of the two antigenic types (K and L). The value of $-b_0$ (determined from the Moffitt-Yang equation) of two type K Bence-Jones proteins was found to increase steeply up to 25 per cent 2-chloroethanol concentration (as shown in Fig. 7.42). In contrast, two type L proteins showed a small increase in $-b_0$ up to 50 per cent 2-chloroethanol, followed by a steep increase above this concentration. The two types of protein can also be distinguished by differences in their a_0 values at different concentrations of 2-chloroethanol. Thus, the type L Bence-

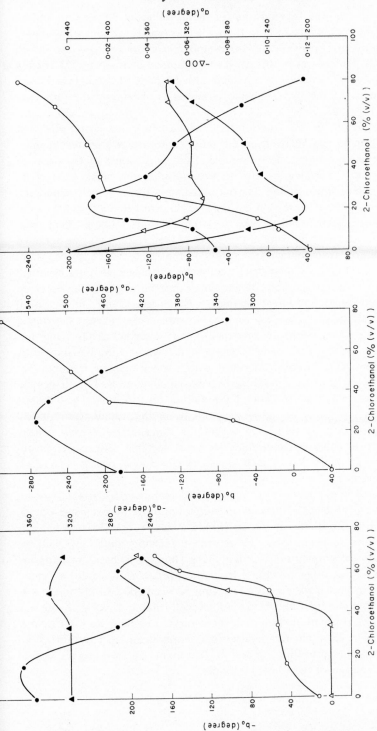

FIG. 7.42. (a) Effect of solvent composition on the values of a_0 and b_0 of Bence-Jones proteins (type L). a_0, closed symbols; b_0, open symbols. Solvent: 2-chloroethanol: water mixtures. Circles: Bence-Jones protein 'Ba'. Triangles: Bence-Jones protein 'Ki'. Measurements at 25° C. (b) Effect of solvent composition on the values of a_0 and b_0 of Bence-Jones proteins (type K). Solvent: 2-chloroethanol: water mixtures. Bence-Jones protein 'Na'. Measurements at 25° C. Symbols as in (a). (c) Variation of the values of a_0 (●), b_0 (○), OD at 293 mμ (△) and OD at 285 mμ (▲) of Bence-Jones protein 'Lo' (type K) with solvent composition in 2-chloroethanol: water mixtures. Measurements at 25° C. (Reproduced by courtesy of Drs. K.Hamaguchi and S.Migita from *Journal of Biochem.* (1964), **56**, 512.)

Jones proteins showed two maxima for the a_0 values at 25 per cent and 60 per cent 2-chloroethanol concentrations whereas type K proteins showed only one maximum, at 25 per cent 2-chloroethanol concentration (as is also shown in Fig. 7.42). Differences in the ratios of the optical densities at 293/285 mμ in guanidine hydrochloride or urea can also be used to distinguish Bence-Jones proteins of the two antigenic types, as is shown by the difference spectra in Fig. 7.42.

Using change in specific rotation ($[\alpha]_D$) as a guide, it has been found that for many proteins the change from the native to denatured state results in an increase in laevo-rotation. For example, from $[\alpha]_D$, values of the order of $-10°$ to $-60°$ for native proteins to values within the range of $-60°$ to $-120°$ after denaturation [409]. The optical rotatory dispersion characteristics of many proteins (i.e. those with less than 40 per cent helix in their structure) have, however, been found to obey the simple Drude relationship. Consequently, a more useful measure of the extent of their folding may be obtained by determining their optical rotatory constant (λ_c), which provides an approximate estimate of their helical content. Jirgensons [355] has classified proteins into three groups, according to the change in this parameter observed following detergent and urea treatment. The largest, and most typical group, comprises proteins (e.g. serum albumin, pepsinogen), showing a decrease in λ_c from about 249 mμ to 215 mμ; a second group comprises proteins (e.g. ovalbumin, ribonuclease, lysozyme) whose λ_c values show little variation upon denaturation. The third group (which includes the immunoglobulins, β-lactoglobulin and several enzymes) is characterized by an increase in λ_c from below 215 mμ to about 250 mμ upon denaturation. Thus, despite the compact structures of the *native* proteins in this group, their optical rotatory dispersion constants fall within the range (210–230 mμ) usually encountered for denatured molecules. Hence, it becomes necessary to postulate that the configuration of such molecules comprises *atypical polypeptide chain arrangements*.

This reasoning applies to the structure of γG globulins, where the evidence of a complete absence of helical structures obtained by extensive optical rotatory dispersion studies on human [355, 356, 384], rabbit [357], and bovine [358] γG globulins is supported by deuterium exchange data [359], and the demonstration of a high proline content [357]. Thus, on the basis of an approximately zero value of b_0 (obtained from the Moffitt-Yang equation) and a λ_c value (from the Drude equation) ranging between 200 and 217 mμ, it was concluded that the light and heavy polypeptide chains of γG globulin lack any helical conformation. It is then necessary to explain how the spatial arrangement of these chains (depicted diagrammatically in two dimensions in the models shown in Figs. 7.6 and 7.37) accounts for the observed optical rotatory properties of the whole molecules.

Callaghan & Martin [360] have interpreted the results of their studies of the optical rotatory dispersion of human γG globulin (crude, ether and ethanol, fractions) under varying conditions (including the presence of 2-chloroethanol) as evidence of compensating right-handed α helix and β structures. According to this idea, the α helical regions are located in the Fc portions of the molecule (thus accounting for its ease of crystallization), whilst the β form is found in the F(ab)$_2$ region (where, due to close apposition of four polypeptide chains, maximal occurrence of hydrogen bond formation is likely). It has not, however, proved possible to demonstrate the presence of α helix in isolated Fab and Fc sub-units of rabbit γG globulin. This is indicated by the low b_0 values of the sub-units [330, 357] and by their minimum mean residue rotation values (near 230 mμ) [330], which were of the order of $-12,000$ to $-20,000°$ in contrast to the minimum value of $-2000°$ shown by random coils. Furthermore, the absence of an absorption peak in the vicinity of 1610 to 1640 cm^{-1} in the infra-red spectrum of whole rabbit γG globulin in D$_2$O suggests that β structures are also absent [361].

An alternative explanation of the anomalous optical rotatory dispersion behaviour of γG globulins, attributing the effect to the presence of equal amounts of right- and left-handed helices, is considered unlikely [361], in view of the constancy of the b_0 value observed when normal rabbit γG globulin is denatured by urea. Nor is it likely that a deficiency in amino-acid composition is the factor restricting α helix formation, in view of the findings that 2-chloroethanol (2 M) [356, 357] and sodium dodecyl sulphate (0·2 M) [361] can induce the formation of such a structure.

On the basis of optical rotatory dispersion studies on a sodium sulphate sub-fraction of a commercial preparation of normal rabbit γG globulin (which showed a somewhat low λ_c value of 195 mμ), supported by spectroscopic measurements in the infra-red and ultra-violet regions, deuterium exchange measurements and acid-base titration, Gould *et al* [361] concluded that these solvent-induced changes are similar to those changes involving hydrophobic bonding which are believed to occur in β-lactoglobulin. Hence, these investigators concluded that hydrophobic bonding (involving the presence of serine and threonine in high proportion), and disulphide bridging, play principal roles in maintaining the three-dimensional structure of rabbit γG globulin. The existence of 'some periodically organized regions', which are not α helices, and probably not β conformations, is not excluded, however. It is also important to take into account the potential contributions of the carbohydrate moiety (and especially of the sialic-acid residues) located in the Fc portion of the molecule.

The precise location of such organized regions within the molecule must await the results of further structural analyses, and will rely ultimately on the findings from X-ray diffraction analyses (which are now being undertaken on certain γG globulins and fragments which have been isolated in a crystalline form). Meanwhile, Edelman & Galley [362] have postulated a topographical model (shown in Fig. 7.43), based on the known size and shape of the γG antibody globulin molecular envelope (referred to earlier), and on analysis [74] of the composition of the polypeptide chains and fragments (isolated as a result of papain and pepsin cleavage), summarized in the classic Porter schematic model (see Fig. 7.6). It is assumed in the Edelman & Gally [362] model

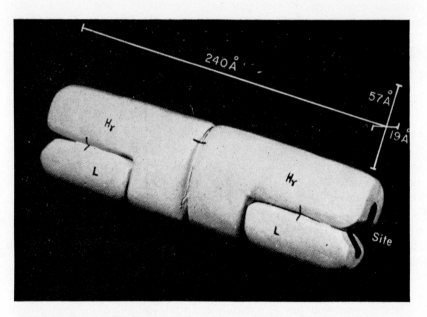

Fig. 7.43. Model of the γG globulin antibody molecule (molecular dimensions taken from Kratsky *et al* [334]). Hγ, heavy polypeptide chain. L, light polypeptide chain. Single lines drawn on model represent interchain disulphide bonds.

(Reproduced by courtesy of Drs. G.M.Edelman and J.A.Gally from *Proc. nat. Acad. Sci.* (*Wash*). (1964), **51**, 846.)

that the bivalent antibody molecule is symmetrical with respect to the polypeptide chains contributing to the combining sites, and that both the heavy and light chains are involved in such activity (as was indicated by methods employed in the characterization of the active sites, outlined in section B3). It also adopts the dimensions of the light chain calculated from the low-angle X-ray data [363] for the dimensions (74·8 × 48·3 × 21·0 Å) of a Bence-Jones protein (a λ chain dimer of 43,000 mol. wt.). The dimensions of the assumed antigen-combining sites were those determined from a study of specific anti-dextran antibodies [364].

There are obvious limitations to such a general model. For instance, the two half-molecules (comprising the light-heavy chain pair) are shown linked by a single inter-heavy chain disulphide bridge, although, as indicated in section B, there is substantial evidence for the existence of other conformational forms of γG globulin (probably with differing arrangements of disulphide bridges, accounting for their different susceptibility to proteolytic degradation). Moreover, the partially flexible 'tripartite' structure referred to earlier is not taken into account. In attempting to explain any such degradation mechanism, it is necessary to depict the maintained structural integrity and stability of the isolated Fc fragments, as indicated, for example, by the observation that papain degradation fails to lead to the exposure of new antigenic determinants within the Fc portion of the rabbit γG globulin molecule.

Obviously, the manner of folding of the polypeptide chains within the γG globulin molecule has a profound influence on its biological activities. Measurement of optical rotatory dispersion provides a means of assessing the extent of this folding under varying conditions. Thus, for example [365], it has been used to demonstrate that the complete denaturation (i.e. maximum unfolding, as indicated by a $[m']_{365}$ value of $-336°$) of Fab fragments of rabbit antibody molecules (by treatment with 7·5 M guanidine for 12 hours), is reversible, suggesting that the stable conformation of the antigen-combining sites is governed by the amino-acid sequence within the constituent heavy and light chains. This conclusion has since been supported by the demonstration [366] of substantial recovery of the antigen (ribonuclease)-combining capacity of Fab fragments of rabbit antibody on reoxidation following complete unfolding and *cleavage of all of its disulphide bonds* by reduction. The recovery of specific activity of Fab fragments of rabbit antibody directed against the DNP-haptenic group has been similarly observed [367]. The failure to detect any antibody activity in a sample of *non-specific* antibody Fab fragment when reoxidized in the presence of a 100-fold excess of ε-N-DNP-lysine is interpreted as further evidence against the hypothesis that antigen-directed formation of disulphide (or non-covalent) bonds is responsible for antibody specificity.

The experimental conditions adopted in a typical reversible denaturation experiment were as follows: a solution (0·4 mg/ml) of Fab fragment (I or II), isolated from rabbit anti-DNP antibody, was exposed for 4 hours at room temperature to 6 M guanidine hydrochloride in tris-acetate buffer (pH 8·6, I = 0·1) containing EDTA (0·001 M) and 2-mercaptoethanol (0·1 M). Complete reduction of the disulphide bonds was demonstrated by S-carboxymethylation of a sample of reduced protein, followed by quantitative amino-acid analysis (as indicated previously, in section B2). Reoxidation of reduced protein was accomplished by cooling to 5° C and diluting to yield a solution of protein (concentration about 4 μg/ml) in tris-acetate buffer (pH 8·6, I = 0·05) containing EDTA (0·001 M) and 2-mercaptoethanol (0·003 M), which was maintained at 5° C for approximately 18 hours. The solution was slowly stirred, at room temperature, for approximately 20 hours, concentrated (by vacuum dialysis) to about one-fifth its original volume, and dialysed (against tris-acetate buffer, pH 8·6, I =0·05). It was further concentrated (vacuum dialysis), dialysed against sodium acetate buffer (pH 5·5, I = 0·05), heated briefly at 35–40° C and clarified by centrifugation. This treatment resulted in the recovery of about half of the original protein, part of the remainder being insoluble at pH 5·5 (due, supposedly, to polymerization following interchain disulphide bond formation). Antibody (anti-DNP) activity was determined by titrating the Fab fragment with ε-N-DNP-lysine and measuring the quenching of fluorescence (see Chapter 12) resulting from the binding of the DNP group [368] (assuming the fluorescence would be completely quenched if the antibody were fully (100 per cent) active).

Although the recoveries of antibody activity thus determined are relatively low (i.e. 11–24 per cent, compared with nearly 100 per cent for ribonuclease and lysozyme activity), the yield has been greater than would have been expected on a statistical basis, if reoxidation of disulphide bonds had occurred randomly. Moreover, recovery of such activity has not been previously convincingly demonstrated for any protein (e.g. insulin) comprising more than one type of polypeptide chain. This raises the question of the role of inter-chain disulphide bridges within the antibody molecule. It is possible that the single disulphide link between the C-terminal end of the light chain, and the heavy chain of the Fab portion of the molecule (i.e. the Fd region) serves as an anchor, permitting the apposition of key amino-acid residues exposed in both chains as a result of their specific folding (controlled by intra-disulphide bonding). Moreover, the results of hybridization experiments [414], in which γG globulin molecules have been re-formed by reoxidation *in vitro* from a variety of heavy and light chains (including the pairing of chains from different species) suggests that the conformation of the Fab fragment might also be maintained by amino-acid interaction in a modulating region (presumably within the C-terminal part of the light chain), the amino-acid sequence of which has been shown to be common to chains of different origin (cf. similar findings in haemoglobins, insulins). In any such consideration of the nature of the folding of the polypeptide chain within the γG globulin molecule, it is important to treat the molecule *as a whole*, i.e. not to neglect the contribution of the Fc portion, which might influence the folding of the Fab regions containing the antigen-binding sites. Conversely (as will be indicated in the next section), antigen combination by the Fab regions can alter the folding of the heavy chains within the *Fc* part of the molecule (as revealed by changes in optical rotation of the antibody molecule) and this can lead to the induction of new biological activities (through an allosteric transition occurring within the γG globulin molecule).

(b) Sub-units of γM globulin

As mentioned already, the enzyme degradation procedures (outlined in section B1), which have provided much insight into the structure of γG globulins, have proved less rewarding in the attempted characterization of γM globulins. For instance, Harboe [370] has employed two peptide digestion procedures in attempts to isolate well-defined fragments from human γM globulins (isolated from Waldenström macroglobulinaemic sera by zone-electrophoresis followed by zone-centrifugation). In one procedure, the protein, dissolved in 0·15 M citric acid-phosphate buffer, pH 4·0, was digested with pepsin at 37° C (using an enzyme–protein ratio of 1 : 50 w/w). The reaction was stopped after varying time-intervals by adjusting to pH 8·0 with tris-HCl buffer and the digest dialysed against large volumes of buffered saline, pH 8·0, for 24 hours at 0° C. Alternatively, after dialysis against critic acid-phosphate buffer, pH 4·0 at 4° C, protein (100 mg) was incubated with pepsin (in a ratio of 1 : 10 w/w) at 37° C as before. Subsequent dialysis was continued, under identical conditions, for 48 hours. Finally, the digestion mixture was dialysed in the cold for 24–48 hours against large volumes of buffered saline.

The peptic digestion of human γM globulin in this way produced considerably less non-dialysable material (about 22 per cent) than was obtained by similar treatment of human γG globulin, where 62 per cent of non-dialysable material (i.e. F(ab')$_2$ fragment) was recovered [370]. γM fragments, antigenically distinct from γG peptic digestion fragments, were isolated by zone-centrifugation in a sucrose density gradient. Fragments from γM globulin antibodies (rheumatoid factors and cold agglutinins) failed, however, to show any antibody activity, this having been destroyed by the peptic digestion procedures adopted.

Miller & Metzger [447] have reported recently the separation of fragments of mol. wt. 47,000 and 114,000 respectively from a human Waldenström γM globulin and its sub-unit (γMs), by gel filtration (on Sephadex G100) of tryptic digests (produced by hydrolysis with diisopropylfluorophosphate trypsin, in a 1 : 100 enzyme : protein weight ratio at 25° C in tris buffer, pH 8·0 for 6–18 hours). On the basis of the composition of their reductive cleavage products and the similarity of these fragments to those obtainable by enzymatic digestion of γ_2G globulins, it has been suggested that they be referred to as Fabμ and F(ab')$_2\mu$ respectively.

Sub-units (6S) separated by Onoue *et al* [371] from highly purified *rabbit* γM globulin antibody (directed against the p-azo-phenyl-arsonate group), by reduction and alkylation, showed essentially the same number of hapten-binding sites and the same binding constant as those for intact γM antibody molecules. Isolation of the sub-units was achieved by the following procedure: to a solution (1·8 ml) of γM globulin antibody (purified by a specific immuno-adsorbant procedure), at a concentration of 1·63 mg/ml, was added 2 M

2-mercaptoethanol to give a final concentration of 0·105 M; after reacting at room temperature for 40 minutes, and at 4° C for 16 hours, the reduced protein was cooled in an ice-bath and alkylated by the addition of 10 per cent excess of 1 M iodoacetamide in 3 M tris-HCl buffer, pH 8·2; after reacting for 30 minutes, excess reagents were removed by dialysis against 0·5 M NaCl, buffered at pH 8·0 and 0·02 M borate.

The sub-units prepared by this procedure possessed a sedimentation coefficient ($S_{20,w}$) of 5·5S (at 1·16 mg/ml). If their molecular weight is assumed to be similar to that of intact γG globulin molecules (i.e. 140,000–160,000) and the molecular weight of the whole antibody is taken as 1,000,000, then equilibrium dialysis data can be interpreted as indicative of *six* binding sites per γM globulin antibody molecule. This implies that the 6S sub-unit represents a univalent fragment of γM antibody (just as the Fab papain digestion product represents a univalent fragment of γG antibody). Thus, the loss of haemagglutinating or precipitating activity of reduced (but not alkylated) γM antibodies can be restored by reoxidation, whereupon the sub-units reassociate with restoration of 'polyvalency'.

The possession of multiple binding sites is undoubtedly responsible for some of the properties which differentiate γM from γG antibodies. Thus, as Onoue *et al* [371] have suggested, it is possible that the reported higher affinity of rabbit γM haemagglutinins for erythrocytes is due to the ability of two (or more) agglutinin molecules to combine with more than one antigenic determinant on the erythrocyte surface. Obviously, steric factors would have a strong influence in such an interaction. The methods applied to the characterization of the tertiary structure of γG globulin molecules (outlined in the previous section) can be expected to find wide application in the study of such effects. Here, however, it is also necessary to take into account the influence on biological activity of the arrangement of the 7S sub-units (each comprising two heavy-light chain pairs), linked by disulphide bridges, i.e. it is necessary to consider also the *quaternary* structure of the molecule. A useful analogy is the study of the contribution of one of the polypeptide chain sub-units to the overall conformation (and therefore properties) of the haemoglobin molecule. The two pairs of polypeptide chains of haemoglobin (i.e. α and β) are not linked, however, by disulphide bridges. If the γG globulin molecule is assumed to comprise two repeatable units (i.e. heavy-light-chain pairs), the γM globulin molecule can be considered (on the basis of the observations of Onoue *et al* [371]) to be composed of twelve such units (with, of course, characteristic heavy chains differing from those of γG globulin). Accurate molecular weight determinations (carried out by Lamm & Small [372]) have now provided evidence, however, that rabbit γM globulin molecules comprise *five* sub-units of approximate molecular weight 180,000 (or presumably, ten heavy-light chain pairs).

γM globulins (and their sub-units) were isolated from the sera of rabbits immunized with *Salmonella enteritidis* endotoxin by a multistage- procedure involving preparative ultracentrifugation of antiserum containing added KBr (to remove lipoprotein), preparative electrophoresis for 25–50 hours at 150–600 mA on a column of formalated ethanolysed cellulose in an LKB unit (5800 A, size 60) in veronal buffer, pH 8·6, I 0·05 (in order to separate the α_2-macroglobulin), gel filtration through a column (120 × 5·7 cm) of 3·5 per cent polyacrylamide gel, and, finally, zone-centrifugation in a linear (5–28 per cent) sucrose gradient (for 26 hours at 23,000 rev/min, −5° C, in a SW25-1 rotor). The product (10–15 mg yield from 100 ml serum) was ultracentrifugally homogeneous, but contained a small amount of un-identified contaminant in the β_1 immunoelectrophoretic region. Molecular weight determinations, by the rapid equilibrium method of Yphantis (see Chapter 4) on the γM globulin in 5 M guanidine hydrochloride, gave a value of 850,000. Its constituent heavy and light chains were isolated by extensive reductive treatment, in the following manner: solutions (0·1–1 per cent) of the protein in a concentrated tris-HCl buffer (pH 8·2) were reduced by the addition of 2-mercaptoethanol to 0·3 M, and finally, solid guanidine hydro-chloride to 6·7 M (final molarity of buffer 0·5 M). It was found that the addition of reagents in this order eliminated the appearance of the small and variable first peak, observed when dry protein was dissolved directly in guanidine hydrochloride in tris-HCl buffer. After reduction at 0° C for 15 minutes, alkylation was accomplished by the addition of an equal volume of 1 M tris-HCl buffer, 3–4 M guanidine hydrochloride and iodoacetamide (twice recrystallized from ethanol and petroleum ether) to 0·36 M, so that the final solution contained protein (1 per cent) in 5·1–5·2 M guanidine hydrochloride. In an alternative alkylation procedure, only an equimolar amount of iodo-acetamide was added, after which the protein was reduced a second time by the addition of 2-mercaptoethanol to a final concentration of 0·3 M, and alkyla-tion repeated using a 10 per cent excess of solid iodoacetamide. The heavy and light chains thus dissociated from the γM globulin preparations were isolated at room temperature by gel filtration through Sephadex G200 in 5 M guanidine hydrochloride. Column effluents were monitored at 280 mμ, and the appro-priate fractions concentrated by ultrafiltration in Visking tubing (0·390 in. flat and 0·002 in. thick), using a pressure of 1 atmosphere for heavy chains and approximately 0·5 atmosphere for light chains (which may pass through the dialysis tubing at the higher pressure).

Several important technical considerations emerged. These included the need to use guanidine hydrochloride of the highest purity and, as this reagent extracts UV-absorbing material from tygon and rubber tubing, polyethylene tubing should be used. It was also found that the flow-rate decreased with time unless the effluent were passed *upwards* through the column. Sephadex

G200, which had been 'fined' ten to twenty times with water, and allowed to soak in 5 M guanidine for 3–4 days, was used for packing the column, and flow-rates of 1·0–1·5 ml/cm^2 per hour were obtained. Loading was facilitated by a density-stabilizing procedure (whereby the sample solution was of a slightly higher density than the solution in the column) and was followed by the application of 5–10 per cent of the column volume of a still denser solution (5·5–5·6 M guanidine). Material eluted from the Sephadex G200 column ahead of the heavy chain peak (to a varying extent in different experiments) was thought to comprise a non-disulphide bonded aggregate of heavy and light chains.

The heavy and light chains isolated in the other peaks were found to have molecular weights of approx. 70,000 and 22,000–23,000 respectively. Apart from its larger molecular weight, γM globulin heavy chain was shown to differ grossly from γG globulin heavy chain, by comparative peptide mapping, and chemical analysis of amino-acid and carbohydrate constituents. Similar comparative analyses provided further evidence of the close similarity of the light chains of the two types (γM and γG) of rabbit immunoglobulin (demonstrated by other investigators [109, 188, 372, 449]).

The larger sub-units (comprising two pairs of heavy and light chains) were isolated by partial reduction and alkylation according to the procedure of Deutsch [374]. This involves reduction in phosphate buffer (pH 7·4, I = 0·2) by 0·1 M 2-mercaptoethanol at room temperature for 10–16 hours. The 2-mercaptoethanol was removed, either by gel filtration through Sephadex G25 equilibrated with the phosphate buffer, or by extensive dialysis against the same buffer. Alkylation was achieved by dialysing the reduced protein against 0·02 M iodoacetamide in the phosphate buffer. As already mentioned, the molecular weight of these sub-units was found to be 180,000 (comprising two heavy chains, mol. wt. 70,000 and two light chains, mol. wt. 22,500).

A similar approach was employed in earlier studies by Miller & Metzger [8, 9], on the characterization of a purified *human* γM macroglobulin preparation isolated by chromatography on agar gel (as described by Salvatore *et al* [375]) from the plasma of a patient with macroglobulinaemia. The intact molecule was found to have a molecular weight of 890,000. Sub-units (similar to those first described by Deutsch & Morton [376] and termed 'γMs') were obtained in ultracentrifugally homogeneous form as follows: γM globulin was degraded rapidly (to the extent of about 85 per cent) by reaction with 0·05 M cysteine in tris-HCl buffer (pH 8·6) for 8 minutes at 25° C, and alkylated by the addition of a 10 per cent excess of iodoacetamide. The mixture was applied to a column (80 × 3·2 cm) of Sephadex G200, effecting a separation of the sub-unit from the residual parent γM globulin molecules. The molecular weight of the sub-unit was estimated to be 185,000 (i.e. 16 per cent higher than that determined simultaneously for the 7S γG globulin molecule). This value is only 4 per cent higher than that expected, if the human γM globulin unit is made up of *five* equivalent sub-units. On the other hand, errors in the molecular weight determinations amounting to ± 20 per cent would be necessary if a four or six sub-unit structure were postulated.

Thus, as was indicated schematically in Fig. 7.1, the human γM globulin molecule appears to resemble the *rabbit* γM antibody molecule studied by Onoue *et al* [371] in possessing *five* sub-units (each presumably comprising, as in the rabbit γM globulin, two 'heavy-light chain pairs'). As mentioned in Chapter 4, however, pathological γM globulins have been observed (by statistical analysis) to fall into two structural groups, having mean $S_{20,w}$ values of 17·0S and 18·3S; and faster sedimenting (29S and 38S) γM components are frequently observed in macroglobulinaemic sera. It is, therefore, quite conceivable that some types of human γM globulin molecule comprise smaller or greater numbers of γMs sub-units.

Further evidence for the five sub-units (γMs) structure of human γM globulin was obtained from studies [9] of the distribution of disulphide bonds within the molecule. The number of disulphide bonds reduced per mole of γM globulin during its conversion to γMs units was followed by evaluating sedimentation patterns, and by concomitant analysis of the sulphydryl groups liberated by reacting these with 5,5'-dithio-bis-(2-nitrobenzoic acid). The protein, in 0·2 M tris-HCl buffer, was reduced at 25° C for 60 minutes by several different reagents; 0·2 M 2-mercaptoethanol at pH 8·2; 0·05–0·5 M cysteine at pH 8·6; 0·001–0·027 M dithiothreitol, pH 8·6. The distribution of released sulphydryl groups with respect to the heavy and light chains of γMs sub-units, after alkylation with ^{14}C-iodoacetamide, was determined by gel filtration on Sephadex G100 in 1 N propionic acid (when 22–28 per cent yield of light chains was indicated). The γM globulin thus reduced in aqueous solution yielded forty-nine to fifty new sulphydryl groups (per molecule of γM globulin transformed to its γMs sub-units), forty of these being associated with the heavy chains, and ten with the light chains. These findings are interpreted as strong support for the five sub-unit (20-chain) model (which possibly incorporates a thermodynamically stable pentameric ring structure).

As already indicated, the precise determination of the disposition of these sub-units within the parent molecules should throw considerable light on the properties of γM globulins. Miller & Metzger [8] are of the opinion that the apparently weak (non-covalent) interactions between the γMs units (compared with the interaction between constituent polypeptide chains) might permit some degree of rotational freedom about the inter-sub-unit disulphide bonds (which would be consistent with the unusually high frictional ratio shown by the γM globulin molecule). Moreover, preliminary depolarization of fluorescence studies [448] have provided evidence in support of this idea (as well as indicating flexibility within the sub-units themselves). Such flexibility of similar univalent sub-units comprising γM antibodies could account for the greater haemagglutinating efficiency of these antibodies than γG antibodies (whose combining capacity is probably more restricted by limitations imposed by the steric configuration of the antigenic determinants on the cell surface). As in the case of rabbit γM antibodies, initial studies on human γM antibodies (e.g. rheumatoid factor) suggested that the molecules possibly possessed six combining sites (thus attributing the 22S peak observed in the ultracentrifugal patterns of rheumatoid arthritic sera to a complex between 19S antibody and six 7S γG globulin 'antigen' molecules [377].)

(c) Sub-units of γA globulin

Similar studies on γA globulin are impeded by the tendency of this protein to occur in multiple molecular forms, and by the difficulty of isolating these in monodisperse distribution. One such (10S) protein has, however, been isolated by Deutsch [374], in relatively pure form and in 70 per cent yields from the serum of a patient with multiple myeloma (containing 79 per cent of 10S material) by a combination of cold ethanol fractionation and ion-exchange chromatography on both CM- and DEAE-celluloses. The molecular weight was calculated from sedimentation ($S_0 = 9.70$S) and diffusion ($D_0 = 2.06 \times 10^7$ cm^2 sec^{-1}) data, to be 424,000, and its axial ratio (a/b) was calculated as 20 (assuming the molecule to be an unhydrated prolate ellipsoid). Papain digestion of the purified protein (with 0.3 per cent of its weight of cysteine-activated papain) for 20 hours at pH 5.0 and 37° C degraded it into a 3.4S component (showing a single boundary on free solution electrophoresis at pH 8.57, of similar mobility to the parent molecule [378]). Vertical starch-gel electrophoresis, however, revealed a series of bands, all with higher anodic mobilities and of similar antigenicity (as revealed by gel-diffusion analysis in a second dimension). Reduction of the purified γA globulin with 0.1 M 2-mercaptoethanol at pH 7.4 converted it to 6.25S (S_0) material, which was stabilized by alkylation (by dialysis against 0.02 M iodoacetamide at pH 7.4). This material was calculated (from S_0 and D_0 data) to have a molecular weight of 190,000 and was assumed, therefore, to represent *half-molecules* of the parent γA globulin. Its molecular weight is close to that found by Miller & Metzger [8] for the γMs sub-unit of γM globulin (as mentioned earlier), suggesting that, like the γM heavy chain, the γA heavy chain is somewhat larger than the heavy chain of γG globulin. This assumes, of course, that the γA globulin molecule isolated by Deutsch [374] comprises two sub-units, each composed of two heavy-light chain pairs (as indicated in Fig. 7.1). It is possibly of some significance in this connection that (like the parent γA globulin) the reduced and alkylated material (i.e. 6.3S sub-unit, designated 'monomer' by Deutsch) is converted to 3.5S fragments when treated with 1 per cent of cysteine-active papain (at pH 5). Moreover, ageing of the parent γA globulin (and its 6·3S sub-units) at 0–2° C, under essentially sterile conditions, leads to breakdown into slower sedimenting components (ranging from 1·5 to 5·5S) which showed reactions of identity when analysed by starch-gel electrophoresis [378].

The extensive aggregation (to multiple molecular components) undergone at pH 5·0 by parent γA globulin and its reduction product is attributed to an unusual reactivity of sulphydryl groups, because alkylated protein failed to aggregate [374]. These aggregation products are likened to the multiple components observed sedimenting between the 7S and 19S peaks in certain multiple myeloma sera (as indicated by Fig. 4.1). Reduction of the native γA globulin by 0·1M 2-mercaptoethanol at neutral pH was found to cleave fourteen to fifteen out of a total of fifty-five disulphide bonds (assuming a protein molecular weight of 420,000), about five of the bonds reforming after removal of the reducing agent.

Attempts [374] to aggregate the native and the reduced ('monomer') material by the use of the bifunctional mercurial reagent, bis-acetoxy-mercurimethyldioxane, under conditions which effect dimerization of serum albumin [411], were unsuccessful.

Ishizaka *et al* [379] isolated human antibody γA globulin (by the method of Vaerman *et al* [380]) from the sera of individuals who had been immunized by two weekly injections of blood-group A substance. These investigators have provided evidence of a reduction in the anti-A haemagglutinating activity of a polymerized form (sedimenting between 7S and 19S) when this was incubated at pH 8·0 for 2 hours at room temperature with 0·1 M 2-mercaptoethanol, and subsequently alkylated by dialysing against 0·02 M iodoacetate for 24 hours. Excess reagents were removed by dialysing against 0·1 M borate buffer (pH8·5)-saline for 48 hours. The 7S sub-unit dissociation products, isolated by density-gradient ultracentrifugation (as described in Chapter 4), retained some haemagglutinating activity, however. Moreover, 2-mercaptoethanol reduction, followed by alkylation, depressed the haemagglutination titre of the 7S monomeric form of anti-A γA antibody globulin. Hence, on the basis of these findings, and those of Rawson & Abelson [381], it cannot yet be concluded that polymerized forms of γA globulin antibody are composed of "univalent" 7S sub-units (as are γM antibodies). Nevertheless, as in the case of the γM antibodies, there is evidence to suggest that the possession of multiple sub-units in a relatively flexible conformation is responsible for the polymer type of γA globulin antibodies showing high agglutinating efficiency.

Further characterization of the tertiary and quaternary structures of γA globulin antibodies by the methods already outlined can be expected to explain such properties. It should also throw further light on other types of γA globulin, such as a horse anti-p-azophenyl-β-lactoside antibody [382] which has been found to be non-precipitating, despite the possession of two binding sites per antibody molecule (based on a molecular weight of 150,000) and a marked avidity for the specific hapten. Conformational studies will also be needed to explain observations [382, 383] that the γA globulin antibody molecule is incapable of fixing complement. The role of carbohydrate in the conformation of human γA globulin and its multiple molecular forms may be of significance, in view of the enhanced overall carbohydrate content of this immunoglobulin (about five times that of human γG globulin) and particularly its elevated sialic-acid content (see Table 7.6).

2. Conformational changes associated with aggregation of γG globulin molecules

The techniques employed in the elucidation of the conformation of immuno-globulin molecules and their sub-units also find application in the determination of the structural changes accompanying *aggregation*. Such changes have been shown to have an important influence on the biological properties of the γG globulin molecule, both in its role as an immunogen and as an antibody. As will be indicated, measurement of optical rotation has proved particularly valuable in the quantitation of such changes.

(a) Non-specific aggregation of γG globulins

As indicated in section B3, the non-specific aggregation of the γG globulin of human and certain other animal species (e.g. rabbit) leads to the induction of skin-reactive and complement-fixing properties, besides making it precipitable by rheumatoid factor. Consequently, the presence of such material renders therapeutic γG globulin preparations unsafe for intravenous injection in humans. Determinations of the optical rotatory dispersion constant (λ_c) provides a useful guide to the presence of such denatured material. Native human γG globulin (prepared by batch DEAE-cellulose chromatography, for instance) shows values within the range 200–205 mμ [385]. Essentially similar values (200–207 mμ) were shown by preparations of rabbit and chicken γG globulins, isolated by the same procedure [385]. Other preparative procedures, involving salt or ethanol precipitation, appear to favour the formation of high molecular weight aggregates (20–40S), whilst the subjection of γG globulin to aqueous solutions of low ionic strength leads to the formation of the 10S dimeric form (referred to earlier).

Indeed, *in vitro* precipitation of rheumatoid factor was first achieved by the use of a Cohn fraction II preparation of human γG globulin (presumably owing to its contamination with aggregate [386]), In later studies [387], soluble aggregates suitable for rheumatoid factor precipitation tests were prepared by heating preparations of γG globulin at 63° C for an arbitrary length of time (usually 20–30 minutes). This, and other treatments (such as acid, alkali, urea, ultrasonic and repeated freezing and thawing) were employed by Milgrom & Witebsky [388] and McCluskey *et al* (389) to denature γG globulins, thereby rendering them auto-immunogenic. No attempt was made, however, to ascertain the nature and extent of the conformational

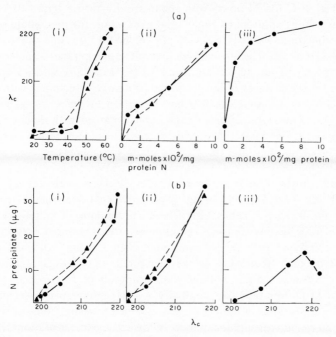

Fig. 7.44

(a) Effect of various forms of denaturation on the rotatory dispersion constant (λc) of two preparations (DEAE-cellulose chromatographic fractions) of human γG globulin. (i) Effect of incubation at various temperatures; (ii) treatment with various concentrations of NaOH; (iii) treatment with various concentrations of sodium dodecyl sulphate (SDS).

(b) Relationship between precipitability with rheumatoid factor and optical rotatory dispersion constant (λc) of human λG globulin preparations denatured by (i) heat treatment; (ii) NaOH treatment; (iii) SDS treatment, as shown in (a) above.

(Reproduced from C.S.Henney and D.R.Stanworth, *Immunology* (1965) **9**, 139.)

changes induced by such treatments, a matter of prime importance if it is assumed possible that similar changes occurring to the human γG globulin *in vivo* are responsible for evoking the immune response observed in certain human disease states (e.g. rheumatoid arthritis).

Determination of the optical rotatory dispersion constant (λ_c) as undertaken by Henney & Stanworth [123] affords a means of *quantitating* the extent of tertiary structural changes induced by various denaturation procedures. This is illustrated in the curves in Fig. 7.44a, which illustrate the effect on γG globulin (1 per cent w/v) solutions of (a) heating at varying temperatures for 20 minutes, or treating with various concentrations of (b) NaOH or (c) sodium dodecylsulphate. The denatured protein solution (0·5 ml) was allowed to interact at 4° C for 24 hours with rheumatoid arthritic serum (0·3 ml) in a reaction volume adjusted to 5 ml with 0·15 M saline, the precipitate recovered by centrifugation, washed (×2) with pre-cooled 0·15 M saline and dissolved in 0·1 N NaOH (1 ml). The nitrogen content of the precipitate was determined by analysing an aliquot by a modification of the Folin procedure [76]. Results indicated that the ability of the denatured proteins to precipitate with rheumatoid factor was in approximately linear relation to the λ_c values (shown in Fig. 7.44b). The atypical form of the curve obtained with detergent-treated γG globulin at the highest detergent/protein ratios could be attributed to the formation of micelles, and the absence of 20–40S aggregates.

An alternative method of measuring the extent of denaturation is afforded by the estimation of the increase in free sulphydryl groups (by the colori-metric method of Jocelyn [122], using bis-(5-carboxy-4-nitrophenyl)disulphide). This is illustrated in Table 7.21, where the amount of sulphydryl groups liberated after heating *human* γG globulin at various temperatures for 10 minutes is compared with the λ_c value (and with various biological activities induced by such treatment). In the denatured state, corresponding to a λ_c value of 220 mμ, the γG globulin (containing about 15 per cent of 20–40S aggregates) showed 0·50 free sulphydryl ($-$SH) groups per molecule of protein. The appearance of these groups is assumed to result from the rupture of labile inter-chain disulphide bonds following the denaturation treatment. Substantial evidence has been obtained to suggest that such bonds are located in the Fc portion of the γG globulin molecule. It is assumed that some of the sulphydryl groups liberated become involved in intermolecular disulphide bridging, resulting in the formation of the 20–40S aggregates. This could occur by a process similar to that considered by Deutsch [374] to account for the aggregation of γA globulin sub-units (mentioned earlier). It is possible, too, that the 20S aggregates of human γG globulin constitute a thermodynamically stable conformation resembling that of γM globulin, which is thought to comprise a pentameric arrangement of 7S sub-units.

Human γG globulin, aggregated by heat-treatment or by coupling with bis-diazotized benzidine (BDB), evokes a typical weal and erythema reaction (reaching a maximum after 10 minutes) within 5 minutes of intradermal injection into normal humans [391, 396]. A definite reaction was observed at a level of aggregate corresponding to 0·25 μg of nitrogen, whereas a dose of untreated human γG globulin as high as 32 μg of nitrogen failed to evoke a positive reaction. In the heat treatment, a 2 per cent solution of human γG globulin (pooled Cohn fraction II, Lederle) was heated for 20 minutes at 63° C. The aggregated γG globulin was separated by precipitation with 0·36 M sodium sulphate solution, dissolved in borate-buffered saline (pH 8·0) and dialysed against the same buffer. The method of preparing BDB-aggregated γG globulin was as follows: benzidine hydrochloride (100 mg) was dissolved in 0·25 N HCl (10 ml) and cooled to 0° C in an ice-water bath. Pre-cooled 0·5 M sodium nitrite solution (2 ml) was slowly added with stirring. Aliquots (0·1 ml) of the resultant BDB solution were added to ice-cold 1 per cent solutions (10 ml) of the γG globulin, and the pH adjusted to 8·5. After 15–60 minutes at 0° C (with occasional mixing, when the solutions became slightly opalescent), the reaction (between the γG globulin and BDB) was stopped by the addition of tyrosine (2 mg). The mixtures were then dialysed against saline for 2 days and centrifuged at 3000 rev/min for 30 minutes, to remove insoluble precipitates. The supernatant (containing the benzidine-azo-γ-globulin) was centrifuged at 70,000 g for 5 hours (in a Spinco Model L preparative ultracentrifuge) in order to separate the aggregated γG globulin, which was recovered from a gelatinous pellet (together with 0·5 ml of contaminating solution), by dissolving in borate-buffered saline.

Further investigations are required to define the conformational changes induced by aggregation of γG globulin molecules by these procedures. The observation that the activity of aggregated γG globulin was dependent upon the animal species from which the γG globulin was derived suggests that such changes are influenced by the *primary* structure of the molecule. For instance [391], neither aggregated bovine nor aggregated chicken γG globulin showed skin reactivity (in guinea-pigs), whilst the activity shown by aggregated horse γG globulin was less than that induced by aggregated human and rabbit γG globulins. The influence of primary structure is also suggested by the recent findings of Morse [392], who (by means of semi-quantitative testing for precipitin formation and complement fixation) found that eleven out of a total of eighteen human γG globulin myeloma proteins were not aggregated by heating at various concentrations (0·15 to 10 mg/ml) in barbitone buffer (pH 8·6, I = 0·05) at 63° C for 10–15 minutes; nor was aggregation effected by treatment with 2-mercaptoethanol (1 : 100 v/v) in 6 M urea in 0·1 M tris-HCl buffer, pH 8·1 followed, after reduction for 1 hour at room temperature, by dialysis overnight at 4° C against tris buffer (1 litre)±0·2 M iodoacetamide. The relative inactivity of heat-treated γG globulins of certain other vertebrate species, such as chicken and horse, cannot be attributed to a similar inability to aggregate, however, as these proteins showed λ_c values after heat denaturation treatment comparable to those of human γG globulin in the fully denatured form [385].

Denaturation treatment of human γG globulin by 2-mercaptoethanol in urea (as applied by Edelman *et al* [387]) effects more extensive structural changes than are induced by the denaturation treatments (heat, alkali, etc.) already outlined. This is indicated by sulphydryl estimation, and is also reflected in the apparent destruction of the conformation responsible for the skin reactivity induced by the milder forms of treatment. The biological activities of human γG globulin preparations aggregated by heat or by 2-mercaptoethanol in urea, are compared in Table 7.24 (taken from Henney [385]). The denaturation treatments employed were as follows: solutions of human γG globulin (1 g per cent) in 0·1 M phosphate buffer, pH 7·5, containing 0·15 M NaCl were made 0·1 M with respect to 2-mercaptoethanol and 6 M with respect to urea. After reacting at room temperature (18° C) for 1 hour, the reaction mixture was dialysed extensively against 0·1 M phosphate buffer (pH 7·5, containing 0·15 M NaCl). Ultracentrifugal analysis of the product revealed a similar composition to that shown by the heat-denatured (63° C for 10 minutes) human γG globulin, i.e. about 20 per cent of aggregated

TABLE 7.24

Some biological properties of 2-mercaptoethanol-urea denatured and heat denatured human γG globulin (Reproduced by courtesy of Dr C.S.Henney from [385])

Activity	Mercaptoethanol-urea denatured γG globulin	Heat denatured γG globulin
μg/N pptd. on addition of 5 mg protein to 0·5 ml RA serum	32	43
Per cent human complement fixed by 100 μg protein	88	97
Minimum skin reactive dose (μg N)	>100	5

material was observed, comprising approximately equal amounts of 10S component and polydisperse component of mean sedimentation coefficient of the order of 25S. Optical rotatory dispersion measurements indicated λ_c values of the order of 220 mμ for the 2-mercaptoethanol–urea denatured material, whilst its content of free sulphydryl groups (1·1 moles sulphydryl per mole γG globulin) was appreciably higher than that evoked by heat denaturation (namely, 0·5 mole sulphydryl per mole γG globulin). As is shown by the data in Table 7.24, the 2-mercaptoethanol–urea aggregates paralleled the heat aggregates in their capacity to precipitate rheumatoid factor and to fix human complement *in vitro*. On the other hand, only the latter aggregates possessed the ability to elicit increased vascular permeability in guinea-pig skin (suggesting that this activity demands a greater degree of structural rigidity within the Fc region, probably maintained by disulphide bridges in the heat aggregates, as the findings of Ishizaka [294] also indicate).

The interesting observation of Milgrom & Witebsky [388] (since confirmed by other investigators [385, 389]) that rabbit antiserum raised against denatured autologous γG globulin reacted more readily with native *human* γG globulin suggests that new immunogenic determinants are exposed by aggregation processes. Moreover, Biro & Garcia [393] have provided evidence that human γG globulin can be non-immunogenic in heterologous systems, unless administered in *aggregated* form. Rabbits injected intravenously (5 mg protein, weekly) with aggregate-free human γG globulin failed to produce any detectable precipitating or non-precipitating antibody; they became, instead, immunologically unresponsive to human γG globulin. Perhaps structures to which the animal is not tolerant appear as a result of *an unfolding of the polypeptide chains on aggregation*. In this connection, it is possible that the usual procedure for eliciting production of rabbit antibodies against human γG globulin, by subcutaneous injection of the protein mixed with complete Freund's adjuvant, is successful because here too the antigen is being administered in an aggregated state (brought about by *in vitro* mixing with the adjuvant [394]).

Recent observations by Gill & Kunz [395] on the immunogenicity of synthetic polypeptide aggregates are of possible relevance. These investigators showed that the formation of an aggregate between a non-immunogenic synthetic polypeptide (poly D-Glu^{57} D-Lys^{43} or poly D-Glu^{52} D-Lys^{33} D-Tyr^{15}) and methylated bovine serum albumin rendered the former immunogenic in heterogeneously-bred New Zealand white rabbits. Thus it was concluded that aggregate formation enhances the amount of antibody formed by a 'poor' immunogen, but not the amount elicited by a 'good' immunogen.

Efforts to raise antiserum (in rabbits and monkeys) against *new* antigenic determinants exposed as a result of the aggregation of human γG globulin have so far proved unsuccessful [394].* Hence, it is a matter for speculation whether active sites appear within the Fc regions of aggregated γG globulin molecules as a result of the juxtaposition of heavy chains from adjacent molecules. This could account for the induction of activity (e.g. complement fixation, skin reactivity) following aggregation of heavy chains (within Fc fragments) by coupling through bis-diazotized benzidine (or by heat or other treatment). It has been suggested that such structural alterations lead to 'toxic configurations' [294]. Furthermore (as will be indicated in the next section), similar configurational changes within the Fc region are induced in antibody γG globulin molecules, *following combination with specific antigen*.

(b) Specific aggregation of γG globulin
The electron-microscopic findings of Feinstein & Rowe [349] suggested that combination of γG globulin with specific antigen results in a conformational

---

* Henney (personal communication) had recently succeeded, however, in raising antibodies in guinea-pigs directed against such determinants.

change within the antibody molecule. Measurement of the changes in optical rotation occurring in the antibody γG globulin molecule as a result of the formation of *soluble* complexes with antigen [350] provides convincing evidence in support of such structural alteration. Furthermore, Robert & Grabar [397] have reported a slow but significant liberation of sulphydryl groups (less than one group per molecule) following antigen–antibody precipitation. As in the case of the structural alterations encountered in the formation of non-specific aggregates, it seems likely [294] that configurational changes result mainly from interaction between the Fc fragments of the antibody molecules (brought into apposition as a result of combination with specific antigen). Moreover, the 'antigen-linked aggregates' show biological properties similar to those induced in certain γG globulins as a result of non-specific aggregation (namely complement fixation, skin reactivity, rheumatoid-factor reactivity).

In employing measurement of optical rotation as an index of the degree of alteration induced in the antibody molecule, it is necessary to determine the specific rotations of equivalent mixtures of the antigen and *normal* γG globulin. Thus, the specific optical rotation ($[\alpha]_D$) of soluble bovine serum albumin (BSA)–anti-(BSA) complex preparations (in borate-buffered saline, pH 8·4, I $= 0\cdot15$) was determined at 589 mμ, and compared with a control mixture of BSA and normal γG globulin [398]. The specific rotation of the complex preparation was significantly different from that of the BSA-normal γG globulin mixture (when tested at the same BSA/γG globulin ratio).

The technique employed by Ishizaka & Campbell [398] in the analysis of the complexes is as follows: γG globulin fractions isolated from rabbit anti-BSA sera (by repeated precipitation at pH 7·8 with ammonium sulphate at 33 per cent saturation) were mixed with amounts of antigen (BSA) corresponding to the equivalence point and maintained at 4° C for 48 hours, when the precipitates, recovered by centrifugation and washed ($\times$3) with cold saline, were suspended in a saline solution containing an excess of antigen (approximately twice the weight of antibody present). The suspension was gently mixed at 4° C for 72 hours, and centrifuged to remove traces of residue. The soluble complexes were freed from most of the excess antigen by precipitation with 50 per cent saturated ammonium sulphate (at pH 7·8), and the precipitates redissolved in, and dialysed against, 5 per cent borate buffer (pH 8·4), containing 0·9 per cent NaCl. The final preparation (designated 'VI' in Table 7.25, showing the results) contained 20·3 mg protein/ml. Complexes of variable composition (designated 'VI$_0$', 'VI$_1$', 'VI$_2$', 'VI$_3$' and 'VI$_4$') were prepared from this material by the addition of an equal volume of saline (VI$_0$) or saline containing 6·8, 23·7, 50·8 and 99·3 mg BSA/ml respectively. Equilibration was achieved by storage at 4° C for periods of 14–20 days. The total ratios of antigen/antibody were determined by free-boundary electrophoresis (in a Perkin-Elmer Model 38 electrophoresis apparatus) at pH 2·35.

Dialysis against glycine–HCl buffer (pH 2·35, I = 0·1) for 24 hours prior to electrophoresis ensured dissociation of the complexes. Electrophoretic analysis of the complexes in barbitone–NaCl buffer (pH 8·5, I = 0·3) permitted the determination of the relative concentrations of free antigen and of soluble complexes. Measurements of optical rotation were made at 589 mμ on samples of complexes, and on mixtures of solutions of BSA with normal human γG globulin as controls, after dialysis against borate-buffered saline (pH 8·4, I = 0·15) for 24 hours.

TABLE 7.25

Specific rotation of soluble BSA–anti-BSA complex preparations. (Reproduced by courtesy of Drs K.Ishizaka and D.H.Campbell from *J.Immunol* (1959) **83,** 318)

Preparation	pH	Total Ag/ total Ab (weight)	$-[\alpha]_{D(obs)}$	$-[\alpha]_{D(calc)}$
BSA	8·4	100 : 0	59·5 ± 0·5	
Normal γ globulin		0 : 100†	42·9 ± 0·4	
Complex VI_0		36·9 : 63·1	60·0 ± 1·0	49·0
Complex VI_1		52·7 : 47·3	59·7 ± 0·08	51·7
Complex VI_2		70·9 : 29·1	58·7 ± 0·8	54·7
Complex VI_3		82·0 : 18·0	57·9 ± 0·7	56·5
Complex VI_4		89·3 : 10·7	57·8 ± 0·7	57·4
BSA + normal γ globulin		36·9 : 63·1†	48·9 ± 0·3	49·0
BSA	2·35	100 : 0	72·7 ± 0·5	
Normal γ globulin		0 : 100†	63·7 ± 0·5	
Complex VI_0		36·9 : 63·1	66·2 ± 0·7	66·4

† Weight ratio of BSA/normal γ globulin
(from [398])

The results obtained from such an analysis (reproduced from Ishizaka & Campbell [398]) are shown in Table 7.25. Values are included for the specific rotations of the complex preparations, calculated from the total BSA/γG globulin ratio and the specific rotations of BSA and of normal γG globulin (on the assumption that normal γG globulin and anti-BSA antibody globulin have the same optical activity, and that soluble antigen–antibody complexes exhibit an optical activity equal to the *sum* of the individual contributions of the antigen and antibody concerned). As will be noted, the observed and calculated values for the specific rotation of the mixture of BSA with normal γG globulin were identical. On the other hand, the observed values for the specific rotations of the soluble complex preparations (at pH 8·4) were more negative (laevorotatory) than the corresponding calculated values. Moreover, it was found that there was a negligible difference between the experimental and calculated values for $[\alpha]_D$ of the antigen–antibody complex VI_0 at pH 2·35 (under which conditions, the complex was shown to be completely dissociated) thus providing additional evidence that the observed increase in laevorotation is a result of antigen–antibody combination.

TABLE 7.26

Specific optical rotation changes induced in rabbit antibody γG globulin by combination with specific antigen (Reproduced from C.S.Henney and D.R.Stanworth *Nature, Lond.* (1966) **210**, 1071 [350])

Antigen	Antigen/ antibody weight ratio	Specific optical rotation at 589·5 mμ		
		Immune complexes	Antigen-non-antibody γG globulin mixture	Difference
BSA	1·9	−64·6	−58·8	+5·8
	2·4	−61·0	−59·3	+1·7
	3·2	−60·4	−59·8	+0·6
	4·5	−60·6	−60·3	+0·3
	9·1	−61·0	−61·1	−0·1
Ferritin	2·7	−40·2	−31·9	+8·3
	4·1	−35·2	−30·9	+4·3
	5·4	−33·8	−30·3	+3·5
	6·8	−30·2	−29·9	+0·3
	13·6	−28·3	−29·0	−0·7
	19·0	−28·6	−28·7	−0·1

Heat denaturation of human γG globulin (50° C for 10 minutes) produced a rise in specific optical rotation at 589·5 mμ of 9·8°

The complexes formed in antigen excess (e.g. Ag_3Ab_2) which show this effect are those which demonstrate the biological activities referred to earlier (i.e. reactivity with guinea-pig skin, complement fixation). In contrast, no evidence of a change in laevorotation was observed to accompany the formation of the biologically inactive Ag_2Ab complex. An increase of laevorotation was observed, however, on formation of skin-reactive soluble complexes comprising polyvalent synthetic precipitating dyestuff-hapten (resorcinol-R'_3) and its homologous rabbit antibody, whereas no change in specific rotation accompanied the formation of a simple hapten (sodium arsanilate)–antihapten complex.

In interpreting such findings as indicative of specific alteration of the conformation of the antibody molecules, it is important to exclude the possibility that the observed increase in laevorotation is due to antigen denaturation. The observations of Henney & Stanworth [350, 415] are probably significant in this connection. These investigators have shown that *new immunogenic determinant groups* are exposed following combination between rabbit antibody and specific antigen in the formation of soluble complexes (of the Ag_3Ab_2 type). These were demonstrated by immunizing rabbits *of the same allotype* as the animals donating the antibody for the preparation of antigen–antibody complex. This procedure overcame the objection to similar findings by Najjar *et al* [399, 400], on the grounds that these represented isologous antibody formation. Moreover, the formation of the soluble complexes demonstrating such an effect resulted in significant increases in laevorotation (as shown in Table 7.26). These results include complexes of BSA/anti-BSA formed over a range of antigen/antibody ratios varying from 1 to 2·5; and complexes of horse ferritin –anti (horse ferritin) comprising a range of antigen/antibody ratios varying from 1 to 20.

It is interesting to note that the combination of rabbit antibody with the horse ferritin antigen leads to structural alterations within the antibody molecule of appreciably greater magnitude than those evoked by combination of specific antibody with the smaller BSA antigen. Moreover, whereas the anti-(BSA/anti-BSA) complex serum reacted with only two of thirty various native rabbit γG globulin preparations (both of which contained high molecular weight aggregates and 10S material), the anti- (ferritin/anti-ferritin) complex antiserum reacted not only with native rabbit γG globulins but it also reacted readily with *native human γG globulins*. It is possibly of some significance in connection with this observation, which parallels the findings of Milgrom & Witebsky [388] using antiserum directed against non-specifically altered autologous rabbit γG globulin (mentioned earlier), that the extent of alteration (indicated by an increase in laevorotation at 589·5 mμ at pH 8·3) induced in the anti-ferritin antibody as a result of combination with ferritin at the lowest antigen/antibody ratio used (i.e. 2·7) was of a similar order of magnitude to that produced by heat-denaturation (50° C for 10 minutes) of human γG globulin (which was accompanied by an increase in laevorotation of 9·8°). Preliminary evidence has been obtained, however, to suggest that the former (specific) alteration process leads to an unfolding in both the Fd and Fc regions of the heavy chain, and is not confined to the Fc portion of the molecule, as appears to result from non-specific aggregation. This could possibly be interpreted as indirect evidence that the Fd portion of the γG globulin antibody molecule is involved in antigen combination, its conformation being modified when combination occurs with the large ferritin antigen molecule (which comprises numerous identical sub-units).

L

This illustrates how measurements of optical rotation are beginning to provide valuable information about γG globulin aggregation processes, which are of considerable significance in immune reactions. It also emphasizes the importance of considering the molecule as a whole, since interactions occurring in one region (e.g. the Fab segment) can obviously have profound effects on the conformation of another region (e.g. the Fc segment). In other words, just as in enzymes, it is considered likely that allosteric transitions lead to changes in the biological activities of antibody molecules.

References

[1] COHEN S. & PORTER R.R. (1964) Structure and biological activity of immunoglobulins. *Adv. Immunol.* **4**, 287

[2] FUDENBERG H.H. (1965) The immune globulins. *Ann. Rev. Microbiol.* **19**, 301

[3] FRANKLIN E.C. (1964) The immune globulins—their structure and function, and some techniques for their isolation. *Progr. All.* **8**, 58

[4] NISONOFF A. & THORBECKE F.J. (1964) Immunochemistry. *Ann. Rev. Biochem.* **33**, 355

[5] ISLIKER H., JACOT-GUILLARMOD H. & JATON J.C. (1965) The structure and biological activity of immunoglobulins and their sub-units. *Physiol. Ergib.* **56**, 67

[6] FAHEY J.L. (1962) Heterogeneity of γ-globulins. *Adv. Immunol.* **2**, 41

[7] PORTER R.R. (1962) The structure of gamma globulins and antibodies. In *Basic Problems of Neoplastic Disease*, p. 177, ed. GELLHORN A. & HIRSCHBERG E. New York: Columbia Univ. Press

[8] MILLER F. & METZGER H. (1965) Characterization of human macroglobulins. I. The molecular weight of its subunit. *J. biol. Chem.* **240**, 3325

[9] MILLER F. & METZGER H. (1965) Characterization of human macroglobulins. II. Distribution of disulphide bonds. *J. biol. Chem.* **240**, 4740

[10] HEREMANS J.F. (1960) *Les globulins sériques du systéme gamma.* Brussels: Arscia S.A.

[11] CEPPELLINI R. *et al* (1964) Nomenclature of human immunoglobulins. *Bull. World Health Organ.* **30**, 447

[12] ROWE D.S. & FAHEY J.L. (1965) A new class of human immunoglobulins. I. A unique myeloma protein. *J. exp. Med.* **121**, 121

[13] KORNGOLD L. & LIPARI R. (1956) Multiple-myeloma proteins. I. Immunological studies. *Cancer* **9**, 183

[14] MANNIK M. & KUNKEL H.G. (1963) Two major types of normal 7S γ-globulin. *J. exp. Med.* **117**, 213

[15] BERNIER G.M. & PUTNAM F.W. (1963) Monomer-dimer forms of Bence-Jones proteins. *Nature, Lond.* **200**, 223

[16] HARBOE M. & DEVERILL J. (1964) Immunochemical properties of cold haemagglutins. *Scand. J. Hemat.* **1**, 223

[17] FRANKLIN E.C. & FUDENBERG H.H. (1964) Antigen heterogeneity of human Rh antibodies, rheumatoid factors and cold agglutinins. *Arch. biochem. Biophys.* **104**, 433

[18] FAHEY J.L. & GOODMAN H. (1964) Antibody activity in six classes of human immunoglobulin. *Science* **143**, 588

[19] TERRY W.D. & FAHEY J.L. (1964) Subclasses of human γ₂-globulin based on differences in the heavy polypeptide chains. *Science* **146**, 400

[20] GREY H.M. & KUNKEL H.G. (1964) H chain subgroups of myeloma proteins and normal 7S γ-globulin. *J. exp. Med.* **120**, 253

[21] LICHTER E.A. (1964) Thyroglobulin antibody activity in the γ-globulins, γA, γB, and γC of human serum. *Proc. Soc. exp. Biol. Med.* **113**, 555

[22] TAKATSUKI K. & OSSERMAN E.F. (1964) Structural differences between two types of 'heavy chain' proteins and myeloma globulins of corresponding types. *Science* **145**, 498

[23] FRANKLIN E.C., FUDENBERG H.H., MELTZER M. & STANWORTH D.R. (1962) The structural basis for genetic variations of normal human γ-globulins. *Proc. nat. Acad. Science. (Wash.)* **48**, 914

[24] LAWLER S.D. & COHEN S. (1965) Distribution of allotypic specificities on the peptide chains of human gamma-globulin. *Immunology* **8**, 206

[25] MELTZER M., FRANKLIN E.C., FUDENBERG H.H. & FRANGIONE B. (1964) Single peptide differences between γ-globulins of different genetic (Gm) types. *Proc. nat. Acad. Sci. (Wash.)* **51**, 1007

[26] FAHEY J.L. (1961) Immunochemical studies of twenty mouse myeloma proteins. Evidence for two groups of proteins similar to gamma and beta-2A globulins in man. *J. exp. Med.* **114**, 385

[27] FAHEY J.L. (1961) Physico-chemical characterization of mouse myeloma proteins. Demonstration of heterogeneity for each myeloma globulin. *J. exp. Med.* **114**, 399

[28] FAHEY J.L., WUNDERLICH J. & MISHELL R. (1964) The immunoglobulins of mice. I. Four major classes of immunoglobulins. 7S γ_2—,7S γ_1—,γ_1A (β_2A) and 18S γ_1M. *J. exp. Med.* **120**, 223

[29] WUNDERLICH J., MISHELL R. & FAHEY J.L. (1964) The immunoglobulins of mice. II. Two sub-classes of mouse 7S γ_2-globulins: γ_{2a} and γ_{2b}-globulins. *J. exp. Med.* **120**, 243

[30] KABAT E.A. & MAYER M.M. (1962) *Experimental Immunochemistry*, 2nd edition. Springfield, Illinois: Thomas

[31] HILL W.C. & CEBRA J.J. (1964) Horse anti-SI immunoglobulins. I. Properties of γM-antibody. *Biochemistry* **4**, 2575

[32] ONOUE K., YAGI Y. & PRESSMAN D. (1966) Isolation of rabbit IgA antihapten antibody and demonstration of skin-sensitizing activity in homologous skin. *J. exp. Med.* **123**, 173

[33] YAGI Y., MAIER P., PRESSMAN D., ARBESMAN C.E. & REISMAN R.E. (1963) The presence of the ragweed-binding antibodies in the β2A-, β2M- and γ-globulins of the sensitive individuals. *J. Immunol.* **91**, 83

[34] FEINSTEIN A., GELL P.G.H. & KELUS A.S. (1963) Immunochemical analysis of rabbit gamma-globulin allotypes. *Nature, Lond.* **200**, 653

[35] BRAMBELL F.W.R. (1966) The transmission of immunity from mother to young and the catabolism of immunoglobulins. *Lancet* **ii**, 7473

[36] TADA T. & ISHIZAKA K. (1965) Arthus type inflammation with γM antibody. *J. Immunol.* **96**, 112

[37] THORBECKE G.J., BENACERRAF B. & OVARY Z. (1963) Antigenic relationship between two types of 7S guinea-pig γ-globulin. *J. Immunol.* **91**, 670

[38] WHITE R.G., JENKINS G.C. & WILKINSON P.C. (1963) The production of skin-sensitizing antibody in the guinea-pig. *Int. Arch. All.* **22**, 156

[39] SCHUURS A.H.W.M., VAN ES.L. & PONDMAN K.W. (1965) Separation of skin-sensitizing and complement-fixing antibodies from guinea-pig anti-bovine insulin sera. *Immunochemistry* **2**, 67

[40] BENACERRAF B., OVARY Z., BLOCH K.J. & FRANKLIN E.C. (1963) Properties of guinea-pig 7S antibodies. I. Electrophoretic separation of two types of guinea-pig 7S antibodies. *J. exp. Med.* **117**, 937

[41] NUSSENZWEIG V. & BENACERRAF B. (1964) Studies on the properties of fragments of guinea-pig γ_1 and γ_2 antibodies obtained by papain digestion and mild reduction. *J. Immunol.* **93**, 1008

[42] BAKER A.R., BLOCH K.J. & AUSTEN K.F. (1964) *In vitro* passive sensitization of chopped guinea-pig lung by guinea-pig 7S antibodies. *J. Immunol.* **93**, 525

[43] BERKEN A. & BENACERRAF B. (1966) Properties of antibodies cytophilic for macrophages. *J. exp. Med.* **123**, 119

[44] OVARY Z., BLOCH K.J. & BENACERRAF B. (1964) Identification of rabbit, monkey and dog antibodies with P C A activity for guinea-pigs. *Proc. Soc. exp. Biol. Med.* **116**, 840

[45] OVARY Z. (1960) Reverse passive cutaneous anaphylaxis in the guinea-pig with horse, sheep or hen antibodies. *Immunology* **3**, 19

[46] BINAGHI R.A., BENACERRAF B., BLOCH K.J. and KOURILSKY F.M. (1964) Properties of rat anaphylactic antibody. *J. Immunol.* **92**, 927

[47] MOTA I. (1964) The mechanism of anaphylaxis. I. Production and biological properties of 'mast cell sensitizing' antibody. *Immunology* **7**, 681

[48] NUSSENZWEIG V. & BINAGHI R.A. (1965) Heterogeneity of rat immunoglobulins. *Int. Arch. All.* **27**, 355

[49] PATTERSON R. & SPARK D.B. (1962) The passive transfer to normal dogs of skin-reactivity, asthma and anaphylaxis from a dog with spontaneous ragweed pollen sensitivity. *J. Immunol.* **88**, 262

[50] PATTERSON R., PRUZANSKY J.J. & JANIS B. (1964) Biologic activity of canine non-precipitating and precipitating antibody. *J. Immunol.* **93**, 51

[51] FIREMAN P., VANNIER W.E. & GOODMAN H.C. (1963) The association of skin-sensitizing antibody with the β_2A-globulins in sera from ragweed-sensitive patients. *J. exp. Med.* **117**, 603

[52] VAERMAN J.P., EPSTEIN W., FUDENBERG H.H. & ISHIZAKA K. (1964) Direct demonstration of reagin activity in purified γ_1A-globulin. *Nature, Lond.* **203**, 1046

[53] ISHIZAKA K., ISHIZAKA T. & HATHORN E.M. (1964) Blocking of Prausnitz-Küstner sensitization with reagin by 'A-chain' of human γ_1A globulin. *Immunochemistry* **1**, 197

[54] STANWORTH D.R. (1965) The structure of reagins. *Int. Arch. All.* **28**, 71

[55] ISHIZAKA K., ISHIZAKA T. & HORNBROOK M.M. (1966) Physico-chemical properties of human reaginic antibody. IV. The presence of a unique immunoglobulin as a carrier of reaginic activity. *J. Immunol.* **97**, 75

[56] ZWAIFLER N.J. & BECKER E.L. (1965) Rabbit passive cutaneous anaphylaxis. *Fed. Proc.* **24** (Abstr. 677), 250

[57] SELA M. & MOZES E. (1966) Dependence of the chemical nature of antibodies on the net electrical charge of antigens. *Proc. Nat. Acad. Sci. (Wash.)* **55**, 445

[58] GERGELY J., STANWORTH D.R., JEFFERIS R., NORMANSELL D.E., HENNEY C.S. & PARDOE G.I. (1966) Structural studies of immunoglobulins. I. The role of cysteine in papain hydrolysis. *Immunochemistry* **4**, 101.

[59] ONOUE K., YAGI Y. & PRESSMAN D. (1964) Multiplicity of antibody proteins in rabbit anti-p-azobenzene arsonate sera. *J. Immunol.* **92**, 173

[60] ROCKEY J.H., KLINMAN N.R. & KARUSH F. (1964) Equine antibody. I. 7S β_{2A} and 10S γ_1 globulin components of purified anti-β-lactoside antibody. *J. exp. Med.* **120**, 589

[61] SCHULTZE H.E., HAUPT H., HEIDE K., HEIMBURGER N. & SCHWICK H.G. (1965) Comparative investigations of purified diphtheria and tetanus-T components and their fragments. *Immunochemistry* **2**, 273

[62] ALLEN P.Z., SRISINHA S. & VAUGHAN J.H. (1965) Immunochemical studies on equine antibodies to human γ_2-globulin. *J. Immunol.* **95**, 918

[63] BURTIN P. (1960) *L'analyse immunoelectrophoretique; ses applications aux milieux biologiques humains*, Ed. GRABAR P. & BURTIN P. Paris: Masson

[64] WALTON K.W., ROWE D.S., SOOTHILL J.F. & STANWORTH D.R. (1963) An investigation of methods of isolation of β_2M globulin (Syn: Iota protein, 19S γ globulin, γ_1-macroglobulin, β_2M globulin) and its association with iso-agglutinin activity, together with preliminary observations on other macroglobulins of slow electrophoretic mobility in normal human serum. *Immunol.* **6**, 305

[65] HENNEY C.S. & STANWORTH D.R. (1965) The reactivity of rheumatoid factor with serum 7S γ-globulins of various species. *Protides of Biol. Fluids (XIth Coll.)* **11**, 155, ed. PEETERS. H. Amsterdam: Elsevier

[66] BUTLER V.H. & VAUGHAN J.H. (1964) Hemagglutination by rheumatoid factor of cells coated with animal gamma globulins. *Proc. Soc. exp. Biol. Med.* **116**, 585

[67] ROBBINS J.B., RIMON A., MOZES E. & SELA M. (1967) Correlation between net charge of antigens and electrophoretic mobility of immunoglobulin M antibodies. *Nature, Lond.* **213**, 1013.

[68] PORTER R.R. (1959) The hydrolysis of rabbit γ-globulin and antibodies with crystalline papain. *Biochem. J.* **73**, 119

[69] PORTER R.R. & PRESS E.M. (1962) Immunochemistry. *Ann. Rev. Biochem.* **31**, 625

[70] EDELMAN G.M., HEREMANS J.F., HEREMANS M. TH. & KUNKEL H.G. (1960) Immunological studies of human γ-globulin. Relation of the precipitin lines of whole γ-globulin to those of the fragments produced by papain. *J. exp. Med.* **112**, 203

[71] HSIAO S. & PUTNAM F.W. (1961) The cleavage of human γ-globulin by papain. *J. biol. Chem.* **236**, 122

[72] FRANKLIN E.C. (1960) Structural units of human 7S gamma globulins. *J. clin. Invest.* **39**, 1933

[73] FRANKLIN E.C. & STANWORTH D.R. (1961) Antigenic relationships between immune globulins and certain paraproteins in man. *J. exp. Med.* **114**, 521

[74] FOUGEREAU M. & EDELMAN G.M. (1965) Corroboration of recent models of the γG immunoglobulin molecule. *J. exp. Med.* **121**, 373

[75] MÜLLER-EBERHARD H.J. (1960) A new supporting medium for preparative electrophoresis. *Scand. J. Clin. Lab. Invest.* **12**, 33

[76] LOWRY O.H., ROSEBROUGH N.J., FARR A.L. & RANDALL R.J. (1951) Protein measurement with the Folin phenol reagent. *J. biol. Chem.* **193**, 265

[77] JACKSON A. & KEOGH R.W. (1966) Personal communication

[78] NISONOFF A., WISSLER F.C. & WOERNLEY D.L. (1959) Mechanism of formation of univalent fragments of rabbit antibody. *Biochem. Biophys. Res. Comm.* **1**, 318

[79] NISONOFF A., WISSLER F.C. & LIPMAN L.N. (1960) Properties of the major component of a peptic digest of rabbit antibody. *Science* **132**, 1770

[80] NISONOFF A., WISSLER F.C., LIPMAN L.N. & WOERNLEY D.L. (1960) Separation of univalent fragments from the bivalent rabbit antibody molecule by reduction of disulphide bonds. *Arch. biochem. Biophys.* **89**, 230

[81] NISONOFF A., MARKUS G., & WISSLER F.L. (1961) Separation of univalent fragments of rabbit antibody by reduction of a single, labile, disulphide bond. *Nature, Lond.* **189**, 293

[82] CEBRA J.J., GIVOL D., SILMAN H.I. & KATCHALSKI E. (1961) A two-stage cleavage of rabbit γ-globulin by a water-insoluble papain preparation followed by cysteine. *J. biol. Chem.* **236**, 1720

[83] JAQUET H. & CEBRA J.J. (1965) Comparison of two precipitating derivatives of

rabbit antibody. Fragment I dimer and the product of pepsin digestion. *Biochemistry*, **4**, 954

[84] UTSUMI S. & KARUSH F. (1965) Peptic fragmentation of rabbit γG-immunoglobulins. *Biochemistry* **4**, 1766

[85] POULIK M.D. (1966) F'c fragments of immunoglobulins. *Nature, Lond.* **210**, 133

[86] HEIMER R. (1966) The Fd' fragment of human γG immunoglobulin. *Immunochemistry* **3**, 81

[87] UTSUMI S. & KARUSH F. (1966) Personal communication

[88] PUTNAM F.W., EASLEY C.W. & LYNN L.T. (1962) Site of cleavage of γ-globulins by papain. *Biochem. biophys. Acta* **58**, 279

[89] HANSON L.A. & JOHANSSON B.G. (1963) Isolation of immunologically active fragments of normal human γG globulin after tryptic degradation. *Clin. chim. Acta* **8**, 66

[90] HANSON L.A. & JOHANSSON B.G. (1963) Unpublished results quoted in ref. 89, *Clin. chim. Acta* **8**, 66

[91] SKVARIL F. (1960) Changes in outdated human γ-globulin preparations. *Nature, Lond.* **185**, 475

[92] JAMES K., HENNEY C.S. & STANWORTH D.R. (1964) Structural changes in 7S γ-globulins. *Nature, Lond.* **202**, 563

[93] CONNELL G.E. & PAINTER R.H. (1966) Fragmentation of immunoglobulin during storage. *Canad. J. Biochem.* **44**, 371

[94] PAINTER R.H., WALCROFT M.J. & WEBER J.C.W. (1966) The efficacy of fragmented immune serum globulin in passive immunization. *Canad. J. Biochem.* **44**, 381

[95] SCHROHENLOHER R.E. (1963) The degradation of human γ-globulin by trypsin. *Arch. biochem. Biophys.* **101**, 456

[96] SCHROHENLOHER R.E. (1964) Studies of the mechanism of the degradation of human γ-globulin by trypsin. *Arch. biochem. Biophys.* **107**, 163

[97] POULIK M.D. & SHUSTER J. (1964) Heterogeneity of H-chains of myeloma proteins. Susceptibility to papain and trypsin. *Nature, Lond.* **204**, 577

[98] POULIK M.D. & SHUSTER J. (1965) Role of cysteine in the production of Fc and F'c sub-components of γG myeloma globulins. *Nature, Lond.* **207**, 1092

[99] DEUTSCH F.F., STIEHM E.R. & MORTON J.I. (1961) Action of papain on human serum globulins. *J. biol. Chem.* **236**, 2216

[100] GOODMAN J.W. (1965) Heterogeneity of rabbit γG-globulin with respect to cleavage by papain. *Biochemistry* **4**, 2350

[101] EDELMAN G.M. & POULIK M.D. (1961) Studies on structural units of the γ-globulins. *J. exp. Med.* **113**, 861

[102] FLEISCHMAN J.B., PAIN R. & PORTER R.R. (1961) Reduction of γ-globulins. *Arch. biochem. Biophys.* **Suppl. 1**, 174

[103] UTSUMI, S. & KARUSH F. (1964) The subunits of purified rabbit antibody. *Biochemistry* **3**, 1329

[104] MILSTEIN C. (1966) Variations in amino acid sequence near the disulphide bridges of Bence-Jones proteins. *Nature, Lond.* **209**, 370

[105] EDELMAN G.M. & BENACERRAF B. (1962) On structural and functional relations between antibodies and gamma-globulins. *Proc. nat. Acad. Sci. (Wash.)* **48**, 1035

[106] FLEISCHMAN J.B., PORTER R.R. & PRESS E.M. (1963) The arrangement of the peptide chains in γ-globulin. *Biochem. J.* **88**, 220

[107] SMALL P.A., KEHN J.E. & LAMM M.E. (1963) Polypeptide chains of rabbit gamma globulin. *Science* **142**, 393

[108] MARLER E., NELSON C.A. & TANFORD C. (1964) The polypeptide chains of rabbit γ-globulin and its papain-cleaved fragments. *Biochemistry* **3**, 279

[109] COHEN S. (1963) Properties of the peptide chains of normal and pathological human γ-globulins. *Biochem. J.* **89**, 334

[110] SOBER H.A. & PETERSON E.A. (1958) Protein chromatography on ion exchange cellulose. *Fed. Proc.* **17**, 1116

[111] OLINS D.E. & EDELMAN G.M. (1962) The antigenic structure of the polypeptide chains of human γ-globulin. *J. exp. Med.* **116**, 635

[112] LAMM M.E., NUSSENZWEIG V. & BENACERRAF B. (1966) Isolation of purified H and L polypeptide chains from guinea-pig γ₂-immunoglobulin after mild reduction. *Immunology* **10**, 309

[113] KOSHLAND M., ENGLBERGER F.M. & SHAPANKA R. (1966) Location of amino acid differences in the subunits of three rabbit antibodies. *Biochemistry* **5**, 641

[114] COHEN S. (1965) Separation of the κ and λ chains of normal human immunoglobulins. *Biochem. J.* **95**, 13P

[115] PALMER J.L., NISONOFF A. & VAN HOLDE K.E. (1963) Dissociation of rabbit gamma globulin into subunits by reduction and acidification. *Proc. nat. Acad. Sci. (Wash.)* **50**, 314

[116] PALMER J.L. & NISONOFF A. (1964) Dissociation of rabbit γ-globulin into half-molecules after reduction of one labile disulphide bond. *Biochemistry* **3**, 863

[117] NISONOFF A. & DIXON D.J. (1964) Evidence of linkage of univalent fragments of half-molecules of rabbit γ-globulin by the same disulphide bond. *Biochemistry* **3**, 1338

[118] MILSTEIN C. (1965) Interchain disulphide bridge in Bence-Jones proteins and γ-globulin B-chains. *Nature, Lond.* **205**, 1171

[119] BROWN J.R. & HARTLEY B.S. (1963) The disulphide bridges of chymotrypsinogen-A. *Biochem. J.* **89**, 59P

[120] CECIL R. & STEVENSON G.T. (1965) The disulphide bonds of human and rabbit γ-globulins. *Biochem. J.* **97**, 569

[121] HONG R. & NISONOFF A. (1965) Relative labilities of the two types of interchain disulphide bond of rabbit γG immunoglobulins. *J. biol. Chem.* **240**, 3883

[122] JOCELYN P.C. (1962) The effect of glutathione on protein sulphydryl groups in rat liver homogenates. *Biochem. J.* **85**, 480

[123] HENNEY C.S. and STANWORTH D.R. (1965) The reactivity of rheumatoid factor with human gamma G globulin. *Immunology* **9**, 139

[124] KARUSH F., KLINMAN N.R. & MARKS R. (1964) An assay method for disulphide groups by fluorescence quenching. *Anal. Biochem.* **9**, 100

[125] FRANĚK F. & LANKÄS V. (1963) The reactivity of disulphide bonds in pig γ-globulin. *Coll. Czech Chem. Communic.* **28**, 245

[126] GUNEWARDENA P. & COOKE K.B. (1966) 1,4-dithiothreitol as a reagent for the reductive degradation of human γG globulin. *Biochem. J.* **99**, 8P

[127] WITKOP B. (1962) Cleavage of peptide bonds wih cyanogen bromide. *J. biol. Chem.* **237**, 1856

[128] HOFMANN T. (1964) Cyanogen bromide cleavage of trypsinogen. *Biochemistry* **3**, 356

[129] CAHNMANN H.J., ARNON R. & SELA M. (1965) Active fragments obtained by cleavage of rabbit antibody with cyanogen bromide. *J. biol. Chem.* **240**, 2762

[130] GIVOL D. & PORTER R.R. (1965) The C-terminal peptide of the heavy chain of the rabbit immunoglobulin IgG. *Biochem. J.* **97**, 32C

[131] GOLDBERGER R.F. & ANFINSEN C.B. (1962) The reversible masking of amino groups in ribonuclease and its possible usefulness in the synthesis of the protein. *Biochemistry* **1**, 401

[132] MERIGAN T.C., DREYER W.J. & BERGER A. (1962) A technique for the specific cleavage of arginyl bonds by trypsin. *Biochem. biophys. Acta* **62**, 122

314   *Antibodies*

[133] HILL R.L. (1965) Hydrolysis of proteins. *Adv. in Protein Chem.* **20**, 37

[134] SMITHIES O. (1959) An improved procedure for starch-gel electrophoresis. Further variations in the serum proteins of normal individuals. *Biochem. J.* **71**, 585

[135] SMITHIES O. (1955) Zone electrophoresis in starch gels. Group variations in the serum proteins of normal human adults. *Biochem. J.* **61**, 629

[136] ORSTEIN L. (1962) *Disc Electrophoresis.* Rochester (N.Y.): Eastman Kodak Co.

[137] POULIK M.D. (1964) Structural sub-units of proteins: A study by two-dimensional starch-gel electrophoresis. *Protides of Biol. Fluids (XIIth Coll.)* **12**, 400, ed. PEETERS. H. Amsterdam: Elsevier

[138] BLACK J.A. & LEAF G. (1965) Action of cyanogen bromide on horse heart cytochrome C and horse heart myoglobin. *Biochem. J.* **96**, 693.

[139] COHEN S. & PORTER R.R. (1964) Heterogeneity of the peptide chains of γ-globulin. *Biochem. J.* **90**, 278

[140] VAERMAN J.P., FUDENBERG H.H., VAERMAN C. & MANDY W.J. (1965) On the significance of the heterogeneity in molecular size of human serum γA-globulins. *Immunochemistry* **2**, 263

[141] FEINSTEIN A. (1966) Use of charged thiol reagents in interpreting the electrophoretic patterns of immune globulin chains and fragments. *Nature, Lond.* **210**, 135

[142] FEINSTEIN A. (1964) Electrophoretic behaviour of rabbit gamma-globulin fragments and chains. *Nature, Lond.* **202**, 1298

[143] WIEME R.J. (1959) An improved technique of agar-gel electrophoresis on microscope slides. *Clin. chim. Acta* **4**, 317

[144] STANWORTH D.R. & FRANKLIN E.C. (1964) Unpublished observations quoted in ref. 3.

[145] SPACKMAN D.H., STEIN W.H. & MOORE S. (1958) Automatic recording apparatus for use in the chromatography of amino acids. *Anal. Chem.* **30**, 1190

[146] GRANT P.T. & SIMKIN J.L. (1965) Structure and biosynthesis of carbohydrate-polypeptide polymers. *Ann. Reports on the progress of Chemistry* **61**, 491

[147] GOODMAN J.W. (1964) Immunologically active fragments of rabbit gamma globulin. *Biochemistry* **3**, 857

[148] MORETTI J., BOUSSIER G. & JOYLE M.F. (1958) A new method of purification of proteins by electrophoresis in starch gel. *Bull Soc. Chim. Biol.* **40**, 59

[149] CONSDEN R., GORDON A.H. & MARTIN A.J.P. (1944) Qualitative analysis of proteins: a partition chromatographic method using paper. *Biochem. J.* **38**, 224

[150] SVENNERHOLM L. (1956) The quantitative estimation of cerebrosides in nervous tissue. *J. Neurochem.* **1**, 42

[151] DISCHE Z. & SHETTLES L.B. (1951) A new spectrophotometric test for the detection of methyl pentoses. *J. biol. Chem.* **192**, 579

[152] WINZLER R. (1960) Glycoproteins. *Plasma Proteins* **1**, 309, ed. PUTNAM F.W. New York: Acad. Press

[153] METZGER H. & SINGER S.J. (1963) Binding capacity of reductively fragmented antibodies to the 2,4-dinitrophenyl group. *Science* **142**, 674

[154] DOOLITTLE R.F. & SINGER S.J. (1965) Tryptic peptides from the active sites of antibody molecules. *Proc. nat. Acad. Sci. (Wash.)* **54**, 1773

[155] JEFFERIS R. & STANWORTH D.R. Application of gel filtration with Gilford monitoring to the isolation and preliminary analysis of peptide fragments of γG globulins. (In Press). Proc. 5th Amino Acid Coll.

[156] Carnegie P.R. (1965) A peptide mapping technique for the estimation of molecular size. *Nature, Lond.* **206**, 1128

[157] CARNEGIE P.R. (1965) Estimation of molecular size of peptides by gel filtration. *Biochem. J.* **95**, 9P

[158] BALLIEUX R.E., SEBENS T. & MUL N.A.J. (1967) Thin layer peptide mapping. *Protides of Biological Fluids, (XIVth Colloquium)* **14**, 527 ed. Peeters H. Amsterdam Elsevier

[159] INGRAM V.M. (1958) The comparison of normal and sickle cell hemoglobins by finger-printing *Biochim. biophys. Acta* **28**, 539

[160] KÖIW E. & GRÖNWALL A. (1952) Staining of protein-bound carbohydrates after electrophoresis of serum on filter paper. *Scand. J. Clin. Lab. Invest.* **4**, 244

[161] CLAMP J.R. & PUTNAM F.W. (1964) The carbohydrate prosthetic group of human γ-globulin. *J. biol. Chem.* **239**, 3233

[162] MOWERY D.P. (1957) Ferricyanide and a modified periodate chromatographic spray for reducing and non-reducing sugars. *Anal. Chem.* **29**, 1560

[163] CARSTEN M.E. & PIERCE J.G. (1963) Chemical studies on thyrotropin preparations and related pituitary gonadotropins. *J. biol. Chem.* **238**, 1725

[164] MOORE S., COLE R.D., GUNDLACH H.G. & STEIN W.H. (1960) In *Symp. on Proteins*, p. 52. 4th Internat. Congr. of Biochem. ed: NEURATH H. & TUPPY H. New York: Pergamon Press

[165] ANFINSEN C.B. & HABER E. (1961) Studies on the reduction and reformation of protein disulphide bonds. *J. biol. Chem.* **236**, 1361

[166] HIRS C.W.H. (1956) The oxidation of ribonuclease with performic acid. *J. biol. Chem.* **219**, 611

[167] KIMMEL J.R., KATO G.K., PAIVA A.C.M. & SMITH E.L. (1962) Tryptic digestion of papain. I. Isolation and sequences of peptides from the oxidized protein. *J. biol. Chem.* **237**, 2523

[168] SMITH E.L., KIMMEL J.R. & LIGHT P. (1959) The effect of residual peroxide on enzymic digestion of oxidized papain. *Biochim. biophys. Acta* **32**, 561

[169] HEMMINGS W.A. (1958) Protein selection in the yolksac splanchnopleura of the rabbit. The total uptake estimated as loss from the uterus. *Proc. roy. Soc.* (B) **148**, 76

[170] ATFIELD G.N. & MORRIS C.J.O.R. (1961) Analytical separations by high-voltage paper electrophoresis: Amino acids in protein hydrolysates. *Biochem. J.* **81**, 606

[171] BAGLIONI C. (1961) An improved method for the fingerprinting of human hemo-globin. *Biochim. biophys. Acta* **48**, 392

[172] EASLEY C.W. (1965) Combinations of specific colour reactions useful in the peptide mapping technique. *Biochim. biophys. Acta* **107**, 386

[173] PARTRIDGE S.M. (1948) Filterpaper partition chromatography of sugars. *Biochem. J.* **42**, 238

[174] KIMMEL J.R., KATO G.K., PAIVA A.C.M. & SMITH E.L. (1962) Tryptic digestion of papain. II. The preparation of oxidized papain. *J. biol. Chem.* **237**, 2525

[175] FRANGIONE B. & FRANKLIN E.C. (1965) Structural differences of human immuno-globulins. I. Differences in the primary structure of heavy chains of normal and patho-logic G, A and M immunoglobulins. *Arch. biochem. Biophys.* **111**, 603

[176] PUTNAM F.W. (1962) Structural relationships among normal human γ-globulins, myeloma globulins and Bence-Jones proteins. *Biochim. biophys. Acta* **63**, 539

[177] BERNIER M., TOMINAGA K., EASLEY C.W. & PUTNAM F.W. (1965) Structural studies of the immunoglobulins. II. Antigenic and chemical properties of γA myeloma globulins. *Biochemistry* **4**, 2072

[178] PUTNAM F.W. & EASLEY C.W. (1965) Structural studies of the immunoglobulins. I. The tryptic peptides of Bence-Jones proteins. *J. biol. Chem.* **240**, 1626

[179] SCHWARTZ J.H. & EDELMAN G.M. (1963) Comparison of Bence-Jones proteins and L-polypeptide chains of myeloma globulins after hydrolysis with trypsin. *J. exp. Med.* **118**, 41

[180] SANGER F. (1945) The free amino groups of insulin. *Biochem. J.* **39**, 507

[181] BAGLIONI C., LA VIA M. & VENTRUTO V. (1965) A study of immunoglobulin structure. I. Fingerprinting of amino-ethylated Bence-Jones proteins. *Biochim. biophys. Acta* **111,** 479

[182] GITLIN D. & MERLER E. (1961) A comparison of the peptides released from related rabbit antibodies by enzymatic hydrolysis. *J. exp. Med.* **114,** 217

[183] KOSHLAND M.E. & ENGLBERGER F.M. (1963) Differences in the amino acid composition of two purified antibodies from the same rabbit. *Proc. nat. Acad. Sci. (Wash.)* **50,** 61

[184] KOSHLAND M.E., ENGLBERGER F.M. & SHAPANKA R. (1964) Differences in the amino acid composition of a third rabbit antibody. *Science* **143,** 1330

[185] FRANGIONE B. & FRANKLIN E.C. (1965) Structural studies of human immunoglobulins. Differences in the Fd fragments of the heavy chains of G-myeloma proteins. *J. exp. Med.* **122,** 1

[186] HEIMBERGER N., HEIDE K., HAUPT H. & SCHULTZE H. E. (1964) Bausteinanalysen von Humanserumproteinen. *Clin. chim. Acta* **10,** 293

[187] CRUMPTON M.J. & WILKINSON J.M. (1963) Amino acid compositions of human and rabbit γ-globulins, and of the fragments produced by reduction. *Biochem. J.* **88,** 228

[188] CHAPLIN H., COHEN S. & PRESS E.M. (1965) Preparation and properties of the peptide chains of normal human 19S γ-globulin (IgM). *Biochem. J.* **95,** 256

[189] WEIR R.C. & PORTER R.R. (1966) Comparison of the structure of the immunoglobulins from horse serum. *Biochem. J.* **100,** 63

[190] SPIES J.R. & CHAMBERS D.C. (1948) Chemical determination of tryptophan. *Anal. Chem.* **20,** 30

[191] MOORE S. (1963) On the determination of cystine as cysteic acid. *J. biol. Chem.* **238,** 235

[192] LEGGETT-BAILEY J. (1967) *Techniques in Protein Chemistry.* 2nd Ed. Amsterdam: Elsevier

[193] HIRS C.H.W., STEIN W.H. & MOORE S. (1956) Peptides obtained by tryptic hydrolysis of performic-acid-oxidized ribonuclease *J. biol. Chem.* **219,** 623

[194] GUIDOTTI G., HILL R.J. & KONIGSBERG W. (1962) The structure of human hemoglobulin. II. The separation and amino acid compositions of the tryptic peptides from the α- and β-chains. *J. biol. Chem.* **237,** 2184

[195] MOORE S. & STEIN W.H. (1954) A modified ninhydrin reagent for the photometric determination of amino acids and related compounds. *J. biol. Chem.* **211,** 907

[196] CATRAVAS G. (1964) Automated method for separation, hydrolysis and detection of peptides. *Anal. Chem.* **36,** 1146

[197] CHERNOFF A.I. & PETTIT H. (1965) The amino acid composition of hemoglobin. VI. Separation of the tryptic peptides of hemoglobin Knoxville No. 1 on Dowex 1 × 2 and Sephadex. *Biochim. biophys. Acta* **97,** 47

[198] EDMAN P. and SJOQUIST J. (1956) Identification and semi-quantitative determination of phenyl thiohydantoins. *Acta chem. Scand.* **10,** 1507

[199] FRAENKEL-CONRAT H., HARRIS I. J. & LEVY A.L. (1955) Recent developments in terminal and sequence studies in peptides and proteins. *Meth. biochem. Analysis* **2,** 359

[200] GRAY W.R. & HARTLEY B.S. (1963) A fluorescent end-group reagent for proteins and peptides. *Biochem. J.* **89,** 59P

[201] PORTER R.R. & PRESS E.M. (1965) N-terminal peptides of the heavy chain of immunoglobuling. *Biochem. J.* **97,** 32P

[202] MARGOLIASH P. (1962) Amino acid sequence of chymotryptic peptides from horse heart cytochrome-C. *J. biol. Chem.* **237,** 2161

[203] NIU C.I. & FRAENKEL-CONRAT H. (1955) Determination of C-terminal amino acids and peptides by hydrazinolysis. *J. Am. chem. Soc.* **77,** 5882.

[204] LOCKER A. (1954) C-terminal groups in myosin, tropomyosin and actin. *Biochim. biophys. Acta* **14**, 533

[205] KONIGSBERG W. & HILL R.J. (1962) The structure of human hemoglobin. III. The sequence of amino acids in the tryptic peptides of the α-chain. *J. biol. Chem.* **237**, 2457

[206] TITANI K., WHITLEY E., AVOGADRO L. & PUTNAM F.W. (1965) Immunoglobulin structure: Partial amino acid sequence of a Bence-Jones protein. *Science* **149**, 1090

[207] HILSCHMAN N. & CRAIG L.C. (1965) Amino acid sequence studies with Bence-Jones proteins. *Proc. nat. Acad. Sci. (Wash.)* **53**, 1403

[208] PIGGOT P.J. & PRESS E.M. (1966) C-terminal peptide of the heavy chain of normal human immunoglobulin G. *Biochem. J.* **99**, 16P

[209] PRESS E.M., PIGGOT P.J. & PORTER R.R. (1966) The N- and C-terminal amino acid sequences of the heavy chain from a pathological human immunoglobulin IgG. *Biochem. J.* **99**, 356

[210] NAUGHTON M.A. & DINTZIS H.M. (1962) Sequential biosynthesis of the peptide chains of hemoglobin. *Proc. nat. Acad. Sci. (Wash.)* **48**, 1822

[211] PRESS E.M. (1966) The chemical structure of heavy chains. Paper read at Royal Society (London) meeting on 'The Chemistry and Biology of Immunoglobulins', London, June 1966

[212] HILL R.L. (1966) Chemical structure of heavy chains. Paper read at Royal Society (London) meeting on 'The Chemistry and Biology of Immunoglobulins', London, June 1966

[213] WEIR R.C. & PORTER R.R. (1966) The antigen-binding capacity of the peptide chains of horse antibodies. *Biochem. J.* **100**, 69

[214] CIOLI D. & BAGLIONI C. (1966) Origin of structural variation in Bence-Jones proteins. *J. Mol. Biol.* **15**, 385

[215] SMITH E.L. & JAGER B.V. (1952) The characterization of antibodies. *Ann. Rev. Microbiol.* **6**, 207

[216] ROSEVEAR J.W. & SMITH E.L. (1958) Structure of glycopeptides from a human γ-globulin. *J. Am. chem. Soc.* **80**, 250

[217] ROSEVEAR J.W. & SMITH E.L. (1961) Glycopeptides I. Isolation and properties of glycopeptides from a fraction of human gamma globulin. *J. biol. Chem.* **236**, 425

[218] MCFADDEN M.C. & SMITH E.L. (1953) The free amino-groups of γ-globulins of different species. *J. Am. chem. Soc.* **75**, 2784

[219] BLIX G. (1948) The determination of hexosamines according to Elson and Morgan. *Acta chem. Scand.* **2**, 467

[220] DISCHE Z. & SHETTLES L.B. (1948) A specific color reaction of methyl pentoses and a spectrophotometric micromethod for their determination. *J. biol. Chem.* **175**, 595

[221] WERNER I. & ODIN L. (1952) On the presence of sialic acid in certain glycoproteins and in gangliosides. *Acta Soc. Med. Uppsal.* **57**, 230

[222] DISCHE Z. (1947) A new specific color reaction of hexuronic acids. *J. biol. Chem.* **167**, 189

[223] ROTHFUS J.A. & SMITH E.L. (1963) Glycopeptides. IV. The periodate oxidation of glycopeptides from human γ-globulin. *J. biol. Chem.* **238**, 1402

[224] CHATTERJEE A.K. & MONTGOMERY R. (1962) The carbohydrate of ovomucoid. *Arch. biochem. Biophys.* **99**, 426

[225] EYLAR E.H. & JEANLOZ R.W. (1962) Oligosaccharides from the α₁-acid glycoprotein of human plasma. *J. biol. Chem.* **237**, 622

[226] DISCHE Z. & BORENFREUND E. (1949) A specific colour reaction for glycolic aldehyde. *J. biol. Chem.* **180**, 1297

[227] KLEVSTRAND R. & NORDAL A. (1950) A spraying reagent for paper chromatograms which is apparently specific for ketohexoses. *Acta chem. Scand.* **4**, 1320

[228] PARDOE G.I. The carbohydrates of human γG globulin. To be published

[229] STACEY M., BARKER S.A., PARDOE G.I. & HOPTON J.W. (1963) *Improvements Relating to the Production of Enzymes.* British patent 29641/63

[230] BARKER S.A., PARDOE G.I., STACEY M. & HOPTON J.W. (1963) Sequential enzyme induction: A new approach to the structure of complex mucoproteins. *Nature, Lond.* **197**, 231

[231] EDELMAN G.M., BENACERRAF B. & OVARY Z. (1963) Structure and specificity of guinea-pig 7S antibodies. *J. exp. Med.* **118**, 229

[232] FRANĚK F. & NEZLIN R.S. (1963) Recovery of antibody-combining activity by interaction of different peptide chains isolated from purified horse antitoxins. *Folia Microbiol. (Prague)* **8**, 128

[233] FARAH F.S., KERN M. & EISEN H.N. (1960) The preparation and some properties of purified antibody specific for the 2,4-dinitrophenyl group. *J. exp. Med.* **112**, 1195

[234] EISEN H.N. (1964) Preparation of purified anti-2,4-dinitrophenyl antibodies. *Methods in Med. Res.* **10**, 94

[235] GROSSBERG A. & PRESSMAN D. (1964) Purification of anti-p-azobenzoate antibodies. *Methods in Med. Res.* **10**, 103

[236] EISEN H.N. (1964) Equilibrium dialysis for measurement of antibody-hapten affinities. *Methods in Med. Res.* **10**, 106

[237] UTSUMI S. & KARUSH F. (1963) The separation of purified rabbit antibody into subunits. *Fed. Proc.* **22** (Abstract 2008), 496

[238] NISONOFF A. & PRESSMAN D. (1958) Heterogeneity and average combining constants of antibodies from individual rabbits. *J. Immunol.* **80**, 417

[239] GOLDSTEIN I.J., HAMILTON J.K. & SMITH F. (1959) Reduction of the products of periodate oxidation of carbohydrates. X. Methylation studies on amylopectin polyalcohol. *J. Am. chem. Soc.* **81**, 6252

[240] VELICK S.F., PARKER C.W. & EISEN H.N. (1960) Excitation energy transfer and the quantitative study of the antibody hapten reaction. *Proc. nat. Acad. Sci. (Wash.)* **46**, 1470

[241] GIVOL D. & SELA M. (1964) Isolation and fragmentation of antibodies to polytyrosyl gelatin. *Biochemistry* **3**, 444

[242] PRESSMAN D. & NISONOFF A. (1959) Studies on the combining site of anti-p-azobenzoate antibody. Loss of precipitation and binding capacities through different mechanisms on acetylation. *J. Immunol.* **83**, 138

[243] PRESSMAN D., STELOS P. & GROSSBERG A. (1961) Retention of rabbit antibody activity during acetylation. *J. Immunol.* **86**, 452

[244] JOHNSON A., DAY E.D. & PRESSMAN D. (1960) The effect of iodination on antibody activity. *J. Immunol.* **84**, 213

[245] ELLIOTT M., ENGLBERGER F.M. & GADDONE S.M. (1962) The effect of iodination on the binding of hapten to arsonic acid. *J. Immunol.* **89**, 517

[246] KOSHLAND M.E., ENGLBERGER F.M. & GADDONE S.M. (1963) Identification of tyrosine at active site of anti-p-benzene arsonic acid antibody. *J. biol. Chem.* **238**, 1349

[247] PRESSMAN D., NISONOFF A., RADZIMSKI S. & SHAW A. (1961) Nature of the active site of antibenzoate antibodies: Further evidence for the presence of tyrosine. *J. Immunol.* **86**, 489

[248] GROSSBERG A.L., RADZIMSKI G. & PRESSMAN D. (1962) Effect of iodination on the active site of several antihapten antibodies. *Biochemistry* **1**, 391

[249] RAY W.J. & KOSHLAND D.E. (1962) Identification of amino acids involved in phosphoglucomutase action. *J. biol. Chem.* **237**, 2493

[250] WOLFSY L., METZGER H. & SINGER S.J. (1962) Affinity labelling. A general method for labelling the active sites of antibody and enzyme molecules. *Biochemistry* **1**, 1031

[251] METZGER H., WOFSY L. & SINGER S.J. (1963) Affinity labelling of the active sites of antibodies to the 2,4-dinitrophenyl hapten. *Biochemistry* **2**, 979

[252] BAKER B.R., LEE W.W., TONG E. & ROSS L.O. (1961) Potential anti-cancer agents. LXVI. Non-classical antimetabolites. III. 4-(iodoacetamido)-salicylic acid, an exoalkylating irreversible inhibitor of glutamic dehydrogenase. *J. Am. Chem. Soc.* **83**, 3713

[253] LAWSON W.B. & SCHRAMM H.J. (1962) Modification of a methionine residue near the active site of chymotrypsin. *J. Am. Chem. Soc.* **84**, 2017

[254] PRESSMAN D. & ROHOLT O.A. (1961) Isolation of peptides from an antibody site. *Proc. nat. Acad. Sci. (Wash.)* **47**, 160C

[255] ROHOLT O.A., RADZIMSKI G. & PRESSMAN D. (1963) Antibody combining site. The B polypeptide chain. *Science* **141**, 726

[256] ROHOLT O.A., SHAW A. & PRESSMAN D. (1962) Chemical differences between antibody fragments as shown by paired label studies. *Nature* **196**, 773

[257] WOFSY L. & SINGER S.J. (1963) Effects of the amidination reaction on antibody activity and on the physical properties of some proteins. *Biochemistry* **2**, 104

[258] INMAN F.P. & NISONOFF A. (1966) Reversible dissociation of fragment Fc of rabbit γG immunoglobulin. *J. biol. Chem.* **241**, 322

[259] GROSSBERG A.L. & PRESSMAN D. (1960) Nature of the combining site of antibody against a hapten bearing a positive charge. *J. Am. Chem. Soc.* **82**, 5478

[260] PRESSMAN D., NISONOFF A. & RADZIMSKI G. (1961) Specific anion effects with antibenzoate antibody. *J. Immunol.* **86**, 35

[261] BENNICH H. (1966) To be published

[262] SELA M., GIVOL D. & MOZES E. (1963) Resolution of rabbit γ-globulin into two fractions by chromatography on diethylaminoethyl-Sephadex. *Biochim. biophys. Acta* **78**, 649

[263] YEMM E.W. & COCKING E.C. (1955) The determination of amino acids with ninhydrin. *Analyst* **80**, 209

[264] SEIJEN H.G. & GRUBER M. (1963) Structure of γ-globulins and antibodies. *J. molec. Biol.* **7**, 209

[265] FLEISCHER S., HARDIN R.L., HOROWITZ J., ZIMMERMAN M., GRESHAM I., TURNER I.E., BURNETT J.P., STARY Z. & HAUROWITZ Z. (1961) Composition of antibodies against acidic and basic azo proteins. *Arch. biochem. Biophys.* **92**, 329

[266] MANDY W.J., STAMBAUGH M.K. & NISONOFF A. (1963) Amino acid composition of univalent fragments of rabbit antibody. *Science* **140**, 901

[267] FLODIN J. & PORATH P. (1964) Zone electrophoresis on starch columns. *Biochim. biophys. Acta* **13**, 175

[268] BASSETT E.W., TANENBAUM S.W., PRYZWANSKY K., BEISER S.M. & KABAT E.A. (1965) Studies on human antibodies. III. Amino acid composition of four antibodies from one individual. *J. exp. Med.* **122**, 251

[269] PIEZ K.A. & MORRIS L.A. (1960) A modified procedure for the automatic analysis of amino acids. *Anal. Biochem.* **1**, 187

[270] HEIMER R., WOODS K.R. & ENGLE R.L. (1962) Amino acid analysis of rheumatoid factors and normal gamma globulins. *Proc. Soc. exp. Biol. Med.* **110**, 496

[271] TURNER M.W. & ROWE D.S. (1966) A naturally occurring fragment related to the heavy chains of immunoglobulin G in normal human urine. *Nature, Lond.* **210**, 130

[272] BARKER S.A., PARDOE G.I., STACEY M. & HOPTON J.W. (1964) Degradation of type XIV *Pneumococcus* polysaccharide by induced enzymes. *Nature, Lond.* **204**, 938

[273] AVIGAD G., AMARAL D., ASENSIO C. & HORECKER B.L. (1962) The *D*-galactose oxidase of *Polyporus circinatus. J. biol. Chem.* **237**, 2736

[274] SVENNERHOLM L. (1956) The determination of hexosamines with special reference to nervous tissues. *Acta Soc. Med. Uppsal.* **61**, 287

[275] NOLAN C. & SMITH E.L. (1962) Glycopeptides. II. Isolation and properties of glyco-peptides from rabbit γ-globulin. *J. biol. Chem.* **237**, 446

[276] NOLAN C. & SMITH E.L. (1962) Glycopeptides. III. Isolation and properties of glyco-peptides from a bovine globulin of colostrum and from fraction II-3 of human globulin. *J. biol. Chem.* **237**, 453

[277] BRAMBELL F.W.R., HEMMINGS W.A. & OAKLEY C.L. (1959) The relative transmission of natural and pepsin-refined homologous antitoxin from the uterine cavity to the foetal circulation in the rabbit. *Proc. Roy. Soc.* (B) **150**, 312

[278] BRAMBELL F.W.R. (1958) The passive immunity of the young mammal. *Biol. Rev. Cambridge Phil. Soc.* **33**, 488

[279] GITLIN D., ROSEN F.S. & MICHAEL J.G. (1963) Transient 19S gamma globulin deficiency in the newborn infant, and its significance. *Pediatrics* **31**, 197

[280] HITZIG VON W.H. (1957) Die physiologische Entwicklung der Immunoglobuline (Gamma und Beta₂-globuline). *Helv. Paed. Acta* **12**, 596

[281] OVARY Z., FUDENBERG H.H. & KUNKEL H.G. (1960) Anaphylactic reactions in the skin of the guinea-pig with high and low molecular weight antibodies and gamma globulins. *J. exp. Med.* **112**, 953

[282] FRANKLIN E.C. & OVARY Z. (1963) On the sensitizing properties of some normal and pathologic human immune globulins and fragments obtained by papain or pepsin digestion. *Immunology* **6**, 434

[283] ROCKEY J.H. & KUNKEL H.G. (1961) Studies of the rabbit antibodies which sensitize red blood cells for agglutination by rheumatoid factors. *Arthr. and Rheum.* **4**, 449

[284] GOODMAN J.W. (1963) Antigenic determinants in fragments of gamma globulin from rabbit serum. *Science* **139**, 1292

[285] COHEN S. & GORDON S. (1965) Dissociation of κ- and λ-chains from reduced human immunoglobulins. *Biochem. J.* **97**, 460

[286] TODD C.W. (1963) Allotypy in rabbit 19S protein. *Biochim. Biophys. Res. Comm.* **11**, 170

[287] FEINSTEIN A. (1963) Character and allotypy of an immune globulin in rabbit colo-strum *Nature, Lond.* **199**, 1197

[288] TARANTA A. & FRANKLIN E.C. (1961) Complement fixation by antibody fragments. *Science* **134**, 1981

[289] AMIRAIAN K. & LEIKHIM E.J. (1961) Interaction of fragment III of rabbit gamma globulin and guinea-pig complement. *Proc. soc. Exp. Biol. Med.* **108**, 454

[290] SCHUR P.H. & BECKER E.L. (1963) Complement-fixing properties of pepsin-treated rabbit and sheep antibodies. *Science* **141**, 361

[291] REISS A.M. & PLESCIA O.J. (1963) Fixation of complement to fragments of antibody. *Science* **141**, 812

[292] CEBRA J.J. (1963) In *Conceptual Advances in Immunology and Oncology*, p. 270. New York: Harper

[293] BLOCH K.J., KOURILSKY F.M., OVARY M.D. & BENACERRAF B. (1963) Properties of guinea-pig 7S antibodies. III. Identification of antibodies involved in complement fixation and hemolysis. *J. exp. Med.* **117**, 965

[294] ISHIZAKA K. (1963) Gamma globulin and molecular mechanisms in hypersensitivity reactions. *Progr. All.* **7**, 32

[295] HUMPHREY J.H. & DOURMASHKIN R.R. (1965) Electron microscope studies of immune cell lysis. In *Complement*, p. 175. ed. WOLSTENHOLME G.E.W. & KNIGHT J., London: Churchill

[296] BORSOS T. & RAPP H.J. (1965) Complement fixation on cell surfaces by 19S and 7S antibodies. *Science* **150**, 505

[297] STANWORTH D.R. & HENNEY C.S. (1967) Some biological activities associated with the 10S form of human γG globulin. *Immunology* **12**, 267

[298] ISHIZAKA K., ISHIZAKA T. & BANOVITZ J. (1965) Biological activities of aggregated γ globulin. VII. Minimum size of aggregated γ-globulin or its piece-III required for the induction of skin reactivity and complement fixation. *J. Immunol.* **94**, 824

[299] PIKE R.M. & SCHULZE M. (1961) The distribution of antibodies for erythrocytes in chromatographic fractions of early and late immune sera. *Immunology* **4**, 425

[300] WIEDERMANN G., MIESCHER P.B. & FRANKLIN E.C. (1963) Effect of mercaptoethanol on complement-binding ability of human 7S gamma globulin. *Proc. Soc. exp. Biol. Med.* **113**, 609

[301] HEIMER R., LEVIN F.M., PRIMACK P., CORCAS J.M. & NOZENZO C. (1962) Inhibition of complement fixation by human serum. *J. Immunol.* **89**, 382

[302] ISHIZAKA K., ISHIZAKA T. & BANOVITZ J. (1965) Complement-fixing activity of rabbit antibody reconstructed from half-molecules. *Proc. Soc. exp. Biol. Med.* **118**, 507

[303] ISHIZAKA K. & ISHIZAKA T. (1964) Molecular basis of passive sensitization. II. The role of fragment II of γ-globulin and its disulphide bonds in passive sensitization and complement fixation. *J. Immunol.* **93**, 59

[304] HENNEY C.S., STANWORTH D.R. & JEFFERIS R. (1967). Studies on low molecular weight peptides derived from human γG globulin II. Identification of rheumatoid-factor reactive peptides in proteolytic digests. To be published

[305] HEMMINGS W.A. & JONES R.E. (1962) The occurrence of macroglobulin antibodies in maternal and foetal sera of rabbits, as determined by gradient centrifugation. *Proc. Roy. Soc.* (B) **157**, 27

[306] PARASKEVAS F. & GOODMAN J.W. (1965) Components of fraction III and pepsin-digested fraction III from papain-digested rabbit γ-globulin. *Immunochemistry* **2**, 391

[307] GOCKE D.J. & OSLER A.G. (1965) *In vitro* damage of rabbit platelets by an unrelated antigen–antibody reaction I. General characteristics of the reaction. *J. Immunol.* **94**, 236

[308] TERRY W.D. (1966) Skin sensitising activity related to γ-polypeptide chain-characteristics of human IgG. *J. Immunol.* **95** 1041

[309] SCHUR P.H. & BECKER E.L. (1963) Pepsin digestion of rabbit and sheep antibodies. The effect on complement fixation. *J. exp. Med.* **118**, 891

[310] ISHIZAKA K., ISHIZAKA T. & SUGAHARA T. (1962) Biological activity of soluble antigen–antibody complexes. VII. Role of an antibody fragment in the induction of biological activities. *J. Immunol.* **88**, 690

[311] ROWLEY D., THOENI M., & ISLIKER H. (1965) Opsonic requirements for bacterial phagocytosis. *Nature, Lond.* **207**, 210

[312] OVARY Z. & KARUSH F. (1961) Studies on the immunologic mechanism of anaphylaxis. II. Sensitizing and combining capacity *in vivo* of fractions separated from papain digests of antihapten-antibody. *J. Immunol.* **86**, 146

[313] LIACOPOULOS M., HALPERN B.N., LIACOPOULOS P. and PERRAMANT M.F. (1963) Comportment des γ-globulines et des fractions I et III de Porter en tant qu'antigènes dans l'anaphylaxie passive *in vitro*. *Compt. Rend. Soc. Biol.* **157**, 76

[314] SPIEGELBERG H.L. & WEIGLE W.O. (1965) The catabolism of homologous and heterologous 7S gamma globulin fragments. *J. exp. Med.* **121**, 323

[315] FAHEY J.L. & ROBINSON A.G. (1963) Factors controlling the serum γ-globulin concentration. *J. exp. Med.* **118**, 845

[316] SCHULTZE H.E. & SCHWICK G. (1962) Neue möglichkeiten intravenöser Gamma-globulin Applikationen. *Dtsch. Med. Wschr.* **87**, 1643

[317] FRANKLIN E.C. (1961) The interaction of rheumatoid factors and gamma globulins. Proc. Xth Internat. Congr. Rheumatol. Rome (communications). *Minerva Med.* **2**, 804

[318] HENNEY C.S. & STANWORTH D.R. (1964) Reaction of rheumatoid factor with the isolated polypeptide chains of human 7S γ-globulin. *Nature, Lond.* **201**, 511

[319] OSTERLAND C.K., HARBOE M. & KUNKEL H.G. (1963) Anti γ-globulin factors in human sera revealed by enzymatic splitting of anti-Rh antibodies. *Vox. Sang.* **8**, 133

[320] GOODMAN J.W. (1961) Reaction of rheumatoid sera with fragments of papain digested rabbit γ-globulin. *Proc. Soc. exp. Biol. Med.* **106**, 827

[321] MORRIS J.G. (1963) Interference with uptake of guinea-pig agglutinins in mice due to fractions of papain-hydrolysed rabbit γ-globulin. *Proc. Roy. Soc.* (B) **157**, 160

[322] POPE C.G. (1963) Development of knowledge of antitoxins. *Brit. Med. Bull.* **19**, 230

[323] SMILEY J.D. & HORTON H. (1965) Isolation and study of the function of human γ2-globulin glycopeptide. *Immunochemistry* **2**, 61

[324] ISLIKER H.C., JACOT-GUILLARMOD H. & THOENI M. (1962) Reversible inactivation of γ1M globulins. Anticomplementary activity and tissue affinity of human γ-globulin. Paper presented at NAS/NRC Symposium on Gamma-globulin, Washington, D.C. 1962.

[325] ROBERT B. (1963) In *Protides of Biol. Fluids (XIth Coll.)* **11**, 152, Ed. PEETERS H. Amsterdam: Elsevier.

[326] EYLAR E.E. (1965) On the biological role of glycoproteins. *J. Theor. Biol.* **10**, 89

[327] DYKES P.W., DAVIES J.W.L., RICKETTS C.R. & STANWORTH D.R. (1966) The effect of plasma concentration on the catabolic rate of human serum albumin. Proceedings of Conference on Problems connected with the Preparation and Use of Labelled Proteins in Tracer Studies. Pisa, 1966

[328] KERN M., HELMREICH E. & EISEN H.N. (1961) The solubilization of microsomal antibody activity by the specific interaction between the crystallizable fraction of γ-globulin and lymph-node microsomes. *Proc. nat. Acad. Sci. (Wash.)* **47**, 767

[329] GOODMAN J.W. & GROSS D. (1963) Studies on fragments of rabbit γ-globulin. *J. Immunol.* **90**, 865

[330] NOELKEN M.E., NELSON C.A., BUCKLEY C.E. & TANFORD C. (1965) Gross conformation of rabbit 7S γ-immunoglobulin and its papain-cleaved fragments. *J. Biol. Chem.* **240**, 218

[331] EPSTEIN W.V. & GROSS D. (1964) Naturally occurring human antibody to Bence-Jones proteins. *J. exp. Med.* **120**, 733

[332] IRREVERRE F. (1965) A modified Sakaguchi spray. *Biochim. biophys. Acta* **111**, 551

[333] BOYD W.C. (1954) The proteins of immune reactions. *The Proteins* **2**, 755, ed. NEURATH H. & BAILEY K. New York: Acad. Press

[334] KRATSKY O.G., POROD A., SEKORA A. & PALETTA B. (1955) Determination of the shape of gamma globulin by means of the X-ray low angle method. *J. Polymer Sci.* **16**, 163

[335] HALL C.E., NISONOFF A. & SLAYTER H.S. (1959) Electron microscopic observations of rabbit antibodies. *J. Biophys. Biochem. Cytol.* **6**, 407

[336] HÖGLUND S. & LEVIN O. (1965) Electron microscopic studies of some proteins from normal human serum. *J. molec. Biol.* **12**, 866

[337] HÖGLUND S. (1966) A study of the γG and γM molecules. *Proc. VIth Int. Congress Electron Microsc. Kyoto, Japan*

[338] PALADE G.E. (1952) A study of fixation for electron microscopy. *J. exp. Med.* **95**, 285

[339] BACKUS R.C. & WILLIAMS R.C. (1950) The use of spraying methods and of volatile suspending media in the preparation of specimens for electron microscopy. *J. Appl. Physics* **21**, 11

[340] HALL C.E. (1960) Measurement of globular protein molecules by electron microscopy. *J. Biophys. Biochem. Cytol.* **7**, 613

[341] BRADLEY D.E. (1954) Evaporated carbon films for use in electron microscopy. *Brit. J. Appl. Phys.* **5**, 65

[342] ROWE A.J. (1966) Some comments on Höglund and Levin's electron micrographs of human serum proteins. *J. molec. Biol.* **16**, 553

[343] SPENCER M. (1959) The preparation of carbon films for electron microscopy. *J. Biophys. Biochem. Cytol.* **6**, 125

[344] ALMEIDA J., CINADER B. & HOWATSON A. (1963) The structure of antigen–antibody complexes. A study by electron microscopy. *J. exp. Med.* **118**, 327

[345] EASTY G.C. & MERCER E.H. (1958) Electron microscopic studies of the antigen–antibody complex. *Immunology* **1**, 353

[346] KLECZKOWSKI A. (1961) Serological behaviour of tobacco mosaic virus and of its protein fragments. *Immunology* **4**, 130

[347] LAFFERTY K.J. & OERTELIS S.J. (1961) Attachment of antibody to influenza virus. *Nature, Lond.* **192**, 764

[348] ELEK S.D., KINGSLEY-SMITH B.V. & HIGHAM W. (1964) The interaction of antigen and antibody in agglutination. *Immunology* **7**, 570

[349] FEINSTEIN A. & ROWE A.J. (1965) Molecular mechanisms of formation of an antigen–antibody complex. *Nature, Lond.* **205**, 147

[350] HENNEY C.S. & STANWORTH D.R. (1966) Effect of antigen on the structural configuration of homologous antibody following antigen–antibody combinations. *Nature, Lond.* **210**, 1071

[351] ASAHI M., TSUZURAHARA K., NAKAJIMA S. & YAMAMURA Y. (1966) Tryptic digestion of rabbit γ-globulin. *J. Biochem.* **59**, 89

[352] MOFFITT W. & YANG J.T. (1956) The optical rotatory dispersion of simple polypeptides. I. *Proc. nat. Acad. Sci. (Wash.)* **42**, 596

[353] URNES P. & DOTY P. (1961) Optical rotation and the conformation of polypeptides and proteins. *Adv. in Protein Chem.* **16**, 401

[354] HAMAGUCHI K. & MIGITA S. (1964) Optical rotatory and ultraviolet spectral properties of Bence-Jones proteins. *J. Biochem.* **56**, 512

[355] JIRGENSONS B. (1963) Optical rotatory dispersion and conformation of various globular proteins. *J. biol. Chem.* **238**, 2716

[356] IMAHORI K. & MOMOI H. (1962) Globulin and myeloma. The structural characterization of γ-globulin and myeloma protein. *Arch. biochem. Biophys.* **97**, 236

[357] WINKLER M. & DOTY P. (1961) Some observations on the configuration and precipitating activity of antibodies. *Biochim. biophys. Acta* **54**, 448

[358] TANFORD C., BUCKLEY C.E., DE P.K. & LIVELY E.P. (1962) Effect of ethylene glycol on the conformation of γ-globulin and β-lactoglobulin. *J. biol. Chem.* **237**, 1168

[359] BLOUT E.R., DE LOZÉ C. & ASADOURIAN A. (1961) The deuterium exchange of water-soluble polypeptides and proteins as measured by infra-red spectroscopy. *J. Am. chem. Soc.* **83**, 1895

[360] CALLAGHAN P. & MARTIN W.H. (1963) Optical rotatory dispersion and the conformation of human γ-globulin. *Biochem. J.* **87**, 225

[361] GOULD H.J., GILL T.J. & DOTY P. (1964) The conformation and the hydrogen ion equilibrium of normal rabbit γ-globulin. *J. biol. Chem.* **239**, 2842

[362] EDELMAN G.M. & GALLY J.A. (1964) A model for the 7S antibody molecule. *Proc. nat. Acad. Sci.* (*Wash.*) **51**, 846

[363] HOLASEK A.O., KRATSKY O., MITTELBACH P. & WAWRA H. (1963) Small-angle X-ray scattering of Bence-Jones proteins. *J. molec. Biol.* **7**, 321

[364] KABAT E.A. (1960) The upper limit for the size of the human anti-dextran combining site. *J. Immunol.* **84**, 82

[365] BUCKLEY, C.E., WHITNEY P.L. & TANFORD C. (1965) The unfolding and renaturation of a specific univalent antibody fragment. *Proc. nat. Acad. Sci.* (*Wash.*) **50**, 827

[366] HABER E. (1964) Recovery of antigenic specificity after denaturation and complete reduction of disulphide in a papain fragment of antibody. *Proc. nat. Acad. Sci.* (*Wash.*) **52**, 1099

[367] WHITNEY P.L. & TANFORD C. (1965) Recovery of specific activity after complete unfolding and reduction of an antibody fragment. *Proc. nat. Acad. Sci.* (*Wash.*) **53**, 524

[368] NOELKEN M.E. & TANFORD C. (1964) Unfolding and renaturation of a univalent antihapten fragment. *J. biol. Chem.* **239**, 1828

[369] BAVANDUN S., KISTLER P., JENNET P. & ISLIKER H. (1962) Intravenous administration of γ-globulin. *Vox Sang.* **7**, 157

[370] HARBOE M. (1965) Pepsin-splitting of γM globulins and high molecular weight antibodies. *Scand. J. clin. Invest.* **17**, Suppl. 84 233

[371] ONOUE K., YAGI Y., GROSSBERG A.L. & PRESSMAN D. (1965) Number of binding sites of rabbit macroglobulin antibody and its sub-units. *Biochemistry* **4**, 401

[372] LAMM M.E. & SMALL P.A. (1966) Polypeptide structure of rabbit immunoglobulins. II. γM immunoglobulins. *Biochemistry* **5**, 267

[373] CARBONARA A.O. & HEREMANS J.F. (1963) Subunits of normal and pathological $γ_{1A}$-globulins ($β_{2A}$-globulins). *Arch. biochem. Biophys.* **102**, 137

[374] DEUTSCH A.F. (1963) Molecular transformations of a $γ_1$ globulin of human serum. *J. molec. Biol.* **7**, 662

[375] SALVATORE G., SALVATORE M., CAHNMANN H.J. & ROBBINS J. (1964) Separation of thyroidal iodoproteins and purification of thyroglobulin by gel filtration and density gradient centrifugation. *J. biol. Chem.* **239**, 3267

[376] DEUTSCH H.F. & MORTON J.I. (1958) Human serum macroglobulins and dissociation units. *J. biol. Chem.* **231**, 1107

[377] FRANKLIN E.C., EDELMAN G.M. & KUNKEL H.G. (1959) Studies on high molecular weight gamma globulins and their complexes in rheumatoid arthritis. *Immunity and Virus Infections*, p. 92, ed. NAJJAR V.A. New York: Wiley

[378] DEUTSCH H.F. (1964) Molecular transformations of human serum. II. Immunochemical studies. *J. Immunol.* **93**, 879

[379] ISHIZAKA K., ISHIZAKA T. & LEE E.H. (1965) Immunochemical properties of human $γ_A$ isoagglutinin II. The effect of reduction and alkylation. *J. Immunol.* **95**, 771

[380] VAERMAN J.P., HEREMANS J.F. & VAERMAN C. (1963) Studies of the immune globulins of human serum I. A method for the simultaneous isolation of the three immune globulins ($γ_{ss}$, $γ_{1M}$ and $γ_{1A}$) from individual small serum samples. *J. Immunol.* **91**, 7

[381] RAWSON A.J. & ABELSON N.M. (1964) Studies of blood group antibodies. VI. The blood group isoantibody activity of $γ_A$ globulin. *J. Immunol.* **93**, 192

[382] KLINMAN N.R., ROCKEY J.H. & KARUSH F. (1964) Valency and affinity of equine nonprecipitating antibody to a haptenic group. *Science* **146**, 401

[383] HEREMANS J.F., VAERMAN J.P., CARBONARA A.O., RODHAIN J.A. & HEREMANS M.TH. (1963) $γ_{1A}$ Globulin ($β_{2A}$globulin): its isolation, properties, fractions and

pathology. *Protides of Biol. Fluids (Xth Coll.)* **10**, 108, ed. PETEERS H. Amsterdam: Elsevier.

[384] EDELHOCH H. LIPPOLOT R.E. & STEINER R.F. (1962) Structural transitions in antibody and normal γ-globulins. I. Molecular properties. *J. Am. chem. Soc.* **84**, 2133

[385] HENNEY C.S. (1965) Biological characteristics of structurally altered γG gobulin. Ph.D. Thesis, University of Birmingham

[386] EPSTEIN W., JOHNSON A.M. & RAGAN C. (1956) Observations of a precipitin reaction between serum of patients with rheumatoid arthritis and a preparation (Cohn fraction II) of human gamma globulin. *Proc. Soc. exp. Biol. Med.* **91**, 235

[387] EDELMAN G.M., KUNKEL H.G. & FRANKLIN E.C. (1958) Interaction of the rheumatoid factor with antigen–antibody complexes and aggregated gamma globulin. *J. exp. Med.* **108**, 105

[388] MILGROM F. & WITEBSKY E. (1960) Studies of the rheumatoid and related factors. I. Autoimmunization of rabbits with γ-globulin. *J. Amer. Med. Assoc.* **174**, 56

[389] McCLUSKEY R.T., MILLER F. & BENACERRAF B. (1962) Sensitization to denatured autologous γ-globulins. *J. exp. Med.* **115**, 253

[390] NEUTRA M. & LEBLOND C.P. (1966) Synthesis of the carbohydrate of mucus in the Golgi complex, as shown by electron microscope radiography of goblet cells from rats injected with glucose-^{3}H. *J. Cell. Biol.* **30**, 119

[391] ISHIZAKA K., ISHIZAKA T. & SUGAHARA T. (1961) Biological activities of aggregated γ-globulin. III. Production of Arthus-like reactions. *J. Immunol.* **86**, 220

[392] MORSE J.H. (1965) The aggregation of γ-myeloma protein. *J. Immunol.* **95**, 722

[393] BIRO C.E. & GARCIA G. (1965) The antigenicity of aggregated and aggregate-free human gamma globulin for rabbits. *Immunology* **8**, 411

[394] HENNEY C.S. & STANWORTH D.R. (1966) Unpublished observations

[395] GILL T. & KUNZ H. (1966) The immunogenicity of polypeptide aggregates. Personal communication.

[396] CHRISTIAN C.L. (1960) Studies of aggregated γ-globulin. II. Effects *in vivo. J. Immunol.* **84**, 117

[397] ROBERT B. & GRABAR P. (1957) Dosage des groupements thiol protéiniques dans des réactions immunochimiques. *Ann. Inst. Pasteur* **92**, 56

[398] ISHIZAKA K. & CAMPBELL D.H. (1959) Biological activity of soluble antigen–antibody complexes. V. Change of optical rotation by the formation of skin-reactive complexes. *J. Immunol.* **83**, 318

[399] NAJJAR V.A. & FISHER J. (1956) The mechanism of antibody–antigen interaction. *Biochim. biophys. Acta* **20**, 158

[400] NAJJAR V.A., SIDBURY J.B. & FISHER J. (1957) Further studies on the mechanism of antibody–antigen interaction. *Biochim. biophys. Acta* **26**, 114

[401] NELSON C.A., NOELKEN M.E., BUCKLEY C.E., TANFORD C. & HILL R.L. (1965) Comparison of the tryptic peptides from rabbit γ-globulin and two specific rabbit antibodies. *Biochemistry* **4**, 1418

[402] BOLTON C.H., CLAMP J.R., DAWSON G. & HOUGH L. (1965) The quantitative analysis of glycopeptides and glycoproteins by gas-liquid chromatography. *Carbohydrate Res.* **1**, 333

[403] ARWIDI B. & SAMUELSON O. (1965) Partition chromatography of sugars on ion-exchange resins. *Svensk Kem. Tidskr* **77**, 84

[404] SELL S. (1964) Evidence for species differences in the effect of serum γ-globulin concentration on γ-globulin catabolism. *J. exp. Med.* **120**, 967

[405] LARSSON L.I. & SAMUELSON O. (1965) An automated procedure for separation of monosaccharides on ion exchange resins. *Acta chem. Scand.* **19**, 1357

[406] STANWORTH D.R. (1966) Mechanism of reactivity of rheumatoid factor with structurally altered and unaltered immunoglobulins. *Ann. Rheum. Dis.* **25,** 475

[407] WEBER G. & WAHL P. (1967) In preparation

[408] INMAN F.P. & NISONOFF A. (1966) Reversible dissociation of fragment Fc of rabbit γG immunoglobulin. *J. biol. Chem.* **241,** 322

[409] DJERASSI C. (1960) *Optical Rotatory Dispersion*. Series in Advanced Chemistry. New York: McGraw Hill & Co., Inc.,

[410] YANG J.T. & DOTY P. (1957) The optical rotatory dispersion of polypeptides and proteins in relation to configuration. *J. Am. chem. Soc.* **79,** 761

[411] EDSALL J.T., MAYBURY R.H., SIMPSON R.B. & STRAESSLE R. (1954) Dimerization of serum mercaptalbumin in presence of mercurials. II. Studies with a bifunctional organic mercurial. *J. Am. chem. Soc.* **76,** 3131

[412] HENNEY C.S., PARDOE G.I. & STANWORTH D.R. (1967) Influence of terminal carbohydrate units on interaction of aggregated γG globulin and rheumatoid factor. To be published

[413] WARREN L. (1959) The thiobarbituric acid assay of sialic acids. *J. biol. Chem.* **234,** 1971

[414] EDELMAN G.M., OLINS D.E., GALLY J.A. & ZINDER N.D. (1963) Reconstitution of immunologic activity by interaction of polypeptide chains of antibodies. *Proc. nat. Acad. Sci. (Wash.)* **50,** 753

[415] HENNEY C.S., STANWORTH D.R. & GELL P.G.H. (1965) Demonstration of the exposure of new antigenic determinants following antigen–antibody combination. *Nature, Lond.* **205,** 1079

[416] LARSSON L.I., RAMNAS O. & SAMUELSON O. (1966) Separation of sugar derivatives by partition chromatography on ion exchange resins. *Anal. Chim. Acta* **34,** 394

[417] HILL R.L., DELANEY R., LEBOVITZ H.E. & FELLOWS R.E. (1966) Studies on the amino acid sequence of heavy chains from rabbit immunoglobulin IgG. *Proc. Roy. Soc.* (B) **166,** 159

[418] BERNIER G.M. & PUTNAM F.W. (1964) Myeloma proteins and macroglobulins: Hall-marks of disease and models of antibodies. *Progr. Hemat.* **4,** 160

[419] LI Y.T. (1966) Presence of α-D-mannosidic linkage in glycoproteins. *J. biol. Chem.* **241,** 1010

[420] MARTENSSON L. (1966) Gm genes and γG molecules. *Acta Univ. Lund.* **II,** No. 3. Univ. of Lund

[421] FUDENBERG H.H., FEINSTEIN D., MCGEHEE W. & FRANKLIN E.C. (1966) Molecular localization of Gm(a) and Gm(b) factors. *Vox Sang.* **11,** 45

[422] FRANGIONE B., FRANKLIN E.C., FUDENBERG H.H. & KOSHLAND M.E. (1966) Structural studies of human γG myeloma proteins of different antigenic subgroups and genetic specificities. *J. exp. Med.* **124,** 715

[423] SELL S. (1966) Immunoglobulin M allotypes of the rabbit. Identification of a second specificity. *Science* **153,** 641

[424] NIRENBERG M., LEDER P., BERNFIELD M., BRIMACOMBE R., TRUPIN J., ROTTMAN F. & O'NEAL C. (1965) RNA codewords and protein synthesis. VII. On the general nature of the RNA code. *Proc. nat. Acad. Sci. (Wash.)* **53,** 1161

[425] HOOD L.E., GRAY W.R. & DREYER W.J. (1966) On the mechanism of antibody synthesis: A species comparison of L-chains. *Proc. nat. Acad. Sci. (Wash.)* **55,** 826

[426] TITANI K., WHITLEY E. & PUTNAM F.W. (1966) Immunoglobulin structure: Variation in the sequence of Bence-Jones proteins. *Science* **152,** 1513

[427] BAGLIONI C., ZONTA L.A., CIOLI D. & CARBONARA A. (1966) Allelic antigenic factor Inv(a) of the light chains of human immunoglobulins. Chemical basis. *Science* **152,** 1517

[428] MORRIS C.J.O.R. (1966) Separation of peptides. *B.M. Bull.* **22**, 168

[429] EASTOE J.E. (1966) Amino acid analysis of glycoproteins. In *Glycoproteins*, p. 112, ed. GOTTSCHALK A. & NEUBERGER A. Amsterdam: Elsevier

[430] NORTHCOTE D.H. (1966) Separation of carbohydrates and mucoid substances. *B.M. Bull.* **22**, 180

[431] NEUBERGER A. & MARSHALL R.D. (1966) Methods for the qualitative and quantitative analysis of the component sugars. In *Glycoproteins*, p. 190, ed. GOTTSCHALK A. & NEUBERGER A. Amsterdam: Elsevier

[432] CRISPIN SMITH J., BERNSTEIN G., SURKS M.I. & OPPENHEIMER J.H. (1966) A method of preparative starch gel electrophoresis. *Biochim. biophys. Acta* **115**, 81

[433] KATZ A.M., DREYER W.J. & ANFINSEN C.B. (1959) Peptide separation by two-dimensional chromatography and electrophoresis. *J. biol. Chem.* **234**, 2897

[434] ARNASON B.G, ST CYR C. DE VAUX & GRABAR P. (1963) Immunoglobulin abnormalities of the thymectomized rat. *Nature, Lond.* **199**, 1199

[435] PRESS E.M. (1965) Carbohydrate heterogeneity in rabbit 7S γ-globulin. In *Symposium on Molecular and Cellular Basis of Antibody Formation*, p. 93, ed. STERZL J. Prague: Czechoslovak Acad. Sci.

[436] MÜLLER-EBERHARDT H.J., KUNKEL H.G. & FRANKLIN E.C. (1956) Two types of γ-globulin differing in carbohydrate content. *Proc. Soc. exp. Biol. Med.* **93**, 146

[437] HEIDE K., HAUPT H. & SCHMIDTBERGER R. (1962) Über den Kohlenhydratgehalt von Proteinen des menschlichen γ-Globulinkomponentensystems. *Behringwerk-Mitteil.* **37**, 3

[438] REISFELD R.A. & SMALL P.A. (1966) Electrophoretic heterogeneity of polypeptide chains of specific antibodies. *Science* **152**, 1253

[439] GOLD E.R., MANDY W.J. & FUDENBERG H.H. (1965) Relation between Gm(f) and the structure of the γ-globulin molecule. *Nature, Lond.* **207**, 1099

[440] NEUTRA M. & LEBLOND C.P. (1966) Radioautographic comparison of the uptake of galactose-^{3}H and glucose-^{3}H in the Golgi regions of various cells secreting glycoproteins and mucopoly-saccharides. *J. Cell. Biol.* **30**, 137

[441] LABAT J. & BERGER N. (1966) Étude de la rupture des liaisons neuraminosidiques de glycoprotéines sériques humaines. *Ann. Biol. Clin.* **24**, 839

[442] ROWE D.S. (1961) Chromatographic separation and salting-out of the slow-migrating component of digests of human γ-globulin. *Protides of the Biol. Fluids (IXth Coll.)* **9**, 101, ed. PEETERS H. Amsterdam: Elsevier

[443] BAGLIONI C. & CIOLI D. (1966) A study of immunoglobulin structure. II. The comparison of Bence-Jones proteins by peptide mapping. *J. exp. med.* **124**, 307

[444] KUNKEL H.G. & PRENDERGAST R.A. (1966) Subgroups of γA immune globulins. *Proc. Soc. exp. Biol. Med.* **122**, 910

[445] VAERMAN J.P. & HEREMANS J.F. (1966) Subclasses of human immunoglobulin A based on differences in the alpha polypeptide chains. *Science* **152**, 647

[446] TERRY W.D. & ROBERT M.S. (1966) Antigenic heterogeneity of human immunoglobulin A proteins. *Science* **153**, 1007

[447] MILLER F. & METZGER H. (1966) Characterization of a human macroglobulin. III. The products of tryptic digestion. *J. biol. Chem.* **241**, 1732

[448] METZGER H., PERLMAN R.L. & EDELHOCH H. (1966) Characterization of a human macroglobulin. IV. Studies of its conformation by fluorescence polarization. *J. biol. Chem.* **241**, 1741

[449] SMALL P.A. & LAMM M.E. (1966) Polypeptide chain structure of rabbit immunoglobulins. *Biochem.* **5**, 259

[450] ROWE D.S. (1962) The separation and antigenic characteristics of some fractions

of papain digests of human serum gamma globulins and the antigenic relationships of human gamma globulins with the gamma globulins of some other mammalian sera. *Immunol.* **5,** 533

[451] McDuffie F.C., Oikawa T. & Nishi I. (1965) Reactivity of rheumatoid factor with rabbit γ-globulin. *J. Immunol.* **95,** 614

[452] Binaghi R.A. & de Merlo E.S. (1966) Characterization of rat IgA and its non-identity with the anaphylactic antibody. *Int. Arch. All.* **30,** 589

[453] Press E.M. & Porter R.R. (1966) Immunoglobulins, in Glycoproteins, p. 395. Ed: Gottschalk A. & Neuberger A. Amsterdam: Elsevier

[454] Press E.M., Givol D., Piggot P.J., Porter R.R. & Wilkinson J.M. (1966) The chemical structure of the heavy chains of rabbit and human immunoglobulin G (IgG). *Proc. Roy. Soc.* (B) **166,** 150

[455] Zwaifler N.J. & Becker E.L. (1966) Rabbit anaphylactic antibody *J. Exp. Med.* **123,** 935

[456] Normansell D.E. & Stanworth D.R. (1966) Ultracentrifugal studies of the reactions of rheumatical factor with native human γG globulin. *Immunol.* **10,** 527

CHAPTER 8

Genetic Studies on γ Globulin with Particular Reference to Man

SYLVIA D. LAWLER

Introduction

The existence of genetically determined differences in human and rabbit γ globulins has been known for the past 10 years. In 1961 the investigators then working on man agreed on a nomenclature [1], and in 1962, those interested in rabbits did the same [2]. The genetics of human γ globulin is continuing to unfold in such a way that semantic difficulties are still a problem. The general term for these γ globulin differences is allotypy. Allotypic specificity is not the same for all the normal members of one species.

The allotypes in rabbits are determined by precipitation in agar gel using the serum of immunized rabbits. The differences are determined by genes at two independent loci *a* and *b* and at least three alleles are involved at each locus. By use of a similar method γ globulin allotypes have also been discovered in the mouse, guinea-pig, and baboon [3]. It is likely that genetic polymorphism is a feature of the γ globulin of all species.

Antisera used in the determination of allotypes in laboratory animals have usually been obtained by immunization with antigen–antibody complexes. One animal is immunized with *Proteus vulgaris* (× 19) to make antibacterial antibody. This antibody is used to coat *Proteus vulgaris* which is then injected into another animal in which the antibody with allotypic specificity is to be prepared. Some workers have reported successful immunizations in rabbits [4], and in mice [5], using serum with Freund's adjuvant.

Discovery of the Gm groups

In man, however, the γ globulin groups are determined by a method involving the inhibition of the agglutination of antibody-coated cells. The discovery of the groups was made by Grubb in 1956 [6] when he observed that 'In the determination of the amount of γ globulin in sera from six patients with hypogammaglobulinaemia by inhibition of the agglutinating effect of Coombs's reagent it was observed that one of the sera diluted up to 1/20 in saline agglutinated the red cells coated with "incomplete" anti-Rh used in this procedure'. The serum that agglutinated the cells was taken from an Rh-positive boy with acquired hypogammaglobulinaemia, and it did not contain anti-Rh. This observation led Grubb to test other sera for this capacity to agglutinate sensitized cells. The results he then observed are shown in Table 8.1.

Grubb distinguished two types of agglutinating sera, a rheumatoid arthritic type and a non-rheumatoid arthritic type. *The rheumatoid arthritic type* of agglutination could be inhibited by pooled γ globulin and by the serum of about 60 per cent of normal individuals. On the other hand in the *non-rheumatoid arthritic type* the agglutinates were less firm but the reaction could not be inhibited by pooled γ globulin.

At about the same time the agglutination of red cells coated with antibody by certain human sera was also observed in other laboratories [7, 8].

TABLE 8.1

	Healthy persons	Miscellaneous diseases	Rheumatoid arthritis
Number tested	333	291	51
Number of sera agglutinating coated cells only	1	13	8
Percentage	0·3	4·5	15·7

Frequency of agglutinating factors in the serum of sick or healthy people taken from Grubb [6].

The observation that normal human sera could be divided into two types, those that did and those that did not inhibit agglutination of coated red cells by rheumatoid arthritic sera showed the existence of human γ globulin groups. Exploring the possibility further Grubb & Laurell [9] showed that the inhibitor was in the γ globulin fraction. They designated the inhibitory sera Gm(a+) and the non-inhibitory Gm(a−) and found that the two types were distributed in the Swedish population thus: Gm(a+) 59·7 per cent and Gm(a−) 40·3 per cent. In family studies they established the hereditary nature of the groups and found that the data fitted the theory of unfactorial inheritance and that the character was independent of sex and certain blood groups. The frequency of the Gm(a+) phenotype among Eskimos was found to be 95 per cent. Thus in the original papers the foundations were laid for further study of the groups from the serological and genetical points of view.

The genetics of the serum groups

After the discovery of the Gm(a) factor the evidence that it was controlled by a gene expressed in the heterozygote was confirmed by many workers [10, 11, 12]. These studies demonstrated that the Gm(a) factor is not associated with

TABLE 8.2

Gm and Inv factors

Gm(a)	Grubb 1956 [6]
Gm(b)	Harboe 1959 [13]
Gm(x)	Harboe & Lundevall 1959 [14]
Gm-like = c	Steinberg *et al* 1960 [20]
Gm(r)	Brandtzaeg *et al* 1961 [16]
Gm(e)	Ropartz *et al* 1962 [23]
Gm(p)	Waller *et al* 1963 [37]
Inv(a)	Ropartz *et al* 1961 [24]
Inv(b)	Steinberg *et al* 1962 [25]
Inv(1)	Ropartz *et al* 1962 [23]

the following blood groups, ABO, MNS, Rh, P, Le, K, Lu, or Fy or with the haptoglobin locus.

In the next few years additional Gm factors and another locus determining γ globulin allotypes were described and these are listed in Table 8.2.

TABLE 8.3

Common Gm phenotypes in Caucasian populations

Phenotype	Possible genotype
Gm(a+b−x+)	Gm^{ax}/Gm^{ax} or Gm^{ax}/Gm^{a}
Gm(a+b−x−)	Gm^{a}/Gm^{a}
Gm(a+b+x+)	Gm^{ax}/Gm^{b}
Gm(a+b+x−)	Gm^{a}/Gm^{b}
Gm(a−b+x−)	Gm^{b}/Gm^{b}

In 1959 two new factors within the Gm system were discovered in Norway [13, 14]. One of these factors Gm(b) appeared to be determined by an allele of Gm(a), the other Gm(x) was associated with Gm(a), Gm(a+) individuals being of two types either (x+) or (x−). Thus Gm(x) could be fitted within the Gm locus by postulating a third allele Gm^{ax}. The common phenotypes in Caucasian populations are given in Table 8.3.

The gene frequencies in the United Kingdom are $Gm^a 0.270$ $Gmax$ 0.115 Gm^b 0.615 [15]. The frequency of the different phenotypes in various populations of Western Europe does vary but only within narrow limits.

The Gm(r) factor, discovered in 1961 [16], occurs in association with Gm(a) in Europeans. Of 413 individuals who were Gm(a+) 90 per cent were Gm(r+) whilst no Gm(a−) individuals were found to be Gm(r+). The relationship to Gm(x) was not defined precisely but all 44 Gm(x+) individuals were Gm (r+).

When Negroid populations came to be investigated it was found that, in the absence of white admixture, everyone typed Gm(a+b+) and consequently two parents both of this phenotype always produced children who, if Caucasian, would have been classified as heterozygotes. These results fitted within the *Gm* system by postulating an additional allele at the locus, Gm^{ab}, which is capable of producing both Gm(a) and Gm(b) substances [17, 18, 19].

It was thus at an early stage in the development of the subject that the great importance of studying different populations became apparent.

In 1960 yet another Gm factor was discovered and named Gm-like [20]. The original studies of the factor did not enable the authors to be certain about its genetic control because the factor was discovered in Negroes, and since almost all of them are Gm(a+b+x−) it was not possible to find segregating families. In later studies [21] evidence was obtained that Gm-like in Negroes may be determined by an allele Gm^{abc} at the Gm locus which determines the factors Gm(a) (b) and like. Although the Gm-like factor had never previously been detected in Caucasians a white woman permanently resident in England has formed an incomplete anti-D antibody that can be used for the detection of the Gm-like factor [22]. Several members of the family were shown to be Gm-like positive but the factor, although similar to, was not identical with the one found in Negroes.

Gm(e)—this is a factor, related to Gm(b), more frequent in Caucasians than in Negroes, the discovery of which first indicated the complexity of the Gm(b) antigens [22].

Gm(p)—this factor, described in 1963 [37], is much commoner in Caucasians (86·8 per cent positive) than in Negroes (39·9 per cent positive). It appears to be independent of Inv(a), Gm(a) (x) and (c) but insufficient data were available to define its relationship to Gm(b). Data from family studies were compatible with the inheritance being controlled by a gene expressed in the heterozygote.

Rare alleles

A few families have been described in Caucasians which do not fit the simple interpretation of allelic inheritance of Gm(a) and Gm(b) but they could be explained by postulating an allele negative for both Gm(a) and Gm(b), Gm−. Three such families have been investigated which where related to each other so that it is likely that the identical silent allele was present in each of the families [27].

The combination Gm(a−x+) undoubtedly exists in Caucasians implying the existence of an allele Gm^{bx} [28, 29].

The Inv system

The Inv system is inherited independently of the Gm system and three factors belonging to it have been recognized. These are Inv(a) [23], Inv(b) [24] and Inv(1) [22]. Family studies [23, 24, 25] fit the theory of a tri-allelic system, Inv^1, Inv^{1a} and Inv^b. The phenotypes distinguishable when all the reagents

TABLE 8.4

The Inv system

Phenotypes
Inv(1+a+b+)
Inv(1+a−b+)
Inv(1+a+b−)
Inv(1+a−b−)
Inv(1−a−b+)

are available are shown in Table 8.4. The phenotype Inv(1−a+) has never been observed and the frequency of Inv(1+a−) is less than 1 per cent.

Population studies

The sera for determining the Inv factors are not so plentiful as those for the Gm system, so fewer population studies have been made. In Europe, however, it is known that the Inv(a+) phenotype has a frequency ranging between 11 and 20 per cent [30, 31]. In Negroid populations the frequency of Inv(a+) individuals is higher—about 48 per cent.

Population studies of the distribution of the Gm(a+) factors have been extensive. The frequency of Gm(a+) individuals in Western Europe varies between 38 per cent in the Ferrara district of Italy [32] and 67 per cent in Lapland [33]. On the other hand almost all non-white populations so far tested have been, with a few exceptions, 100 per cent Gm(a+). The Gm^{ax} allele is present in Whites, American Indians, Japanese and Chinese and Australian aborigines but it is generally agreed to be absent in Negro populations in which there has been no white admixture. The Gm-like factor,

Gm(c), is characteristic of Negroes. A good review of the racial distribution has been given by Steinberg [34].

The Gm(b) factor

It is the Gm(b) factor that is the most complex and the interpretation of the genetic control of this factor has given rise to some interesting arguments [35].

It is only in Caucasian populations that the presence of Gm(a) and Gm(b) substances appears to be controlled by allelic genes. In all other populations except in Australian aborigines from the Western Desert where Gm(b) appears to be absent[34], if there is a single Gm locus, Gm(b) is produced by an allele that also produces Gm(a). As more investigations have been made it has become apparent that there is a diversity in the expression of the Gm(b) factor which, on an allelic hypothesis, is produced by the following alleles: Gm^b in Caucasoids, Gm^{ab} or Gm^{abc} in Negroids and in other races different Gm^{ab} alleles.

Using seven different anti-Gm(b) antisera for the detection of Gm(b), that gave identical reactions in all but two French Gm(b+) individuals, evidence was obtained [35] of three different patterns of reaction amongst Japanese, and the factors were defined as Gm(bα), Gm(bβ) and Gm(bγ).

Steinberg & Goldblum [36] have suggested the following system of nomenclature for the Gm(b) factor:

Gm(b¹) = original Gm(b) factor described in Whites.
Gm(b²) = Gm(b) present in Whites but absent in Negroes. This factor was originally designated by Steinberg & Wilson as Gm(b^w) [21].
Gm(b³) = ⎫
Gm(b⁴) = ⎬ Factors present in Whites but absent in some Negroes.

The commoner Gm(b) alleles and their antigenic products in this scheme are as follows:

Gm^b	1, 2, 3, 4
Gm^{ab} (Negroes)	{ 1, 3, 4 { 1, 4
Gm^{abc} (Negroes)	1
Gm^{ab} (Mongoloids)	1, 2, 3, 4
$Gm^{ab(3)}$	3

The scheme is shown in detail in Table 8.5 which is taken from Steinberg & Goldblum [36].

Three reports of a new genetic determinant Gm(f) have been made [38, 39, 40]. Kunkel *et al* [39] have suggested that the Gm(f) factor is controlled by genes at a different locus from the other Gm factors. The question has recently been raised by Steinberg [41] 'is Gm(f) the same as Gm(b²)' in which case, of course, only a single Gm locus is required. In order to discuss the arguments about the relationship of Gm(f) to the other Gm factors it is necessary to deal next with the distribution of Gm substances throughout the γ globulin molecule.

Distribution of the allotypic substances in the γ globulin molecule

The terminology used for the immunoglobulins in this section was published in the *Bulletin of the World Health Organization* (vol. 30, page 447), by a representative group of workers. This new nomenclature has been presented and discussed by Cohen [42].

TABLE 8.5

Reactions of the more common alleles in Negroids, Mongoloids and Caucasoids with the Gm(b) antibodies and a suggested nomenclature

	Allele		Antibody	Draves	Da	Th	Bu
Race	Current terminology	Suggested terminology	Antigen detected	$Gm(b^1)$	$Gm(b^2)$	$Gm(b^3)$	$Gm(b^4)$
Negroid	Gm^{ab}	$Gm^{ab(1, 3, 4)}$		+	−	+	+
	Gm^{ab}	$Gm^{ab(1, 4)}$		+	−	−	+
	Gm^{abc}	$Gm^{ab(1)c}$		+	−	−	−
Mongoloid	Gm^a	Gm^a		−	−	−	−
	Gm^a	$Gm^{ab(3)}$		−	−	+	−
	Gm^{ax}	Gm^{ax}		−	−	−	−
	Gm^{ab}	$Gm^{ab(1, 2, 3, 4)}$		+	+	+	+
Caucasoid	Gm^a	Gm^a		−	−	−	−
	Gm^{ax}	Gm^{ax}		−	−	−	−
	Gm^b	$Gm^{b(1, 2, 3, 4)}$		+	+	+	+

Steinberg and Goldblum [36]

Studies of the distribution of Gm and Inv factors throughout the immunoglobulins have shown that Gm specificity is confined to IgG [43] and that Inv factors are present in IgG, IgA and IgM [44, 45]. When human γ globulin is split by digestion with papain by the method of Porter [68], Gm(a) and (b) specificity is detected in the Fc (fast) fragment whilst the Fab (slow) fragment carries the Inv antigens [44, 46].

By reduction of disulphide bonds γ globulin can be separated into two types of chains, heavy and light [47]. The international group have suggested that the heavy chains of the three classes of immunoglobulins should be designated γ, α and μ. When human γ globulin is separated into chains by the method of the Fleishman *et al* [48], Gm(a) and (b) activity is retained by the heavy chain and Inv activity by the light [49]. In the rabbit the Fc fragment consists of heavy chains [48] and so this is in accordance with the presence of Gm activity in the Fc fragment and the heavy chains in man.

The model proposed for the structure of IgG immunoglobulin by Porter [50], and the distribution of Gm and Inv factors is shown in Fig. 8.1.

According to this model the IgG molecule is composed of two heavy and two light chains. When the molecule is split by papain digestion the Fc fragment is composed of part of the A chains, and the Fab fragment consists of

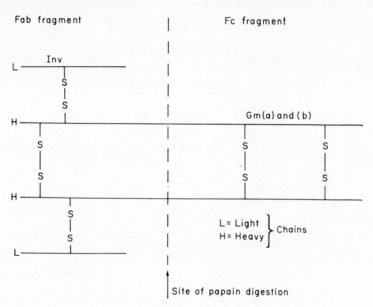

FIG. 8.1. Diagrammatic structure of IgG (Porter [50]) showing the location of Gm(a), (b) and Inv specificities.

the other part of the heavy chains and the two light chains, that part of the A chain in the Fab fragment is the Fd fragment.

Myeloma proteins and macroglobulins

Large amounts of protein may be produced by tumours of the plasma cell series having, in different tumours, the properties of IgG, IgA or IgM. The proteins produced by these tumours are usually homogeneous in marked contrast to the heterogeneity of normal γ globulin. These proteins can be readily purified thus yielding adequate amounts for study. Studies on such proteins have confirmed that Gm sites are present only in IgG, because purified A-myeloma or M-macroglobulin does not carry Gm specificity [43, 45, 51].

The Inv antigens on the other hand have been detected on A-myeloma, M-macroglobulin and on Bence-Jones proteins [44, 45].

The consensus of opinion now is that G-myeloma proteins even in a Gm (a + b +) individual, produce either Gm(a) or Gm(b) or neither but not both. Myeloma proteins probably correspond to an individual normal protein and presumably are formed by a single clone of cells.

Up to this point wherever Gm(b) activity has been mentioned reference has been made to the original Gm(b) factor of Harboe, Gm(b^1) according to Steinberg. The Gm(b^2) factor differs from all other Gm factors in that it is present on the Fab fragment of papain split γ globulin, and it cannot be detected on isolated heavy or light chains. If the heavy and light chains are recombined then the Gm(b^2) activity is restored [52]. These observations have led Polmar & Steinberg [52] to postulate that the Gm(b) antigen depends on quaternary structure of γ globulin. Similarly Gm(f) activity has been recovered in the Fab fragment [53].

On genetical and serological grounds Steinberg [41], has argued that the more recently described Gm(f) factor represents a rediscovery of Gm(b^2). He based this view on tests of 255 serum samples from people of different ethnic groups. All the tests gave concordant results.

The possibility exists that Gm(p) is also the same as Gm(f) and (b^2) because myeloma proteins having both activities have been described. On the other hand Gm(p) activity is recoverable in the Fc fragment like other Gm determinants whereas Gm(f) is unique in being present on Fab fragments. Gm(p) is undoubtedly a factor within the Gm(b) mosaic of antigens. Similarly it is not possible in the present state of knowledge to assess the relationship of the Gm(e) factor to the other antigens included in the Gm(b) complex.

Märtensson [40] has examined a number of myeloma proteins and found that such proteins if active show only a single Gm specificity Gm(a), Gm(b) or Gm(f). Kunkel et al [34] found that G-myeloma proteins can be divided into four groups using antibodies prepared against γ H chains. All Gm(f +) or (a +) proteins give positive reactions with one of the antibodies (anti-We), and all the (b +) with another (anti-Vi). Kunkel et al postulate that this could be explained by an allelic relationship between Gm^a and Gm^f at the We locus, and a closely linked locus Vi for Gm^b and hitherto unidentified alleles. On this hypothesis the genetic situation of the Gm locus is beginning to rival that of Rh in complexity. Countering these arguments and defending the single locus hypothesis Steinberg [41] has pointed out that a possible explanation may be that a Gm(b^1) cannot be formed in the absence of the Vi antigenic site and that the We antigenic site may be necessary for Gm(a) and (b^2). There are certain parallels for such a situation in the human blood groups. Another similar situation may be operating in light chain synthesis. Separated light chains from Bence-Jones proteins can be classified into two types formerly named Type 1 and Type 2, now K and L, and Inv activity is found, rarely if ever, in Type L and frequently in Type K [41]. The conflict over the number of loci involved in the control of the synthesis of Gm substances may ultimately be resolved by further biochemical and family studies.

Biochemical basis of allotypy

In an attempt to define the structural basis for allotypic differences Fudenberg *et al* [54] have made peptide maps of tryptic hydrolysates of Fc fragments of normal IgG. A single peptide present in Gm(a+) H chains and Fc fragments was not found in corresponding preparations from Gm(a−) individuals. The possibility therefore exists that the serological differences in the Gm system may reflect the substitution of but a single amino acid.

Gm groups and transfusion

In the early stages of work on these groups, although the tests were based on standard immunological inhibition technique, some doubt existed as to whether the Gm–anti-Gm reactions were classical antigen–antibody reactions. The anti-Gm agglutinators which originally were found only in patients with rheumatoid arthritis and certain other diseases were therefore referred to as 'reagins'. The evidence against the immunologic nature of the reactions was as follows:

(1) Clinically, there was no reaction when γ globulin of a particular group was transfused into a patient who had the appropriate anti-Gm agglutinator [55], or when rheumatoid factor was given to normal subjects [56].

(2) The survival time of γ globulin in subjects with anti-Gm reagents was the same as in normal subjects [55].

Evidence has now accumulated that the Gm factors are in fact antigenic. The anti-Gm agglutinators have been shown to have the physical and chemical properties of an immunoglobulin, and in the majority of cases the Gm agglutinator is iso-specific and not auto-specific [57, 58]. It has also become apparent that Gm agglutinators may appear in the sera of people who have had multiple transfusions. For example, Allen & Kunkel [59] described their findings in 24 children all of whom had had at least three transfusions. The serum of 17 of these children contained agglutinating substances active against Gm factors not present in their own serum. Each of these agglutinators was active against a single Gm factor and proved to be a useful reagent for typing. Similarly Vierucci [60] in studying 73 children with Cooley's anaemia some of whom required frequent transfusions, found Gm(a) (b) or (x) agglutinators in 43 per cent. The frequency of the occurrence of these anti-Gm substances was proportional to the number of transfusions received. Experimental transfusion of blood of incompatible Gm type did not produce any reaction in four patients with anti-Gm in the serum. Substances with anti-Inv(a) specificity were looked for but not found by Allen & Kunkel [59].

It is therefore difficult to escape the conclusion that these Gm agglutinators have been produced by immunization of the recipient against foreign Gm substances in the donor's serum.

By a very interesting family study Fudenberg & Fudenberg [61] have managed to show that Gm factors can be responsible for iso-immunization during pregnancy. Serum samples from the mother of four children were tested for agglutinators during each pregnancy. During and after these pregnancies resulting in a Gm(a−) infant no anti-Gm activity was detected in the serum. However anti-Gm(a) activity became detectable at the beginning of third trimester of the fourth pregnancy; subsequently this activity disappeared, and the infant when tested at the age of 3 months proved to be Gm(a+). This case demonstrates that a foetus can synthesize γ globulin by the seventh month of gestation and that such γ globulin can immunize a mother against Gm factors that she herself lacks.

So that it now has to be accepted that Gm factors are immunogenic. The argument used formerly that anti-Gm activity is only found in patients with rheumatoid arthritis is no longer tenable not only because of these demonstrations of its formation after transfusion. In 1959 Grubb [33] had already commented that sera with anti-Gm activity could be found with a frequency of about 1/2000 in normal people. Ropartz *et al* [62] screened 12,000 blood donors living in the area of Seine-Maritime, France, and found 9 anti-Gm(a) sera and 1 anti-Gm(x) and pointed out certain serological differences between these Ragg (rheumatoid agglutinator) and SNagg (serum-normal agglutinator) sera.

Steinberg & Wilson [63] examined the mothers of the donors of SNagg sera. In eight such cases the donors, who had not been transfused, lacked the factor for which they had the agglutinator whereas their mothers were positive for this factor. These observations invite the conclusion that the donors had been immunized by the maternal γ globulin, and thus that intra-uterine exposure to Gm antigens does not produce immune tolerance.

Techniques for determining γ globulin factors

The principles of the methods used are as follows. Gamma globulin of the appropriate type is fixed on to human red cells. These cells are then capable of being agglutinated by the corresponding anti-Gm agglutinator. This agglutination reaction can be inhibited by normal human serum which

M

contains the Gm factor under test. The method is represented schematically in Table 8.6.

Choice of red cells

In Gm testing the red cell acts as a passive carrier of γ globulin of the appropriate type. Therefore if anti-D antibodies are being used any group O Rh-positive cells can be chosen provided that they can be coated with an adequate amount of γ globulin. It is known that Rh-positive red cells of different genotypes vary in the number of their antigenic sites and that a greater amount of anti-D is taken up by homozygous than by heterozygous cells [64]. Among the Rh genotypes the R_2R_2 (cDE/cDE) red cell has a more powerful D antigen than any other cell apart from those of rare donors who are heterozygous or homozygous for the –D– complex. Most workers therefore choose to

TABLE 8.6

Testing for the Gm(a) factor

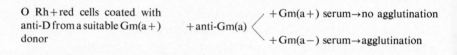

| O Rh+red cells coated with anti-D from a suitable Gm(a+) donor | +anti-Gm(a) | +Gm(a+) serum→no agglutination |
| | | +Gm(a−) serum→agglutination |

work with a readily available 'homozygous' cell. R_1R_1 (cDE/cDE) or R_1R_2 (CDe/cDE), the most suitable red cell for a particular Gm system, usually has to be worked out by trial and error.

Selection of anti-Rh sera

The Rh antibody provides a source of γ globulin of appropriate type. The specificity of the antibody is really of no consequence but most people work with anti-D antibodies because they are sufficiently strong to coat the red cells adequately for the test. Antibodies with specificities other than anti-D can be used if they are sufficiently potent [65]. To be useful for Gm typing an antibody must be active by the routine Indirect Coombs Test at a titre of at least 1/64, and its content of saline agglutinin should be negligible. The serum of the donor of the anti-D must contain the appropriate factor in the test system. For example, in testing for the Gm(a) factor the anti-D's must come from donors of the Gm type Gm(a+). Although anti-D from a Gm(a+b+) donor may well fix Gm(a) or Gm(b) factors to the red cells the best results are usually obtained with antibodies from Gm(a+b−) donors for Gm(a) typing and from Gm(a−b+) donors for Gm(b) typing. In the case of testing for the Gm(x) factor the antibody used comes from a Gm(a+x+) donor because only in rare instances does Gm(x) occur in the absence of Gm(a). The fact that an anti-D antibody has a high titre and is of the appropriate type does not necessarily mean that it will be a useful antibody in the test system. A particular antibody may be useful with some anti-Gm reagents but not with others. Sometimes an anti-D serum can be used successfully for typing for more than one Gm factor.

The amount of antibody used for coating the cells depends on the strength of all the reagents in the system. For testing for Gm(a), (b) and (x) factors, for which there is no particular difficulty in finding suitable reagents most people work with proportions of the order of: 1 vol. of packed cells, 1 vol. of anti-D to 10 vols. of saline.

It is difficult to give exact figures for the chance of finding suitable reagents when screening anti-D sera. The yield of suitable reagents from one series of anti-D sera sent to my laboratory by the late Dr Ivor Dunsford is shown in Table 8.7.

TABLE 8.7

Screening for suitable reagents for Gm typing.
No. of anti-D sera screened, 166.
No. of useful reagents:
   Gm(a) 14
   Gm(b) 11
   Gm(x) 3

The agglutinators
As has been said already the earliest work on Gm factors was done using sera from patients with rheumatoid arthritis (Ragg). The successful reagents came from patients who gave high scores in tests used for the detection of the rheumatoid factor and were most reliable when the donor did not carry the Gm factor for which they had the agglutinator. Certain difficulties were encountered in the use of Ragg sera, part of the problem being the frequent occurrence of prozones shown in serial dilutions of Ragg sera when tested against Rh-sensitized cells. Within the Gm system this has been ascribed to the simultaneous occurrence in the same individual of a Gm factor and the corresponding agglutinator. However this cannot be the complete explanation because prozones have been observed within the Gm system even when these conditions do not operate [66].

It is now known that suitable agglutinators for Gm typing can be found in normal sera (Inv reagents are found only in normal sera). The agglutinators in normal sera have a certain advantage over Ragg sera. When typing is done with Ragg sera it is quite usual to find inhibition with the normal sera under test if it is used at high concentration. So the difference between positive and negative is a quantitative one. When using SNagg sera there is no non-specific inhibition even with undiluted normal sera [62].

When screening for agglutinators the serum should be tested in serial dilutions against suitable sensitized red cells. If there is an agglutination then one or two dilutions of the agglutinator are selected and these are then tested against serial dilutions of serum of known Gm and Inv type to see whether the agglutination can be specifically inhibited. Only if the results are satisfactory with a panel of normal sera of known type can the reagents be regarded as suitable for typing.

The actual technique for performing the inhibition test varies in different laboratories, but when giving results of Gm and Inv tests the workers always state the quantities of anti-D used for cell sensitization, the dilution(s) of the agglutinator, and the dilutions of the sera being typed. The sensitized cells must always be washed (3 times) and tested with Coombs's reagent before use.

Methods

(1) In the original method described by Grubb & Laurell in 1956 [9] the tests are run in round-bottomed tubes 80 mm by 8 mm (Kahn Tubes) using:

0·12 ml in serial dilution of the serum being tested;
0·12 ml of suitably diluted agglutinator is added to each tube.

This mixture is left to stand on the bench for 15 minutes. The following controls are required:

(a) 0·12 ml Ragg serum diluted as above +0·12 ml normal saline;
(b) 0·12 ml of each serum under test diluted 1/4+0·12 ml normal saline;*
(c) 0·25 ml normal saline.

To each tube is then added 0·25 ml of a 0·4 per cent suspension of sensitized red cells. The tubes should be left to stand at room temperature for 4–6 hours. The results are read by looking at the pattern of the settled cells with the naked eye before and after gentle shaking (sometimes a concave mirror may be found useful for reading the patterns).

This method has the disadvantage of taking a long time and it is sometimes difficult to distinguish between weak agglutination and a negative result.

(2) Harboe & Lundevall [14] prefer to use carefully cleaned glass slides 25×6 cm on which rings have been made with paraffin wax. One drop of diluted Ragg serum is mixed with one drop of a serial dilution of normal serum. This mixture is kept at room temperature and then one drop of a suspension of sensitized red cells is added. Appropriate controls are included

* Phosphate buffered saline was used by Grubb & Laurell [9], this is not essential.

(see (1)). The slides are agitated slowly for 5 minutes, left undisturbed, and placed in a moist chamber. The results are read under the low power of a microscope.

(3) An improvement of method (2), since making paraffin rings is obviously tedious, is recommended by Steinberg [34].

The test is done in a depression of a glass micro-flocculation test slide. One drop of normal serum to be typed is mixed with one drop of appropriately diluted Ragg or SNagg serum. The mixture is shaken at 60 rev/min for about 5 minutes. One drop of 0·3 per cent suspension of sensitized cells is added to the mixture which is then placed in a moist chamber at room temperature for about 45 minutes. The mixture is again shaken for about 5 minutes and the reaction read at 45, 90 or 120 × under a dissecting binocular microscope.

(4) Podliachouk *et al* [67] have described their method which is essentially the same as (3). The serum to be tested is diluted in tubes. One drop of each dilution is mixed, by a circular movement, with one drop of the selected dilution of the appropriate agglutinator in a depression of a slide made of 'plexiglas'. After 20 minutes at bench temperature one drop of a suitable suspension of red cells is added 0·5 per cent for Gm(a), (b) and (x). The contents of the depressions are mixed well by a circular movement of the slide which is then covered by aluminium to prevent evaporation. The readings are made 10–20 minutes later by observing, with the naked eye, the appearance of the red cells when the slide is gently tilted. The experiment is controlled as in (1).

(5) Ropartz & Lenoir [69] give the details of their method which is similar to (3) and (4).

The reactions are set up on plastic tiles and incubated at room temperature, in a moist chamber. (The tile is covered by a damp cloth and the cloth is prevented from touching the cell suspensions by a plastic grid.) The readings are made half an hour after adding the sensitized cells and the tile is rocked.

(6) Märtensson [40] describes a tube method in which the tubes are spun before reading.

0·06 ml of the sample to be tested, 0·03 ml of a suitably diluted agglutinator and 0·03 ml of a 2 per cent suspension of sensitized cells are mixed in round-bottomed test tubes. After standing for 1 hour at room temperature the tubes are centrifuged for 45 seconds and then read immediately for agglutination with the naked eye. The washing fluid is isotonic phosphate-buffered NaCl (pH 7·2). Conventional controls are included.

(7) Disagglutination (Lawler [12]). This method depends on the fact that the reaction between sensitized cells and anti-Gm is reversible. Suitably sensitized Rh + ve cells are agglutinated on a white porcelain blood grouping tile. The sera to be typed are added in serial dilution to the agglutinated cells, the mixture is stirred, the tile is rocked. If the serum being tested contains the

factor being tested for, the agglutinates disperse, but if it does not the agglutinates reappear. The test is controlled by including sera of known type, positive and negative, by testing each serum diluted 1/4 against the sensitized cells to make sure that the individual being tested does not have an agglutinator, and by observing the sensitized cells in saline only.

This method gives reliable results but the reagents have to be potent because the addition of agglutinator to sensitized cells must produce clumps that are clearly visible to the naked eye otherwise it is pointless to proceed to the second part of the test. The advantages of disagglutination are, it is reasonably economical in the amounts of reagents required, it is very simple, and many observations can be made simultaneously. Its disadvantages are that it is not so sensitive as the tube method. It can be used for Gm(a) (b) (x) (c) and Inv (a) typing but thus far not for Inv(b) typing.

The methods in use in various laboratories in 1960 have been documented by Ropartz [70].

Gm typing of blood stains

The successful typing of dried blood stains for Gm factors has been reported. Nielsen & Henningsen [71] recorded correct typing of experimental stains on linen, nylon, cotton, silk and wool. The Gm grouping was performed by making eluates of the stains and testing titrations of these for Gm(a) (b) and (x) activity using Ragg agglutinators. If the stains were kept dry there was no deterioration up to 11 weeks. If the fabrics were kept in a moist chamber the Gm activity deteriorated. Control experiments on unstained fabrics are obviously essential. Duços *et al* [72] recommend placing the stained material in direct contact with suitably diluted Gm agglutinator, and testing the serum for agglutinating activity before and after absorption. These workers found that they could test stains that were at least 10 years old but that with such old stains SNagg agglutinators were preferable to Ragg. Both methods work well with fresh stains taken under experimental conditions.

The Gm groups are not generally used in forensic medicine. As far as blood stains are concerned it is clear that much work will have to be done on stains on different materials, taken and kept under varying conditions before the results can be reliable enough for application in particular cases. Another difficulty for forensic laboratories is to obtain adequate supplies of reliable reagents.

For this reason and also because of the complicated genetical situation at the Gm locus these groups have not been generally applied to cases of disputed paternity in the United Kingdom.

The use of animal sera for Gm typing

Antibodies with anti-Gm specificity can be produced by immunizing Rhesus monkeys with human γ globulin [73, 74]. In response to immunization with pooled γ globulin Gm(a) and Gm(b) specificity can be detected—and anti-Gm(c) may be produced [74]. Since the anti-D reagents in current usage for detecting the Gm(x) factor also fix Gm(a) to the red cells it has not been possible to decide whether Rhesus monkeys can produce anti-Gm(x).

In an experiment in which two Rhesus monkeys were immunized with purified IgG from a Gm(a + b − x −) donor and another three with Gm(a − b + x −) IgG, one of the animals produced an anti-Gm(a) which has proved useful as an accessory typing reagent. No satisfactory anti-Gm(b) reagents were obtained [89].

Although attempts have been made nobody has yet succeeded in producing antibodies for detecting the antigens determined by the Inv locus in experimental animals [73, 74, 31].

Gm groups and rheumatoid arthritis

In view of the fact that the rheumatoid factor is associated with the presence of anti-Gm agglutinators, it is pertinent to enquire what relationship there is between rheumatoid arthritis and the Gm groups. Various workers have studied the distribution of Gm types in patients with rheumatoid arthritis. The conclusion reached is that the distribution of Gm phenotypes does not differ significantly from that in normal controls drawn from the population of which the patient is a member. Earlier studies were confined to the estimation of the Gm(a +) phenotype [75, 76, 66, 77, 67, 78, 79]. The distribution of Gm(a) (b) and (x) has been studied by Deicher & Schupp [80] and of Gm(a) (b) and (c) by Podliachouk *et al* [81]. There is a single conflicting report of a higher incidence of the Gm(a +) phenotype amongst patients with rheumatoid arthritis than in normal controls [82].

Part of the problem lies in the difficulty of typing sera containing an agglutinator. One way of destroying the agglutinating factors is to heat the diluted serum (1/4) at 63° C for 10 minutes. The serum should be diluted because changes in Gm phenotype have been observed when normal serum is heated undiluted to 63° C for half an hour and then tested with Ragg agglutinators [83]. An alternative method of typing rheumatoid sera is to prepare the euglobulin fraction by the method of Svartz & Schlossmann [84] and to separate the supernatant by centrifugation, put it in dialysis tubing and to allow it to concentrate by drying in a jet of air. This fraction, 'pseudoglobulin', contains all the protein not precipitated in the euglobulin fraction and can be used for Gm typing. Tests in parallel on this fraction and on sera, previously heated at a dilution of $\frac{1}{4}$, gave identical results with 32 sera [85]. The euglobulin fraction can be used to test for agglutination activity.

Application of the Gm and Inv groups to linkage and gene localization studies

The Gm and Inv loci provide genetic markers for classical linkage studies. From this point of view the Gm(a) and (b) factors are most informative in Caucasian families, and Negroid families can give more information on the Inv system because of a more favourable distribution of the phenotypes. To be maximally useful for a linkage investigation the frequency of alleles in a two-allelic system not showing dominance need to be approximately equal. Systems like Inv, for example, where the frequency of the Inv $(1+a+b+)$ individual in Caucasians is only of the order of 11 per cent require the collection of a large number of families because most of them will consist of parents each of whom is Inv$(1-a-b+)$. Family studies that have already been made indicate that the Gm locus is not within measurable distance of the loci for: ABO, MNS, Rh, P, Kell, Duffy, Haptoglobin, Inv and red cell acid phosphatase [11, 25, 32, 86, 87].

The Gm and Inv groups can also be part of the battery of characters that may be applied to the problem of gene localization by use in families showing chromosomal anomalies. In a family in which certain members carried a translocation chromosome made up of a large and a small acrocentric chromosome (D (13–15) and G (21–22Y) group chromosome), Zergollen *et al* [88] have obtained evidence to suggest linkage with the Gm group. This means that the possibility exists that the Gm locus is carried on one of the chromosomes that fused to form the translocation chromosome.

Summary

Allotypy is probably a property of many species. In man individual genetically determined differences in γ globulin are detected by a serological method involving the inhibition of the agglutination of antibody-coated human red cells. The agglutinators are found in the serum of patients with rheumatoid arthritis (Ragg) and rarely in the serum of normal donors (SNagg). Agglutinators may appear in the serum of patients who have had multiple transfusions. In the unravelling of the genetic control of the groups anthropological and biochemical studies have been of importance. The inheritance of the Gm system can be interpreted on the basis of a single locus with multiple alleles. Recent immunochemical evidence suggests that more than one genetic site may be involved in the Gm system. The Inv system is inherited independently of the Gm system, there being a single locus with at least three alleles. When IgG is split by papain, Gm(a) and (b) activity is recovered in the Fc fragment and Inv in the Fab fragment. Inv is expressed in all classes of immunoglobulin,

Gm only in IgG. When IgG is separated into heavy and light chains Gm(a) and (b) specificity is present in the heavy chains and Inv in the light.

Addendum

Since this chapter was completed several new discoveries about the Gm system have been made. The immunochemical evidence supports the contention that the Gm factors are controlled by at least two, possibly three, genetic sites, defining a site as a segment of a DNA molecule determining one polypeptide chain. These sites may residue within the boundaries of a single classical gene defined as a unit of hereditary material. The integration of the biochemical and genetical studies of the Gm groups is well discussed by Martensson, L. in 'Genes and immunoglobulins', Editorial, *Vox Sang.* (1966), **11**, 521–545.

A standard nomenclature for Gm and Inv factors has been suggested (*Bull. Wld. Hlth. Org.* (1964) **30**, 447–450). It is shown below:

TABLE 8.8

Notation for the factors at the Gm locus

Original	New
a	1
x	2
b^w and b^2	3
f	4
b and b^1	5
c	6
r	7
e	8
p	9
b^x	10
b^β	11
b^γ	12
b^3	13
b^4	14

Notion for the factors at the Inv locus

Original	New
l	1
a	2
b	3

M*

References

[1] GRUBB R. (1961) A notation for the Gm groups. *Nature, Lond.* **189**, 845–846

[2] DRAY S., DUBISKI S., KELUS A., LENNOX E.S. & OUDIN J. (1962) A notation for allotypy. *Nature, Lond.* **195**, 785–786

[3] KELUS A. & MOOR-JANKOWSKI J.K. (1961) Serum protein antigens of hereditary character. In *Protides of the Biological Fluids*, pp. 193–199, ed. PEETERS H. Amsterdam–New York: Elsevier

[4] DRAY S. & YOUNG, GLENDOWLYN O. (1958) Differences in the antigenic components of sera of individual rabbits as shown by induced isoprecipitins. *J. Immunol.* **81**, 142–149

[5] DUBISKI S. & CINADER B. (1963) A new allotypic specificity in the mouse (MuA₂). *Nature, Lond.* **197**, 705

[6] GRUBB R. (1956) Agglutination of erythrocytes coated with 'incomplete' anti-Rh by certain rheumatoid arthritic sera and some other sera. The existence of human serum groups. *Acta path. microbiol. Scand.* **39**, 195–197

[7] MILGROM F., DUBISKI S. & WOZNICZKO G. (1956) Human sera with 'anti-anti-body'. *Vox Sang.* **1**, 172–183

[8] WALLER, MARION V. & VAUGHAN J.H. (1956) Use of anti-Rh sera for demonstrating agglutination activating factors in rheumatoid arthritis. *Proc. Soc. exp. Biol. Med.* **92**, 198–200

[9] GRUBB R. & LAURELL, ANNA-BRITA (1956) Hereditary serological human serum groups. *Acta path. microbiol. Scand.* **39**, 390–398

[10] MOULLEC J., KHERUMAIN R., SUTTON E. & ESPAGNON P. (1956) Contribution à l'étude du facteur de groupe Gmᵃ du plasma humain. *Rev. Hémat.* **11**, 512–518

[11] LINNET-JEPSON P., GALATIUS-JENSEN F. & HAUGE M. (1958) On the inheritance of the Gm serum group. *Acta Genet.* **8**, 164–196

[12] LAWLER, SYLVIA D. (1960) A genetical study of the Gm groups in human serum. *Immunology* **3**, 90–94

[13] HARBOE M. (1959) A new haemagglutinating substance in the Gm system, anti-Gm. *Nature, Lond.* **183**, 1468–1469

[14] HARBOE M. & LUNDEVALL J. (1959) A new type in the Gm system. *Acta path. microbiol. Scand.* **45**, 357–370

[15] LAWLER, SYLVIA D. & LELE, KUSUM (1961) Some comments on the Gm serum groups. *Proc. 8th Congr. Europ. Soc. Haematol.* No. 220. Karger, Basel–New York, 1962

[16] BRANDTZAEG B., FUDENBERG H. & MOHR J. (1961) The Gm(r) serum group. *Acta Genet.* **11**, 170–177

[17] STEINBERG A.G., STAUFFER, RACHEL & BOYER S.H. (1960) Evidence for a Gmᵃᵇ allele in the Gm system of American Negroes. *Nature, Lond.* **188**, 169–170

[18] ROPARTZ C., RIVAT L. & LENOIR J. (1961) Fréquence des facteurs Gm(a), Gm(b), Gm(x), Gm-like et Inv chez quatre cents noirs Africains. *Rev. Franç. Etudes Clin et Biol.*, **5**, 814–816

[19] BOYER S.H. & WATSON-WILLIAMS E.J. (1961) The γ-globulin, Gmᵃᵇ, in Nigerians. *Nature, Lond.* **190**, 456

[20] STEINBERG A.G., GILES, BRENDA D. & STAUFFER, RACHEL (1960) A Gm-like factor present in Negroes and rare or absent in whites: its relation to Gmᵃ and Gmˣ. *Am. J. Human Genet.* **12**, 44–51

[21] STEINBERG A.G. & WILSON, JANET A. (1963) Studies on hereditary gamma globulin

factors: evidence that Gm(b) in Whites and Negroes is not the same and that Gm-like is determined by an allele at the Gm locus. *Am. J. Human Genet.* **15**, 96–105

[22] STEINBERG A.G., STAUFFER, RACHEL & DUNSFORD I. (1963) Studies on hereditary gamma globulin factors: detection of the factor Gm-like in a white family. *Vox Sang.* **8**, 51–57

[23] ROPARTZ C., RIVAT L. & ROUSSEAU P.Y. (1962) Deux nouveaux facteurs dans les systèmes héréditaires de gamma-globuline: Le Gm(e) et l'Inv(l). *Proc. 9th Congr. Int. Soc. Blood transf., Mexico*, pp. 455–458. Karger, Basel–New York, 1964

[24] ROPARTZ C., LENOIR J. & RIVAT L. (1961) A new heritable property of human sera: The Inv factor. *Nature, Lond.* **189**, 586

[25] STEINBERG A.G., WILSON, JANET A. & LANSET, SUZANNE (1962) A new human gamma globulin factor determined by an allele at the Inv locus. *Vox Sang.* **7**, 151–156

[26] RITTER H., ROPARTZ C., ROUSSEAU P.Y., RIVAT L. & BÄHR M.L. (1964) Zur Formal genetik und Populations genetik des Gammaglobulin— Polymorphismus Inv, Merkmale Inv(l) und Inv(a). *Acta Genet.* **14**, 15–24

[27] STEINBERG A.G. (1962) Evidence for a Gm allele negative for both Gm(a) and Gm(b). *Vox Sang.* **7**, 89–92

[28] HENNINGSEN K. & NIELSEN J.C. (1961) A rare phenotype within the Gm system. *Nature, Lond.* **192**, 476–477

[29] ROPARTZ C., ROUSSEAU P.Y. & RIVAT L. (1962) Un deuxième exemple du phenotype Gm($a-x+$) pouvant confirmer l'hypothèse de l'existence d'un allèle Gm^{bx}. *Vox Sang.* **7**, 375–378

[30] ROPARTZ C., RIVAT L., ROUSSEAU P.Y., BAITSCH H. & VAN LOGHEM J. (1963) Les systèmes Gm et Inv en Europe. *Acta Genet.* **13**, 109–123.

[31] LOPEZ V. & BÜTLER R. (1965) The Inv groups in Switzerland with remarks on the methods of detection. *Vox Sang.* **10**, 314–319

[32] ADINOLFI M., MARONE A., OLIVELLI F., POLOSA P. & SINISCALCO M. (1960) Dati sulla genetica dei gruppi gamma-globulinici nell'Uomo. Atti Accad naz Lincei Rc *Sci. fis. mat. nat.*, **28**, 390–395.

[33] GRUBB R. (1959) Hereditary gamma globulin groups in man. In *Ciba Foundation Symposium on Biochemistry of Human Genetics*, pp. 264–273. London: Churchill Ltd.

[34] STEINBERG A.G. (1962) Progress in the study of genetically determined human gamma globulin. Types (The Gm and Inv groups) In *Progress in Medical Genetics* **2**, 1–33, ed. STEINBERG A.G. & BEARN A.G. New York: Grune & Stratton

[35] ROPARTZ C., RIVAT L. & ROUSSEAU P.Y. (1963) Le Gm(b) et ses problèmes. *Vox Sang.* **8**, 717–723

[36] STEINBERG A.G. & GOLDBLUM R. (1965) A genetic study of the antigens associated with the Gm(b) factor of human gamma globulin. *Am. J. Human Genet.* **17**, 133–147

[37] WALLER, MARION, HUGHES R.D., TOWNSEND J.I., FRANKLIN E.C. & FUDENBERG H. (1963) New serum group, Gm(p). *Science* **142**, 1321–1322

[38] GOLD E.R., MARTENSSON L., ROPARTZ C., RIVAT L. & ROUSSEAU P.Y. (1965) Gm(f)— a determinant of human γ-globulin. Preliminary communication. *Vox Sang.* **10**, 299–302

[39] KUNKEL H.G., ALLEN J.C., GREY H.M., MARTENSSON L. & GRUBB R. (1964) A relationship between the chain groups of 7S γ-globulin and the Gm system. *Nature, Lond.* **203**, 413–414

[40] MARTENSSON L. (1964) On the relationship between the γ-globulin genes of the Gm system. *J. exp. Med.* **120**, 1169

[41] STEINBERG A.G. (1965) Comparison of GM(f) with Gm(b^2) Gm(b^w) and a discussion of their genetics. (In press).

[42] COHEN S. (1965) Editorial. Nomenclature of human immunoglobulins. *Immunology* **8,** 1–5

[43] FAHEY J.L. & LAWLER, SYLVIA D. (1961) Gm factors in normal γ-globulin fractions, myeloma proteins and macroglobulins. *J. nat. Cancer Inst.* **27,** 973–981

[44] FRANKLIN E.C., FUDENBERG H., MELTZER M. & STANWORTH D.R. (1962) The structural basis for genetic variations of normal human γ-globulins. *Proc. nat. Acad. Sci. (Wash.)* **48,** 914–922

[45] HARBOE M., OSTERLAND C.K., MANNIK M. & KUNKEL H.G. (1962) Genetic characters of human γ-globulins in myeloma proteins. *J. exp. Med.* **116,** 719–738

[46] HARBOE M., OSTERLAND C.K. & KUNKEL H.G. (1962) Localization of two genetic factors to different areas of γ-globulin molecules. *Science* **136,** 979–980

[47] EDELMAN G.M. & BENACERRAF B. (1962) On structural and functional relations between antibodies and proteins of the gamma-system. *Proc. nat. Acad. Sci. (Wash.)* **48,** 1035–1042

[48] FLEISCHMAN J.B., PAIN R.H. & PORTER R.R. (1962) Reduction of γ-globulins. *Arch. biochem. Biophys.* **Suppl., 1,** 174–180

[49] LAWLER, SYLVIA D. & COHEN S. (1965) Distribution of allotypic specificities on the peptide chains of human gamma globulin. *Immunology* **8,** 206–212

[50] PORTER R.R. (1962) The structure of γ-globulins and antibodies. In *Basic Problems of Neoplastic Disease*, pp. 177–194, ed. GELLHORN A. & HIRSCHBERG E. Columbia Press, New York University

[51] MARTENSSON L. (1961) Gm characters of M components. *Acta Med. Scand.*, **170,** **Suppl. 367,** 87–93

[52] POLMAR S.H. & STEINBERG A.G. (1964) Dependence of a Gm(b) antigen on the quaternary structure of human gamma globulin. Science **145,** 928–929

[53] KRONVALL G. (1965) Gm(f) activity of human gamma globulin fragments. *Vox Sang.* **10,** 303–313

[54] FUDENBERG H.H., STIEHM E.R., FRANKLIN E.C., MELTZER M. & FRANGIONE B. (1964) Antigenicity of hereditary human gamma globulin (Gm) factors—Biological and biochemical aspects. *Cold Spring Harbor Symposium on Quantitative Biology* **29,** 463–472

[55] GRUBB R. (1961) The Gm groups and their relationship to rheumatoid arthritis serology. *Arth. & Rheumat.* **4,** 195–202

[56] HARRIS, JEAN & VAUGHAN J.H. (1961) Transfusion studies in rheumatoid arthritis. *Arth. & Rheumat.* **4,** 47–55

[57] FUDENBERG H.H. & KUNKEL H.G. (1961) Specificity of the reaction between rheumatoid factor and gamma globulins. *J. exp. Med.* **114,** 257–278

[58] FUDENBERG H.H. & FRANKLIN E.C. (1965) Rheumatoid factors and the etiology of rheumatoid arthritis. *Ann. N.Y. Acad. Sci.* **124,** 884–895

[59] ALLEN J.C. & KUNKEL H.G. (1963) Antibodies to genetic types of gamma globulin after multiple transfusion. *Science* **139,** 418–419

[60] VIERUCCI A. (1965) Gm groups and anti-Gm antibodies in children with Cooley's anaemia. *Vox Sang.* **10,** 82–93

[61] FUDENBERG H.H. & FUDENBERG, BETTY R. (1964) Antibody to hereditary human gamma-globulin (Gm) factor resulting from maternal-foetal incompatibility. *Science* **145,** 170–171

[62] ROPARTZ C., LENOIR J., HEMET Y. & RIVAT L. (1960) Possible origins of the anti-Gm sera. *Nature, Lond.* **188,** 1120–1121

[63] STEINBERG A.G. & WILSON, JANET A. (1963) Hereditary globulin factors and immune tolerance in man. *Science* **140,** 303–304

[64] MASOUREDIS S.P. (1960) The $Rh_0(D)$ genotype and red cell $Rh_0(D)$ antigen content. *Science* **131**, 1442

[65] WIEL, Th. W.M. VAN DE & DORFMEIJER H. (1959) Reumatöide arthritis en erfelijke serumgroepen. *Nederl. tijdschr. genesk.*, **103**, 2314–2319

[66] HARBOE M. (1960) Relationship between Gm types and haemagglutinating substances in rheumatoid sera. *Acta. path. microbiol. Scand.* **50**, 89–105

[67] PODLIACHOUK, LUBA, JACQUELINE F. & EYQUEM A. (1962) Étude des substances anti-Gm dans les rhumatismes inflammatoires chroniques. *Ann. Inst. Pasteur* **103**, 59–74

[68] PORTER R.R. (1959) The hydrolysis of rabbit γ-globulin and antibodies with crystalline papain. *Biochem. J.* **73**, 119–126

[69] ROPARTZ C. & LENOIR J. (1960) Les antiglobulines humaines présentes dans les sérums de sujets normaux II—Frequénce et caractéristiques sérologiques. *Rev. Hémat.* **15**, 40–51

[70] ROPARTZ C. (1960) Les groupes seriques Gm état actual de la question. *Revue fr. Etude clin. biol.*, **9**, 933–945

[71] NIELSEN J.C. & HENNINGSEN K. (1963) Experimental studies on the determination of the Gm groups in blood stains. *Medicine, Science & Law*, **3**, (3), 49–58

[72] DUCOS J., RUFFIÉ J. & VARSI M. (1962) Mise en évidence des antigènes Gm^a, Gm^b, Gm^x dans les taches de sang sec. *Vox Sang.* **7**, 722–731

[73] HESS M. & BÜTLER R. (1962) Anti-Gm specificities in sera of Rhesus monkeys immunized with human gamma globulin. *Vox Sang.* **7**, 93–95

[74] ALEPA, F.P. & STEINBERG A.G. (1964) The production of anti-Gm reagents by Rhesus monkeys immunized with pooled human gamma globulin. *Vox Sang.* **9**, 333–339

[75] EYQUEM A., PODLIACHOUK, LUBA & JACQUELINE F. (1958) Relation entre le facteur serique Gm^a et la gravité de la polyarthrite chronique évolutive. *Ann. Inst. Pasteur* **95**, 753–756

[76] GRUBB R. (1958) Interactions between rheumatoid arthritic sera and human gamma globulin. *Acta Haemat.* **20**, 246–252

[77] PODLIACHOUK, LUBA, EYQUEM A. & JACQUELINE F. (1960) Obervations sur certaines propriétés du facteur sérique Gm^a. *Ann. Inst. Pasteur* **99**, 224–240

[78] ROPARTZ C., ROUSSEAU P.Y. & RIVAT L. (1962) Le système de γ-globuline, Gm, dans une population de la Seine-Maritime. *Revue fr. Étud. clin. biol.* **7**, 847–855

[79] JACQUELINE, F., PODLIACHOUK, LUBA & EYQUEM A. (1964) Les anticorps du système sérique Gm au corps de la polyarthrite chronique évolutive. *Presse méd.* **72**, 2205–2208

[80] DEICHER H. & SCHUPP E. (1963) Frequenzen von Gm-serum-Gruppen bei der primär-chronischen Polyarthrites. *Z. Rheumaforsch* **22**, 69–76

[81] PODLIACHOUK, LUBA, JACQUELINE F., EYQUEM A., EVRARD M.C. & BEAUD R. (1965) The serum factors Gm(a), Gm(b), Gm(x) and Gm-like in patients with chronic rheumatic affections. *Vox Sang.* **10**, 188–194

[82] JULKUNEN H. & TIILIKAINEN ANYA. (1959) Importance of an increased gamma globulin level in the determination of Gm groups in collagen diseases. *Ann. rheum. dis.* **18**, 318–321

[83] STEINBERG A.G. & STAUFFER RACHEL. (1962) Effect of heat on the serum factors Gm^a, Gm^b, Gm^x and Gm-like. *Nature, Lond.* **187**, 791–792

[84] SVARTZ N. & SCHLOSSMANN K. (1954) A serum cold precipitable haemagglutinating factor in rheumatoid arthritis. *Acta. Med. Scand.* **149**, 83–89

[85] WALLER, MARION & LAWLER, SYLVIA D. (1962) A study of the properties of the Rhesus antibody (R_1) diagnostic for the rheumatoid factor and its application to Gm grouping. *Vox Sang.* **7**, 591–606

[86] MAKELA O., ERIKSSON A.W. & LEHTOVAARA RAIMO. (1959) On the inheritance of the haptoglobin serum groups. *Acta. Genet.* **9,** 149–166

[87] CONNEALLY P.M., NEVO, SARAH, CLEGHORN T.E., HARRIS H., HOPINSON D.A., ROBSON, ELIZABETH B., SPENCER N. & STEINBERG A.G. (1965) Linkage studies with the human red blood cell, acid phosphatase locus *Am. J. Hum. Genet.,* **17,** 109–110

[88] ZERGOLLERN LJILJANA, HOEFNAGEL D., BENIRSCHKE K. & CORCORAN, PATRICIA A. (1964) A patient with Trisomy 21 and a reciprocal translocation in the 13–15 group. *Cytogenetics* **3,** 148–158

[89] COTES, P. MARY, HUMPHREY J.H. & LAWLER, SYLVIA D. (1963). Unpublished observations.

SECTION 2
Antigens

CHAPTER 9

The Separation and Purification of Bacterial Antigens

I.W. SUTHERLAND

Introduction

The general description of preparative methods for bacterial antigens presents several problems. Because of the considerable dissimilarity of components of different bacterial species, methods of wide application in this field are relatively rare. In only a few cases do numerous methods for extraction or purification of a particular bacterial antigen exist, but in these instances the method or methods of widest applicability have been outlined here. Where possible, approximate yields have been given for some of the products; most of these figures are based on evaluation tests performed in the author's laboratory. As a guide, an overnight aerobic static fluid culture of a non-exacting bacterial species such as *Escherichia coli* in the stationary phase may be expected to yield 1·0 mg dry bacterial cells per ml of growth medium. Shaking of the culture fluid during growth should increase the cell yield twofold. To avoid contamination with antigenic constituents from the culture medium, it is usually preferable to employ a completely synthetic medium or a simple laboratory medium such as nutrient broth. However, this is not possible with many of the more nutritionally exacting bacterial species. When a more complex medium is used, antigenic material can sometimes be excluded by overlaying the solid medium with a layer of sterile cellophane on which the bacteria are then grown. Alternatively, the bacteria may be grown within a dialysis sac surrounded by liquid medium. These methods are only possible when the only active constituents of the medium are all freely diffusible. Preliminary experiments are frequently of value in determining whether an increased yield of the antigen under study can be obtained by slight alterations of the culture medium; this is most often the case in the production of exotoxins and other extracellular antigens.

It is probably unnecessary to stress that special precautions are required when handling bacteria, but other precautions are also needed. Slight bacterial contamination of preparations during handling can be obviated by the addition of thiomersalate* (1 in 10,000) or phemeride† (1 in 10,000). The use of such agents should be carefully noted as it is sometimes difficult

---

* Eli Lilley & Co., Basingstoke, England.   † Parke, Davis & Co., Hounslow, England.

to remove traces from the final antigenic product. Many bacteria contain enzymes that can depolymerize other constituents following disruption of the cell. These present no significant problems if the antigen is prepared by some rapid procedure, but such enzymes may be a greater nuisance during more lengthy procedures under mild conditions of temperature at neutral pH. If the antigen to be extracted is thermostable, mild heating may be used to inactivate these enzymes.

Extracellular antigens

Extracellular protein antigens
Many bacterial products of immunological importance occur extracellularly; they diffuse into the surrounding medium after production by the bacterial cells. Among the most important are those that function as exotoxins or as extracellular enzymes. They can be separated from the bacteria by centrifugation of liquid cultures. Inevitably, numerous extracellular products are synthesized and, in addition, some cell autolysis liberates intracellular components into the medium. Thus the material under examination requires to be separated from a variety of other compounds. Ideally, the microorganisms would be grown in a completely synthetic liquid medium so that constituents of the medium can then be removed by dialysis of the centrifuged culture supernatants. However, in many cases the bacteria are more exacting and require a complex medium for growth but many species will grow in nutrient broth which is free of antigenic constituents although not completely diffusible. Under these circumstances, culture supernatants are first dialysed against water or dilute buffer until all diffusible matter is removed. At this stage, large volumes may be involved and these can be reduced considerably by surrounding the dialysis membranes with a very concentrated solution of polyethylene glycol (average molecular weight 20,000) as recommended by Kohn [32]. After 24–48 hours in the cold, the volumes should have been reduced to one tenth or less of the original, thus simplifying further procedures.

The separation of the non-diffusible material into its different components is essentially a problem in preparative protein chemistry. As there is such a wide variation in the properties of bacterial extracellular proteins, this can be no more than a guide to their purification. The subject is more fully covered in several of the standard reference books [15, 17, 10, 11]. It must be remembered that exotoxins are frequently extremely thermolabile and may also be inactivated by extremes of pH and by the presence of oxygen. They tend to become even less stable as they are purified and care must be taken to control these variables during purification procedures. A suggested outline purification might be: (i) ammonium sulphate fractionation; (ii) chromatography on an anion exchange cellulose or dextran; (iii) chromatography on cation exchange cellulose or dextran; (iv) preparative electrophoresis.

Ammonium sulphate fractionation
After reduction in volume, followed by brief dialysis against a suitable buffer (e.g. 0·05 M phosphate buffer, pH 7·0), the supernatant fluid is centrifuged at 50,000 g for 15–30 minutes at 4° C and the deposit of particulate material discarded. To the cold solution, 11·5 g of finely powdered ammonium sulphate per 100 ml is added slowly with gentle stirring. The resulting solution is 20 per cent saturated with respect to ammonium sulphate. Any precipitate formed is removed by centrifugation at 10,000 g for 15 minutes at 4° C. The supernatant fluid is retained for addition of further salt. The precipitate can be dissolved in a small volume of phosphate buffer and dialysed free of ammonium sulphate at 4° C. In the same manner, a series of saturation steps and resultant fractions can be obtained. Steps of 20, 40, 60 and 80 per cent saturation may be suitable, or the intervals may be smaller. The amounts of solid ammonium sulphate required can be deduced from the nomogram prepared by Dixon [13]. The recovery of the precipitates obtained during ammonium sulphate fractionation is easiest when a swing-out head is used for centrifugation.

The use of the ion exchange material
Before employing ion exchange chromatography, one should ascertain the range of pH over which the material under examination is stable and active. Any incidental information, such as the isoelectric point, will also be useful. This can be determined by electrophoresis in a series of buffers of different pH and observation of the pH value at which the material remains at the origin due to its overall neutral charge. If the isoelectric point is higher than the desired starting pH, the material of choice for the next stage of purification is an anion exchanger, e.g. diethylaminoethyl (DEAE-)-cellulose or DEAE-Sephadex. Conversely, if the isoelectric point is below the starting pH value, a cation exchange material should be used, e.g. carboxymethyl (CM-)-cellulose or CM-Sephadex. The advantages of using the substituted dextran (Sephadex) lie in their molecular sieving effects which can be utilized at the same time as their ion exchange capacity. Thus, by using a suitable form of Sephadex gel, materials of similar charge but of differing molecular weight may be separated.

The type of ion exchange material and the geometry of the column to be used must be considered carefully. Flocs give much slower flow rates than do powders and the latter are usually preferable. The highest resolution is obtained with long, narrow columns. As the flow rate through these is very slow, the choice will probably involve a compromise to give acceptable resolution coupled with a moderate flow rate. These columns are most readily made by inserting sintered glass disks into water-jacketed condensers of effective length 40×2 cm or 20×1 cm. The size of the column and the amount of absorbent used will obviously depend on the amount of material to be chromatographed. It is important that the columns should not be overloaded because this causes loss of resolution and poor separation of the fractions. The capacity of the ion exchange materials tends to vary from batch to batch and the manufacturer's instructions and data should be consulted. The actual conditions of chromatography should first be determined by small-scale pilot experiments in test-tubes. The charge on the molecule and hence its affinity for the exchanger can be altered by altering the pH of the eluting buffer. Alternatively, the affinity of the protein for the substituted cellulose or dextran is reduced by increasing the salt concentration. Either method, or a combination of both, may be used. The changes in the eluting fluid can be produced stepwise or they can be achieved by means of a gradient device (q.v.).

Method. The selected ion exchange material, say DEAE-cellulose (10 g) is suspended in 400 ml of N NaOH in a beaker, stirred for 5 minutes and allowed to sediment. As much of the fluid as possible is removed by decantation. The remainder is filtered off using a Buchner funnel and filter flask. The cellulose is then suspended in 400 ml of N HCl and recovered immediately by filtration. It is re-suspended in NaOH, filtered and thoroughly washed with distilled water and then with the starting buffer. It is finally suspended in about 200 ml of the starting buffer and the slurry is de-aerated in a stoppered filter flask by the application of suction from a water pump at 700 mmHg pressure for 15–30 minutes. The column (20×1 cm) is now prepared. A small pad of glass wool is inserted over the sintered glass disk and the absorbent is poured in and packed down with a glass plunger. At no time should the column be allowed to dry out. The starting buffer is pumped through the column by a micro-pump, and the flow rate is checked. Several buffers are available; for pH values of the order of 5·0 , 7·0 and 8·0, acetate, phosphate and tris buffers respectively are suitable and can be used with a starting molarity of 0·01–0·02 M. The sample is incorporated in a small volume (1–3 ml) of the buffer and this is carefully applied to the top of the column, then 100 ml of the buffer is pumped through. The gradient is now started; a suitable set-up is shown in Fig. 9.1. A tightly stoppered flask can be used as the mixing vessel, containing initially say 400 ml of the starting buffer and a magnetic stirrer cased in glass or plastic. Several types of micro-pump are available and a flow rate of 20–30 ml per hour should prove satisfactory. With DEAE-cellulose equilibrated against 0·1 M phosphate buffer (pH 7·0) as the starting buffer, a gradient of increasing salt concentration from 0 to 1·0 M sodium chloride is suggested. Similarly, a pH gradient from 4·8 to 5·6 using 0·02 M acetate buffer may be suitable with CM-cellulose. When an ultraviolet-scanning device is applied to the eluate, identification of those fractions containing protein is relatively simple. Alternatively, comparison of the percentage transmission at wavelengths of 280 and 260 μ made manually on a spectrophotometer, or protein estimations by the Folin technique reveal which tubes in the fraction collector contain protein and therefore which should be tested for biological activity.

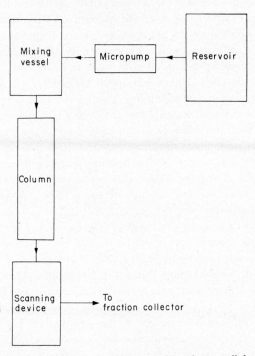

FIG. 9.1. A schematic assembly for gradient elution of extracellular proteins from ion exchange material.

After ion exchange chromatography, the product may be pure enough for use. If not, it can be purified further by electrophoresis on paper or gel followed by elution from the supporting matrix.

Flagella
The importance of bacterial flagella in the serology of genera such as the *Salmonellae* has long been noted. In the preparation of such antigens in a pure state, the main problem is to detach them from the bacterial cells without undue disintegration of the bacteria, so that contamination with cell components is avoided or minimized. Usually some form of vigorous shaking is employed, followed by differential centrifugation to separate the bacteria

from the detached flagella. Although the flagella may be subsequently purified by dissociation with acid, followed by re-polymerization of the flagellar protein 'flagellin' [31], such preparations were still found to be frequently contaminated with small amounts of lipopolysaccharide [1].

Isolation and purification

It is preferable to use young bacterial cells grown in liquid culture; a 6–8 hour culture in nutrient broth is suitable. The bacteria are harvested by centrifugation and washed once with 0·9 per cent (w/v) sodium chloride solution. Care should be taken, as some bacterial species lose their flagella very readily. The cells are then suspended in a small volume of saline or of borate buffer (0·1 M, pH 7·6; see [24]). The suspension is treated for 15–20 minutes in a tissue homogenizer or in a Mickle tissue disintegrator [37] without glass beads. The cells are recovered by centrifugation at 4000 g for 20 minutes in an angle centrifuge, and they should be extracted twice more in the homogenizer. The combined supernatant fluids are centrifuged at 5000 g for 25 minutes in a swing-out head to remove any residual bacteria. The flagella are sedimented by centrifugation at 75,000 g for 45 minutes in the Spinco model L preparative ultracentrifuge, again using a swing-out rotor. The colourless deposit is suspended in saline containing merthiolate (1 in 100,000). The yield represents about 1·0–1·5 per cent of the dry weight of the bacteria. The next stage in the preparation is the disassociation of the flagella and their re-aggregation at neutral pH. The suspension is acidified with 1/20 volume of 1·0 N HCl and allowed to stand at room temperature for 30 minutes. The mixture is then centrifuged at 80,000 g for 60 minutes in the ultracentrifuge. The supernatant fluid is carefully removed and neutralized with 1·0 N NaOH. Polymerization of the flagellar protein is achieved by the addition of 2 volumes of cold saturated (70 per cent w/v) ammonium sulphate solution. After standing for 16 hours at 4° C, the mixture is centrifuged at 20,000 g for 15 minutes and the supernatant fluid is discarded. The deposit is suspended in a small volume of distilled water, dialysed free of ammonium sulphate and lyophilized. In a typical experiment with a strain of *Escherichia coli*, the final product represented 0·4 per cent of the original dry weight of bacteria and contained 1·3 per cent polysaccharide [Sutherland, unpublished results]. Examination in the electron microscope showed the presence of typical flagellar filaments and confirmed the absence of other structures.

Exopolysaccharides

Exopolysaccharides comprise those polysaccharides which are secreted outside the bacterial cell wall and cell membrane. They are thus distinguishable from other polysaccharides, such as the lipopolysaccharides of Gram negative bacteria, which are integral components of the cell walls.

These extracellular polysaccharides of bacteria form an important group of substances because of their position at the cell surface. While much work has been done on the immunochemistry of those produced by pneumococcal species (e.g. [28]), exopolysaccharides from various other bacterial genera have also been studied [41, 23]. The pure polysaccharides are probably haptens and not true antigens, but antisera can frequently be prepared against them by the injection of the whole bacterial cultures or by the use of adjuvants. Alternatively, the polysaccharide may be coupled to a protein carrier prior to injection into the experimental animal. The method of preparation and purification of the extracellular polysaccharides must depend on their physical state; they may be present as loose slime or as discrete capsules surrounding the bacterial cells. In the latter instance, some slime will always be found due to dissolution of capsular material. The two forms may be distinguished by examination of wet India ink films [19].

The bacteria should be grown under conditions that allow maximal polysaccharide production. For species such as *Klebsiella aerogenes* this involves nitrogen limitation in the presence of excess carbon source, low incubation temperature (20–25° C) and good aeration [20]. The best yields of exopolysaccharides are obtained from growth on solid media. Where large amounts of polysaccharide are required, the use of enamel trays for bacterial culture is recommended. These trays (39·5 × 30 cm), covered with aluminium or steel lids (40 × 30 cm), are sterilized in the hot air oven at 160° C for 1 hour. The chosen medium (1 l.) is sterilized, melted, poured into the trays and allowed to solidify. A liquid culture (50 ml) of the bacteria is then poured over the entire surface of the medium. Unfortunately, agar contamination may result from this method of culture. Where this is a problem, it can be obviated by overlaying the medium with a layer of sterile cellophane. Alternatively liquid media can be used. But, as with growth on cellophane, the yield of exopolysaccharide is greatly reduced.

Isolation of slime
The liquid culture, or a saline suspension of culture material from solid medium, is centrifuged at 10,000 *g* in an angle centrifuge for 30–60 minutes. Although such conditions of centrifugation are normally satisfactory for the deposition of the capsulate bacterial cells, some variants such as *K. aerogenes* A3(S1) [55], produce a very viscous polysaccharide slime. To obtain adequate separation of bacterial cells and polysaccharide in such cases, prolonged centrifugation at higher speed, e.g. 2–3 hours at 25,000 *g* may be required. The supernatant solutions containing slime polysaccharide are poured into 2–3 volumes of cold (−20° C) acetone and the mixture stirred vigorously with a glass rod. The crude polysaccharide can then be obtained as a fibrous mass wound round the rod.

In a few cases, the polysaccharide does not precipitate immediately and the mixture may be left overnight at $-20°$ C for complete sedimentation to occur; a few crystals of solid sodium acetate may be added to assist precipitation. The fibrous mass is removed from the acetone and dried under vacuum over phosphorous pentoxide (yield ca. 1·5 g/litre of solid medium for *K. aerogenes* A3(Sl)).

Purification of the polysaccharide is achieved by deproteinization according to the method of Sevag [48]. In this process it is important that a dilute solution of the polysaccharide is used. It is dissolved to a concentration of 0·5 per cent (w/v) in acetate buffer containing 4 per cent (w/v) sodium acetate and 2 per cent (v/v) acetic acid. To each 100 ml of the mixture are added 20 ml chloroform and 4 ml butanol and this is then shaken vigorously for 30 minutes. The turbid preparation is poured into a separating funnel and allowed to stand until the aqueous and organic phases have separated. The lower, organic layer together with the precipitate at the interface are poured off and discarded. To achieve complete removal of proteinaceous material, repetition of this procedure three times or more with the aqueous solution of polysaccharide may be necessary. The yield of polysaccharide represents about 50 per cent of the original product. The final aqueous solutions are centrifuged, dialysed against tap water and distilled water and freeze-dried.

An alternative method of deproteinization is to employ the phenol extraction procedure described for preparation of lipopolysaccharides. This method can be used for some bacterial exopolysaccharides but the acidity of the phenol may cause partial hydrolysis of others.

If several polysaccharides are produced simultaneously by the same strain of bacterium, further separation may be necessary. This can be accomplished by fractional precipitation with ethanol, or by treatment with quaternary ammonium salts [46, 47]. A further possible contamination may be by lipopolysaccharide. This can be removed by ultracentrifugation for 4 hours at 100,000 g. In this way, three different antigenic polysaccharides have been separated from *Escherichia coli* preparations [26, 41].

Isolation of capsular material
The presence of extracellular polysaccharide in the form of a capsule presents rather more difficulties in purification than do slime polysaccharides. Prior to decapsulation, slime may be removed by washing the packed capsulate cells twice with distilled water containing 1 per cent formalin. Subsequently, the cells are suspended in several volumes of distilled water, the pH adjusted to neutrality and the suspension heated at 100° C for 15 minutes to decapsulate the bacteria. Alternatively, the capsules may be removed with alkali after fixation of the cells with 1 per cent (v/v) formaldehyde solution for 15 minutes at room temperature [18]. Sodium hydroxide is added to the cell suspension

to a concentration of 1 per cent (w/v). The mixture is stirred at room temperature for 30 minutes and then carefully neutralized with 1·0 N HCl.

Deposition of the bacterial cells and purification of the polysaccharide following the boiling or the alkali extraction is accomplished by the same methods as are used for the isolation of slime polysaccharides. As the methods of isolation of the capsular polysaccharides are, of necessity, relatively drastic, the likelihood of contamination with other materials is high and subsequent purification is essential, especially as lipopolysaccharide is a probable contaminant. Both slime and capsular polysaccharides are highly hygroscopic; even freeze-dried preparations may contain up to 15 per cent of water.

Cell walls

The importance of preparing bacterial cell walls, free from other antigenic material of intracellular origin, is appreciated when the immunogenic role of these structures is studied. Cell wall preparations active in protecting experimental animals against subsequent experimental infection have been obtained from numerous bacterial species, e.g. *Brucella abortus* [25] and *Bordetella pertussis* [40, 52]. Numerous methods are available for the preparation of bacterial cell walls and a detailed discussion of these may be found in the monograph by Salton [44].

Before attempting to make bacterial cell wall preparations, two points should be borne in mind regarding their structure and their production. (i) In Gram positive bacteria, the cell wall and the cell membrane are distinct entities which can be separated relatively easily. In Gram negative bacteria the two components form an integral structure and the separation of one from the other is extremely difficult. Usually this can only be achieved by selective destruction of one component, possibly by enzymic hydrolysis or alternatively by drastic chemical methods. (ii) The bacteria must be cultured under conditions that favour production of the antigen under investigation. This is probably most important in genera such as *Salmonella* which readily undergo the 'Smooth'(S) to 'Rough'(R) antigenic variation. Thus Collins [9] observed such variation on increasing the dilution rate and hence the growth rate, of *Salmonella enteritidis* in continuous culture.

The most widely applicable methods of cell wall preparation are those involving mechanical disruption of the whole bacteria. These methods can be separated, on the one hand, into relatively simple procedures such as (a) grinding with abrasives in a mortar and pestle, and on the other, into those methods which require specialized apparatus. In this latter category may be included: (b) ultrasonic disintegration; (c) disruption in a pressure cell; and (d) shaking with small glass beads (ballotini). The physical properties of the bacterial cell can be exploited in further methods such as heat disruption, freezing and thawing, or osmotic lysis.

(a) *Grinding*. The bacteria, in the form of a thick paste (say 40–50 mg dry weight/ml) are cooled and added to an equal volume of polishing alumina (grade 3/50) carborundum powder or coarse sand in a chilled mortar. Grinding by hand is performed for 10–15 minutes. This method has the advantage that it can be performed without any danger of localized heating. It may therefore be especially valuable when dealing with very labile antigens. The main drawback is the limited number of bacterial species that are broken by grinding and the poor reproducibility of the method.

(b) *Ultrasonic disintegration*. The two most commonly used disintegrators are probably those manufactured by M.S.E. Ltd.* and by The Raytheon Corporation.† The disintegration of bacteria with the former equipment has been studied in detail by Hughes [30]. Numerous species of bacteria are highly susceptible to ultrasonic disruption, but others, especially certain cocci, are completely resistant. Other disadvantages of the method are localized heating and aeration of the bacterial suspension. The cell walls are reduced to a highly fragmented state which may also be undesirable for some experimental purposes. The optimal duration of exposure to ultrasonic irradiation is dependent on the apparatus, the volume and the concentration of the bacterial suspension, the bacterial species and the physiological state of the cells. Optimal breakdown is usually achieved when a suspension in distilled water of cells (ca. 10 mg dry weight/ml) grown on solid medium is used. Bacteria grown in liquid medium, or suspended in physiological saline or other salt solutions, are more resistant to disintegration. When a probe of the M.S.E.-Mullard type is used, some cooling can be achieved by surrounding the sample tube with ice or other coolant. The Raytheon instrument is cooled by running water.

(c) *Pressure cell*. When relatively small quantities of bacteria are to be disrupted, the Hughes press [29] is extremely useful. On a larger scale, the press described by Edebo [21] has proved satisfactory. In each case, the bacteria, in the form of a frozen paste, are compressed and passed through a small orifice into a second chamber where expansion, and hence cell rupture, occurs. The fact that low temperatures are employed may be advantageous in minimizing denaturation and in reducing the activity of cell-degrading enyzmes.

(d) *Mechanical disintegration*. A heavy suspension of washed bacteria (10–20 mg dry weight/ml) is cooled and added to an equal volume of small glass beads (No. 12 grade ballotini) in a Mickle cell. The mixture is shaken for 5–15 minutes in the Mickle disintegrator, after which the beads are removed

* M.S.E. Ltd., London, England.
† Raytheon Corporation, Waltham, Mass., U.S.A.

by passage through a coarse sintered glass filter. (After thorough washing, in concentrated nitric acid and in distilled water, the beads can be re-used.)

Although specialized attachments such as that for the International Centrifuge [50] are available, the Mickle tissue disintegrator probably remains the most useful apparatus for the preparation of bacterial cell walls on a scale of 2–3 g. The disadvantages of this equipment's small capacity (approximately 20 ml) have been overcome recently by the late Professor Weidel and his colleagues in Tübingen [personal communication]. These workers have developed an apparatus of the same type possessing twelve to fifteen vessels with a total capacity of approximately 160 ml. Pre-cooling of the bacterial suspension, together with the use of the disintegrator in the cold, result in minimal heating of the cells.

Separation of bacterial cell walls after cell disintegration
Three methods are available for the separation of cell walls from unbroken cells and other disintegration products: (i) differential centrifugation; (ii) density gradient centrifugation; (iii) fractionation in liquid two phase systems. Combinations of these three methods are also possible.

(i) Differential centrifugation provides a rapid and simple method, giving at least a preliminary isolation of the cell walls. The conditions of centrifugation used will normally depend on the size of the cells of the particular bacterial species. Unbroken cells of *Bordetella pertussis*, a species of relatively small cell size ($1.5\,\mu \times 0.5\,\mu$), were removed by centrifugation at 2500 *g* in an angle centrifuge for 15 minutes, while the cell walls were subsequently recovered by centrifugation at 10,000 *g* for 15 minutes [52]. In general, the unbroken cells remaining after disintegration of most bacterial species are removed by centrifugation at 2500–3500 *g* for 10–15 minutes while the cell walls are deposited by centrifugation at 8000–12,000 *g* for 20–30 minutes. Such preparations are still contaminated with small quantities of unbroken cells together with adherent cell membrane and intracellular components. If lower yield is acceptable, more exact fractionation can be accomplished.

(ii) Density gradient centrifugation can also be used to separate cell walls from other material. The standard methods for sucrose gradients, as applied to other biological fields, are suitable for this. Using centrifuge tubes of dimensions 25 mm × 170 mm a gradient from 10–40 per cent (w/v) sucrose should prove satisfactory. With such tubes it is possible to apply 1–4 ml of broken cell suspension and obtain good separation. As an alternative to sucrose gradients, glycerol gradients have been employed in the isolation of cell walls from *Brucella abortus* [25, 43]. The actual gradients used may be prepared by layering solutions of different concentration within the tubes or by utilizing a gradient machine [8].

(iii) Another possible method of cell wall isolation stems from investigations of aqueous polymer two-phase systems by Albertsson [2]. A system containing phosphate buffer (30·69 g, K_2HPO_4; 16·86 g, KH_2PO_4, per 100 ml, pH 7·1) and polyethylene glycol (PEG) of molecular weight 4000 was used. The broken cells were contained in 70·4 ml water; PEG (11·2 g) and buffer (36·1 g) were added. After shaking at 20° C, the two phases were separated in a separating funnel. In this system, cell walls from *Aerobacter* species moved to the phosphate-rich phase.

Subsequent treatment of the cell walls

Following any of the isolation procedures outlined above, bacterial cell walls, even of Gram positive species, will be contaminated with adherent cytoplasmic material. Much of this can be removed by thorough washing; the cell walls are suspended in 2·0 M sodium chloride solution and stirred at 0° C for 60 minutes. After centrifugation at 10,000 *g* for 20 minutes the supernatant fluid is discarded. This process is repeated once. The preparation is then similarly washed twice with cold distilled water. The product thus obtained may be sufficiently pure for use without any further purification, especially if it is derived from Gram positive bacteria. However, in many cases, further treatment may be necessary. This usually takes the form of enzymic digestion and/or treatment with detergent to solubilize any membranous impurities.

The three most useful enzymes for the purification of the bacterial cell walls are trypsin, pepsin and ribonuclease. Care in the choice of enyzmes is required as digestion with trypsin or with pepsin may destroy desired protein components. Digestion with trypsin and ribonuclease may be performed simultaneously. The cell walls, at a concentration of approximately 1 per cent (w/v), are suspended in phosphate buffer (0·05 M, pH 8·0). Ribonuclease and trypsin are then added to give a final concentration of 500 μg/ml of each, and the mixture is incubated, with stirring, at 37° C for 2–3 hours. The cell walls are recovered by centrifugation at 10,000 *g* and thereafter they are washed twice with distilled water. Digestion with pepsin is performed in 0·02 N HCl using the enzyme at a concentration of 500 μg/ml. The mixture is incubated at 37° C for 12–18 hours. After recovering the cell walls by centrifugation, they are washed at least twice with distilled water.

An alternative or an adjunct to enzymic treatment is the use of surface-active agents. Shafa & Salton [49] suggested the use of sodium dodecyl sulphate (syn. sodium lauryl sulphate) to disaggregate the cell walls of Gram negative bacteria. The cell walls are suspended in a 0·2 per cent (w/v) solution of the detergent such that the concentration of walls in the suspension is approximately 1 per cent (w/v), and stirred at 37° C for 30 minutes. The cell walls are recovered and subsequently washed with distilled water as detailed above.

Initially, washed cell walls comprise 15–20 per cent of the bacterial cell mass. This proportion may vary depending on the physiological state of the cells. The yield is reduced to approximately half by tryptic and ribonuclease digestion or by detergent treatment, but the yield from a combination of the procedures is more difficult to assess. In the case of *Bordetella pertussis*, treatment with detergent, followed by trypsin, produced material comprising about 5 per cent of the dry weight of whole cells [52].

Somatic antigens of Gram negative bacteria
The cell walls of Gram negative bacteria contain numerous antigens, among which are the complexes of lipoprotein, polysaccharide and lipid that have been variously termed somatic antigens, O antigens and endotoxins. For many purposes, extraction of the lipopolysaccharide components is all that is necessary (q.v.), but it is also possible to extract and isolate the whole somatic antigen complex. Although extraction with diethylene glycol proved to be very effective for smooth strains of *Shigella dysenteriae* [39], the method is of very limited applicability. The use of trichloracetic acid, as originally suggested by Boivin & Mesrobeanu [7] can be applied to a number of bacterial species, but it should be noted that the yield may vary considerably with the strain under examination. In particular, rough strains yield much less material than do the corresponding wild type or smooth strains. With these provisions, the trichloracetic acid extraction method is outlined below.

Procedure. Dry bacteria are suspended (2 per cent w/v) in cold distilled water at 0–4° C. An equal volume of 1·0 N trichloracetic acid at the same temperature is added and the mixture is stirred for 3 hours in the cold. The cell debris is then removed by centrifugation at 12,000 g for 30 minutes and the supernatant solution is dialysed for 48 hours against running tap water to remove the trichloracetic acid. As the material is relatively thermostable, the solution of non-diffusible material can be concentrated by distillation under reduced pressure until it contains about 1 per cent (w/v) of solid material. To each 100 ml of solution, 50 ml of cold ethanol is added and any resultant precipitate is removed by centrifugation at 12,000 g for 30 minutes. The deposit is discarded. A further 35 ml of cold ethanol is added per 150 ml of supernatant solution and the mixture is left for 12–16 hours in the cold. The somatic antigen is precipitated at this stage and is recovered by centrifugation at 12,000 g for 30 minutes, washed with ethanol and dried under vacuum over phosphorous pentoxide.

Lipopolysaccharides
The lipopolysaccharides found in the cell walls of Gram negative bacteria are antigens whose importance as determinants of the surface specificities

of these micro-organisms is reflected by the very large bibliography on the subject. The role played by the lipopolysaccharides in the serology of the genus *Salmonella* and the intriguing properties of these substances have been the subject of numerous studies by Kauffmann, Lüderitz, Neter, Staub, Westphal and others. In particular, the chemical and serological properties of lipopolysaccharides have been recently reviewed [13, 36, 51].

The classical method for the preparation of bacterial lipopolysaccharides is that of Westphal, Lüderitz and Bister [54]; whole bacteria are extracted with 45 per cent (w/v) phenol at 60° C. On centrifugation at 0° C, a diphasic mixture is obtained in which the upper aqueous layer contains the lipopolysaccharide while the lower phenolic layer contains protein. However, several other substances in addition to lipopolysaccharide are present in the upper aqueous solution. These include nucleic acid, glycogen and other intracellular storage products of polysaccharide nature. Moreover, in certain cases, soluble polysaccharides with serological activity may also be present in the aqueous phase. These last substances, found in the RI type of *Salmonella* 'rough' mutant and reacting with antisera to the corresponding 'smooth' strains, were detected by Beckmann, Subbaiah & Stocker [6], in RI mutants of *Salmonella minnesota* and *Salmonella typhimurium*.

To permit the preparation of purer lipopolysaccharides, several modifications of the original procedure have been developed. Thus, Davies [12] employed ultracentrifugation to sediment the lipopolysaccharide while other compounds were left in solution. The use of cell walls as starting material also minimizes the amount of contaminating nucleic acid and other intracellular components. The original extraction procedure, which involves relatively drastic conditions, has been shortened from 30 minutes to 5 minutes without any significant reduction in the yield of lipopolysaccharide [35]. These refinements are incorporated in the following method for the extraction and isolation of lipopolysaccharides.

Method. The most suitable starting materials are (i) an acetone powder preparation of the bacteria, or (ii) a cell wall preparation. In the former case, the bacteria are harvested by centrifugation and washed twice with saline (0·85 per cent w/v NaCl). The cells are then suspended at a concentration of approximately 10 mg dry weight/ml in cold distilled water. This thick suspension is poured into 10 volumes of cold acetone (−20° C) and left for 60 minutes; during this time the bacteria should sediment. As much as possible of the yellowish supernatant fluid is then removed by decantation. The residue is poured on to a Buchner funnel and washed with a further 5 volumes of cold acetone under suction. A final washing with diethyl ether has been used by some authors but may not prove necessary. The cells are transferred to a desiccator and dried under vacuum in the presence of phosphorous pentoxide. Before use, the acetone powder should be thoroughly ground in a mortar.

Extraction. The dry bacteria (or cell walls) are suspended at a concentration of approximately 6 per cent (w/v) in water and the mixture is stirred in a wide-necked Erlenmeyer flask in a water bath at 65° C. Stirring is continued until the contents of the flask are at 65° C. An equal volume of 90 per cent (w/v) aqueous solution of phenol at the same temperature is then added and stirring is continued for 5 minutes. The flask is removed from the water bath and the contents cooled to 0–5° C, then centrifuged at approximately 2000 *g* for 60 minutes in the swing-out head of a refrigerated centrifuge at 0° C. The mixture is very caustic and it is preferable to use metal or polystyrene tubes for this centrifugation. Following centrifugation, the upper aqueous layer is carefully removed without removing the proteinaceous precipitate at

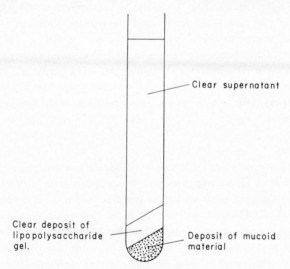

Clear supernatant

Clear deposit of lipopolysaccharide gel.

Deposit of mucoid material

FIG. 9.2. The purification of lipopolysaccharide by ultracentrifugation.

the interface. This can be achieved by applying *gentle* suction to the mouthpiece of a glass wash-bottle fitted with a fine nozzle. The material at the interface, and the lower, phenolic layer are discarded. The aqueous solution is dialysed for 48 hours against running tap water, concentrated to about $\frac{1}{4}$ volume under reduced pressure and lyophilized. Alternatively, the lipopolysaccharide may be precipitated by pouring the solution into 10 volumes of cold acetone at −20° C. The yield represents 5–10 per cent of the dry weight of the original cells.

Purification. The crude lipopolysaccharide is dissolved in water to give a 3 per cent (w/v) solution and centrifuged at 100,000 *g* for 4 hours in the Spinco model L preparative ultracentrifuge. The clear supernatant fluid is discarded and the sedimented gel of lipopolysaccharide (Fig. 9.2) should be carefully removed with a small spatula, resuspended in half the original volume of distilled water and recentrifuged. This entire ultracentrifugation procedure is repeated once more, making three times in all, and the final sediment of lipopolysaccharide is suspended in a small amount of distilled water and freeze-dried. The yield is normally of the order of 0·5–2·0 per cent of the dry weight of the original cells.

Polysaccharide preparation. Lipid-free polysaccharide hapten may be prepared from the lipopolysaccharide by hydrolysis with 1 per cent (v/v) acetic acid [14]. Although the time of hydrolysis required to free the polysaccharide from the associated lipid A may vary for different bacterial species, 30 minutes at 100° C was found to be adequate for lipopolysaccharides of some *Salmonella* species [53]. Aliquots of the lipopolysaccharide (200 mg) in 20 ml of 1 per cent (v/v) acetic acid are heated in test-tubes fitted with ground glass stoppers. Hydrolysis is continued at 100° C for 30 minutes. The contents of the tubes are centrifuged at low speed (500 *g*) on a bench centrifuge to remove the lipid A precipitate. The supernatant solution is dialysed against several volumes of glass-distilled water at 4° C for 48 hours and freeze-dried. The yield is about 30–40 per cent of the lipopolysaccharide starting material.

Teichoic Acids

The predominant role of the lipopolysaccharides as antigenic determinants in the cell walls of Gram negative bacteria appears to be paralleled, in many cases, by the teichoic acids in Gram positive bacteria. The observations of Mitchell & Moyle [38] that cell envelopes of *Staphylococcus aureus* contain unusually large amounts of phosphorus, led eventually to the discovery of the group of polyol phosphates that have been termed the 'teichoic acids'. Subsequently, Baddiley and his co-workers [4] isolated teichoic acids of differing chemical composition from a number of Gram positive bacteria, using either whole bacteria or cell walls as the starting material. Although Lilly [34] reported the presence of material resembling teichoic acid in a strain of *Escherichia coli* there has been no further confirmation of the presence of compounds of this type in the Gram negative bacterial cell.

The exact role of the teichoic acids in the cell walls of Gram positive bacteria has yet to be completely elucidated, but they are nevertheless of immunological importance. Thus Elliott [22] showed that the group D streptococcal antigen was a teichoic acid, while other workers showed that in *Staphylococcus aureus* (strain Copenhagen) and in *Lactobacillus* species certain serological properties are determined by the presence of teichoic acids [5, 45].

The method of isolation of teichoic acids initially developed by Baddiley and his colleagues involved prolonged treatment of the bacterial cell walls with cold trichloracetic acid. Following suggestions that the long exposure to low pH values might cause some degradation of the polyol phosphates, the time of extraction was decreased. As a result, lower yields were obtained. Recently, an alternative procedure was proposed [3] and this obviates exposure to reagents at low pH values. In the author's laboratory, both methods have proved satisfactory in the extraction of teichoic acids from the cell walls of a *Bacillus* species.

Method 1. Trichloracetic acid extraction. Bacterial cell walls (1·0 g) are suspended in 40 ml of an aqueous solution of trichloracetic acid (10 per cent w/v) and the suspension is stirred at 4° C for 70 hours. The insoluble residues are removed from the mixture by centrifugation at 5000 g for 30 minutes and washed with an additional 20 ml of cold trichloracetic acid solution. The extract and washings are combined and ether-soluble material is removed by shaking vigorously with three successive batches of equal volumes of diethyl ether to the aqueous solution. The aqueous layer from the final extraction is freeze-dried. It is dissolved in 100 ml of 10 per cent (w/v) trichloracetic acid solution and the teichoic acid is precipitated by the addition of 200 ml of cold ethanol. The precipitate is recovered by centrifugation at 5000 g for 20 minutes, washed with ethanol, then with ether, and finally lyophilized.

Method 2. An aqueous solution containing sodium acetate (60 per cent w/v) and phenylhydrazine hydrochloride (40 per cent w/v) is prepared. Care must be taken as this solution is highly toxic to the skin. The pH value of the solution is adjusted to neutrality with aqueous ammonia. Bacterial cell walls are then suspended in the solution to a concentration of 5 per cent (w/v). The mixture is stirred vigorously at 80° C for 30 minutes. After cooling to room temperature, the residual debris is removed by centrifugation at 10,000 g for 30 minutes. The supernatant solution is dialysed against distilled water for 48 hours in the cold and freeze-dried.

Bacterial cell membranes

The isolation of the cell membrane from bacterial cells is simplest with those species that are highly susceptible to the enzyme lysozyme. This digests the mucopeptide of the cell wall and leaves an osmotically fragile *protoplast* or *spheroplast* in Gram positive and Gram negative species respectively. When such enzymic digestion in an osmotically stabilized medium is followed by transfer to distilled water, the cells lyse and the membrane fraction can be recovered by centrifugation. Lysozyme sensitivity is greatest in young cells (6–8-hour cultures) and synchrony of the cell cultures may also increase the proportion of sensitive cells, especially in the case of gram negative bacterial species. Other enzymes similar in their mode of action to lysozyme may be used. Thus, Goldfarb and his colleagues [27] used an enzyme from the bacteriophage T2 to digest the cell walls of *E. coli* and produce osmotically fragile spheroplasts. Unfortunately, removal of the cell wall by such enzymes is incomplete in Gram negative cells and the resulting membrane fractions are heavily contaminated with cell wall components. Osmotically sensitive cells of enteric bacteria have also been produced by growing the cells under conditions that interfere with cell wall synthesis. This is achieved by exposing the growing bacteria to media containing penicillin, sucrose and magnesium ions [33]. As with lysozyme, only the mucopeptide is removed, thus leaving other cell wall components to contaminate the cell membranes.

Method 1. The young Gram positive cells are washed free of medium components and suspended in 0·03 M phosphate buffer (pH 7·0) containing 0·2 M sucrose. Lysozyme is added to give a final concentration of 0·5 mg/ml. The suspension is incubated at 37° C for 10–30 minutes. The proportion of protoplasts can be determined by examination of wet films in the phase contrast microscope and determination of the number of spherical cells in relation to the number of rod-shaped bacteria. When the enzyme action is complete, the protoplasts are recovered by centrifugation at 5000 *g* for 20 minutes in a refrigerated centrifuge. The deposit is shaken thoroughly in distilled water to lyse the protoplasts, and the membranes are then recovered by centrifugation at 10,000 *g* for 15 minutes. They are washed once with 1·0 M sodium chloride solution and then two to three times with distilled water.

Method 2. The method applied to Gram negative cells is essentially that described by Repaske [42]. The washed bacteria are suspended in 0·03 M tris buffer (pH 8·0) together with Versene (EDTA) (pH 7·5; 0·27 mg/ml) and lysozyme (17 μg/ml), and the mixture is incubated at 37° C for 10–30 minutes. The membranes are thereafter prepared for osmotic shock and isolated as detailed above for Gram positive cells.

For organisms which are insusceptible to lysozyme or similar enzymes it is possible to isolate small amounts of cell membrane material following disruption of the cells by ultrasonic irradiation. Centrifugation at relatively low speed deposits the cell walls and unbroken cells, while centrifugation at 10,000 *g* for 30 minutes sediments portions of the cell membranes. These can then be washed with sodium chloride solution and with distilled water as above.

Intracellular components

After disintegration of bacterial cells and the removal of cell wall and cell membrane constituents, the residual intracellular material can be divided into particulate and soluble matter. The former can be isolated in the ultra-centrifuge, while the soluble antigens can be purified by methods similar to those used for the purification of extracellular protein antigens (see p. 356).

Method. The cells are washed and disintegrated by ultrasonic irradiation or by treatment in the Mickle disintegrator. Fragments of the cell walls or the membrane are removed by centrifugation at 10,000 g for 10 minutes. Further high speed centrifugation at 25,000; 50,000 and 100,000 g can be used to fractionate the smaller particulate matter. The final supernatant fluid contains the soluble material and this can be subjected to such procedures as ammonium sulphate fractionation, and ion exchange chromatography.

In investigations of this sort, the material that is of interest may be present in very small quantities. In the preparation and analysis of such substances, microanalysis and small-scale preparative procedures may be required. Thus, the chromatographic methods listed earlier might have to be scaled down using smaller columns, flasks and other pieces of apparatus, while electro-phoresis might usefully be performed on the microscope slide ($7\cdot5 \times 2\cdot5$ cm) covered with agar or other supporting medium.

References

[1] ADA G.L., NOSSAL G.J.V., PYE J. & ABBOT A. (1964) Antigens in Immunity. I. Preparation and properties of flagellar antigens from *Salmonella adelaide*. *Austr. J. exp. Biol.* **42**, 267

[2] ALBERTSSON P.-A. (1958) Particle fractionation in liquid two-phase systems. *Biochim. biophys. Acta* **27**, 378

[3] ARCHIBALD A.R. & BADDILEY J. (1965) The extraction of teichoic acids from bacterial cell walls with phenylhydrazine, and its significance for the nature of their linkage with glycosamino-peptides. *Biochem. J.* **95**, 19c

[4] ARMSTRONG J.J., BADDILEY J., BUCHANAN J.G., CARSS B. & GREENBERG G.R. (1958) Isolation and structure of ribitol phosphate derivatives (teichoic acids) from bacterial cell walls. *J. chem. Soc.* p. 4344

[5] BADDILEY J. & DAVISON A.L. (1961) The occurrence and location of teichoic acids in lactobacilli. *J. gen. Microbiol.* **24**, 295

[6] BECKMANN I., SUBBAIAH T.V. & STOCKER B.A.D. (1964) Rough mutants of *Salmonella typhimurium*. 2. Serological and chemical investigations. *Nature, Lond.* **201**, 1299

[7] BOIVIN A. & MESROBEANU L. (1933) Technique pour la preparation des polyosides microbiens specifiques. *C.R. Soc. Biol.* **113**, 490

[8] BRITTEN R.J. & ROBERTS R.B. (1960) High resolution density gradient sedimentation analysis. *Science* **131**, 32

[9] COLLINS F.M. (1964) The effects of the growth rate on the composition of *Salmonella enteritidis* cell walls. *Austr. J. exp. Biol.* **42**, 255

[10] COLOWICK S.P. & KAPLAN N.O. (1955) *Methods in Enzymology. I. Methods of Extraction of Enzymes from Animal Tissues*, p. 25. New York: Academic Press

[11] COLOWICK S.P. & KAPLAN N.O. (1962) *Methods in Enzymology V. Column Chromatography of Proteins: Substituted Celluloses*, p. 3. New York: Academic Press

[12] DAVIES D.A.L. (1958) The smooth and rough somatic antigens of *Pasteurella pseudo-tuberculosis. J. gen. Microbiol.* **18**, 118

[13] DAVIES D.A.L. (1960) Polysaccharides of gram-negative bacteria. *Adv. Carbohydrate Chemistry* **15**, 271

[14] DAVIES D.A.L., MORGAN W.T.J. & RECORD B.R. (1955) Studies in immunochemistry. 15. The specific polysaccharide of the dominant 'O' somatic antigen of *Shigella dysenteriae. Biochem. J.* **60**, 290

[15] DAVIS R.J. & CLAPP C.E. (1961) Preparation of purified polysaccharides from *Rhizobium. Appl. Microbiol.* **9**, 519

[16] DIXON M. (1953) A nomogram for ammonium sulphate solutions. *Biochem. J.* **54**, 457

[17] DIXON M. & WEBB E.C. (1964) *Enzymes*, pp. 28–50. London: Longmans

[18] DUDMAN W.F. & WILKINSON J.F. (1956) Composition of extracellular polysaccharides of aerobacter–klebsiella strains. *Biochem. J.* **62**, 289

[19] DUGUID J.P. (1951) The demonstration of bacterial capsules and slime. *J. Path. Bact.* **63**, 673

[20] DUGUID J.P. & WILKINSON J.F. (1953) The influence of cultural conditions on poly-saccharide production by *Aerobacter aerogenes. J. gen. Microbiol.* **9**, 174

[21] EDEBO L. (1960) A new press for disruption of micro-organisms and other cells. *J. biochem. microbiol. Techn. Eng.* **2**, 453

[22] ELLIOTT S.D. (1962) Teichoic acid and the group antigen of group D streptococci. *Nature, Lond.* **193**, 1105

[23] ERIKSEN J. (1965) Immunochemical studies on some serological cross-reactions in the *Klebsiella* group. 13. Serological investigation of the cross-reaction of *Klebsiella* type 3(C), *Klebsiella aerogenes* strain B 1076/48 and *Enterobacter* strain 349. *Acta path. scand.* **64**, 527

[24] ERLANDER S.R., KOFFLER H. & FOSTER J.F. (1960) Physical properties of flagellin from *Proteus vulgaris*, a study involving the application of the Archibald sedimentation principle. *Arch. biochem. Biophys.* **90**, 139

[25] FOSTER J.W. & RIBI E. (1962) Immunological role of *Brucella abortus* cell walls. *J. Bact.* **84**, 258

[26] GOEBEL W.F. (1963) Colanic acid. *Proc. nat. Acad. Sci. (Wash.)* **49**, 464

[27] GOLDFARB D.M., ZUEV V.A. & GERSHANOVITCH V.N. (1964) Spheroplasts of *Escherichia coli* obtained by the lytic enzyme isolated from phage T_2. *Nature, Lond.* **204**, 1331

[28] HEIDELBERGER, M. (1960) Structure and immunological specificity of polysaccharides. *Prog. Chem. org. nat. Prod.* **18**, 503

[29] HUGHES D.E. (1951) A press for disrupting bacteria and other micro-organisms. *Brit. J. exp. Path.* **32**, 97

[30] HUGHES D.E. (1961) The disintegration of bacteria and other micro-organisms by the MSE-Mullard ultrasonic disintegrator. *J. biochem. microbiol. Techn. Eng.* **3**, 405

[31] KOBAYASHI T., RINKER J.N. & KOFFLER H. (1959) Purification and chemical properties of flagellin. *Arch. biochem. Biophys.* **84**, 342

[32] KOHN J. (1959) A simple method for concentrating fluids containing protein. *Nature, Lond.* **183**, 1055

[33] LEDERBERG J. (1956) Bacterial protoplasts induced by penicillin. *Proc. nat. Acad. Sci. (Wash.)* **42**, 574

[34] LILLY M.D. (1962) Cell-wall precursors in *Escherichia coli. J. gen. Microbiol.* **28**, 2P

[35] LUDERITZ O., RISSE H.J., SCHULTE-HOLTHAUSEN H., STROMINGER J.L., SUTHERLAND I.W. & WESTPHAL O. (1965) Biochemical studies of the S–R mutation in *Salmonella minnesota. J. Bact.* **89**, 343

[36] LUDERITZ O., STAUB A.M. & WESTPHAL O. (1966) Immunochemistry of O and R antigens of *Salmonella* and related *Enterobacteriaceae. Bact. Rev.* **30,** 192

[37] MICKLE H. (1948) Tissue disintegrator (part II). *J. Roy. Microscop.* **68,** 10

[38] MITCHELL P. & MOYLE J. (1951) The glycerophospho-protein complex envelope of *Micrococcus pyogenes. J. gen. Microbiol.* **5,** 981

[39] MORGAN W.T.J. (1937) Studies in immunochemistry. II. The isolation and properties of a specific antigenic substance from *B. dysenteriae* (Shiga). *Biochem. J.* **31,** 2003

[40] MUNOZ J., RIBI E. & LARSON C.L. (1959) Antigens of *Bordetella pertussis*. I. Activities of cell walls and protoplasm. *J. Immunol.* **83,** 496

[41] ØRSKOV I., ØRSKOV F., JANN B. & JANN K. (1963) Acidic polysaccharide antigens of a new type from *Escherichia coli* capsules. *Nature, Lond.* **200,** 144

[42] REPASKE R. (1956) Lysis of gram-negative bacteria by lysozyme. *Biochim. biophys. Acta* **22,** 189

[43] RIBI E. & HOYER B.H. (1960) Purification of Q fever Rickettsiae by density gradient sedimentation. *J. Immunol.* **85,** 314

[44] SALTON M.R.J. (1964) *The Bacterial Cell Wall.* Amsterdam: Elsevier

[45] SANDERSON A.R., JUERGENS W.G. & STROMINGER J.L. (1961) Chemical and immuno-chemical structure of teichoic acid from *Staphylococcus aureus* (Copenhagen). *Biochem. Biophys. Res. Commn.* **5,** 472

[46] SCOTT J.E. (1960) Aliphatic ammonium salts in the assay of acidic polysaccharides from tissues. *Methods of Biochemical Analysis* **8,** 145

[47] SCOTT J.E. (1965) Fractionation by precipitation with quaternary ammonium salts. In *Methods in Carbohydrate Chemistry* **5,** 38, ed. WHISTLER R.L. New York: Academic Press

[48] SEVAG M.G. (1934) Eine neue physikalische Entweissungs-methode zur Darstellung biologisch wirksamer Substanzen. *Biochem. Z.* **273,** 419

[49] SHAFA F. & SALTON M.R.J. (1960) Disaggregation of bacterial cell walls by anionic detergents. *J. gen. Microbiol.* **22,** 137

[50] SHOCKMAN G.D., KOLB J.J. & TOENNIES G. (1957) A high speed shaker for the disruption of cells at low temperatures. *Biochim. biophys. Acta* **24,** 203

[51] STAUB A.M. & RAYNAUD M. (1964) Connaissances actuelles sur la nature chimique des antigenes presents dans les Salmonella. In *The World Problem of Salmonellosis,* p. 143, ed. VAN OYE E. The Hague: W. Junk

[52] SUTHERLAND I.W. (1963) The protective activity of components of *Bordetella pertussis* cell walls. *Immunology* **6,** 246

[53] SUTHERLAND I.W., LUDERITZ O. & WESTPHAL O. (1965) Studies on the structure of lipopolysaccharides of *Salmonella minnesota* and *Salmonella typhimurium* R strains. *Biochem. J.* **96,** 439

[54] WESTPHAL O., LUDERITZ O. & BISTER F. (1952) Uber die Extraktion von Bakterien mit Phenol-Wasser. *Z. Naturforsch.* **7B,** 148

[55] WILKINSON J.F., DUDMAN W.F. & ASPINALL G.O. (1955) The extracellular polysaccharide of *Aerobacter aerogenes* A3(S1) (*Klebsiella* type 54). *Biochem. J.* **59,** 446

CHAPTER 10

Preparation of Antigens from Animal Viruses

G. APPLEYARD & H.T. ZWARTOUW

Introduction

The behaviour of viruses as antigens is important for a variety of reasons. The immune reaction that is stimulated by a viral infection is usually beneficial to the host since it aids recovery from disease and increases resistance to reinfection with the same virus. The antibodies responsible for protection are those that neutralize infectivity by combining with certain essential antigens of the virus particle. Other non-neutralizing antibodies may also be produced and, although these are not known to play any part in combating infection, the detection of their presence is frequently useful to the diagnostician or epidemiologist.

A different reason for considering viruses as antigens is the usefulness of immunological techniques for the study of virus structure and multiplication. This arises from the fact that the specificity of a viral antigen depends upon the viral nucleic acid that codes for it and not upon the cell in which it is synthesized. So it is possible by means of an anti-viral serum to distinguish virus-specific products of infection from host cell components. The main precaution to be observed in such tests is that the antiserum does not contain antibodies to host constituents as well as virus; this is achieved most conveniently by preparing the serum against virus grown in a completely different tissue or, if this is not possible, by absorbing the serum with host tissue.

There are two kinds of viral antigen. Some antigens are structural components of the virus, and will be referred to as 'virus particle antigens'. Others are separate from and smaller than the virus particles; these will be called 'soluble antigens' although it is appreciated that the term 'soluble' has no precise meaning. Soluble antigens may be further subdivided into those that are also present in the virus particle and those that occur exclusively in the soluble form; the first group are probably virus components synthesized in excess whereas the second may be enzymes required for virus multiplication. Soluble antigens not present in the virus particle have been demonstrated so far only with the poxviruses. But it now seems likely that some of the enzymes concerned in replication of the nucleic acid (both RNA and DNA)

376

of several virus groups are virus-specific. If this is so, such enzymes should be demonstrable as soluble viral antigens that are not virus particle components.

All the known viral antigens are simple or conjugated proteins. Purification of soluble antigens is therefore primarily a problem of protein fractionation. A recent account of the various methods available in this field is given by Sober *et al* [1]. The preparation of antigens from virus particles raises a different problem. Methods must be found to disrupt the virus without at the same time destroying the specificity of the antigens. However, an antigen that can be obtained from a suspension of purified virus will be almost free from contaminating host material; if obtained in good yield, it is likely to provide a better starting-point for purification than the corresponding antigen in an extract of infected tissues. With some antigens, of course, this choice between two sources is not available.

The degree of purity desirable in an antigen depends upon the purpose for which it is required. For some purposes, e.g. use as a diagnostic antigen, it may be sufficient that the antigen is free from other viral antigens and the presence of host materials is unimportant. Other procedures, e.g. determination of the amino-acid composition of an antigen, would require an antigen of the greatest possible purity. These considerations will affect the method of purification that is chosen.

In this chapter we describe the preparation of antigens from poxviruses, adenoviruses, myxoviruses and foot-and-mouth disease virus. The methods used with these four groups exemplify the kinds of approach that should prove to be profitable with other viruses that have so far been studied less extensively. Since the authors' own experience has been predominantly with the poxviruses, the techniques used with this group are described in most detail.

POXVIRUSES

Nature of the antigens

The poxviruses comprise a number of subgroups which are distinguished mainly by their antigenic constitution and host range. The most important subgroup contains the viruses of vaccinia, variola, alastrim, cowpox, rabbit-pox, ectromelia and monkeypox all of which cross-react and appear to contain very similar antigens. Viruses of different subgroups do not cross-react directly but all poxviruses are believed to possess a common internal antigen [2]. This shared antigen was extracted from the virus particles with hot alkali and was originally thought to be a nucleoprotein. More recent evidence, to be discussed later, suggests that it may be a protein that does not contain nucleic acid.

Vaccinia is by far the most extensively studied poxvirus because of the relative ease with which large quantities of this virus can be grown and purified. Like the other members of the group, vaccinia is a large virus which has a very complex morphology [3, 4] and consists of about 90 per cent protein. The virus particle would, therefore, be expected to contain a number of different antigens. Early work, reviewed by Smadel & Hoagland [5], demonstrated the existence of four viral antigens. However, more recent investigations have shown that the antigenic composition of the poxviruses is considerably more complex than was previously supposed. This is in contrast to evidence on the chemical composition for it is now believed that some substances, once considered suggestive of a rudimentary respiratory system, are not essential components of the virus [6].

Early nomenclature of antigens
The original nomenclature of vaccinia virus antigens [5] is still widely quoted so it will be described first and then related to more recent evidence.

LS antigen
This soluble antigen was responsible for the serological activity of infected tissue extracts after virus particles had been completely removed by centrifugation and filtration. The antigen possessed two specificities which were apparently on a single molecule; one of these specificities was labile (L) and the other stable (S) to heat. LS antigen was also present as a surface component of the virus particle from which it spontaneously dissociated.

NP antigen
The nucleoprotein antigen comprised about half the weight of the virus particle but was not present in 'soluble antigen'. It contained the virus DNA and was obtained in solution by treating purified virus with sodium hydroxide solution at 56° C.

X agglutinogen
Some antisera that had been adsorbed with both LS and NP antigens were still able to agglutinate virus particles. The existence of antigen 'X' on the virus surface was therefore postulated.

Protective antigen
As none of the above antigens was able to elicit neutralizing antibody or immunity to infection, a further 'protective antigen' was apparently present in the virus.

Present knowledge of the antigens
The antigens are conveniently divided into those found as soluble antigens and those found in the virus particle. The investigation of both these groups has been greatly assisted by the technique of immunodiffusion which is able to differentiate the individual components in a complex mixture of antigens.

Soluble antigens
The first immunodiffusion studies revealed up to nine precipitin lines when extracts of infected tissues were reacted with the appropriate antiserum [7, 8]. This number has been considerably increased by using more concentrated antigen preparations and the more sensitive micro-immunodiffusion technique of Crowle [9]. Seventeen precipitin lines were produced by the soluble antigens of vaccinia [10] and twenty by that of rabbitpox [11]. The difference in number produced by the two viruses is not to be regarded as significant, for both figures are provisional and may be increased when further advances are made in methods of antigen detection.

When vaccinia virus soluble antigen is heated for half an hour at 60° C, about half the components are inactivated whereas the others remain detectable by immunodiffusion [10]. The original concept of the single LS antigen thus accounted for the collective behaviour of a large number of antigens some of which were more heat-labile than the others.

Contrary to former belief, one component of poxvirus soluble antigen is able to react with neutralizing antibody [12]. Injection of soluble antigen into rabbits also elicits neutralizing antibody and produces some immunity to infection [13]. The 'protective antigen' responsible for these effects appears to be a protein of molecular weight between 100,000 and 200,000 [14]. This antigen has not been correlated with a precipitin line in immunodiffusion tests. The biological significance of the other components of soluble antigen is less certain; this problem is discussed later.

Virus particle antigens
Vaccinia virus particles are too large to produce lines in an immunodiffusion test. However, the artificial disruption of purified virus liberates a number of antigens that are detectable by this technique. The NP antigen of earlier workers was obtained by treating the virus with hot 0·04 N sodium hydroxide [15]. This relatively drastic treatment produced a marked clarification of concentrated virus suspensions but it still left a large insoluble fraction and the dissolved material was partially degraded. Recently it has been shown that treatment at a lower temperature and less alkaline pH releases antigens that give more and stronger precipitin lines in immunodiffusion tests, even though the procedure dissolves a smaller proportion of the virus [16]. These serologically active extracts contain little or no nucleic acid. Subsequent treatment

N*

of the virus at higher pH values does extract the viral DNA together with more protein but these later extracts do not produce precipitin lines. Thus it appears that the NP or nucleoprotein antigen was an artefact due to the simultaneous extraction from the virus of DNA, inactive protein and partially degraded precipitinogens.

Material resembling that extracted by the milder alkaline treatment is

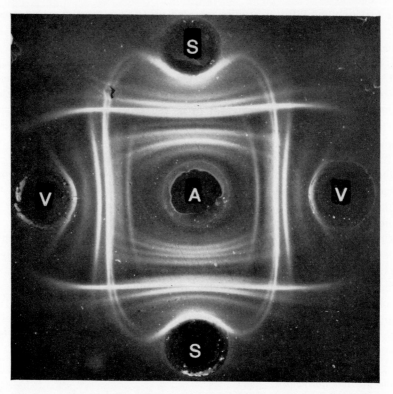

FIG. 10.1 Immunodiffusion pattern of vaccinia virus antigens. Complete vaccinia antiserum was placed at the central position A, soluble antigens at S and a solution of virus particle antigens at V.

slowly released during prolonged incubation of purified virus suspensions. This autodegradation is almost complete after 3 days at 37° C but the same antigens can be liberated more rapidly and conveniently by digestion of the virus with a small amount of a protease such as trypsin [16].

The soluble materials obtained from the virus particles by these three methods are similar and produce up to eight lines in immunodiffusion tests but they represent only 20 per cent of the total viral nitrogen. Solutions containing more viral material do not produce any further precipitin lines but such solutions can only be obtained by more drastic procedures. Hence it is possible that some antigens of the virus particle have yet to be obtained in an active 'soluble' form.

Relationship between soluble and virus particle antigens

Vaccinia soluble antigens and the antigens from the virus particle have been compared directly by immunodiffusion [10]. Most of the lines produced by the virus particle antigens link only with weak soluble antigen lines and the dominant soluble antigen lines do not correspond to any of the virus particle

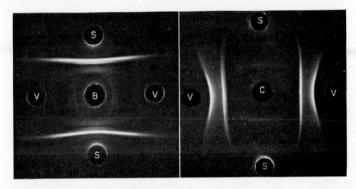

FIG. 10.2. Comparison of immunodiffusion patterns of vaccinia virus antigens obtained with different antisera. Soluble antigen antiserum was placed at the central position B, virus particle antiserum at the central position C, soluble antigens at S and a solution of virus particle antigens at V.

components (Fig. 10.1). Confirmation of the difference between the two sets of antigens is obtained by using antisera prepared against virus-free soluble antigens or against inactivated purified virus. Neither type of antiserum is as effective for producing precipitin lines as antiserum prepared against infective virus. Nevertheless, the patterns of lines produced by these antisera emphasize the general difference between the two sets of antigens (Fig. 10.2). Tests with antiserum to inactivated virus also indicate the presence of antibody to a ninth virus particle antigen that is not detectable in the virus extracts; it is revealed as a precipitin line when the antiserum reacts with soluble antigen.

As many of the soluble antigens do not appear to be virus precursor material, some other function can be attributed to them. Cells infected with poxviruses are known to form increased amounts of at least two enzymes (thymidine kinase and DNA polymerase) that are concerned in the synthesis of DNA and there is some evidence that these enzymes are produced under the influence of the viral rather than the host cell genome [17, 18, 19]. It is therefore possible that some of the soluble antigens are virus-induced enzymes which are essential for virus synthesis but are not incorporated into the mature particles.

Haemagglutinin
The erythrocytes of certain fowls are agglutinated by extracts of tissues infected with many poxviruses. Haemagglutination is not caused by the virus itself but by a smaller particle, about 65 mμ in diameter, containing phospholipid [20, 21]. Some reports [22, 23] have indicated the existence of two haemagglutinins of different sedimentation characteristics, but only one

TABLE 10.1
Vaccinia virus antigens

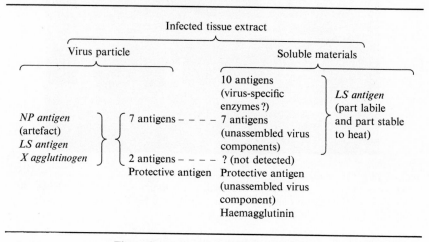

The early nomenclature is shown in italics.

of these appears to be virus-specific. It has also been suggested that the active material is polydisperse [24]. Vaccinia haemagglutinin may be formed at the host cell surface; antiserum prevented its appearance in tissue culture while not affecting the intracellular formation of virus particles [25]. Some strains of vaccinia and rabbitpox viruses do not produce any haemagglutinin. Thus the haemagglutinin may be regarded as a rather ill-defined lipid–protein complex which arises at the cell surface as a non-essential by-product during the replication of some strains of virus.

Summary
Our present knowledge of the antigens of vaccinia virus is represented in Table 10.1.

Preparative methods

Growth of virus

Poxviruses are able to replicate in a wide range of animal cells and this is exemplified by the following three systems which have been used to prepare antigens. Titres may be increased if the virus has been 'adapted' to a particular host system by serial passage. After replication, most of the virus remains inside the infected cells so it is necessary to break these open. Large particles of debris are then removed from the infected tissue extracts by low-speed centrifugation (800 g for 10 minutes).

In chorioallantoic membranes (*CAM*)

This method has been used with minor variations for many of the poxviruses [2, 7, 8, 26, 27, 28, 29]. Typically, fertile hens' eggs are incubated for 11 or 12 days to obtain well-developed CAM which are 'dropped' by forming an artificial air sac and then infected via a hole in the shell with 10^3–10^4 pock-forming units of virus. After 2 or 3 days at 37° C, the infected area of each CAM is collected and disrupted in buffer (1 ml of 0·004 M phosphate–citrate pH 7·4 per CAM) with a high-speed homogenizer.

In tissue culture

This method has been used for vaccinia and rabbitpox viruses in HeLa cells [14, 29, 30] and it should be of more general application. Monolayer cultures are infected by adding about 5 pock- (or plaque-) forming units per cell and adsorbing the virus from a minimal volume of medium during 1 hour at 37° C. Growth medium is then added (about 1 ml per 10^6 cells) and the cultures incubated for 24 hours at 37° C. The infected cells, which often become loosened, are shaken or scraped off the glass surface into the medium and collected by centrifugation (200 g for 10 minutes). The cells are resuspended in a small volume (4×10^7 cells per ml) of phosphate-buffered saline (pH 7·4) and disrupted by ultrasonication.

In tissue cultures, the 'early antigens' can be obtained preferentially by preventing completion of the growth cycle. This is achieved by harvesting the cells a short time after infection, by ultraviolet-irradiating the infecting virus, or by adding inhibitors such as sodium azide or isatin β-thiosemicarbazone [31].

In rabbit skin

This procedure is especially suitable for vaccinia virus [5]. The hair is removed from the back and sides of rabbits with razor and soap to leave the skin clean and reasonably sterile. Vaccinia virus (10 ml of 10^8 pock-forming units per ml) is put dropwise on to the skin while the surface is lightly scratched with the edge of a fine wire gauze or a fine wire brush (suede leather brush). A uniform 'blush' should be produced on the skin without bleeding. After 3 days, the animals are killed and the infected area of skin removed and pinned out tightly on a board. The surface of the skin is moistened with about 10 ml of buffer (0·004 M phosphate–citrate pH 7·8 with 0·1 per cent sodium azide to inhibit growth of bacteria) and gently scraped with a blunt blade so that the material already oozing from the infected vesicles is completely expressed. The fluid and curd-like material are gathered and two further scrapings each with 10 ml of buffer are carried out. The infected cells are easily disrupted and scraping too vigorously adds unwanted tissue pulp to the virus material. After shaking with glass beads to disperse the material uniformly in the buffer, the larger particles are removed by centrifugation and the supernatant fluid retained. The sediment can be re-extracted by shaking with glass beads and buffer.

Soluble antigens

Virus particles are sedimented from the infected tissue extract by high-speed centrifugation to leave the soluble antigens (and soluble host-cell material) in the supernatant fluid. Less than 1 per cent of the total virus remains in the supernatant after centrifugation at 35,000 g for 30 minutes. If complete removal of virus particles is essential (e.g. when required to immunize with soluble antigens specifically) the preparation must be filtered. Membrane filters (a.p.d. 300–350 mμ) are preferable to Seitz pads but some adsorption of precipitin line components occurs even on membranes [10].

Purification of individual soluble antigen components has not yet been achieved. The acid precipitation method for 'isolation' of LS antigen [32] produces only slight separation of the antigens forming different precipitin lines. A partial separation of some of these antigens has been achieved by chromatography on DEAE-cellulose, CM-cellulose and calcium phosphate [14].

Virus particle antigens

Purification of virus

Poxviruses have usually been purified by centrifugation and this procedure is best carried out by rate zonal sedimentation in a density gradient [27, 30]. As the viruses are aggregated by salt solutions, sucrose is used to form the density gradient and the virus is suspended in very dilute buffer (0·004 M sodium phosphate–sodium citrate) at a slightly alkaline pH (7·8). The virus sediment, obtained after centrifugation of an infected tissue extract, is first dispersed by ultrasonication to form an opalescent suspension in dilute buffer (one-tenth of the volume of the original fluid). Suitable density gradients for 3 × 1 in. tubes can be prepared by successively layering 6 ml each of 60, 50, 40 and 30 per cent (w/v) sucrose in dilute buffer followed by 6 ml of the resuspended virus. After centrifugation in a swinging bucket rotor (Spinco SW-25) at 39,000 g for 20 minutes, the virus forms an opalescent zone in the 50 per cent sucrose (Fig. 10.3). As some sediment collects at the bottom of the tube, the virus zone is removed via the top of the tube with a pipette. This process is aided by lowering a perforated disk into the gradient and locating it successively at the boundaries of each required zone. The corresponding zones containing purified virus from a number of tubes are combined, diluted with two volumes of buffer and the virus deposited by centrifugation (35,000 g for 60 minutes). Removal of the sucrose is completed by further washing in the centrifuge (35,000 g for 30 minutes) with buffer followed by water. Finally, the virus is suspended in water and stored frozen at $-60°$ C.

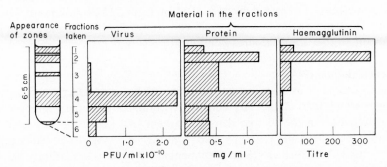

Fig. 10.3. Separation of vaccinia virus, haemagglutinin and protein impurity after centrifugation in a sucrose density gradient. (This figure was originally published in [30] *The Journal of General Microbiology*)

Purity is checked most satisfactorily by examining the virus in the electron microscope. When thawed out, the stored virus is sometimes flocculated. This does not matter if antigens are to be dissolved from the virus particles as the treatments involved rapidly disaggregate the particles. For other purposes, ultrasonication in 0·004 M phosphate–citrate pH 7·8 or in 0·01 M ammonium bicarbonate (which can be volatilized for electron microscopy) is generally satisfactory. Dry weight or total nitrogen determinations can be used to measure the concentration of virus for subsequent work. Dried vaccinia virus contains 14·7 per cent nitrogen [6].

Dissolving antigens from the virus particles [16]

A suspension of purified virus (0·1 per cent dry weight) in 0·01 M sodium phosphate buffer pH 8·0 with 0·001 per cent crystallized trypsin is incubated at 37° C for 3 hours. The insoluble material is removed by centrifugation

(30,000 *g* for 15 minutes is sufficient for small volumes) to leave a clear solution containing about 20 per cent of the viral nitrogen.

Two other methods produce similar materials. In the first, virus in dilute buffer at pH 7·5–8·0 with 0·1 per cent sodium azide (to prevent growth of any contaminating organisms) is incubated at 37° C for 72 hours. In the second, virus in buffer at pH 10·5 (e.g. 0·1 M glycine + NaOH) is incubated at 37° C for 30 minutes.

Non-infective virus particles

Two methods appear to be equally suitable for the preparation of non-infective whole virus particle antigens for subsequent preparation of antisera [10]. Purified virus suspensions (0·13 per cent dry weight) are either treated with formaldehyde (0·4 per cent) for 1 hour at 20° C or irradiated for 5 minutes as a thin layer (1·7 mm) at a distance of 34 cm from a 15 W Phillips ultraviolet lamp. The treated virus may be mixed with 1·5 volumes of Freund's complete adjuvant so that the final virus concentration is 0·05 per cent dry weight.

Haemagglutinin (HA)

When vaccinia virus is sedimented from infected tissue extracts, as described above, about half of the HA activity is obtained with the impure virus. Centrifugation in the sucrose density gradient [30] leaves the HA near the top of the gradient and well separated from the virus (Fig. 10.3). Attempts to purify the HA by further velocity sedimentations in sucrose density gradients appear to confirm the polydisperse nature of this substance. It does, however, form a band in potassium tartrate gradients under sedimentation equilibrium conditions (39,000 rev/min in Spinco rotor SW-39 for 6 hours) [33]. The HA can be adsorbed on DEAE-cellulose [34].

ADENOVIRUSES

Nature of the antigens

The known antigens of the adenoviruses are (i) a group-specific antigen, (ii) a toxic factor, and (iii) a type-specific antigen. The antigens have received a variety of other designations which are summarized in Table 10.2. All three antigens occur in soluble form, and recent studies with adenovirus type 5 [35, 36] have shown that they are also constituents of the virus particles.

The soluble group-specific antigen is demonstrated by complement fixation or immunodiffusion tests. It carries a specificity that is common to all mammalian adenoviruses and is one of the distinguishing features of this group. It is possible, however, that the group-specific antigen is not identical in all virus serotypes, for the antigens of types 4 and 5 have been found to differ in their behaviour on DEAE-cellulose [37]. In the virus particle, all but twelve of the 252 capsomeres consist of group-specific antigen, which is a spherical protein with a diameter of 8 mμ [36].

The soluble toxic factor is responsible for the early cytopathic effect that is seen in tissue cultures after the inoculation of crude adenovirus preparations. It can also be demonstrated by immunodiffusion and complement-fixation tests and shows subgroup specificity, one such subgroup containing the virus types 1, 2, 4, 5 and 6. Treatment with trypsin destroys the toxic activity and subgroup specificity and converts the toxic factor to a substance indistinguishable from type-specific antigen [38]. Electron microscopy shows that the toxic factor consists of a spherical head 8 mμ in diameter attached to a tail 20 mμ long and 2 mμ wide with a 4 mμ knob on the end. In the virus particle it occurs as the twelve capsomeres at the vertices of the icosohedral structure with the tails extending outwards from the virus surface [36].

TABLE 10.2

Nomenclature of adenovirus antigens

Authors	Group-specific antigen	Type-specific antigen	Toxic factor
Klemperer & Pereira [45]	A	C	B
Wilcox & Ginsberg [37]	L	E	T
Brandon & McLean [78]	3	1	2

The type-specific antigen is responsible for the specificity of the twenty-eight human and several animal virus serotypes that are distinguished by neutralization tests. In its soluble form, the antigen fixes complement and forms a precipitin line with homotypic antiserum. Morphologically it appears to be identical with the tail of the toxic factor and in the virus particle it exists only as a part of this antigen [36].

Preparative methods

Growth of virus

Since adenoviruses do not in general infect laboratory animals, they are grown in tissue culture. HeLa and KB cells usually give high virus yields. The infected monolayer cultures are incubated until the cytopathic effect shows that all cells are producing virus. The time required varies from about 2 days, if the ratio of infecting virus to cells approaches unity, to a week or more with lower multiplicities of infection. Both soluble antigens and virus particles tend to remain intracellular. The medium is therefore discarded and a concentrated suspension of the infected cells (about 10^6 per ml) in 0·01 M phosphate buffer pH 7 is disrupted by a homogenizer, ultrasonication or freezing and thawing. The larger cell debris is removed by low-speed centrifugation (800 *g* for 10 minutes) and the clarified material is used for the preparation of soluble antigens or virus.

Soluble antigens

Separation of the three recognized soluble antigens can be achieved by electrophoresis in agar [39]. A more satisfactory method is chromatography on DEAE-cellulose with varied concentrations of sodium chloride as the eluant. The crude preparation of virus and antigens is dialysed overnight against 0·01 M buffer (phosphate, acetate or borate) of the required pH and is then applied to the DEAE-cellulose. A column 1 cm in diameter and 10 cm in height contains about 1 g dry weight of adsorbent and may be loaded with about 50 mg protein. Elution is carried out by gradient or stepwise increases in sodium chloride concentrations. The technical aspects of chromatography on substituted celluloses are described by Petersen & Sober [40]. After elution, the effluent fractions are tested for virus infectivity, for early toxic activity in tissue culture [41], and for complement fixation with homotypic rabbit antiserum (reacts with all antigens) and heterotypic rabbit antiserum (reacts with group-specific antigen and with toxic factor of the same subgroup). If an antiserum against purified type-specific antigen is already available, this can be used to titrate the type-specific antigen directly. Immunodiffusion in agar is also a useful, though less quantitative, test.

The soluble antigens are eluted before the virus and produce fairly well-defined peaks of activity. Their behaviour varies according to the pH of the eluting fluid so that antigens that overlap at one pH may prove to be easily separable at another [37]. Virus infectivity elutes later and often gives a diffuse peak and poor total recovery. The reported elution characteristics of some types of adenovirus and their antigens are given in Table 10.3.

The separation of antigens by a single chromatographic run is unlikely to be complete. Appropriately pooled fractions should therefore be chromatographed at least once more. Chromatography at two different pH values may be necessary to separate all three antigens. For example, Wilcox & Ginsberg [37] found that chromatography of adenovirus type 5 antigens at pH 7·2 separated the group-specific antigen (eluted late) from a mixture of the type-specific antigen and toxin (eluted early); the latter antigens could then be separated from each other by chromatography at pH 5·2. It should be emphasized that the antigens prepared in this way, although probably monospecific when tested against adenovirus antiserum, are likely to be contaminated with protein from the host cells.

Virus particle antigens

The group-specific and type-specific antigens occur in about equal amounts in the soluble material [46], but the virus particles contain predominantly the group-specific antigen. Disrupted virus is therefore likely to be a more useful source of group-specific antigen than of either of the other two.

The virus must first be purified. The procedure used by Wilcox & Ginsberg [46] with adenovirus type 5 produced a virus suspension that contained about 10^{11}–10^{12} plaque-forming units per ml and no detectable host cell or virus

TABLE 10.3

Elution of adenoviruses and their soluble antigens from DEAE-cellulose

| Reference | Serotype | pH of eluant | NaCl concentration (M) reported for elution of | | | |
			Group-specific antigen	Type-specific antigen	Toxic factor	Virus infectivity
42	1	8·1			0·2	0·45
43	1	7·2	0·2	0·0	0·1	0·4
43	2	7·2	0·2	0·0	0·1	0·4
44	2	7·2	0·5		0·25	>0·5
45	2	6·5	0·3	0·05		
42	3	8·1				0·25
37	4	7·2	0·08	0·08		0·2
37	4	5·2	0·0	0·12		
37	5	7·2	0·26	0·08	0·12	0·4
37	5	5·2	0·16	0·0	0·16	
45	5	6·5	0·3	0·05	0·2	>0·5
42	8	8·1				0·25

soluble antigens. The method consists of precipitation with 30 per cent methanol at $-25°$ C, two treatments with fluorocarbon and two or three equilibrium sedimentations in a caesium chloride density gradient; the virus particles form a band at a mean buoyant density of 1·3349. The virus can also be purified on a density gradient of rubidium chloride [47].

The purified virus is disintegrated at pH 10·5 by dialysing the suspension for 4 days against 0·1 M carbonate–bicarbonate buffer at 4° C [46]. The slightly opalescent suspension becomes clear and the resulting solution contains viral nucleic acid and the three antigens. Final separation of antigens obtained from the virus has not been reported but it should be possible to achieve this by chromatography on DEAE-cellulose.

MYXOVIRUSES

Nature of the antigens

The myxoviruses may be divided into two subgroups, the distinguishing features of which have been summarized by Waterson [48]. Subgroup 1 consists of the true influenza viruses, types A, B and C, while subgroup 2 includes the viruses of Newcastle disease, mumps, parainfluenza 1, 2, 3 and 4, and probably also measles and respiratory syncytial viruses. With only a few exceptions, the myxoviruses of both groups possess (i) a ribonucleoprotein antigen, (ii) a haemagglutinin and (iii) a neuraminidase.

The ribonucleoprotein antigen is the internal component of the virus particle. It occurs as a tightly coiled helix, which has a diameter of 9 mμ in subgroup 1 and 18 mμ in subgroup 2 viruses. An apparently identical antigen is found free in infected tissues, and is then referred to as soluble (or 'S') antigen. The nucleoprotein antigen in its soluble form is responsible for the specificity of the three influenza virus types that is shown by complement fixation.

The haemagglutinin consists of surface projections that radiate from the lipoprotein membrane of the virus. The membrane itself is probably derived, at least in part, from host cell material. Serologically, the haemagglutinin shows strain specificity within the influenza virus types. It is identical, or very closely associated, with the strain-specific 'V' antigen that is detected by complement fixation and with the antigen that elicits virus-neutralizing antibody. It does not occur naturally as a soluble antigen separate from the virus particle.

The neuraminidase, like the haemagglutinin, is present on the virus surface. The enzyme splits N-acetylneuraminic acid from the mucoprotein receptor substance of cells and is responsible for the spontaneous elution of adsorbed virus from erythrocytes.

Preparative methods
Growth of virus

Most myxoviruses grow to high titre in the allantoic cavity of 10–12 day fertile hens' eggs. A suitable inoculum is 0·1 ml of a 1 in 100 dilution of infected allantoic fluid. The eggs are incubated for 24 or 48 hours to obtain the maximum titre of haemagglutinin. They are then chilled to 4° C and the allantoic fluid is harvested by suction.

The virus can be partially purified by adsorption on to erythrocytes. This is achieved by the addition of a 2 per cent suspension of washed human, guinea-pig or fowl erythrocytes to the allantoic fluid, or by tearing the chorioallantoic membranes at the time of harvest so that the vessels of the embryo bleed into the fluid. After 1 hour at 4° C, the erythrocytes are sedimented by centrifugation, washed once with cold saline, and resuspended in about one-tenth the original volume of saline at pH 7. Virus is eluted by incubating the erythrocyte suspension at 37° C. Complete elution may take up to 6 hours, but it is considerably hastened by the addition of 50 units per ml of receptor destroying enzyme from Vibrio cholerae (RDE). The erythrocytes are removed by centrifugation, and the supernatant fluid then contains the concentrated and partially purified virus. The virus can be further concentrated, if required, by centrifugation at 30,000 g for 1 hour.

Influenza viruses can also be purified by column chromatography, either alone or following preliminary purification by adsorption to erythrocytes. Miller & Schlesinger [49] used columns of aluminium phosphate gel mixed with silica gel as a supporting material to purify several virus strains. Virus adsorbs to the column more readily than most of the impurities and can then be eluted by increasing the phosphate concentration and pH. The Melbourne strain, for example, is adsorbed from 0·125 M phosphate at pH 6·6 and eluted by 0·25 M phosphate at pH 7·2. Cellulose phosphate columns were used by Laver [50] to purify the Lee strain of virus. In this method, the virus suspended in 0·1 M phosphate at pH 7·1 passes directly through the column whereas most of the impurities are adsorbed.

Nucleoprotein antigen
The purest nucleoprotein antigen is obtained from the virus particles. Hoyle [51] first demonstrated that type A influenza virus (DSP strain) could be disrupted by ether to yield nucleoprotein antigen and haemagglutinin, and Schäfer & Zillig [52] obtained similar results with fowl-plague virus. The method was studied in detail by Lief & Henle [53], using PR8 and other strains of type A virus, and has since been employed successfully with a wide range of myxoviruses. The purified virus suspension is mixed with half its volume of peroxide-free ether. The mixture is agitated for 2 hours at room temperature, either continuously with a magnetic stirrer or intermittently by vigorous shaking about every half-hour. When the aqueous and ether phases are separated by centrifugation, the denatured lipoprotein material of the virus collects at the interface. The aqueous layer is taken and nitrogen is bubbled gently through it to evaporate the last traces of ether. Haemagglutinin is removed from the solution by repeated adsorption with guinea-pig erythrocytes at 4° C; the first batch of erythrocytes used for adsorption can also act as a source for preparation of haemagglutinin (v.i.). Finally, the nucleoprotein antigen may be concentrated by centrifugation at 80,000 g for 6 hours, followed by resuspension of the deposit in a small volume and clarification at 6000 g for 10 minutes [54].

A richer source of nucleoprotein antigen is the soluble antigen from infected chorioallantoic membranes [55]. After growth of virus in eggs as described above, the chorioallantoic membranes are homogenized in saline (1–2 ml per membrane) and the suspension is clarified by low-speed centrifugation. The virus particles are then removed by high-speed centrifugation or by repeated adsorption with erythrocytes until haemagglutinin is no longer detectable. The antigen prepared in this way has only a single viral specificity but is grossly contaminated with cellular material.

Haemagglutinin

The haemagglutinin, unlike the nucleoprotein antigen, can be prepared only from virus particles. Purified virus is disrupted with ether, as for the preparation of nucleoprotein antigen. The haemagglutinin is separated by adsorption to a 2 per cent suspension of erythrocytes at 4° C; ether treatment sometimes reduces the haemagglutinating activity for fowl cells relative to that for guinea-pig cells, so the use of guinea-pig cells is preferable. The haemagglutinin is eluted from the erythrocytes at 37° C, with the help if necessary of RDE. One further cycle of adsorption and elution is usually sufficient to free it from detectable nucleoprotein antigen. The final elution is made into a small volume of fluid, and the haemagglutinin is concentrated further, if required, by centrifugation at 80,000 *g* for 6 hours.

Treatment with ether probably causes partial destruction of the haemagglutinin from some myxoviruses, though this may be masked by an increase in activity caused by disaggregation of the haemagglutinating particles. Norrby [56] found that if measles virus was stirred for 5 minutes with 0·125 per cent Tween 80 before exposure to ether, the yield of haemagglutinin was considerably higher than from virus treated with ether alone. This was attributed to stabilization of the haemagglutinin by Tween. The effect of this modified procedure on the yield of haemagglutinin from other myxoviruses has not been reported.

Laver [57] examined ether-treated influenza virus (Lee strain) under the electron microscope and concluded that the virus particles were only partially disintegrated. The detergent sodium dodecyl sulphate (SDS) is a considerably more efficient agent for the disruption of at least some strains of influenza virus [57, 58]. To effect disruption, the purified and concentrated virus is mixed with SDS at a final concentration of 2 per cent and maintained at room temperature for 10 minutes. Further action of the detergent is then stopped by precipitating it with potassium chloride in the cold [58] or by diluting the mixture 1 in 250 [57]. A major disadvantage of SDS for the preparation of haemagglutinin is that it inactivates the haemagglutinin of some virus strains. Thus, the haemagglutinin from Lee virus was inactive, that from MEL virus attached to red cells but did not agglutinate them, while that from BEL virus remained active. Sodium deoxycholate may be safer in this respect for it efficiently disrupted the Lee strain of virus without damaging the haemagglutin [57]. The effect of detergents on the serological activity of the nucleoprotein antigen has not been tested.

Neuraminidase
The haemagglutinin obtained by ether treatment of myxoviruses has neuraminidase activity, for it can elute spontaneously from erythrocytes at 37° C. It was thought for some time that the neuraminidase and haemagglutinating activities might be properties of the same virus component. However, it is now known that neuraminidase, free from haemagglutinin, can be released from influenza virus particles by treatment with trypsin [59, 60]. To obtain neuraminidase from the Lee strain, the purified and concentrated virus (10^4–10^6 haemagglutinating units per ml) is incubated for 10 minutes with 0·1 per cent crystalline trypsin at 37° C and pH 7·2 [60]. These conditions are chosen to give maximum liberation of enzyme with minimum thermal inactivation. The virus particles are removed by centrifugation, and the supernatant fluid then contains the neuraminidase together with the trypsin used in its preparation.

Neuraminidase is also liberated from virus particles by treatment with 2 per cent SDS or deoxycholate, and can be partially separated from the other products of virus disruption by electrophoresis on cellulose acetate [57]. But SDS inactivates the neuraminidase of some strains of virus, and the product obtained by the complete disruption of virus with detergent is clearly more difficult to purify than that set free by tryptic digestion.

FOOT-AND-MOUTH DISEASE VIRUS

Nature of the antigens

Tissues that are infected with foot-and-mouth disease (FMD) virus contain two viral antigens. The '25 mμ antigen' (sedimentation coefficient 140) consists of the whole virus particles, both infective and non-infective. The 7 mμ antigen (sedimentation coefficient 14) is non-infective, and may be composed of free viral capsomeres. Recently a third antigen, intermediate in size, has been described [61] but its nature is unknown.

The 25 mμ and 7 mμ antigens give rise to separate precipitin lines when they react in immunodiffusion tests with complete virus antiserum [62]. Nevertheless, the two antigens are closely related, for material apparently identical with the natural 7 mμ antigen is produced by degradation of the 25 mμ

particles. This relationship is confirmed by the observations that 25 mμ antigen removes those antibodies which combine with 7 mμ antigen in complement-fixation and immunodiffusion tests [63, 64], and conversely that 7 mμ antigen removes neutralizing antibody directed against infective 25 mμ particles [65].

There are seven serological types of FMD virus, namely A, O, C, S.A.T. 1, S.A.T. 2, S.A.T. 3 and Asia 1. The 25 mμ antigen is almost completely type specific, with the excepton that sera collected soon after infection may show some cross-neutralization between the three European types (A, O and C) [66]. The 7 mμ antigen is predominantly type specific, though considerable cross-complement fixation occurs between the European types.

It may be noted here that the relationship between the D and C antigens of poliovirus [67, 68] resembles in many ways that between the 25 mμ and 7 mμ antigens of FMD virus. The main difference is that the non-infective C antigen of poliovirus consists of particles of the same size as the potentially infective D antigen, even though the particles have lost most of their RNA and may be defective in other ways.

Preparative methods
Growth of virus
FMD virus can be grown to high titre in guinea-pig plantar pads or bovine tongues, in explants of bovine tongue, or in primary cultures of bovine or pig kidney cells. The most satisfactory host for production of the virus is the BHK 21 (baby hamster kidney) continuous cell line [69, 70]. Roller bottle cultures of BHK 21 cells are inoculated with a high multiplicity of virus (1 to 5 pfu per cell) in a small volume of medium (about 1 ml per 10^7 cells). The cultures are incubated on a roller drum at 37° C for 7 hours. The bulk of both types of antigen is found in the medium which contains between 10^9 and 10^{10} pfu/ml of infective virus [71].

Preparation of 25 mμ antigen
As the two viral antigens differ considerably with respect to their sedimentation coefficients, they are readily separated by centrifugation [72]. To obtain 25 mμ antigen, the medium from infected cultures is first clarified by centrifugation. The antigen is then purified by two cycles of sedimentation (35,000 rev/min for 1 hour) and clarification (10,000 rev/min for $\frac{1}{2}$ hour). After each sedimentation, the antigen is resuspended in 0·04 M phosphate buffer pH 7·6 with the aid of sonication. The use of small volumes of resuspending fluid enables the antigen to be concentrated as desired.

As an alternative method, 25 mμ antigen can be freed from 7 mμ antigen by treatment of the crude virus preparation with fluorocarbon [73]. One volume of Arcton 113 (Imperial Chemical Industries Ltd) is added to two volumes of virus suspension. The mixture is either shaken in a stoppered bottle for 1 hour or 'blended' at 14,000 rev/min for 2 minutes, and is then centrifuged (2000 rev/min for 5 minutes). The upper aqueous layer is taken and the extraction procedure is repeated until no solid material is seen at the fluid interface after centrifugation. The final product contains the original amount of 25 mμ antigen but no detectable 7 mμ antigen. As the 25 mμ antigen is readily degraded to 7 mμ antigen, all preparative procedures should be carried out as far as possible at a temperature below 4° C and a pH no lower than 7·4.

Preparation of 7 mμ antigen

The 7 mμ antigen is most easily separated from 25 mμ particles by centrifugation. After one clarifying centrifugation, the virus preparation is centrifuged twice at 35,000 rev/min for 1 hour, the upper two-thirds of the supernatant fluid being retained each time [72]. The material obtained in this way is free from detectable 25 mμ antigen but is presumably contaminated with protein from the host cells and medium.

Purer 7 mμ antigen can be prepared by disruption of the previously purified virus (25 mμ antigen). When the virus is heated for $\frac{1}{2}$ hour at 56° C, it is converted to 7 mμ antigen [74] and viral RNA [75]. A similar result is achieved by exposing the virus suspension to pH 6 for about 10 minutes [76]. Further purification of the antigen prepared in this way has not been reported but it should be possible by ordinary methods of protein fractionation. It is known, for example, that the 7 mμ antigen of type O virus adsorbs to DEAE-cellulose and is eluted by 0·05 M sodium chloride at pH 7·6 [77].

References

[1] SOBER H.A., HARTLEY R.W., CARROLL W.R. & PETERSEN E.A. (1965) Fractionation of proteins. In *The Proteins*, Vol. 3, pp. 1–97, ed. NEURATH H. New York and London: Academic Press

[2] WOODROOFE G.M. & FENNER F. (1962) Serological relationships within the poxvirus group: An antigen common to all members of the group. *Virology* 16, 334

[3] WESTWOOD J.C.N., HARRIS W.J., ZWARTOUW H.T., TITMUSS D.H.J. & APPLEYARD G. (1964) Studies on the structure of vaccinia virus. *J. gen. Microbiol.* 34, 67

[4] BYKOVSKY A.F. (1964) Changes in the envelope of vaccinia virus during ontogenesis. *Acta virol. Prague* 8, 490

[5] SMADEL J.E. & HOAGLAND C.L. (1942) Elementary bodies of vaccinia. *Bact. Rev.* 6, 79

[6] ZWARTOUW H.T. (1964) The chemical composition of vaccinia virus. *J. gen. Microbiol.* 34, 115

[7] GISPEN R. (1955) Analysis of poxvirus antigens by means of double diffusion. A method for direct serological differentiation of cowpox. *J. Immunol* 74, 134

[8] RONDLE C.J.M. & DUMBELL K.R. (1962) Antigens of cowpox virus. *J. Hyg., Camb.* **60,** 41

[9] CROWLE A.J. (1958) A simplified micro double-diffusion agar precipitin technique. *J. lab. clin. Med.* **52,** 784

[10] WESTWOOD J.C.N., ZWARTOUW H.T., APPLEYARD G. & TITMUSS D.H.J. (1965) Comparison of the soluble antigens and virus particle antigens of vaccinia virus. *J. gen. Microbiol.* **38,** 47

[11] APPLEYARD G. & WESTWOOD J.C.N. (1964) The growth of rabbitpox virus in tissue culture. *J. gen. Microbiol.* **37,** 391

[12] APPLEYARD G. (1961) An immunizing antigen from rabbitpox and vaccinia viruses. *Nature, Lond.* **190,** 465

[13] APPLEYARD G. & WESTWOOD J.C.N. (1964) A protective antigen from the poxviruses. II. Immunisation of animals. *Brit. J. exp. Path.* **45,** 162

[14] APPLEYARD G., ZWARTOUW H.T. & WESTWOOD J.C.N. (1964) A protective antigen from the pox-viruses. I. Reaction with neutralizing antibody. *Brit. J. exp. Path.* **45,** 150

[15] SMADEL J.E., RIVERS T.M. & HOAGLAND C.L. (1942) Nucleoprotein antigen of vaccine virus. I. A new antigen from elementary bodies of vaccinia. *Archs. Path.* **34,** 275

[16] ZWARTOUW H.T., WESTWOOD J.C.N. & HARRIS W.J. (1965) Antigens from vaccinia virus particles. *J. gen. Microbiol.* **38,** 39

[17] KIT S., PIEKARSKI L.J. & DUBBS D.R. (1963) Induction of thymidine kinase by vaccinia-infected mouse fibroblasts. *J. molec. Biol.* **6,** 22

[18] MCAUSLAN B.R. (1963) The induction and repression of thymidine kinase in the pox virus-infected HeLa cell. *Virology* **21,** 383

[19] APPLEYARD G. & ZWARTOUW H.T. (1965) The effect of p-fluorophenylalanine on the replication of rabbitpox virus and its nucleic acid. *J. gen. Microbiol.* **38,** 429

[20] BURNET F.M. (1946) Vaccinia haemagglutinin. *Nature, Lond.* **158,** 119

[21] CHU C.M. (1948) Studies of vaccinia haemagglutinin. I. Some physico-chemical properties. *J. Hyg., Camb.* **46,** 42

[22] GILLEN A.L., BURR M.M. & NAGLER F.P. (1950) Recovery of two distinct haemagglutinins of vaccinia virus. *J. Immunol.* **65,** 701

[23] YOUNGER J.S. & RUBENSTEIN G. (1962) Separation and characterization of haemagglutinins from chorioallantoic membranes of embryonated eggs infected with vaccinia virus. *Virology* **16,** 272

[24] BRIODY B.A. (1951) A 'unitarian' view of vaccinia haemagglutinin. *Yale J. Biol. Med.* **24,** 1

[25] ODA M. (1963) Vaccinia virus–HeLa cell interaction. I. The effect of immune serum on the production of infective virus, complement-fixing antigen and haemagglutinin. *Virology* **20,** 552

[26] DOWNIE A.W. & MACDONALD A. (1950) A study of the pox viruses by complement fixation and inhibition of complement fixation methods. *J. Path. Bact.* **62,** 389

[27] JOKLIK W.K. (1962) The purification of four strains of poxvirus. *Virology* **18,** 9

[28] NOYES W.F. (1962) The surface fine structure of vaccinia virus. *Virology* **17,** 282

[29] MARQUARDT J., HOLM S.E. & LYCKE E. (1965) Immuno-precipitating soluble vaccinia virus antigens. *Arch. ges. Virusforsch.* **15,** 178

[30] ZWARTOUW H.T., WESTWOOD J.C.N. & APPLEYARD G. (1962) Purification of pox viruses by density gradient centrifugation. *J. gen. Microbiol.* **29,** 523

[31] APPLEYARD G., WESTWOOD J.C.N. & ZWARTOUW H.T. (1962) The toxic effect of rabbitpox virus in tissue culture. *Virology* **18,** 159

[32] SHEDLOVSKY T. & SMADEL J.E. (1942) The LS-antigen of vaccinia. II. Isolation of a single substance containing both L- and S-activity. *J. exp. Med.* **75**, 165

[33] MCCREA J.F., EPSTEIN R.S. & BARRY W.H. (1961) Use of potassium tartrate for equilibrium density-gradient centrifugation of animal viruses. *Nature, Lond.* **189**, 220

[34] MCCREA J.F. & O'LOUGHLIN J. (1959) Separation of vaccinia haemagglutinin from infectious virus particles by chromatography on DEAE columns. *Virology* **8**, 127

[35] WILCOX W.C., GINSBERG H.S. & ANDERSON T.F. (1963) Structure of type 5 adenovirus. II. Fine structure of virus subunits. Morphologic relationship of structure subunits to virus-specific soluble antigens from infected cells. *J. exp. Med.* **118**, 307

[36] VALENTINE R.C. & PEREIRA H.G. (1965) Antigens and structure of the adenovirus. *J. mol. Biol.* **13**, 13

[37] WILCOX W.C. & GINSBERG H.S. (1961) Purification and immunological characterization of types 4 and 5 adenovirus soluble antigens. *Proc. nat. Acad. Sci. (Wash.)* **47**, 512

[38] PEREIRA H.G. (1960) Antigenic structure of non-infectious adenovirus materials. *Nature, Lond.* **186**, 571

[39] PEREIRA H.G., ALLISON A.C. & FARTHING C.P. (1959) Study of adenovirus antigens by immunoelectrophoresis. *Nature, Lond.* **183**, 895

[40] PETERSON E.A. & SOBER H.A. (1962) Column chromatography of proteins: Substituted celluloses. In *Methods in Enzymology*, Vol. 5, pp. 3–27, ed. COLOWICK S.P. & KAPLAN N.O. New York and London: Academic Press

[41] PEREIRA H.G. (1958) A protein factor responsible for the early cytopathic effect of adenoviruses. *Virology* **6**, 601

[42] HARUNA I., YAOI H., KONO R. & WATANABE I. (1961) Separation of adenovirus by chromatography on DEAE-cellulose. *Virology* **13**, 264

[43] KASEL J.A. & HUBER M. (1964) Relationship of the adenovirus erythrocyte-receptor-modifying factor to the type-specific complement-fixing antigen. *Proc. Soc. exp. Biol., N.Y.* **116**, 16

[44] PHILIPSON L. (1960) Separation on DEAE-cellulose of components associated with adenovirus reproduction. *Virology* **10**, 459

[45] KLEMPERER H.G. & PEREIRA H.G. (1959) Study of adenovirus antigens fractionated by chromatography on DEAE-cellulose. *Virology* **9**, 536

[46] WILCOX W.C. & GINSBERG H.S. (1963) Structure of type 5 adenovirus. I. Antigenic relationship of virus-structure proteins to virus-specific soluble antigens from infected cells. *J. exp. Med.* **118**, 295

[47] GREEN M. (1962) Studies on the biosynthesis of viral DNA. *Cold Spring Harb. Symp. quant. Biol.* **27**, 219

[48] WATERSON A.P. (1962) Two kinds of myxovirus. *Nature, Lond.* **193**, 1163

[49] MILLER H.K. & SCHLESINGER R.W. (1955) Differentiation and purification of influenza viruses by adsorption on aluminium phosphate. *J. Immunol.* **75**, 155

[50] LAVER W.G. (1962) The structure of influenza viruses. 1. N-terminal amino acid analyses. *Virology* **18**, 19

[51] HOYLE L. (1952) Structure of the influenza virus. The relation between biological activity and chemical structure of virus fractions. *J. Hyg., Camb.* **50**, 229

[52] SCHÄFER W. & ZILLIG W. (1954) Über den Aufbau des Virus-Elementarteilschens der klassischen Geflugelpest. *Zeitsch. Naturforsch.* **9b**, 779

[53] LIEF F.S. & HENLE W. (1956) Studies on the soluble antigen of influenza virus. I. The release of S antigen from elementary bodies by treatment with ether. *Virology* **2**, 753

[54] HOYLE L., HORNE R.W. & WATERSON A.P. (1961) The structure and composition of myxoviruses. II. Components released from the influenza virus particle by ether. *Virology* **13**, 448

[55] LIEF F.S. & HENLE W. (1959) Methods and procedures for the use of complement-fixation technique in type- and strain-specific diagnosis of influenza. *Bull. Wld. Hlth. Org.* **20**, 411

[56] NORRBY E. (1962) Haemagglutination by measles virus. 4. A simple procedure for production of high potency antigen for haemagglutination-inhibition (HI) tests. *Proc. Soc. exp. Biol., N.Y.* **111**, 814

[57] LAVER W.G. (1963) The structure of influenza viruses. 3. Disruption of the virus particle and separation of neuraminidase activity. *Virology* **20**, 251

[58] LAVER W.G. (1964) Structural studies on the protein subunits from three strains of influenza virus. *J. molec. Biol.* **9**, 109

[59] MAYRON L.W., ROBERT B., WINZLER R.J. & RAFELSON M.E. (1961) Studies on the neuraminidase of influenza virus. I. Separation and some properties of the enzyme from Asian and PR8 strains. *Arch. Biochem. Biophys.* **92**, 475

[60] NOLL H., AOYAGI T. & ORLANDO J. (1962) The structural relationship of sialidase to the influenza virus surface. *Virology* **18**, 154

[61] PLANTROSE D.N. & RYAN J.K.O. (1965) A 65S particle containing viral protein in cells infected with foot-and-mouth disease virus. *Virology* **26**, 372

[62] BROWN F. & CRICK J. (1958) Application of agar gel precipitin tests to the study of the virus of foot-and-mouth disease. *Virology* **5**, 133

[63] BRADISH C.J., BROOKSBY J.B. & TSUBAHARA H. (1960) The complement-fixation test in studies of components of the virus system of foot-and-mouth disease and its antibodies. *J. gen. Microbiol.* **22**, 392

[64] CARTWRIGHT B. (1962) A study of the antibodies in guinea-pigs infected with foot-and-mouth disease virus. *J. Immunol.* **88**, 128

[65] BRADISH C.J., FARLEY J.O. & FERRIER H.E.N. (1962) Studies on the nature of the neutralization reaction and the competition for neutralizing antibody between components of the virus system of foot-and-mouth disease. *Virology* **18**, 378

[66] BROOKSBY J.B., GALLOWAY I.A. & HENDERSON W.M. (1948) Strains of virus of foot-and-mouth disease recovered from outbreaks in Mexico. Serum neutralization tests. *Proc. Soc. exp. Biol., N.Y.* **69**, 74

[67] LEBOUVIER G.L., SCHWERDT C.E. & SCHAFFER F.L. (1957) Specific precipitates in agar with purified poliovirus. *Virology* **4**, 590

[68] LEBOUVIER G.L. (1959) Poliovirus D and C antigens: Their differentiation and measurement by precipitation in agar. *Br. J. exp. Path.* **40**, 452

[69] MOWAT G.N. & CHAPMAN W.G. (1962) Growth of foot-and-mouth disease virus in a fibroblastic cell line derived from hamster kidneys. *Nature, Lond.* **194**, 253

[70] POLATNICK J. & BACHRACH H.L. (1964) Production and purification of milligram amounts of foot-and-mouth disease virus from baby hamster kidney cell cultures. *Appl. Microbiol.* **12**, 368

[71] BRADISH C.J. (1965) Personal communication

[72] BRADISH C.J., HENDERSON W.M. & KIRKHAM J.B. (1960) Concentration and electron microscopy of the characteristic particle of foot-and-mouth disease. *J. gen. Microbiol.* **22**, 279

[73] BROWN F. & CARTWRIGHT B. (1960) Purification of the virus of foot-and-mouth disease by fluorocarbon treatment and its dissociation from neutralizing antibody. *J. Immunol.* **85**, 309

[74] BRADISH C.J. & BROOKSBY J.B. (1960) Complement fixation studies of the specificity

of the interactions between components of the virus system of foot-and-mouth disease and its antibodies. *J. gen. Microbiol.* **22,** 405

[75] BACHRACH H.L. (1964) Foot-and-mouth disease virus: Structure and mechanism of degradation as deduced from absorbance temperature relationships. *J. molec. Biol.* **8,** 348

[76] RANDRUP A. (1954) Ultracentrifugation of the virus of foot-and-mouth disease. IV. Splitting of the greater complement-fixing particle. *Acta Path. Microbiol. Scand.* **34,** 366

[77] BROWN F. & CARTWRIGHT B. (1959) Fractionation of the virus of foot-and-mouth disease by chromatography on DEAE-cellulose. *Biochim. biophys. Acta* **33,** 343

[78] BRANDON F.B. & MCLEAN I.W. (1962) Adenovirus. *Adv. Virus Research* **9,** 157

CHAPTER 11

Preparation of Antigens from Tissues and Fluids

D.A.L. DAVIES

Introduction

Antigens are recognized by their reaction with antibody in some observable way, and are differentiated by the high order of specificity of these reactions.

Thus it has been found that antigens may be essentially protein, carbohydrate, lipid or nucleic acid, or some complex of these. There are, therefore, few general methods for extracting and purifying antigens and this chapter is made up largely of examples, with references judged to lead to the variety of methods that have been used successfully. Antigens are very frequently used in impure form, for example in vaccines, because it may not matter in the context of a particular operation that non-antigenic substances are also present and it may not cause interference for antigens other than that required or being studied to be present also. On the other hand it would often lead to clearer conclusions if pure antigens could be made available for study.

Antigen is used here to describe a property of one molecular species and not loosely as one frequently reads: 'Sheep red cells were used as antigen . . .'; this means that sheep red cells were used as source or carrier of one or more of the many antigens they possess. The theme of this chapter is that of operations leading to purification of antigens and identification of their specific antigenic determinant groups; an antigenic molecule may have few or many such groups of one kind or of many different kinds. Each different kind may be studied separately but are not physically separable without splitting the molecule. The methods used in the preparation and purification of serum proteins (including antibodies) that have their own particular antigenic features (as seen by some other individual of the species or of some other species) have been discussed in section 1.

Test systems
Methods for the detection of antigenic components are dealt with in detail in section 3, but antigens cannot be discussed without some consideration of assay procedures. Once detected, a test system is required to follow the increase in specific activity on purification and serve as a guide to the value

400

of a particular step. The method of detection may itself be quantitated, e.g. if an agar-diffusion line leads to the recognition of a new antigen this can be adapted to a dilution end-point assay, at least until such time as information has been gained to lead to a more precise method. A unit of specific activity has also to be established, preferably on a dry-weight basis if sufficient material is available, otherwise, for example, on total protein or total carbohydrate; this may be in units of haptenic activity, and immunogenicity may have to be established independently.

Test systems may not be wholly immunological; to study an antigenic hormone it may be convenient to follow its physiological effect. If a desired product is already known to have some characteristic chemical constituent it may be more convenient, rapid and accurate to measure such a component chemically, e.g. the neuraminic-acid content of a glycoprotein where this contributes to the specificity. However, at some stage an immunological test is involved. Immunogenic activity measured by an *in vivo* method is necessary at least at some stages, but to follow activity on purification by direct measure-ment of an immune response on the part of an animal is inherently imprecise, because neither antibody production nor induction of an immune state that is not clearly associated with a humoral response are related in a simple way to the amount of antigen injected. Antibody, once produced, can be measured accurately, however, by a variety of methods.

Inhibition assays *in vitro* frequently provide good precision in measurement of specific activity once an antibody is available, but it should be borne in mind that this is no measure of immunogenicity. The use of serial 1:2 dilu-tion steps of inhibitor is a much-used design and frequently adequate with relatively impure preparations, but once an antigen preparation is 50 per cent pure it is necessary to take it to 100 per cent purity to gain one more dilution of activity in an inhibition assay. It is therefore preferable to be able to interpolate a 50 per cent end-point, e.g. by spectrophotometric measurement of released haemoglobin on haemolysis, or release of radioactivity on cytolysis [1].

In the interpretation of specificity in inhibition assays, material obtained by degradation of the antigen being studied is likely to give the most straight-forward results; cross-reaction due to material of known composition from heterologous sources frequently gives valuable information on the likelihood of the presence of particular structures, particularly in the carbohydrate field [2] if putative inhibitors are related in structure to known components of the antigen. Otherwise anomalous results may also be obtained; thus 3-*O*-methyl-D-fucose and 3-*O*-methyl-L-fucose give equal inhibition in assays for human blood group 'H' substance (using eel serum natural 'O' cell haemag-glutinins) [3]; this is due to a similar molecular shape-profile as can be seen from molecular models [4].

There is a class of immunologically active substances which, in spite of normally adequate precautions for lability, do not show the expected increases of specific activity on removal of impurities. This is true for a number of cell-surface-located antigenic specificities that have proved to be glycolipid haptens on release from the cell. The difficulty can be overcome by providing a 'carrier' to give adequate anchorage and the necessary orientation of the lipid soluble–water soluble axis for reaction with antibody. Suitable carriers are, for example, phrenosin for Forssman hapten [5], cholesterol/lecithin emulsion for cytolipins [6] and the inactive lipid fractions previously removed during the purification in the case of human A-B-O active glycolipids of erythrocytes [7]. This is likely to be a feature of importance in future studies as glycolipids are probably responsible for many more cell-surface specificities, including some already recognized and not yet chemically defined.

Another feature of test systems is that quite different conclusions might be drawn from different kinds of tests applied to the same substance. An obvious one already referred to is that a highly active inhibitor in an *in vitro* assay may prove to have lost activity as determined by test for its direct immunogenic response. Spleen is a better source of transplantation antigen in the mouse than liver as determined by testing for ability to hasten the rejection of allogeneic skin grafts, but compared by induction of specific tolerance liver is a better source than spleen [8]. Studies of microbial antigens are further advanced in some respects than studies in higher animals: the dermotropic mould *Trichophyton rubrum* produces a glycopeptide responsible for the hypersensitivity of infected individuals; the peptide moiety is the cause of the delayed type response but the immediate type response is due to the carbohydrate component. Thus the latter effect only is labile to treatment with periodate, while the former only is labile to proteolysis [9]. One should generalize and take the view that a variety of tests should be applied in following the activity of any antigen if such are available.

Stability

Information about stability is desirable at an early stage, as it may give some clue to the chemical nature of the antigen and hence to likely purification procedures and to the conditions of treatment that maintain full activity. The primary structure of proteins is chemically rather stable as most peptide bonds are hydrolysed only by 6 normal mineral acid for several hours at 100° C. In peptides specificities may be due to particular exposed amino acids [10] and are relatively stable. However, as antigens, globular proteins are very labile because specificity involves tertiary structure and conformation [11] so that interference with hydrogen bonding may severely alter or destroy specificity and immunogenicity. There are exceptions; ribonuclease is unusually stable to heat and will withstand 100° C for 15 minutes [12]; γ globulin is exceptional in that its specificity will withstand normal acetic acid at 2° C for several days.

Polysaccharides are basically somewhat less stable chemically than proteins in their primary structure, glycosidic bonds are generally hydrolysed by normal acid at 100° C in a few hours. But carbohydrate specificity is more akin to that of peptides and is due to the configuration of sugar residues at or near the non-reducing ends of the polysaccharide chains. They are generally heat stable (100° C for 30 minutes or more); some links are particularly stable; for example, those of chitin have been shown to survive for 500 million years since Cambrian times. However, the lability of carbohydrate specificity generally is that of their primary structure and exceptionally this may be relatively labile; for example, neuraminic acid is very acid labile [13] and *O*-acetyl groups are very alkali labile. Both of these provide specific immunological determinants in the human M,N blood-group antigens [14] and in many bacterial-specific polysaccharides [15] respectively. Proteins may be adequately stable for maintenance of activity initially in the presence of other macromolecular material and become labile, even in the cold, after some purification, particularly if kept in dilute solution. An adequately buffered inert protein 'carrier' may then be necessary and/or a reducing environment (e.g. cysteine).

Proteolytic enzymes may be used to show the essentially protein nature of an antigen, but may destroy the immunogenicity (depending on the particular test system employed) of a glycoprotein whose specificity is due to the carbohydrate. Whereas proteases can be used in this way, especially those that are relatively non-specific (e.g. pronase) [16], non-specific carbohydrases are not available; preparations from molluscan digestive glands are the least specific and most likely to degrade an unknown carbohydrate; these are mixtures of more specific carbohydrases that are still inadequately characterized.

As antigens lipids are mostly labile, release from the cell is usually sufficient to render them haptenic only, as they are probably not covalently linked but held by solubility features in a particular orientation in the cell membranes. The haptens have the lability features of the carbohydrate residues to which the specificity is most often due. However, there are purely lipid specificities (e.g. cardiolipin) [17] and also lipid structures labile to dilute periodate such as adjacent hydroxyl groups or hydroxyl and amino groups (e.g. sphingosine).

If a material is essentially stable, cold-room working is desirable because stable material may be quickly degraded by enzymic impurities until a stage when these have been removed, unless suitable enzyme inhibitors can be added. It is also impracticable with many sources of material to avoid microbial contamination which cold working helps to control.

Sources of material

Recent trends in immunology suggest some precautionary comments on

o

selecting starting material for recovery of antigens. It is clear that almost all individuals of a species differ from one another by polymorphisms and allotypy to give individual specificity, of which histocompatibility or transplantation specificity form a part, except in the case of monozygotic siblings and inbred strains of animals (mainly rodents and birds). The two exceptions differ from one another to the extent that inbred animals are identical and homozygous whereas monozygotic twins are identical with normal heterozygosity. Pooling of products from several individuals is therefore precluded for some kinds of study such as work on blood-group polymorphisms, serum-protein allotypy, and isozymes (enzymes having the same enzymic properties) may have different features (electrophoretic, antigenic) if derived from different tissues of the same individual. Blood-group distributions are well documented for man [18] and many animal species [19]. Pooling products from different sexes even in inbred strains of animals is clearly ruled out for some studies; thus there is a 'Y' sex-linked histocompatibility antigen(s) in mice [20] and in rats [21]; also, for example, male rats have a component in the soluble fraction of liver-cell homogenates, identified in DEAE-column effluents, not found in females [22]. One may be confined, then, to the products of one individual or to one kind of tissue from carefully selected individuals. The same kind of problem arises in studies of tumour specificity, e.g. different specificities are found in different tumours induced with the same carcinogen in the same inbred line of mice [23]. Otherwise large amounts of material may be obtained by pooling if the situation is carefully considered.

For satisfactory handling in purification, solubility is a most helpful feature and the soluble antigens of tissue fluids, particularly those of blood serum, are the most thoroughly studied. Other tissue fluids generally provide a source of a variety of antigens in addition to those of serum, e.g. cerebrospinal fluid, tears, sweat, cyst fluids, pleural and ascitic fluids. In recent years cell-bound specificities have proved of much importance and solubilization has become a problem; the methods for separating components of mixtures of essentially insoluble but quasi-stable suspensions have relatively poor resolution, e.g. density separations, although this method is improved by the latest techniques [24]. However, a single property, such as density, is most unlikely to yield a homogeneous material and generally a number of other features are used to achieve separations such as size, charge, solubility, etc.

For soluble products of a particular tissue the whole tissue is removed and extracted in some appropriate way, salivary glands for some glycoproteins [25], endocrine glands for hormones, etc. Otherwise cell suspensions may be prepared, to be handled thereafter in ways similar to those used for cells that are already free. Both normal and malignant cells may sometimes be more conveniently obtained from tissue culture than directly from the animal [26]. Free cells again have been most thoroughly studied because of ease of access and relative homogeneity of cell type whereas most tissues yield several different kinds of cell often not easily separated. Erythrocytes have received the most attention but are possibly the least representative of mammalian cells. Leucocytes have become popular as a source of specificities not represented or poorly represented on erythrocytes; lymphocytes are easily obtained from lymph nodes, thymus and spleen or by cannulation of the thoracic duct; polymorphonuclear cells can be mobilized in the peritoneum by previous injection of starch, Kupffer cells separated from the liver by collagenase treatment [27] and peripheral leucocytes by quick water lysis of erythrocytes and subsequent separation into cell types by passage through a glass-bead column or one of a variety of methods described [28]. Platelets can be obtained in quantity also [29]. In mice a variety of strain-specific ascites tumours are available which are much used in immunological work, some of these yield up to 250 g (dry wt.) of tumour cells from 1000 mice [30].

The age of development of an animal or a cell may need to be considered even if essentially unrelated to the nature of the project, because different antigens appear at different stages in development [31]. Some of these items are considered in more detail below.

Recovery of antigens from fluids

Most body fluids have a background 'serum protein' composition. Sweat has been studied and found to contain serum components and antigens not detected in serum as judged from agar immunodiffusion, but not yet characterized [32]. The composition of milk is well known for larger mammals, of particular interest is the presence of a series of oligosaccharides containing the sugar residues of antigenic determinants present in many glycoproteins of the body including the blood-group mucoids [33]; a method for milking mice has been described [34]. Saliva and tears contain blood-group mucopolysaccharides if the individuals are 'secretors'; there is a phenotypic interaction between secretor status and Lewis blood group although they are not genetically linked [18]. The secretor situation in non-human primates has also been studied [35]. Fluids held in the foetal membranes have been analysed and that of eggs, for example chick allantoic fluid has a blood group 'A' related antigen and influenza virus haemagglutination inhibitor, which is a similar substance but contains neuraminic acid [36]. Antigenic components of urine have been described [37].

In disease states the fluids contain an interesting assemblage of antigens in addition to abnormal serum components, which are keys to the nature of so many bodily disorders. Ovarian cysts are a rich source of mucoids and a classical source of blood-group mucopolysaccharides; enough material may sometimes be obtained from one individual to isolate, purify and chemically characterize the material. In this way the A.B.H. (O) . AB and Le^a

mucopolysaccharides were described, that have a carbohydrate moiety providing blood-group specificity containing D-galactose, L-fucose, *N*-acetyl-D-glucosamine and *N*-acetyl-D-galactosamine, and a peptide component which lacks the aromatic amino acids [38]. Similar materials having *N*-acetyl-neuraminic acid have activity as influenza virus haemagglutination inhibitors; in man only the *N*-acetyl derivative is found, some other animals also have *N*-glycolyl-neuraminic acid, which may provide different antigenic determinants. Ovarian cysts have been induced in animals by feeding thiourea and injecting oestradiol.

Hydatid cysts caused by *Echinococcus granulosus* have proved to be a source of human blood group P substance that is also a mucopolysaccharide probably having a galactose specificity [39]. Pleural fluid from a case of cholecystitis was shown to possess serum proteins and also acidic mucopolysaccharides in common with some urinary components. These were recovered by phosphotungstic-acid precipitation from the perchloric-acid soluble fraction [40].

Ascitic fluid provides a convenient source of antigens available in man in large quantities but little studied. Useful amounts can be induced in rodents by non-specific irritation, e.g. injection of Freund's adjuvant intraperitoneally [41]. Tumour-induced ascitic fluid has been more extensively studied, some relatively non-specific ascites tumours will grow readily in any mouse strain (e.g. Ehrlich, Krebs, and many others) for most inbred lines there are also strain-specific ascites tumour lines that will, however, in some cases override histocompatibility barriers if inoculated in larger amounts. The fluid is basically normal serum at about half the concentration of normal serum proteins and in the volumes obtainable is thus an excellent source of mouse serum proteins. In addition there are cell-derived materials from the tumour cells at later stages of tumour growth [42] recognizable by hetero-antisera, and tumour-specific components [43]. Also present is an antigen always found where active cell-growth is in progress but not yet characterized [44], oedema fluid from burns is also a source of this material.

Recovery of antigens from free cells

Erythrocyte antigens have been most studied because of their ready availability and ease of handling. Immunological studies of haemoglobins are well advanced [45], as the substances can easily be purified in adequate quantities for structural work [46] and genetic variants are available for comparison. The general antigenic characters of erythrocyte stroma have also been recorded and methods fully described [47]. For surface-located specificities, detected by haemagglutination or haemolysis, there is a volume of data but these cells are not a good source of all the antigenic molecules they carry. It seems that the erythrocyte is a particularly good vehicle for allowing detection of its specificities but the amounts of material present are really very small, and in some instances (e.g. Le^a) are only adsorbed from surrounding fluid. The A.B. and H, Le^a and P substances were characterized as mucopolysaccharides from cyst fluids; only recently have materials carrying ABO characters been separated from red cells themselves. Rh specificity can be found associated with an insoluble fraction [48] derived from erythrocyte stroma and has yet to be solubilized; mucoids have been extracted with phenol and shown to carry MN, S and T specificities [49]. However ABO-reactive material is not present in erythrocyte stroma in mucopolysaccharide form but as sphingolipid, where the sugar residues characteristic of the polysaccharide moiety of the mucoid are linked directly to sphingosine. Methods of preparation are therefore quite different, the materials being extractable with chloroform/methanol mixtures and may be fractionated by standard lipid procedures [50]. The Forssman hapten has also proved to be glycolipid and a fractionation process has been described for extraction from sheep erythrocytes [5]. It should be noted that the isolated specific glycolipids are not antigenic but are haptens; methods have been described, however, for linking them chemically to proteins to make antigens having the specificity of the glycolipids [51].

In mice the specificities of the stronger (H-2) transplantation antigens are present on erythrocyte surfaces but extraction has not been achieved and their molecular form in that location is not known. From other sources (e.g. lymphoid cells) they have been successfully purified. On the erythrocyte surface some H-2 specificities are so sparse that using γG isoantibody the sites barely allow adjacent antibody molecules to bind complement for lysis, and most non-H-2 specificities are not detectable.

Lymphoid cells are included in this section because they yield suspensions of free cells by merely pressing through a screen. They provide a most important source of antigens, particularly of isoantigens concerned in histoincompatibility; most red cell antigens appear to be present but there are many others in addition. Leucocyte typing for histocompatibility testing in man has yet to clarify the immunogenetic systems involved, but lipoprotein extracts appear to carry some of the specificities [52]. In rodents inbred strains have allowed extensive studies and extracts of spleen cells, lymph node lymphocytes and thymocytes have been made by standard cell fractionation methods [53] and more recently by gentle elution methods [54] to give lipoproteins carrying strong (H-2) and weaker (non H-2), sex-linked and tumour-specific isoantigens. The resolution of the mixed lipoprotein fraction is only now beginning with the advent of solubilization procedures [55]. Some isoantigens that are largely confined or at least very strongly represented in a particular tissue (e.g. θC3H in mouse brain) are also present on thymocytes which appear to have a very complete antigenic makeup. A limitation in this field is that for species where no inbred lines are available, work is limited to cells from one individual and future success may depend on tissue culture as source, the transplantation antigens having been shown to be a stable character on prolonged life of cells in culture.

The methods for separating different kinds of leucocytes will become of increasing importance because there is ample evidence that different kinds of leucocytes have their own specific antigens. There is, for example, a thymocyte-specific antigen (TL antigen in the mouse) [56], and in man neutrophil granulocytes have their own antigen distinguishing them from other white cells [57].

Methods are available for recovering and purifying platelets, that also have a range of antigens detected but amounts of material are limiting for extraction work [29].

Ascites tumour cells have proved to be a very convenient source of cell-bound antigens in mice, human malignant ascitic fluid is much less cellular. In rodents the cells provide larger amounts of material than can conveniently be obtained otherwise, and antigens from these cells have been extensively studied; these are most often substances that are normal constituents of the host species. Strain-specific ascites tumours also provide a source of tumour-specific antigens and harvested at a suitable time after inoculation have advantages over solid tumours that become necrotic centrally. Tumour specificities have been found in insoluble lipoprotein fractions of the cells but in one instance (TL) has also been solubilized. The cell population includes a proportion, sometimes high, of leucocytes, which are sometimes separable from the tumour cells, e.g. on a sucrose density gradient. A number of tumour banks have been established to provide strain-specific transplantable tumours, including ascites tumours. Antigens of these cells have generally been studied following cell fractionation to show location in particular subcellular fractions. A series of glycolipid haptens have also been described, called cytolipins, that appear to have tissue specificity [6]; for these, lipid extraction and purification procedures have been used.

Use of whole tissue

There is no choice but to use whole tissue as source for many studies of tissue-specific antigens, although some tissues secrete antigenic material of interest, e.g. the various mucins, nasal, gut-lining, cervical, bronchial, etc. [58]. Likewise the hormones that in some cases are recoverable from fluids (e.g. urine) but otherwise the tissue of origin has to be used [59]. For other tissues no generalizations can be made as the tissue-specific components are probably a variety of different kinds of substances for which extraction procedures have to be worked out individually. A great deal of study has gone into this kind of work and almost all tissues have already proved to yield specific substances, though few have been purified. In some cases tissue specificity is self-evident for a known functional component, e.g. thyroglobulin, but in some cases it is not yet clear what role such substances play. Usually tissue is ground in the cold in an extracting solvent with or without cell breakage to give a starting material whose antigenic makeup may often be assessed initially by gel diffusion using absorbed heteroantisera, but for antigenic material bound to insoluble fractions, complement fixation is useful.

Dissociation of cells and tissue culture
Some tissue are easily dissociated, for the more difficult ones various methods have been described. Collagenase has been referred to [27] for obtaining pure suspensions of Kupffer cells from the liver. Liver is easily dissociated by gentle homogenization but only gives a suspension of intact cells at a pH below 7·0. Treatment with proteolytic enzymes is much used to separate cells from more closely knit tissues or those having more connective-tissue structure. Trypsin alone or trypsin/versene is a frequent choice, pronase has also been used successfully [60]. However, some damage is done by using enzymes in this way; it has been shown that a peptide containing neuraminic acid is released by trypsin though it is not known if this is a determinant residue of an antigen [61]. For some virus receptors, having neuraminic acid as a component, removal proteolytically or by neuraminidase is followed by quite rapid repair [62]. However, these methods should be treated with caution in immunological work.

Tissue culture as a source of cells is now very frequently used [63]; for monolayers, trypsin/versene is usually used to obtain cell suspensions, the hazards have to be weighed up against those of mechanical damage done by the alternative of magnetic scraping. Antigenic changes do occur in the course of life of tissue cultures and a definitive lifespan seems established [64] short of malignant transformation that is again accompanied by antigenic changes.

Cell fractionation
These procedures have been adequately reviewed [65] and in their standard form have been used in studies of antigens localized in different subcellular fractions. Cells are disrupted by homogenization in a Potter Elvehjem-type apparatus, by high-speed blending or by decompression in suspension in 0·25 M sucrose. Subcellular fractions are then recovered by differential centrifuging and zonal centrifuging; Ficoll has advantages over sucrose for density gradients as it is of high molecular weight and isotonicity can be maintained with salts.

Many studies have been made with good preparations of clean nuclei, nucleoli and nuclear membranes have also been obtained [66]. Liver is a convenient source; for cells with very large nuclei satisfactory homogenization in the plunger-type apparatus requires critical plunger clearances [67]. Mitochondria have their own particular antigens [68] but not extensively studied compared with the advanced work on their enzyme systems. They contain no glycolipid and no H-2 transplantation antigens in the mouse [53]; attempts to show antigenicity of cytochrome C have not been successful [69]. It is difficult to obtain a lysosomal fraction free from mitochondria and microsomes; although structurally similar to external-type membrane they have an antigenic dissimilarity [70]. The absolute amount of lysosomal material can be increased by non-specific stimulation of animals with, for example, BCG. The microsome fraction has been studied antigenically, especially for isoantigens in mice [53] purification and separation of rough and smooth vesicles is well documented [71]. The soluble fraction remaining after highest speed centrifuging has a variety of antigens that have been studied mainly by agar-diffusion methods [42].

The external membrane is the most difficult part of the cell to recover uncontaminated with other structural cell material (erythrocytes excepted). At the same time it is perhaps the most interesting and important from the immunological point of view because it is accessible for detection of antigenic specificities exposed on the surface of the intact cell and these specificities are probably the functional structures, of the otherwise featureless cholesterol/lecithin/protein surface, mediating reactions of the cell with its environment. One approach for preparing external membrane is through homogenization, followed by fractionation of subcellular particles. Clearly the external membrane breaks up into fragments of a range of sizes that form vesicles, on account of the lipid/protein basic structure, in the same way that the membranes of the endoplasmic reticulum form microsomes. The bulk of external membrane-derived vesicles sediments in the region between mitochondria and microsomes—the lyosome region—but well spread into the adjacent fractions [72]. For particular cell types, membrane preparations have been made in other ways, from muscle cells by shearing [73], from liver cells [74], etc. 'Ghosts' of cells can be made by treatment with hypertonic salt [75]. A good yield of surface-derived material containing all of a variety of antigens sought was obtained by treatment with hypotonic salt to a level insufficient to give cell rupture, the conditions differing markedly for different cell types [54]. Another successful method that gives clean membranes (from 'L' cells) results from gentle shearing following treatment to toughen the membrane; this has been done in several ways, such as with dilute zinc chloride [76]. It is not clear what damage the heavy metal ion might inflict upon protein antigens, but so far no surface-located specificities have been clearly attributed to protein structure.

The preservation of tissue-culture cell lines and transplantable tumour cells is by suspension in glycerol/serum or dimethylsulphoxide/serum mixtures, slow freezing (1–2° C per minute) to about −40° C and storage at −80° C (CO_2) or −196° C (liquid nitrogen). Cell suspensions in physiological saline may be freeze dried and resuspended substantially intact for antigenic studies [54].

Solubilization

Many important antigenic specificities present in structural parts of cells, including the external membranes, prove to be bound to insoluble lipoproteins on primary isolation, e.g. a number of tissue-specific antigens, histocompatibility and other isoantigens. Insolubility, however, is related to the solvents used and the human blood-group specific and other glycolipid haptens appeared to be bound to the insoluble fraction of red cells only because aqueous solvents had previously been used. For cases not falling into this class, insolubility precludes proper purificaton and characterization of the molecules concerned because of the paucity of methods available for separating components of such mixtures, density separations being almost the only means available. Release of antigens in soluble form from lipoproteins has been achieved by detergent action [77] though some specificities are labile to such conditions; ultrasonic treatment may also be effective where antigenic components are not co-valently linked into the lipoprotein complex. Otherwise enzymic treatment shows promise, e.g. for transplantation antigens, release can be effected by treatment with snake venom (by its phospholipase A) [78] by autolysis (presumed to be proteolytic) or by controlled proteolysis with ficin or papain [55]. By the latter means an immunogenic soluble monodisperse molecular species is released that can be satisfactorily purified. For isoantigens and tissue-specific antigens whose specificity might be due to protein structure, there is a variety of proteolytic enzymes available of very limited specificity of action, which might release immunogenic material without degrading the product required.

General purification methods

General methods can only be mentioned briefly as they are the standard methods for purifying biological macromolecules and are described in numerous textbooks and symposia. In the last decade most of the analytical procedures for demonstrating homogeneity of molecular species have become preparative methods of high resolving power.

Initially it is frequently the most economical step to make a concentration of the desired activity by ultracentrifugation or precipitation to reduce volumes as much as possible. Thereafter column separations offer a wide range of conditions; gel filtration (non-adsorptive) can be used to remove larger and/or smaller inactive molecules than those carrying the required activity; this can be done with charged or uncharged molecules. Then there

o*

are the ion exchange adsorption methods with DEAE-substituted polymers for negatively charged materials and CM-substituted polymers for positively charged molecules, using increases in ionic strength of eluting solvent to release in turn those components of mixtures weakly adsorbed and subsequently those more strongly adsorbed. For substances with a suitably convenient isoelectric point, both DEAE and CM may be used at different pH. Other substituted functional groups are useful mainly for antigens that are more highly charged and/or stable outside the physiological range of pH. Electrophoretic methods in stabilized media have succeeded the essentially analytical free-solution methods where only leading and trailing components could be clearly separated. Thus preparative procedures employing polyacrylamide gel and starch or acetylated cellulose columns are available. Ultracentrifugal methods are essentially differential (enrichment procedure) or zonal (clear separation) both available in continuous-flow machinery. These have been dealt with in detail in section 1. A suitable sequence for these methods has to be determined for each individual case.

Combined methods can be very effective, e.g. electrophoresis in an ion exchange molecular sieve, logically however the conditions can only be arrived at after defining the conditions for each of the component methods individually.

For carbohydrates there are methods based on removal of proteins by denaturation either by shaking with solvents (e.g. amyl alcohol) [79] or using phenol. In the preparation of blood-group mucopolysaccharides 90 per cent phenol has been used to dissolve protein, in most cases the active material remains in the insoluble fraction [38]. A method used for preparation of bacterial lipopolysaccharides (see Chapter 9) makes use of 45 per cent aqueous phenol, giving one phase at 60° C and separating into water and phenol phases at 0° C; the phenol phase contains deatured protein, DNA remains insoluble, polysaccharide and RNA are in the water phase and can be separated in various ways (ethanol precipitation, ultracentrifugation, ion exchange) [80]. Acidic and neutral polysaccharides can be separated by precipitation with cetavlon [81].

Enzymes, that can subsequently be removed, are also used in purification if the desired antigen is clearly unaffected by such treatment, e.g. to remove RNA or DNA, or protein from carbohydrate (pronase, trypsin, papain). Carbohydrate is more difficult to remove from other compounds by this means for lack of suitable enzymes, molluscan digestive enzymes have not been adequately characterized and include proteinases, other mucinases are present in bacteria [82].

Immunological methods have likely applications for the future; some of the antibody can frequently be recovered from an antigen–antibody complex but antigen can only rarely be recovered free from antibody, except by proteolytic destruction of the antibody for carbohydrate antigens or carbohydrate-precipitating haptens, this would be applicable also to nucleic acids.

There are, however, filtration methods in which mixed antigens are passed over antisera lacking antibody for the desired antigen in the mixture, this may be done by immunodiffusion in gels [83], or using columns where antibody is bound to an insoluble matrix [84] (see Chapter 5).

Methods that have been used for a selection of antigens will be found in the following papers: liver [85], kidney [86], heart [87], pancreas [88], brain [89], thyroid [90], adrenal [91], pituitary [92], blood-group mucopolysaccharides [38, 93], mucins [58], blood-group glycolipids [94], cytolipins [6], transplantation antigens [54, 55], Forssman antigen [5].

Examination of fractionated products

Only when a product is demonstrably not inhomogeneous by all available criteria is analysis meaningful, and only in such a state can the physiological properties of molecular species be surely established. Several classical methods for demonstrating homogeneity have become preparative procedures and are therefore not applicable when the latter have been used. Immunological homogeneity can be shown by careful use of gel-diffusion methods, but this is a negative approach and a more critical procedure is to immunize animals with the product and test the antisera against the starting material, to find if only antibody reacting with the purified product has been induced.

For determining the chemical nature of the specific antigenic determinant groups of carbohydrates, the classical methods of carbohydrate chemistry are available, used with serological inhibition tests employing fragments isolated by partial hydrolysis (chemical or enzymic) of the antigen [95]; sugar analysis on a micro scale can be achieved by thin-layer chromatography or gas chromatography of the trimethylsilyl derivatives [96]. For proteins, work on antigenic determinants is most advanced with the rather small number of smaller proteins whose amino-acid sequence is known; here the tertiary structure is highly involved [12] although there are example where particular amino acids are of major importance [97]. Few studies have been recorded for tissue antigens other than those of serum, haemoglobin and hormones.

It turns out that apart from enyzmes, many proteins adequately examined prove to have substantial amounts of carbohydrate, in many cases it is not clear what antigenic role is played by the two parts. Examples are the immunoglobulins (Chapter 7), thyroglobulin [98], ceruleoplasmin [99] and ovalbumin [100].

Progress in studies of glycolipid haptens has been referred to earlier, purification methods are essentially lipid methods, but study of the specific immunological determinants in most cases falls to the field of carbohydrate chemistry. However, there exist also purely lipid haptens with no carbohydrate component, e.g. cardiolipin [17]. Immunological studies of nucleic acids have only a short history but clearly are to be of great significance in the immediate future. Preparation and purification of nucleic acids is well documented [101]. Antibodies have been prepared against RNA and DNA and having purine and pyrimidine directed specificity [102]; naturally occurring nucleic-acid antibody is of significance in lupus erythematosus [103] (see also Chapter 26).

References

[1] SANDERSON A.R. (1965) Quantitative titration, kinetic behaviour and inhibition of cytotoxic mouse isoantisera. *Immunology* **9**, 287–300; WIGZELL H. (1965) Quantitative titrations of mouse H-2 antibodies using Cr^{51} labelled target cells. *Transplantation* **3**, 423

[2] WATKINS W.M. & MORGAN W.T.J. (1952) Neutralization of the anti-H agglutinin in eel serum by simple sugars. *Nature Lond.* **169**, 825

[3] SPRINGER G.F. & WILLIAMSON P. (1962) Immunochemical significance of L- and D-fucose derivatives. *Biochem. J.* **85**, 282

[4] KABAT E.A. (1962) Structural similarities of methylated D- and L-fucose derivatives as seen in three-dimensional models. *Biochem. J.* **85**, 291

[5] MEGLI E.C. & MALLETTE M.F. (1964) Aggregation and activity of Forssman hapten in dilute aqueous solutions. *J. Immunol.* **92**, 961; DIEHL J.E. & MALLETTE M.F. (1964) Nature of the Forssman hapten from sheep erythrocytes. *J. Immunol.* **93**, 965

[6] RAPPORT M.M. & GRAF L. (1964) Serological activity of cytolipin H (lactocytoside). *Nature, Lond.* **201**, 879

[7] KOŚCIELAK J. (1963) Blood group A specific glycolipids from human erythrocytes. *Biochim. biophys. Acta* **78**, 313

[8] HILGERT I. & KRIŠTOFOVÁ H. (1966) Tolerance inducing capacity of cell free spleen and liver extracts of various immunogenicity. *Folia Biol.* (in press)

[9] BARKER S.A., CRUICKSHANK C.N.D., MORRIS J.H. & WOOD S.R. (1962) The isolation of trichophytin glycopeptide and its structure in relation to the immediate and delayed reactions. *Immunology* **5**, 627

[10] SELA M. (1965) Immunological studies of synthetic polypeptides. *Advanc. Immunol.* **5**, 29

[11] CRUMPTON M.J. (1966) The molecular basis of the serological specificity of proteins with particular reference to sperm whale myoglobin. In *Antibodies to Biologically Active Proteins*, ed. CINADER B. Oxford: Pergamon Press

[12] CARTER B.G., CINADER B. & ROSS C.A. (1961) Immunochemical analysis of the multiple forms of bovine ribonuclease. *Ann. N.Y. Acad. Sci.* **94**, 1004

[13] GIBBONS R.A. (1963) The sensitivity of neuraminosidic linkage in mucosubstances towards acid and towards neuraminidase. *Biochem. J.* **89**, 380

[14] HOTTA K. & SPRINGER G.F. (1964) Blood group N specificity and sialic acid. *Sangre* **9**, 183

[15] STAUB A.M. (1964) The role of the polysaccharide moiety in determining the specificity and immunological activity of the O antigen complex of Salmonellae. In *Bacterial Endotoxins*, Symp. Inst. Microbiol., Rutgers, ed. LANDY & BRAUN. New Brunswick: State University Press

[16] NOMOTO M., NARAHASHI Y. & MURAKAMI M. (1960) A proteolytic enzyme of *Streptomyces griseus. J. Biochem., Tokyo* **48**, 593–602, 906–918

[17] DE HAAS G.H. & VAN DEENEN L.L.M. (1965) Chemical structure and serological activity of synthetic and natural cardiolipin. *Nature, Lond.* **206**, 935

[18] RACE R.R. & SANGER R. (1962) *Blood Groups in Man*, 4th ed. Oxford: Blackwell Scientific Publications

[19] COHEN C. (ed.) (1962) Blood groups in infrahuman species. *Ann. N.Y. Acad. Sci.* **97**, 1

[20] ELKINS W.L. (1964) Decreased immunogenicity of a transplantation antigen in hosts sensitized to other isoantigens of its cellular vehicle. *J. Immunol.* **92**, 275

[21] ZEISS I.M., NISBET N.W. & HESLOP B.P. (1962) A male antigen in rats. *Transpl. Bull.* **30**, 49

[22] BOND H.E. (1960) A sex-associated protein in liver tissues of the male rat. *Biochem. biophys. Res. Commun.* **3**, 53

[23] GLOBERSON A. & FELDMAN M. (1964) Antigenic specificity of benzo[a]pyrene-induced sarcomas. *J. natl. Cancer Inst.* **32**, 1229

[24] SCHUEL H. & ANDERSON N.G. (1964) Studies on isolated cell components fractionated in the zonal ultracentrifuge. *J. cell. Biol.* **21**, 309

[25] TSUIKI S., HASHIMOTO Y. & PIGMAN W. (1961) Bovine submaxillary mucin. *Nature, Lond.* **189**, 399

[26] MANSON L.A., FOSCHI G.V., DOUGHERTY T. & PALM J. (1964) Microsomal lipoproteins as transplantation antigens. *Ann. N.Y. Acad. Sci.* **120**, 251; MANNICK J.A., GRAZIANI J.T. & EGDAHL R.H. (1964) A transplantation antigen recovered from cell culture medium. *Transplantation* **2**, 321

[27] GARVEY J.S. (1961) Separation and *in vitro* culture of cells from liver tissue. *Nature, Lond.* **191**, 972

[28] BOYUM A. (1964) Separation of white blood cells. *Nature, Lond.* **204**, 793

[29] WOODSIDE E.E., THERRIAULT D.G. & KOCHOLATY W. (1964) Lipids of human platelets and their action on the blood coagulation process. *J. Hematol.* **24**, 76

[30] DAVIES D.A.L. (1962) The isolation of mouse antigens carrying H-2 histocompatibility specificity. *Biochem. J.* **84**, 307

[31] EDIDIN M. (1964) Transplantation antigen levels in the early mouse embryo. *Transplantation* **2**, 627–637; FLICKINGER R.A. (1962) Embryological development of antigens. *Advanc. Immunol.* **2**, 309

[32] JIRKA M. & MASOPUST J. (1963) Immunochemical behaviour of proteins in human sweat. *Biochim. biophys. Acta* **71**, 217

[33] KUHN R. (1958) Les oligosaccharides du lait. *Bull. Soc. Chem. biol., Paris* **40**, 297

[34] MCBURNEY J.J., MEIER H. & HOAG W.G. (1964) Device for milking mice. *J. lab. clin. Med.* **64**, 485

[35] WIENER A.S. (1965) Blood groups of chimpanzees and other non-human primates. *Trans. N.Y. Acad. Sci.* **27**, 488

[36] SPRINGER G.F. & TRITEL H. (1962) Blood group A active substances in embryonated chicken eggs and their relation to egg-grown virus. *Science* **138**, 687

[37] DINH B.L., TREMBLAY A. & DUFOUR D. (1965) Immunochemical study of rat urinary proteins. *J. Immunol.* **95**, 574

[38] WATKINS W.M. (1966) Blood group specific substances. In *Glycoproteins*, pp. 462, ed. GOTTSCHALK. Amsterdam: Elsevier

[39] MORGAN W.T.J. & WATKINS W.M. (1964) Blood group P1 substance: (1) Chemical properties. *Proc. 9th Congr. int. Soc. Blood Transfusion*, 1962, pp. 225

[40] FISCHEL C.W. (1960) Mucopolysaccharides of serum and pleural fluid. *Nature, Lond.* **186**, 804

[41] LIEBERMAN R., MANTEL N. & HUMPHREY W. (1961) Ascites production in 17 mouse strains. *Proc. Soc. exp. Biol., N.Y.* **107**, 163

[42] BOYLE W., DAVIES D.A.L. & HAUGHTON G. (1963) Mouse tissue cell antigens: Some properties of cell bound components. *Immunology* **6**, 499

[43] DAVIES D.A.L. (1963) Occurrence of 'X' antigenic specificity in histocompatibility antigens prepared from mouse leukaemic cells. *Brit. J. exp. Path.* **44**, 546

[44] HAUGHTON G. (1962) Some cell-bound, species specific antigens of mouse ascites-tumor cells. *Ann. N.Y. Acad. Sci.* **101**, 131; TAL C. (1965) The nature of the cell membrane receptor for the agglutination factor present in the sera of tumour patients and pregnant women. *Proc. nat. Acad. Sci. (Wash.)* **54**, 1318

[45] OVARY Z. (1964) Antigenicity of hemoglobin and its constituents. *Immunochemistry* **1**, 241

[46] BRAUNITZER G., HILSE K., RUDLOFF V. & HILSCHMANN N. (1964) The hemoglobins. *Advanc. Protein Chem.* **19**, 1

[47] MICHELI A. & GRABAR P. (1961) Étude immunochimique des hémolysats de globules rouges humains. *Ann. Inst. Pasteur* **100**, 569

[48] WOLFF I. & SPRINGER G.F. (1964) Attempts to characterize the Rh antigen. *Fed. Proc.* **23**, No. 2

[49] UHLENBRUCK G. (1964) Erythrocyte mucoids. *Vox Sang.* **9**, 377

[50] GRAY G.M. (1965) The isolation and partial characterization of the glycolipids of BP8/C3H ascites sarcoma cells. *Biochem. J.* **94**, 91

[51] TAKETOMI T. & YAMAKAWA T. (1963) Immunochemical studies of lipids; preparation and immunological properties of synthetic psychosine-protein antigens. *J. Biochem., Tokyo* **54**, 444

[52] BRUNING J.W., VAN LEEUWEN A. & VAN ROOD J.J. (1964) Purification of leucocyte group substances from human placental tissue. *Transplantation* **2**, 649; RAPAPORT F.T., DAUSSET J., CONVERSE J.M. & LAWRENCE H.S. (1965) Biological and ultra-structural studies of leucocyte fractions as transplantation antigens in man. *Transplantation* **3**, 490

[53] HERBERMAN R. & STETSON C.A. (1965) The expression of histocompatibility antigens on cellular and subcellular membranes. *J. exp. Med.* **121**, 533

[54] DAVIES D.A.L. (1966) Mouse histocompatibility isoantigens derived from normal and from tumour cells. *Immunology* **11**, 115

[55] NATHENSON S.G. & DAVIES D.A.L. (1966) Solubilization and characterization of mouse histocompatibility antigens from membrane derived lipoprotein. *Proc. nat. Acad. Sci. (Wash.)* **56**, No. 2

[56] BOYSE E.A., OLD L.J. & STOCKERT E. (1966) The TL (thymus leukemia) antigen: A review. *Proc. Int. Congr. Immunopathol., Monaco.* Stuttgart: Schwabe & Co.

[57] LALEZARI P. (1966) The distribution patterns of leucocyte antigens in various blood cells and body tissue. In *Histocompatibility Testing.* Copenhagen: Munks-gaard

[58] GIBBONS R.A. & ROBERTS G.P. (1963) Some aspects of the structure of macro-molecular constituents of epithelial mucus. *Ann. N.Y. Acad. Sci.* **106**, 218

[59] HUMPHREY J.H. (1963) Hormones as antigens: Clinical significance and immuno-logical methods of assay. In *Clinical Aspects of Immunology,* Chap. 20, ed. GELL P.G.H. & COOMBS R.R.A. Oxford: Blackwell Scientific Publications

[60] GWATKIN R.B.L. & THOMPSON J.L. (1964) A new method for dispersing the cells of mammalian tissues. *Nature, Lond.* **201**, 1242

[61] LANGLEY O.K. & AMBROSE E.J. (1964) Isolation of a mucopeptide from the surface of Ehrlich ascites tumour cells. *Nature, Lond.* **204**, 53

[62] MARCUS P.I. & HIRSCH D. (1963) Renewal of a normal surface component: Cellular receptors for virus attachment. *J. cell Biol.* **19**, 47A

[63] CHARNEY J. & CORIELL L.L. (1964) Demonstration, purification and partial characterization of abnormal (HSL) antigens in stable human cell lines. *J. nat. Cancer Inst.* **33**, 285

[64] HAYFLICK L. (1965) The limited *in vitro* lifetime of human diploid cell strains. *Exp. cell Res.* **37**, 614

[65] DEDUVE C. & GRANT J.R. (ed.) (1963) *Methods of Separation of Subcellular Structural Components.* Cambridge University Press

[66] MURAMATSU M., SMETANA K. & BUSCH H. (1963) Quantitative aspects of isolation of nucleoli of the Walker carcinosarcoma and liver of the rat. *Cancer Res.* **23**, 510

[67] ALDRIDGE W.N., EMERY R.C. & STREET B.W. (1960) A tissue homogenizer. *Biochem. J.* **77**, 326–327; WEBSTER G.R. & SMITH A.T. (1964) A note on the construction of a modified tissue homogenizer. *Biochem. J.* **90**, 64

[68] D'AMELIO V., MUTOLO V. & BARBARINO A. (1963) Immunological and electrophoretic analysis of rat liver mitochondria and other cellular fractions. *Exp. Cell. Res.* **29**, 1; PINCKARD R.N. & WEIR D.M. (1966) Antibodies against the mitochondrial fraction of liver after toxic liver damage in rats. *Clin. exp. Immunol.* **1**, 33

[69] STORCK J., TIXIER R. & UZAN A. (1964) Immunological investigations of cytochrome C. *Nature, Lond.* **201**, 835

[70] WEISSMAN G. (1964) Lysosomes, analytical review. *J. Hematol.* **24**, 594; QUIE P.G. & HIRSCH J.G. (1964) Antiserum to leucocyte lysosomes. *J. exp. Med.* **120**, 149

[71] OKADA T.S. & SATO A.G. (1963) Production of a highly specific antiserum against a particular subfraction, separated from kidney microsomes. *Nature, Lond.* **197**, 1216; WHITBECK E.G. & ROSENBERG L.T. (1964) Antigenic properties of microsomes from guinea pig spleen, liver and lymph nodes. *Immunology* **7**, 363

[72] WALLACH D.F.H. & KAMAT V.B. (1964) Plasma and cytoplasmic membrane fragments from Ehrlich ascites carcinoma. *Proc. nat. Acad. Sci. (Wash.)* **52**, 721

[73] McCOLLESTER D.L. & SEMENTE G. (1964) Membrane isolation and cytoskeletal breakdown. *Biochim. biophys. Acta* **90**, 146

[74] TAKEUCHI M. & TERAYAMA H. (1965) Preparation and chemical composition of rat liver cell membranes. *Exp. Cell Res.* **40**, 32

[75] HAUGHTON G. & DAVIES D.A.L. (1962) Tissue cell antigens: Antigens of mouse tumour cell ghosts. *Brit. J. exp. Path.* **43**, 488

[76] WARREN L., GLICK M.C. & NASS M. (1966) The isolation of animal cell membranes. In *The Specificity of Cell Surfaces*, Symp. Soc. gen. Physiol.

[77] KANDUTSCH A.A. & STIMPFLING J.H. (1963) Partial purification of tissue isoantigens from a mouse sarcoma. *Transplantation* **1**, 201

[78] KANDUTSCH A.A., JURGELEIT H.C. & STIMPFLING J.H. (1965) The action of snake venom on an isoantigenic lipoprotein from a mouse sarcoma. *Transplantation* **3**, 748

[79] STAUB A.M. (1965) Removal of proteins, Sevag method. In *Methods in Carbohydrate Chemistry*, pp. 5–6, ed. WHISTLER. New York: Academic Press

[80] WESTPHAL O., LÜDERITZ O. & BISTER F. (1952) Uber die Extraktion von Bacterien mit Phenol/Wasser. *Z. Naturf.* **7b**, 148

[81] SCOTT J.E. (1960) Aliphatic ammonium salts in the assay of acidic polysaccharides from tissues. In *Methods of Biochemical Analysis*, pp. 146–197, ed. GLICK D. New York: Interscience Publ. Inc.

[82] FORMAL S.B., LOWENTHAL J.P. & GALINDO E. (1958) Serological study of the mucinases from *Shigella flexneri*. *J. Bact.* **75**, 467

[83] ABELEV G.I., PEROVA S.D., KHRAMKOVA N.I., POSTNIKOVA Z.A. & IRLIN I.S. (1963) Production of embryonal α-globulin by transplantable mouse hepatomas. *Transplantation* **1**, 174

[84] WELIKY N. & WEETALL H.H. (1965) The chemistry and use of cellulose derivatives for the study of biological systems. *Immunochemistry* **2**, 293

[85] SOLITZEANU D., YAGI Y. & PRESSMAN D. (1963) Separation of an antigenic fraction from rat liver responsible for the formation of liver localizing antibodies. *J. Immunol.* **90**, 424

[86] STEBLAY R.W. (1965) Some immunological properties of human glomerular basement membrane. *J. Immunol.* **95**, 517

[87] KAPLAN M.H. & CRAIG J.M. (1963) Immunologic studies of heart tissue. *J. Immunol.* **90**, 725; FINCK, H. (1965) Immunochemical studies of myosin. *Biochim. biophys. Acta* **111**, 208

[88] METZGAR R.S. (1964) Immunologic studies of pancreas-specific isoantigens. *J. Immunol.* 176

[89] MILGROM F., TUGGAC M., CAMPBELL W.A. & WITEBSKY E. (1964) Thermostable ethanol—insoluble antigens of brain. *J. Immunol.* **92**, 82; REIF, A.E. & ALLEN J.M.V. (1964) The AKR thymic antigen and its distribution in leukemias and nervous tissue. *J. exp. Med.* **120**, 413

[90] ROITT I.M., JONES H.E.H. & MILLS G.L. (1965) The activity of different fractions of homologous thyroid extract in the production of allergic thyroiditis in the rat. *Immunology* **9**, 281

[91] BARNETT E.V., DUMONDE D.C. & GLYNN L.E. (1963) Induction of antoimmunity to adrenal gland. *Immunology* **6**, 382–402; SHULMAN S., MILGROM F. & WITEBSKY E. (1964) Immunological studies on adrenal glands. *Immunology* **7**, 605

[92] MILGROM F., TUGGAC M. & WITEBSKY E. (1965) Organ-specific antigens of liver, testicle and pituitary. *J. Immunol.* **94**, 157

[93] MORGAN W.T.J. (1965) Blood group specific muco-polysaccharides. In *Methods in Carbohydrate Chemistry*, pp. 95–98, ed. WHISTLER. New York: Academic Press; COOK G.M.W. & EYLAR E.H. (1965) Separation of the M and N blood-group antigens of the human erythrocyte. *Biochim. biophys. Acta* **101**, 57

[94] HAKOMORI S. (1965) Substances containing amino sugars in blood cells and in hemopoietic organs. In *The Amino Sugars*, Vol. 2A, pp. 353–379, ed. JEANLOZ R.W. & BALAS E.A. New York: Academic Press

[95] REGE V.P., PAINTER T.J., WATKINS W.M. & MORGAN W.T.J. (1964) Isolation of a serologically active, fucose-containing, trisaccharide from human blood group Le^a substance. *Nature, Lond.* **204**, 740

[96] OATES M.D.G. & SCHRAGER J. (1965) The use of gas-liquid chromatography in the analysis of neutral monosaccharides in hydrolysates of gastric mucopolysaccharides. *Biochem. J.* **97**, 697

[97] ANDERER F.A. (1963) Preparation and properties of an artificial antigen immunologically related to tobacco mosaic virus. *Biochim. biophys. Acta* **71**, 246

[98] MURTHY P.V.N., RAGHUPATHY E. & CHAIKOFF I.L. (1965) Studies on thyroid proteins. 1. Isolation and properties of a glycopeptide from sheep thyroglobulin. *Biochemistry* **4**, 611; SPIRO R.G. & SPIRO M.J. (1965) The carbohydrate composition of the thyroglobulins from several species. *J. biol. Chem.* **240**, 997

[99] JAMIESON G.A. (1965) Studies on glycoproteins. 1. The carbohydrate portion of human ceruleoplasmin. *J. biol. Chem.* **240**, 2019

[100] MONTGOMERY R., LEE Y.C. & WU Y. (1965) Glycopeptides from ovalbumin.

Preparation, properties and partial hydrolysis of the asparaginyl carbohydrate. *Biochemistry* **4,** 566

[101] KIRBY K.S. (1964) Isolation and fractionation of nucleic acids. *Progr. nucleic acid Res.* **3,** 1–31

[102] BUTLER V.P., STUART M.D., TANENBAUM S.W. & BEISER S.M. (1965) A study of the cross reactivity of antipurin-6-oyl serum with deoxyribonucleic acid (DNA). *J. exp. Med.* **121,** 19; SEAMAN E., LEVINE L. & VAN VUNAKIS H. (1965) Immunochemical studies on bacteriophage deoxyribonucleic acid. *Biochemistry* **4,** 2091; PLESCIA O.J., PALCZUK N.C., CORA-FIGUEROA E., MUKHERJEE A. & BRAUN W. (1965) Production of antibodies to soluble RNA. *Proc. nat. Acad. Sci. (Wash.)* **54,** 1281

[103] HOLBOROW E.J. (1963) Systemic lupus erythematosus. In *Clinical Aspects of Immunology*, pp. 677–693, ed. GELL & COOMBS. Oxford: Blackwell Scientific Publications; SELIGMANN M. (1964) Antinuclear antibodies in disseminated lupus erythematosus. In *Immunological Methods*, pp. 417–442, ed. ACKROYD. Oxford: Blackwell Scientific Publications

Methods for the study and demonstration of antigen–antibody interaction

PART A

PRIMARY INTERACTION

CHAPTER 12

Spectrofluorometric Methods

CHARLES W. PARKER*

Introduction

In the past decade a plethora of new techniques and instruments have become available for biological research. The spectrofluorophotometer is one of the most useful recent additions to the scientific armamentarium. Fluorometric procedures which are simple and sensitive have been developed for the quantitation of a wide variety of substances of biologic importance [1]. The rapidly increasing employment of fluorometry can be attributed to several inherent advantages of fluorometric measurements: (i) They have a high degree of sensitivity, far greater, for example, than that of absorption spectrophotometry [2]. (ii) Fluorescence provides a marker by which the behaviour of a fluorescent molecule in a complex mixture can be studied. (iii) Fluorescence intensity is strongly influenced by the local molecular environment. Changes in fluorescence can provide qualitative information about protein denaturation and sensitive and precise information about inter-molecular complex formation. (iv) Fluorescence polarization is greatly influenced by molecular size. Changes in polarization can be used as a measure of intermolecular reactions in which aggregation occurs [3].

The sensitivity of fluorometry has been well illustrated in fluorometric microchemical methods for measuring enzymes as pioneered by Lowry and his colleagues [4]. By refinements of these techniques Lowry and his colleagues [5] and Rotman [6], working independently, have been able to detect the activity of single enzyme molecules. In the study by Rotman, β-D-galactosidase

* Supported by Grants 5-K3-AI-9881, 2 TI AI 219 and AI 04646 from the U.S. Public Health Service.

423

was measured by following the hydrolysis of the fluorogenic substrate, 6-hydroxyfluoran β-D-galactopyranoside, in micro-droplets under the fluorescence microscope. Fluorescence intensity was measured with a sensitive microphotometer. Under the assay conditions employed it was possible to detect as few as 2×10^6 molecules of hydrolysed substrate. Fluorometric techniques utilizing an antibody activity are less sensitive than those in which a catalytic function is involved. Nonetheless, fluorescence can provide a new and highly useful dimension in the measurement of antibody.

Immunologists have utilized fluorescence primarily as a label for antibody in fluorescence microscopy studies [7]. In this technique information is obtained from the distribution of antibody fluorescence. It can be inferred that local accumulation of antibody is due to the formation of complexes with antigen (for details of these methods see Holborow & Johnson, Chapter 16). In the procedures described in this chapter antigen–antibody reactions are measured in solution by a change in the intensity or polarization of fluorescence. Fluorescence may be derived from tryptophane residues of the antibody itself, as in the method of fluorescence quenching of purified antibody by hapten. Alternatively, fluorescence may originate from fluorescent haptens or protein antigens labelled with fluorescent markers.

The greater part of the discussion will be devoted to fluorescence quenching of purified antibody and to polarization of antigen or hapten fluorescence. While these two techniques are of recent origin they have been examined in sufficient detail to be considered as established procedures for measurement of antigen–antibody reactions. In principle, enhancement of hapten fluorescence on combination with antibody provides a third method for the quantitation of antigen–antibody interactions. In recent studies in this laboratory a workable enhancement system has been developed and the results are so promising that it now appears that fluorescence enhancement may prove to be the most useful of the three systems.

The general nature of fluorescence

In the application of established spectrofluorometric techniques a detailed knowledge of the theoretical basis for fluorescence is not requisite. None the less, any attempt to read relevant literature and develop new methodology necessitates some familiarity with terminology and at least a rudimentary understanding of the nature of the phenomenon. The general discussion of fluorescence presented here is necessarily brief. For further information discussions by Weber & Teale [8], Weber [9] and Udenfriend [1] are highly recommended.

Fluorescence is brought about by the absorption of ultraviolet light.

When molecules absorb light their electronic energy level is raised. In non-fluorescent molecules the absorbed energy is dissipated by collision with near-by molecules and other non-radiative processes. In fluorescent molecules, the energy is emitted as light at a higher wavelength than that absorbed. Energy derived from the incident light is termed the excitation or activation energy.

In characterizing the fluorescence of a substance one can begin by finding that combination of absorption and emission wavelengths which produces maximal fluorescence. The activation (excitation) spectrum is a plot of fluorescence intensity measured at the wavelength of maximal fluorescence versus

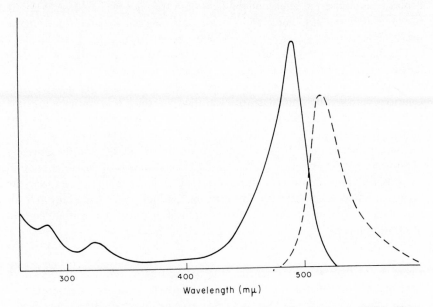

Fig. 12.1. Absorption and emission spectra of sodium fluorescein at pH 7·1. The scale of the ordinate is arbitrary and the two spectra cannot be compared directly. Taken from J.E.Fothergill [ref. 10, p. 7].

activation wavelength. The activation spectrum corresponds very closely to the absorption spectrum. The shape of the fluorescence spectrum is independent of the exciting wavelength. With some fluorescent molecules the fluorescence spectrum is a mirror image of absorption spectrum. More commonly, there is only one fluorescence band corresponding to the mirror image of the absorption band of longest wavelength (the principal absorption band) [8]. This is illustrated in the emission spectrum of sodium fluorescein (Fig. 12.1).

Most fluorescent molecules squander a substantial portion of their activation energy in non-radiative processes. The quantum yield of fluorescence, Q, is the ratio of quanta of energy emitted to quanta of energy absorbed. Values of Q for many substances of biologic interest have been tabulated by Udenfriend [1]. Rhodamine B, fluorescein and 1-dimethylaminonaphthalene-5-sulphonic acid (DANS), molecules commonly used in fluorescence studies, have values in the range of 0·4–0·92. Measured intensity of fluorescence will of course depend on the molar absorbance of the fluorescent molecule, its concentration, the intensity of the incident light, cell geometry and photometer sensitivity, as well as the quantum yield. Fluorometry differs in this respect from absorption spectrometry in that absorbance is essentially determined by concentration and the length of the light path through the solution. With the use of an intense light source and a highly sensitive photometer, fluorometric measurements can become extremely sensitive [4].

The quantum yield of a substance in solution can be estimated by relating its fluorescence intensity to that of a reference for which Q is known. The comparison is made in the same instrument at the same activation band using solutions with similar optical densities. If the absorption and emission maxima of the two substances do not correspond closely, correction factors must be applied [11, 12].

There is a finite interval between the absorption of energy and the emission of fluorescence. The average lifetime of the excited state is of the order of 10^{-8} seconds for most fluorescent molecules [13]. It is customary to express the excited lifetime mathematically in terms of r, which is the time required for fluorescence intensity to fall to $1/e$ (or 0·365) of its initial value after removal of exciting light:

$$I = I_0 e^{-t/r} \tag{1}$$

where I_0 is fluorescence intensity during excitation and I is fluorescence intensity at time t after excitation is stopped [1]. Thus the diminution of fluorescence with time is a first-order process analogous to radioactive decay.

Knowledge of the magnitude of r is useful in selecting the most appropriate fluorescent molecules for polarization studies. A direct measure of r is possible using special instrumentation [13]. An indirect approximation of r can be obtained by determining changes in fluorescence polarization with medium viscosity and temperature and applying appropriate formulae [3] (see below). The calculation requires an independently obtained value for the rotational relaxation time of the fluorescent molecule. One may also approximate r from the intensity of the principal absorption band as obtained by integration [14]. Competitive processes which reduce the quantum yield of fluorescence, reduce the value of r proportionately. The actual excited lifetime, r, is given by:

$$r = Qr_0 \tag{2}$$

where r_0 is the maximal excited lifetime and Q is the quantum yield [8].

Protein fluorescence

Nearly all proteins exhibit fluorescence in the ultraviolet region. The potentially fluorescent amino-acid residues in proteins are phenylalanine, tyrosine and tryptophane. The fluorescence maxima of the free amino acids are at 282, 303 and 350 mμ respectively with quantum yields of 3·5, 21 and 20 per cent [8]. In proteins containing all three amino acids the fluorescence spectrum is essentially that of tryptophane. Even in human serum albumin which contains only one tryptophane residue and eighteen tyrosines [15] contributions by

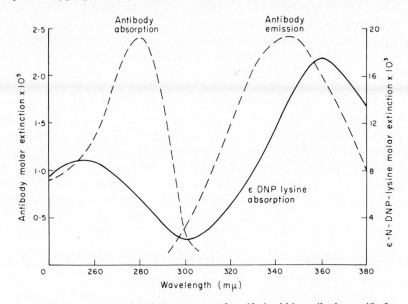

FIG. 12.2. Absorption and emission spectra of purified rabbit antibody specific for the DNP group – – – – – and the absorption spectrum of ε-N-DNP-lysine ———. By convention antibody emission is made equal in intensity to antibody absorption although the quantum yield of fluorescence is about 20 per cent [18].

tyrosine are relatively minor [16]. The emission maximum of proteins containing tryptophane varies between 330 and 350 mμ, depending on the protein and the solvent in which it is examined. The quantum yield of tryptophane fluorescence in various proteins ranges from 0·04 to 0·3 [17], the latter value in excess of the quantum yield of free tryptophane. The absorption and fluorescence spectra of rabbit γ globulin, which is a tryptophane containing protein are shown in Fig. 12.2. The quantum yield of tryptophane fluorescence in this protein is about 0·2 [18]. In proteins which contain tyrosine and phenylalanine but no tryptophane the emission spectrum is that of tyrosine with a maximum at or near 305 mμ [8]. Proteins differ in the extent of polarization of emitted light as well as fluorescence maxima and quantum yield [17]. Changes in these three parameters under conditions which produce protein denaturation provide information on alterations of the internal structure of proteins.

Excitation energy transfer

Electronically excited tyrosine and tryptophane residues in proteins are able to transfer excitation energy to a second molecule attached to the protein, a phenomenon known as excitation energy transfer [18, 19, 20, 21]. Transfer is possible when the absorption spectrum of the acceptor overlaps the emission spectrum of the donor. The transfer takes place via resonance interaction between the two molecules without direct molecular contact or emission of radiation [19, 20]. One might consider the acceptor molecule as analogous to a tuning-fork which is set into sympathetic vibration by a near by tuning-fork, vibrating at an appropriate frequency. The attachment of the acceptor molecule to the protein may be via a covalent bond [21] or a reversible bond, as exemplified by antibody–hapten and albumin–dye interactions [18]. When the acceptor molecule is non-fluorescent, excitation energy transfer results in diminution of protein fluorescence. The non-fluorescent ligand dissipates the energy by non-radiative processes. When the acceptor molecule is fluorescent, quenching of protein fluorescence is accompanied by excitation of acceptor fluorescence (sensitized fluorescence) [21]. Because changes in fluorescence are determined by the extent of ligand-binding fluorescence quenching and sensitized fluorescence can provide very useful quantitative data on antibody–hapten and albumin–dye interactions.

In the method of fluorescence quenching which was originally described by Velick, Parker & Eisen [18], the binding of a chromophoric hapten by antibody causes a marked diminution of antibody tryptophane fluorescence. The requirement that the hapten must absorb in the region of protein fluorescence emission in order to produce quenching largely limits the method to ligands which absorb in 300–360 mμ region.* The most extensive studies utilizing fluorescence quenching for the study of antibody–hapten reactions have been with antibodies to the 2,4-dinitrophenyl (DNP) group [18, 22, 23, 24]. Most DNP derivatives have a high degree of absorbancy in the 350 mμ region as exemplified by ε-N-DNP-lysine (Fig. 12.2). An important advantage

---

* However, the range of useful absorption is extended if the absorption spectrum of the ligand is shifted during interaction with antibody. For example, DNP toluene, which absorbs maximally at 250 mμ and has no appreciable absorbance at 350 mμ quenches the fluoresence of DNP specific antibody efficiently. On binding of the ligand to antibody there is a new absorption peak at 300 mμ and significant absorbance up to 360 mμ [23].

of the DNP system in fluorescence quenching studies is the availability of a method for obtaining highly purified antibody in reasonable yield [25]. Moreover, as a result of the widespread use of the DNP group in the study of the primary amino-acid sequence of proteins, many DNP amino acids are commercially available.

The degree of diminution of antibody fluorescence produced by small DNP ligands is remarkable. ε-N-DNP-lysine (Fig. 12.4), which can come in physical contact with only a small number of amino acids in the antibody site, can quench the fluorescence of purified guinea-pig anti-DNP antibody to the extent of 85 per cent [26].* This requires the transfer of energy from excited tryptophane residues in remote areas of the antibody molecule to the acceptor DNP group. Based on the theoretical treatment of Förster, transfer is generally believed to take place by resonance dipole interactions of acceptor molecules with excited donor molecules [19, 20]. According to Förster's formulation, the likelihood of transfer should: (i) Decrease with the 6th power of the distance between donor and acceptor. (ii) Be dependent on the mutual orientation of donor and acceptor molecules. (iii) Increase with increases of r, the lifetime of the excited state of the donor. (iv) Vary with the extent of overlap between donor emission and acceptor absorbance. (v) Vary with the molar extinction coefficient of the acceptor in the region of overlap.

The probability that quenching will occur can be expressed mathematically by the term r_c, which is the critical distance at which an excited molecule has an equal chance of emitting fluorescence or transferring excitation energy to the ligand. If it is assumed that the donor and acceptor molecules are randomly oriented and measurements are in aqueous solution then:

$$(r_c)^6 = \frac{9 \cdot 5 \times 10^{-34} \cdot r \cdot J\bar{v}}{\bar{v}_0{}^2} \tag{3}$$

r is the lifetime of the excited state of the donor; $\bar{v}_0$ is the arithmetic mean of the wave numbers of the absorption and fluorescence maxima of the donor; $J\bar{v}$ is the integral of the spectral overlap of the acceptor and donor; its terms include the molar extinction coefficient of the acceptor and the intensity of emission of the donor.† Because the probability of transfer decreases with the

---

* DNP groups are capable of quenching the fluorescence of other proteins provided reversible association takes place. For example, a single DNP group can quench 90 per cent of the fluorescence of avidin [27].

† Since r_c varies with the sixth root of the molar extinction coefficient of the acceptor in the region of overlap, ligands with relatively low absorbance in the 300–350 mμ range quench relatively well. For example, DNP toluene and DNP lysine in combination with antibody differ five-fold in absorbance in the region of tryptophane emission but quench protein fluorescence to the same degree. Lipoic acid with a molar extinction coefficient of only 117 at 330 mμ quenches avidin fluorescence to the extent of 50–60 per cent [27].

6th power of the distance, transfers over distances much larger than r_c are unlikely. Using the above formula it is possible to predict the approximate distance of excitation energy transfer for a given donor acceptor pair. There has been reasonably good agreement between predicted values of r_c and the experimentally observed values in proteins [14]. Obviously, perfect agreement cannot be expected since the distribution of donor and acceptor molecules is not random.*

Green has calculated that r_c is a distance of about 37 Å for the ε-N-DNP-lysine-tryptophane system [27]. Since γ globulin is a large protein and the probability of transfer falls off rapidly with distance, tryptophane residues in the general area of the antibody site should be especially susceptible to quenching. In accord with this expectation it has been found that the two antibody sites on 7S γ globulin titrate independently, indicating that a ligand at one site does not affect tryptophane residues associated with the other site [18]. If it is assumed that each of the 20–26 tryptophane residues of 7S rabbit γ globulin [26] fluoresce equally, each hapten molecule must capture the excitation energy of 8–11 tryptophane molecules. The univalent proteolytic fragments of antibody (Porter's pieces I and II) are quenched to a somewhat greater extent than whole antibody [26]. This suggests that in intact antibody, tryptophane residues in the piece III portion of the molecule (without combining sites) are quenched relatively poorly by the ligand.

Fluorescence quenching of purified antibody

In addition to the DNP system useful degrees of quenching have been observed with antibodies to benzylpenicillenate, p-azobenzenearsonate and trinitrophenyl [18, 26, 29]. The absorption maxima of the homologous haptens are at 328, 330 and 350 mμ respectively. The description of the method presented here will be limited to the DNP system. Titrations are performed with highly purified antibody. While the fluorescence of purified antibody may be diminished more than 80 per cent by ligand, if a globulin fraction containing 90 per cent 'normal' globulin and 10 per cent antibody were used, the diminution in fluorescence would be only 8 per cent [22]. This small change would not permit accurate evaluation of antibody binding.

The preparation of purified anti-DNP antibody for fluorescence quenching studies has been described in detail by Eisen and his colleagues [25, 30]. In brief, animals are immunized with a DNP-protein conjugate, usually

---

* Randomness is best approximated in the special case of intramolecular transfer from tryptophane to acceptor groups covalently bound to the same protein. This relationship exists provided the protein is relatively large and the groups on the protein with which the acceptor combines are distributed evenly and possess similar reactivity [28].

DNP-bovine γ globulin. Purification is accomplished by formation of a specific precipitate with antigen, elution of antibody from the precipitate by means of hapten at neutral pH and removal of free hapten. The precipitating antigen may be DNP-bovine γ globulin or another DNP protein. Precipitates are formed at equivalence and washed thoroughly with saline. Hapten elution is generally carried out with 0·1 M 2,4-dinitrophenol, in the presence of streptomycin sulphate. The streptomycin prevents solubilization of the precipitating antigen. Dinitrophenol is removed on a Dowex-1 column and by dialysis. Recoveries are usually about 25 per cent and antibody purity as determined by precipitability is in excess of 90 per cent. Better recoveries are possible with haptens which have a higher affinity for antibody than dinitrophenol but removal of hapten from the final product is much more difficult.

Published experimental results with fluorescence quenching of antibody have been obtained with spectrofluorophotometers equipped with monochromators in the incident and emitted beam. The antibody solution is activated at 290 mμ and fluorescence is measured in arbitrary units at 350 mμ. It is also possible to use filter fluorometers, provided an adequate light source and suitable filters are available. The fluorometer should be equipped with a shutter to protect the protein and hapten from incident ultra-violet radiation except during the short interval required for reading. Because protein fluorescence varies with temperature, a jacketed cell connected to a constant-temperature water pump will improve the accuracy of titrations. The theoretical sensitivity of the fluorometer is not realized in practice because of fluctuations in the light source, resulting in variable readings at high sensitivity settings, and significant solution blanks. The latter are due to solvent fluorescence and light-scattering effects. The level of antibody recommended below provides reproducible titrations. It is subject to modification with improved instrumentation.

Titrations are usually made in cuvettes containing 1·0 ml antibody solution at a concentration of 40 μg antibody per ml [24]. The suitability of a given buffer solution for titration can be evaluated by determining blank values. At neutral pH both 0·15 M NaCl– 0·01 M phosphate, pH 7·4, and 0·15 M NaCl–0·01 M tris, made with ordinary distilled water, have usually given satisfactory blank values. Fluorescence readings are obtained in arbitrary units, the instrument setting being adjusted so that initial readings of about 70–80 (out of 100) are obtained. This permits one to follow the fall in fluorescence down to readings of 15–20 without changing the setting on the machine. When a stable fluorescence value has been obtained (after temperature equilibration is established) increments of 0·01–0·02 ml of hapten are added, measuring fluorescence after each addition [18]. Once gentle mixing has been accomplished (glass stirring rod) fluorescence readings can be taken immediately. For a solution of antibody at 40 μg/ml a concentration of hapten from

6–20 mμM/ml is chosen, the value depending on the association constant. Additions of hapten are continued until 0·2 ml of hapten solution have been added. It is convenient to make additions with a 0·2 ml pipette which is filled at the beginning of the titration. With practice the solution can be retained in the pipette while shutter adjustments, stirring and recording are done with the opposite hand. After each titration a solvent fluorescence blank is determined.

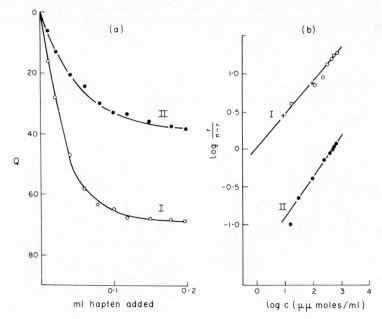

FIG. 12.3. Fluorometric titrations of an anti-dinitrophenyl antibody preparation with ε-DNP-lysine (curves I) and with 2,4-dinitrotoluene (curves II). Data for I are from Table 12.1. In (a), ordinate values correspond to col. 3 and abscissa to col. 1 in Table 12.1. In the Sips plots (b), the first three points of the titration for I are ignored since no free hapten can be determined for them by the method of calculation used. K_a for I is $5 \times 10^8 - 1 \times 10^9$ L/M, and for II is 2×10^6 L/M; a, for I is 0·5 and for II is 0·6. Taken from Eisen [24].

In order to calculate binding constants it is necessary to determine the diminution in antibody fluorescence when essentially all antibody sites are occupied by hapten (termed maximal quench or Qmax) [24]. In theory Qmax can be established by performing titrations at high concentration of hapten (e.g. 300–600 mμM/ml). Under the titration conditions described above this would produce a final hapten concentration which is several hundred times the antibody concentration. The problem is that when the absorbance of hapten at the activation wavelength approximates the antibody absorbance there is considerable non-specific reduction in fluorescence. It is necessary to compare antibody quenching with that obtained with 'normal' globulin or tryptophane at similar instrument settings and fluorescence intensity. The value of Qmax, obtained by difference, is subject to some uncertainty. Another approach is to do parallel determinations of the association constant

TABLE 12.1

Representative fluorometric titration of antibody with homologous hapten*

Hapten added, ML	Fluor. arbitrary units	Quench†	Hapten bound, mμmoles‡	Free hapten conc. M/L × 10ν (c)	Ratio: moles hapten bound/ mole antibody (r)
0	71·8	—	—	—	—
0·01	60·5	16·3	(0·099)‖	(−0·036)	—
0·02	52·5	27·9	(0·169)	(−0·045)	—
0·04	39·5	47·1	(0·286)	(−0·036)	—
0·06	31·9	58·3	0·353	0·017	1·608
0·08	28·2	63·6	0·386	0·102	1·753
0·10	26·9	65·1	0·395	0·205	1·794
0·12	25·1	67·5	0·410	0·298	1·862
0·15	24·1	68·4	0·415	0·448	1·886
0·18	23·5	68·6	0·416	0·593	1·893
0·20	23·0	69·0	0·419	0·684	1·903

* Purified rabbit antibody specific for dinitrophenyl group titrated with ε-DNP-lysine. Antibody solution: 1·0 ml with 0·22 mμmoles antibody, based on absorbance at 278 mμ, E cm^1 for antibody of 15·5, and mol. wt. 180,000. Hapten concentration: 6·2 mμmoles/ml based on absorbance at 360 mμ and molar absorbancy of 17,530. Solvent: 0·1 M tris-Cl, pH 7·6; temp. 30° C. From plot in Fig. 12.3, K_o, the average intrinsic association constant, is between 5×10^8 L/M and 1×10^9 L/M; a, the Sips index of heterogeneity, is 0·5.

† Fluorescence is corrected for the solvent (blank) fluorescence (6·0) and for the volume of hapten solution added, then normalized to the initial stable fluorescence (71·8 ≡ 100) and deducted from 100.

‖ The values in parentheses (cols. 4 and 5) are obviously inconsistent; see text for considerations of their possible significance.

‡ (Quench/Qmax) × (total antibody in mμmoles) × (2). Qmax for this system was taken as 72.

Taken from Eisen [24].

K_a by equilibrium dialysis (for details of the procedure see Pinckard & Weir, Chapter 14). Qmax is taken to be the value which gives the best fit for the two methods. By both procedures the Qmax for rabbit anti-DNP antibody is 72 per cent [23].

A representative titration is shown in Table 12.1 and Fig. 12.3a. Fluorescence values are corrected for dilution and the solvent blank and related to the initial fluorescence value, which is taken to be 100 per cent.* At a given total hapten concentration the ratio of the observed quench to Qmax is taken as the fraction of antibody sites occupied. Since the total antibody concentration is known, the concentration of free and bound antibody sites is readily calculated. The free hapten concentration is determined by the difference. K_a, the association constant in L/M, is given by:

$$K_a = \frac{(Ab\text{-}H)}{(Ab_f)\,(C)} \tag{4}$$

where Ab-H is bound hapten or occupied antibody sites, C is unbound hapten, and Ab_f is free antibody sites, all expressed in M/L.

Due to antibody heterogeneity values of K_a vary at different points on the curve. An average value for K_a and an index of antibody heterogeneity can be obtained from a Sips plot of log r/n−r against log C [24, 31] (Fig. 12.3b), where n is antibody valence (taken to be 2) and r is moles of hapten bound per mole of antibody. By inspection of equation (4) it is evident that K_a is equal to the reciprocal of the free hapten concentration when half the antibody sites are occupied. In the graph this is the point at which log r/n−r = 0; a, the heterogeneity index, is given by the regression coefficient or slope. In theory it can assume values from 1 (homogeneity) to 0 (maximal heterogeneity).

Not infrequently an anomalous result is obtained in the early part of the titration curve. Usually this takes the form of quenching in excess of the calculated theoretical maximum for the amount of hapten added [25]. In calculating such curves one can choose to neglect the excess quenching and assume that hapten is completely bound. An observation of a different sort has been noted with certain DNP peptides which exhibit better quenching in later portions of the curve than they do early [32]. In the case of early excess quenching it might be postulated that certain antibody molecules with one site occupied by hapten are being quenched excessively due to partial extension of quenching into the unoccupied site. This would result in excessive quenching early but Qmax would not be affected. Observations with univalent antibody fragments, however, also indicate some degree of excess quenching [26]. Presumably, therefore, these observations are indicative of heterogeneity of antibody sites in regard to Qmax. Whatever the explanation, there appears to be excellent correspondence between fluorescence quenching and other methods in regard to the relative binding constants of various haptens with DNP antibody. In the use of fluorescence quenching with other ligands, however, an independent substantiation of binding constants by equilibrium

* Calculations can be performed by a digital computer (IBM-7072) according to a programme developed by Mr Richard A.Dammkoehler and Mr Thomas L.Gallagher of the Computer Centre of Washington University, St Louis, Missouri [24].

dialysis seems desirable. Once correspondence has been established the highly convenient fluorometric assay can be employed with considerable confidence.

Titrations by fluorescence quenching have their greatest accuracy where the average antibody affinity is in the range of $10^6 - 10^8$ [22]. With antibodies of low affinity and hapten concentrations which do not non-specifically diminish fluorescence, relatively few antibody sites are occupied. On the other hand attenuation of antibody fluorescence at high hapten concentrations limits the accuracy of titrations at this level. The problem with antibodies of very high affinity has to do with quenching curves which are too close to the theoretical maximal to permit accurate determination of free hapten and free antibody. In theory antibodies of high affinity could be titrated more accurately in very dilute solution. In practice fluorometer instability and solvent blanks preclude this.

A special advantage of fluorescence quenching is the ease and rapidity of the measurement. This permits the study of antibody hapten interactions under a variety of conditions of pH, temperature and ionic strength where prolonged equilibration would complicate the interpretation. Using a stopped-flow technique, Day *et al* [33] were able to utilize fluorescence quenching to study the kinetics of the antibody–hapten reaction. It could be shown that equilibrium between rabbit antibody to DNP and DNP ligands was reached within a small fraction of a second.

While the bulk of fluorescence quenching studies have employed 7S antibody and univalent hapten, the technique is applicable to univalent antibody fragments and hapten or hapten-substituted proteins [18]. The method has been useful in the study of the effects of reduction and enzymatic digestion on antibody binding. One of the early demonstrations that 3·5S antibody fragments are univalent was by the fluorometric technique [18].

The requirement for a hapten which absorbs in the 300–350 mμ region does restrict the applicability of the fluorescence quenching method. Extension of the method to haptens without absorbance in the 300–400 mμ range may be possible by the introduction of substituents with the requisite absorption. Whether the efficiency of transfer will approximate the situation in which antibody specificity is for the quenching group remains to be established. Moreover, because the fluorescence quenching technique is dependent on the distribution and orientation of tryptophane residues in the antibody molecule, the extent of quenching with a given ligand cannot be anticipated. Tanenbaum *et al* [34] have reported that antibodies to β-D-galactosyl-phenylazo and β-D-glucosyl-phenylazo residues have little or no tryptophane in univalent antibody fragments obtained by proteolysis. Presumably in this circumstance, useful degrees of fluorescence quenching would not be obtained even if the homologous ligands were attached to an accessory structure with absorbance in the 300–350 mμ system.

P

The first quantitative studies of the antibody–hapten reaction in a soluble system were performed by equilibrium dialysis [35] (Chapter 14). Equilibrium dialysis continues to be the most straightforward procedure for determining equilibrium constants. Unlike fluorescence quenching it can be performed with γ globulin fractions rather than purified antibody. Unlike fluorescence quenching, any hapten which can be conveniently measured in dilute solution can be used. Disadvantages of equilibrium dialysis relative to the fluorometric procedure are the relatively large amount of antibody required, the greater amount of labour, and the delay before equilibrium is established. In principle, equilibrium dialysis can be performed with antibody affinities in the range of 10^7–10^{10} as well as in the usual range of 10^5–10^6. In practice radioactive haptens of very high specific activity are required and serious problems may arise in synthesis. The fluorescence quenching method permits accurate titrations with antibodies which have an affinity in the range of 10^6–10^8.

The most noteworthy advantages of the fluorescence quenching technique are its convenience and the minute amounts of antibody required. It permits the routine measurement of antibody affinity in physical and biological studies on antibody [22]. Using fluorescence quenching it has been learned that the range of affinities of DNP antibody extends at least from 10^5–10^9 [18, 23, 36]. Even purified antibody preparations from single animals display substantial binding heterogeneity with variations in K_a of at least several orders of magnitude [31, 23]. It has been shown that the average affinity of anti-DNP antibody increases with time after immunization [23]. While the basis for the variations in antibody affinity is not known, it is clear that in the full characterization of an antibody a description of its affinity (or average affinity) is desirable.

The importance of considering the role of antibody affinity in allergic responses deserves further discussion. Biological reactions mediated by antibody are triggered by the formation of antigen–antibody complexes. From formula (4) it can be seen that at limiting concentrations of antibody and antigen, the concentration of complex should be roughly proportional to K_a [37]. It has been demonstrated that 'high affinity antibodies' mediate immediate hypersensitivity responses under circumstances in which similar concentrations of low affinity antibody are inactive [36, 38]. These observations provide experimental validation for the assumption that biologic reactivity should be a function of affinity as well as concentration.

In view of the ability of high affinity antibody to complex with antigen in low concentration the possibility has to be considered that manifestations of hypersensitivity might be produced by antibodies in very low concentrations in serum. Karush and Eisen have postulated that delayed hypersensitivity responses are mediated by serum antibodies in concentrations too low to measure by current techniques [37]. One characteristic of delayed reactions is a requirement for the protein of the immunizing conjugate as well as the hapten moiety. It was suggested that there can be combined antigenic determinants comprised of hapten and contiguous areas of protein which by summation provide high affinities of interaction with antibody [37].

The possibility that antibody specificity extends beyond the haptenic group to adjacent amino acids on the protein carrier is subject to direct experimental attack. The approach taken in our laboratory has been to use synthetic DNP tetra- and pentapeptides as antigens [32]. DNP-specific antibody has been purified in the usual way using as precipitating antigen a DNP protein in which the peptide portion is absent. It has been possible to demonstrate that amino-acid side chains several residues distant from the DNP group can contribute substantially to antibody binding. While these observations help to establish the existence of relatively large antigenic determinants, there is no proof at this time that the antibodies involved can produce delayed hypersensitivity responses.

Sensitized fluorescence

Sensitized fluorescence is a special form of fluorescence enhancement due to excitation energy transfer. It occurs where fluorescent ligands which absorb in the region of tryptophane emission are bound to protein. Diminution of protein fluorescence is observed, analogous to what occurs with non-fluorescent ligands. Whereas non-fluorescent ligands dissipate the transferred excitation energy, the fluorescent ligand may be excited to exhibit its own characteristic fluorescence. This effect is best observed by excitation near the excitation maximum of the protein. Ligand fluorescence will be derived in part from direct activation and in part from resonance transfer of excitation energy from the protein. The component of fluorescence due to transfer is termed sensitized fluorescence.

A suitable molecule for the study of sensitized fluorescence in proteins is the 1-dimethylaminonapthalene-5-sulphonamido (DANS) group [3, 21] (Fig. 12.4). It has an absorption maximum where tryptophane fluorescence is maximal and an absorption minimum where the protein absorbs maximally. Moreover, it emits fluorescence at 520 mμ, a region where there is essentially no protein fluorescence. Demonstration of sensitized fluorescence has been possible with a number of covalent conjugates of DANS with various proteins and transfer efficiencies of close to 100 per cent have sometimes been observed [21].

Results in this laboratory with rabbit antibodies specific for DANS indicate that sulphonamides of DANS (DANS-amide and ε-DANS-lysine) undergo strikingly increasing fluorescence when they are bound to antibody

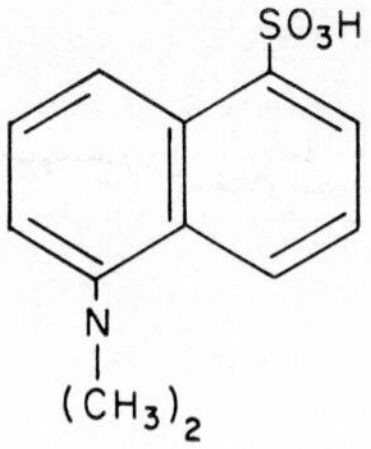

DANS

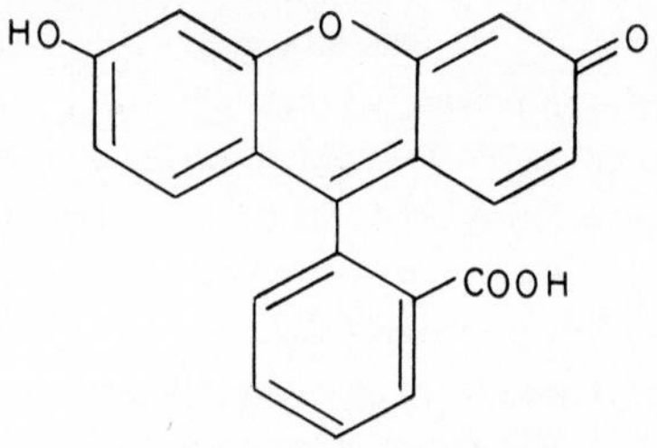

Fluorescein

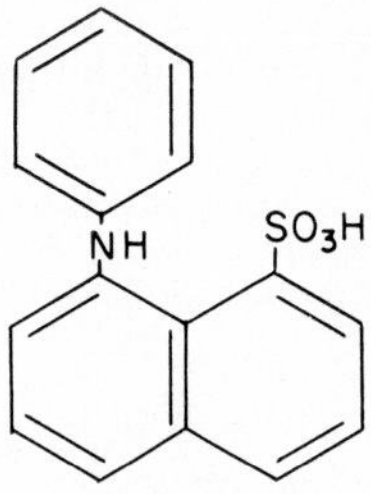

ANS

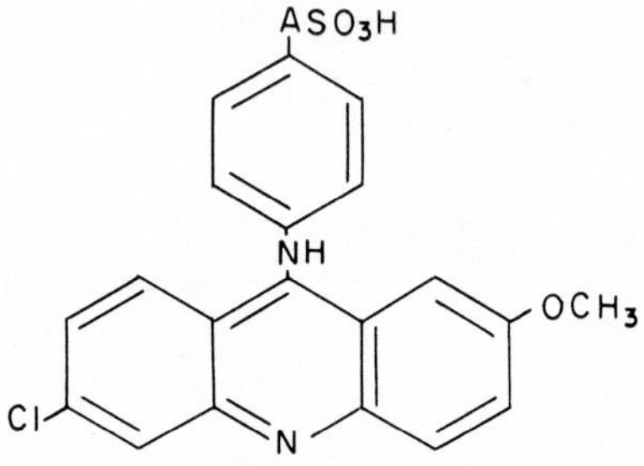

AcR

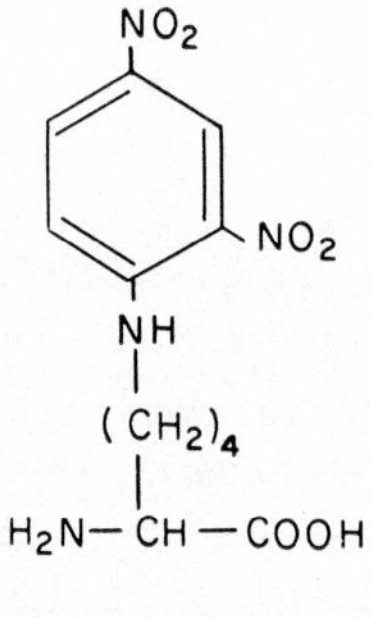

ε—N—DNP—Lysine

FIG. 12.4. Structural formulae.

DANS, 5-dimethylamino-1-naphthalene sulphonic acid (in DANS amide there is an SO_2NH_2 at the 1 position); ANS, 1-anilino-8-naphthalene-sulphonic acid; AcR, 2-methoxy-6-chloro-9-acridyl)-N-p-aminobenzene arsonic acid; ε-N-DNP-lysine, ε-N-2,4-dinitrophenyl-L-lysine.

[39a, b]. That this increase can be due at least in part to excitation energy transfer is evident from the appearance of a new activation maximum at 290 mμ (Fig. 12.5), where unbound DANS-amide has an absorption minimum. The shape of the excitation spectrum depends on the ratio of anti-DANS antibody to normal γ globulin. If the ratio is low the nonspecific γ globulin absorbs much of the excitation energy at 290 mμ. In this case the excitation maximum will be 340 mμ. The absorption maximum of antibody-bound DANS-amides. Interference by nonspecific protein absorption

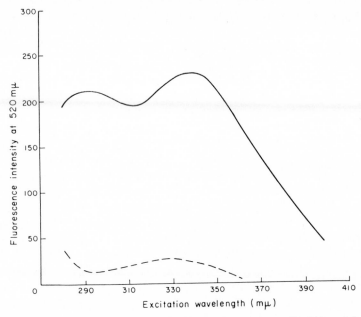

FIG. 12.5. The excitation spectrum of DANS amide with 'normal' rabbit γ globulin – – – – – and with rabbit antibody to DANS ———. Fluorescence is measured in arbitrary units at 520 mμ. The curves are corrected for protein emission.

is greatly reduced at this wavelength. In addition to a change in the excitation spectrum there is a shift in the fluorescence maximum to 480 mμ, where free DANS-amides have little fluorescence. There is also a marked increase in fluorescence quantum yield on excitation between 250 and 400 mμ. The increase in quantum yield at wavelengths at which excitation energy transfer from the proteins is minimal can be ascribed to sequestration of DANS molecules in non-polar antibody sites. This form of fluorescence enhancement is discussed in the next section. A more detailed description of the titration of anti-DANS antibody by fluorescence enhancement is given below.

Sensitized fluorescence has also been utilized by Velick and others in the study of enzyme-coenzyme complexes [40]. Velick was able to follow the reversible binding of reduced diphosphopyridine nucleotide (DPNH) to apoglyceraldehyde-3-phosphate dehydrogenase and a variety of other DPN-linked dehydrogenases by means of changes in DPNH fluorescence. DPNH has an absorption maximal at 340 mμ and emits fluorescence in the 400–500 mμ region. The curves shown in Fig. 12.6 are the fluorescence excitation spectra of free and bound DPNH. When DPNH is complexed with lactic dehydrogenase the excitation spectrum in the 280 mμ region corresponds closely with the absorption spectrum of the protein indicating excitation energy transfer. The polarization of the fluoresence of bound DPNH activated 280 mμ differs in sign from the fluorescence of directly excited DPNH. This indicates that there is one specific energy level of DPNH involved in transfer and another in direct excitation.

Fluorescence enhancement of non-planar molecules

There is a general class of organic molecules which exhibit very little fluorescence in aqueous solution but assume a high degree of fluorescence on binding to albumin and denatured proteins [41]. This behaviour occurs with acridines and napthalene sulphonic acids which are substituted with aniline or aniline derivatives. Two examples (2-methoxy-6-chloro-9-acridyl)-N-p-amino-benzene arsonate (abbreviated AcR) and 8-anilino-1-naphthalene sulphonate (abbreviated ANS) are shown in Fig. 12.4. Failure to observe fluorescence is apparently due to angulation of the aniline ring out of the plane of the remainder of the conjugated system. Such non-planar molecules are fluorescent in apolar solvents but are highly susceptible to quenching in polar solvents such as water. The basis for the assumption of fluorescence on binding to protein is not fully understood. It presumably is due to sequestration of a critical portion of ring system away from molecules of solvent [42]. The increment in fluorescence on binding to albumin can be at least several hundred-fold. For example, ANS bound to bovine serum albumin has a fluorescence quantum yield of about 0·75, whereas the unbound molecules have a quantum yield of about 0·004 [43].

Attempts to utilize molecules like ANS in the study of antibody have been very sparse. Berns & Singer [42] studied fluorescence enhancement of AcR with antibody to p-azobenzene-arsonate. While augmentation of fluorescence was observed, it was less than 5 per cent of that obtained with bovine serum albumin. This result suggested that in order for striking enhancement to occur, antibody specificity should be to the naphthalene or acridine portions of the molecule rather than the aniline portion. In a brief report Winkler described fluorescence enhancement of anilino-naphthalenes with antibodies to 1-azo-4-naphthalene sulphonic acid. However, no data were given in regard to the fluorescence quantum yield and no attempt was made to correlate the results of fluorometric titrations with quantitative precipitin titres or equilibrium dialysis.

Current studies in this laboratory indicate that rabbit antibodies to 1-azo-

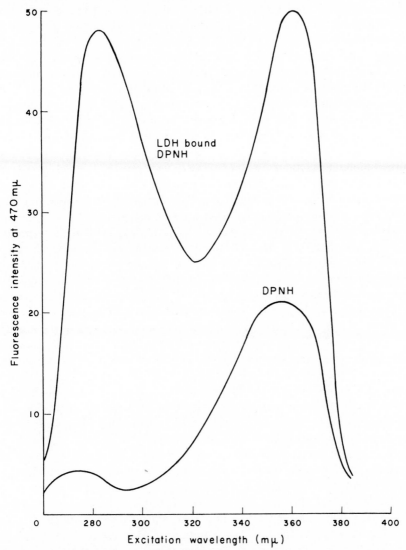

FIG. 12.6. The excitation spectrum of DPNH (reduced diphosphopyridine nucleotide) in the presence and absence of lactic dehydrogenase (LDH). Fluorescence intensity is measured in arbitrary units at 470 mμ. Taken from Velick [40].

4-naphthalene sulphonic acid and its 1,8 isomer cause a striking increase in 1, 4 or 1, 8 ANS fluorescence comparable in magnitude to the increase observed with serum albumin [44]. Rabbit antibodies to DANS (see above) augment ε-DANS-lysine fluorescence to nearly the same extent [39a]. Fluorescence enhancement studies are carried out with γ globulin fractions. In titrations with anilinonaphthalene sulphonates highly purified γ globulin is required. This can be obtained by preliminary salt fractionation with sodium or ammonium sulphate followed by CM-cellulose or DEAE-chromatography. Even pure γ globulins bind ANS to some extent but the degree of fluorescence enhancement and the association constant for the interaction is very low compared with that of specific antibody. The binding of DANS haptens by albumin and other non-globulin serum proteins is much weaker than ANS binding. This is an important advantage of the DANS system over the ANS system in studies on antibody. Titrations of anti-DANS antibody can be carried out with relatively crude γ globulin fractions; normal globulin fractions obtained by two successive $(NH_4)_2 SO_4$ precipitations at 33 or 40 per cent of saturation produce little nonspecific increase in DANS-amide fluorescence. Highly purified normal γ globulin does not bind DANS haptens at all under the usual titration conditions.

Titrations of anti-DANS and anti-ANS antibodies with their respective haptens differ mainly in the activation and emission wavelengths which are used. In DANS titrations activation is at 340 mμ and emission is measured at 480 mμ. Activation and emission wavelengths for 8–1 ANS titrations are at 365 and 470 mμ respectively. Where 4–1 ANS is the ligand fluorescence is measured at 415 mμ. The titration procedure is similar in many respects to that described in the section on fluorescence quenching of purified antibody. One millilitre of a solution of globulin in 0·15 M NaCl 0·01 M PO_4 is added to a clean dry cuvette. The total protein concentration can vary over a wide range but if the 280 mμ absorbance is greater than 5·0 high protein fluorescence blanks are obtained. The proportion of the total globulin fraction which is anti-DANS antibody varies widely and a preliminary titration may be necessary to establish the optimal titration conditions. Where the actual concentration of anti-DANS antibody is known from an earlier titration or an independent assay for antibody, titrations are usually carried out at an antibody concentration of about 30 μg/ml. After temperature equilibration protein and solvent blanks are determined. A standard solution of ε-DANS-lysine in buffer, usually at a concentration of 26 mμmoles/ml, is read intermittently during the titration in order to detect fluctuations in machine sensitivity. The standard solution is also used to readjust the sensitivity of the instrument before each titration so that the magnitude of the fluorescence readings will be comparable in different titrations (see below).

A typical titration is shown in Table 12.2. A relatively dilute solution of ε-DANS-lysine (or another DANS-amide) is added in 0·01–0·03 ml increments up to a volume of 0·2 ml. For titrations involving 30 μg of antibody a solution which contains 6 mμmoles of ε-DANS-lysine/ml is usually employed. It is sometimes advantageous to use several solutions containing different concentrations of ε-DANS-lysine in this portion of the titration curve so that a maximal range of values of R (the ratio of moles of hapten bound/mole of antibody) is obtained. This is especially desirable in dealing with antibodies of relatively low affinity. After the addition of the initial

TABLE 12.2

A representative titration of antibody by fluorescence enhancement

Volume of hapten solution added	mμmoles hapten added	Total hapten concentration mμmoles/ ml (H)	Fluor. arbitrary units (F)	Bound hapten fluor. (BF)	Bound hapten mμmoles/ ml	Assn. constant L/M × 10⁻⁶
0·00			110			
0·01	0·06	0·059	280	170·9	0·056	51·4
0·02	0·12	0·118	440	331·7	0·109	43·7
0·04	0·24	0·231	685	577·9	0·190	21·9
0·06	0·36	0·340	828	721·6	0·238	14·5
0·08	0·48	0·444	905	789·9	0·263	11·3
0·10	0·60	0·545	955	849·0	0·280	10·4
0·12	0·72	0·643	990	884·1	0·291	9·58
0·15	0·90	0·783	1020	914·1	0·302	9·37
0·18	1·08	0·915	1020	914·0	0·302	8·53
0·20	1·20	1·000	1040	934·0	0·308	9·89
0·24	17·20	13·87	1350	1350·0	0·342	—
0·28	33·20	25·94	1480	970·0	0·320	—

0·2 ml of ε-DANS-lysine, two additions of 0·04 ml of a 4×10^{-4} M solution of ε-DANS-lysine are made completing the titration. The final concentration of ε-DANS-lysine is usually 26 mμmoles/ml or higher, approximately eighty times the concentration of antibody. This very high ratio of hapten to antibody assures virtual saturation of antibody sites at the end of the titration.

In interpreting fluorescence enhancement curves it is necessary to know the relative fluorescence of free and bound hapten. These are designated as Ff and Fb respectively and are expressed in terms of the number of arbitrary fluorescence units given by the free or bound hapten at a concentration of 1 mμmoles/ml. For most preparations of anti-DANS antibody the ratio of

Fb/Ff is about 150–200 to 1. Ff is determined from the ε-DANS-lysine standard solution (see legend to Table 12.2). Ff in arbitrary fluoresence units and could easily vary from titration to titration. It is convenient to select an arbitrary constant value for Ff and adjust the fluorometer sensitivity setting so that this value is obtained in each titration.

The determination of Fb can be made (1) on the basis of the initial slope of the titration curve (where the antibody concentration is not known), or (2) on the basis of the total increase in fluorescence (after a correction for free hapten fluorescence and solution blanks (see Table 12.2), at the end of the titration (where the antibody concentration is known [39b]).

1. Where the antibody concentration is not known. In order to determine Fb it is necessary to obtain a titration in which the first four to five 0·01 ml additions of hapten produce a linear increase in fluorescence (after blank and volume corrections). This is the region of the curve where hapten concentration is low relative to antibody concentration and essentially all of the added hapten is bound. With animals immunized with antigen in complete adjuvant antibodies obtained 2 weeks or more after immunization can be titrated at approximately 100 μg of antibody/ml with a 2 mμmoles/ml solution of ε-DANS-lysine. With antibodies of low affinity relatively high concentrations of antibody may have to be used in order to obtain linearity in the early part of the titration curve.

2. Where the antibody concentration is known. By dividing the bound hapten fluorescence (FB, Table 12.2) at the end of the titration by the antibody concentration (corrected for dilution) an average Fb is obtained. Antibody concentration as determined by quantitative preciptitin analysis may be somewhat lower than the value obtained by equilibrium dialysis or fluorescence enhancement (see Table 12.2). This is probably due to failure to obtain precipitation of all the antibody present. For this reason equilibrium dialysis may be the better method for determining antibody concentration. However, it is difficult to be certain of saturation of all the antibody sites unless antibody affinity is reasonably high so that neither technique is entirely satisfactory.

The major potential problem in determining association constants by fluorescence enhancement is the possibility of heterogeneity of antibody with respect to Fb. Fb does vary with time after immunization, clearly indicating that anti-DANS antibody molecules can have markedly different Fbs. However, several lines of evidence indicate that Fb heterogeneity is ordinarily not of a magnitude which precludes using fluorescence enhancement to obtain useful information about antibody concentration and affinity: (1) Fbs determined from the initial slope and average Fbs based on antibody concentration correlate well. Moreover, by suitably designed filtrations at high concentrations of antibody it can be shown that Fb is about the same when 5, 10, 20, 40, 60 and 80 per cent of antibody sites are occupied by hapten. (2) Association constants and number of binding sites obtained by equilibrium dialysis correlate well with results of fluorescence enhancement. (3) Highly purified rabbit anti-DANS antibodies are found to have 2·0 binding sites/molecule by fluorescence enhancement using a value for Fb determined from the initial slope.

Fluorescence enhancement would appear to have many potential applications in the study of antibody hapten interactions. It has the convenience and sensitivity of the fluorescence quenching assay but does not require specifically purified antibody. Therefore, the entire antibody population can be studied. It can be used in the study of γM antibody [39b] and in combination with fluorescence polarization provides information about molecular size and configuration. It serves as a semi-quantitative assay for antibody at very low concentrations in the range of 1–5 μg of antibody protein/ml. At such low concentrations of antibody the determinations of Fb by initial slope is not possible. Whether animals immunized without adjuvant would develop enhancement of the magnitude exhibited by animals given antigen in adjuvant remains to be established. To date studies with anti-DANS antibody have been limited to rabbits and guinea-pigs.

Another application for fluorescence enhancement might be in the study of the biosynthesis of antibody. An intriguing possibility would be the use of ANS or DANS to detect antibody formation at the cellular level. Jerne & Nordin [45] and Ingraham & Buzzard [46] have devised a highly useful technique in which lymph-node cells from animals immunized with sheep erythrocytes are suspended in a semi-solid medium containing sheep erythrocytes and complement. Cells forming erythrocyte antibody produce localized areas of haemolysis (Chapter 33). It is possible to detect small numbers of antibody producing cells in a large population of lymphoid cells. Work is in progress in our laboratory to develop an analogous fluorescent system involving the incorporation of ANS into a semi-solid medium containing lymphoid cells from animals immunized to 1-azo-4-naphthalane sulphonic acid. While the information obtainable by fluorescence enhancement and red-cell lysis is qualitatively similar, in theory the fluorescence technique could provide better quantitation and probably greater sensitivity. Moreover, unlike red-cell lysis which is primarily a function of 19S antibody, fluorescence enhancement would not require a specialized antibody function which is distributed unevenly among the three classes of immunoglobulins.

Fluorescence polarization

Before discussing applications of fluorescence polarization to the study of antibody let us consider briefly the physical basis for this phenomenon and how it can furnish information on molecular interactions. Light can be resolved with a polarizing lens or prism into rays with their electrical vectors in a single plane. Fluorescent solutions which are excited with vertically polarized or natural light emit partially polarized fluorescence as viewed at right-angles to the incident beam. Excitation with vertically polarized light is illustrated diagrammatically in Fig. 12.7. The vertically polarized light is vibrating in the plane of the paper along OX and is propagated in direction

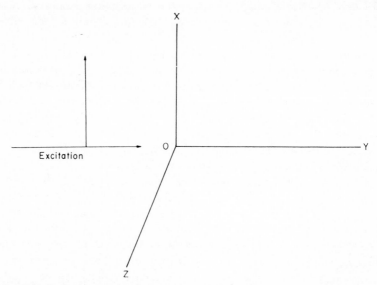

FIG. 12.7. Excitation with vertically polarized light vibrating along OX and propagated in direction OY. Observation is along OZ, at right-angles to OX and OY. Taken from Feofilov [47].

OY, at right-angles to OX. Observation is along OZ, normal to both OX and OY (towards the reader). P, the degree of polarization of fluorescence, is given by the formula:

$$P = \frac{F_V - F_H}{F_V + F_H} \tag{5}$$

where F_V is fluorescence intensity with the analyser prism positioned vertically (parallel to OX) and F_H is the fluorescence intensity with the analyser prism in the horizontal position (parallel to OY). P_P, the extent of polarization of fluorescence with polarized incident light, is related to P_L, the polarization of fluorescence with natural incident light, by the formula:

$$P_L = \frac{P_P}{2 - P_P} \quad [48] \tag{6}$$

For all possible positive values of P_P (0 to $\frac{1}{2}$) P_P is greater than P_L. Despite the greater magnitude of P_P, unpolarized radiation is often employed for excitation because of its greater intensity.

Polarization of fluorescence is due to the fixed relationship between molecular orientation and the absorption and emission of fluorescence. Specific regions of the fluorescent molecule are concerned with absorption and emission; they are termed absorption and emission oscillators respectively, referring to the fact that the involved areas become oscillating electrical dipoles

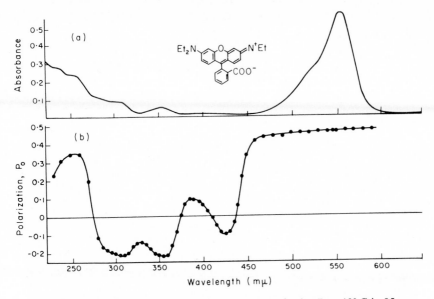

FIG. 12.8. Absorption and polarization spectra of rhodamine B at 10° C in 95 per cent glycerol, 5 per cent water. Emission observed at 573 mμ. Taken from Chen & Bowman [49].

during activation of fluorescence [8]. Data obtained by fluorescence polarization studies are consistent with the interpretation that fluorescent molecules contain several absorption oscillators (one for each electronic transition state) oriented at various angles with a single emission oscillator. Because of the presence of several axes of absorption in complex molecules, polarization varies with the activation wavelength as illustrated by the polarization spectrum of rhodamine B (Fig. 12.8). Maximal polarization is generally observed at the principal absorption band. At shorter wavelengths negative polarization may be observed (e.g. maximal polarization is obtained in the direction of propagation of exciting light). Interpolated between regions of maximal positive and negative polarization are transition zones corresponding to involvement of more than one electronic transition [8]. In many organic molecules there are complexities in the polarization spectrum which do not correspond to changes in the absorption spectrum. Tryptophane-containing proteins exhibit subleties in their polarization spectra, as compared with free tryptophane, apparently due to the local tryptophane environment.

Fluorescent molecules have a preferred orientation for excitation, depending on the position of the absorption oscillator(s) which is (are) being excited. In a solution of randomly oriented fluorescent molecules, polarized light will preferentially excite molecules positioned so that their absorption oscillators are parallel to the plane of polarization, as illustrated in Fig. 12.9. As the

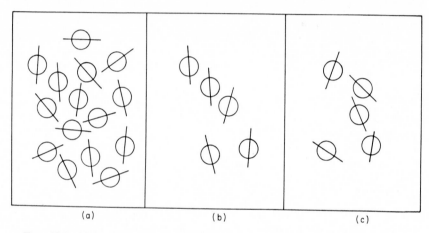

(a)   (b)   (c)

FIG. 12.9. The relationship between Brownian motion and depolarization of fluorescence. Taken from Weber [9].

Protein molecules in solution are represented by ϕ. As shown in (a) they are randomly oriented. Excitation by polarized light preferentially excites molecules lying parallel to one another (b). By the time fluorescence is emitted, excited molecules have become partially disoriented (c) resulting in partial depolarization of fluorescence.

direction of a molecule deviates from the position of maximal excitation the likelihood of excitation decreases. Once a molecule is excited, the location of the emission oscillator will specify the direction of the fluorescent beam. Provided the position of the molecule at the time of excitation is partially retained at emission, the molecule will exhibit 'memory' [14] and fluorescence will be partially polarized.

The extent to which fluorescent molecules polarize fluorescence is influenced by a number of factors. While we will be primarily concerned in our subsequent discussion with the effects of Brownian motion on polarization we will briefly consider other causes of depolarization first. (i) A molecule, fixed in position, can absorb light from one direction and emit light in a new direction. The extent of deviation from the theoretical polarization maximum depends on the mutual orientation of the absorption and emission oscillators [13]. The maximal polarization value for a given molecule, in the absence of all other causes for depolarization, is termed the principal polarization (P_0). (ii) Partially aligned molecules may be excited; the likelihood of excitation is related to the (cosine)^2 of the angle between the plane of the excitation beam and the plane of the absorption oscillator [9, 47]. (iii) In a single macromolecule containing a number of fluorescent molecules, oriented randomly, there may be transfer of excitation energy to molecules with a new spatial orientation. Evaluation of depolarization of fluorescence constitutes a valuable technique for demonstration of excitation energy transfer in proteins [21]. (iv) Radiative transfer of the excited state where fluorescence is absorbed and re-emitted is another, generally less important cause for depolarization [50]. It differs from excitation energy transfer which is a non-radiative process. In studies where radiative transfer must be eliminated, reabsorption of fluorescence is minimized by using solutions as thin layers (in the range of 30 μ).

If intermolecular transfer is minimized and excitation is in the principal absorption band, polarization can assume values near the theoretical maximum. Under these conditions the extent of polarization is primarily a function of rotational Brownian motion. Molecules in solution change in position continually by translational and rotational movement. The extent of this motion is dependent on molecular size and shape as well as the physical properties of the medium. Small molecules in aqueous solution may undergo such rapid rotational diffusion that they assume a random orientation between the time of excitation and emission. Under these conditions fluorescence will be completely depolarized. With larger molecules the molecular orientation at excitation is partially preserved at emission and fluorescence is partially polarized (Fig. 12.9). If a fluorescent molecule interacts with another molecule of any size and the complex has some rigidity, polarization of fluorescence will increase.

The equation of Perrin expresses fluorescence polarization as a function of the fluorescent molecule, the lifetime of its excited state and solvent temperature and viscosity [51]:

$$\frac{1}{P} = \frac{1}{P_0} + \left(\frac{1}{P_0} - \frac{1}{3}\right)\left(\frac{RT}{V}\right)\frac{r}{n} \tag{7}$$

P is observed polarization (vertically polarized light, observed at a right-angle); P_0 is the maximal polarization; R is the gas constant; T is absolute temperature; n is viscosity (poise); r is the mean lifetime of the excited state and V is the molar volume of the fluorescent molecule. The quantity V is a function of molecular size, shape and state of hydration. In rigid spherical molecules

V is directly related to the rotational relaxation time, ρ (the time required for an average molecule to move through an angle, θ, the cosine of which is 0·365). In proteins the relationship between V and ρ is more complex and cannot be completely described by a simple model. The behaviour of most proteins is adequately approximated by treating them as ellipsoids rotating about their three principal axes.

The effect of temperature and viscosity is readily evaluated by measuring P at different temperatures in aqueous solutions containing glycerol or propylene glycol in various proportions. For many proteins there is a linear relationship between $1/P$ and T/n. $1/P_0$ is given by the intercept on the ordinate as illustrated in Fig. 12.10. The regression coefficient or slope is related to both R and V and if either is known the other can be estimated. Deviations from linearity occur for a variety of reasons which include marked molecular asymmetry and internal rotation within the protein molecule.

The relationship between r, v and p in equation (7) provides a basis for selecting fluorescent molecules suitable for following protein–protein interactions. The value of r and of V, before and after complex formation, will determine the extent of change in polarization on aggregation. It has been found that DANS and fluorescein, with values of r of about 1·3 and $0·5 \times 10^{-8}$ seconds respectively, afford useful degrees of polarization with proteins in the molecular weight range of 5000–200,000. Most studies of fluorescence polarization involving proteins have been with these two molecules.

Fluorescence polarization in quantitation of antigen antibody reactions

It is the influence of molecular size and shape on fluorescence polarization which makes this technique useful in the study of antibody–antigen and antibody–hapten interactions. If a small fluorescent hapten ($MW < 1000$) becomes bound to 7S antibody (MW 160,000) there will be a marked reduction in its rotational diffusion and a corresponding increase in fluorescence polarization. Easily measurable changes in polarization also can be obtained when fluorescent protein antigens combine with antibody. As discussed above, the extent of the change depends on the fluorescent oscillator and its mean lifetime in the excited state as well as the molecular weight of the protein and the nature of the antigen–antibody complexes which form.

The most frequent immunological application of fluorescence polarization has been to study the reactions of protein antigens with their respective antibodies. In order to follow changes in antigen fluorescence in a complex mixture of proteins, the antigen is labelled with a fluorescent molecule which absorbs and emits in regions of the spectrum where other groups on protein do not interfere. As few as 1–4 molecules of the fluorescent marker per molecule of protein are required for useful degrees of fluorescence. At this level of substitution it is generally possible to prepare conjugates in which protein antigenicity is not appreciably altered. In a protein containing many groups able to react with the labelling agent it is generally justifiable to assume that fluorescent label is randomly distributed and is unaffected by local protein environment.

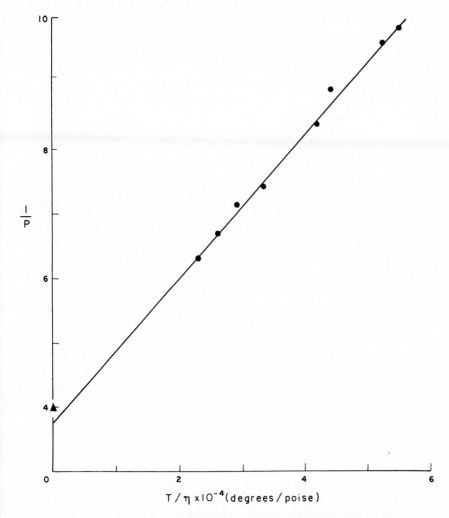

Fig. 12.10. Perrin plot for fluorescence polarization of β-anthryl conjugate of bovine serum albumin at 0·12 mg/ml. Activation at 380 mμ, emission at 461 mμ. Various points along the abscissa were obtained by varying the temperature and glycerol content of the protein solution. Taken from Chen & Bowman [49].

Commonly used fluorescent labelling agents in polarization studies are fluorescein isothiocyanate (FITC) and 1-dimethylaminonaphthalene-5-sulphonyl chloride (DANS chloride). The structures of fluorescein and DANS are shown in Fig. 12.4. Under weakly alkaline conditions these two reagents react predominantly with protein lysyl residues forming thiourea and sulphonamido linkages respectively. Because DANS chloride and FITC have low water solubility coupling to protein is relatively inefficient. Variations in the coupling procedure include adding the fluorescent reagent as a solid, as a solution in acetone, or in the dry state adsorbed to diatomaceous earth or cellulose [13]. Since the labelled protein must function as an antigen, denaturation must be kept to a minimum. Volumes of organic solvent in excess of 5 per cent of the total volume of aqueous protein solution should be avoided and additions should be made slowly with constant stirring by a magnetic bar. Conjugations usually are carried out at 0–4° C. The use of bicarbonate–carbonate buffers in the pH range of 8–9 avoids excess alkalinity while permitting reactions to be completed within 6–24 hours. High degrees of protein labelling are undesirable since fluorescence is not necessarily correspondingly increased and considerable alteration in protein structure may result. Desirable ratios of coupling agents to protein are in the range of 0·01–0·1 mg per mg of protein. They depend in considerable measure on the purity and physical form of the fluorescent material. For example, Goldberg has noted that crystalline fluorescein isothiocyanate couples to protein with several times the efficiency of the amorphous form of the isothiocyanate [7]. Protein concentration, stirring efficiency and duration of reaction also influence the degree of conjugation obtained.

Conjugates must be freed of non-covalently bound fluorescent material and aggregated protein. The bulk of the unconjugated dye is eliminated by dialysis; final traces can be removed on Sephadex G25 columns. The adequacy of removal of unbound dye is evaluated by constancy of fluorescence polarization, by chromatography, or by reapplication to Sephadex. Aggregation between protein molecules is undesirable for it increases the effective molecular weight, giving high polarization values [52]. Aggregated protein can be removed on Sephadex G75 or G100, by passage through a bacterial filter [52] or by ammonium sulphate fractionation.

The number of fluorescent molecules/molecule of protein can be estimated from the dry weight and the absorption spectrum as compared with the unsubstituted protein. DANS groups have an absorption maximum in the 330–360 mμ region. The ε-DANS derivative of lysine has a molar extinction coefficient of $4\cdot74 \times 10^3$ at 330 mμ [39b] and this figure can be used as a standard in calculating the DANS concentration. The calculation involves the assumption that nearly all the DANS residues on protein are bound to ε-amino groups and that the absorption of the free amide provides an accurate reference. The absorption spectrum of a DANS-protein conjugate is shown in Fig. 12.11. The molar extinction coefficient of fluorescein groups is about 50×10^3 at 490 mμ.

Most fluorescence polarization studies have been carried out with modified light-scattering photometers or improved polarization fluorometers. Recently Chen and Bowman have described the use of polarizing filters with large apertures which are readily adapted to commercially available spectrofluorophotometers and which have excellent transmission properties [49]. Two coated quartz lenses are mounted vertically and horizontally in a sliding filter holder which is positioned in the incident beam. Two polaroid

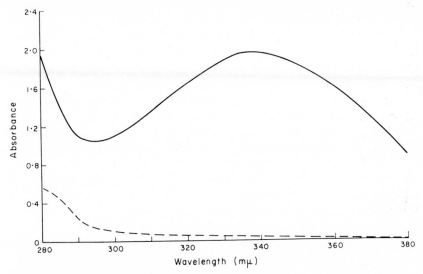

FIG. 12.11. Absorption spectra of human serum albumin – – – – – and DANS substituted human serum albumin ———, each at 1 mg/ml in water. Using DANS lysine as a reference (see text) the conjugate contains about 30 DANS groups per molecule of protein.

discs mounted similarly are positioned at a right-angle in the incident beam. While it is convenient to position the analyser lens between the cell and the monochromator grating, values of p must be corrected for the effect on the latter on polarization. The correction factor is readily obtained by measuring fluorescence intensities with the analysers oriented vertically and horizontally and the incident beam horizontally polarized (I_{HV} and I_{HH} respectively). In theory G, the ratio of I_{HV} to $I_{HH'}$, should be 1 (i.e. fluorescence should not be polarized), since observation is along the electrical vector of the incident beam. In practice, with the Aminco-Bowman spectrofluorophotometer, values of G range between 0·75 and 1·0 [40]. The correction factor G varies with the emission wavelength and the size of the slit used in the emission beam. The degree of polarization, P, using vertically polarized incident light is then given by:

$$P = \frac{I_{VV} - GI_{VH}}{I_{VV} + GI_{VH}} \tag{8}$$

The concentration of antibody for titrations is kept within the range where antigen and antibody form soluble complexes. Even small amounts of turbidity will give spurious fluorescence readings. While the limiting antibody concentration will vary with the antigen/antibody system and the duration of immunization it will usually be in the range of 5–20 μg antibody protein [53]. Proteolytic fragments of antibody can be evaluated at a higher concentration. In the absence of quantitative information on antibody concentration suitable dilutions can be determined empirically. In order to evaluate antibody affinity, titrations can be carried out at several different antibody concentrations (covering a five- to ten-fold range). It is desirable to use purified globulin fractions of antibody rather than whole serum. Fluorescent molecules bind non-specifically to serum albumins, requiring the use of correction factors in calculating binding data if serum is used. Satisfactory globulin fractions have been obtained by precipitation with ammonium sulphate or by DEAE-cellulose fractionation (see Stelos, Chapter 1 and Fahey & Terry, Chapter 3). After dialysis, filtration through a sintered glass funnel may be necessary in order to eliminate turbidity. Satisfactory buffers for dilution of antibody and antigen include 0·15 M NaCl, 0·01 M PO_4 and 0·15 M NaCl, 0·01 M tris chloride.

A stock antigen solution at concentration of the order of $1–10 \times 10^{-7}$ M is used for fluorescein conjugates [53]. The exact concentration will vary depending on antibody concentration, affinity and the ratio of antigen to antibody at equivalence. Some fluorescent antigens give unstable fluorescence readings in very dilute solution. The addition of 0·05 per cent normal globulin can be used to stabilize the protein [53].

The antigen is added in small increments to the antibody solution until about 0·2 volumes have been added. The titration should cover a range from antibody excess to relatively far antigen excess. Antigen fluorescence also is evaluated in buffer alone and with 'normal' γ globulin. Excitation may be with unpolarized or vertically polarized light, ordinarily at the principal absorption band. Readings are taken with the analyser in the vertical and horizontal positions. In contrast to fluorescence quenching, establishment of equilibrium is not instantaneous. A delay of 8–10 minutes between additions may be necessary to ensure equilibration [53]. Since fluorescence polarization varies with temperature, and titrations are relatively time-consuming, care is required that the solution remain at constant temperature throughout the titration.

Polarization is calculated from equation (5). Corrections are made for solvent and normal globulin blanks and for changes of polarization caused by the emission monochromator (see previous section). Representative titrations are shown in Fig. 12.12 and Table 12.3. The data here, taken from Dandliker *et al* [53], were obtained with rabbit antibody to ovalbumin and fluorescein-labelled ovalbumin. As expected, the polarization of antigen increases with antibody concentration.

The quantitative interpretation of binding data obtained by fluorescence polarization is still under development. The only extensive mathematical

TABLE 12.3

Titration of fluorescein-labelled ovalbumin with antibody to ovalbumin. The data, shown graphically in Fig. 12.12, are taken from Dandliker *et al*. Antibody concentration is 3·3 μg/ml. Calculations are based on the values of Pf, Pb, Qf and Qb given in Fig. 12.12. Ff is free antigen, and Fb is bound antigen. Ag$_{max}$ is taken as the total concentration of antibody sites, based on precipitin analyses and using 160,000 and 2 as antibody molecular weight and valence

P	0·276	0·262	0·252	0·244
Ab sites M/L × 10⁸	4·1	4·1	4·1	4·1
AG conc. M/L × 10⁸	0·83	1·71	3·44	6·83
Agb/Agf	2·78	1·01	0·49	0·23
Agb M/L × 10⁸	0·61	0·86	1·14	1·28
Agf M/L × 10⁸	0·22	0·85	2·30	5·55

treatment to date is that of Dandliker and his colleagues [53]. In their formulation it is assumed that all fluorescent molecules bound to antibody can be described with a single polarization value. There are then only two species of fluorescent molecules, bound and free. The ratio of Fb, the fraction of antigen bound, to Ff, the fraction of antigen free, is given by:

$$\frac{Fb}{Ff} = \frac{Qf\,(P-Pf)}{Qb\,(Pb-P)} \tag{9}$$

where P is the experimentation value for polarization, Pf is polarization of free antigen, Pb is polarization of bound antigen and Qf and Qb are the fluorescence intensities of free and bound antigen respectively as given by the sum of the horizontal and vertical fluorescence intensities ($I_V + I_H$). Pf is readily obtained since it is the polarization of antigen fluorescence in the absence of antibody. Pb cannot be measured directly because it is the polarization value when all the antigen is bound and this condition is not realized experimentally. As shown in Fig. 12.12, the maximal experimental values for P are in the region of far antibody excess, at relatively high antibody concentrations. Pb can be estimated graphically by extrapolation of the titration curve to infinitely high antibody concentration (intersection with the ordinate). A better estimate of Pb can be obtained by plotting the maximal titration values of P (termed p′) at several antibody concentrations against P′ − Pb/(AB)

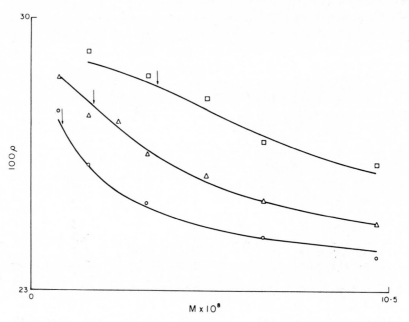

FIG. 12.12. Titration of antibody to ovalbumin with fluorescein-labelled ovalbumin. Taken from Fig. 9 in Dandliker *et al* [53]. Antibody concentrations (μg/ml) are calculated from precipitation with native ovalbumin: ○—3·3, △—6·6, □—13·2. Solid curves are plotted using Pf = 0·234, Pb = 0·293, Qf = 4·36, Qb = 3·9 and values for K_0, a, and Pb max which give the best fit for the experimental data, as determined by computer [53].

where AB, the antibody concentration, is expressed in any convenient units [53]. Pb is given by the intercept of the line joining the experimental points with ordinate.

The apparent equilibrium constant, K_0, can be calculated by a Sips distribution using data obtained from the precipitin curve as the basis for antibody concentration [53].

$$\text{Log Agf} = \frac{1}{a} \log \left(\frac{\text{Agb}}{\text{Ag}_{max} - \text{Agb}} \right) - \log K_0 \qquad (10)$$

where Agf is the concentration of free antigen (M/L), Agb is the concentration of bound antigen (M/L), Ag_{max} is maximal concentration of antigen which can be bound (equivalent to twice the antibody concentration, expressed in M/L) and a is the heterogeneity index [32]. One can determine K_0 and a by a plot of log $(Agb)/(Ag_{max} - Agb)$ against log Agf (an analogous graph using fluorescence quenching data is shown in Fig. 12.3b).

While a quantitative approach to polarization data is highly desirable, several inherent limitations in the use of fluorescence polarization to calculate the equilibrium constants of antigen antibody interactions require

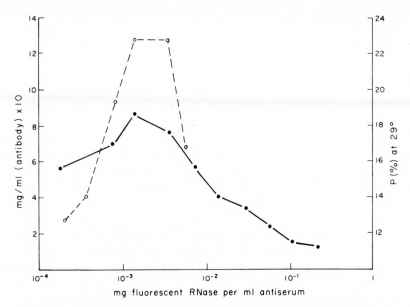

FIG. 12.13. A fluorescence polarization titration of antibody to ribonuclease with fluorescein-labelled ribonuclease ●—●—●, compared with standard precipitin reaction ○—○. The p value for free antigen is 0·11. After Haber *et al* [52, Fig. 2].

consideration: (i) Clearly it is an approximation to view all bound antigen molecules as a single species. Actually a number of different complexes, represented by the general formula Ag_xAb_y are formed. Each presumably has its own unique polarization value. A mathematical treatment of the relationship between relative amounts of antigen and antibody and aggregate size has been derived by Goldberg [54]. By analogy with the precipitin reaction maximal polarization might occur in the equivalence zone, where the largest aggregates are formed. In practice, Haber & Bennett [52] have observed polarization maxima at equivalence ratios of antigen to antibody as shown in Fig. 12.13 but similar peaks are absent from the titration curves of Dandliker *et al* [53]. From the data given by the latter authors it appears that relatively few antibody sites are occupied in this portion of the curve. It is doubtful that under these conditions the distribution of antigen–antibody complexes will correspond to ratios observed in the precipitin reaction or in soluble complexes formed at higher concentrations of antigen and antibody. More probably, Ag_1Ab_1 complexes predominate throughout most of the titration. If this is the case, the approximation that all bound antigen can be represented by a single polarization value is reasonable. In view of the different results of Haber and Bennett with other antigen–antibody systems, however, the method of Dandliker *et al* for handling experimental data may not be applicable to all antigen–antibody reactions. (ii) In the graphical determination of K_0 by the Sips distribution in Fig. 12.13, less than 50 per cent of the total antibody sites are occupied at any given point. Calculation of K_0 here involves the implicit assumption that the fraction of antibody titrated is representative of the total antibody population. Since sizeable proteins contain at least several different antigenic determinants this assumption cannot be entirely valid. If very large amounts of antigen are used in an attempt to titrate all antibody sites the contribution of bound antigen to the total fluorescence is too small to measure accurately. (iii) Antigenic size (or more strictly the molar volume of antigen) determines the extent of change in p on interaction with antibody. Antigens employed have included the B chain of insulin, ribonuclease, ovalbumin and bovine serum albumin, ranging in molecular weight from 3000 to about 70,000. Larger antigens will require fluorescent markers with larger values for r, but the best choice is not clear at present.

In summary it seems evident that the nature of the polarization curve will vary depending on antigen valence and molecular weight and antibody concentration and affinity. Calculation of association constants by this method must be regarded as highly provisional. To date there has not been a study directly comparing binding data obtained by fluorescence polarization with that obtained in other soluble systems. The comparison would have to be made with the same antibody preparation since antibodies vary greatly in affinity depending on the method of immunization. A good antigen for this purpose might be insulin or growth hormone. Highly sensitive chromato-electrophoretic techniques for measuring the interactions of these antigens with their respective antibodies are available (see Chapter 18). In lieu of validation of K_0 values by independent methods, fluorescence polarization should none the less provide a useful, empirical assay for comparing antibodies formed at different times and in different animals to the same antigen.

The calculation of association constants by fluorescence polarization is more straightforward with univalent antibody fragments or fluorescent haptens. In these systems antibody concentration is not limited and the classes of molecular complexes which can form are much more restricted. While proteolytic procedures for production of univalent antibody fragments are well standardized the possibility of modification of antibody during digestion has to be considered. Quantitation of the reaction of antibody with univalent fluorescent haptens by fluorescence polarization does not have this drawback and it should be a useful supplement to presently available techniques.

Despite the potential value of fluorescence polarization in the study of antibody hapten reactions, it is in the area of protein–anti-protein interactions where there is the greatest need for new methodology. The standard technique for the measurement of antibody is the quantitative precipitin assay. In the presence of reasonable amounts of antibody the precipitin technique permits the precise measurement of antibody concentration. What the two-phase system fails to provide is information about the dynamic equilibrium between antigen and antibody. Moreover, the formation of an insoluble complex is dependent on antigen and antibody bivalence and is subject to variations in pH and ionic strength. Despite the advantages in the measurement of antigen–antibody interactions in a soluble system, quantitation in such systems is often not entirely satisfactory. Available methods include ultracentrifugation, electrophoresis, chromatography and fluorescence polarization [55]. In the first three systems cited the analysis of antigen–antibody mixtures involves the physical separation of individual components of the mixture. During separation, some dissociation and re-equilibration of antigen–antibody complexes occurs. In systems characterized by relatively weak interaction between antigen and antibody misleading information about original equilibrium conditions is obtained. Fluorescence polarization avoids this problem in that the reaction mixture is analysed directly. This advantage as well as convenience of the fluorometric titration is balanced by difficulties in precise quantitation of binding. While fluorescence polarization is undoubtedly a useful supplement to the other methods, more information is needed before its relative value is clearly defined.

References

[1] UDENFRIEND S. (1962) *Fluorescence Assay in Biology and Medicine*. New York: Academic Press

[2] THEORELL H. (1958) Kinetics and equilibria in the liver alcohol dehydrogenase system. In *Advances in Enzymology*, Vol. XX, p. 31, ed. NORD F.F. New York: Interscience Publishers

[3] WEBER G. (1952) Polarization of the fluorescence of macromolecules. 2. Fluorescent conjugates of ovalbumin and bovine serum albumin. *Biochem. J.* **51,** 155

[4] LOWRY O.H. (1957) Micromethods for the assay of enzymes. In *Methods in Enzymology*, Vol. IV, p. 366, ed. COLOWICK S.P. & KAPLAN N.O. New York: Academic Press

[5] LOWRY O.H., PASSONNEAU J.V., SCHULZ D.W. & ROCK M.F. (1961) The measurement of pyridine nucleotides by enzymatic cycling. *J. biol. Chem.* **236,** 2746

[6] ROTMAN B. (1961) Measurement of activity of single molecules of B-D-galactosidase. *Proc. nat. Acad. Sci.* **47,** 1981

[7] MCDEVITT H.O. & COONS A.H. (1964) Methods for preparation of fluorescent proteins. In *Methods in Medical Research,* Vol. 10, p. 142, ed. EISEN H.N. Chicago: Year Book Medical Publishers

[8] WEBER G. & TEALE F.W.J. (1965) Interaction of proteins with radiation. In *The Proteins,* Vol. III, p. 466, ed. NEURATH H. New York: Academic Press

[9] WEBER G. (1953) Rotational Brownian motion and polarization of the fluorescence of solutions. In *Advances in Protein Chemistry,* Vol. VII, p. 416, ed. ANSON M.L., BAILEY K. & EDSALL J.T. New York: Academic Press

[10] FOTHERGILL J.E. (1964) In *Fluorescent Protein Tracing,* pp. 4–53, ed. NAIRN R.C. Baltimore: Williams & Wilkins Company

[11] PARKER C.A. & REES W.T. (1960) Correction of fluorescence spectra and measurement of fluorescence quantum efficiency. *Analyst* **85,** 587

[12] CHURCHICH J.E. (1965) Fluorescence properties of pyridoxamine-5-phosphate. *Biochim. et Biophys. Acta* **102,** 208

[13] STEINER R.F. & EDELHOCH H. (1962) Fluorescent protein conjugates. *Chem. Reviews,* p. 457

[14] SELIGER H.H. & MCELROY W.D. (1965) *Light: Physical and Biological Action,* p. 80. New York: Academic Press

[15] TRISTRAM G.R. & SMITH R.H. (1963) Amino acid composition of certain proteins. In *The Proteins,* Vol. I, p. 46, ed. NEURATH H. New York: Academic Press

[16] STEINER R.F. & EDELHOCH H. (1963) The ultraviolet fluorescence of proteins. *Biochim. et Biophys. Acta* **66,** 341–355

[17] WEBER G. (1960) Fluorescence-polarization spectrum and excitation energy transfer in proteins. *Biochem. J.* **75,** 345

[18] VELICK S.F., PARKER C.W. & EISEN H.N. (1960) Excitation energy transfer and the quantitative study of the antibody hapten reaction. *Proc. nat. Acad. Sci. (Wash.)* **46,** 1470

[19] FÖRSTER T. (1960) Transfer mechanisms of electronic excitation. *Discussions of the Faraday Society,* Vol. 27, pp. 7–17

[20] FÖRSTER T. (1960) Transfer mechanisms of electronic excitation energy. *Radiation Research,* **Supplement 2,** pp. 326–339

[21] STRYER L. (1960) Energy transfer in proteins and polypeptides. *Radiation Research,* **Supplement 2,** pp. 432–451

[22] PARKER C.W. (1963) Antibody–hapten reactions as measured by a spectrofluorometric method. In *Conceptual Advances in Immunology and Oncology,* p. 191. New York: Hoeber Medical Division of Harper & Row

[23] EISEN H.N. & SISKIND G.W. (1964) Variations in affinities of antibodies during the immune response. *Biochemistry* **3,** 996

[24] EISEN H.N. (1964) Determination of antibody affinity for haptens and antigens by means of fluorescence quenching. In *Methods in Medical Research,* Vol. X, p. 115, ed. EISEN H.N. Chicago: Year Book Medical Publishers

[25] FARAH F.S., KERN M. & EISEN H.N. (1960) The preparation and some properties of purified antibody specific for the 2,4-dinitrophenyl group. *J. exp. Med.* **112,** 1195

[26] LITTLE J.R. & EISEN H.N. Personal communication

[27] GREEN N.M. (1964) Avidin quenching of fluorescence by dinitrophenyl groups. *Biochem. J.* **90,** 564–568

[28] WEBER G. & TEALE F.J.W. (1959) Electronic energy transfer in haem proteins. *Discussions Faraday Soc.* Vol. 27, 134

[29] PARKER C.W., SHAPIRO J., KERN M. & EISEN H.N. (1962) Hypersensitivity to penicillenic acid derivatives in humans with penicillin allergy. *J. exp. Med.* **115**, 789–810

[30] EISEN H.N. (1964) Preparation of purified anti 2,4-dinitrophenyl antibodies. In *Methods in Medical Research*, Vol. X, p. 94, ed. EISEN H.N. Chicago: Year Book Publishers

[31] NISONOFF A. & PRESSMAN D. (1958) Heterogeneity of average combining constants of antibodies from individual rabbits. *J. Immunol.* **80**, 417

[32] PARKER C.W., GODT S.M. & JOHNSON M.C. (1966) The antibody response to a 2,4-dinitrophenyl peptide. *Biochemistry* **5**, 2314

[33] DAY L.A., STURTEVANT J.M. & SINGER S.J. (1963) The kinetics of the reactions between antibodies to the 2,4-dinitrophenyl group and specific haptens. *Annals New York Acad. Sci.* **103**, 611

[34] TANENBAUM S.W., BEISER S.M. & BASSETT E.W. (1965) Amino acid composition of antibodies from individual rabbits. *Fed. Proc., Abstracts, 49th Annual Meeting, Atlantic City, New Jersey.*

[35] EISEN H.N. & KARUSH F. (1949) The interaction of purified antibody with homologous hapten, antibody valence and binding constant. *J. Am. chem. Soc.* **71**, 363

[36] PARKER C.W., KERN M. & EISEN H.N. (1962) Polyfunctional dinitrophenyl haptens as reagents for elicitation of immediate-type allergic skin responses. *J. exp. Med.* **115**, 803

[37] KARUSH F. & EISEN H.N. (1962) A theory of delayed hypersensitivity based on the determinant role of humoral antibody. *Science*, **136**, 1032

[38] OVARY Z. (1963) In vitro and in vivo interactions of anti-hapten antibodies with monovalent and bivalent haptens. In *Conceptual Advances in Immunology and Oncology*, p. 206. New York: Hoeber Medical Division of Harper & Row

[39a] PARKER C.W. (1966) Fluorescence enhancement in the study of antibody hapten reactions. *Federation Proceedings* **25**, 247 (Abstract 329)

[39b] PARKER C.W., GODT S. & JOHNSON M.C. In preparation

[40] VELICK S.F. (1958) Fluorescence spectra and polarization of glyceraldehyde-3-phosphate and lactic dehydrogenase coenzyme complexes. *J. biol. Chem.* **233**, 1455

[41] WEBER G. & LAWRENCE D.J.R. (1954) Fluorescent indicators of adsorption in aqueous solution and on the solid phase. *Biochem. J.* **56**, xxxi

[42] BERNS D.S. & SINGER S.J. (1964) A fluorescence study of specific and nonspecific dye–protein interactions. *Immunochemistry* **1**, 209

[43] WEBER G. & YOUNG L.B. (1964) Fragmentation of bovine serum albumin by pepsin. I. The origin of the acid expansion of the albumin molecule. *J. biol. Chem.* **239**, 1415

[44] YOO T.J. & PARKER C.W. (1966) Spectrofluorometric studies in hapten–anti-body interaction. *Biophysical Society, 10th Annual Meeting, February* 1966 p. 78 (Abstract)

[45] JERNE N.K. & NORDIN A.A. (1963) Plaque formation in agar by single antibody-producing cells. *Science* **140**, 405

[46] INGRAHAM J.S. & BUSSARD A. (1964) Application of a localized hemolysin reaction for specific detection of individual antibody-forming cells. *J. exp. Med.* **119**, 667

[47] FEOFILOY P.P. (1961) *The Physical Basis of Polarized Emission*, p. 43. New York: Consultants Bureau

[48] LAURENCE D.J.R. (1957) Fluorescence techniques for the enzymologist. In *Methods in Enzymology*, Vol. IV, p. 174, ed. COLOWICK S.P. & KAPLAN N.O. New York: Academic Press

[49] CHEN R.F. & BOWMAN R.L. (1965) Fluorescence polarization: Measurement with ultraviolet-polarizing filters in a spectrophotometer. *Science* **147**, 729

[50] WEBER G. (1960) Fluorescence-polarization spectrum and electronic energy transfer in tyrosine, tryptophan, and related compounds. *Biochem. J.* **75,** 335

[51] WEBER G. (1952) Polarization of the fluorescence of macromolecules. 1. Theory and experimental method. *Biochem. J.* **51,** 145

[52] HABER E. & BENNETT J.C. (1962) Polarization of fluorescence as a measure of antigen–antibody interaction. *Proc. nat. Acad. Sci. (Wash.)* **48,** 1935

[53] DANDLIKER W.B. *et al* (1964) Application of fluorescence polarization to the antigen–antibody reaction theory and experimental method. *Immunochemistry* **1,** 165

[54] GOLDBERG R.J. (1952) A theory of antibody reactions. I. Theory for reactions of multivalent antigens with bivalent and univalent antibody. *J. Am. chem. Soc.* **74,** 5715

[55] SINGER S.J. (1965) Structure and function of antigen and antibody proteins. In *The Proteins*, 2nd edition, Vol. 3, p. 269, ed NEURATH H. New York: Academic Press

CHAPTER 13

The Ammonium Sulphate Method to Measure Antigen-binding Capacity

PERCY MINDEN & RICHARD S.FARR

Introduction and general principles

Most antibody tests measure the capacity of an antiserum to produce secondary effects of a primary antigen–antibody interaction such as precipitation and complement fixation rather than measure the capacity of an antiserum to bind antigen. The value and importance of measuring antigen-binding capacity rather than the amount of antibody nitrogen (N) in the precipitate became apparent when it was recognized that some populations of antibodies do not precipitate spontaneously even in the presence of optimal proportions of antigens [1, 2]. In addition, it has been shown that the presence or absence of complement affects spontaneous precipitation of antibody [3, 4]. Since the primary antigen–antibody interaction must somehow control the extent of the secondary effects, methods to measure antigen-binding capacity *per se* are necessary to compare antibody content with antibody function.

In 1949, Eisen & Karush [5] measured the primary binding between antiserum and haptenes by means of equilibrium dialysis, but this approach cannot be applied to the larger non-dialysable protein antigens. The ammonium sulphate test fulfils the need for a primary binding test suitable for certain non-dialysable antigens because it measures the capacity of antisera to combine with soluble macromolecular antigens and detects both precipitating and non-precipitating antibody. The original antigen employed was bovine serum albumin (BSA) and the test is based on the principle that ^{131}I-labelled bovine serum albumin (I*BSA) is soluble in 50 per cent saturated ammonium sulphate (SAS/2), whereas soluble I*BSA antigen–antibody complexes are insoluble under the same conditions. When a constant amount of I*BSA is added to serial dilutions of anti-BSA, a point is reached when antigen excess is achieved, spontaneous precipitation of I*BSA-antibody aggregates cannot occur and equilibrium in solution is established as represented by the following equation:

$$I^*BSA + Ab \underset{kd}{\overset{ka}{\rightleftharpoons}} I^*BSA.Ab$$

463

when I*BSA represents one of the several antigen sites on a given I*BSA molecule and Ab represents one combining site on an antibody molecule. Upon addition of an equal volume of saturated ammonium sulphate (SAS), the soluble I*BSA.Ab complexes are precipitated, and I*BSA not bound to antibody remains in the supernatant. The use of ammonium sulphate was suggested by studies of the purification of antigen–antibody complexes by Singer & Campbell [6]. This fractionation procedure does not appreciably alter the proportions of I*BSA which are bound to antibody or in solution prior to the addition of SAS because SAS markedly inhibits the formation and dissociation of I*BSA–antibody complexes [7–9]. The precipitated radio-activity which this test measures is an indication of *antigen-binding capacity* rather than the amount of antigen or antibody *spontaneously* precipitated and results are expressed as μg I*BSA nitrogen (N) bound/ml of undiluted serum.

The principle of labelling protein antigens with ^{131}I was introduced by Eisen & Keston [10], who measured antigen radioactivity in the precipitate of a standard precipitin test. Talmage & Maurer [11], extended these observations and measured the antigen-precipitating capacity of antisera by determining the amount of ^{131}I-labelled antigen in a precipitate when 80 per cent of the antigen added to the test serum was involved in the antigen–antibody precipitate. The antigen-precipitating capacity, or the P-80 test, which is also described below, is a modification of the procedure originally reported by Talmage and Maurer. In contrast to the ammonium sulphate test, the P-80 test yields information comparable to the quantitative precipitin test but specifically measures the amount of antigen N in the precipitate rather than attempting to measure antibody N. Expressing precipitating antibody levels in terms of antigen-precipitating capacity rather than antibody N eliminates the variables which occur when different antisera contain inconstant mixtures of antibody molecules with different molecular weights and nitrogen content.

This chapter will describe the details of both the ammonium sulphate and the P-80 tests, and special attention will be given to those conditions where the ammonium sulphate test will detect antibody in the absence of antigen-precipitating capacity. In addition, a description will be given of modifications of the ammonium sulphate test that have been developed to (a) detect the presence of circulating antigen–antibody complexes *in vivo* [12, 13], (b) quantitate and discriminate between trace amounts of identical or cross-reacting antigen groups [14–18] and (c) to study the rates of association and dissociation of antigen–antibody complexes [7–9, 19, 20]. BSA has been used as the antigen for many of the examples and much of the experimental work cited in this section. Reference will be made, however, to a number of experiments where this procedure has been applied with varying degrees of success to detect and measure antibodies to other antigens [17, 18, 21–27].

Detailed technical procedure

Reagents and procedure needed to perform the ammonium sulphate and P-80 tests
Reagents
1. Borate buffer, pH 8·3–8·5, ionic strength $= 0·1$.
    6·184 grammes boric acid.
    9·536 grammes borax (sodium tetraborate).
    4·384 grammes sodium chloride.
    Make up to 1 litre with distilled water.
2. Normal serum (1 : 10). Add one part normal serum to nine parts borate buffer. *Use serum from the same species being tested for antibody.*
3. Normal serum (1 : 100). Add one part normal serum to ninety-nine parts borate buffer. Normal homologous serum is needed to serve as a protein carrier for antibody [7].
4. Saturated ammonium sulphate (SAS). Store at 4° C with crystals remaining in the flask to prevent the solution from becoming supersaturated. Filter before using.
5. 50 per cent saturated ammonium sulphate. Add one part SAS to one part borate buffer.
6. Stock I*BSA solution. Prepare trace labelled I*BSA (see Freeman, Chapter 17) containing approximately one molecule of iodine per molecule of albumin and having a specific activity of 2–3 $\mu c/\mu g$ N. The nitrogen content of the stock I*BSA should be carefully determined and will contain 90–100 μg I*BSA N/ml when prepared as previously described [28–30]. After iodination and dialysis, the stock antigen should contain less than 3 per cent free ^{131}I as measured by precipitation of the protein with 10 per cent trichloroacetic acid.
7. Specific activity counting standards. Using volumetric glassware, dilute an aliquot of the stock I*BSA with normal serum (1 : 100) to the desired concentration in the range to be used for the test antigen. Pipette 1 ml aliquots of this carefully diluted stock antigen into 8 ml Wasserman tubes (13×100 mm) and mark the nitrogen content/ml on the label.
8. Test antigen. Dilute another aliquot of the stock I*BSA solution with normal serum (1 : 100) to the exact concentrations desired for the test antigen. This is usually between 0·04–4·0 μg N/ml.
9. Trichloroacetic acid (TCA). 20 per cent aqueous solution.

Antiserum dilutions and experimental tubes
1. First dilution. Add one part antiserum to nine parts borate buffer to make a 1 : 10 dilution. In practice, this is usually 0·5 ml antiserum added to 4·5 ml borate buffer.

2. Subsequent dilutions. Make serial 1 : 3, or 1 : 5 dilutions with normal serum (1 : 10); e.g. add 1·0 ml of previous dilution to 2·0 or 4·0 ml of normal serum (1 : 10). Use separate volumetric pipettes for each dilution.
3. Experimental tubes. Pipette duplicate 0·5 ml aliquots from each dilution into 8 ml Wasserman tubes (13 × 100 mm). A single volumetric pipette may be used for each serum by starting with the most dilute solution and rinsing the pipette in the next highest concentration.

Controls for each experiment
1. Normal serum controls. To each of four tubes, add 0·5 ml aliquots of normal serum (1 : 10). These tubes will receive both I*antigen and SAS.
2. Protein bound ^{131}I controls. To two tubes add 0·5 ml aliquots of normal serum (1 : 10). These tubes will receive TCA, but not SAS.
3. Antigen-added controls. Four tubes will be used to receive antigen only. These tubes will not receive serum, or SAS, but will be used as counting standards.
4. Add 0·5 ml of labelled antigen to *all* of these control tubes. Promptly mix and store the control tubes under the same conditions used to incubate the experimental tubes.

Addition of antigen
Pipette 0·5 ml of labelled antigen into all experimental tubes. Promptly mix the tubes well and incubate overnight at 4° C. If incubation is carried out for a longer period of time, significant evaporation occurs and tubes must be stoppered.

For ammonium sulphate test
*Precipitation of I*BSA–antibody complexes with ammonium sulphate*
1. Keep all reagents and tubes at 4° C.
2. Add 1·0 ml SAS to experimental tubes and the normal serum control tubes only. Mix immediately. No more than 1–2 minutes should elapse between the addition of SAS and mixing of the tube. SAS has a greater specific gravity than the other reactants and will settle to the bottom of the tube unless vigorous agitation is used. Until satisfied that complete mixing is being routinely attained, check for schlieren (wavy) lines in each tube. *Improper mixing following the addition of SAS is the most common souce of error encountered with this method.*
3. After addition of SAS, incubate at 4° C for 30 minutes.
4. Centrifuge for 30 minutes at 4° C in a refrigerated centrifuge at 2000 rev/ min.

5.   Decant and discard the supernatants. Blot the tubes on absorbent towels to take up the remaining drops on the edge of the tubes.

6.   Wash these precipitates by adding 3 ml of 50 per cent SAS. Shake tubes to resuspend the precipitates.

7.   Centrifuge tubes immediately at 4° C for 30 minutes at 2000 rev/min. Decant and blot as in step No. 5.

8.   Add 1·0 ml of 20 per cent TCA to the two protein-bound ^{131}I control tubes. Centrifuge for 30 minutes at 2000 rev/min, decant and discard the supernatant.

Counting and calculating procedure

1.   Using a γ detector, determine the counts per minute (count/min) in the specific activity counting standards (Std), the antigen-added control tubes (Ag-add), the normal serum control precipitate tubes (NsPpt), the protein bound I^{131} control (TCAPpt), and the experimental precipitate tubes (ExPpt). Repeat a given set of tubes if the count/min in one of the duplicates differs more than ± 5 per cent of the other.

2.   Average the data, subtract background and make the following calculation:

$$\text{per cent protein bound } {}^{131}\text{I} = \frac{\text{count/min in TCAPpt}}{\text{count/min in Ag-add}} \times 100.$$

The antigen should be used only if this value is greater than 97 per cent.

3.   Calculate the μg I*BSA N in the antigen-added control as follows:

$$\frac{\text{count/min in Ag-add}}{\text{count/min in Std}} \times \mu\text{g I*BSA N in Std} = \frac{\mu\text{g I*BSA N in Ag-add}}{= \text{AgN}.}$$

4.   The total amount of I*BSA in the precipitate is partly antibody bound and partly non-antibody bound. The small amount of non-antibody bound I*BSA that is non-specifically precipitated by ammonium sulphate in either normal serum or in an antiserum must be accounted for in each individual determination. *This amount is proportional to the amount of I*BSA in the supernatant which is entirely non-antibody bound and is not proportional to the total amount of test antigen added.* Accordingly, the non-antibody bound I*BSA in a given experimental precipitate cannot be corrected for by merely subtracting the amount of I*BSA in the control normal serum precipitate. Instead, to accurately correct for non-antibody bound I*BSA in a given experimental precipitate, the data may be readily corrected in a manner which has been previously described in detail [7].

     Subsequently, however, another method for calculating data has evolved and is recommended because of its greater simplicity. This new method is also based on the fact that I*BSA in the supernatant is directly proportional to the total amount of non-antibody bound I*BSA in a given mixture.* The simplified stepwise procedure may be carried out as as follows:

a. Subtract the count/min in the NsPpt from the count/min of the Ag-add, to obtain the count/min of the normal serum supernatant (NsSup).

b. Subtract the count/min in the ExpPpt from the count/min of the Ag-add, to obtain the count/min in the experimental supernatant (ExSup).

c. Divide the count/min in the ExSup by the count/min in the NsSup and multiply by 100 to obtain the per cent count/min non-antibody bound. This is the per cent Ag-add in the supernatant (per cent S) and the method of calculation has automatically corrected this value for the amount of non-antibody I*antigen non-specifically present in each experimental precipitate.

d. Subtract the per cent S from 100 to obtain the per cent Ag-add in the precipitate (per cent P) or the per cent Ag-add which is specifically bound to antibody.

5. Plot the per cent P versus the reciprocal of the antiserum dilution on semi-logarithmic paper. The per cent P is plotted on the linear axis and the reciprocal of the antiserum dilution is plotted on the log axis. An example of this step is illustrated in Fig. 13.1.

6. From these plots, determine the reciprocal dilution of antiserum which would have precipitated exactly 33 per cent of the antigen added. Designate this dilution as the ABC-33 end-point. In the example shown in Fig. 13.1, this is 420.

7. Since 0·5 ml of the antiserum dilution designated as the ABC-33 end-point would have specifically precipitated 33 per cent of the I*BSA N used for the test, the ABC-33 value is calculated as follows:

(ABC-33 end-point) (2) (0·33) (AgN) = I*BSA N bound/ml undiluted serum at the antigen concentration employed.

* The authors wish to thank Dr James H.Day, Department of Medicine, Queen's University, Kingston, Ontario, Canada, for this valuable simplification which was derived as follows:

$$\frac{\text{Count/min of (Ag-add)}}{\text{Count/min of (NsSup)}} = \frac{\text{Total non-antibody bound count/min in experimental tube}}{\text{Count/min of (ExSup)}}$$

$$\text{Total non-antibody bound count/min in experimental tube} = \frac{\text{(ExSup) (Ag-add)}}{\text{(NsSup)}} = \frac{\text{Count/min of experimental supernatant, adjusted}}{}$$

$$\text{Per cent Ag-added in adjusted supernatant} = \frac{\frac{\text{(ExSup) (Ag-add)}}{\text{(NsSup)}}}{\text{Ag-add}} \times 100 = \frac{\text{ExSup}}{\text{NsSup}} \times 100 = \text{per cent S}$$

100 − per cent S = per cent P or per cent Ag-add specifically bound to antibody.

For example, if 0·5 ml of a 1 : 420 dilution of antiserum bound 33 per cent of 0·02 μg I*BSA N, the ABC-33 is $420 \times 2 \times 0.33 \times 0.02 = 5.54$ μg I*BSA N bound/ml undiluted serum. Also, for reasons described below, the concentration of antigen used for a given test should be indicated by a subscript such as:

$$\text{ABC-33} @ 0.02 \ \mu g = 5.54 \ \mu g \ \text{I*BSA N/ml.}$$

8. The 33 per cent precipitation end-point was arbitrarily selected because spontaneous precipitation does not occur at this degree of antigen excess, but enough of the ^{131}I activity is in the precipitate to permit accurate counting procedures. Using the 33 per cent end-point, multiple tests

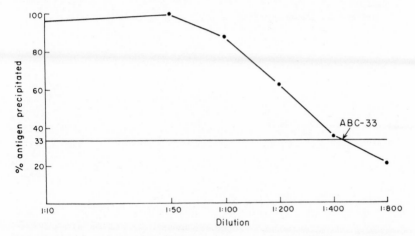

FIG. 13.1. Per cent of I*BSA antigen precipitated after the addition of SAS by a number of dilutions of a single antiserum. Curve indicates that the ABC-33 end-point or the dilution of antiserum that would precipitate 33 per cent of the antigen added is 1 : 420.

performed with the same antigen on a single antiserum are highly reproducible. The average per cent of the antigen-added in the precipitate should have a standard deviation of the mean of less than 3 per cent. Because of spontaneous precipitation, end-points with more than 33 per cent of the antigen in the precipitate are not recommended. End-points with 20 or 25 per cent of the antigen in the precipitate are satisfactory but should be designated as ABC-20 or ABC-25.

For P-80 test

1. Antiserum dilutions, experimental tubes, controls and addition of antigen are carried out as for the ammonium sulphate test above, except that

1·0 ml aliquots of antisera are used, and the addition of SAS is omitted. Incubation is carried out for 6 days at 4° C with daily agitation. Tubes should be stoppered during incubation to prevent evaporation.

2. After 6 days of incubation, centrifuge tubes at 2000 rev/min in a refrigerated centrifuge for 30 minutes at 4° C. Decant supernate from precipitate, count tubes in a γ detector and calculate as described above for the ammonium sulphate test with the following differences.

Calculation Procedure

For the P-80 test the end-point selected is that point near equivalence, in slight antigen excess where 80 per cent of the antigen-added is precipitated

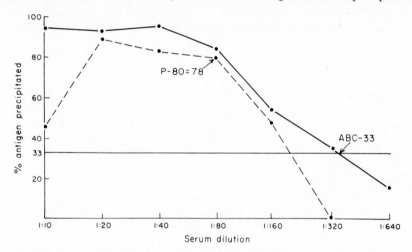

FIG. 13.2. Per cent of I*BSA antigen precipitated spontaneously (P-80) and per cent precipitated after the addition of SAS (ABC-33) by a number of dilutions of the same antiserum. Curves indicate that the P-80 end-point or the dilution of antiserum needed to precipitate 80 per cent of the antigen added is 1 : 78. The ABC-33 end-point is 1 : 340.

and the P-80 values are expressed as the μg I*BSA N precipitated/ml of undiluted serum. This is determined by multiplying the reciprocal of the dilution of antiserum needed to precipitate 80 per cent of the antigen-added by (0·8) (μg I*BSA N added). In addition, a designation is included to indicate the μg I*BSA N used and the total volume of a particular test. Figure 13.2 illustrates the determination of a P-80 and an ABC-33 end-point in a single antiserum. Note that the concentration of antiserum needed to precipitate 80 per cent of the antigen-added occurred both in the areas of antibody excess (antiserum dilution of 1 : 20) and antigen excess (antiserum dilution of 1 : 78) with this particular antiserum. This phenomenon of soluble antigen–antibody complexes in the zone of antibody excess is a variable occurrence, more frequently noted with human as compared to rabbit antisera, and it is important that the P-80 end-point be selected at the antiserum dilution where antigen is in excess. In the example shown in Fig. 13.2, 1·0 ml of a 1 : 78 dilution of antiserum precipitated 80 per cent of 0·02 μg I*BSA N and the P-80 $= 78 \times 1 \times 0.80 \times 0.02 = 1.25$ μg I*BSA N *precipitated*/ml undiluted serum. As indicated in Fig. 13.2, 0·5 ml of a 1 : 340 dilution of the same antiserum bound 33 per cent of 0·02 μg I*BSA N after the addition of SAS, and the ABC-33 $= 340 \times 2 \times 0.33 \times 0.02 = 4.49$ μg I*BSA N *bound*/ml undiluted serum.

Critical considerations for the ammonium sulphate test

Effect of ammonium sulphate on antigen–antibody bonds in solution

A number of experiments have demonstrated that antibody globulin does not release, exchange or bind appreciable amounts of labelled or unlabelled BSA after the addition of SAS/2 and the antigen–antibody equilibrium appears to be 'frozen' under these conditions [7–9]. It is also probable that the SAS/2 does not 'freeze' the equilibrium instantaneously and that partial re-equilibration can occur during part of the 30 minutes needed to precipitate the antigen-antibody complexes with ammonium sulphate [7–9].

Effect of heat labile serum components upon the primary antigen–antibody interaction

The effect of heat labile normal rabbit serum (NRS) components upon the precipitation of antigen–antibody complexes by SAS/2 in rabbits was studied since all dilutions for the ammonium sulphate test were made in 1 : 10 NRS and non-specific serum proteins such as complement aid the spontaneous precipitation of antibody in the presence of antigen [3, 4]. Accordingly, to test the effect of heating either the diluents or the antiserum at 56° C for 2 hours, four triplicate sets of NRS antibody were prepared in such a way that one set contained unheated sera, one set contained heated 1 : 10 NRS and unheated anti-BSA, one set contained heated anti-BSA and unheated 1 : 10 NRS, and the last set contained heated 1 : 10 NRS and heated anti-BSA [7]. SAS/2 was added to each group and the procedure carried out as described above. The results presented in Table 13.1 showed no differences in the per cent of I*BSA precipitated in any of the four groups. This was verified when assays of rabbit anti-HSA sera were performed with and without ethylene-diamine-tetra-acetic acid sodium salt (EDTA) [31]. The latter compound was used to chelate divalent cations, thereby minimizing those interactions involving complement and conglutinin [32, 33].

Applications

To compare antigen-binding capacity with antigen-precipitating capacity in rabbits

The complete antigen-binding and antigen-precipitating curves of three rabbit anti-BSA sera with very different characteristics are illustrated in Figs. 13.3, 13.4, and 13.5. Figure 13.3 is characteristic of early primary response antisera collected within 2 weeks of the first antigenic stimulation. Figure 13.4 is typical of most secondary response antisera (pattern #1) and Fig. 13.5 is typical of a minority of antisera following a second antigen stimulation

TABLE 13.1

The effect of heating anti-BSA and/or the normal rabbit serum diluent on the antigen-binding capacity

| | Experimental procedure | | | | Per cent of original I*BSA in precipitate with two dilutions of antisera and I*BSA | |
| | Diluent | | Anti-BSA | | 1 : 100+0·25 μg | 1 : 400+0·125 μg |
Group	Heated	Unheated	Heated	Unheated	I*BSA	I*BSA
I		+		+	40·1	22·0
II	+			+	39·4	21·0
III		+	+		39·8	21·7
IV	+		+		38·5	22·0

Basic experimental plan:

$$0.5 \text{ ml Ag}+0.5 \text{ ml Ab} \xrightarrow[\text{days}]{2} 1 \text{ ml SAS/2} \xrightarrow[\text{min}]{30} \text{centrifuge.}$$

This table is reproduced from FARR R.S. (1958) *J.I.D.* **103**, 239 [7], courtesy of the University of Chicago Press, Chicago, Illinois.

(pattern #2). The ordinates represent μg I*BSA N precipitated/ml undiluted serum on identical samples of serum by both the P-80 and the ammonium sulphate tests. The open circles represent the μg I*BSA N precipitated with SAS/2 and the closed circles represent the I*BSA N spontaneously precipitated. In the zone of antibody excess, the SAS/2 data resembles the spontaneous precipitin curve, but in the zone of antigen excess it is apparent that the SAS/2 precipitated otherwise soluble I*BSA–antibody complexes.

When the early primary antiserum (Fig. 13.3) reached the point of maximum spontaneous antigen precipitation more than 50 per cent of the antigen remained in the supernatant. This was in contrast to the secondary response antiserum (pattern #1, Fig. 13.4) which reached the point of maximum

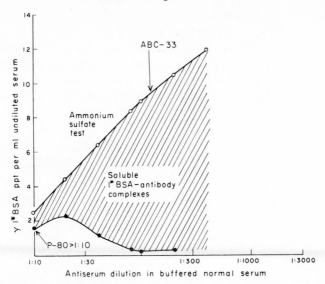

FIG. 13.3. Early primary antiserum. The precipitation of I*BSA in the presence of anti-BSA with and without the addition of SAS. Reproduced from [7], courtesy of the University of Chicago Press, Chicago, Illinois.

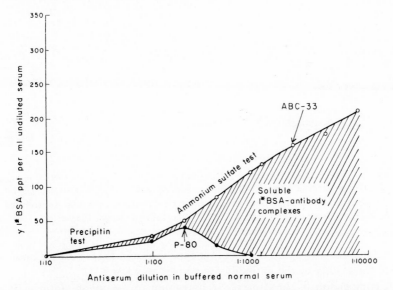

FIG. 13.4. Secondary (pattern #1) antiserum. The precipitation of I*BSA in the presence of anti-BSA with and without the addition of SAS. This pattern is typical of most rabbit antisera and is occasionally observed in human antisera. Reproduced from [7], courtesy of the University of Chicago Press, Chicago, Illinois.

spontaneous antigen precipitation when only 14 per cent of the antigen remained in the supernatant. In both systems, 100 per cent of the unprecipitated antigen at the point of maximum spontaneous antigen precipitation was bound to antibody in the supernatant as demonstrated by the SAS/2 data [7]. This situation with regard to maximum spontaneous antigen precipitation was described in detail by Talmage & Maurer [11] and they

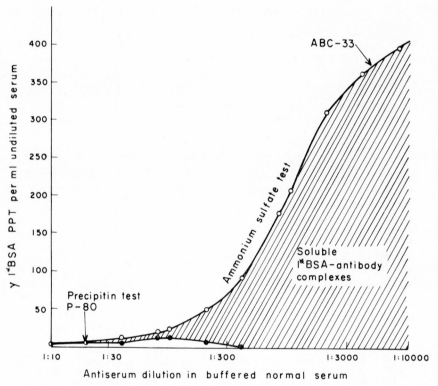

FIG. 13.5. Secondary (pattern #2) antiserum. The precipitation of I*BSA in the presence of anti-BSA with and without the addition of SAS. This pattern is occasionally observed in rabbit antisera and is more typical of human antisera. Reproduced from [7], courtesy of the University of Chicago Press, Chicago, Illinois.

postulated that precipitin curves of the type shown in Fig. 13.3 were observed when the avidity of the antibody for antigen was low.

A comparison of the capacity of antiserum to precipitate antigen (P-80) with the capacity of the same antiserum to bind antigen (ABC-33) can be used as an index of the antigen-precipitating efficiency of an antiserum and expressed as a P-80 : ABC ratio. Figure 13.4 illustrates an antiserum with relatively high antigen-precipitating efficiency typical of most rabbit antisera but occasionally observed in human antisera. Figure 13.5 illustrates an antiserum with relatively low antigen-precipitating efficiency occasionally observed in rabbit antisera but which is more typical of human antisera.

To demonstrate specificity of antigen–antibody reaction

The specificity of a primary antigen–antibody reaction may be established by testing the capacity of unlabelled antigens to suppress the binding of the I* antigen to a specific antiserum. Trace amounts of unlabelled antigen will cause complete inhibition of I*antigen binding if the unlabelled antigen is identical to the I*antigen. Other unrelated or cross-reacting unlabelled antigens lack all or part of this inhibiting capacity. These principles were used to demonstrate the specificity of the trace amounts of I*BSA binding observed in many human sera studied for the presence or absence of detectable anti-BSA [14]. In the experimental procedure employed, duplicate 2 ml aliquots of a 1 : 10 dilution of the test serum in borate buffer were prepared. A 0·5 ml aliquot of borate buffer containing 1 mg unlabelled BSA per ml was added to one of the duplicate samples and 0·5 ml of borate buffer without unlabelled antigen to the other. After a 10 minute incubation period at room temperature, 0·5 ml of a solution containing 0·02 μg I*BSA N was added to both control and experimental tubes. The resulting 3 ml mixtures were incubated overnight at 4° C, two 1 ml aliquots were taken from each tube and 1 ml of SAS was added to each tube. After 30 minutes, the samples were centrifuged, washed and counted. The calculation of the per cent antigen precipitated was determined by the ratio of counts/min in the precipitate to the total counts/min in the I*BSA N initially added. The per cent of I*BSA precipitated in the tubes containing the additional unlabelled BSA was subtracted from the per cent I*BSA precipitated in the tubes without the unlabelled BSA added. A serum was considered to have anti-BSA activity when the difference between the control and experimental tubes was greater than 5 per cent. The specificity of the I*BSA binding observed in the human sera was further studied by adding the following unlabelled proteins to the antiserum prior to the addition of the I*BSA: (a) fat-free milk; (b) crystalline alphalactalbumin (ALA); (c) bovine γ globulin (BGG); (d) ovalbumin; (e) insulin; (f) pertussis vaccine; (g) diphtheria and tetanus toxoid; (h) poliomyelitis vaccine; and (i) influenza vaccine. Aliquots of 0·5 ml of 1 mg/ml unlabelled BSA or 0·5 ml of fat-free milk completely inhibited the reaction between I*BSA and antibody. BGG and ALA inhibited the reaction to a lesser extent due to trace amounts of BSA present in the BGG and ALA. In contrast, no effect was observed following addition of ovalbumin which has no shared antigenic groups with BSA [21]. There was no inhibition when diphtheria and tetanus toxoids, poliomyelitis and influenza vaccine, or insulin were added to the sera

Q*

prior to the labelled antigen, although a slight but unexplained inhibition of I*BSA binding occurred with pertussis vaccine.

A micro-method modification of the above procedure has also been devised to detect anti-BSA in small fractions following separation of serum proteins by sucrose density gradient ultracentrifugation [34]. Specifically, 0·2 ml of a gradient fraction was diluted with 0·3 ml of 1 : 5 NRS. Duplicate 0·1 ml aliquots of the diluted gradient were mixed with either 0·1 ml of borate buffer or 0·1 ml of borate buffer containing 1 mg of unlabelled BSA/ml in micro-conical tubes. Following 30 minutes of incubation, a 0·1 ml aliquot containing 0·001 μg I*BSA N/ml in 1 : 100 NRS was added to each tube. After incubating overnight, 0·3 ml of SAS was added to each micro-tube, and the samples centrifuged, washed and counted. With the micro-method, the presence of antibody is indicated only if the difference between the control and experimental tubes is greater than 10 per cent.

To discriminate between trace amounts of homologous and heterologous cross-reacting antigenic groups
Inhibition studies were employed by Linscott to detect contamination of commercial rabbit albumin (RSA) preparations with BSA [15]. Serial dilutions of rabbit antiserum to BSA were incubated with I*BSA in the presence of an excess of certain unlabelled commercial RSA preparations. I*BSA bound to antibody globulin was precipitated with SAS and detected in a scintillation counter. As a result of competition between I*BSA and unlabelled BSA in the RSA samples, more antiserum was needed to bind a given amount of labelled BSA in the presence of contaminated RSA than in controls lacking RSA. By comparison, no significant inhibition occurred with uncontaminated RSA prepared by Linscott. The inhibition curves presented in Fig. 13.6 demonstrated the contamination of RSA with BSA and further illustrated the quantitative attributes of this method. To aliquots of a dilution of antiserum sufficient to bind 60 per cent of the I*BSA added, 0·5 ml aliquots of increasing amounts of unlabelled RSA or BSA were added as a blocking agent. After 18 hours, I*BSA was added to each tube and the ^{131}I content of each resulting precipitate determined. A sufficient quantity of either BSA or commercial RSA completely blocked the reaction between labelled BSA and antiserum to BSA. Slopes of the curves were quite similar and from the amount of RSA required to produce 50 per cent inhibition it was possible to calculate that the three RSA preparations examined contained as little as 0·35 to 0·54 per cent BSA.

Cross-reactivity between grass and ragweed pollens was described as a result of similar studies with an I*ragweed (I*RW)–anti-ragweed (RW) system and suggested that grass pollen contained molecular groups that could bind anti-RW [16]. Inhibition studies illustrated that RW extract markedly

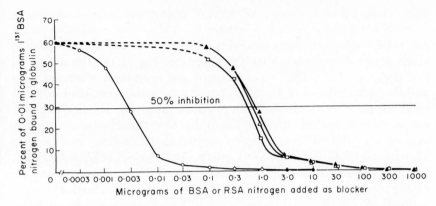

Fig. 13.6. Inhibition of reaction between ^{131}I-labelled BSA (I*BSA) and antibody to BSA by commercial rabbit serum albumin (RSA) preparations and by BSA. Ordinate: per cent of I*BSA (0·01 μg of nitrogen) bound to antibody globulin. Abscissa: log of amount of unlabelled BSA or RSA added to block the reaction (μg of nitrogen). Reproduced from [15], courtesy of the American Association for the Advancement of Science, Washington D.C.
    ○ BSA Blocker. □ RSA #4 Blocker. △ RSA #R51 Blocker. ▲ RSA #3517 Blocker.

inhibited the binding of I*RW but unlabelled grass pollen extract also caused significant though lesser inhibition (see Fig. 13.7). At I^{50}, or the end-point at which 50 per cent of the specific binding of I*RW by an antiserum was inhibited, 0·0005 μg ragweed pollen N was as effective as 0·15 μg grass pollen

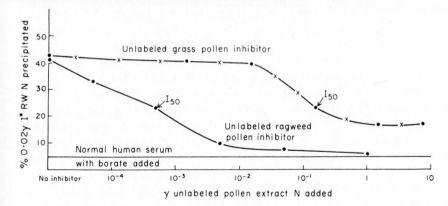

Fig. 13.7. Inhibition of ^{131}I-ragweed–anti-ragweed serum interaction by the addition of graded quantities of unlabelled grass and ragweed pollen extracts. Reproduced from [16], courtesy of the C.V.Mosby Co., St Louis, Missouri.

N or, expressed another way, 300 units of grass pollen were as effective as 1 unit of RW pollen. Differences between the RW and grass inhibition curves also ruled out the possibility that cross inhibition was due to contamination of the grass extracts with actual RW pollen (see Fig. 13.7). With unlabelled RW pollen inhibitor, there was an orderly and progressive effect that went on to complete inhibition. In the grass pollen inhibitor curve, inhibition was never complete. This is characteristic of similar rather than identical antigenic groups because had this inhibition been due to contamination of the grass mixture with RW antigen, complete inhibition should have been possible after the addition of enough grass pollen. These curves suggest, therefore, that grass extract was itself free of actual ragweed. These principles also were employed extensively by Weigle *et al* [35–39] to study the effects of passive antibody, X-radiation and the influence of heterologous and altered serum protein antigens upon the development and termination of immunological tolerant states in rabbits. An inhibition-test system used in the manner described above is a more sensitive indicator of the presence of trace amounts of homologous antigen or a cross-reacting antigen than a direct test. This increased sensitivity is attained because it is possible to add a great excess of unrelated unlabelled antigen without affecting I*antigen binding, but even trace amounts of related unlabelled antigen will cause changes in the amount of I*antigen bound.

To study association and dissociation rates

Some of the qualitative changes in antisera that have been observed during the course of immunization in several antigen–antibody systems [7, 19, 20, 40, 41] can be ascribed to an increase in strength of the union between antigen and antibody while other qualitative changes are due to differences in the physical and chemical properties of the different classes of immunoglobulins in a given antiserum. Some of these qualitative differences may be demonstrated by comparing rates of association and dissociation of antigen–antibody complexes between early and late antisera [7, 8, 19].

The ammonium sulphate test lends itself to kinetic studies of this type because: (a) SAS/2 rapidly stops the action between antigen and antibody; (b) utilization of I*BSA as test antigen allows low concentrations of reactants to be used; and (c) the precipitation of antigen–antibody complexes with the ammonium sulphate test allows easy calculation of free and bound antigen.

The rates of association and dissociation of antigen–antibody complexes may be studied by:

(a) Association rate measurement: An antibody dilution should be selected so that only 40 per cent of the I*antigen will be bound when I*BSA and antibody are incubated together at 4° C and equilibrium is reached. Equal aliquots of I*BSA and the appropriately diluted antiserum are mixed at 4° C and duplicate 1 ml aliquots are pipetted into tubes containing 1 ml of SAS at selected time intervals such as 5, 10, 20, 30, 40 and 60 minutes after the initial mixing. The last aliquots are taken 18 hours after the initial mixing to determine the amount of antigen bound at equilibrium. All samples are centrifuged, washed, counted and calculated as described above.

(b) Dissociation rate measurement: Similar to the procedure to study association rates, the dilution of antibody is determined which will bind only 40 per cent of the I*antigen when equilibrium is reached. Equal aliquots of I*BSA and the appropriate dilutions of antibody are then incubated together

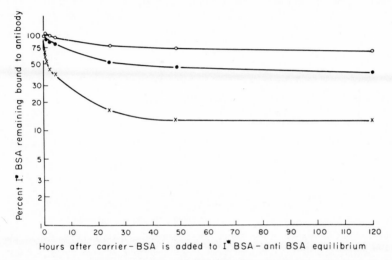

Fig. 13.8. The dissociation time of I*BSA–antibody bonds in solution when unlabelled carrier BSA was added to I*BSA-antibody equilibrium. Reproduced from [7], courtesy of the University of Chicago Press, Chicago, Illinois.

○ Secondary response pattern #1. ● Secondary response pattern #2. × Early primary response.

overnight at room temperature at 25° C or at 4° C. After equilibrium is reached, a large excess of unlabelled BSA is then added and the dissociation of I*BSA-anti-BSA complexes followed by observing the rate of decline of radioactive antigen in the ammonium sulphate precipitates over a period of time. This is calculated at various time intervals after the addition of the unlabelled BSA. This laboratory usually uses 5 and 30 minutes, 1, 2, 4, 24, 48 and 120 hours. The amount of I*BSA bound without the addition of excess BSA provides the 100 per cent antibody bound I*BSA value. Figure 13.8 is an example of such an experiment where the I*BSA remaining bound to globulin is plotted against the time the I*BSA–antibody complexes were in the presence of excess unlabelled BSA [7]. These results indicate the diversity of antibody with respect to the strength of antigen–antibody bonds in each of three antisera tested because a uniform population of antibodies would have resulted in a first-order reaction and the curves presented in Fig. 13.8 would have been straight lines. These three antisera contained various proportions of at least two antibody populations: one of which dissociated rather freely from the I*BSA during the first hours of the experiment and another with a half dissociation time of greater than 100 hours. The experiment presented in Fig. 13.8 was performed at 4° C and the rates of dissociation would have been more rapid had the experiment been performed at 25° C as were some of the data to be presented below.

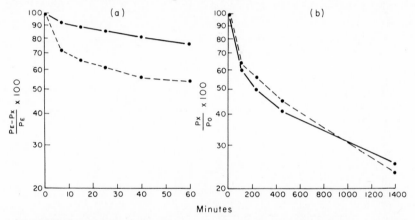

FIG. 13.9. Comparison of the rate of association and dissociation of rabbit 7S and 19S anti-BSA. Antibody was obtained 7 days following an injection of 2 mg of alum-precipitated BSA. 7S and 19S antibody were separated by density gradient ultracentrifugation. Reproduced from [19].
(a) Association (0° C). (b) Dissociation (24° C). ———— 19S anti-BSA antibody. ----- 7S anti-BSA antibody.

Figures 13.9 and 13.10 compare data obtained from both association and dissociation rate studies reported by Grey [9, 19]. Figure 13.9 represents the kinetic characteristics of 19S and 7S antibody from a single rabbit serum collected 7 days after immunization. For association times, the ordinate is

$$\frac{Pe\text{-}Px}{Pe} \times 100.$$

Pe is the per cent antigen bound at equilibrium and Px is the per cent bound at time x after the addition of antigen. At time 0, Px would be zero and

$$\frac{Pe\text{-}Px}{Pe} \times 100$$

would equal 100. For dissociation times, the ordinate is Px/Po × 100. Po is the per cent bound at equilibrium, and Px is the per cent I*BSA specifically bound by antibody at time x after the addition of unlabelled BSA. At time 0, Px = Po and Px/Po = 100. The 7S antibody had a faster rate of association than did the 19S antibody, whereas the dissociation rates of 7S and 19S were the same.

Figure 13.10 compares the I*BSA association and dissociation rates of unfractionated antiserum and of two antibody fractions separated according to electrical charge by continuous flow curtain electrophoresis. Fraction 16, collected from the anode end of the globulin with capacity to bind I*BSA,

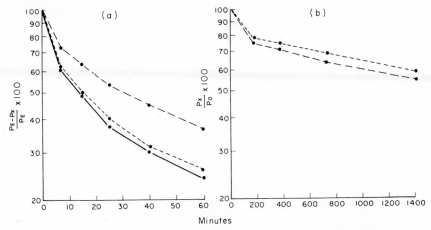

Fig. 13.10. Rates of association and dissociation of antiserum after fractionation by continuous flow electrophoresis. Fraction 9 represents antibody that was nearer the cathode and Fraction 16 was closer to the anode. Reproduced from [9], courtesy of Williams & Wilkins Co., Baltimore, Maryland.
    (a) Association (0° C). (b) Dissociation (24° C). ——— Whole serum. ..... Fraction 9. – – – – – Fraction 16.

had slower association rates for I*BSA than either the antibody population in whole serum or the antibody in fraction 9 which was collected nearer the cathode. In contrast, there was little if any difference in the rates of dissociation from I*BSA by the antibody in whole serum or in either fraction. The data in Fig. 13.9 and 13.10 indicate that the rates of association and dissociation among antibody populations can vary independently of one another. The differences in Fig. 13.9 appear to be due to molecular size while the differences in Fig. 13.10 were concerned with molecular charge.

To study the changing effect of antigen dilution upon the ABC-33
The effect of antigen dilution on the ABC-33 has also been used as an index

to measure qualitative differences in the antibody responsible for binding I*BSA. This dilution effect can be conveniently expressed as a ratio of antigen concentrations; e.g. ABC-33 @ 0·02 μg/1·0 ml and ABC-33 @ 0·2 μg/1·0 ml or as a percentage if this fraction is multiplied by 100. Antisera collected during the first 2 weeks of a primary antibody response in rabbits were found to be greatly affected by dilution whereas antisera collected later were less

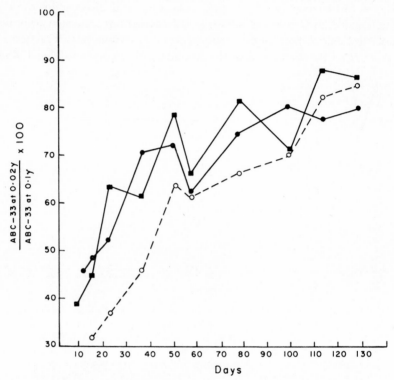

FIG. 13.11. The changing effect of antigen dilution upon the ABC-33 in rabbit antisera immunized by several procedures. Reproduced from [34].
    ● Oral. 0·1 per cent BSA in the drinking water daily between day 0 and day 105.
    ■ Subcutaneous. 7 mg BSA in incomplete Freund's adjuvant on day 0.
    ○ Intravenous. 100 mg BSA in saline on day 0 and day 63.

affected [7]. This changing quality is well demonstrated in Fig. 13.11 in which Rothberg *et al* [34] observed the changing effect of dilution in rabbit antisera obtained following three different kinds of immunization procedures.

An ABC-33 @ 0·02 μg I*BSA N/ml usually represents a minimal binding capacity and if the antibody involved is greatly affected by dilution, even the ABC-33 @ 0·1 or 0·2 μg may appear deceptively low if compared to the ABC-33 determined at higher antigen concentrations. Without a K value for calculating the total ABC-33, it is necessary to determine the ABC-33 at higher antigen concentrations if a maximum binding capacity is desired. An ABC-33 value represents the amount of I*antigen bound to antibody at the time ammonium sulphate was added, but does not reflect the number of unoccupied antibody sites in equilibrium with the I*antigen–antibody complexes. For this reason, similar to equilibrium dialysis, it may be desirable to obtain ABC determinations with more than one concentration of test antigen to detect the presence or absence of unoccupied antibody sites in solution at the

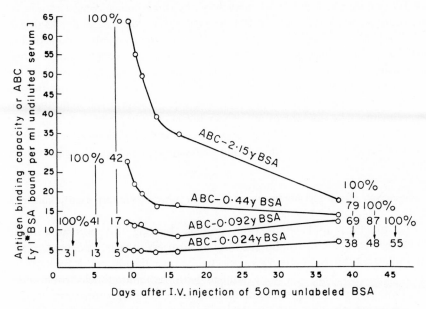

FIG. 13.12. The ABC-33 as determined with four concentrations of ^{131}I-labelled BSA (I*BSA) after a single intravenous injection of BSA on day 0. Reproduced from [7], courtesy of the University of Chicago Press, Chicago, Illinois.

ABC-33 end-point. If most of the available antibody sites are bound to antigen at an ABC-33 end-point, an increase in concentration of test antigen will not increase the ABC-33. On the other hand, if a significant proportion of the total number of antibody sites are unoccupied and dissociated from the I*antigen–antibody complexes at the ABC-33 end-point, an increase in concentration of test antigen will increase the ABC-33 value. In practice, the ABC-33 is usually greater but never less when the concentration of test antigen is increased. As a general rule, a marked discrepancy between ABC-33 @ 0·02 and 0·2 μg indicates the presence of a large proportion of antibody with a rapid dissociation rate.

Figure 13.12 is a graphic illustration of the considerations discussed above.

ABC-33 data were determined after four concentrations of I*BSA were used to study binding of rabbit antisera obtained between days 9 and 38, after immunization with a single injection of BSA. After the initial burst of antibody production, most of the loss of binding capacity involved the ability of anti-serum to bind the more concentrated solutions of I*BSA, whereas at the lower concentrations of antigen of 0·024 and 0·092 μg the ABC-33 values were generally unchanged and even increased between days 17 and 38 [7]. The percentile values represented at either end of the graph represent the effect of dilution on the ABC-33 when each of the three higher concentrations of test antigen were used for the 100 per cent value. More recently, Mulligan *et al* and Osler *et al* [31, 42], cognizant of this problem, have studied maximum ABC-33 values obtained by holding the antibody level constant and adding increasing amounts of I*antigen. This modification has the advantage of determining antigen-binding capacity under conditions approaching infinite antigen excess for a given anti-serum and will be helpful for some types of experiments. The amount of antigen in the precipitate, however, represents only a small per cent of the total antigen added and caution must be exercised under these circumstances in handling such data on a per cent P or per cent S basis.

Comparison of antigen-binding capacity with other commonly used laboratory tests

Other practical applications of a primary binding test become evident if antisera are examined simultaneously by a variety of tests, as demonstrated in Table 13.2. Fifteen human sera selected because they bound I*BSA by the ammonium sulphate test were studied with radioimmunoelectrophoresis, the P-80 precipitin test, microimmunodiffusion, haemagglutination, passive cutaneous anaphylaxis and the Prausnitz-Küstner passive transfer skin test for reaginic activity [43]. Radioimmunoelectrophoresis, another method for studying primary binding, was the only other test that detected antibodies to I*BSA in each of the fifteen human sera. There was considerable variation among all other techniques with regard to their capacity to detect and measure anti-BSA activity. Haemagglutination was positive in ten of the fifteen sera, passive cutaneous anaphylaxis was positive only in the rabbits used as controls and reaginic activity was present in four of the twelve human sera tested. Of the fourteen sera studied for antigen-precipitating capacity (P-80) seven showed no detectable precipitating anti-BSA, three reached a P-80 end-point, and four had only trace amounts of precipitating activity. There was poor correlation between the amount of circulating anti-BSA measured by the ammonium sulphate test and the precipitating activity found by the P-80 test. The human serum with the highest ABC-33 value of 11 μg had no detectable precipitating activity.

TABLE 13.2

Comparison of methods for determination of antibody in human and rabbit sera

	Human sera, No.															Rabbit sera[a]	
	1	2	3	4	5	6	7	8	9	10	11	12	13	14	15	a[b]	b[c]
ABC-33 at 0·02 µg I*BSA N/ml	11·6	6·07	5·02	4·62	2·77	1·52	1·24	0·96	0·96	0·77	0·66	0·45	0·37	0·34	0·31	3·83	5·94
Radioimmuno-electrophoresis																	
Anti-whole serum	+	+	+	+	+	+	+	+	+	+	+	+	+	+	+	+	+
Anti-γA	+	+	+	+	−	−	−	−	−	−	+	−	−	−	−	?	?
Anti-γM	−	−	−	−	−	−	−	−	−	−	−	−	−	−	−	?	?
Anti-γG	+	+	+	+	+	+	+	+	+	+	+	+	+	+	+	+	+
Per cent antigen precipitated	−	>80	36·4	>80	>80	−	63·3	32·9	−	46·4	−	−	−	−	−	<80	>80
P-80 at 0·02 µg I*BSA N/ml	−	0·70	−	1·28	0·32	−	−	−	−	−	−	−	−	−	−	0·67	2·24
P-80/ABC-33	−	0·11	−	0·28	0·12	−	−	−	−	−	−	−	−	−	−	0·17	0·38
Haemagglutination	1/64	1/32	1/256	1/512	1/256	1/16	0	1/32	1/64	1/32	1/128	0	0	0	0	1/4096	1/2048
Gel diffusion	−	−	+	+	*[d]	−	−	−	−	−	−	−	−	*[d]	−	+	+
PCA	−	−	+	+	−	−	−	−	*[d]	−	−	*[d]	−	−	−	+	+
P-K	+	*[d]	+	+	−	−	−	−	*[d]	−	−	*[d]	+	−	−	*[d]	*[d]
Age	17	17	8	18	6	10	39	3	61	46	3	44	34	8	78		
Diagnosis[e]	1	1,2	1	1	1	3	4	3	5	3	3	6	1,3	1,3	4		

[a] Diluted 1 : 10.

[b] Immunized by i.v. route.

[c] Immunized by oral route.

[d] Asterisk indicates not examined.

[e] Diagnosis of patients with symptoms unrelated to milk and beef: 1 = allergic rhinitis, 2 = regional enteritis, 3 = bronchial asthma, 4 = neurodermatitis, 5 = hypertension, 6 = functional bowel disorder.

This Table is reproduced from Minden et al (1966) J. Immunol. 96, 180 [43], courtesy of Williams & Wilkins Co., Baltimore, Maryland.

Most of the human anti-BSA sera had lower precipitating efficiencies than the two rabbit antisera shown in Table 13.2 or most of the twenty additional samples of the rabbit anti-BSA previously studied in this respect [7]. Seventy-five per cent of normal children under 16 years of age were shown to have circulating antibodies to BSA as measured by the ammonium sulphate test [14] whereas when gel diffusion was the test system, this was 10 per cent or less [44, 45]. This low precipitating efficiency may be a characteristic of the human species and not limited to the anti-BSA system. Grey observed low precipitating efficiency in human antisera when the antigen was ^{131}I-labelled M-12 streptococcal extract [27], and the same observation was made when the antigen was ^{131}I-ragweed [46].

When the ammonium sulphate test, the P-80 and the erythrocyte haemagglutination techniques were used by Samuelson *et al* to study the immunosuppressant effects of acriflavine in rabbits, variations of antibody efficiencies were frequently noted in different antisera [47]. P-80 values and anti-BSA haemagglutinating capacities of the individual sera did not reflect the binding capacities of antisera as noted by the ABC-33. In a number of animals the ammonium sulphate test was positive at a time when the P-80 and haemagglutination tests were negative, indicating the hazards of reliance on a secondary manifestation type of antibody test. In no instance did a serum demonstrate haemagglutination or precipitating activity when the ammonium sulphate test was negative.

Many investigations dealing with the sequential synthesis of different molecular weight antibodies to BSA have been based on the passive haemagglutination technique. As a consequence, early primary antisera were considered to consist predominantly of 19S antibodies [48–50]. However, when serum from a rabbit immunized to BSA was fractionated by sucrose gradient ultracentrifugation and each fraction tested for antibody by the ammonium sulphate technique and haemagglutination, Grey found binding activity associated with the 7S globulins as well as the macroglobulins as early as 7 days after immunization [19]. These early 7S antibodies which bound I*BSA had very low haemagglutinating efficiency and were not detected by haemagglutination. Similar observations have since been noted by Benedict [51] and Rothberg *et al* [34].

To detect antibody in species where precipitating antibody is difficult to detect
As indicated previously, most rabbits immunized to BSA produce antisera with high precipitating efficiency as compared to similar human antisera [27, 43, 46]. Low precipitating efficiency has also been noted in a number of other species. The antibody response of rats immunized to heterologous serum protein is generally poor if measured by the precipitin reaction while a considerable response may be shown by the ammonium sulphate technique. This was

illustrated in a study where Long-Evans and Holtzman rats and New Zealand White rabbits were immunized with BSA, and the anti-BSA sera characterized by antigen-binding capacity and the P-80 precipitin test. In general, the rat anti-BSA sera had lower ABC values than did rabbit antisera obtained at the same stage of immunization. In addition, however, Holtzman anti-BSA sera showed almost no spontaneous precipitation and, although the Long-Evans anti-BSA did precipitate I*BSA to some extent, it had markedly lower precipitating efficiency as compared to the usual rabbit anti-BSA [52]. Similar studies have shown a considerable anti-BSA response by mice and guinea-pigs when antibodies were measured by the ammonium sulphate technique instead of precipitin reactions [53]. The measurement of antigen binding with the ammonium sulphate test has been utilized to study a number of characteristics of the immune responses of guinea-pigs and rats by Weigle & Dixon [54] and for the study of immune tolerance in newborn mice by other investigators [55, 56]. Mitchison used this system to define the conditions of treatment that would lead to immunization or paralysis of CBA mice [57].

To detect circulating antigen–antibody complexes in vivo

Although experimental serum sickness has long been a laboratory model for the study of a variety of human diseases of hypersensitive etiology, the possible mechanisms by which antigen–antibody reactions produced lesions of this disease were not, until recently, clearly understood. By means of the ammonium sulphate test, Dixon *et al* demonstrated that soluble antigen–antibody complexes occurred *in vivo* at the same time that serum sickness occurred [12, 13]. Figure 13.13 illustrates the sequence of immunologic and morphologic events that occur subsequent to the injection of a large dose of serum protein antigen (I*BSA) into a rabbit. Throughout the response to an injection of I*BSA it was possible to determine the amount of circulating I*BSA combined with antibody in the form of soluble antigen–antibody complexes. Simultaneous with the appearance of detectable antigen–antibody complexes in the circulation, there was a sharp drop in complement and the appearance of morphologic lesions in the heart, blood vessels, joints and kidneys. The period of development of morphologic manifestations of serum sickness is indicated by the shaded area in Fig. 13.13. It was thus possible to establish that these complexes circulating in the body fluids played a key role in the initiation of the inflammatory responses that resulted in the development of the lesions of serum sickness.

Use of ammonium sulphate test with other antigens

Although originally developed for use in the BSA–anti-BSA system, this method has also been used with varying degrees of success with other antigens. Some of these are: ten additional mammalian albumins [17, 18]; egg albumin

[21]; alphalactalbumin [22]; type-specific streptococcal M protein [27]; crude [23] and purified antigen [24] derived from ragweed pollens; somatic antigen from Gram-negative bacteria [25] and a protein fraction of rabbit spinal cord [26].

Limitations

The following criteria must be met when using ammonium sulphate fractionation to accurately quantitate antigen-binding capacity: (a) the labelled

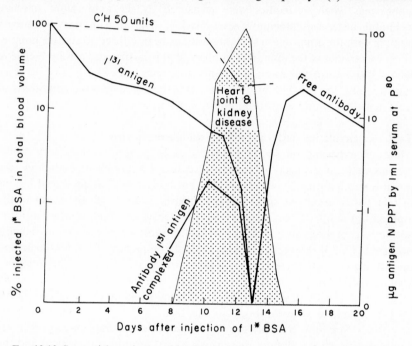

Fig. 13.13. Serum sickness in the rabbit. Simultaneous appearance of soluble antigen-bovine serum albumin. Reproduced from [13], courtesy of Academic Press Inc., New York.

antigen must be a homogeneous population of molecules immunologically unaltered by the isotope labelling procedures; (b) the labelled antigen must be soluble in 40–50 per cent saturated ammonium sulphate; (c) it must be determined that the fractionation procedure has no appreciable effect upon the equilibrium that had been established between free and antibody-bound antigen prior to the addition of SAS/2; (d) it is desirable, but not necessary, that the isotope employed emits γ radiation because the counting procedure for other isotopes such as S35 and C14 are more time consuming.

The criteria set forth represent the ideal circumstances as exemplified by the use of I*BSA as the test antigen. On the other hand, the method can sometimes yield useful information even when these criteria cannot be met. Under such circumstances, the limitations involved when using the antigen in question should be well defined and the data cannot be calculated in the manner described above for I*BSA [23, 27].

Other primary antigen–antibody tests

The ammonium sulphate test is only one of the primary binding types of antigen–antibody tests which are currently available to solve a particular problem. Each test has certain advantages and limitations which makes one or another the test of choice in a given set of circumstances. Some of these, like the ammonium sulphate test, give quantitative information. These are: (a) equilibrium dialysis [5, 58] (see Chapter 14), (b) precipitation of antigen-antibody complexes with anti-human globulin [59–62]; (c) fluorescence polarization [63, 64] (see Chapter 12); (d) paper electrophoresis [65]; (e) ^{131}I-labelled eluates [66]; (f) differential sedimentation of labelled antigens in the presence of antibody [67]; fluorescence quenching [68] (see Chapter 12).

Other primary binding tests give qualitative information and are powerful tools for the identification and localization of proteins and/or organs where antigen–antibody reactions may take place. These are: (a) direct immunofluorescence [69] (see Chapter 16); (b) radioimmunoelectrophoresis [70] (see Chapter 6); and (c) free boundary electrophoresis [71].

References

[1] HEIDELBERGER M. & KENDALL F.E. (1935) A quantitative theory of the precipitin reaction. III. The reaction between crystalline egg albumin and its homologous antibody. *J. exp. Med.* **62,** 697
[2] KABAT E.A. & HEIDELBERGER M. (1937) A quantitative theory of the precipitin reaction. V. The reaction between crystalline horse serum albumin and antibody formed in the rabbit. *J. exp. Med.* **66,** 229
[3] MAURER P.H. & TALMAGE D.W. (1953) The effect of complement in rabbit serum on the quantitative precipitin reaction. *J. Immunol.* **70,** 135
[4] WEIGLE W.O. & MAURER P.H. (1957) The effect of complement on soluble antigen–antibody complexes. *J. Immunol.* **79,** 211
[5] EISEN H.N. & KARUSH F. (1949) The interaction of purified antibody with homologous hapten. Antibody valence and binding constant. *J. Am. chem. Soc.* **71,** 363
[6] SINGER S.J. & CAMPBELL D.H. (1952) Physical chemical studies of soluble antigen–antibody complexes. I. The valence of precipitating rabbit antibody. *J. Am. chem. Soc.* **74,** 1794

[7] FARR R.S. (1958) A quantitative immunochemical measure of the primary interaction between I*BSA and antibody. *J. Infect. Dis.* **103**, 239

[8] TALMAGE D.W. (1960) The kinetics of the reaction between antibody and bovine serum albumin using the Farr method. *J. Infect. Dis.* **107**, 115

[9] GREY H.M. (1963) Studies on the heterogeneity of the rate of combination of antibody with antigen. *J. Immunol.* **91**, 90

[10] EISEN H.N. & KESTON A.S. (1949) The immunologic reactivity of bovine serum albumin labeled with trace amounts of radioactive iodine (I^{131}). *J. Immunol.* **63**, 71

[11] TALMAGE D.W. & MAURER P.H. (1953) I^{131} labeled antigen precipitation as a measure of quantity and quality of antibody. *J. Infect. Dis.* **92**, 288

[12] DIXON F.J., VASQUEZ J.J., WEIGLE W.O. & COCHRANE C.G. (1958) Pathogenesis of serum sickness. *AMA Archives of Path.* **65**, 18

[13] DIXON F.J. (1963) The role of antigen–antibody complexes in disease. *The Harvey Lecture Series* **58**, 21. New York: Academic Press

[14] ROTHBERG R.M. & FARR R.S. (1965) Anti-bovine serum albumin and anti-alpha lactalbumin in the serum of children and adults. *Pediatrics* **35**, 571

[15] LINSCOTT W.D. (1963) Contamination of commercial rabbit albumin preparations by bovine albumin. *Science*, **142**, 1170

[16] LIDD D. & FARR R.S. (1963) Similarities between antigens derived from ragweed pollen and from other botanical sources. *J. Allergy* **34**, 48

[17] WEIGLE W.O. (1961) Immunochemical properties of the cross-reactions between anti-BSA and heterologous albumins. *J. Immunol.* **87**, 599

[18] WEIGLE W.O. (1962) Biological properties of the cross-reactions between anti-BSA and heterologous albumins. *J. Immunol.* **88**, 9

[19] GREY H.M. (1964) Studies on changes in the quality of rabbit-bovine serum albumin antibody following immunization. *Immunology*, **7**, 82

[20] TALMAGE D.W. (1957) The primary equilibrium between antigen and antibody. *Ann. of the N.Y. Acad. Sc.* **70**, 82

[21] WEIGLE W.O. & MCCONAHEY P.J. (1962). The serological cross-reaction between bovine serum albumin and anti-ovalbumin. *J. Immunol.* **88**, 121

[22] ROTHBERG R.M. & FARR R.S. (1965) Antibodies in rabbits fed milk and their similarities to antibodies in some human sera. *J. Allergy*, **36**, 450

[23] LIDD D. & FARR R.S. (1962) Primary interaction between I^{131} labeled ragweed pollen and antibodies in the sera of humans and rabbits. *J. Allergy* **33**, 45

[24] LIDD D. & CONNELL J.T. (1964) Specific binding of an I^{131}-labeled ragweed pollen fraction by sera of untreated ragweed-sensitive humans. *J. Allergy* **35**, 289

[25] FRETER R. (1962) Influence of various antibody characteristics on the titration of 0 antibodies by different methods. *J. Infect. Dis.* **111**, 25

[26] KIBLER R.F. & BARNES A.E. (1962) Antibody studies in rabbit encephalomyelitis induced by a water-soluble protein fraction of rabbit cord. *J. exp. Med.* **116**, 807

[27] GREY H.M. (1962) Studies on the binding between streptococcal M protein and antibody. *J. exp. Med.* **115**, 671

[28] TALMAGE D.W., DIXON F.J., BUKANTZ S.C. & DAMMIN G.J. (1951) Antigen elimination from the blood as an early manifestation of the immune response. *J. Immunol.* **67**, 243

[29] WEIGLE W.O. & DIXON F.J. (1959) The antibody response of lymph node cells transferred to tolerant recipients. *J. Immunol.* **82**, 516

[30] MCCONAHEY P.J. & DIXON F.J. (1966) A method of trace iodination of proteins for immunologic studies. *Int. Arch. of Allergy and Appl. Immunol.* **29**, 185

[31] MULLIGAN J.S. JR., OSLER A.G. & RODRIGUEZ E. (1966) Weight estimates of rabbit antihuman serum albumin based on antigen-binding capacity. *J. Immunol.* **96**, 324

[32] MAYER M.M., OSLER A.G., BIER O.G. & HEIDELBERGER M. (1946) The activating effect of magnesium and other cations on the hemolytic function of complement. *J. exp. Med.* **84**, 535

[33] LEON M.A. (1957) Role of cations in conglutination and in formation of properdin zymposan complex from bovine serum. *Proc. Soc. exp. Biol. Med.* **96**, 202

[34] ROTHBERG R.M., KRAFT S.C. & FARR R.S. (1966) A comparison of oral with parenteral bovine serum albumin immunization in rabbits. Manuscript in preparation

[35] WEIGLE W.O. (1962) Termination of acquired immunological tolerance to protein antigens following immunization with altered protein antigens. *J. exp. Med.* **116**, 913

[36] WEIGLE W.O. (1964) The effect of x-radiation and passive antibody on immunologic tolerance in the rabbit to bovine serum albumin. *J. Immunol.* **92**, 113

[37] WEIGLE W.O. (1965) The antibody response in rabbits to previously tolerated antigens. *Ann. of the N.Y. Acad. Sc.* **124**, 1333

[38] LINSCOTT W.D. & WEIGLE W.O. (1965) Induction of tolerance to bovine serum albumin by means of whole body x-radiation. *J. Immunol.* **94**, 430

[39] DIETRICH F.M. & WEIGLE W.O. (1964) Immunologic unresponsiveness to heterologous serum proteins induced in adult mice and transfer of the unresponsive state. *J. Immunol.* **92**, 167

[40] TALIAFERRO W.T., TALIAFERRO L.G. & PIZZI A.K. (1959) Avidity and intercellular transfer of homolysin. *J. Infect. Dis.*, **105**, 197

[41] JERNE N.K. & AVENGO P. (1956) The development of the phage-inactivating properties of serum during the course of specific immunization of an animal; reversible and irreversible inactivation. *J. Immunol.* **76**, 200

[42] OSLER A.G., MULLIGAN J.S. JR. & RODRIGUEZ E. (1966) Weight estimates of rabbit antihuman serum albumin based on antigen-binding and precipitin analyses. Specific hemagglutinating activities of 7S and 19S components. *J. Immunol.* **96**, 334

[43] MINDEN P., REID R.T. & FARR R.S. (1966) A comparison of some commonly used methods for detecting antibodies to bovine serum albumin. *J. Immunol.* **96**, 180

[44] HEINER D.C., SEARS J.W. & KNIKER W.T. (1962) Multiple precipitins to cow's milk in chronic respiratory disease. *Amer. J. Dis. Child.* **103**, 634

[45] HOLLAND N.H., HONG R., DAVIS N.C. & WEST C.D. (1962) Significance of precipitating antibodies to milk proteins in the serum of infants and children. *J. Pediat.* **61**, 181

[46] LIDD D. & FARR R.S. Unpublished observations

[47] SAMUELSON J.S., KRAFT S.C. & FARR R.S. (1965) The contrasting immunosuppressant effects of acriflavine and dietary restriction. *J. Immunol.* **95**, 1013

[48] FAHEY J.L. (1962) Heterogeneity of γ-globulins. *Advances in Immunology* **2**, 42. New York and London: Academic Press

[49] UHR J.W. (1964) The heterogeneity of the immune response. *Science* **145**, 457

[50] NISONOFF A. & THORBECKE G.J. (1964) Immunochemistry. *Ann. Rev. Biochem.* **33**, 355. Palo Alto, California: Annual Reviews Inc.

[51] BENEDICT A.A. (1965) Sensitivity of passive hemagglutination for assay of 7S and 19S antibodies in primary rabbit anti-bovine serum albumin sera. *Nature* **206**, 1368

[52] MCCARTER J.H. & FARR R.S. (1962) A comparison between rat and rabbit anti-BSA. *Fed. Proc.* **21**, 30 (Abstract)

[53] FARR R.S. (1957) Antibody response of rats, mice, and guinea pigs to bovine serum albumin as measured by the antigen binding capacity test. *Fed. Proc.* **16**, 412 (Abstract)

[54] WEIGLE W.O. & DIXON F.J. (1957) The elimination of heterologous serum proteins and associated antibody responses in guinea pigs and rats. *J. Immunol.* **79**, 24

[55] TERRES G. & HUGHES W.L. (1959) Acquired immune tolerance in mice to crystalline bovine serum albumin. *J. Immunol.* **83**, 459

[56] SERCARZ E.E. & COONS A.H. (1963) The absence of antibody-producing cells during unresponsiveness to BSA in the mouse. *J. Immunol.* **90**, 478

[57] MITCHISON N.A. (1964) Induction of immunological paralysis in two zones of dosage. *Proc. of Royal Soc. of London. Biological Sciences*, Series B, **161**, 275

[58] NISONOFF A. & PRESSMAN D. (1958) Heterogeneity and average combining constants of antibodies from individual rabbits. *J. Immunol.* **80**, 417

[59] FEINBERG R. (1956) Detection of nonprecipitating antibody with radioiodinated antigen. *Fed. Proc.* **15**, 586 (Abstract)

[60] SKOM J.H. & TALMAGE D.W. (1958) The role of nonprecipitating insulin antibodies in diabetes. *J. clin. Invest.* **37**, 787

[61] FARR R.S. & BLOCH H. (1960) The binding capacity of tuberculous human serum for I^{131} labeled tubercle bacilli. *Am. Rev. Resp. Dis.* **82**, 687

[62] PRUZANSKY J.J., PATTERSON R. & FEINBERG S.M. (1962) Binding of ragweed antigen labeled with iodine-131 by sera of untreated allergic subjects. *Nature* **195**, 1113

[63] DANDLIKER W.B., SCHAPIRO H.C., MEDUSKI J.W., ALONSO R., FEIGEN G.A. & HAMRICKS J.R. JR. (1965) Application of fluorescence polarization to the antigen–antibody reaction. *Immunochemistry* **1**, 165

[64] DANDLIKER W.B., HALBERT S.P., FLORIN M.C., ALONSO R. & SCHAPIRO H.C. (1965) Study of penicillin antibodies by fluorescence polarization and immunodiffusion. *J. exp. Med.* **122**, 1029

[65] BERSON S.A., YALOW R.S., BAUMAN A., ROTHSCHILD M.A. & NEWERLY K. (1956) Insulin-I^{131} metabolism in human subjects: Demonstration of insulin binding globulin in the circulation of insulin treated subjects. *J. clin. Invest.* **35**, 170

[66] BARNES A. & FARR R.S. (1963) The influence of race and phenotype on the erythrocyte D antigen studied by I^{131}-labeled anti-D. *Blood* **21**, 429

[67] FARR R.S. (1959) A specific binding capacity between normal human serum and beef albumin. *Fed. Proc.* **18**, 566 (Abstracts)

[68] VELICK S.F., PARKER C.W. & EISEN H.N. (1960) Excitation energy transfer and the quantitative study of the antibody hapten reaction. *Proc. nat. Acad. Sci. (Wash.)* **46**, 1470

[69] COONS A.H. & KAPLAN M.H. (1950) Localization of antigen in tissue cells. II. Improvements in a method for the detection of antigen by means of fluorescent antibody. *J. exp. Med.* **91**, 1

[70] YAGI Y., MAIER P., PRESSMAN D., ARBESMAN, C.E. & REISMAN R.E. (1963) The presence of the ragweed-binding antibodies in the B_2A, B_2M and γ-globulins of the sensitive individuals. *J. Immunol.* **91**, 83

[71] FARR R.S., CAMPBELL D.H. & VINOGRAD J. (1963) Electrophoretic boundary disturbances as a test for antigen–antibody interaction and some observations on the production of non-specific boundary disturbances. *J. Immunol.* **90**, 619

CHAPTER 14

Equilibrium Dialysis and Preparation of Hapten Conjugates

R.N.PINCKARD & D.M.WEIR

Introduction

Equilibrium dialysis is not a recent advance in immunochemical methodology; the technique was first developed in 1932 by Marrack & Smith [1] and by Haurowitz & Breinl [2] as a direct method for studying the primary interaction between antibody and hapten. The method was modified in 1949 by Eisen & Karush [3] into a procedure which today is of primary importance not only for studies on the interaction of antibody and hapten but as a tool to study changes in the antibody-combining site after chemical treatment or enzymatic digestion of the antibody molecule. Figure 14.1 illustrates the basis of the technique. The upper cell shows the distribution of antibody and hapten molecules at time zero. The cell is divided into two compartments separated by a cellophane membrane which allows only the hapten molecules to pass through in either direction; the antibody molecules, because of their large size, are contained within the inner compartment. The lower cell represents the same cell but after equilibrium has been established. The concentrations of free or unbound hapten on both sides of the cellophane membrane are the same; however, there are a greater number of hapten molecules in the inner compartment because in addition to the free hapten molecules there are hapten molecules which are bound to antibody. By determining the concentration of bound hapten as a function of the free hapten concentration and with the aid of the following equations, the average intrinsic association constant (K_0) of the interaction between antibody and hapten can be determined experimentally. The value of K_0, as will be seen later, is of paramount importance in the elucidation of the nature of the antibody- and antigen-combining sites and of the forces involved in their union.

Chemical equilibria and antibody–hapten interaction

We begin with a consideration of the theoretical aspects of single and multiple equilibria. This discussion is directed primarily towards the reader without

493

Antigen–Antibody Interactions

an extensive mathematical knowledge and will employ, as far as possible, algebraic equations giving definitions without derivation for the more complex concepts. It is intended not only for the laboratory worker planning to perform equilibrium dialysis but also for those who wish to obtain a general outline of the subject so that reports in which the technique is employed may be more readily assessed.

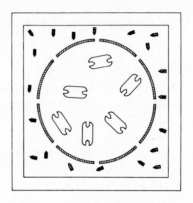

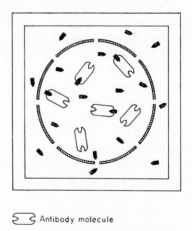

⊋⊂ Antibody molecule

➡ Hapten molecule

FIG. 14.1. Schematic representation of equilibrium dialysis showing the distribution of antibody and hapten molecules before and after equilibrium is established. The upper cell shows such a distribution at time zero; the lower cell shows the distribution at equilibrium. Note that there are a greater number of hapten molecules in the inner compartment of the lower cell because in addition to the free hapten molecules there are also hapten molecules which are bound to antibody.

The concepts applied to equilibrium dialysis can be formulated in a number of ways and workers in different laboratories have used a variety of procedures for plotting and analysing their data. The two methods to be described and compared in this chapter are the one described by Karush [4, 5], Method A, and that of Nisonoff & Pressman [6], Method B. The present description of the application of chemical equilibria to antibody–hapten interaction is necessarily brief and the reader may wish to consult other sources in conjunction with this report [7, 8, 9, 10, 11, 36].

Consider first the situation where an antibody molecule (Ab) with a single combining site (i.e. a univalent antibody molecule) reacts with a univalent hapten (H).

$$Ab + H \rightleftharpoons AbH \tag{1}$$

According to the law of mass action the rate of formation of the antibody–hapten complex (AbH) is proportional to the concentration of the reactants, (Ab) and (H). The rate of formation of the AbH complex is thus equal to $K_1(Ab)(H)$ where K_1 is a constant. Similarly the dissociation rate of the AbH complex is equal to $K_2(AbH)$. At equilibrium the rate of formation is equal to the rate of dissociation and therefore

$$K_1(Ab)(H) = K_2(AbH) \tag{2}$$

Setting the quotient K_1/K_2 by definition equal to the association constant K, the simple equation of chemical equilibria is obtained,

$$\frac{K_1}{K_2} = K = \frac{(AbH)}{(Ab)(H)} \tag{3}$$

From Eq. 3 it follows that

$$K(Ab)(H) = (AbH) \tag{4}$$

The total concentration of antibody molecules (Ab_t) is equal to the sum of the concentrations of antibody molecules which are bound to hapten (AbH), and the concentration of free or unbound antibody molecules (Ab) as is shown in Eq. 5,

$$(Ab_t) = (Ab) + (AbH) \tag{5}$$

This assumes that the antibody is univalent; later in the chapter the discussion will be expanded for an antibody molecule possessing n number of combining sites. Eq. 5 can be rewritten as

$$(Ab) = (Ab_t) - (AbH) \tag{6}$$

Substituting the value of (Ab) from Eq. 6 into Eq. 4,

$$K(H)[(Ab_t) - (AbH)] = (AbH) \tag{7}$$

After multiplying out the left-hand side of Eq. 7 and rearranging,

$$K(H)(Ab_t) = (AbH)[1 + K(H)] \tag{8}$$

Dividing both sides of Eq. 8 by $(AB_t)[1 + K(H)]$,

$$\frac{(AbH)}{(Ab_t)} = \frac{K(H)}{1 + K(H)} \tag{9}$$

The ratio of $(AbH)/(Ab_t)$ is the number of moles of bound hapten per mole of antibody and represents that fraction of antibody molecules that are bound to hapten; this ratio will be denoted as R. Thus Eq. 9 becomes,

$$R = \frac{K(H)}{1 + K(H)} \tag{10}$$

Eq. 10 is essentially the same as the one derived by Langmuir [12] and is a statement of the law of mass action. Eq. 10 is, however, ultimately modified to give two related methods for expressing the binding data.

Method A
Before generalizing Eq. 10 which expresses the relation of an antibody molecule possessing a single combining site to an equation which relates to an antibody molecule with n number of combining sites, it must first be assumed that each antibody-combining site has the same intrinsic affinity for the hapten. If this is assumed, it can be shown [7] that Eq. 10 becomes

$$R = \frac{nK(H)}{1 + K(H)} \tag{11}$$

This expression can be made suitable for graphic representation by multiplying each side of Eq. 11 by $[1 + K(H)]$ and rearranging,

$$R = -RK(H) + nK(H) \tag{12}$$

Finally dividing by (H),

$$\frac{R}{(H)} = -RK + nK \tag{13}$$

Graphing $R/(H)$ vs. R using a Scatchard plot [13] it can be seen from the slope-intercept form shown in Fig. 14.2 that

$$y = R/(H)$$
$$x = R$$
$$\text{Slope} = -K$$
$$y \text{ intercept} = nK$$
$$x \text{ intercept} = n.$$

By inspection of Eq. 13 and Fig. 14.2 it can be seen that it is necessary to determine experimentally (i) the total concentration of antibody molecules (Ab_t), (ii) the concentration of bound hapten (AbH) and (iii) the concentration of free hapten (H). The determinations of (i) and (ii) are required to calculate R since R is equal to $(AbH)/(Ab_t)$. Because the total concentration of antibody molecules must be known prior to plotting the binding data, a specifically purified antibody preparation must be used in the equilibrium dialysis cell. The valence of the antibody molecule is determined by extrapolating the binding curve to the x axis as $(H) \to \infty$, i.e. as $R/(H) \to 0$. In the experimental situation, then, a series of equilibrium dialysis cells must be

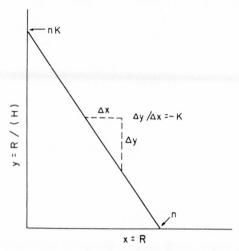

FIG. 14.2. Slope-intercept form of Eq. 13 which is used to plot the binding data in Method A.

assembled with constant amounts of purified antibody in one compartment and varying concentrations of hapten over at least a forty-fold range in the other compartment.

Method B

Instead of deriving the association constant K with respect to the antibody molecule as was done in Method A, Method B determines the association constant with respect to the antibody-combining site which as a result eliminates the n term. This has the advantage that only the free and bound hapten concentrations need be determined experimentally. Specifically purified antibody preparations do not have to be employed to determine the association constant except when the valence of the antibody molecule is also to be determined.

The derivation begins as before following Eqs. 1 through 9 but noting that the terms (AbH) and (Ab$_t$) are the concentration of bound *antibody-combining sites* and the total concentration of antibody-*combining sites* respectively. Thus again Eq. 9 is obtained.

$$\frac{(AbH)}{(Ab_t)} = \frac{K(H)}{1 + K(H)} \tag{9}$$

The equation used to plot the binding data may be directly established by taking the reciprocal of Eq. 9 and thus

$$\frac{(Ab_t)}{(AbH)} = \frac{1 + K(H)}{K(H)} \tag{14}$$

Dividing both sides of Eq. 14 by (Ab$_t$)

$$\frac{1}{(AbH)} = \frac{1 + K(H)}{(Ab_t) K(H)} \tag{15}$$

Expanding the right-hand side of Eq. 15,

$$\frac{1}{(AbH)} = \frac{1}{(Ab_t) K(H)} + \frac{1}{(Ab_t)} \tag{16}$$

This is the equation which is used to plot the binding data; using the slope-intercept form it can be seen from Eq. 16 and Fig. 14.3 that

$$y = 1/(AbH)$$
$$x = 1/(H)$$
$$\text{Slope} = 1/K(Ab_t)$$
$$y \text{ intercept} = 1/(Ab_t).$$

As previously stated, when using Method B only the free and bound hapten concentrations need be determined; the total concentration of antibody-combining sites is determined by extrapolating the binding curve to the y axis as (H)$\rightarrow\infty$, i.e. 1/(H)$\rightarrow$0. However, if a valence determination for the antibody molecule is required a specifically purified antibody preparation must be employed and the valence of the antibody molecule is then equal to the total concentration of antibody-combining sites divided by the number of moles of antibody molecules. Experimentally, as in Method A, a series of equilibrium dialysis cells are assembled keeping the antibody concentration constant in one compartment and varying the concentration of hapten over at least forty-fold range in the other compartment.

Both Eqs. 13 and 16 predict linear relationships between $R/(H)$ vs. R and 1/(AbH) vs. 1/(H) respectively; however, when experimental data are plotted it is found that a linear relationship is not the usual case. As seen in Figs.

14.9 and 14.10 the graph tends to curve away from the y axis using Eq. 13 and tends to curve towards the x axis using Eq. 16. This deviation away from linearity has been taken to be due to heterogenicity of the antibody-combining sites; this can be seen in Figs. 14.9 and 14.10 because as the free hapten concentration is increased the apparent association constant K decreases, as exemplified by the changing slopes of the binding curves. Because of this deviation away from linearity, the association constant cannot be calculated on the basis of the slope of the plotted data. Therefore, some other method must be employed in order to calculate the average intrinsic association

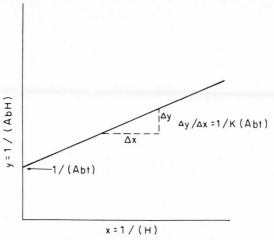

FIG. 14.3. Slope-intercept form of Eq. 16 which is used to plot the binding data in Method B.

constant (K_0); this can be done if it is assumed that the heterogeneity of the antibody–hapten interaction can be described by some type of distribution function. There are two related methods for calculating the value of K_0 and the indices of heterogeneity, which indicate a range and distribution of the association constants, K, about the average intrinsic association constant K_0.

Average intrinsic association constant K_0 and the indices of heterogeneity

Method A
Pauling *et al* [14], studying the inhibition of antigen–antibody precipitation with haptens, employed a Gauss error function with respect to the free energies of combination to describe the heterogeneity of the system. This same formulation has been used by Karush [4, 9, 11] to describe the heterogeneity of binding of antibody to haptens. The distribution function when

R

normalized and expressed in terms of the association constants by the relation given in Eq. 33 is

$$\omega(K) = \frac{1}{\sigma\sqrt{\pi}} \exp(-[\ln(K/K_0)]^2/\sigma^2) \tag{17}$$

where σ is the index of heterogeneity indicating the range and distribution of the values of K (the apparent association as a function of the free hapten concentration) about K_0. From this distribution function it can be shown [4, 7], if it is assumed that each antibody-combining site acts independently and is unaffected by the other combining sites on the same molecule of antibody, that the fraction of antibody-combining sites bound to hapten as a function of the free hapten concentration is given by the equation,

$$\frac{R}{n} = 1 - \frac{1}{\sqrt{\pi}} \int_{-\infty}^{+\infty} \frac{\exp(-t^2)}{1 + K_0(H)\exp(t\sigma)} dt \tag{18}$$

where R/n is the fraction of antibody-combining sites bound to hapten and t equals $\ln(K/K_0)/\sigma$. For convenience we take the reciprocal of Eq. 18 and thus

$$\frac{n}{R} = \frac{1}{1 - f(\lambda)} \tag{19}$$

where

$$f(\lambda) = \frac{1}{\sqrt{\pi}} \int_{-\infty}^{+\infty} \frac{\exp(-t^2)}{1 + K_0(H)\exp(t\sigma)} dt \tag{20}$$

and $\lambda = K_0(H)$. The integral in $f(\lambda)$ can not be evaluated analytically and therefore numerical or graphical integration must be carried out in order to determine $f(\lambda)$. The authors have carried out such procedures as follows. It can be shown from Eq. 20 that

$$f(\lambda) = \frac{1}{2} + \frac{(1 - \lambda^2)}{2\sqrt{\pi}} \int_{-\infty}^{+\infty} \frac{\exp(-t^2)}{1 + 2\lambda\cosh\sigma t + \lambda^2} dt \tag{21}$$

and so

$$f(\lambda) + f\left(\frac{1}{\lambda}\right) = 1 \tag{22}$$

Using this relation it is then necessary to compute the value of the integral only for $0 \leqslant \lambda \leqslant 1$. Then for $\lambda \geqslant 1$,

$$f(\lambda) = 1 - f\left(\frac{1}{\lambda}\right) \tag{23}$$

The integral itself was calculated as

$$\int\limits_{0}^{\infty} \frac{\exp(-t^2)}{1+2\lambda\cosh\sigma t+\lambda^2}\,dt$$

and the values of σ taken between 0 and 4·00 and the values of $1/\lambda$ between 0·000 and 10·000. It was found that if the range of the integration is taken as (0, 5) the remainder is less than 10^{-10}. The numerical value of the integral was found by using repeated Simpson's rule with variable step length. The

TABLE 14.1

$1/K_0$ (H)			n/R values			
	$\sigma = 0·000$	$\sigma = 0·2000$	$\sigma = 0·4000$	$\sigma = 0·6000$	$\sigma = 0·8000$	$\sigma = 1·000$
0·0000	1·000	1·000	1·000	1·000	1·000	1·000
0·1000	1·100	1·101	1·103	1·107	1·113	1·121
0·2000	1·200	1·201	1·205	1·212	1·221	1·231
0·3000	1·300	1·302	1·306	1·314	1·324	1·336
0·4000	1·400	1·402	1·407	1·415	1·425	1·437
0·5000	1·500	1·502	1·506	1·514	1·524	1·536
0·6000	1·600	1·601	1·606	1·613	1·621	1·632
0·7000	1·700	1·701	1·705	1·710	1·717	1·726
0·8000	1·800	1·801	1·803	1·807	1·812	1·818
0·9000	1·900	1·900	1·902	1·904	1·907	1·910
1·000	2·000	2·000	2·000	2·000	2·000	2·000
1·111	2·111	2·111	2·109	2·106	2·103	2·099
1·250	2·250	2·249	2·245	2·239	2·231	2·222
1·429	2·429	2·426	2·419	2·408	2·394	2·378
1·500	2·500	2·497	2·488	2·475	2·459	2·440
2·000	3·000	2·993	2·974	2·945	2·908	2·867
2·500	3·500	3·489	3·459	3·412	3·353	3·286
3·000	4·000	3·985	3·942	3·876	3·793	3·700
3·500	4·500	4·481	4·425	4·339	4·231	4·109
4·000	5·000	4·976	4·907	4·801	4·667	4·516
4·500	5·500	5·472	5·390	5·262	5·101	4·920
5·000	6·000	5·967	5·871	5·723	5·534	5·322
5·500	6·500	6·462	6·353	6·183	5·967	5·723
6·000	7·000	6·958	6·834	6·642	6·398	6·123
6·500	7·500	7·453	7·316	7·101	6·829	6·521
7·000	8·000	7·948	7·797	7·560	7·260	6·919
7·500	8·500	8·443	8·278	8·019	7·690	7·316
8·000	9·000	8·938	8·759	8·478	8·120	7·713
8·500	9·500	9·433	9·240	8·936	8·549	8·108
9·000	10·00	9·929	9·721	9·395	8·978	8·504
9·500	10·50	10·42	10·20	9·853	9·407	8·898
10·00	11·00	10·92	10·68	10·31	9·835	9·293

14.1 *cont.*

$1/K_0$ (H)			n/R values		
	$\sigma = 1{\cdot}200$	$\sigma = 1{\cdot}400$	$\sigma = 1{\cdot}600$	$\sigma = 1{\cdot}800$	$\sigma = 2{\cdot}000$
0·0000	1·000	1·000	1·000	1·000	1·000
0·1000	1·130	1·140	1·151	1·164	1·178
0·2000	1·244	1·258	1·273	1·288	1·305
0·3000	1·350	1·365	1·381	1·397	1·414
0·4000	1·451	1·466	1·481	1·497	1·512
0·5000	1·548	1·562	1·576	1·590	1·603
0·6000	1·643	1·654	1·666	1·678	1·690
0·7000	1·735	1·744	1·753	1·763	1·772
0·8000	1·825	1·831	1·838	1·844	1·850
0·9000	1·913	1·916	1·920	1·923	1·926
1·000	2·000	2·000	2·000	2·000	2·000
1·111	2·095	2·091	2·087	2·083	2·080
1·250	2·213	2·203	2·194	2·185	2·176
1·429	2·361	2·344	2·328	2·311	2·296
1·500	2·420	2·400	2·380	2·361	2·343
2·000	2·823	2·780	2·737	2·696	2·657
2·500	3·216	3·146	3·078	3·013	2·953
3·000	3·602	3·504	3·409	3·319	3·235
3·500	3·982	3·854	3·731	3·615	3·508
4·000	4·357	4·200	4·048	3·905	3·772
4·500	4·730	4·541	4·359	4·188	4·030
5·000	5·100	4·879	4·666	4·466	4·283
5·500	5·468	5·213	4·969	4·741	4·531
6·000	5·834	5·546	5·270	5·012	4·775
6·500	6·198	5·876	5·568	5·280	5·016
7·000	6·561	6·205	5·863	5·545	5·253
7·500	6·923	6·532	6·157	5·808	5·488
8·000	7·284	6·857	6·448	6·068	5·721
8·500	7·644	7·182	6·739	6·327	5·951
9·000	8·003	7·505	7·027	6·584	6·180
9·500	8·362	7·827	7·315	6·839	6·406
10·00	8·720	8·148	7·601	7·093	6·631

values of the integral are known at $\sigma = 0$, and this was used to check the validity of the method. In addition Hermite's quadrature formula was used as a further check for various values of λ and σ. The computation was performed on an English Electric KDF9 computer and the program was written in the Edinburgh University Atlas Autocode. The results are calculated accurate to six decimal places and are shown in Figs. 14.4 and 14.5 and in Table 14.1. It can be seen that whenever $f(\lambda) = 1/2$ (i.e. whenever half of the antibody-combining sites are bound to hapten) the values of $K_0(H) = 1$. This means for any value of σ, K_0 is equal to the reciprocal of the free hapten

$1/K_0$ (H)			n/R values		
	$\sigma = 2\cdot200$	$\sigma = 2\cdot400$	$\sigma = 2\cdot600$	$\sigma = 2\cdot800$	$\sigma = 3\cdot000$
0·0000	1·000	1·000	1·000	1·000	1·000
0·1000	1·192	1·206	1·221	1·236	1·251
0·2000	1·321	1·337	1·354	1·370	1·386
0·3000	1·430	1·446	1·462	1·477	1·492
0·4000	1·527	1·542	1·557	1·571	1·584
0·5000	1·617	1·630	1·643	1·655	1·666
0·6000	1·701	1·712	1·722	1·732	1·742
0·7000	1·780	1·789	1·797	1·805	1·812
0·8000	1·856	1·862	1·868	1·873	1·878
0·9000	1·929	1·932	1·935	1·938	1·940
1·000	2·000	2·000	2·000	2·000	2·000
1·111	2·076	2·073	2·069	2·066	2·063
1·250	2·168	2·160	2·153	2·146	2·139
1·429	2·281	2·268	2·255	2·243	2·232
1·500	2·326	2·310	2·295	2·281	2·268
2·000	2·621	2·587	2·556	2·527	2·501
2·500	2·896	2·844	2·796	2·752	2·712
3·000	3·158	3·087	3·021	2·962	2·908
3·500	3·408	3·318	3·235	3·160	3·092
4·000	3·651	3·540	3·440	3·349	3·266
4·500	3·886	3·755	3·637	3·530	3·433
5·000	4·115	3·964	3·827	3·704	3·594
5·500	4·340	4·168	4·013	3·874	3·749
6·000	4·560	4·367	4·193	4·038	3·899
6·500	4·777	4·562	4·370	4·199	4·045
7·000	4·990	4·754	4·543	4·355	4·188
7·500	5·201	4·943	4·713	4·509	4·327
8·000	5·408	5·129	4·880	4·659	4·463
8·500	5·614	5·312	5·045	4·807	4·597
9·000	5·817	5·493	5·207	4·953	4·728
9·500	6·018	5·672	5·366	5·096	4·857
10·00	6·217	5·850	5·524	5·237	4·984

concentration at which half the concentration of antibody-combining sites are bound to hapten. Thus the value of K_0 can be obtained directly from the experimental data if the value of n is known. The value of σ is obtained by comparing theoretical curves, derived from those shown in Figs. 14.4 and 14.5 and with the aid of Table 14.1, to the experimental points; the index of heterogeneity is taken from the theoretical curve which best fits the experimental points. It should be pointed out that when $\sigma = 0$, $f(\lambda) = 1/1 + K_0(H)$ and Eq. 19 reduces to Eq. 11. For another description of the evaluation of $f(\lambda)$ and the determination of σ see [15, 16].

14.1 *cont.*

$1/K_0$ (H)	n/R values				
	$\sigma = 3.200$	$\sigma = 3.400$	$\sigma = 3.600$	$\sigma = 3.800$	$\sigma = 4.000$
0·0000	1·000	1·000	1·000	1·000	1·000
0·1000	1·266	1·281	1·295	1·310	1·324
0·2000	1·401	1·416	1·431	1·445	1·458
0·3000	1·507	1·521	1·534	1·547	1·559
0·4000	1·597	1·609	1·621	1·632	1·643
0·5000	1·677	1·688	1·698	1·707	1·717
0·6000	1·751	1·759	1·767	1·775	1·782
0·7000	1·819	1·825	1·831	1·837	1·843
0·8000	1·882	1·887	1·891	1·895	1·898
0·9000	1·943	1·945	1·947	1·949	1·951
1·000	2·000	2·000	2·000	2·000	2·000
1·111	2·061	2·058	2·056	2·054	2·052
1·250	2·133	2·128	2·123	2·118	2·113
1·429	2·222	2·212	2·203	2·195	2·187
1·500	2·255	2·244	2·234	2·224	2·215
2·000	2·476	2·454	2·433	2·413	2·396
2·500	2·675	2·641	2·610	2·581	2·555
3·000	2·858	2·813	2·771	2·733	2·699
3·500	3·030	2·973	2·921	2·874	2·831
4·000	3·192	3·124	3·062	3·006	2·955
4·500	3·346	3·267	3·196	3·131	3·071
5·000	3·494	3·404	3·323	3·249	3·182
5·500	3·636	3·535	3·444	3·362	3·287
6·000	3·774	3·662	3·562	3·471	3·388
6·500	3·908	3·785	3·675	3·575	3·486
7·000	4·038	3·904	3·785	3·677	3·580
7·500	4·165	4·020	3·891	3·775	3·670
8·000	4·289	4·134	3·995	3·870	3·758
8·500	4·410	4·244	4·096	3·963	3·844
9·000	4·529	4·352	4·194	4·054	3·928
9·500	4·646	4·458	4·291	4·142	4·009
10·00	4·760	4·562	4·386	4·229	4·088

Method B

Nisonoff & Pressman [6] employed a distribution function which is similar to the one just described; it was first derived by Sips [17] and has the advantage that it can be integrated analytically. Klotz [7] related Sips equation, which was derived for the absorption of a gas on to a solid, to equilibria of proteins and ions in solution and in terms of our previous terminology in Method A is

$$\frac{R}{n} = \frac{[K_0(H)]^\alpha}{1 + [K_0(H)]^\alpha} \tag{24}$$

where α is the index of heterogeneity and $0 \leqslant \alpha \leqslant 1$. Since R is the number of moles of hapten bound per mole of antibody, it follows that R/n is the number of moles of bound hapten per mole of antibody-combining sites or simply represents the fraction of antibody-combining sites bound to hapten and in Nisonoff's terminology is equal to F_b. Substituting F_b into Eq. 24 and taking the reciprocal,

$$\frac{1}{F_b} = \frac{1 + [K_0(H)]^\alpha}{[K_0(H)]^\alpha} \tag{25}$$

or

$$\frac{1}{F_b} = \frac{1}{[K_0(H)]^\alpha} + 1 \tag{26}$$

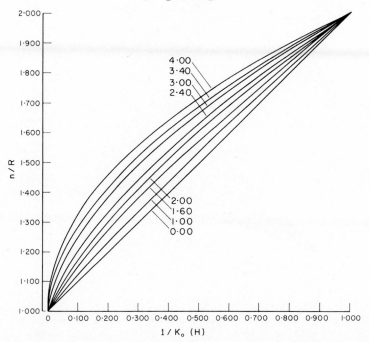

FIG. 14.4. Theoretical curves based upon a Gaussian distribution which were calculated from Eq. 19 for various values of σ in the higher range of binding. Numerical values are given in Table 14.1.

It can be seen from Eq. 26 that K_0 is equal to the reciprocal of the free hapten concentration at which half the antibody-combining sites are bound to hapten, i.e. when $F_b = 1/2$

$$\frac{1}{1/2} = \frac{1}{[K_0(H)]^\alpha} + 1 \tag{27}$$

or

$$\frac{1}{[K_0(\text{H})]^\alpha} = 1 \tag{28}$$

Eq. 28 can also be written

$$\frac{1}{K_0^\alpha(\text{H})^\alpha} = 1 \tag{29}$$

or

$$K_0^\alpha = (\text{H})^{-\alpha} \tag{30}$$

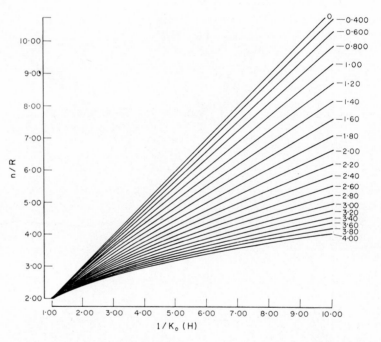

FIG. 14.5. Continuation of the theoretical curves shown in Fig. 14.4 into the lower range of binding. Note that when half the antibody-combining sites are bound with hapten (i.e. when $n/R = 2\cdot00$), $1/K_0(\text{H}) = 1$ or $K_0 = 1/(\text{H})$; this relationship applies for any value of σ.

By raising both sides of Eq. 30 to the $1/\alpha$, taking into consideration that $0 \leqslant \alpha \leqslant 1$,

$$K_0 = \frac{1}{(\text{H})} \tag{31}$$

Therefore K_0 can be obtained from the experimental data as was the case in Method A. The index of heterogeneity α is obtained by using Eq. 26 or Eq. 41

and plotting $1/(AbH)$ vs. $1/(H)^x$, by decreasing the value of α, by small increments from 1, it can be seen that the modified curve will bend upwards towards the y axis. The index of heterogeneity is that value of α which yields a modified curve closest to a straight line. It should be noted that when $\alpha = 1$ Eq. 25 may be transformed into Eq. 16.

Thermodynamics of the antibody–hapten interaction

Many reports involving equilibrium dialysis give the thermodynamic values of the standard free energy change (ΔF°), standard enthalpy change (ΔH°), and the standard entropy change (ΔS°). These values are calculated from the value of K_0 and thus require brief comment; it is necessary to mention that because a value of the average intrinsic association constant is used to calculate the three thermodynamic functions, these will also represent average values. Detailed account of these thermodynamic functions is beyond the scope of this chapter and the reader is referred to standard tests on thermodynamics for further information [18, 19]. For an account of the relationship of thermodynamics to antibody–antigen interaction see the reviews of Karush [9] and Singer [10]; the following is intended solely as a highly simplified description to allow the calculation of ΔF°, ΔH°, and ΔS°.

Standard free energy change may be described as the maximum amount of useful work which can be obtained from a reaction that occurs at constant temperature and pressure and where the products and reactants at equilibrium are all at unit activity, i.e. they are all 1 molal in concentration. Standard free energy change is composed of an enthalpic term and an entropic term given by Eq. 32,

$$\Delta F^\circ = \Delta H^\circ - T\Delta S^\circ \qquad (32)$$

where ΔH°, the standard enthalpy change, and is termed the 'heat content' or 'heat of reaction', and ΔS°, the standard entropy change, represents the amount of energy which is unavailable to perform work.

The value for ΔF° can be obtained directly from the value of K by the relation

$$\Delta F^\circ = -RT \ln K \qquad (33)$$

where R is the universal gas constant ($1\cdot9871$ cal/degree/mole) and T is the absolute temperature (obtained by adding the temperature in $^\circ$C to $273\cdot15$) and $\ln K$ is the natural logarithm of K and is equal to $2\cdot303 \log K$ and therefore

$$\Delta F^\circ = -4\cdot576\, T \log K \qquad (34)$$

The standard enthalpy change ΔH° (in actual practice ΔH° may be considered to be equal to the enthalpy change ΔH) is obtained by the van't

R*

Hoff equation which expresses a relation in the change of the association constant as a function of the absolute temperature.

$$\frac{\mathrm{d}\ln K}{\mathrm{d}T} = \frac{-\Delta H^\circ}{RT^2} \qquad (35)$$

By integrating Eq. 35 between the limits of temperatures from T_1 to T_2,

$$\log \frac{K_2}{K_1} = -\frac{\Delta H^\circ}{2\cdot303\,R}\left(\frac{1}{T_2} - \frac{1}{T_1}\right) \qquad (36)$$

where K_1 and K_2 are the association constants obtained at the absolute temperatures T_1 and T_2 respectively. Solving Eq. 36 for ΔH and simplifying,

$$\Delta H^\circ = \frac{4\cdot576\,(\log K_2 - \log K_1)}{\left(\dfrac{1}{T_1} - \dfrac{1}{T_2}\right)} \qquad (37)$$

It can be seen that by using Eqs. 32, 34 and 37 that ΔS° can be calculated by difference.

Until recently the values of ΔF°, ΔH° and ΔS° have been used to interpret the secondary bonds of antibody–hapten complex formation. Whether these values reflect the true stabilization of the complex is uncertain. Karush [9] in an attempt to clarify the situation has recently proposed the use of the concept of unitary entropy; see Gurney [21]. Another way of viewing the standard entropy change is the degree of disorder of the system; i.e. as a system approaches equilibrium a positive entropy change or an increase in entropy represents a transition of the molecules in the system from a more highly ordered state to a less ordered state. A negative entropy change or a decrease in entropy is the transition of the molecules in the system from a less ordered state to a more highly ordered state. It can be seen from Eq. 1, an antibody molecule combines with a hapten molecule forming a single 'molecule' of the antibody–hapten complex; therefore a decrease in the standard entropy change is to be expected since two molecules combine to form a single complex representing a shift to a more highly ordered state. In the experimental situation, however, the standard entropy change instead of being largely negative is usually minimal or in the positive direction of change. This observation can be partially explained if Eq. 1 is rewritten to include bound water on both the antibody- and antigen-combining sites which is released or altered in configuration upon antibody–hapten combination, thereby satisfying the expected shift to a less ordered state. This modified equation [9] is:

$$\mathrm{Ab}_{(x+n)\mathrm{H_2O}} + \mathrm{H}_{(y+m)\mathrm{H_2O}} \rightleftharpoons \mathrm{Ab}_{(n)\mathrm{H_2O}}H_{(m)\mathrm{H_2O}} + (x+y)\,\mathrm{H_2O} \qquad (38)$$

Because of the role played by bound water molecules in the over-all reaction, the contribution of the water molecules interacting with the antibody and antigen sites as well as the antibody–hapten interaction must be taken into consideration when calculating the values of $\Delta S°$ and $\Delta F°$. As stated previously, Karush [9] has done this by the use of the concepy of unitary entropy. The derived equation for the determination of the unitary entropy change (ΔS_u) is [20],

$$\Delta S_u = \Delta S° + R \ln 55·6 = \Delta S° + 7·98 \tag{39}$$

where $\ln 55·6$ is the natural logarithm of the concentration of water molecules. By incorporating Eq. 39 into Eq. 32, the unitary free energy change is obtained.

$$\Delta F_u = \Delta F° - 7·98\,T \tag{40}$$

These two new values of ΔF_u and ΔS_u may be used to describe more adequately the stabilization of the antibody–hapten complex through secondary bonding.

There is another point which requires mentioning at this time in order to avoid misleading interpretations when relating K_0 values and the respective thermodynamic functions to serologic and biologic reactions. The average *intrinsic* association constant as Singer [10] has recently pointed out '... describes the state of equilibrium of an isolated haptenic or antigenic combining site with an isolated antibody valence...'. This may have profound implications when using multivalent antigens and antibody in as far as to the extent the reaction may tend to go to completion. Although the value of K_0 may be of relatively low magnitude, the extent to which the reaction may proceed to completion in serologic and/or biologic reactions may not be fully reflected in the value of K_0 if the antigen is multivalent. This has been pointed out by Singer & Campbell [22] who showed that

$$K_M = \frac{n\,K_0}{2}$$

where K_M is the association constant of the molecular interaction between a divalent antibody molecule and an antigen molecule possessing n number of combining sites. Thus the valence of the antigen molecule may have pronounced effects upon the extent to which a serologic and/or biologic reaction may tend to go to completion even though the average *intrinsic* association constant is of a low magnitude.

Preparation of hapten–protein conjugates
Although there are numerous methods for coupling haptens to proteins, only the method of coupling through diazo bonds will be discussed. This

method has been used to couple a variety of haptens to proteins via the amino group either on the aliphatic or aromatic portion of the hapten [23]. The reaction site on the protein is important because antibodies of varying specificity could arise due to different side-chain groupings of the amino-acid

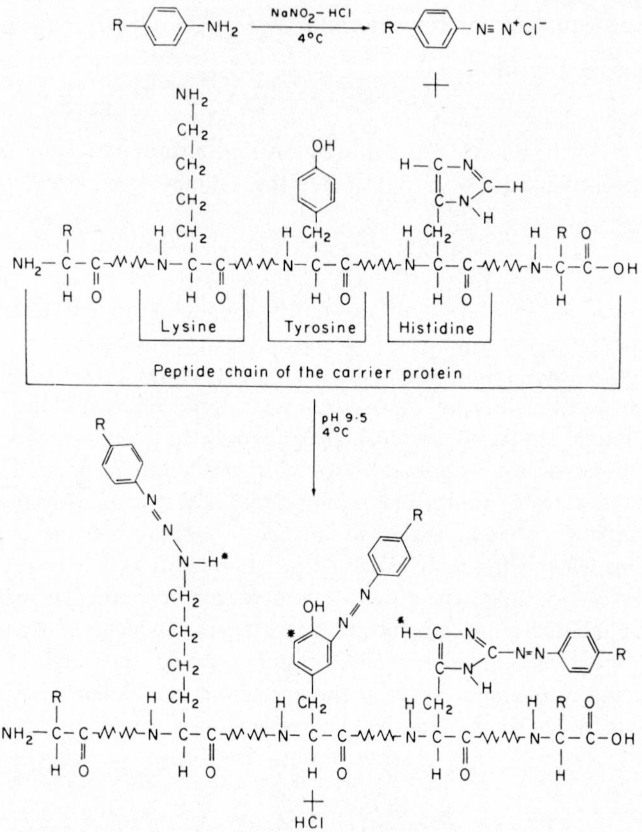

Fig. 14.6. Illustration of the chemical reactions involved when coupling a hapten to a protein carrier via diazo bonds; only the three major substitution reactions are shown. * indicates the other probable sites of coupling.

residues on the protein adjacent to the site of coupling. Generally the tyrosyl and histidyl residues have been implicated in the coupling reaction, each possessing two reactive sites; however, other groups are known to react with diazonium compounds such as the free amino group of glycine, the ε amino group of lysine, −SH groups, and, at three sites on the guanidine group of arginine [8]. One of these groups, the ε amino group of lysine may actually predominate in the reaction. Gelewitz *et al* [24] could detect only approximately one-third of the haptenic substitution using spectrophotometric methods and titration with titanous chloride which determines the number of azo groups as compared to elemental analysis for the hapten itself. They suggested that the hapten could couple into the ε amino group of lysine and form either a triazene or a pentazene structure. More recently Tabachnick & Sobotka [25] found that only 50 per cent of hapten coupled into the tyrosyl and histidyl residues whereas if they acetylated the protein carrier prior to coupling, thus blocking the free amino groups, essentially all of the hapten was bound to tyrosine and histidine. In light of these findings the three main coupling reactions of a diazotized hapten with a carrier protein can be illustrated as is shown in Fig. 14.6.

Although one may wish to couple a number of different haptens to a variety of protein carriers, the procedure is basically the same for any particular combination. The following two points should be helpful when conjugating hapten to proteins: (i) most immunizing antigens have between ten and thirty haptenic groups per protein molecule, (ii) the efficiency of the coupling process is in the order of 20–40 per cent. With these two points in mind approximate calculations of the amounts of hapten and protein necessary to yield the required degree of coupling can be made. This ratio, however, will be a rough estimate and the exact hapten/protein ratio can only be obtained from elemental analysis for the hapten molecule.

Since bovine γ globulin (BGG) has been used quite extensively as the protein carrier, it will be used here as an example of a typical coupling process. Ten grammes of BGG is approximately 0·06 mmoles of protein (assuming a M.W. = 156,000); thus in order to obtain a conjugate with a hapten/protein ratio of 20 (assuming a coupling efficiency of 30 per cent), 4 mmoles of the desired hapten would be used. The figure of 20 is only an approximation.

The 4 mmoles of hapten are diazotized by adding the hapten to 100 ml of 0·1 N HCl and then slowly adding dropwise a 1 per cent solution of $NaNO_2$ with constant stirring at 4° C. The addition of $NaNO_2$ must be carefully controlled because a large excess of HNO_2 is undesirable. This can easily be done by testing the reaction mixture for free HNO_2 by the use of starch-iodide test paper. If there is free HNO_2 present it will oxidize the iodide to free iodine which then reacts with the starch, giving a blue-black colour. The end-point of the addition of the 1 per cent $NaNO_2$ is taken as the first positive starch-iodide test 15 minutes after the last addition of $NaNO_2$.

The coupling reaction is carried out at 4° C between a pH of 9·0 and 9·5 with continuous stirring. The BGG is dissolved in 100 ml of borate buffer (alternatively a carbonate buffer can be used) and the pH is adjusted to 9·5 with 0·1 N NaOH. The diazotized hapten is added slowly to the BGG solution by running it down the side of the reaction beaker (this prevents local excess of acid that might occur by the dropwise addition). The addition is monitored by a pH meter and when the pH of the mixture falls below 7·0, the reaction mixture is adjusted back to pH 9·5 by running 0·1 M NaOH down the side of the beaker. This process is continued until all of the diazotized hapten is added. A final adjustment of the pH is made to 9·0 and mixing continued for 1–2 hours with frequent checks to maintain the pH at 9·0. The mixture is allowed to stand in a refrigerator overnight and then dialysed for 6–8 days against daily 5–7 litre changes of 0·15 M NaCl or borate buffered saline.

Other methods of separating the uncoupled hapten from the azoprotein may be used if desired; for example filtration through Sephadex G25, ammonium sulphate precipitation, or precipitation of the azoprotein at its isoelectric point. The azoprotein is brought up to 500 ml with saline which should result in a protein concentration of 20 mg/ml. The azoprotein is then sterilized by passing through a Seitz filter and stored at −20° C in dark bottles. If precipitating test antigens are to be prepared, an acetone precipitation [6] is recommended to ensure complete removal of an unbound hapten.

Method of immunization

The method of immunization depends largely upon how the anti-haptenic antibody is to be used. If one wishes to study the affinity of antibodies towards various haptens, it is advisable to inject the smallest amount of antigen which will produce a measurable immune response. Karush [9, 26] has pointed out that if large amounts of antigen are injected it is quite probable that the high-affinity antibodies will be selectively removed from the circulation and the value of K_0 may represent a population of low-affinity antibody. This possibility may account for the thousand-fold difference in the association constants arrived at by Cartsen & Eisen [27] and by Velick *et al* [29] for the same ε-N-2,4-dinitrophenyllysine (DNP) hapten. The first group used an antigen with 8 DNP molecules/BGG molecule, while the second group used an antigen containing 55 DNP molecules/BGG molecule; and in addition the first group gave sixteen i.v. injections of 1·5 mg of alum-precipitated antigen while the second gave a single injection of 5 mg in Freund's adjuvant. In light of this and other reports (see ref. 36) there is clearly a need for standardization of the hapten/protein ratio of the immunizing antigen, the amount of antigen injected and the duration of the immunization schedule.

Purification of the antisera

If Method B is to be used and only the K_0 and index of heterogeneity measured, a simple γ globulin preparation by sodium sulphate precipitation is needed. The method of Kekwick [29] is used and generally three precipitations are required, carried out at 18 per cent, 14 per cent, and 14 per cent weight Na_2SO_4/vol. The sodium sulphate fractionation is necessary since many haptens will bind non-specifically to albumin. If oligosaccharide haptens are used, fractionation is generally not necessary since albumin-binding is negligible.

If Method A is used or if Method B is used to determine the valence of the antibody, a specifically purified antibody preparation is needed. There have been numerous methods used for this purpose largely depending upon what hapten is employed (see Stelos, Chapter 5).

The question may arise whether specific purification of the antibody may lead to a selection of a certain population of antibody. It seems likely that this in fact would occur. In the first step of specific precipitation of the antibody with the test antigen, low-affinity antibody may not be present in the precipitate. Also when the complexes are dissociated the antibody with high affinity may remain bound to the antigen and hence be lost. This possibility should always be kept in mind and tested for in each particular situation. In the case of p-azobenzoate Nisinoff & Pressman [6] found the purified antibody had the same value of K_0 and α as did the γ globulin fraction of the same antisera within the experimental error of the test.

Equilibrium dialysis
From the earlier theoretical discussion of chemical equilibria related to antibody–hapten interaction, it was noted that a series of equilibrium dialysis cells must be set up with constant amounts of antibody and varying the hapten concentration over a forty-fold range. The design of the equilibrium dialysis cell is dependent upon the method which is used to determine the free and bound hapten concentrations; these methods are in turn dependent upon what hapten is employed. There are two general methods for calculating the concentration of hapten in solution. The first method is to use the molar extinction coefficient at the absorption spectrum maximum of a coloured hapten. More recently the use of radioactive labelled haptens have been employed which have certain advantages over the first method.

When using the molar extinction coefficient of the hapten, generally only the free hapten concentration in the non-protein portion of the cell can be determined. This is because either the protein may interfere with accurate absorption measurements, or the hapten which is bound to antibody may exhibit either a spectral shift in its absorption curve and/or a change in the molar extinction coefficient [4]. Therefore the only way to determine the amount of hapten specifically bound to antibody is by noting the decrease in the initial hapten concentration of the protein-free side of the cell over and above that which is observed in an identical cell containing normal γ globulin. Using this method for determining the free and bound hapten concentration, a cell of the design reported by Carsten and Eisen is advisable [27].

The equilibrium dialysis cell consists of two top portions of 2–5 ml screw-capped vials; the cut edges are heated, flared out and ground down so that the two sections form a tight seal when joined together (see Fig. 14.7). The volume of each half of the cell should be slightly greater than 1 ml. A piece of cellophane which has been prewashed for 24 to 48 hours in order to remove bound glycerine is blotted and placed between the two sections of the cell after the ground edges have been lightly covered with silicone grease. The cell is then assembled and all of the joints are sealed with paraffin wax to

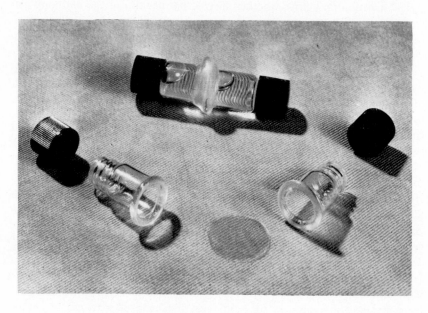

FIG 14.7. Equilibrium dialysis cell of the type designed by Cartsen & Eisen [27]. The assembled cell is joined together with paraffin wax; alternatively clamps may be used in order to ensure stability of the cell.

prevent leaks. To one side of the cell add 1·00 ml of the desired hapten solution, and to the other side of the cell add one of the following: the buffer control—1·00 ml of buffer, the normal γ globulin control—1·00 ml of normal γ globulin which is equal in protein concentration to the antibody preparation, or 1·00 ml of the antibody solution. A small air bubble should be trapped in both sides of the cell; this air bubble facilitates mixing during the equilibration period. For a single point of a binding curve three cells must be set up; (i) a buffer control which is used to determine whether equilibrium has been established and also the amount of hapten which is absorbed to the cellophane; (ii) a normal γ globulin control which serves to determine the amount of hapten non-specifically bound to γ globulin, and (iii) a cell containing the antibody solution to be tested. At least duplicate, and if possible triplicate, cells should be run; therefore, to obtain a binding curve containing ten experimental points at least sixty cells would be required.

From the above it can be seen that to prepare a single binding curve would be a laborious task. This may be overcome to some extent by employing radioactive labelled haptens which eliminate many of the mechanical difficulties in the procedure just described. Many labelled haptens may be obtained commercially; alternatively there are procedures described by which certain radioactive labelled haptens may be prepared in the laboratory. For instance ^{35}S-labelled sulphanilic acid [31] prepared by the sulphonation of analine with ^{35}S-labelled sulphuric acid, or ^{131}I-labelled p-iodobenzoic acid may be prepared by the method of isotope exchange [32]. When radioactive haptens are employed, the bound hapten concentration may be determined directly from the protein side of the equilibrium dialysis cell; the number of counts obtained from the protein side represents the sum of the free and bound hapten concentrations. Thus the bound hapten concentration may be determined by subtracting the free hapten concentration which is obtained by counting the protein free side of the cell and correcting for non-specifically bound hapten using the normal γ globulin control. Because the bound hapten concentration can now be determined directly, an equilibrium dialysis cell of the design previously described is not required. Instead, small dialysis bags containing the protein solution are used, and are dialysed against a single pool of free hapten [6, 35]. It should be mentioned that spectrophotometric methods can also be used in this procedure if the spectral shift can be quantitated so that the bound hapten concentration can be determined from the protein side [4] or if the absorption of the protein side is compared to known values of bound hapten at particular protein and free hapten concentrations [33, 34].

The dialysis bags are made from $\frac{1}{4}$ inch dialysis tubing. For each hapten concentration nine bags will be needed: three for the antibody solution, three for the normal γ globulin control, and three for the buffer control. The tubing is cut into 3 to 4 inch pieces and washed continuously for 24 to 48 hours prior to use. After washing, a knot is tied in one end of the tubing and tested for possible leaks. The bags are then filled with approximately 0·5 ml of the desired solution; this can best be accomplished if a piece of $\frac{1}{4}$ inch glass tubing is inserted into the open end of the dialysis tubing and the solution delivered through it with a Pasteur pipette. The bag is tied off with a soft piece of string, care being taken to trap a small air bubble inside the bag. Different coloured strings may be used to aid in the identification of the various bags. After the bags are completed, all nine are placed into a 50 ml bottle which is filled with the desired hapten concentration and the top of the bottle sealed, leaving an air bubble to aid mixing (see Fig. 14.8). To obtain by this procedure a binding curve containing ten experimental points only ten bottles are necessary.

The cells of either design are placed in a water bath at the desired temperature which is thermostatically controlled to within $\pm 0.1°$ C. The cells are rotated at 5–6 rev/min for from 24 to 48 hours, or for whatever time is needed to establish equilibrium. When equilibrium is reached duplicate or triplicate samples are volumetrically taken from the protein and non-protein sides of the cells and the free and bound hapten concentrations determined; it is extremely

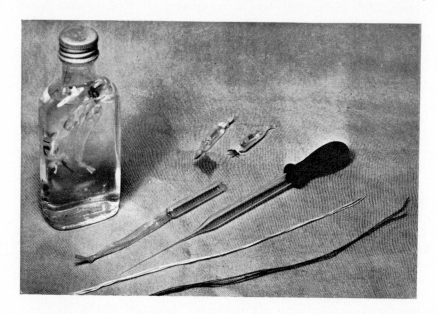

FIG. 14.8. Equilibrium dialysis apparatus employing small cellophane bags [35]. A total of nine bags are placed into the 50 ml bottle which contains the desired hapten concentration; six bags are used for the buffer and normal γ globulin controls and three bags are used for the antibody preparation.

important to determine if the protein concentration of the cell has remained constant and this can be done by taking readings at 280 mμ. The values of (AbH) must be corrected when there is a change in the protein concentration.

A few final points regarding the buffer systems are worth noting. It is important to guard against possible microbial contamination during the experiment, especially if runs are being made at high temperatures. Some haptens are themselves bacteriostatic. If this is not so, either sterile solutions must be employed or a suitable antibiotic added. Borate buffers may be used as these tend to retard microbial growth.

The pH and ionic strength of the buffer system employed are also important. Karush [4] has pointed out that at a pH of 8·5 there may be an electrostatic repulsion between the negatively charged antigen and antibody molecules which might result in non-specific effects upon the value of K_0. Velick *et al* [28] reported that K_0 values were relatively insensitive to changes in either pH or ionic strength when studying the DNP–anti-DNP interaction by the method of fluorescent quenching. Generally two buffer systems have been used: (i) a saline–phosphate buffer pH 7·4, $\Gamma/2 = 0·16$ [4], and (ii) a saline–borate buffer pH 8·0, $\Gamma/2 = 0·16$ [6].

Practical aspects of plotting binding data

This last section has been written so that the reader can follow through the calculations of the values of K_0, n, and indices of heterogeneity using Methods A and B. The data were taken from a report by Nisonoff & Pressman [6].

TABLE 14.2

$(H) \times 10^6$	$(AbH) \times 10^6$	$1/(H) \times 10^{-5}$	$1/(AbH) \times 10^{-5}$	R	$R/(H) \times 10^{-3}$
2·32	3·06	4·31	3·27	0·437	188
2·36	3·08	4·24	3·25	0·440	186
4·57	4·36	2·19	2·29	0·623	136
4·58	4·20	2·18	2·38	0·600	131
9·21	6·7	1·09	1·49	0·957	104
9·42	6·5	1·06	1·54	0·929	98·6
18·8	8·6	0·532	1·16	1·23	65·4
19·0	9·2	0·526	1·09	1·31	68·9
43·0	12·2	0·233	0·820	1·74	40·5
43·4	12·2	0·230	0·820	1·74	40·1
68·6	12·3	0·146	0·813	1·76	25·7
69·0	11·9	0·145	0·840	1·70	24·6
92·6	14·4	0·108	0·694	2·06	22·2
95·0	14·3	0·105	0·699	2·04	21·5

The antibody tested was specifically purified rabbit anti-p-azobenzoate; the data taken was that from Rabbit D. The test hapten was p-iodobenzoate; ^{131}I was incorporated into the hapten molecule by the method of isotope exchange [32]. The concentration of the purified antibody from Rabbit D was $7·0 \times 10^{-6}$ molar.

The experimental data are given in the first two columns of Table 14.2.

The third and fourth columns are the reciprocal values of (H) and (AbH) which are used when plotting by Method B, and the plot is shown in Fig. 14.10. The R values in column 5 are determined by dividing the values of

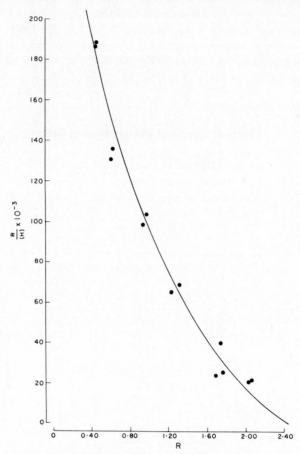

FIG. 14.9. Plot of the experimental data from Rabbit D [6] by Method A. The points are experimental and the curve is theoretical based upon the Gaussian distribution and derived from Table 14.2. See Table 14.1 for the numerical values of the data.

(AbH) by the concentration of antibody molecules, $7 \cdot 0 \times 10^{-6}$ M. Columns 5 and 6 are used when plotting by Method A shown in Fig. 14.9.

The calculation of K_0 from Figs. 14.9 and 14.10 is a relatively simple operation. The binding curves shown in Figs. 14.9 and 14.10 are extrapolated to the x axis and y axis respectively as (H)→∞. If Method A is used, the extrapolated R value is divided by 2 giving that point where half of the antibody-combining sites are bound to hapten and the corresponding value of $R/(H)$ is obtained. From these two values of $R/2$ and $R/(H)$ the value of $1/(H)$ is calculated giving the value of K_0. From Fig. 14.9 it is shown that the extrapolated value of R is equal to 2·46 and thus $R/2 = 1·23$ and the corresponding value of $R/(H)$ is $72·4 \times 10^3$ litres/mole; therefore $K_0 = 1/(H) = 72·4 \times 10^3/1·23 = 5·89 \times 10^4$ litres/mole.

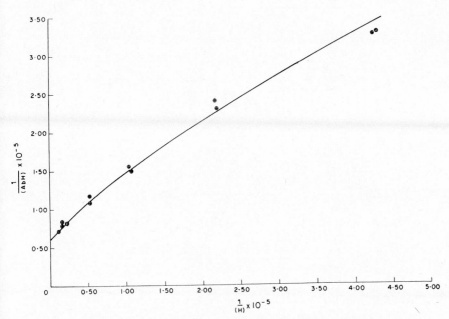

FIG. 14.10. Plot of the experimental data from Rabbit D [6] by Method B. The points are experimental and the curve is theoretical based upon the Sips distribution shown in Eq. 41. See Table 14.1. for the numerical values of the data.

When using Method B it can be seen from Fig. 14.10 that the extrapolated value of $1/(AbH)$ or $1/(Ab_t)$ is $0·580 \times 10^5$ litres/mole. Because this is a reciprocal plot the value of $1/(Ab_t)$ is multiplied by 2 giving the reciprocal value of half the total concentration of antibody-combining sites or $1·16 \times 10^5$ litres/mole. The corresponding value of $1/(H)$ is $0·589 \times 10^5$ litres/mole or $K_0 = 5·89 \times 10^4$ litres/mole. The value of n is obtained by dividing the total concentration of antibody-combining sites by the molar concentration of antibody molecules; $n = 17·24 \times 10^{-6}/7·0 \times 10^{-6} = 2·46$. Thus, as expected, both Methods A and B arrive at the same values of K_0 and n.

The indices of heterogeneity are determined as follows. For Method A the above values of K_0 and n are used to derive a series of theoretical curves for various values of σ from Table 14.2. The index of heterogeneity is that value of σ which yields a theoretical which best fits the experimental data. The curve drawn in Fig. 14.9 was derived from a value of $\sigma = 1\cdot80$. Figure 14.11

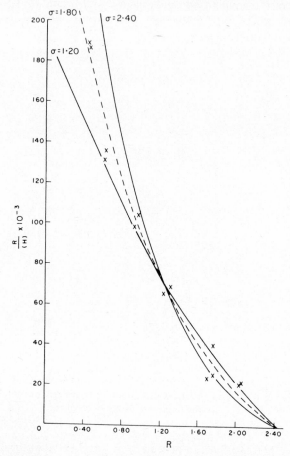

FIG. 14.11. Similar plot as in Fig. 14.10 but for various values of σ. Note that the theoretical curve derived when $\sigma = 1\cdot80$ best fits the experimental points.

shows theoretical curves for different values of σ and it can be seen that $\sigma = 1\cdot80$ gives the best fit.

When using Method B the experimental values of $1/(H)$ are raised to the fractional exponent α which can be varied from 0 to $1\cdot00$. The index of heterogeneity is that value of α which yields a modified curve of $1/(AbH)$ vs. $1/(H)\alpha$ closest to a straight line. Figure 14.12 shows such a plot for three values of α and a value of 0·80 gives the best straight line. The curve drawn in Fig. 14.10 is theoretical and was derived from the Sips equation using a value of 0·80 for α.

Although the preceding description is at first sight relatively straightforward, errors in the calculation of K_0 and n may arise if one extrapolates the binding curves by an inappropriate method. It can be seen in both 14.9 and 14.10 that a small variation in the extrapolated point of R or $1/(AbH)$ may have quite a large effect upon the values of K_0 and n, a larger effect being noted in

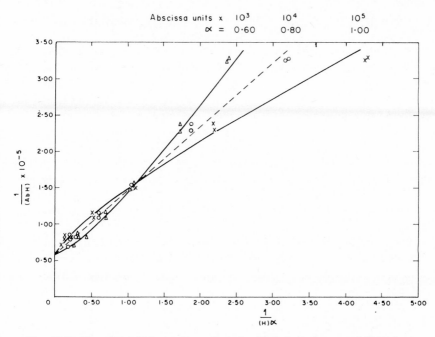

FIG. 14.12. Plot of Eq. 41 for various values of α. Note that when α = 0·80 the best straight line is obtained and this value is taken as the index of heterogeneity.

the more heterogeneous antisera. In view of these possible pitfalls this last section will be devoted to a discussion of the extrapolation procedure.

In an earlier section it was shown that in order to obtain a value of the *average* intrinsic association constant K_0 for a heterogeneous population of antibody-combining sites, either a Gaussian or Sips distribution function had to be assumed and theoretically there should be one and only one theoretical curve which should fit a particular set of binding data. There is undoubtedly much argument which could be raised against these last two points. First, simply due to experimental error it would be anticipated that a number of theoretical curves could be fitted equally well to a particular set of binding data. Second, the Gaussian and/or Sips distributions may not adequately describe the distribution of the apparent association constant K about K_0 thereby giving a value of K_0 which does not correspond to the apex of a more applicable distribution function and therefore not representing the actual value of the *average* intrinsic association constant. Unfortunately this last point has not been adequately tested, either because theoretical curves have not been compared to the experimental data, or because the binding curves have been measured over a small range of free hapten, e.g. only a ten-fold range.

Upon inspection of a set of binding data it is very tempting to use a linear form of extrapolation when plotting by either Method A or B. If the antibody population is relatively homogeneous the extrapolated point is likely to be correct; however, with a relatively heterogeneous antibody population linear extrapolation may not yield the best point and therefore the best values of K_0 and n. Because it has been assumed that both the Gaussian and Sips distributions are reasonably correct, these distribution functions themselves should be able to be used in aiding the extrapolation of the binding curves as $(H) \to \infty$. In fact, it is possible to process the binding data solely on a mathematical basis thereby eliminating graphing errors. The following suggestions are time-consuming because an iterative procedure is used; however, with the increased availability of computer services, a relatively simple program may be written thus eliminating the time-consuming, repetitive procedure described here.

The following discussion although placing more emphasis upon the more flexible Sips equation can be applied with some modification to the Gaussian distribution. Instead of deriving theoretical curves from Table 14.2 using the three variables K_0, n and σ, the Sips equation can be used in effect with only one variable, α; K_0 and n may be calculated from an equation modified from Eq. 26. By transforming Eq. 26 into the form of Eq. 16,

$$\frac{1}{(\text{AbH})} = \frac{1}{(\text{Ab}_t)\,K_0^\alpha\,(\text{H})^\alpha} + \frac{1}{(\text{Ab}_t)} \tag{41}$$

This equation is the one used in Fig. 14.12 to obtain the index of heterogeneity α. It should also be pointed out that the Sips equation may be applied to a Scatchard plot used in Method A.

The following is a suggested method for obtaining the values of K_0, (Ab_t) and α which best agree to theoretical values of K_0, (Ab_t) and α obtained from Eq. 41. The calculated experimental values of $1/(\text{H})$ and $1/(\text{AbH})$ are recorded on graph paper. If a straight line can be drawn through all of the points, the antibody is homogeneous and there is no difficulty in extrapolating; however, this is not the usual case. If the experimental points do not lie on a straight line, the Sips equation is used to determine the approximate value of α which yields, by visual inspection, a modified curve closest to a straight line. When this is completed, the best straight line through the points $1/(AbH)$ vs. $1/(H)^\alpha$ is determined by the method of least squares. The total concentration of antibody-combining sites (Ab_t) and value of K_0 can then be determined by the y intercept and slope of the line respectively. These values, however, are only a first approximation. There are certain complications, inherent in the method of least squares, which can arise at this point and therefore another method is needed to cross-check the values of K_0 and (Ab_t) obtained by the method of least squares, to see whether they agree with theoretical considerations of the Sips distribution. Dr Nisonoff [35] has suggested such a procedure which compares theoretical values of (AbH), obtained by the Sips equation, with the experimental values of (AbH). The approximated values of K_0, (Ab_t) and α, obtained by the method of least squares, together with the experimental values of (H) are substituted into either Eq. 26 or Eq. 41 and the theoretical values of (AbH) obtained. These theoretical values of (AbH) are then subtracted from the corresponding experimental values of (AbH) and the difference squared. The sums of the squares of the differences between the theoretical values of (AbH) and the experimental values of (AbH) are then determined. After this is done the entire procedure is repeated using a value of α which is ± 0.01 of the first approximation and the corresponding values of K_0 and (Ab_t) are obtained once again by the method of least squares. This is continued until values of α, K_0 and (Ab_t) are obtained which give the smallest value of the sums of the squares of the difference between the theoretical values of (AbH) and experimental values of (AbH).

The authors and Dr Nisonoff [35] are of the opinion that more emphasis should be placed upon the values of (AbH) at the higher free hapten concentrations (i.e. where greater than 40 per cent of the total concentration of antibody-combining sites are bound to hapten) because it is this portion of the curve which most markedly affects the value of K_0. Therefore it is recommended that the above procedures also be carried out for those points where greater than 40 per cent of the antibody-combining sites are bound to hapten. In our experience this last determination has aided in choosing between several values of α which give equal values for the sums of the squares of the difference between the theoretical values of (AbH) and experimental values of (AbH) when employing all of the points on the binding curve.

The method described above has been employed for the example in this chapter. After studying a wide range of values for K_0, (Ab_t) and α, it has been concluded that the values which best satisfy the above theoretical considerations of the Sips distribution are $K_0 = 5.89 \times 10^4$ litres/mole, $(Ab_t) = 17.24 \times 10^{-6}$ moles/litre, and $\alpha = 0.80$. The sums of the squares of the differences between the theoretical values of (AbH) and experimental values of (AbH)

for all fourteen points and the six points representing the highest free hapten concentration respectively are $3 \cdot 25 \times 10^{-12}$ moles^2/litre^2 and $2 \cdot 89 \times 40^{-12}$ moles^2/litre^2. This procedure is unfortunately time-consuming, but with a little experience of the method, the entire procedure should take no more than from 1 to 2 hours using a desk calculator, and it is felt that this method is a satisfactory and accurate way of processing binding data. If one plans extensive work employing equilibrium dialysis, a computer could relieve the worker of much of the burden of calculation.

It should be stressed once again that at present it is not known whether either the Gaussian and/or Sips distributions adequately describe the heterogeneity of the antibody–hapten interaction. In the authors' experience within the experimental error for determining the free and bound hapten concentrations, both distribution functions appear to be close approximations; however, the number of data processed have been relatively small.

It is suggested that reports which employ equilibrium dialysis should give detailed account of the method(s) for extrapolating and if possible give the raw experimental data. If this is done, various reports may be more easily correlated with one another which will enable a standardized method for extrapolation to be developed. Lastly, it is felt that there is a need to analyse statistically the experimental data with respect to experimental errors and such analysis used to calculate the average intrinsic association constant and indices of heterogeneity.

Acknowledgments

The authors thank Mr D. Kershaw of the Edinburgh University Department of Computer Science without whose help the calculation of Table 14.1 would not have been possible.

We wish to thank Dr Alfred Nisonoff for advice concerning the Sips distribution, for helpful comment on the last section of this chapter and for allowing us to use the data from Rabbit D as an example.

References

[1] MARRACK J. & SMITH F.C. (1932) Quantitative aspects of immunity reactions: The combination of antibodies with simple haptens. *Brit. J. expt. Path.* **13,** 394

[2] HAUROWITZ F. & BREINL F. (1933) Chemische Untersuchung der spezifischen Bindung von Arsanil—Eiweiss und Arsanilsäure an Immunserum. *Z. Physial. Chem.* **214,** 111

[3] EISEN H.N. & KARUSH F. (1949) The interaction of purified antibody with homologous hapten. Antibody valence and binding constant. *J. Am. chem. Soc.* **71,** 363

[4] KARUSH F. (1956) The interaction of purified antibody with optically isomeric haptens. *J. Am. chem. Soc.* **78**, 5519

[5] KARUSH F. (1957) The interaction of purified anti-B-lactoside antibody with haptens. *J. Am. chem. Soc.* **79**, 3380

[6] NISONOFF A. & PRESSMAN D. (1958) Heterogeneity and average combining constants of antibodies from individual rabbits. *J. Immunol.* **80**, 417

[7] KLOTZ I.M. (1953) Proteins interactions. In *The Proteins*, Vol. I, Part B, ed. NEURATH H. & BAILEY K. New York: Academic Press Inc.

[8] KABAT E.A. & MAYER M.M. (1961) *Experimental Immunochemistry*, 2nd edition. Springfield, Illinois: C.C.Thomas

[9] KARUSH F. (1962) *Immunologic Specificity and Molecular Structure in Advances in Immunology*, Vol. 2, ed. TALIAFERRO W.H. & HUMPHREY J.H. New York: Academic Press

[10] SINGER S.J. (1965) Structure and function of antigen and antibody proteins. In *The Proteins*, Vol. III, 2nd edition, ed. NEURATH H. New York: Academic Press

[11] KARUSH F. (1959) Quantitative measurement of heterogeneity among antibodies. In *Mechanisms of Hypersensitivity*, ed. SHAFFER J.H., LE GRIPPE G.A., & CHASE M.W.J. London: A. Churchill Ltd

[12] LANGMUIR I. (1918) The absorption of gases on plane surfaces of glass, mica and platinum. *J. Am. chem. Soc.* **40**, 1361

[13] SCATCHARD G. (1949) The attractions of proteins for small molecules and ions. *Ann. N.Y. Acad. Sci.* **51**, 660

[14] PAULING L., PRESSMAN D. & GROSSBERG A.L. (1944) The serological properties of simple substances. VII. A quantitative theory of the inhibition by haptens of the precipitation of heterogeneous antisera with antigens, and comparisons with experimental results for polyhaptenic simple substances and for azoproteins. *J. Am. chem. Soc.* **66**, 784

[15] KARUSH F. & SONENBERG M. (1949) Interaction of homologous alkyl sulfates with BSA. *J. Am. chem. Soc.* **71**, 1369

[16] KARUSH F. (1950) Heterogeneity of binding sites of bovine serum albumin. *J. Am. chem. Soc.* **72**, 2705

[17] SIPS R. (1949) On the structure of a catalyst surface. *J. Chem. Phys.* **16**, 490

[18] KLOTZ I.M. (1957) *Energetics in Biochemical Reactions*. New York: Academic Press

[19] EDSALL J.T. & WYMAN J. (1958) *Biophysical Chemistry*, Vol. I, Chapter 4, Thermodynamics. New York: Academic Press

[20] KAUZMAN W. (1959) *Adv. in Protein Chem.* **14**, 1. *Some Factors in the Interpretation of Protein Denaturation*, ed. ANFINSEN C.B., ANSON M.L., BAILEY K. & EDSALL J.T. New York: Academic Press

[21] GURNEY R.W. (1953) *Ionic Processes in Solution*. New York: McGraw-Hill

[22] SINGER S.J. & CAMPBELL D.H. (1953) Physical chemical studies of soluble antigen–antibody complexes. II. Equilibrium properties. *J. Am. chem. Soc.* **75**, 5577

[23] LANDSTEINER K. (1946) *The Specificity of Serological Reactions*, revised edition. Cambridge, Mass.: Harvard University Press

[24] GELEWITZ E.W., RIEDEMAN W.L. & KLOTZ I.M. (1954) Some quantitative aspects of the reaction of diazonium compounds with serum albumin. *Arch. Biophys.* **53**, 411

[25] TABACHNICK M. & SOBOTKA H. (1960) Azoproteins. II. A spectrophotometric study of the coupling of diazotized arsanilic acid with proteins. *J.B.C.* **235**, 1051

[26] KARUSH F. & EISEN H.N. (1962) A theory of delayed hypersensitivity. *Science* **136**, 1032

[27] CARSTEN M.E. & EISEN H.N. (1955) The specific interaction of some dinitrobenzenes with rabbit antibody to dinitrophenyl, bovine-γ-globulin. *J. Am. chem. Soc.* **77**, 1273

[28] VELICK S.F., PARKER C.W. & EISEN H.N. (1960) Excitation energy transfer and the quantitative study of the antibody hapten reaction. *Proc. nat. Acad. Sci. (Wash.)* **46**, 1470

[29] KEKWICK R.A. (1940) The serum proteins in multiple myelomatosis. *Biochem. J.* **34**, 1248

[30] SINGER S.J., FOTHERGILL J.E. & SHAINOFF J.R. (1960) A general method for the isolation of antibodies. *J. Am. chem. Soc.* **82**, 565

[31] CAMPBELL D.H., GARVEY J.S., CREMER N.E. & SUSSDORF D.H. (1963) *Methods in Immunology.* New York: W.A.Benjamin, Inc.

[32] BLAU M., JOHNSON A.C. & PRESSMAN D. (1958) p-Iodobenzoyl groups as a paired label for in vivo protein distribution studies: Specific localization of anti-tissue antibodies. *International Journal of Applied Radiation and Isotopes*, **3**, 217

[33] NISONOFF A. & PRESSMAN D. (1958) Heterogeneity of antibody sites in their relative combining affinities for structurally related haptens. *J. Immunol.* **81**, 126

[34] NISONOFF A. & PRESSMAN D. (1959) Studies on the combining site of anti-p-azobenzoate antibody. Loss precipitation and binding capacities through different mechanisms on acetylation. *J. Immunol.* **83**, 138

[35] NISONOFF A., Personal communication

[36] EISEN H.N. & SISKIND G.W. (1964) Variations in affinities of antibodies during the immune response. *Biochemistry* **3**, 996

CHAPTER 15

Immunoferritin Technique for the Identification of Antigens by Electron Microscopy

GIUSEPPE A.ANDRES, KONRAD C.HSU &
BEATRICE CARRIER SEEGAL

A. Introduction

Coons developed the immunofluorescein technique in which antibody labelled with fluorescein is used as an immunologic tool to identify antigens within tissues [1, 2]. He described this technique as a visible microprecipitin test [3]. When the fluorescein-labelled antibody is brought into contact with its corresponding antigen in smears of cells or in tissue sections it is specifically bound and the microprecipitin reaction can be seen by viewing the slide with the ultra-violet light microscope. The brilliant green areas of fluorescence identify sites of the antigen–antibody reaction. This technique has added a new dimension to the field of immunology.

In almost the same period of time the study of the fine structure of cells by electron microscopy has made great progress. Since the resolution of the electron microscope is much greater than that of the light microscope it is obviously desirable to label and thus render visible individual antibody molecules so as to identify antigen in cells at the molecular level.

Singer [4] conjugated globulins with an electron-dense marker, ferritin, without loss of immunologic activity. The introduction of this method extended the usefulness of the visible microprecipitin test to the identification and localization of antigens at the ultrastructural level.

B. Preparation of ferritin-conjugated antibody

I. *Coupling agent*

Two protein molecules can be coupled together by the use of a bifunctional reagent of low molecular weight under conditions which favour the reaction with protein molecules. Singer [4] first employed metaxylylene diisocyanate (XC) and later suggested toluene 2,4-diisocyanate (TC) [5], each in a two-step reaction. Sri Ram *et al* [6] used p,p'-difluoro-m,m'-dinitrodiphenyl sulphone (FNPS) in a one-step procedure. Other agents such as toluene-2-isocyanate-4-

isothiocyanate, 3-methoxydiphenylmethane-4,4′diisocyanate [5], benzidine di-isocyanate, 1,5-naphthalenedisulphonyl chloride [7] and 3,6-bis (acetato-mercurimethyl) dioxane (AMMD) [8] have been tested for use in the two-stage procedure. Borek & Silverstein [7] and Isliker *et al* [8] have found that the yields with XC are higher and give more satisfactory results. XC* is a clear colourless solution free of precipitates. Polymerization sometimes occurs during storage, however, and is indicated by precipitation. Under such circumstances the compound must be redistilled before use. To minimize polymerization, which is rapid when the reagent is exposed to air, XC should be transferred immediately in 0·1 ml amounts to melting-point capillary tubes, sealed and stored at 4° C.

II. *Purification of immune globulin*
Since only part of the globulin is conjugated, specific antisera of high titre are essential. If the serum contains unwanted antibodies, it is necessary to remove them by absorption with appropriate antigens. The globulin fraction of the antiserum is then separated by precipitation in 1·436 M sodium sulphate [9]. Further purification of the globulin can be accomplished by using a column of DEAE-cellulose to separate γG (7S) and γM (19S) [10]. Both γG and γM have been satisfactorily labelled. Fragments I and II, obtained by papain digestion, have been also coupled to ferritin [8].

III. *Purification of ferritin*
Ferritin is an iron-containing protein that is characterized by its high electron density. It has a protein shell, with a diameter of 100–120 Å, which envelops an inner core of ferric hydroxide micells of 55–60 Å in diameter [11]. The molecular weight of ferritin is approximately 750,000 [12]. Its iron content averages 23 per cent. Despite the low atomic number of iron as compared with that of mercury or uranium [13, 14] the 2000–3000 atoms of iron in a molecule of ferritin confer a very high electron density [15]. Ferritin can be obtained from many animal sources. Although commercial horse spleen ferritin solution of good quality can be purchased from many suppliers, it must be further purified in order to get the fraction that yields optimum results in electron microscopy.

(a) *Recrystallization*. Ferritin is purified by recrystallization and repreciptation. In the first step the concentrated ferritin solution is diluted to a 1 to 2 per cent solution with 2 per cent ammonium sulphate, pH 5·85. The pH is critical. Twenty per cent cadmium sulphate is added until a final concentration of 5 per cent cadmium sulphate is reached in the diluted ferritin solution. The mixture is placed in the cold for 2 hours or more to complete crystallization. After centrifugation the brown supernatant fluid containing non-

* Polysciences, Inc., Rydal, Penn.

crystallizable ferritin is discarded. The dark-coloured crystals are redissolved in 2 per cent ammonium sulphate and the solution is again centrifuged to remove any insoluble material. The clear supernatant fluid is decanted and the ferritin is recrystallized in 5 per cent cadmium sulphate. The crystallization procedure should be repeated until microscopic examination shows only typical orange-brown ferritin crystals as illustrated in Fig. 15.1. Usually five to seven recrystallizations are required.

(b) *Reprecipitation*. The purified ferritin crystals are redissolved in 2 per cent ammonium sulphate and amorphous ferritin is precipitated three times with

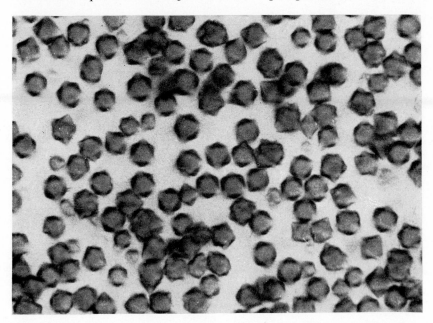

Fig. 15.1. Crystalline horse spleen ferritin purified by repeated recrystallization with cadmium sulphate. Magnification 560×.

ammonium sulphate at 50 per cent saturation. This procedure removes the free cadmium ions and also converts ferritin into a stable form. After adding a small amount of water to the final precipitate, the concentrated suspension is dialysed against running cold water until it is salt free, and then against 0·05 M phosphate buffer, pH 7·5, in the cold overnight.

(c) *Ultracentrifugation*. The purified cadmium-free ferritin is ultracentrifuged at 100,000 g for 2 hours. The upper three-quarters of the fluid in the centrifuge tube, which is colourless, is discarded. The pellet and the suspension of concentrated ferritin of high iron content in the bottom quarter of the tube will be completely dissolved after incubation overnight at 4° C.

(d) *Sterilization.* The concentrated purified ferritin is sterilized by passing it through a millipore filter. Sterile ferritin solution stored at 4° C remains stable for years but it cannot be frozen or lyophilized without deterioration.

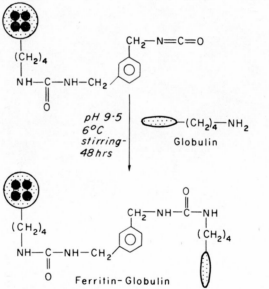

Fig. 15.2. Diagram illustrating the conjugation of ferritin to globulin in a two-step reaction with XC as the coupling agent.

IV. *Conjugation of ferritin with globulin in a two-step process*

XC and TC are the coupling agents which are currently in use for the preparation of ferritin–globulin conjugates. XC has been more extensively employed and Fig. 15.2 shows the reaction of this reagent with ferritin and globulin. The two-step procedure is carried out as follows:

(a) *First stage.* The coupling agent is first linked to ferritin by forming the ferritin-XC-mono-ureido or ferritin-TC-mono-ureido-substituted compound through one of its isocyanate groups and the ε amino group of ferritin.

1. XC. The purified ferritin is mixed, in an ice-bath, with 0·05 M phosphate buffer pH 7·5 and 0·3 M borate buffer pH 9·5 in volumes calculated to achieve a final concentration of 20–25 mg per ml of ferritin in 0·1 M borate buffer. XC is added to the mixture in the proportion of 0·1 ml per 100 mg of ferritin. The mixture is stirred vigorously in an ice-bath on a magnetic stirrer for 45 minutes and then is centrifuged at 4° C and 1500 *g* for 30 minutes. The clear brown supernatant fluid is pipetted off and placed in an ice-bath for 1 hour to complete the reaction.

2. TC. The procedure in the preparation of TC conjugates differs from that used with XC conjugates (see above) in some important details. TC, being solid when stored under refrigeration, is first melted at room temperature and then added to a 2–2·5 per cent solution of purified ferritin in 0·05 M phosphate buffer pH 7·5 in the proportion of 0·1 ml per 100 mg of ferritin. The mixture is stirred in an ice-bath on a magnetic stirrer for 25 minutes. It is then centrifuged at 4° C and 1500 *g* for 30 minutes. The supernatant fluid is pipetted off and placed in an ice-bath for 1 hour.

(b) *Second stage.* The ferritin intermediate obtained either from XC (B IV a 1) or TC (B IV a 2), is then conjugated with the antibody through ureido linkage of the remaining unreacted isocyanate groups with ε amino groups of the globulin.

Immune globulin is added to the reacted ferritin solution, containing the ferritin-intermediate, in the proportion of 1 part of globulin to 4 parts of ferritin by weight. Fresh borate buffer is added to maintain 0·1 molarity and pH 9·5. When XC is used in the first stage, the mixture is stirred gently with a magnetic stirrer for 48 hours at 4° C. If TC is used in the first stage, the mixture is stirred for 1 hour at 37° C.

The yield of ferritin-globulin depends upon the presence of the unreacted isocyanate group in the ferritin-intermediate and its subsequent reaction with the second protein. Portions of both antibody and ferritin in the reaction mixture remain unconjugated.

V. *Removal of the unconjugated antibody*

The mixture of ferritin-conjugate, unconjugated protein and unconjugated ferritin is centrifuged three times at 100,000 *g* for 4½ hours each time. After each run the heavier conjugated protein and unconjugated ferritin, which form a pellet, are resuspended in 0·05 M phosphate buffer at pH 7·5. The pellet obtained after the final run is incubated with a small amount of phosphate buffer at 4° C overnight. The resulting solution is passed through a bacterial millipore filter and stored at 4° C in a sterile container. Conjugates thus

S

stored for over a year have given satisfactory results. As will be seen later, no detectable unconjugated antibody remains in these preparations. The same results may be achieved by sucrose density gradient centrifugation [16].

VI. *Removal of unconjugated ferritin*
Conjugated globulin can be separated from unconjugated ferritin by continuous-flow or starch-block electrophoresis and recovered by ultracentrifugation [7]. In the experience of the authors, however, unconjugated ferritin has not interfered with the specific binding of the conjugate.

VII. *Conjugation of ferritin with globulin in a single-step process*
Sri Ram *et al* [6] have used p,p′-difluoro-m,m′-dinitro diphenyl sulphone (FNPS) as the coupling agent in a single-step procedure for the conjugation of ferritin with antibody. After a thorough study of factors important in the use of this reagent, they recommended the following procedure: To a mixture of 160 mg of rabbit globulin and 460 mg of ferritin, cold 2 per cent aqueous sodium carbonate is added to constitute a 4 per cent protein solution. Then 5 mg of FNPS in 1 ml of chilled acetone is added and stirred in the cold (2–4° C) for 24 hours. Subsequently after exhaustive dialysis against normal saline the mixture is centrifuged to remove a small precipitate.

C. Testing conjugate before use in electron microscopy

Many factors can affect the success of immunoferritin experiments by electron microscopy. Negative findings may result from an antiserum of insufficient titre, unsatisfactory labelling of the antibody or inadequate treatment of the specimen with the ferritin conjugate. It is recommended that one or both of the following tests be applied to the conjugates before they are used.

I. *Immunoelectrophoretic analysis*
Ferritin-conjugated globulin is faster than γ globulin and slower than the ferritin–xylylene intermediate in its electrophoretic mobility. Borek & Silverstein [7] reported that the electrophoretic mobilities of the components of a crude ferritin–rabbit antiovalbumin conjugate at pH 8·6 were as follows:

Component	Mobility $\times 10^5$ $cm^2\ V^{-1}\ sec^{-1}$
Rabbit γ globulin (slow, colourless)	1·49
Conjugate (intermediate, coloured)	4·54
Treated ferritin (fast, coloured)	6·85
Untreated ferritin	4·47

Isliker *et al* [8] reported that, as demonstrated with a rabbit anti-ferritin serum, treatment with XC confers on ferritin a high electrophoretic mobility which is due to significant binding of isocyanate groups with concomitant increase of the negative charge of ferritin. After the second stage (incubation with γ globulin) the electrophoretic mobility of the conjugate is reduced to that of the native ferritin. The non-coupled but XC-treated ferritin retains its high

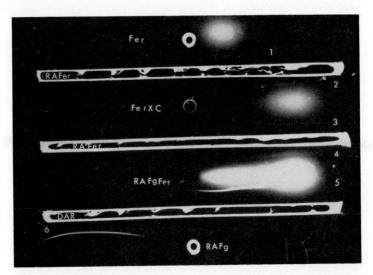

FIG. 15.3. Agar gel slide 2 × 3 in. Ferritin (Fer) in top well; ferritin-XC derivative (FerXC) in second well; ferritin conjugate, containing ferritin-labelled rabbit antibody to human fibrinogen (RAFgFer) and FerXC in third well; unlabelled rabbit antibody (RAFg) in bottom well. These preparations were electrophoresed for 2 hours and 15 minutes at 11 mA, pH 8·2. The pattern developed in 18 hours against antibody to ferritin (RAFer in top and middle troughs) and duck antibody to rabbit globulin (DAR in bottom trough). Slide photographed unwashed. Blobs in agar gel represent positions to which reagents containing ferritin migrated in electrophoretic field.

mobility. By immunoelectrophoretic analysis it can be ascertained whether the 'ferritin conjugate' is present and whether the conjugated antibody is still reactive with its specific antigen. This is illustrated in Figs. 15.3 and 15.4.

Figure 15.3 shows the pattern of an immunoelectrophoretic analysis of pure ferritin (Fer) in the top well; ferritin-XC-derivative (FerXC) in the second well; ferritin conjugate containing ferritin-labelled rabbit antibody to human fibrinogen (RAFgFer) and FerXC in the third well; and unlabelled rabbit antibody to human fibrinogen* (RAFg) in the bottom well. These

* The antiserum to human fibrinogen was prepared and absorbed with lyophilized aged human serum in the laboratory of Dr Gorstein, New York University School of Medicine.

four reactants were subjected to electrophoresis for 2·25 hours. The top and middle troughs were then filled with antiserum to ferritin prepared in the rabbit (RAFer) and the bottom trough was filled with duck antiserum to rabbit globulin (DAR). After 18 hours of incubation lines of precipitation appeared as follows:

(a) Arc 1 produced by Fer against RAFer in the β region;

(b) Arcs 2 and 3 developed by FerXC against RAFer in the albumin area;

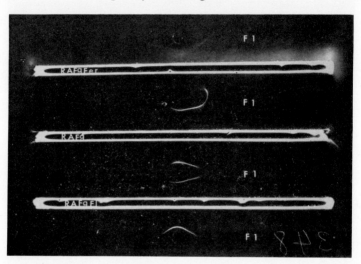

FIG. 15.4. Agar gel slide 2 × 3 in. Human serum Fraction I (FI) in four central wells was electrophoresed for 2 hours and 15 minutes. The line of precipitation developed in 3 days against ferritin-conjugated antibody against human fibrinogen (RAFgFer in top trough), unlabelled antibody (RAFg in middle trough) and fluorescein-labelled antibody (RAFgFl in bottom trough). Slide photographed after 1 week washing. Agar gel still retained some brownish tint of ferritin. Lines of precipitation with reagents containing ferritin were brownish in colour.

(c) A biphasic line of precipitation, Arc 4, between RAFgFer and RAFer, wherein the more rapid component exhibits the same mobility as Arcs 2 and 3, and represents FerXC, and the slower component in the β region corresponds to Arc 5, produced by RAFgFer against DAR, and represents the conjugated antibody (Arc 5 would have extended to the cathodal region of γ globulin if there were any unconjugated antibody in RAFgFer); and

(d) Arc 6 developed by the unconjugated RAFg against DAR in the normal γ position.

Figure 15.4 shows that the labelled antibody is still reactive with its specific antigen. After electrophoresis of Cohn's human serum Fraction I in the four central wells, the upper trough was filled with RAFgFer, the middle trough with RAFg and the bottom trough with fluorescein-labelled antibody to human fibrinogen (RAFgFl). The precipitin arcs indicate that the ferritin-conjugated antibody, the fluorescein-labelled antibody and the unlabelled antibody to human fibrinogen all reacted with the specific antigen, fibrinogen.

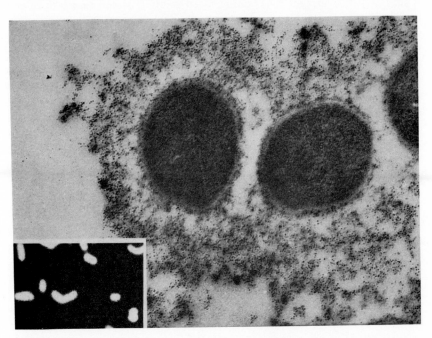

Fig. 15.5. The main picture is an electron micrograph of pneumococci type 18 treated with fluorescein-ferritin doubly labelled specific antibody. Capsular material swollen as a result of the reaction with antibody. Ferritin-labelled antibody molecules are distributed throughout the capsule. Magnification 60,000 ×. The inset is a picture of pneumococci type 18 stained with fluorescein-ferritin doubly labelled antibody as seen with ultra-violet light microscope. Magnification 800 ×.

II. *Studies with immunofluorescein technique in relation to the immunoferritin technique*

(a) *Sequential labelling of antibodies with ferritin fluorescein.* Rabbit antibodies to Group A β haemolytic streptococcus, pneumococcus type 2, pneumococcus type 18, [17] *Veillonella* endotoxin, [18] and reovirus, [19] as well as duck antibody to rabbit globulin, [20] have been sequentially labelled with fluorescein and ferritin. In the procedure of doubly labelling the antibody, the ferritin-conjugated globulin can be labelled with fluorescein by using fluorescein isothiocyanate according to the method of Riggs & Marshall [21, 22] (see Holborow & Johnson, Chapter 16). After dialysing the resulting mixture in 0·05 M phosphate buffer, pH 7·5, in the cold until no fluorescence is seen in ultra-violet light, it is centrifuged sequentially three times at 100,000 *g* for 4½ hours each time in the same manner as described in B V above. After the final run a small quantity of phosphate buffer is added to the pellet which is kept at 4° C overnight. The homogenized solution is then passed through a bacterial millipore filter and stored at 4° C in sterile containers.

Alternatively, fluorescein-labelled immune globulin, after being passed through a Sephadex column [23], can be substituted for the unlabelled globulin to react with the ferritin–xylylene intermediate in the conjugation procedure (B IV b). This product is dialysed, centrifuged and recovered as in the case of singly labelled ferritin conjugate. Irrespective of which label is conjugated to the globulin first, immunologic activity is maintained. Immunoelectrophoretic analyses and other immunologic tests have confirmed the observation that the immune globulins are conjugated to both labels without loss of specific activity. Moreover, these preparations are as specific in immunofluorescent and immune electron microscopic studies as are the singly labelled antibodies. Figure 15.5 is an electron micrograph of pneumococcus type 18 treated with its specific fluorescein-ferritin-labelled antibody. Capsular material is swollen as a result of its reaction with antibody. Ferritin-labelled antibody molecules are distributed throughout the capsule. The inset shows a smear of the organism, stained with the doubly labelled reagent and examined by ultra-violet light. The pairs and short chains of pneumococci are fluorescent. This technique of doubly labelling the antibody permits the relatively simple method of immunofluorescence to be used as a screen in selecting optimal conjugates of ferritin and antibody for subsequent study by electron microscopy [24].

(b) *Usefulness of immunofluorescence studies as an adjunct to immunoferritin studies.* The objective of the immunoferritin technique is to localize the sites of antigen–antibody reaction in the fine structure of the tissue, but electron microscopic study without previous knowledge derived from the immuno-fluorescein technique at the level of light microscopy is often difficult to interpret. The general area of tissue where the antigen–antibody reaction takes place can first be sought with the fluorescent antibody. The potency and specificity of the antiserum used in the investigation can be readily determined with the immunofluorescent technique. A variety of controls can be easily run with the simple method of immunofluorescence. Therefore, it is recommended that a thorough study by the immunofluorescein technique should precede most experiments in which electron microscopy is used.

D. Treatment of specimens with ferritin-conjugated antibody

Three factors must be considered in the preparation of specimens for treatment with ferritin-conjugated antibody: the maintenance of cellular fine structure; the preservation of antigenic determinants; and the penetration of large ferritin molecules into the cells. The ideal solution to the problems would be to stain embedded thin sections directly before examining them in the electron microscope. The usual embedding procedure, however, either greatly diminishes or eradicates the capacity of the antigen to react with antibody [25, 26]. The commonly used embedding polymers and the copper grids also show an electrostatic attraction which causes non-specific binding of ferritin molecules [26, 27]. Consequently, the method usually employed is to prefix the specimen in reagents which do not affect the antigenic determinants but still preserve the fine structure sufficiently for electron microscopic evaluation.

I. *Pre-fixation*

Among the fixatives that have been tried, only a few have proved to be satisfactory. *Osmium tetroxide* [28], usually employed in conventional electron microscopy, has been shown to rapidly destroy the specificity of most, if not all, antigens [25, 29, 30]. To date only certain antigenic determinants of bacteria have been reported to be unaffected by osmium fixation [26]. *Potassium permanganate* has been found to denature all antigens tested [26]. Two per cent *acrolein* so damages the antigen that very faint fluorescence results in specimens fixed for 10 minutes [19]. Exposure to 6·5 per cent *glutaraldehyde* for 20 minutes reduces the capacity of antigens in renal tissue to react with antibody and seems to prevent adequate penetration of the conjugates [31]. In experiments concerning localization of fibrinogen products, however, the tissue has been fixed in 6·5 per cent gluteraldehyde for 10 minutes with fair results [32]. Glutaraldehyde in a concentration of 1·0 per cent reduces binding of fluorescent antibody to virus-infected cells after 10 minutes, although exposures for 5 minutes have given satisfactory results [19]. Dilute *formalin*, however, has proved to be the fixative which most adequately fufils the requirements of the immunoferritin technique [25, 29, 30]. Five per cent formalin phosphate, buffered at pH 7·2, when used to pre-fix cultured cells or small pieces of tissue at 0° C, even up to 24 hours, helps to maintain fine structure without inactivating the antigens so far tested. After treatment with the ferritin-conjugated antibody further fixation with osmium tetroxide or with glutaraldehyde followed by osmium is essential in order to preserve fine structure.

Certain studies dealing with the identification of an antibody reaction on cell surfaces may be carried out without pre-fixation [33, 36].

II. *Localization of surface antigens*

The localization of surface antigens in membranes, tissue-cultured cells or suspended cells, may be accomplished by simple immersion in the specific ferritin conjugate for 5–20 minutes at room temperature [37, 34, 38]. Prior fixation in 10 per cent or 0·25 per cent buffered formalin at pH 7·2 is suggested in order to preserve internal structures and in some instances to prevent pinocytosis of the conjugates [25, 27, 39].

III. *Localization of intracellular antigens in free cells*

Ferritin-labelled antibody, due to its large size, does not penetrate untreated cells [29]. In order to open the plasma membranes and make the cells permeable to the conjugates several methods have been employed. One technique that has given satisfactory results in staining intracellular antigen is the follow-

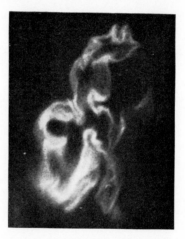

Fig. 15.6. A small fragment of renal cortex from the kidney of a rat injected with rabbit anti-rat kidney serum. The specimen was fixed at 0° C in 5 per cent formalin buffered with phosphates at pH 7·2, cut by hand under a dissecting microscope, and stained with fluorescein-labelled duck antibody to rabbit globulin. The fluorescence is evident. Magnification 1400× [Andres G.A. *et al*, 30].

ing [29]: The cells are fixed for 5 minutes in 5 per cent formalin buffered with phosphates at pH 7·2, frozen in a carbon dioxide-ethyl alcohol bath, and cut, while still frozen, in a cryostat. The thawed sections, 10 μ thick, are immersed in the ferritin-conjugated antibody at room temperature for 10–30 minutes and then washed three times with cold buffer, centrifuged at 3800 rev/min for 5 minutes, fixed in glutaraldehyde and in osmium tetroxide, dehydrated, and embedded in plastic. Sufficient opening of the cellular membranes may be obtained for tissue-cultured cells simply by freezing and thawing [40]. In another method that has been proposed, the cells, after formalin fixation, are disrupted by gentle homogenization and then are treated with the conjugates [41]. Pre-treatment of infected cells with 4×10^{-5} digitonin solution in phosphate-buffered saline at pH 7·0 has been reported to be effective in permitting penetration of conjugated anti-reovirus serum [19]. The addition of complement to ferritin-conjugated cytotoxic antibody when applied to the specific substrate increased permeability of the cell membranes [35, 56].

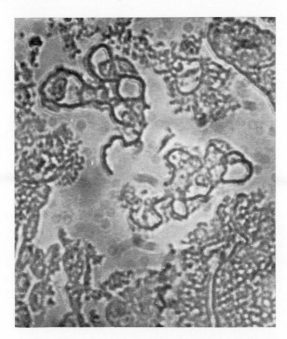

Fig. 15.7. A phase-contrast photograph of methacrylate-embedded renal tissue from the same rat illustrated in Fig. 15.6, but treated with ferritin-conjugated antibody. The picture illustrates the fine fragmentation which is necessary for adequate penetration of the ferritin conjugates. Glomerular parts are in the centre and tubular parts are visible. Magnification 840× [Andres G.A. *et al*, 30].

IV. *Localization of intra- or intercellular antigens in tissue*
Localization of such antigens in solid tissue presents other problems and the following technique has been proposed [42, 30]. Pieces of tissue, not more than 2 × 10 mm, are first fixed for 40–60 minutes at 4° C in 5 per cent formalin buffered with phosphates at pH 7·2, followed by washing in cold buffer. They are then finely minced with a sharp razor blade under the dissecting microscope in the cold room (Fig. 15.6). The mincing may also be performed by using a cutting machine.* The fragments are suspended in test-tubes containing ferritin-conjugated antibodies, and occasionally agitated for 20 minutes at room temperature. After being washed three times in a large

* H. Mickle, Gomshall, Surrey, England.

S*

volume of cold buffer they are centrifuged at 3000 rev/min. The final pellet is fixed for 30 minutes in osmium, or for 20 minutes in glutaraldehyde and then in osmium, dehydrated in graded acetone or ethyl alcohol and embedded in Vestopal W, Araldite or Epon 812 [42, 30]. For isolating particular structures in the tissue, such as glomeruli, 0.5μ sections are cut and stained with toluidine blue, or directly observed in a phase-contrast microscope (Fig. 15.7). The blocks are then trimmed and thin-sectioned for electron microscopy. Although not all cells are opened by the fine cutting technique, penetration of the ferritin-conjugated antibody is sufficient to achieve satisfactory localization of the intra- and intercellular antigens, while the fine structure of the tissue is satisfactorily preserved.

As an alternative to this method of manual sectioning after formalin fixation, the tissue may be quickly frozen in a dry ice–alcohol bath and sectioned in a cryostat at 10–50μ thickness. The sections are then immersed in the ferritin-conjugated antibody, washed, fixed in gluteraldehyde and osmium tetroxide, and finally embedded in plastic [39].

V. *Indirect technique*
Ferritin-labelled antibody is applied directly to specimens in all the techniques described above (D II, III, IV). The indirect or two-layer technique has also been used [36, 43–45]. In this method the specimen is first incubated with unlabelled specific antibody which combines with its homologous antigen in the tissue. After washing off the excess unlabelled antibody it is treated with ferritin-conjugated antibody to γ globulin of the species of animal in which the specific antibody has been prepared. The localization of ferritin indicates the sites of the first antigen–antibody reaction (Fig. 15.16). The indirect method is convenient because only one ferritin conjugate is required for the study of many specific antibodies provided that all of these are prepared in the same species [46]. Another advantage is that a specific antiserum of relatively low antibody titre can still be used effectively in the two-layer technique [7]. The direct technique, however, is generally preferred because it is easier to set up proper controls, and additional manipulations which may produce artefacts are avoided.

VI. *Controls to establish the specificity of the immunoferritin technique*
The controls routinely employed in immunoferritin studies fall into three categories: specific immunologic 'blocking' of the reaction; treatment of the duplicate pieces of tissue with non-specific ferritin conjugates; and treatment of similar but not identical tissue with the specific ferritin conjugates.

(a) 'Blocking' controls are carried out in one of two ways. In the first a duplicate piece of the tissue under study is treated with an unconjugated portion of the specific antibody. After about 30 minutes this is washed off and the tissue is then treated with the ferritin conjugate in the same manner used for the original test. The unconjugated antibody should almost completely block the binding of the conjugated antibody. Because antigen–antibody reactions are in equilibrium, a few of the unconjugated antibodies may be replaced by conjugated antibodies. The second control test, which can be considered to belong in this category, is accomplished by absorbing the specific ferritin-conjugated antibody with the specific antigen. Pieces of the tissue are tested simultaneously with the absorbed and unabsorbed ferritin conjugates. The absorbed conjugate should not be bound in the tissue. This control is only applicable when a suitable preparation of the antigen in question is available.

(b) Treatment with ferritin-labelled antibody not specific for antigens present in the test tissue, is useful to establish the fact that the conditions of the experiment do not promote non-specific binding of ferritin–globulin conjugates. In addition to or in place of the non-specific ferritin–globulin conjugate, pure ferritin, and ferritin-XC-derivative (FerXC) are frequently employed.

(c) The third control is the treatment of similar but not identical tissue with the specific conjugate. Studies of viruses may be controlled by testing the ferritin conjugate on tissues infected with other viruses than the one under investigation. Similarly, heterologous strains of bacteria can be used to establish the specificity of the binding of a conjugate. In the study of diseased tissue such as renal tissue from human glomerulonephritis the specific conjugates used are tested on normal renal tissue and also on renal tissue from patients with renal disease other than glomerulonephritis. The choice of appropriate controls in this category depends on the individual experiment.

E. Applications of the immunoferritin technique

The immunoferritin technique has been in use for 5 years. During this brief period it has been applied to a wide variety of problems which include the identification of viral antigens; the localization of surface antigens on bacteria, red blood cells, ascites tumour cells, sea urchin sperm and eggs; the production by cell of antibodies, basement membranes, enzymes; the structural position of fibrinogen in clot formation; studies on the mechanisms of certain experimental and human diseases. Information concerning experiments in each of these fields of investigation is presented and Table 15.1 summarizes the reports available to date.

I. *Viral structure and development*
Before studies with immunoferritin became possible, morphologic information

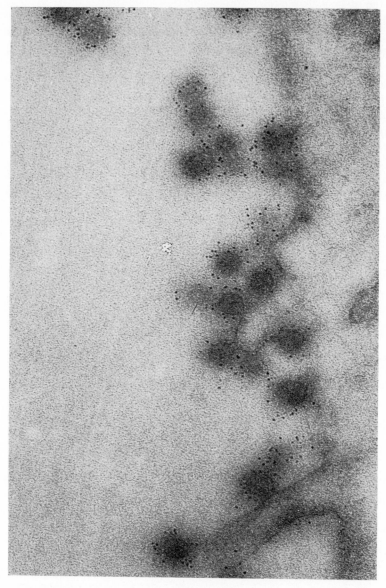

Fig. 15.8. Influenza virus at the surface of an infected epithelial cell of a chick embryo chorioallantoic membrane. Ferritin-conjugated anti-influenza antibody has bound to the viral particles. Magnification 116,400× [Morgan C. *et al*, 34].

FIG. 15.9. Part of the nucleus of an influenza-infected cell treated with specific ferritin-conjugated antibody. The ferritin-labelled antibody was bound to aggregates of dense material indicating that they are composed of, or contain, soluble antigen. Magnification 91,100× [Morgan C. *et al*, 49].

concerning viral structure and development was limited to the terminal stages of viral growth since components could not be recognized before their definitive incorporation into viral particles had occurred. The ferritin antibody

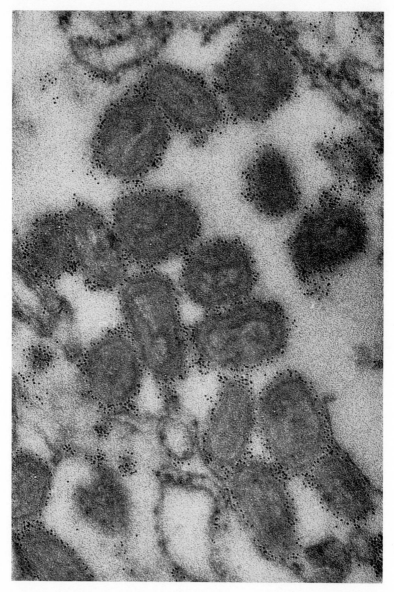

FIG. 15.10. Intracellular vaccinia virus reacted with ferritin-conjugated specific antibody. Magnification 95,000× [Morgan C. *et al*, 29].

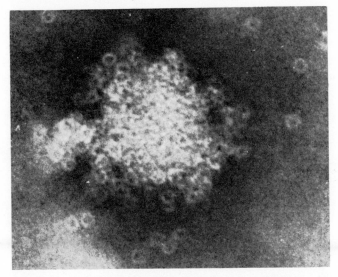

FIG. 15.11. Reovirus particle covered by specific ferritin-conjugated antibody and viewed by negative contrast. Magnification 384,000× [Dales S. *et al*, 19].

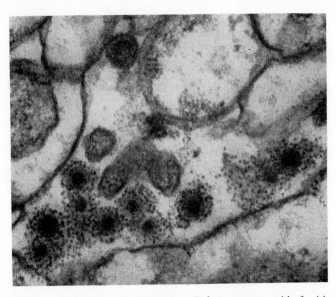

FIG. 15.12. Part of a cell infected with reovirus. Before treatment with ferritin-conjugated antibody the cell was frozen and thawed. Ferritin conjugates are bound to reovirus particles, whereas other components of the cell are uncoated. Magnification 80,000× [Dales S. *et al*, 19].

technique, however, has been successfully used for localizing viral protein in virus-infected cells [47, 48]. Influenza virus was chosen for initial examination because it develops at the surface of the cell. Ferritin-conjugated antibody to PR8 influenza virus was found localized on viral particles lining the cellular surface of chick allantoic membranes (Fig. 15.8) [37, 34]. In other experiments,

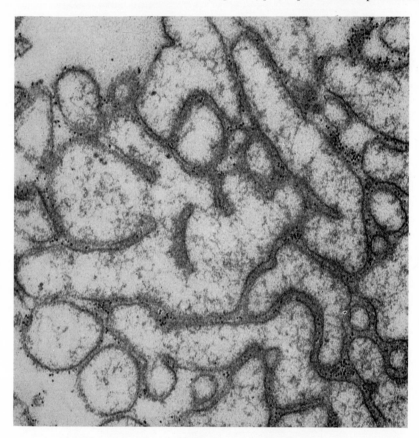

Fig. 15.13. Ascites tumour cell incubated with ferritin-conjugated rabbit antibody against whole ascites tumour cells. The ferritin-labelled antibody is localized along the plasma membrane in a zone of antibody-induced surface foldings. Magnification 68,000× [Easton J.M. *et al*, 56].

exploring the interior of infected cells, aggregates of soluble nucleoprotein, a viral precursor, were identified in the nucleus and in the cytoplasm [40] (Fig. 15.9). Further studies carried out after infection with concentrated inocula showed that the fragments of cytoplasm coated with viral antigen, but devoid of viral components, may constitute the incomplete forms of the virus which contain little nucleic acid and are not infectious [49]. Intracellular localization of vaccinia virus was also demonstrated with specific ferritin-conjugated antibody [29] (Fig. 15.10), or with ferritin-conjugated Porter II fraction of the antibody globulin [8]. The immunoferritin technique has been

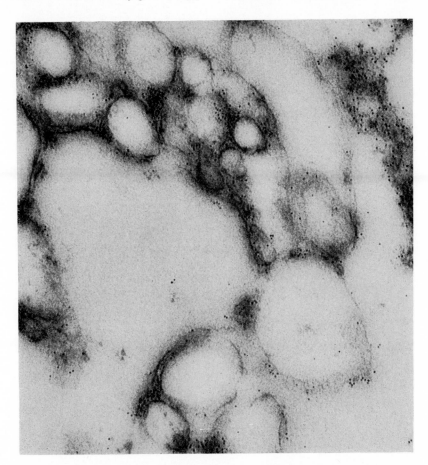

Fig. 15.14. Part of a broken ascites tumour cell incubated with ferritin-conjugated antibody and complement. Ferritin is localized on smooth membrane-bounded profiles. Magnification 75,000× [Easton J.M. *et al.* 56].

employed as well for the identification of T2 phage [50], tobacco mosaic virus [5, 51], equine abortion virus [51], rabies virus [52], and parainfluenza viruses [53] (see Table 15.1). In a study on the development of reovirus its morphogenesis has been related to the presence of mitotic-spindle-tubules and filamentous components of the cytoplasm [19] (Figs. 15.11 and 15.12).

TABLE 15.1

Application of ferritin-conjugated antibody (F-Ab)

Subject of study	Antigen(s) involved	Coupling agent	Treatment with F-Ab	Structures binding F-Ab	References
Viruses	Tobacco mosaic (TMV)	XC	Spray virus and F-Ab on grid	TMV (not control bacteriophage)	Singer & Schick, 1961 [5]
	T2 phage	TC	Infected coli spheroplasts treated with F-Ab	Phage particles in spheroplasts	Lee, 1960 [50]
	Influenza (PR8)	XC	Infected chick membrane treated with F-Ab	Viral particles on membrane cells	Rifkind et al, 1960 [37]
	Vaccinia	XC	Infected Hela cells formalin fixed, frozen and sectioned in cryostat; treated with F-Ab	Virus within as well as without the cells	Morgan et al, 1961 [29]
	Influenza	XC	Infected chick membrane treated with F-Ab	Viral particles	Morgan et al, 1961 [34]
	Influenza	XC	Formalin-fixed membrane frozen, thawed and treated with F-Ab	Dense aggregates in nuclei, dispersed virus in cytoplasm	Morgan et al, 1961 [40]
	Influenza	XC	Infected chick membrane treated with F-Ab	Viral particles as well as fragments of cytoplasm containing viral antigen	Morgan et al, 1962 [49]
	Equine abortion	XC	Infected hamster liver formalin fixed, 1 mm section treated with F-Ab	Nests of virus in nuclear region and in membrane area	Metzger & Smith, 1962 [51]
	TMV		TMV agglutinated with F-Ab	Agglutinated TMV	
	Rabies	XC	Infected tissue culture cells washed with saline; F-Ab added	Viral particles and filaments	Atanasiu et al, 1963 [52]

TABLE 15.1 (*cont.*)

Subject of study	Antigen(s) involved	Coupling agent	Treatment with F-Ab	Structures binding F-Ab	References
	Vaccinia	3 tested XC TC AMMD 1st best	Whole γ globulin or Porter II fragment conjugated. Formalin-fixed infected cells frozen. cut in cryostat and treated with F-Ab	Surface of vaccinia virus binds whole globulin and fragment II	Isliker et al, 1964 [8]
	Parainfluenza 2	XC	Infected amnion cells treated with F-Ab	Viral particles specifically identified	Howe et al, 1965 [53]
	Influenza (PR8)	XC	Infected chick membrane treated over intervals of time with F-Ab to influenza virus and chick membrane	Envelope of PR8 virus binds only F-Ab to the virus; contains little if any host antigen	Duc-Nguyen et al, 1965 [74]
	Reovirus	XC	Frozen and thawed or pre-treated with digitonin then formalin or glutaraldehyde. Pellets of cells cut, treated with F-Ab	Reovirus particles, not spindles	Dales et al, 1965 [19]
Bacteria and fungi	Staphylococcus	XC	Formalin-fixed organisms treated with F-Ab	Cell walls	Smith et al, 1960 [25]
	Candida albicans Klebsiella rhinoscler-atoma	XC	Formalin-fixed organisms treated with F-Ab	C. albicans, cell wall; Klebsiella, mucopoly-saccharide capsule	Metzger & Smith, 1962 [51]
	Streptococcus Pneumococcus	XC	Formalin-fixed organisms treated with specific and non-specific F-Abs	Streptococcus, cell wall; pneumococcus, carbohydrate capsule; each with homologous but not heterologous F-Ab	Hsu, 1962 [54] Hsu et al, 1963 [17] Rifkind et al, 1964 [39]
	S. typhi murium E. coli	TC	F-Ab added to cultures Agglutinated or unagglutinated sediment washed, examined	Each organism bound homologous but not heterologous F-Ab	Shands, 1965 [38]

TABLE 15.1 (*cont.*)

Subject of study	Antigen(s) involved	Coupling agent	Treatment with F-Ab	Structures binding F-Ab	References
	Veillonella parvula	XC	F-Ab added to culture, agglutinated sediment washed, examined	'Outer three-layered membrane'	Mergenhagen, 1965 [18]
Free animal cells	Ascites tumour	XC	F-Ab incubated with cells	Cell membrane	Easton *et al*, 1962 [35]
			F-Ab incubated with complement and cells	Cell membrane and smooth endoplasmic reticulum	Easton *et al*, 1962 [56]
	Sea urchin eggs	XC TC	F-Ab to egg, egg jelly and sperm added to fresh eggs. *Indirect test*: rabbit antibody to same antigens (not conjugated) added to fresh eggs followed by F-Ab to rabbit globulin	F-Ab to egg and jelly bound to specific antigens. Indirect test heavier tagging. F-Ab negative with unfertilized egg	Baxandall *et al*, 1962 [36], 1964 [43]
	Sea urchin spermatozoa		Free sperm and fertilized eggs of sea urchin treated with sperm F-Ab	Sperm in portions of tail and acrosomal region. Fertilized egg in fertilization membrane and cortical 'globules'	Baxandall, 1965 [57]
	Red blood cells	FNPS TC	Washed erythrocytes incubated with F-Abs to A and Rh antigens	F-Ab to A bound only to A cells (heavily tagged). Rh F-Ab localized periodically and much less intensely	Lee & Feldman, 1964 [58]
	Red blood cells	TC	Erythrocytes mixed with F-Abs to A and B blood group antigens. Stroma prepared, placed directly on grids	Cells of groups A and B specifically bind F-Ab	Harris, 1964 [75]

TABLE 15.1 (cont.)

Subject of study	Antigen(s) involved	Coupling agent	Treatment with F-Ab	Structures binding F-Ab	References
Production of proteins	Rat glomerular basement membranes (BM) (in nephrotoxic nephritis)	XC	Bits of renal tissues formalin fixed, sectioned by hand, exposed to F-Ab to injected nephrotoxic rabbit globulin	Glomerular capillary BM and cisternae in epithelial cells, indicating common antigens	Andres *et al*, 1962 [30]
	Yolk sac carcinoma, secreting BM-like material	FNPS	Membranes exposed to F-Ab	Endoplasmic reticulum of secreting cells	Pierce *et al*, 1963 [62]
	Reichert's membrane of mouse	FNPS	Formalin-fixed membranes frozen, sectioned at 30 μ, F-Ab added	Endoplasmic reticulum of parietal yolk sac and other BMs	Pierce *et al*, 1964 [63]
	Plasma cell myeloma globulin C$_3$H mouse	XC	Cells of tumour teased out, pellet frozen, thawed—F-Ab added	Myeloma globulin within cisternae of the endoplasmic reticulum	Rifkind *et al*, 1962 [33]
	Amylase pork pancreas	XC	Formalin-fixed bits of tissue frozen and thawed, F-Ab added	Vesicles and area of the Golgi apparatus	Yasuda, 1965 [64]
Blood coagulation	Fibrinogen	TC	F-Ab to human fibrinogen added to human plasma. Clotting induced by CaCl$_2$	F-Ab shows periodic banding of fibrin. Interval between 195 ± 10 Å	White *et al*, 1964 [32]
	Fibrinogen	TC	F-Ab to human fibrinogen added to platelet-rich human plasma. Clotting induced by CaCl$_2$	F-Ab shows connection between extra-cellular fibrin periodically tagged and intra-platelet material also tagged	White *et al*, 1965 [65]
	Fibrinogen	XC TC	Glutaraldehyde-fixed fresh human clot, homogenized rat muscle containing human clot, treated with F-Ab	Surface of fibrin	Wyllie, 1964 [66]

TABLE 15.1 (*cont.*)

Subject of study	Antigen(s) involved	Coupling agent	Treatment with F-Ab	Structures binding F-Ab	References
	Fibrinogen	TC	Formalin or glutaraldehyde-fixed bits of early fatty lesions of human atherosclerosis; treated with F-Ab to human fibrinogen	Fibrillar and granular material bound F-Ab; not collagen or elastica	Haust *et al*, 1964 [67]
Experimental and human pathology	Nephrotoxic nephritis, glomerular BMs (rat)	XC	Formalin-fixed small pieces of kidney cut by hand; placed in F-Ab to nephro-toxic globulin	BM and BM-like material in epithelial endoplasmic reticulum	Andres *et al*, 1962 [30]
	Serum disease type of nephritis in rabbit produced with bovine serum albumin (BSA)	XC	Formalin-fixed small pieces of kidney cut by hand; placed in F-Ab to BSA and rabbit globulin	F-Ab to BSA bound in glomerular deposits; F-Ab to BSA and rabbit globulin bound to precipitates in capillary lumen	Andres *et al*, 1963 [70]
	Nephrotoxic nephritis glomerular BM (rabbit)	TC	Fresh bits of kidney placed in F-Ab to nephrotoxic globulin	BM	Arhelger, 1963 [68]
	Renal biopsies from patients with acute glomerulo-nephritis	XC	Formalin-fixed small pieces cut by hand; placed in F-Ab to human γ globulin, β_{1c}, and products of T12 streptococcal antigens	F-Ab to γ globulin, β_{1c} in capillary lumen, between mesangial cells, in subendothelial and subepithelial deposits, in Bowman's space and in arteriolar walls F-Ab to type 12 streptococcal products present except in subepithelial deposits	Seegal *et al*, 1965 [71] Andres *et al*, 1966 [72]

TABLE 15.1 (*cont.*)

Subject of study	Antigen(s) involved	Coupling agent	Treatment with F-Ab	Structures binding F-Ab	References
	Amyloid from human liver and spleen; bacteria coated with human γ globulin	XC	Amyloid fibrils and bacteria coated with human γ globulin prepared. F-Ab to human γ globulin added	F-Ab not bound to amyloid fibrils; is bound to bacteria	Paul & Cohen, 1963 [44]
	Rat psoas muscle, cardiac muscle Rabbit extraocular muscle	XC	Formalin fixed, frozen, treated with normal human serum of patients with myasthenia gravis then treated with F-Ab to human γ globulin	Some binding of F-Ab in tissue treated with normal globulin; more binding in tissues treated with myasthenia globulin; in medial A band and peri-Z regions	Douglas et al, 1965 [45]
	β toxin of *Cl. botulinum*	XC	Inject ferritin-conjugated toxin i.v. in mice	Ferritin-labelled toxin localizes in primary and secondary synaptic clefts of post-synaptic apparatus	Zacks et al, 1962 [73]

II. *Bacterial and fungal cell components*

Localization of ferritin conjugates in elements of capsule or cell wall has been reported for several bacterial species and one fungus [25, 54, 17, 38, 51, 55] (see Table 15.1). Figure 15.5 illustrates the reaction of ferritin-conjugated type 18 pneumococcal antibody [54] when mixed with a suspension of the organisms. Diffuse penetration of the conjugate throughout the capsule is apparent. A study on the localization of antigenic sites in the cell wall of *Veillonella parvula*, a human oral strain of Gram-negative coccus, was carried out by

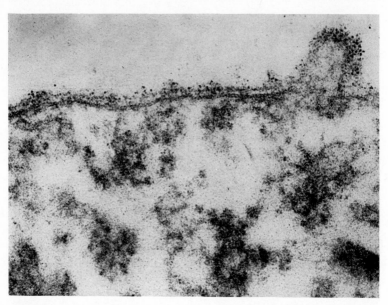

FIG. 15.15. The surface of an unfertilized sea urchin (*Paracentrotus lividus*) egg treated with a ferritin-conjugated γ globulin fraction of an anti-egg serum. One-layer or direct technique. Ferritin-conjugated antibody is localized on the vitelline membrane which is adjacent to the plasma membrane. Magnification 100,000 × [Baxandall J. *et al*, 43].

using ferritin- and fluorescein-ferritin-conjugated antibody to the pure lipopolysaccharide, which is supposed to be the endotoxin, and which was thought to be localized only in the inner layer of the cell wall. It has been shown that the outer three-layered membrane of *Veillonella* is wholly or partially responsible for endotoxin activity and antigenic specificity [18]. Other data are given in Table 15.1.

III. *Surface cellular antigens*

Free cells such as ascites tumour cells, sea urchin eggs and red blood cells have been examined by the immunoferritin technique in various studies.

(a) Ferritin-conjugated antibodies to whole ascites tumour cells localize primarily on the surface of the tumour cell membrane (Fig. 15.13) and within pinocytic vacuoles [35]. After incubation with ferritin-conjugated antibody plus complement, followed by lysis of the cells, cytotoxic antibody penetrated within broken ascites tumour cells (Fig. 15.14) and combined with cell membranes and the smooth membranes of the endoplasmic reticulum [56]. These data favour the concept that antigens contained in membranous structure are most important in the formation of cytotoxic antibodies.

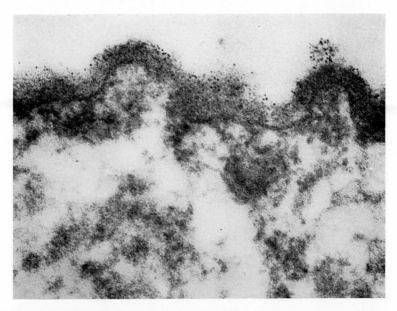

FIG. 15.16. The picture illustrates an application of the two-layer or indirect ferritin-conjugated antibody technique. Sea urchin egg first treated with rabbit anti-egg γ globulin and subsequently with a ferritin-conjugated γ globulin fraction of an antiserum prepared in sheep against rabbit γ globulin. The plasma membrane is tagged by a layer of ferritin-conjugated antibody. The localization of ferritin in this area indicates the site of the first antigen-antibody reaction. Magnification 100,000 × [Baxandall J. *et al*, 36].

(b) The role of specific surface antigenic sites on unfertilized and fertilized sea urchin eggs was explored by studying the antigenic nature of the surface layers of unfertilized eggs [36, 43]. The vitelline membrane proved to be rich in egg antigens, which may be responsible for species specificity and may also constitute specific sperm receptor sites (Fig. 15.15). Ferritin-labelled antibody to sperm of the sea urchin has been used for localizing sperm antigens in sperms and in fertilized eggs of the sea urchin [57]. In the sperm itself the antigenic sites are mainly in the tail filaments. The acrosomal region and the sperm head were also tagged when the plasma membrane was broken. In the fertilized eggs ferritin-labelled antibody was bound in the fertilization membrane and in the cortical 'globules'. The data suggested that most of the antigenic sites detected in the fertilized egg were associated with sperm substances.

(c) Sites and distribution of type A and type Rho(D) antigens on human red

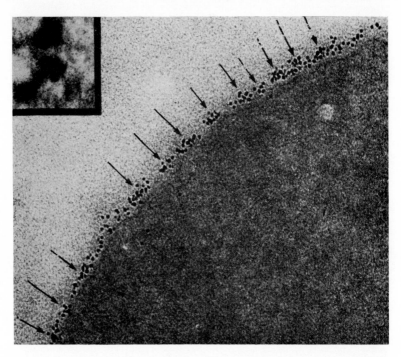

Fig. 15.17. Group A red cell treated with ferritin-conjugated anti-A globulin. Binding of ferritin particles to surface of erythrocyte indicates loci of antigen. Magnification 120,000 × . Insert—one of the ferritin particles has been resolved to five of the six iron micelles. Magnification 950,000 × [Lee R.E. & Feldman J.C., 58].

cells have also been explored [58]. It was seen that ferritin-labelled anti-A serum binds only to A cells and that cells from different individuals bind different amounts of antibody. Ferritin-labelled antibody to A antigen was clustered on such red cells and spaced so as to suggest a pattern of antigenic sites (Fig. 15.17). By contrast the ferritin tagging of Rh positive cells with specific antibody was more discrete (Fig. 15.18). By assuming that 30–50 per cent of the globulin present was labelled with ferritin and that each section was 500 Å thick, the total number of antigenic sites was estimated at from 1000 to 3000 per cell. This was of the same order of magnitude (5000–10,000) as that calculated by studying the quantity of ^{131}I-labelled anti-Rho(D) bound to the red cells [59]. Other data are given in Table 15.1.

IV. *Protein synthesis*

(a) The theory that the basement membranes of epithelia are formed by polymerization of connective tissue ground substance [60] has been a subject of controversy. Recently morphologic studies have shown that the cisternae of endoplasmic reticulum of epithelial podocytes contain material which

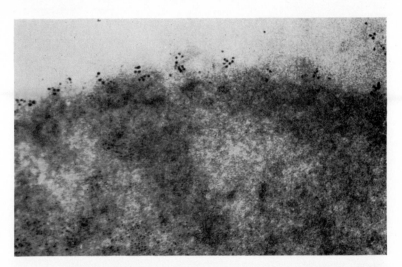

FIG. 15.18. Type O Rho(D) red cell exposed to ferritin-conjugated anti-Rho(D) globulin. By comparison with Fig. 15.17 it may be seen that the receptor sites are much less numerous. Magnification 100,000× [Lee R.E. & Feldman J.C. 58].

resembles the lamina densa of the glomerular basement membrane [61]. This gives support to the hypothesis that the endoplasmic reticulum of epithelial cells may be concerned with synthesis of some components of the glomerular basement membrane.

In rats rendered nephritic by injection of rabbit globulin containing antibody to rat-kidney, it was shown that ferritin-labelled antibody to rabbit globulin localized both in the glomerular capillary basement membrane and in basement membrane-like material contained in the cisternae of the epithelial endoplasmic reticulum [30] (Fig. 15.19). The observation is consistent with the assumption that similar antigens are present in these two structures. Other studies in parietal yolk sac carcinoma of the mouse, which secretes large amounts of basement membrane-like material, showed that

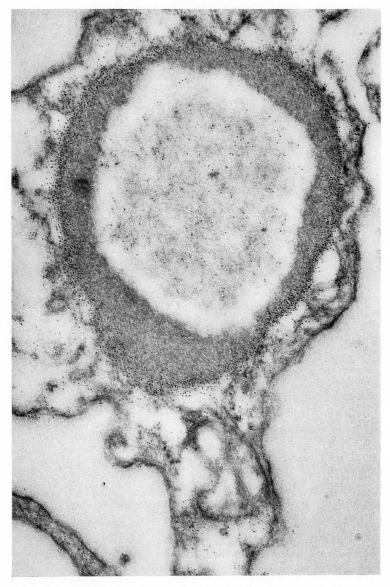

Fɪɢ. 15.19. The micrograph illustrates a fraction of an epithelial cell from the glomerular capillary wall of a rat injected with nephrotoxic rabbit anti-rat kidney serum. The tissue was treated with ferritin-labelled antibody to rabbit globulin. The distended cisterna of the endoplasmic reticulum of this cell contains basement membrane-like material which is concentrated in a peripheral ring. The ferritin-conjugated antibody is bound in this area. Magnification 63,000×.

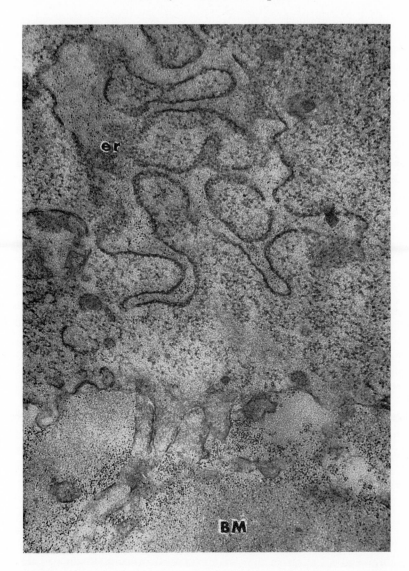

FIG. 15.20. Parietal yolk sac carcinoma cells incubated with ferritin-conjugated antibody to the neoplastic basement membrane-like material, which they secrete. Ferritin-conjugated antibody is seen in the endoplasmic reticulum (er) and in the extracellular basement membrane-like material (BM). Magnification 54,000 × [Pierce G.B. *et al*, 63].

ferritin-labelled antibody to this neoplastic hyaline material localized in the endoplasmic reticulum of the secretory cells [62] (Fig. 15.20). Ferritin-conjugated antibodies to Reichert's membrane, a basement membrane of the mouse embryo, also localized in the endoplasmic reticulum of parietal yolk sac epithelium and in extracellular basement membrane material; further-more, they localized in the basement membrane of the testes, seminal vesicles and visceral yolk sac, but failed to react with collagen and reticulin [63]. All these findings support the view that the epithelial endoplasmic reticulum may be responsible for the synthesis of some components of the basement membranes. Besides, it seems apparent that the basement membranes of different organs share common antigens and do not have an immunologic relationship with the connective tissue.

(b) In an effort to obtain further information on secretory mechanisms of proteins by cells, the localization of 'myeloma globulin' in the plasma cells in a mouse plasma cell tumour has been studied [33]. Antibody to the globulin fraction of sera from tumour-bearing mice was labelled with ferritin. Cells of the tumour were teased into saline and exposed to the conjugate. Myeloma globulin was first seen within cisternae of the endoplasmic reticulum (Fig. 15.21) at a stage of the secretory process when the remainder of the cytoplasm was free of labelled protein. In a further phase this secretory protein could be found also in the cytoplasmic matrix and there was some evidence of partici-pation of the Golgi apparatus in the release of the globulin. Another pathway appeared to be through fragmentation of the peripheral cytoplasm with rupture of distended ergastoplasmic vesicles.

(c) A further cytochemical application of ferritin antibody technique in the study of secretory mechanisms was represented by the intracellular localiza-tion of amylase in pig pancreas [64]. Ferritin-conjugated antibody to pure amylase localized in the Golgi region and at the periphery of zymogen gran-ules located in the apical part of the cells. There was no localization in the ergastoplasmic cisternae or in the ground substance of the cytoplasm.

V. *Blood coagulation*

The ferritin antibody technique has been used to investigate the process of blood coagulation in physiologic and pathologic conditions. The formation of fibrin and its ultrastructure were examined utilizing conjugated ferritin antibody to human fibrinogen. The ferritin-conjugated antibody tagged the fibrin strands at periodic intervals of 195 ± 10 Å (Fig. 15.22). This finding suggests that fibrinogen molecules may line up, end to end, and the resulting filaments become laterally associated in the long axis of the developing fibrin strand [32]. The same ferritin-conjugated antibody to human fibrinogen was incubated with platelet-rich human plasma during clot formation. Electron microscopic study of the clot revealed that the ferritin-conjugated

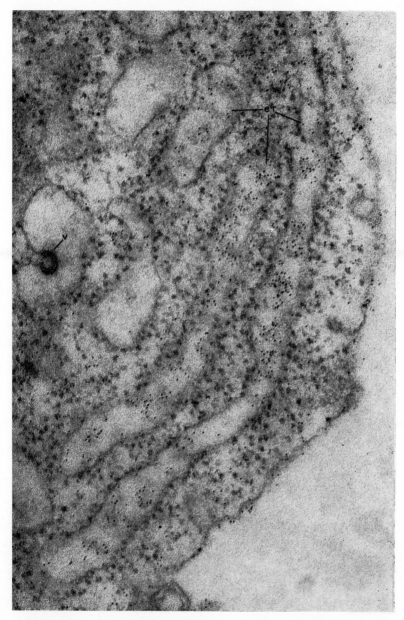

FIG. 15.21. The electron micrograph illustrates a site of production of globulin. A cell from a mouse plasma cell tumour treated with ferritin-conjugated antibody to myeloma globulin is seen. The ferritin-conjugated antibody is mainly localized in the cisternae of the endoplasmic reticulum (er). An ergastoplasmic cisterna contains a virus-like particle (v). Magnification 87,200 × [Rifkind R.A. *et al*, 33].

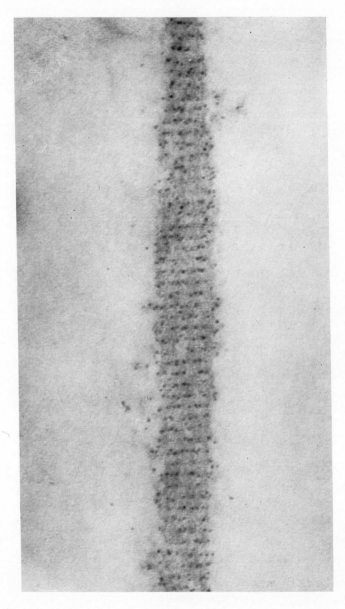

FIG. 15.22. A fibrin strand formed in plasma to which ferritin-labelled antibody to fibrinogen has been added. The periodic binding of the ferritin-conjugated antibody to fibrinogen is seen. The interval between bands is 195 ± 10 Å. Magnification $131,300 \times$ [White J.G. *et al*, 32].

antibody was present in developing fibrin strands and in platelets undergoing viscous metamorphosis. Connections between intracellular material tagged by ferritin-conjugated antibody and extracellular fibrin strands, periodically tagged, were observed (Fig. 15.23). These findings support the opinion that

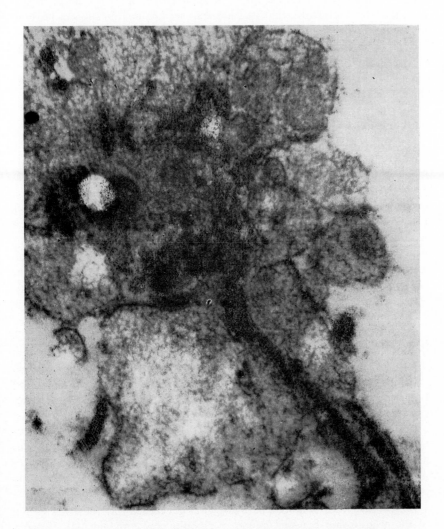

Fig. 15.23. A platelet 10 minutes after clot formation in platelet-rich plasma incubated with ferritin-conjugated antibody to human fibrinogen, The picture shows continuity between fibrinogen products, labelled with ferritin-conjugated antibody, contained within the cell and a fibrin strand forming outside the platelets. Magnification 36,000× [White J.G. *et al*, 65].

T

fibrin strands outside the platelets are related to the alpha granulomere within the altered thrombocytes [65].

Ferritin-conjugated antihuman fibrinogen was found specifically to bind human fibrin in a blood clot in an experimentally produced depot within rat muscle. The preparations did not show the axial periodicity of fibrin. Therefore, the immunoferritin technique has enabled the identification of fibrin or fibrinogen products in the absence of characteristic morphology [66]. These studies have been extended to identify electron-dense fibrillar or granular material observed in early fatty lesions of human atherosclerosis. In the aorta ferritin conjugates specifically localized in the foreign deposits present between the elastica and the smooth muscle cells [67].

VI. *Experimental and human pathology*

(a) In the field of acute glomerulonephritis experimentally produced with nephrotoxic sera or antigen–antibody complexes, the ferritin antibody technique has provided definitive information concerning sites of reaction. In acute glomerulonephritis in the rat, produced with rabbit nephrotoxic sera, the injected globulins are localized in the glomerular basement membrane [30]. Likewise, chicken anti-rabbit kidney serum localizes in rabbit glomerular basement membranes [68]. In membranous glomerulonephritis in rabbits, which follows repeated injections of foreign antigens [69], antigen aggregates were identified in the capillary lumen, in the basement membrane and in the subepithelial deposits of the glomeruli. In rabbits which died of anaphylactic shock, embolic precipitates of antigen–antibody complexes were present in the lumina of the capillaries [70].

(b) Studies of cases of severe acute glomerulonephritis in man have shown that: human γ globulin and β_{1c} (C'3) are localized in foreign material present in capillary lumens, between proliferating cells, in subendothelial and certain subepithelial deposits, in Bowman's space and in the walls of some arterioles; type 12 streptococcal products have been demonstrated in the same areas except in the subepithelial deposits. Figure 15·24 illustrates the localization of ferritin-conjugated antibody to human γ globulin in the basement membrane of a glomerulus from a renal biopsy taken from a patient with glomerulonephritis. The findings support the hypothesis that some forms of severe acute glomerulonephritis in man are the result of inflammatory activity of antigen-antibody complexes in the glomeruli [71, 72].

(c) Another study of human pathology was concerned with the investigation of the relationship between human γ globulin and amyloid [44]. Ferritin-conjugated antibody to γ globulin did not localize in amyloid fibrils isolated from human liver and spleen thus indicating that γ globulin, in an immunologically identifiable form, is not an intrinsic component of the amyloid fibrils.

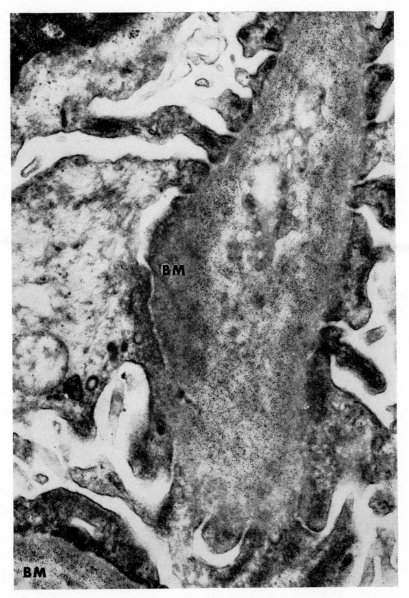

FIG. 15.24. Glomerulonephritis in man. Fragment of kidney cortex treated with ferritin-conjugated antibody to human 7S γ globulin. The conjugate is bound to glomerular basement membrane (BM)—visible in cross and tangential sections—indicating excess of human γ globulin in this area. Magnification 45,000 ×.

(d) A preliminary report on the localization of sera from patients with myasthenia gravis in mammalian skeletal muscle has indicated that such sera are identified by the immunoferritin technique in the medial portion of the A band and the peri-Z regions [45]. This observation is an extension of earlier immunofluorescein studies and is probably the first application of the technique in the field of autoimmune diseases.

(e) An unusual application of ferritin conjugation is described in a study of ferritin-labelled B toxin of *Clostridium botulinum* [73]. Following injection of such toxin into mice, the electron microscopic examination of the intercostal muscles revealed the presence of ferritin-labelled toxin in the primary and secondary synaptic clefts of the post-synaptic apparatus.

Such direct labelling of other antigens may eventually be used to trace their deposition in tissues. Similarly it should be possible to localize the sites of antibody formation by the use of labelled antigens.

F. Conclusion

At present several difficulties limit the useful application of the immunoferritin technique. Improvement and modifications have to be sought in the future. Among the more important would be: a technique which enables higher yield of conjugated antibody; new embedding media which permit direct application of ferritin antibody to the surface of thin sections; a fixative which will hold soluble antigens, such as enzymes or hormones, to their original sites during labelling and processing for electron microscopic examination.

However, in spite of these limitations a wide range of subjects has been opened up for investigation during the past 5 years. By making highly specific immunologic reactions visible electron microscopically, the ferritin antibody technique promises to be an important tool for the study of certain mechanisms operating in health and disease.

Acknowledgments

The authors wish to thank Dr J.Baxandall, Dr S.Dales, Dr J.C.Feldman, Dr B.Goldberg, Dr W.Krivit, Dr C.Morgan, Dr G.B.Pierce, Dr R.A.Rifkind, and their colleagues, for permission to use their electron micrographs. The authors express their deep appreciation and thanks to Dr Councilman Morgan for his generous help and advice. Figures 15.6, 15.7, 15.8, 15.9, 15.13, 15.14 and 15.21 were first published in *The Journal of Experimental Medicine*; Figs. 15.10, 15.11 and 15.12 in *Virology*; Figs. 15.17 and 15.18 in *The Journal* of Cell Biology; Fig. 15.20 in *The American Journal of Pathology*; Figs. 15.22 and 15.23 in *Blood*. The authors are grateful to these journals for permission to republish the photos.

References

[1] COONS A.H., CREECH H.J., JONES R.N. & BERLINER E. (1942) The demonstration of pneumococcal antigens in tissues by the use of fluorescent antibody. *J. Immun.* **45,** 159

[2] COONS A.H., SNYDER J.C., CHEEVER F.S. & MURRAY E.S. (1950) Localization of antigen in tissue cells. IV. Antigens of rickettsiae and mumps virus. *J. exp. Med.* **91,** 31

[3] COONS A.H. (1961) The beginnings of immunofluorescence. *J. Immun.* **87,** 499

[4] SINGER S.J. (1959) Preparation of an electron-dense antibody conjugate. *Nature, Lond.* **183,** 1523

[5] SINGER S.J. & SCHICK A.F. (1961) The properties of specific stains for electron microscopy prepared by the conjugation of antibody molecules with ferritin. *J. Biophys. Biochem. Cytol.* **9,** 519

[6] SRI RAM J., TAWDE S.S., PIERCE G.B. JR. & MIDGLEY A.R. JR., (1963) Preparation of antibody–ferritin conjugates for immune-electron microscopy. *J. Cell. Biol.* **17,** 673

[7] BOREK F. & SILVERSTEIN A.M. (1961) Characterization and purification of ferritin–antibody globulin conjugates. *J. Immun.* **87,** 555

[8] ISLIKER H., LeMAIRE B. & MORGAN C. (1964) The use of ferritin-conjugated antibody-fragments in electron microscopic studies of viruses. *Path. Microbiol.* **27,** 521

[9] STRAUSS A.J.L., SEEGAL B.C., HSU K.C., BURKHOLDER P.M., NASTUK W.L. & OSSERMAN K.E. (1960) Immunofluorescence demonstration of a muscle binding complement-fixing serum globulin fraction in myasthenia gravis. *Proc. Soc. exp. Biol. Med.* **105,** 184

[10] FAHEY J.L. & HORBETT A.P. (1959) Human gamma globulin fractionation on anion exchange cellulose columns. *J. biol. Chem.* **234,** 2645

[11] FARRANT J.L. (1954) An electron microscopy study of ferritin. *Biochem. biophys. Acta* **13,** 569

[12] HOFMAN T. & HARRISON P. (1963) The structure of apoferritin: Degradation into and molecular weight of subunits. *J. molec. Biol.* **6,** 256

[13] PEPE F.A. (1961) The use of specific antibody in electron microscopy. I. Preparation of mercury labeled antibody. *J. Biophys. Biochem. Cytol.* **11,** 515

[14] STERNBERGER L.A., DONATI E.J. & WILSON C.E. (1963) Electron microscopic study on specific protection of isolated Bordetella bronchiseptica antibody during exhaustive labeling with uranium. *J. Histochem. Cytochem.* **11,** 48

[15] SINGER S.J. & McLEAN J.D. (1963) Ferritin–antibody conjugates as stains for electron microscopy. *Lab. Invest.* **12,** 1002

[16] VOGT A. & KOPP R. (1964) Loss of specific agglutinating activity of purified ferritin-conjugated antibodies. *Nature, Lond.* **202,** 1350

[17] HSU K.C., RIFKIND R.A. & ZABRISKIE J.B. (1963) Fluorescent, electron microscopic and immunoelectrophoretic studies of labeled antibodies. *Science* **142,** 1471

[18] MERGENHAGEN S.E., BLADEN H.A. & HSU K.C. (1966) Electron microscopic localization of endotoxin lipopolysaccharide in gram-negative organism. *Ann. N.Y. Acad. Sci.* **133,** 279

[19] DALES S., GOMATOS P.J. & HSU K.C. (1965) The uptake and development of reovirus in strain L cells followed with labeled viral ribonucleic acid and ferritin–antibody conjugates. *Virology* **25**, 193

[20] HSU K.C., SEEGAL B.C. & ANDRES G.A. (1962) Unpublished data

[21] RIGGS J.L., SEIWALD R.J., BURCKHALTER J.H., DOWNS C.M. & METCALF T.C. (1958) Isothiocyanate compounds as fluorescent labeling agents for immune serum. *Am. J. Path.* **34**, 1081

[22] MARSHALL J.D., EVELAND W.C. & SMITH C.W. (1958) Superiority of fluorescein isothiocyanate (Riggs) for fluorescent-antibody technique with a modification of its application. *Proc. Soc. exp. Biol. Med.* **98**, 989

[23] GOLDSTEIN G., SLIZYS I.S. & CHASE M.W. (1961) Studies on fluorescent antibody staining. I. Nonspecific fluorescence with fluorescein-coupled sheep-anti-rabbit globulins. *J. exp. Med.* **114**, 89

[24] HSU K.C., RIFKIND R.A. & ZABRISKIE J.B. (1964) Immunochemical studies with fluorescein and ferritin doubly-labeled antibodies. *J. Histochem. Cytochem.* **12**, 7

[25] SMITH C.W., METZGER J.F., ZACKS S.I. & KASE A. (1960) Immune electron microscopy. *Proc. Soc. exp. Biol. Med.* **104**, 336

[26] SPENDLOVE R.S. & SINGER S.J. (1961) On the preservation of antigenic determinants during fixation and embedding for electron microscopy. *Proc. Nat. Acad. Sci. (Wash.)* **47**, 14

[27] SMITH C.W. & METZGER J.F. (1961) 'Pitfalls' in immune electron microscopy. *Experientia* **17**, 394

[28] PALADE G.E. (1952) A study of fixation for electron microscopy. *J. exp. Med.* **95**, 285

[29] MORGAN C., RIFKIND R.A., HSU K.C., HOLDEN M., SEEGAL B.C. & ROSE H.M. (1961) Electron microscopic localization of intracellular viral antigen by the use of ferritin-conjugated antibody. *Virology* **14**, 292

[30] ANDRES G.A., MORGAN C., HSU K.C., RIFKIND R.A. & SEEGAL B.C. (1962) Electron microscopic studies of experimental nephritis with ferritin-conjugated antibody. The basement membranes and cisternae of visceral epithelial cells in nephritic rat glomeruli. *J. exp. Med.* **115**, 929

[31] ANDRES G.A., ACCINNI L., HSU K.C., ZABRISKIE J.B. & SEEGAL B.C. (1965) Unpublished data

[32] WHITE J.G., KRIVIT W. & VERNIER R. (1964) An ultrastructural investigation of the fibrin clot utilizing ferritin-labeled anti-human fibrinogen antibody. *Blood* **24**, 443

[33] RIFKIND R.A., OSSERMAN E.F., HSU K.C. & MORGAN C. (1962) The intracellular distribution of gamma globulin in a mouse plasma cell tumor (X5563) as revealed by fluorescence and electron microscopy. *J. exp. Med.* **116**, 423

[34] MORGAN C., HSU K.C., RIFKIND R.A., KNOX A.W. & ROSE H.M. (1961) The application of ferritin-conjugated antibody to electron microscopic studies of influenza virus in infected cells. I. The cellular surface. *J. exp. Med.* **114**, 825

[35] EASTON J.M., GOLDBERG B. & GREEN H. (1962) Demonstration of surface antigens and pinocytosis in mammalian cells with ferritin–antibody conjugates. *J. Cell Biol.* **12**, 437

[36] BAXANDALL J., PERLMANN P. & AFZELIUS B.A. (1962) A two-layer technique for detecting surface antigens in the sea urchin egg with ferritin-conjugated antibody. *J. Cell Biol.* **14**, 144

[37] RIFKIND R.A., HSU K.C., MORGAN C., SEEGAL B.C., KNOX A.W. & ROSE H.M. (1960) Use of ferritin-conjugated antibody to localize antigen by electron microscopy. *Nature, Lond.* **187**, 1094

[38] SHANDS J.W. (1965) Localization of somatic antigen on gram-negative bacteria by electron microscopy. *J. Bact.* **90**, 266

[39] RIFKIND R.A., HSU K.C. & MORGAN C. (1964) Immunochemical staining for electron microscopy. *J. Histochem. Cytochem.* **12**, 131

[40] MORGAN C., HSU K.C., RIFKIND R.A., KNOX A.W. & ROSE H.M. (1961) The application of ferritin-conjugated antibody to electron microscopic studies of influenza virus in infected cells. II. The interior of the cell. *J. exp. Med.* **114**, 833

[41] PIERCE G.B. JR., SRI RAM J. & MIDGLEY A.R. JR. (1964) The use of labeled antibodies in ultrastructural studies. *Intl. Rev. Exptl. Path.* **3**, 1

[42] ANDRES G.A., MORGAN C., HSU K.C., RIFKIND R.A. & SEEGAL B.C. (1962) Use of ferritin-conjugated antibody to identify nephrotoxic sera in renal tissue by electron microscopy. *Nature* **194**, 590

[43] BAXANDALL J., PERLMANN P. & AFZELIUS B.A. (1964) Immunoelectron microscope analysis of the surface layers of the unfertilized sea urchin egg. II. Localization of surface antigens. *J. Cell Biol.* **23**, 629

[44] PAUL W.E. & COHEN A.S. (1963) Electron microscopic studies of amyloid fibrils with ferritin-conjugated antibody. *J. Path.* **43**, 721

[45] DOUGLAS S.D., GOTTLIEB A.J., STRAUSS A.J.L. & SPICER S.S. (1965) Electron microscopic localization of striated muscle binding factor in myasthenia gravis by ferritin-labeled antibody. *Fed. Proc.* **24**, 370. Abstract 1335

[46] BAXANDALL J., PERLMANN P. & AFZELIUS B.A. (1963) Immune electron microscopy using a two-layer method of ferritin labeling. *J. Royl. Microsc. Soc.* **81**, 155

[47] MORGAN C., RIFKIND R.A. & ROSE H.M. (1962) The use of ferritin-conjugated antibodies in electron microscopic studies of influenza and vaccina viruses. *Cold Spring Harbour Symp. on Quantitative Biology.* **27**, 57

[48] MORGAN C., RIFKIND R.A. & ROSE H.M. (1963) A new technique for the study of viruses in the electron microscope. *Can. Med. Assoc. J.* **88**, 472

[49] MORGAN C., HSU K.C. & ROSE H.M. (1962) Structure and development of viruses as observed in the electron microscope. VII. Incomplete influenza virus. *J. Exp. Med.* **116**, 553

[50] LEE S. (1960) Ferritin-labeled antibody as an electron stain for phage protein. *Exp. Cell Research* **21**, 249

[51] METZGER J.F. & SMITH C.W. (1962) The application of electron microscopy to the demonstration of antigenic sites in biologic systems. *Lab. Invest.* **11**, 902

[52] ATANASIU P., ORTH G., SISMAN J. ET BARREAU, C. (1963) Identification immunologique, du virion rabique en cultures cellulaires par les anticorps specifiques conjugues a la ferritine. *C.R. Acad. Sci.* (*Paris*) **257**, 2204

[53] HOWE C., ST CYR DE V., MORGAN C. & HSU K.C. (1965) Immunochemical investigation of parainfluenza virus (type 2). *Fed. Proc.* **24**, 379. Abstract 1388

[54] HSU K.C. (1962) *Hereditary, Developmental and Immunologic Aspects of Kidney Disease*, pp. 157–159, ed. METCOFF J. Evanston, Ill.: Northwestern Univ. Press

[55] SMITH C.W. & METZGER J.F. (1962) Demonstration of a capsular structure on Listeria monocytogenes. *Path. Microbiol.* **25**, 499

[56] EASTON J.M., GOLDBERG B. & GREEN H. (1962) Immune cytolysis: Electron microscopic localization of cellular antigens with ferritin–antibody conjugates. *J. exp. Med.* **115**, 275

[57] BAXANDALL J. (1965) Sperm antigens in sperm and fertilized egg. *Electron Microscopy 1964, Proc. III European Regional Conference. Prague 1964*, Vol. B, pp. 463–464, ed. TITLBACH M. Prague: Publishing House of Czechoslovak Acad. Sci.

[58] LEE R.E. & FELDMAN J.C. (1964) Visualization of antigenic sites of human erythrocytes with ferritin–antibody conjugates. *J. Cell Biol.* **23**, 396

[59] MASOUREDIS S.P. (1960) Relation between Rho (D) genotype and quantity of I^{131} anti-Rho (D) bound to red cells. *J. Clin. Invest.* **39,** 1450

[60] GERSH I. & CATCHPOLE H.R. (1949) The organization of ground substance and basement membrane and its significance in tissue injury, disease and growth. *Am. J. Anat.* **85,** 457

[61] FARQUHAR M.G., WISSIG S.L. & PALADE G.E. (1961) Glomerular permeability. I. Ferritin transfer across the normal glomerular capillary wall. *J. exp. Med.* **113,** 47

[62] PIERCE G.B. JR., MIDGLEY A.R. JR. & SRI RAM J. (1963) The histogenesis of basement membranes. *J. exp. Med.* **117,** 339

[63] PIERCE G.B., BEALS T.F., SRI RAM J. & MIDGLEY A.R. (1964) Basement membranes. IV. Epithelial origin and immunologic cross reactions. *Am. J. Path.* **45,** 929

[64] YASUDA K. (1965) Localization intracellulaire d'une enzyme a l'aide d'anticorps marques a la ferritine. *J. de Microscopie* **4,** 169

[65] WHITE J.G., KRIVIT W. & VERNIER R.L. (1965) The platelet–fibrin relationship in human blood clots: An ultrastructural study utilizing ferritin-conjugated anti-human fibrinogen antibody. *Blood* **25,** 241

[66] WYLLIE J.C. (1964) Identification of fibrin with ferritin-conjugated anti-fibrinogen. *Exp. and Mol. Path.* **3,** 468

[67] HAUST D.M., WYLLIE J.C. & MORE R.H. (1964) Electron microscopic demonstration of fibrin with ferritin-conjugated antibody in early fatty lesions of human atherosclerosis. *Circulation* **30,** Supplementum III, 13

[68] ARHELGER R.B., GRENVALL J.A., CARR O.B. JR. & BRUNSON J.C. (1963) Electron microscopic localization of nephrotoxic serum in rabbit glomeruli with ferritin-conjugated antibody. *Lab. Invest.* **12,** 33

[69] DIXON F.J., FELDMAN J.D. & VAZQUEZ J.J. (1961) Experimental glomerulonephritis. The pathogenesis of a laboratory model resembling the spectrum of human glomerulonephritis. *J. exp. Med.* **113,** 899

[70] ANDRES G.A., SEEGAL B.C., HSU K.C., ROTHENBERG M.S. & CHAPEAU M.L. (1963) Electron microscopic studies of experimental nephritis with ferritin-conjugated antibody. Localization of antigen–antibody complexes in rabbit glomeruli following repeated injections of bovine serum albumin. *J. exp. Med.* **117,** 691

[71] SEEGAL B.C., ANDRES G.A., HSU K.C. & ZABRISKIE J.B. (1965) Studies on the pathogenesis of acute and progressive glomerulonephritis in man by immunofluorescein and immunoferritin techniques. *Fed. Proc., Symposia,* **24,** 100

[72] ANDRES G.A., ACCINNI L., HSU K.C., ZABRISKIE J.B. & SEEGAL B.C. (1966) Electron microscopic studies of human glomerulonephritis with ferritin-conjugated antibody. *J. exp. Med.* **123,** 399

[73] ZACKS S.I., METZGER J.F., SMITH C.W. & BLUMBERG J.M. (1962) Localization of ferritin-labeled botulinus toxin in the neuromuscular junction of the mouse. *J. Neuropath. Exp. Neurol.* **21,** 610

[74] DUC-NGUYEN H., ROSE H.M. & MORGAN C. (1966) An electron microscopic study of the changes at the surface of influenza-infected cells as revealed by ferritin-conjugated antibodies. *Virology* **28,** 404

[75] HARRIS G. (1964) Labeling of red cells with ferritin antibody complexes. *Vox Sang.* **9,** 70

CHAPTER 16

Immunofluorescence

E.J.HOLBOROW & G.D.JOHNSON

Introduction

In laboratory practice there are numerous methods available for using the specific reactivity of antibody with antigen to reveal the presence of antibodies in sera and other body fluids or to identify determinant groups in antigens of many different sorts, including those present in tissue cells and bacteria. These methods differ according to the mechanisms by which antigen–antibody interaction is revealed. Thus agglutination, precipitation and ana-phylaxis are classical examples of gross effects produced by antigen–antibody interaction, and more or less immediately visible to the naked eye. Another widely used group of methods exploits various secondary devices, such as antiglobulin serum, or particles or cells passively coated with antigen, as a means of converting to observable form antigen–antibody reactions that by themselves produce no obvious effects, at least when they take place *in vitro*.

In certain types of immunological investigations, however, procedures based on such test-tube reactions are inappropriate because for one reason or another a paramount requirement is recognition of antigen or antibody *in situ* in the tissues. This situation may arise, for example, in studying antibody production in lymphoid tissues at the cellular level, or in tracing the distribution in the body of antigens, whether these are foreign substances introduced into the tissues, or native constituents of the latter. In problems of this type labelled antibody or antigen used as a topographical tracer is an especially valuable tool.

Two different methods of labelling antibody or antigen molecules are in common use, one involving radio-isotopes, the other fluorochromes, and each has its place in immunological studies. Isotopes such as ^{131}I are detectable in very minute amounts, but their use in tracing antigens requires the indirect methods of autoradiography, and the resulting cytological localization may be poor.

Fluorochrome labelling of antibody or antigen on the other hand has distinct advantages in tissue tracing, as discussed below. Fluorochromes are dyes which will absorb radiation, e.g. ultraviolet light, and become excited

T* 571

thereby; the excited molecules are then capable of emitting radiation which ceases almost immediately after withdrawal of the exciting radiation. This effect is called fluorescence. The principal fluorochrome we shall deal with here is *fluorescein*, which is excited by ultra-violet/blue light to emit visible yellow-green light.

Fluorochromes may be converted to derivatives containing chemically active groups such as sulphonyl chloride or isothiocyanate, and in these forms they can be readily coupled or conjugated, with protein. In this way immune serum (or the globulin fraction from such serum in which its antibody activity resides) can be labelled with a firmly attached tracer which becomes highly conspicuous when excited. Such a labelled immune serum (or *conjugate*), properly prepared, retains its specific immunological reactivity so that if it is layered on a tissue section containing the corresponding specific antigen, union between the fluorochrome-conjugated antibody molecules and antigen takes place *in situ* in the tissue. Subsequent washing of the section in saline removes uncombined conjugate, so that on examination the sites of specific union, and hence of antigen localization, appear fluorescent. This immuno-fluorescent technique is due to A.H.Coons, of Harvard Medical School, who published the first account of conjugated antibody in 1941 [1]. Coons & Kaplan [2] showed that fluorochrome labelling allows both direct observation and precise localization of the sites of reaction of antibody; the high intensity of fluorescence produced by fluorescein and by another fluorochrome, lissamine rhodamine B [3], gives them practical value as visual markers of even very small amounts of combined antibody.

It will be readily seen that this type of procedure may be used either with conjugated *antibody* of known specific reactivity in order to detect antigen in the tissue examined, or with tissue containing known *antigen* of known localization in order to test an unknown serum conjugate for the presence of the corresponding antibody.

From these basic procedures immunofluorescent methods for detecting antibody have developed in several ways (see Fig. 16.1). In commonest use is the indirect method, in which tissue sections or cell preparations on slides are treated with the serum under investigation, thoroughly washed, and then tested for any antibody remaining specifically combined with antigen by using a conjugated antiglobulin serum of appropriate species specificity. Immunofluorescent methods are also especially applicable to localization of γ globulin—and indeed specific antibody itself—in cells and tissues. A fluorescent conjugate prepared from antiglobulin serum can be used to show the γ globulin in the cytoplasm of cells of the plasmocyte series in spleen, lymph nodes or any tissue in which antibody-forming cells are present. The chief proviso here is that the tissue sections must be prepared in such a way as to preserve the immunological reactivity of γ globulin molecules as *antigen*.

Further, it is not difficult to see that if the specific reactivity of γ globulin molecules as *antibody* can be preserved, then application of labelled antigen, or of antigen followed by labelled antibody, will pick out the individual antibody-producing cells involved in a particular specific immune response.

A practical difficulty which accompanies immunofluorescent tracing is the occurrence of 'non-specific' fluorescence, that is to say fluorescence on microscopy which is not attributable to specific antigen–antibody interaction. This may be due to autofluorescence of fibres, granules and other components in the tissue examined, often of a colour different from that of the excited

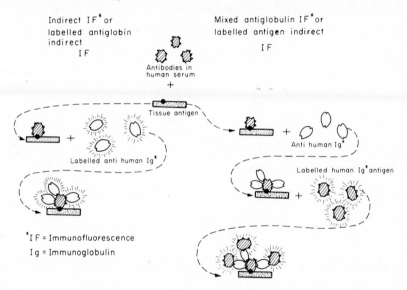

FIG. 16.1. Diagrammatic representation of indirect staining procedures.

fluorochrome; or it may be due to adherence of fluorochrome-labelled protein to components in cells or tissues for reasons unconnected with the specific antigen–antibody interactions under study. The latter unwanted effect is the more troublesome, but may in various ways be prevented or minimized, as described later in this chapter.

General consideration of factors affecting results obtained by immunofluorescent methods

The application of immunofluorescent methods involves the use of four component procedures. These are: (i) the preparation and immunological characterization of the fluorescent reagents; (ii) the preparation in suitable form of the substrate material; (iii) staining methods, and (iv) microscopy under conditions appropriate for observing fluorescence. In addition, equipment for photographing results in colour and in monochrome is virtually essential. These procedures are described in detail below, but some general aspects of preparation of substrates and characterization of conjugates may be discussed here.

Substrate

Although some immunological reactions involving fluorescent reagents may be successfully observed using antigen-carrying particles—such as cells— suspended in fluid medium, the precise localization of antigen–antibody interaction by means of fluorescence is as a rule better visualized under the microscope when a layering procedure on microscope slides is used. The substrate material is prepared and attached to the slide so as to alter as little as possible both its natural structural topography and its immunological reactivity. The use of fixatives may seriously impair or destroy the latter, and it is often necessary to use the substrate unfixed. If the material under examination is taken from an organ or tissue, snap-frozen blocks may be prepared, and sections cut from them on a microtome housed in a low-temperature cryostat cabinet. Frozen sections obtained in this way may be transferred to microscope slides and firmly attached by rapid thawing followed by drying in air. Other substrates may take the form of cell smears or impressions, blood films, or smears of micro-organisms or material containing them, all of which are suitable for testing by immunofluorescence.

The substrate usually contains the antigen involved in the immune reaction under study, but sometimes, as already mentioned, it is itself the source of antibody—as happens, for example, when sections or smears containing lymphoid tissues are to be examined for specific antibody present in cells. Here, especial care must be taken to avoid fixatives that destroy the reactivity of γ globulin as antibody. In investigational work it is therefore wise to proceed cautiously, using at first no fixative. If difficulty is encountered in retaining soluble antigen in the substrate, or as a result of repeated washing the sections or parts of them become detached, the fixing methods described below may be tried. Of these one of the most useful is the cold ethanol fixation of tissue blocks described by Sainte-Marie [4].

The conjugate

In most cases the conjugated reagent used in immunofluorescent work is antibody, but it is not difficult to envisage situations in which labelled *antigen* may be useful in tracing specific antibody in cells; a well-known example is the use of labelled aggregated γ globulin in detecting the cellular distribution of rheumatoid factor in the tissues of rheumatoid arthritis patients. Conjugates may thus be prepared with the object of providing either labelled antigen or labelled antibody. In either case, however, their quality as immunofluorescent reagents depends upon the manner of their preparation and use, especially with regard to optimal labelling and specific immunological reactivity of their constituent molecules.

For convenience of description here, factors affecting the immunofluorescent staining properties of conjugates may be considered from the standpoint of antibody, but in general, similar considerations apply also to antigen conjugates.

The procedure of conjugation consists essentially of bringing together protein and fluorochrome under conditions which allow attachment of the latter to free amino groups on the protein molecules, chiefly those in the lysine side chains. The resulting product contains a markedly heterogeneous collection of molecules, some heavily, some less heavily and some lightly labelled with fluorochrome, some serologically active and some inert. In addition, the reaction solution contains free unconjugated fluorescent material of low molecular weight, and this may be readily removed by dialysis, or by gel filtration. Some of this unreacted material, however, becomes strongly absorbed on to the protein molecules present, and is not removed by these methods [5].

If a conjugate prepared from normal serum is treated in this way, and then used to 'stain' tissue sections, a greater or lesser amount of fluorescent material will be taken up owing to the tendency of labelled protein to adhere non-specifically to tissues. This 'non-specific staining' is one of the major causes of difficulty in interpreting immunofluorescence. In the widely used indirect or 'sandwich' method, where unconjugated serum is applied to the substrate, washed off, and then followed by an antiglobulin conjugate, additional interference may be caused by adherence of some non-antibody protein from the initial serum layer, which is subsequently *specifically* stained by labelled antibodies present in the conjugate. When 'non-specific staining' due to these causes is present, observation and localization of any significant specific staining is rendered difficult and sometimes impossible.

The remedy for such non-specific staining lies in dilution of the reagents. For any conjugate a dilution may be found at which non-specific uptake of the conjugated protein by a given substrate is negligible; to put it another way, non-specific staining due to the conjugate is related directly to its total fluorochrome content. It is thus apparent that in the indirect method there is much advantage in the use of hyperimmune antisera, in which a considerable proportion of the globulin fraction is specific antibody, and experience shows that such hyperimmune conjugates diluted to the point where they give only minimal non-specific staining still contain more than enough labelled antibody to give bright and easily discernible staining of specific antigen in the substrate.

Contrary, then, to an idea implicit in much current immunofluorescent practice, detection of weak positive staining in the presence of non-specific staining in the indirect test is not necessarily improved by using concentrated conjugate; weak staining is in fact rendered clearer by using a 'strong' conjugate appropriately diluted. Consideration shows why this is so. If a serum under test for the presence of a tissue-reactive antibody is of low titre, it will yield only a small amount of antibody γ globulin for specific attachment to antigen present in the substrate. The antibody remaining specifically attached after washing serves as antigen to take up labelled antiglobulin antibody from the conjugate subsequently applied and clearly the amount of antiglobulin antibody then taken up is limited by the number of antibody molecules that have initially secured antigen sites in the substrate. The number of labelled antiglobulin molecules required to combine with all the available antigenic determinants on these antibody molecules depends not only upon the number of these determinants but also upon the concentration of labelled antiglobulin antibody. Since this antiglobulin antibody is in the main divalent, at low concentrations there is a tendency for individual molecules to bridge across where possible between neighbouring determinants. With increasing concentration it becomes more likely that each molecule of antiglobulin antibody in the conjugate will combine with only one antigenic determinant. When saturation point of the available antigenic determinants is reached, nothing is gained by further increasing the concentration of conjugated antibody, and attempts to do so merely increase the likelihood of non-specific uptake. With potent antiglobulin the saturation point is achieved at considerable dilution of the conjugate.

These considerations apply with even greater force to titration of antibodies in sera by the indirect immunofluorescent method. With serial dilution of unconjugated sera under test the amount of non-specific uptake of protein by the substrate rapidly falls off, so that specific staining by subsequently applied conjugate is predominantly staining of specifically reacted antibody, and minimally staining of non-antibody protein. It is obviously important not to mask reactions due to this specific antibody by non-specific staining, which, as discussed above, is due to inadequate dilution of the conjugate, and this is especially important near the end-point of the serum titration where the intensity of specific staining is beginning to fall off. Thus it can hardly be stressed too strongly that reproducible titrations by immunofluorescence demand the use of well-tailored conjugates whose immunological and staining properties have been carefully assessed for specificity; some simple methods of assessment are described in detail below.

When acceptable specificity is achieved, there remains the problem of sensitivity. As pointed out above, the small amount of antibody globulin yielded by a low titre serum, or by the higher dilutions of a serum titration, can take up only as many molecules of labelled antibody as its available antigenic determinants permit. It will be seen, however, that heavily labelled molecules fluoresce more brightly than lightly labelled molecules, and it follows that, provided immunological reactivity remains unimpaired, an antiglobulin conjugate containing highly labelled antibody will provide a more sensitive immunofluorescent tracer than a lightly labelled reagent. Comparisons of titration results obtained with different conjugates should therefore take into account not only their immunological and staining characteristics, but also their mean fluorochrome : protein (F : P) ratios.

When these parameters are defined, attempts to standardize immuno-fluorescent procedures are more likely to meet with success.

PROCEDURES

Fluorescent reagents

The success with which immunofluorescent studies are carried out depends largely on the selection of suitable starting material for the preparation of the fluorescent reagents. As discussed above, these fall into two categories depending on whether the application is intended to demonstrate the location of antigen or antibody. Conjugated antisera for the detection of antigen are of two kinds—those intended for use by the direct staining method which involves the use of fluorescent antiserum specific for the antigen under study, and those employed in the indirect method which are conjugates of antisera to γ globulin capable of combining with the complex formed between antigen present in the substrate and specific antibody.

I. Conjugated antisera
A. *Preparation of antisera*
It is essential to employ very potent antisera, as those which have only moderate activity do not permit the degree of dilution which is desirable in the staining procedure. Suitably potent sera are prepared in animals known to give a good precipitin response—rabbit and goat are most commonly employed for this purpose. We have found the following scheme satisfactory for the production of suitably potent antisera to protein antigens:

A group of six young adult rabbits is given twice-weekly deep subcutaneous (suprascapular) injections of the protein antigen combined with Freund's complete adjuvant. Usually 1 mg of the antigen is given per dose. After the eighth injection the animals are rested for 1 week and a trial bleeding carried out. The neat sera are tested for precipitating activity in capillary tubes with an equal volume of a series of tenfold dilutions of antigen solution. It is usually found that one or two of the rabbits respond better than the others and these are selected for further immunization, the others being discarded. The twice-weekly injections are resumed for several weeks and the animals rested for 1 week. They are then given a single intraperitoneal injection of the antigen solution and bled 1 week later. The serum is best stored in small aliquots in polystyrene tubes at $-20°$ C. Storage at higher temperatures and in the presence of bacteriostatic agents may not be satisfactory.

Commercial antisera against various protein fractions are now available and these undoubtedly fulfil a need where animal immunization is not practicable. However, it must be emphasized that such sera, which may have been intended for other uses, should on no account be used in immunofluorescent studies until they have been adequately assessed both quantitatively and qualitatively as described below.

Indirect staining involves the use of antisera specific for the antibody-containing fractions of serum. The scope of this procecure has been widened by recent studies on the heterogeneity of the immunoglobulin class of proteins, and by the use of specific antisera it is possible to characterize the immunoglobulins involved in any system which can be studied by immunofluorescence without recourse to elaborate fractionation of individual test sera. Thus, rabbit antisera may be prepared which react specifically with IgG, IgA or IgM or against the light peptide chain common to immunoglobulins.

The evaluation of antisera and the determination of their suitability for use as fluorescent reagents must be considered in terms of both potency and specificity.

1. *Quantitative assessment*

The degree to which an antiserum may be diluted and still give visible precipitation with a standard amount of antigen gives some indication of the serum's potency. In order to compare antisera and carry out fluorescent tests at comparable degrees of sensitivity in different antigen–antibody systems it is desirable to use a standardized procedure to determine antibody content. For this purpose an accurate quantitative estimation may be performed but we have found the following simpler method capable of giving very reproducible results. Antisera are titrated in a series of doubling dilutions against a solution containing 1 mg of protein antigen per ml. The test is carried out in 0·9 per cent Ionagar either in Petri dishes, using the Shandon titration die, or when material is limited to small quantities, by pouring a layer of agar on to a standard microscope slide and cutting a pattern consisting of six wells equally spaced round a centre well (2·5 mm diameter, 8 mm between centres of the central and peripheral wells). Doubling dilutions from neat to 1 : 32 of the antiserum are placed in the peripheral wells and the antigen solution is placed in the centre. The test is read after standing at room temperature for 3 days, or 2 days in the case of the micro-method. The highest dilution of the antiserum which gives a visible line of precipitation is taken as the end-point, the reciprocal of this dilution expressing the number of units of precipitating antibody present in 1 ml of the neat serum. Potent antisera usually contain 16–32 units per ml by this method and such sera should be selected for conjugation if possible since problems with non-specific staining will be encountered if weaker antisera are employed owing to their relatively high content of γ globulin lacking specific antiglobulin activity.

2. *Qualitative assessment*
The specificity of the antisera used for conjugation should be established by appropriate testing. In the case of antiglobulin sera intended for use in the indirect staining method this involves analysis by immunoelectrophoresis. Absorption of unwanted antibodies by addition of *solutions* of appropriate antigens should be carried out with caution, for the following reasons. Firstly, it may result in subsequent conjugation of irrelevant material from the solution used for absorption. Secondly, antibody present in combination with antigen in the form of soluble complexes may subsequently dissociate and recombine with insoluble antigen present in the substrate. It is therefore preferable to remove irrelevant antibodies by the addition of insoluble antigen after the antiserum has been conjugated.

B. *Procedure for conjugation of antisera*
Conjugates are usually prepared from a globulin fraction of the antiserum in order to avoid non-specific staining attributable to the presence of a large amount of conjugated albumin and other irrelevant proteins. Although other workers have advocated conjugation of isolated γ globulin fractions obtained by chromatographic separation on DEAE-cellulose, we find that satisfactory fluorescent reagents may be prepared from crude globulin fractions prepared by a simple salting-out procedure, provided that proper consideration be given to the points described below. The method of preparation of the globulin fraction described here is designed to preserve maximum antibody activity rather than provide a chemically pure fraction, and when prepared in this way the albumin-depleted solution contains precipitating antibody activity comparable with that of the original whole serum.

1. *Preparation of globulin fraction*
Add an equal volume of cold saturated ammonium sulphate solution to the chilled serum, and mix thoroughly by pouring backwards and forwards. Refrigerate at 4° C for 30 minutes, centrifuge in the cold and discard the supernate. With some sera the precipitated protein does not pack well in the

tube and it is necessary to centrifuge for about 1 hour at about 3000 rev/min in the M.S.E. Major refrigerated centrifuge. The precipitate is partly redissolved by adding the minimum volume of 0·15 M saline necessary to enable it to be transferred to a dialysis bag. Excessive dilution at this stage is undesirable in view of the final protein concentration required in the conjugate. Dialysis against normal saline is carried out for about 18 hours at 4° C with at least one change. Mechanical aids to dialysis such as the use of magnetic stirrers should be employed cautiously in order to minimize frothing which may bring about denaturation of γ globulin. After dialysis is completed the globulin solution should be almost clear. The small amount of undissolved material consisting of denatured protein is easily removed by brief centrifugation. The protein content of the globulin solution is determined—usually by the Biuret reaction—and its volume measured.

2. Choice of fluorochrome

Most workers prefer to use conjugates made with fluorescein on account of its bright fluorescence emission. It is claimed by Fothergill [6] that derivatives of rhodamine have the advantage of providing better contrast with the blue autofluorescence which is characteristic of many tissues. Other fluorochromes have been advocated but have not found general acceptance. We feel that the intensity obtained with fluorescein outweighs the possible disadvantage of the proximity of its emission wavelength to that of autofluorescence. Following the introduction of the isothiocyanate compound it is possible to carry out the conjugation under simple conditions in an aqueous medium, the fluorochrome itself being stable in powder form provided that it is kept dry. It has been suggested [7] that there would be an advantage in returning to the use of fluorescein isocyanate on account of its higher molar emission. Unfortunately, however, this compound is highly reactive with water and requires to be stored in organic solution, and furthermore, the conjugation mixture involves the use of water-free reagents.

Rhodamine R.B. 200, in the sulphonyl chloride form, is a useful second fluorochrome for simultaneous demonstration of two independent specific immunological reactions. When conjugated with an irrelevant protein it may also be applied as a non-specific fluorescent counterstain (*vide infra*) as described by Smith, Marshall & Eveland [8]. Absorption and emission characteristics of fluorescent conjugates are more fully dealt with in the section on microscopy.

3. Conjugation reaction mixture. (a) *Fluorescein isothiocyanate (FITC)*

Conjugation is carried out at a final protein concentration of 10 mg per ml at pH 9·0. This is accomplished by dilution of the globulin solution to an appropriate volume using isotonic saline solution and carbonate–bicarbonate buffer. The volume of buffer added is equal to one-tenth of the final volume, as shown in the following example. The mixture is prepared in an ice-bath with gentle mechanical stirring and the required amount of fluorescein iso-thiocyanate then added.

Example of conjugation mixture:

5 ml globulin solution containing 20 mg protein per ml (i.e. total protein = 100 mg)
4 ml 0·15 M sodium chloride solution
1 ml carbonate–bicarbonate buffer pH 9·0, 0·5 M (3·7 g $NaHCO_3$ and 0·6 g Na_2CO_3 (anhydrous) made up to 100 ml with distilled water)
5 mg FITC.

Chill the mixture in an ice-bath before adding the dry FITC powder which has been stored in a desiccator over $CaCl_2$. Leave for 18 hours at 4° C with *gentle* mixing to avoid frothing (a magnetic stirrer or rotary mixer as used for blood samples is suitable). Dialyse the solution against several changes of phosphate buffered saline pH 7* until the dialysing fluid no longer shows fluorescence. Store stock conjugate at −20° C, either divided into small aliquots in plastic tubes or lyophilized.

Amount of FITC for conjugation: Between 0·02 mg and 0·08 mg of FITC per 1 mg of protein should be used; 0·08 mg is required only for strong antisera containing at least 16–32 units of precipitating activity. For most antisera the optimum amount is 0·05 mg per 1 mg of protein.

Conjugation reaction mixture. (b) *Rhodamine R.B.* 200
Commercial preparations of this fluorochrome may contain a high proportion of impurity (mostly dextrin) and it is advantageous to remove this by extract-ing the dye with alcohol and reprecipitating with acetone, as follows:

Dissolve 10 g of the dye in about 100 ml of 75 per cent ethanol with warm-ing. Cool, filter through kieselguhr. Wash through with 75 per cent ethanol and concentrate the filtrate to a small volume by evaporation on a water-bath. Add 9 volumes of acetone to precipitate the dye, filter and wash the precipi-tate with acetone. Evaporate to dryness.

Rhodamine is converted to its sulphonyl chloride derivative for conjugation by trituration of 1 g of the purified dye with 2 g of phosphorus pentachloride. 10 ml of acetone are added and the solution is filtered after standing for 5 minutes.

Conjugation is carried out under similar conditions to those used for FITC described above, i.e. in an ice-bath at pH 9. A suitable reaction mixture is as follows:

* 8·5 g NaCl, 0·85 g Na_2HPO_4 (anhydrous) and 0·54 g KH_2PO_4 made up to 1 litre with distilled water. This is referred to throughout as phosphate buffered saline.

1 ml whole serum or globulin solution
1 ml 0·15 M saline
1 ml carbonate–bicarbonate buffer pH 9, 0·5 M
0·1 ml of the acetone solution is added drop by drop with continuous stirring. After mixing overnight in the cold the solution is dialysed and stored as described above for FITC conjugates.

II. Conjugation of antigens
As described above, fluorescent staining may also be carried out using a conjugated solution of antigen rather than of antibody. In the case of protein antigens the conjugate is prepared following the principles outlined for the conjugation of antisera, most of the linkage occurring through the epsilon amino group of lysine. Conjugation of antigenic materials other than proteins can also take place through available OH or SH groups under suitable reaction conditions, e.g. at pH <9. The use of conjugated γ globulin in the mixed indirect technique which has recently been described by Beutner, Holborow & Johnson [9] has renewed interest in labelled antigen.

III. Methods of reducing non-specific staining due to the conjugate
A characteristic feature of fluorescent conjugates is their ability to stain most tissues non-specifically. In order to recognize true specific staining it is therefore necessary to minimize this effect without detriment to the specific activity of the reagent. Consideration of the problems of non-specific staining (NSS) not associated with properties of the conjugate will be found in later sections. It is appropriate to deal here with NSS attributable to the conjugate itself. Extensive work has been carried out on this subject and procedures of varying complexity have been advocated for dealing with the problem.

Purification procedures. The most widely used method for removing components of the conjugate responsible for NSS is absorption with tissue homogenate as originally described by Coons and Kaplan. This empirical procedure not only has the merit of simplicity, but if the absorption is carried out serially two or three times obviates the time-consuming process of dialysis for removal of unreacted dye [10].

Preparation of tissue homogenate.
1. Homogenize the chosen tissue in an equal volume of 0·15 M saline in a Waring blender.
2. Transfer to a large measuring cylinder and precipitate with about 5 volumes of acetone.
3. Remove supernate by suction and wash 3 times with saline by filling the cylinder, allowing the tissue particles to sediment, and removing the supernate.
4. Remove lipids by further washing with acetone.

5. Transfer to Büchner funnel and wash through with acetone.

6. Spread material on filter paper and dry overnight in incubator at 37° C.

7. Grind in a mortar and pass through a fine sieve to remove fibrous particles.

8. Shake in phosphate buffered saline pH 7, distribute in tubes, centrifuge and discard supernatant fluid.

9. Stored in deep freeze, the material keeps indefinitely.

Absorption procedure. One volume of packed homogenate is usually added to about 2 volumes of conjugate. The tube is gently rotated for about 10–20 minutes, preferably in the cold, and then centrifuged. In order to eliminate the highly fluorescent particles adhering to the top of the tube it is advisable to transfer the absorbed conjugate to a second tube and recentrifuge before use.

Choice of tissue for absorption. It is usual to employ a cellular tissue unrelated to the system being studied. For example, rabbit liver is suitable for absorbing conjugates required for studying human antibodies by the indirect staining method. The only proviso is that the absorbing material should not normally contain antigen related to the specific activity of the conjugate.

Unreacted dye may also be removed by passing the conjugate through a column of G50 Sephadex which acts as a 'molecular sieve'. This procedure is equivalent to dialysis but has no advantage other than being less time consuming. Moreover, it is not on its own an adequate treatment for the prevention of non-specific staining of tissue due to the conjugate.

A more elegant procedure for the purification of conjugates involves fractionation of the conjugated material by column chromatography using ion-exchange resins. By this means it is possible to separate globulin fractions of varying degrees of labelling. It has been shown that NSS is associated with strongly labelled protein, and when conjugates are passed through columns of DEAE-cellulose elution with low molarity buffers results in removal of lightly conjugated globulin, the more highly charged heavily conjugated material being retained in the column. Conjugated proteins are not eluted under exactly the same conditions as native proteins and for details of this procedure the papers of Goldstein *et al* [11, 12] and McDevitt *et al* [7] should be consulted.

Dilution procedure

The problem of NSS attributable to the conjugate can be resolved by consideration of the basic components of the conjugate. Recent findings in our laboratory favour the adoption of a simple approach based upon dilution of the conjugate. The following conclusions have been reached following an extensive analysis in collaboration with Dr Ernst Beutner of factors affecting detection of antinuclear factor (ANF) [13] in human sera using an FITC conjugate of rabbit anti-human IgG [14]. They have been confirmed in other systems and appear to be generally applicable.

Specific staining is clearly a function of the antibody activity present in the conjugate associated with a satisfactory degree of labelling. Non-specific staining, on the other hand, is attributable to the presence of unreacted dye, to excessively labelled protein and also to high absolute fluorescein concentration in the solution. We have found that consideration of all these factors is desirable in order to prepare conjugates of maximum efficiency.

Unreacted free dye is readily removable by dialysis against phosphate buffered saline, as described above; the influence of the remaining variables will be considered separately.

A. *Antibody activity.* There has long been uncertainty regarding the relation of the *precipitating* antibody activity of the conjugate to its staining efficacy. Conjugates prepared as described above from potent precipitating antisera can be shown to have retained their precipitating activity by the usual serological techniques. Thus, the antibody content of such conjugates may be demonstrated both qualitatively, e.g. by immunoelectrophoresis and quantitatively by titration in agar against a standard antigen solution as described in IA section 1 above. Potent conjugates usually contain 4 to 16 units of precipitating activity. We have studied the effect of varying the amount of conjugated antibody on the results of titrating a serum containing ANF. It was found that the maximum ANF titre in the patient's serum was obtained as a plateau over a wide range of dilutions of the conjugate extending beyond the maximum dilution which had given visible precipitation in the standard precipitin test described. When several conjugates were compared, it was found that they all gave a similar plateau for ANF titre, sometimes extending to a dilution of the conjugate containing as little as 1 : 16 of the maximum dilution found to give a precipitin line, when titrated against a solution containing 1 mg of human IgG per ml. This is illustrated in Fig. 16.2 showing the titration of a conjugate containing 4 units of precipitating antibody (i.e. giving a precipitin line in the gel-diffusion test at a dilution of 1 : 4 but not at 1 : 8). The maximum ANF titre obtainable with a given serum using this conjugate, viz. 1 : 800, is maintained over a range of conjugate dilutions from 4 units to $\frac{1}{16}$ unit (i.e. from neat conjugate down to a dilution of 1 : 128). Beyond this range the ANF titre obtained drops rapidly.

It is therefore apparent that the potency of the fluorescent reagent in terms of the maximum obtainable antibody titre which it gives by indirect staining *is* a function of its antiglobulin activity but is not directly correlated with precipitating activity.

B. *Absolute FITC concentration.* The concentration of FITC in conjugates prepared by adding 0·05 mg of FITC per mg of protein is of the order 100 μg per ml after dialysis to remove unreacted dye. It has been found that conjugates diluted to contain 5 μg of FITC per ml or less give negligible non-specific staining when applied to tissue sections. On the other hand, solutions containing over 25 μg/ml usually give so much NSS as to render them unusable. FITC levels between 5 μg and 15 μg yield variable amounts of NSS but are usually satisfactory.

It is therefore evident, in view of the findings discussed above relating to antibody activity in the conjugate, that conjugates may be diluted so that they contain an acceptably low level of conjugated fluorochrome yet still possess maximum sensitivity for the detection of titration end-points.

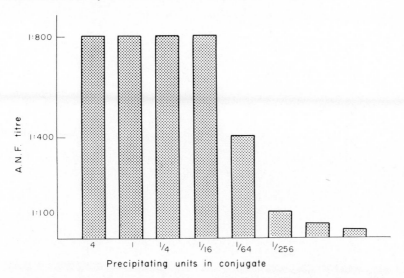

FIG. 16.2. Effect of diluting conjugate on titre of ANF obtained with a given positive serum. Ordinate shows dilutions of conjugate expressed in terms of precipitating units.

Estimation of FITC in conjugates
The relative FITC content of conjugates is determined by measurement of absorption in the spectrophotometer at 492 mμ—the maximum absorption peak of FITC. The reading is corrected to allow for irrelevant absorption (at this wavelength) by subtraction of half the absorption at 320 mμ. Unless this correction is made optical density is not a linear function of the FITC concentration of the conjugate.

Thus, the corrected extinction at 492 mμ = E 492 mμ−½E 320 mμ. This value is converted to FITC concentration by reference to a standard solution of the dye. Using a standard solution of crystalline FITC we have obtained the following extinction coefficient:

$$E_{1\,cm}^{1\,\mu g/ml} \; 492 \; m\mu = 0{\cdot}20$$

The fluorescein concentration of the conjugate is calculated using this coefficient as follows:

$$\text{FITC concentration of conjugate} = \frac{\text{E 492 m}\mu\,(\text{corrected}) \times \text{dilution}}{0\cdot20}\ \mu\text{g/ml.}$$

A dilution of the neat conjugate suitable for spectrophotometry is of the order 1 : 20.

C. *Fluorescein : protein ratio*. As already indicated above, heavily conjugated protein in the conjugate is also a cause of non-specific staining. The

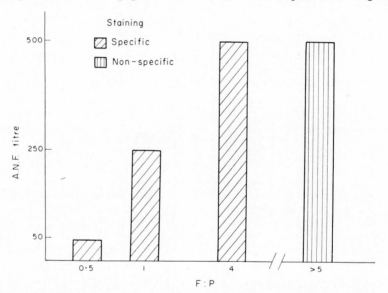

FIG. 16.3. The effect of using conjugates with different mean fluorescein: protein (molar) ratios prepared from a single antiglobulin serum on the ANF titre obtained with a given serum.

relation of both specific and non-specific staining to the overall fluorescein : protein ratio has been studied using conjugates of antisera labelled with different amounts of fluorescein. The results are summarized in Fig. 16.3. Conjugates with F : P ratios over about 5 : 1 appear to be of little value because they give rise to an unacceptably high level of NSS. However, with ratios below this, it appears that the titre of antibody obtained for a particular serum by indirect staining is proportional to the F : P ratio of the conjugate used.

Determination of FITC : protein ratio of conjugate
The ratio of the fluorescein concentration to the protein contained in the

conjugate is obtained from the FITC level as determined above, and the protein as estimated by the Biuret method using a protein standard, spectrophotometer readings being made at 560 mμ. With molecular weights of 390 for FITC and 160,000 for antibody globulin the F : P ratio is estimated according to the following formula:

$$F : P = 0{\cdot}41 \times \frac{\mu g/ml\ FITC}{mg/ml\ protein}$$

A simpler expression for the determination of F : P ratio may be derived by combining the constants relating to the FITC extinction coefficient and the relative molecular weights.

$$F : P = 2{\cdot}06 \times \frac{E\,492\ m\mu\ (corrected)}{mg/ml\ protein}$$

IV. Standardization

It is evident from the foregoing that the problems of establishing adequate specific reactivity for *titration* of antibody by the indirect method, combined with an acceptably low level of NSS can be simply resolved by appropriate dilution of the conjugate in accordance with the above parameters. Furthermore, conjugates adjusted in this way have proved to be equally satisfactory reagents for *screening* sera for the presence of particular antibodies.

The need for standardization in immunofluorescence has long been apparent. Disagreement between different laboratories could evidently be due to variability not only in test materials but also in the basic fluorescent reagent itself. The above considerations suggest an approach to this problem which would make comparisons between different laboratories a functional possibility, for by appropriate analysis and consequent adjustment of the conjugate as outlined it is possible to prepare defined reagents for use in particular systems.

The following is a summary of the minimum requirements for characterization of conjugated antiglobulin sera for use in indirect staining.

A. Serological analysis: 1. Qualitative assessment by immunoelectrophoresis.
2. Quantitative determination of antibody.
B. Chemical analysis: 1. FITC concentration.
2. Protein content.
3. F : P ratio.

On the basis of these measurements it is suggested that the dialysed conjugate should be diluted for use both in screening tests and for titration of antibodies so that it contains:

about $\frac{1}{8}$ unit of precipitating antibody of defined Ig specificity
    FITC concentration 5 μg/ml
    F : P ratio 5 : 1

Under these conditions non-specific staining is negligible and specific staining easily recognized

Note: It is known that commercial preparations of FITC may contain varying quantities of impurity and our findings are based upon experience of conjugates prepared from such samples. When FITC of standard purity becomes available the figures quoted above may require modification.

Substrates

I. *Tissues*

The method of preparation of material for staining by immunofluorescence is determined by the particular antigen/antibody system involved, and in new systems the most suitable procedure should be established by experiment. Fixation, for example by alcohol, results in sections of tissue which are histologically superior to those obtained from unfixed material. On the other hand, such fixed tissue is not suitable for study of antigens soluble in alcohol, e.g. the cytoplasmic antigen in thyroid epithelium which reacts with antibody often present in the serum of patients with thyroiditis. Accordingly it is necessary to consider two types of tissue processing.

    A. *Unfixed tissue.* Slices of tissue up to about 0·5 cm in thickness are placed in polythene bags* which are sealed. A freezing-mixture consisting of solid CO_2 in alcohol is prepared. This may be conveniently stored in a Ewer flask, and kept in a deep-freeze cabinet at $-20°$ C. The tissue is snap-frozen by holding the bag below the surface of the mixture for about 5 minutes. This method results in rapid freezing and is preferable to placing the tissue in contact with dry CO_2. After snap-freezing the bag is stored in a deep-freeze cabinet at a temperature not higher than $-20°$ C, and the tissue is on no account subsequently allowed to thaw. Prolonged storage in an atmosphere of CO_2 is to be avoided as this may result in acidification due to penetration by the gas. When preparing tissue for snap-freezing it is important to consider the desired orientation as this is often difficult to determine when it is frozen. In the case of thin tissues, such as gastric mucosa and synovial membrane, where it is necessary to cut full-thickness sections at right-angles to the surface, a larger area of the tissue may be prepared for study by rolling it in the form of a 'Swiss roll' and cutting sections at right-angles to the long axis.

    Sections of snap-frozen tissue are usually cut in a cryostat which is essentially a refrigerated cabinet maintained at $-20°$ C containing a microtome.

---

* 'Minigrip' bags supplied by Supreme Novelty Co., Vale Road, Finsbury Park, London, N.4, have been found very convenient.

The microtome knife should have an antiroll device, which corrects the tendency of the sections to curl—and consists of a hinged transparent plate which is held in a suitable position parallel to the ground facet of the knife during the cutting operation. This device is necessary because the sections should not be floated out on water in the usual way. The exact positioning of the plate, with regard to both height and angle in relation to the knife, is extremely critical and should be established by trial and error at each location of the knife, otherwise considerable difficulty will be experienced due to the sections failing to slide flatly down the knife surface. The tissue block is frozen on to the microtome chuck by applying the smallest amount of water round its base necessary to effect attachment. The water may be conveniently applied with a blunt-ended pair of forceps which when closed hold a small drop which can be accurately deposited by opening the forceps. A small piece of filter paper frozen to the chuck face below the tissue improves adhesion. It is important that the tissue does not become waterlogged as this results not only in destruction of the cellular architecture by partial thawing and refreezing, but also in diffusion of any water-soluble components which may be associated with immunological activity. This is unavoidable at the base of the tissue block and for this reason very small specimens are not suitable for handling by this procedure. The cut sections are transferred to acid-washed slides kept at room temperature, by bringing the slide close to the knife surface so that the section becomes attached. As the section thaws out it becomes firmly bound to the glass. It is essential to dry out the sections completely, and this process should be accelerated by placing the slide immediately in the air current from an electric fan. The average drying time taken is about 10 minutes. However, some tissues, particularly those from the alimentary tract which are rich in polysaccharide, and also lipid-containing tissues, require at least 30 minutes' drying to ensure that the sections do not become detached during the staining process.

B. *Fixed tissue.* An alternative procedure to the use of snap-frozen material, involving fixation in cold alcohol followed by embedding in paraffin, has proved successful in many studies. This method has been found to preserve reactivity of antibody better than freezing, and the quality of the sections produced is certainly superior. In systems where the immunological activity of the tissue component is not adversely affected by treatment with alcohol, this procedure is the method of choice, thereby obviating the need for a cryostat. The steps in the processing of tissue by this method as described by Sainte-Marie [4] are as follows:

1. Place a block of tissue not more than 5 mm thick into 95 per cent ethanol pre-cooled to 4° C in a well-stoppered container. Return to refrigerator for 1 hour.

2. After hardening trim into slices 2–4 mm thick and return to refrigerator for 15–24 hours at 4° C to complete fixation in 95 per cent alcohol.

3. Dehydrate in four changes of pre-cooled absolute alcohol, 1–2 hours each.

4. Clear by passing through three consecutive baths of pre-cooled xylene for 1–2 hours each at 4° C, and bring the last bath to room temperature.

5. Embed in paraffin at 56° C, passing through four consecutive baths for 1–2 hours each.

6. The blocks are stored at 4° C and may be satisfactory for up to 2 or 3 months.

7. Sectioning is carried out as usual but flotation on water at 40° C should be as brief as possible: after drying at 37° C for half an hour the sections are deparaffinized by placing the slides in two consecutive baths of cold xylene for 10–15 seconds each.

8. Remove the xylene in three baths of cold 95 per cent alcohol (10–15 seconds each), and remove the alcohol by gentle agitation in three baths of fresh cold phosphate-staining buffer, each lasting about a minute.

9. Immunofluorescent staining should be carried out promptly.

This procedure has been found very satisfactory in this laboratory for the demonstration of rheumatoid factor activity in tissues by staining them with heat-aggregated conjugates of γ globulin. It is not, however, suitable for preparing substrates for the detection of antinuclear factor.

Variations of the above procedures may be required in particular situations. For example, in order to demonstrate the presence of antibodies to colloid constituents of the thyroid in the serum of cases of Hashimoto's thyroiditis, it is desirable to fix cryostat sections of snap-frozen thyroid by immersing the slides in 95 per cent ethanol; methanol and acetone have also been employed in this way as fixatives in other systems. In the paraffin-embedding technique also, alternative fixatives may prove superior for some antigens; among those which may be tried are cold ethanol in concentrations varying from 10 to 30 per cent and from 80 to 100 per cent, 95 per cent methanol, absolute acetone and 5 per cent formalin in 95 per cent ethanol.

II. *Other substrates*

The reactivity of antigen or antibody in isolated cells by fluorescent staining has been studied using both cell suspensions and dried smear preparations. By the former method only superficial staining of the cells is likely to occur owing to lack of penetration by the reagents and this produces a characteristic peripheral staining pattern, which is seen both at the margins of free cells and also around clumps of cells. Jankovic [15] and Cohen, Zuelzer & Evans [16] have used this procedure for the demonstration of blood-group antigens on the surface of red blood cells. The staining and washing is carried out in small test-tubes, the cells being recovered by gentle centrifugation and finally suspended in neutral glycerine for examination.

A simpler method of studying cells is by the use of dried smear preparations which give very satisfactory results provided that they are suitably made. An advantage of this method is that the permeability of the cell membranes is increased and this results in better exposure of cell contents to the staining reagents and consequently more uniform staining. We have found that such smears of, for example, whole blood may be successfully used in a variety of systems. Very thin smears are essential and these are made by inclining the spreading slide at not more than 10°. It has been found that smears of more usual thickness tend to show large areas of non-specific staining. Unfixed smears are satisfactory in many systems, but unless they are thoroughly dried many of the cells become detached during staining and are lost during washing. It is therefore desirable to dry the smears with the aid of a fan for at least 30 minutes. As the smear cannot be easily seen after washing it is helpful to mark a small area—about 1 cm in diameter—in the thinnest part of the smear. This test area should not be allowed to become dry after the commencement of the staining procedure. After the final washing the preparation is mounted in buffered glycerine in the usual way.

As in the case of tissue sections it is sometimes an advantage to apply fixatives to the dried smears before staining. In virus studies, for example, the smears of pathological material may be fixed in cold acetone for a few minutes prior to treatment with fluorescent reagents.

It will be evident from the foregoing that it is not possible to describe a method of preparation of material for study by immunofluorescence which is universally applicable. The ideal conditions are determined by the characteristics of the particular system involved and should be determined experimentally according to the principles outlined.

Staining procedures
General considerations
Conjugates standardized as described above should be used whatever staining procedure is adopted. In order to prevent loss by evaporation during staining it is essential to treat the slides in a moist chamber. The time of application of each reagent is usually 30 minutes. Longer exposure than this has not been found to enhance specific staining but does increase the amount of non-specific staining produced. Removal of non-specifically bound reactants is best accomplished by washing the slides in a bath of buffered saline with the aid of a mechanical stirring device. A convenient arrangement is to place them in a carrier supported over a magnetic stirring bar so that there is a continuous circulation of saline. Transfer of free serum or conjugate to the

bath may be avoided by first gently rinsing each slide with saline from a wash-bottle. Phosphate-buffered saline pH 7 is used for washing after treatment with both serum and conjugate and the minimum washing time is 30 minutes. After the application of conjugate, however, more prolonged washing for up to 2 hours is desirable. The stained preparations are finally mounted in glycerine containing 10 per cent by volume of buffered saline pH 7.

It is imperative that the test area on the slide does not become dry at any stage during the entire procedure, as this results in local concentration of salt which produces artefacts on subsequent solution. This is particularly important in systems involving tissue components which are soluble in hypertonic solutions, e.g. nucleoprotein, and must be especially borne in mind when large batches of slides are being processed. In order to minimize dilution of the reagents it is necessary to mop off surplus moisture from the slide with lint-free cloth, avoiding the test area which is left wet. When several slides are to be stained, each slide in turn should be mopped off, treated with the next reagent and returned to the moist chamber. Finally, it must be emphasized that appropriate controls for the particular method should be included in each batch of staining in order to interpret the results correctly.

I. *Direct staining*

This method is appropriate for the demonstration of antigen when potent antiserum is available for conjugation, and also for the demonstration of the sites of antibody formation by the use of conjugated antigen. In both cases the staining procedure is as follows:

Method. 1. Apply conjugate for 30 minutes.
2. Wash in buffered saline for 1 to 2 hours.
3. Mount.

Controls. In order to distinguish staining attributable to specific immunological reaction from non-specific staining, as for example in the demonstration of the presence of antigen in tissue by the use of conjugated antiserum, the following controls are desirable: (1) Pre-treatment of a tissue section with the unconjugated antiserum. This results in specific inhibition of subsequent staining by the conjugated antiserum whereas pre-treatment with unconjugated antiserum of unrelated specificity has no effect. (2) Addition to the conjugate of excess specific antigen which prevents specific staining. (3) Use of conjugated antiserum not directed against the antigen in question.

An interesting application of the direct staining method is the demonstration of rheumatoid factor activity in tissues from rheumatoid patients by the use of conjugated γ globulin aggregated by heat [17]. This is illustrated in Plate 16.1.

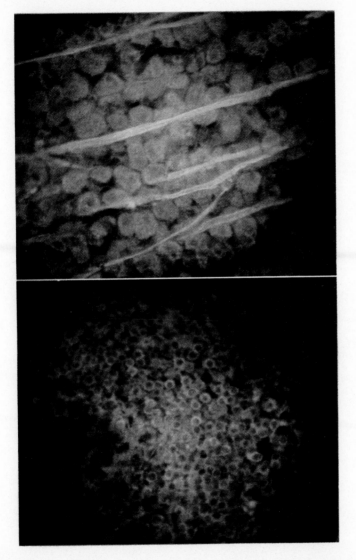

PLATE 16.1. Cryostat section of rat stomach mucosa treated with serum from a case of 'lupoid' hepatitis and anti-human globulin conjugate showing staining of smooth muscle fibres in the mucosa. The patient's serum also contains antibody reacting with gastric parietal cells.

PLATE 16.2. Section of ethanol-fixed lymph node from a case of sero-positive rheumatoid arthritis, stained with heat-aggregated conjugated human γ globulin showing presence of rheumatoid factor in the cytoplasm of plasma cells.

(*Facing page* 592)

II. *Indirect staining*
This involves the use of unconjugated serum, the site of whose reaction is demonstrated by means of labelled antiserum specific for the immunoglobulin participating in the first stage of the reaction. It is therefore possible to use one conjugate for the detection of most antibodies likely to be found in the sera of a particular species; for example, a single conjugated antiserum against human immunoglobulins will serve to detect most human antibodies. The use of this procedure may in fact reveal unexpected or indeed hitherto unrecognized reactions. For example, in the course of screening sera for the presence of the antibody to gastric parietal cell cytoplasm [18] we observed staining of smooth muscle fibres in the sections of stomach. Subsequent work has shown this serological finding to be a feature of lupoid hepatitis which may prove to be of value in differentiating this disease from systemic lupus erythematosus [19]. This is illustrated in Plate 16.2. A further advantage of this system as compared with direct staining is that since the immune complexes are produced in antibody excess there is a geometric increase at each stage in the amount of antibody combined and this results in considerable enhancement of sensitivity. The use of unconjugated serum in the middle layer, however, is an additional source of non-specific staining, and for this reason it is usually desirable to dilute the serum at least 1 : 4.

Method. 1. Apply (diluted) serum . . . 30 minutes.
2. Wash . . . 30 minutes.
3. Stain with labelled antiglobulin serum . . . 30 minutes.
4. Wash . . . 1–2 hours.
5. Mount.

Controls. Since the conjugated antiserum is directed against the globulin of the middle layer, rather than against a component of the first layer, control of staining specificity is usually simpler than in the case of direct staining. Inclusion of slides treated with sera which are known to contain the antibody in question and also with negative sera usually affords adequate control.

III. *Mixed antiglobulin or labelled antigen indirect staining (MIF)*
This procedure, recently described, is a variation of the indirect method. Instead of applying conjugated antiglobulin serum following the antibody-containing serum, however, *unlabelled* antiglobulin is employed followed by conjugated *immunoglobulin*. The advantage of this method over the simpler indirect technique is that whereas in the latter the fluorescent label is attached to globulin regardless of its immunological reactivity as antibody, in the case of MIF only relevant immunologically specific protein is labelled. This method is useful in quantitative studies when it is necessary to work exclusively with fully characterized reagents.

1. Treat with diluted serum . . . 30 minutes.
2. Wash . . . 30 minutes.
3. Treat with antiglobulin serum . . . 30 minutes.
4. Wash . . . 30 minutes.
5. Stain with conjugated immunoglobulin . . . 30 minutes.
6. Wash . . . 1–2 hours.

Controls. As in the indirect method (II) the minimum controls for this procedure require known positive and negative sera in step 1.

Mixed conjugate staining. The above methods may be used for the simultaneous demonstration of two antigens/antibodies by making use of two specific conjugates, one labelled with fluorescein the other with rhodamine. When both conjugates stain the same sites the combination is recognizable as orange-yellow fluorescence. In order to avoid possible interaction between the conjugates it is usually preferable to apply them individually, separated by a brief wash.

Microscopy

The correct interpretation of results obtained by immunofluorescence is largely dependent on the proper use of the microscope used to study the preparations. It is not proposed to describe here in detail the different types of equipment which are now available, and it is too early to assess the relative merits of very recent developments in this field. The basic principles have been well described by Nairn [5]—his book includes an excellent review of fluorescence microscopy and photomicrography, and will be found a useful source of reference. The following brief discussion deals with the principal points of practical importance.

The conventional light source is a high-pressure mercury vapour lamp whose main emission peaks are 365 mμ and 435 mμ, i.e. in the ultra-violet-blue region of the spectrum. This is suitable for the excitation of FITC conjugates which have maximum fluorescence emission at 520 mμ (apple-green). In order to remove unwanted visible light various exciter (primary) filters are used which transmit principally in the ultra-violet-blue region, the particular type being selected according to the following considerations. With light-field microscopy, i.e. using an Abbé-type condenser, only the minimum amount of visible light should be allowed to reach the eye-piece. This is accomplished by using a combination of filters. Visible red, which is passed by most ultra-violet transmitting filters, e.g. Schott UG 1/2·5 mm, is absorbed either by the use of a cell containing copper sulphate solution interposed in the light-path, or by means of an additional red-stopping filter, e.g. Schott BG 12/3 mm. With dark-field microscopy, however, it is possible to use less selective filters and this results in enhanced fluorescence intensity. Thus maximum excitation of FITC-stained preparations is obtainable using blue light as transmitted, for example, by Schott BG 12/2 mm. A considerable disadvantage associated with the use of high-intensity blue light illumination, however, is that the fluoresence emitted by FITC is rapidly bleached and it may therefore be necessary to use a thicker exciter filter, for example BG 12/6 mm during prolonged inspection. An alternative arrangement with dark-field illumination is the use of a high-transmission ultra-violet-passing filter (UG 1/1·5 mm) whose red component is not troublesome in this system. This type of filter, however, tends to produce dull green autofluorescence of tissue sections which gives poor contrast with the apple-green fluorescence produced by specific staining with FITC conjugates. The ideal situation in which the exciting light corresponds to the precise wavelength of the maximum absorption peak of the fluorochrome is not attainable with the filter systems at present available, and it is therefore necessary to decide the most satisfactory compromise by experiment. Secondary filters are necessary between the objective and the eye-piece in order to absorb ultra-violet-blue light, and are either colourless, e.g. Wratten 2B/3 mm sandwiched between 3 mm and 1 mm of Schott GG 13, or pale yellow-green (GG 9/1 mm). A more efficient blue-stopping filter (GG 9/1 mm + OG 1/1·5 mm) is sometimes an advantage when using a blue-passing primary filter. Again, the most suitable combination of primary and secondary filters is best decided by experiment.

It will be apparent from the above that since illumination by very short wave ultra-violet light is not essential for immunofluorescence, ordinary glass optical components are satisfactory. There is therefore no advantage in using quartz optical equipment. Highly satisfactory results may be obtained with a standard research-grade microscope using an appropriate light source and filters as outlined above. The more sophisticated equipment now available for fluorescence microscopy simply provides greater mechanical convenience for rapid interchange of filters, variation of the type of illumination and photomicrography.

Photomicrography
In view of the comparatively low intensity image which is obtained by immunofluorescence as compared with ordinary light microscopy the camera attachment should be designed to receive as much light as possible from the specimen. Photographic equipment which involves the use of a permanently fixed 'beam-splitter' is therefore unsuitable, for it is essential to remove the prism from the light-path during exposures. Using High Speed Ektachrome film with an ASA rating of 160 bright fluorescent images require exposures between 10 seconds and 2 minutes. Prolonged exposure beyond this range is undesirable on account of the fading which occurs, and high-transmission blue-passing exciter filters are precluded for the same reason.

U

References

[1] COONS A.H., CREECH H.J. & JONES R.N. (1941) Immunological properties of an antibody containing a fluorescent group. *Proc. Soc. exp. Biol. (N.Y.)* **47,** 200

[2] COONS A.H. & KAPLAN M.H. (1950) Localization of antigen in tissue cells. II. Improvements in a method for the detection of antigen by means of fluorescent antibody. *J. exp. Med.* **91,** 1

[3] CHADWICK C.S., McENTEGART M.G. & NAIRN R.C. (1958) Fluorescent protein tracers; a simple alternative to fluorescein. *Lancet* **i,** 412

[4] SAINTE-MARIE G. (1962) A paraffin-embedding technique for studies employing immunofluorescence. *J. Histochem. Cytochem.* **10,** 250

[5] NAIRN R.C. (1964) *Fluorescent Protein Tracing,* 2nd edn., Chapter 2. Edinburgh and London: Livingstone

[6] FOTHERGILL J.E. (1964) In *Fluorescent Protein Tracing,* 2nd edn., p. 44, ed. NAIRN R.C. Edinburgh and London: Livingstone

[7] McDEVITT H.O., PETERS J.H., POLLARD L.W., HARTER J.G. & COONS A.H. (1963) Purification and analysis of fluorescein-labelled antisera by column chromatography. *J. Immunol.* **90,** 634

[8] SMITH C.W., MARSHALL J.D. & EVELAND W.C. (1959) Use of contrasting fluorescent dye as counterstain in fixed tissue preparations. *Proc. Soc. exp. Biol. (N.Y.)* **102,** 179

[9] BEUTNER E.H., HOLBOROW E.J. & JOHNSON G.D. (1965) A new fluorescent antibody method: Mixed antiglobulin immunofluorescence or labelled antigen indirect immunofluorescence staining. *Nature, Lond.* **208,** 353

[10] JOHNSON G.D. (1961) Simplified procedure for removing non-specific staining components from fluorescein-labelled conjugates. *Nature, Lond.* **191,** 70

[11] GOLDSTEIN G., SLIZYS I.S. & CHASE M.W. (1961) Studies on fluorescent antibody staining. I. Non-specific fluorescence with fluorescein-coupled sheep anti-rabbit globulins. *J. exp. Med.* **114,** 89

[12] GOLDSTEIN G., SPALDING B.H. & HUNT W.B. (1962) Studies on fluorescent antibody staining. II. Inhibition by sub-optimally conjugated antibody globulins. *Proc. Soc. exp. Biol. (N.Y.)* **111,** 416

[13] HOLBOROW E.J., WEIR D.M. & JOHNSON G.D. (1957) A serum factor in lupus erythematosus with affinity for tissue nuclei. *Brit. med. J.* **ii,** 732

[14] HOLBOROW E.J., JOHNSON G.D. & BEUTNER E.H. To be published

[15] JANKOVIC B.D. (1959) Specific staining of red cell antigens by the use of fluorescein-labelled antibody. *Acta haemat. (Basel)* **22,** 278

[16] COHEN F., ZUELZER W.W. & EVANS M.M. (1960) Identification of blood group antigens and minor cell populations by the fluorescent antibody method. *Blood* **15,** 884

[17] MELLORS R.C., HEIMER R., CORCOS J. & KORNGOLD L. (1959) Cellular origin of rheumatoid factor. *J. exp. Med.* **110,** 875

[18] TAYLOR K.B., ROITT I.M., DONIACH D., COUCHMAN K.G. & SHAPLAND C. (1962) Auto-immune phenomena in pernicious anaemia: Gastric antibodies. *Brit. med. J.* **ii,** 1347

[19] JOHNSON G.D., HOLBOROW E.J. & GLYNN L.E. (1965) Antibody to smooth muscle in patients with liver disease. *Lancet* **ii,** 878

CHAPTER 17

Trace Labelling with Radioiodine

TRISTRAM FREEMAN

Introduction

In many immunological techniques it is useful to be able to follow one or more of the protein constituents and this has been made possible by the trace labelling of single proteins with radioactive isotopes. Proteins tagged in this way can be used to simplify techniques and to increase the accuracy of existing methods. They also permit the assessment of much smaller quantities of reactants than could be detected by non-isotopic methods. However, the fact that the label can be measured with considerable accuracy does not necessarily mean that the overall error is decreased, unless care is taken in preparing the tagged proteins.

In theory it would be desirable to label proteins by replacing a naturally occurring atom with an active one (e.g. carbon, sulphur or tritium). This can be done by feeding an animal, micro-organism or cells in culture (see van Furth, Chapter 6) with suitably substituted amino acids but this would mean a large number of proteins becoming tagged. Since most techniques require a single marked antigen, the chosen active protein would then have to be isolated. An alternative procedure is to label a protein, which has been prepared in a pure state, using an *in vitro* technique to add a foreign atom. Chromium, bromine and iodine have been used. There is now reliable evidence [1, 2, 3] that carefully iodinated proteins, although essentially altered by the addition of an iodine atom, cannot be distinguished from native protein.

The advantages of radioiodine as a trace label are:

1. Labelling can be performed *in vitro*, thus enabling very high specific activities to be reached.

2. The label remains firmly bound to the selected protein and does not exchange with other protein molecules. Even in the body, provided that the thyroid is effectively blocked with an excess of stable iodine (45 mg NaI/day), the iodine label is excreted and is not incorporated into fresh protein.

3. If iodination is performed under carefully controlled conditions, the labelled proteins can be indistinguishable from native protein by either *in vitro* or *in vivo* tests.

The *in vitro* labelling of an isolated protein may easily give a final product that bears little relation to the native protein. Because of the many variables, both in isolation of proteins and in iodination techniques, it is always desirable to check as closely as possible that the labelled protein is sufficiently similar to native protein to give valid data in the system in which it is being used.

For many *in vitro* techniques some denaturation of the protein will not affect its use as a reagent. Labelled human albumin may be so damaged that it will be rapidly rejected from the body and so will give no valid data about the behaviour of native albumin, although the same albumin may retain all its antigenic properties and can be used as a valid tracer for following the fate of this antigen in the laboratory.

Choice of method of iodination

Whenever free iodine comes in contact with protein it will react and enter a tyrosine ring to form mono- or di-iodotyrosine. The iodine may also be utilized to oxidize sulphydril groups and, if present in excess, it may enter into histidine [4]. Only the first reaction, the formation of monoiodotyrosine, has been shown to tag the protein without significant alteration.

There are a number of techniques by which iodine can be liberated in the presence of protein. The three methods described at the end of this chapter have been well tested, each having advantages and all giving a theoretical 100 per cent incorporation of the label.

The iodine monochloride technique described by McFarlane [5, 6] has been widely used to label plasma proteins for metabolic studies in both man and animals, but the method presents difficulties if less than 2–5 mg of protein is available.

The electrolytic method of Rosa [7, 8] and his co-workers requires only small amounts of protein. For low levels of substitution and specific activities it will produce labelled plasma proteins with no evidence of denaturation. However, when very high specific activities are required, the time taken for electrolytic labelling is liable to result in denaturation due to irradiation.

The method utilizing chloramine-T described by Hunter & Greenwood [9], has been widely used for labelling hormones where very high specific activities are required for the immuno-assay technique. This iodination system is suitable for use with very small quantities of protein and is so rapid that radiation damage to the protein molecule can be minimized. This method has not been examined so rigorously as the other two for the absence of denaturation in relation to *in vivo* studies.

Criteria of a good labelled preparation

For the interpretation of data obtained from most techniques using iodine-labelled protein, it is necessary to assume that:

1. There is no free activity.

2. All the activity is attached to a single protein.

3. The labelled protein is not so denatured that it cannot behave in the test system as native protein.

The first requirement (i.e. that all the activity be protein bound) may be examined by techniques such as precipitation of protein with measurement of activity in the supernatant; measurement of activity in a known quantity of dialysate; or measurement of activity in the eluates from a gel-filtration column. All are capable of giving reliable data if a small amount of inactive 'carrier' protein is added to the labelled protein. The use of a gel-filtration system suitable for protein separation (e.g. Sephadex G100, 150 or 200), although it is the most elaborate method, will give data about the homogeneity of the labelled protein as well as about the proportion of non-protein-bound activity; thus, good-quality preparations should give a symmetrical peak, while the presence of polymers or labelled molecules of different size will produce an asymmetry.

The second requirement (i.e. that the activity be in one protein only) can also be examined by *in vitro* techniques. The protein used for iodination should be pure and undenatured, but this ideal is seldom attained. Different proteins have varying avidities for iodine, so an insignificant quantity of a contaminating protein in the unlabelled material may take up a significant proportion of radioactivity. It is, therefore, necessary to examine the distribution of activity after subjecting the protein to fractionation methods such as electrophoresis, gel filtration and chromatography. If contaminating proteins are found, the labelled material may be refractionated, together with fresh, unlabelled whole serum. It is sometimes necessary deliberately to iodinate a mixture of proteins and to refractionate after the iodination. In this way, a single protein may be labelled without ever having been completely isolated.

The final requirement (i.e. that the labelled protein should behave as native protein in the test system) may be more difficult to assess. For much immunological work it is sufficient to show that the labelled antigen or antibody behaves in the same way as the unlabelled material. Since the immunological properties appear to resist denaturation, it is usually possible to satisfy these requirements, even though the protein may be so denatured that it would be rejected by the living organism. For *in vivo* studies the absence of denaturation is more difficult to demonstrate because it is possible to prepare a protein which behaves in an identical fashion to native protein by *in vitro* tests yet is rejected by the body faster than native protein. There seem to be two main types of denaturation when studied in the body [10]. Grossly denatured protein is taken up by the reticulo-endothelial system within a few minutes of its introduction, and then catabolized. Proteins with minor alterations can survive in the body but are catabolized at a faster rate than native protein. Fortunately it has proved difficult to so damage protein molecules that they

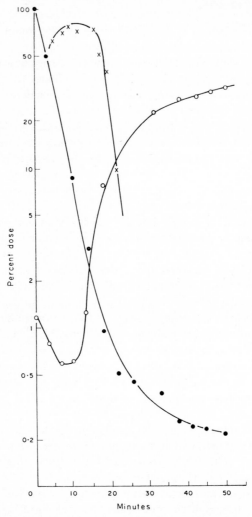

FIG. 17.1. Soluble heat-denatured ^{131}I-albumin in rats. × Activity in the perfused liver. ○ Plasma non-protein-bound activity. ● Plasma protein-bound activity.

are all affected to the same degree, so that a uniform breakdown rate, particularly on the first day, is presumptive evidence for the absence of denaturation.

Causes of denaturation

1. Damage during the procedures necessary for isolation of the protein to be labelled.

2. Faulty iodination.

3. Irradiation damage after iodination.

Denaturation during isolation. It is obvious that a labelled protein can be no better than the material that is selected for labelling. However, this is perhaps the most usual reason for a denatured end-product. Organic solvents and extremes of pH result in damage to the molecule and most commercially available plasma proteins are sufficiently altered to be unusable for *in vivo* work.

Faulty iodination is probably the least common cause of denaturation provided that reasonable care is taken. It has been found that albumin can be labelled to a mean level of five atoms of iodine per molecule and human, rat and rabbit γG globulin to a mean of 1·5 atoms without showing evidence of denaturation by the most rigorous biological tests [10, 11]. However, other protein molecules (e.g. haptoglobin) show evidence of denaturation if labelled above a mean level of 1 atom per 2 molecules. It would seem that no generalizations are possible as to the permissible safe level of iodine substitution.

Radiation damage may be avoided if the specific activities required are moderate. It has been shown that such damage is inversely proportional to the protein concentration so the damage can be reduced by adding, after iodination is complete, an excess of any protein to act as a 'carrier'. Where very high specific activities are required, radiation damage can be minimized by allowing the shortest possible time to elapse between iodination and use and by adding the 'carrier' protein directly after iodination.

Choice of iodine isotope

Two iodine isotopes are available in sufficient purity for contaminants to be ignored. [131]Iodine has a half-life of 8·2 days and is a β and γ emitter. The γ rays from ^{131}I are of moderately high energy (0·36 M.e.V.) which permits the detection of this isotope in deep tissues.

[125]Iodine has a half-life of 57 days and emits γ rays of low energy only. The γ ray energy of these two isotopes differs sufficiently for them to be estimated independently, from a mixed sample, by means of a pulse height analyser. [125]Iodine is the better isotope to use for autoradiography because the lower energy γ emission permits a more precise localization of the source.

Health hazards

Any user of radioactive material should be aware of the dangers involved. A non-touch technique should always be employed and adequate lead shielding used. In none of the iodination methods described is there much risk of active iodine vapour being liberated. However, iodination should be performed in a ventilated fume cupboard and thyroid activity should be checked periodically. In the event of accidental iodine contamination an excess of stable iodine (45 mg NaI) should be taken immediately and continued until the thyroid shows no further activity. Checks should also be made on the contamination of benches and floors. Iodide is best washed with a stable iodine solution, and iodinated protein with saline or dilute (N/10) NaOH.

TABLE 17.1

Decay tables

Days	^{125}I ($t_\frac{1}{2} = 57 \cdot 4$ days $= 0 \cdot 0121$)	^{131}I ($t_\frac{1}{2} = 8 \cdot 14$ days $= 0 \cdot 007096$)	Days	^{125}I ($t_\frac{1}{2} = 57 \cdot 4$ days $= 0 \cdot 0121$)	^{131}I ($t_\frac{1}{2} = 8 \cdot 14$ days $= 0 \cdot 007096$)
1	0·988	0·9183	17	0·814	0·2351
2	0·976	0·8434	18	0·804	0·2159
3	0·964	0·7745	19	0·795	0·1983
4	0·953	0·7113	20	0·785	0·1821
5	0·941	0·6532	22	0·766	0·1536
6	0·930	0·6000	24	0·748	0·1295
7	0·919	0·5510	26	0·730	0·1093
8	0·908	0·5060	28	0·712	0·0922
9	0·897	0·4647	30	0·696	0·0777
10	0·886	0·4268	35	0·654	0·0508
11	0·875	0·3919	40	0·616	0·0332
12	0·865	0·3599	45	0·580	0·0217
13	0·855	0·3305	50	0·546	0·0142
14	0·845	0·3036	55	0·513	0·0092
15	0·834	0·2788	60	0·484	0·0060
16	0·824	0·2560			

Iodine monochloride iodination technique [5]

Reagents required

1. Radioactive iodine free of reducing agent.

2. Iodine monochloride. *Stock solution:* dissolve 150 mg NaI and 108 mg $NaIO_3.H_2O$ in 2·5 ml water; the sodium iodide and iodate used for this should be dried in a desiccator prior to use. Add 1 ml chloroform and one drop (0·035 ml) M/10 NaI to produce a faint pink colour. Dilute with water to give a water phase volume of 10 ml (i.e. 11 ml in all).

Working solution: 1 ml of stock solution plus 22·85 ml 2 M NaCl, 2·06 ml N.NaOH and 22·84 ml water to give a total volume of 48·75 ml. This solution, which is straw coloured, can be kept for months at 4° C and contains 0·42 mg iodine per ml.

3. Buffer solutions:

A. 19 : 1 acid glycine buffer. 19 ml molar glycine in 0·25 M NaCl plus 1 ml N.HCl.

B. 9 : 1 alkaline glycine buffer. 9 ml molar glycine in 0·25 M NaCl plus 1 ml N.NaOH.

C. 8 : 2 alkaline glycine buffer. 8 ml molar glycine in 0·25 M NaCl plus 2 ml N.NaOH.

4. An anion-exchange resin such as Deacidite FF (Permutit Ltd, Gunnersbury Avenue, London). This should be extensively (24 hours) backwashed with tap water to remove small particles. It may then be stored in 0·15 M saline at 4° C until required for use.

5. Iodine-iodate mixture. 150 mg NaI plus 108 mg $NaIO_3$, H_2O in 50 ml water.

6. Normal HCl.

7. Normal NaOH.

8. Thymol blue indicator.

Method

The solution containing a known weight of protein is buffered to pH 9 by adding 8 : 2 alkaline glycine buffer (3C). The precise amount depends on the solution in which the protein is dissolved; for an unbuffered solution 1·5 ml is sufficient. The pH reached may be checked on a tile using thymol blue as an indicator. The protein is now ready for iodination. Some of the active iodine may be utilized in the oxidation of sulphydril groups thus causing a loss of efficiency; this is more pronounced with some proteins than others, depending on the availability of the sulphydrils. Albumin gives only 30–40 per cent incorporation of radioiodine, whereas γG globulin gives 70–80 per cent. Where the presence of sulphydril groups seriously affects the iodination efficiency, these may be preoxidized with stable iodine prior to the introduction of active iodine.

Preoxidation

Because the hydroxyl group of tyrosine is not ionized at pH 4·5, oxidation of sulphydrils can be carried out at this pH without introducing iodine into the tyrosine ring. The protein solution (containing a known weight) is buffered to pH 4·5 using 19 : 1 acid glycine buffer (3A). Free iodine, obtained by adding one drop of N. HCl to an iodide iodate mixture, is added drop by drop until a permanent straw colour is obtained. The protein solution is then passed through an anion-exchange resin to remove the free iodine; the ion-exchange column used now for this process and later for the removal of free

U*

radioactivity should be about 5×0.5 cm and must be washed by passage of about 10 ml of 0·15 M NaCl immediately prior to use. The protein eluate is adjusted to pH 9 by adding N.NaOH until just blue to thymol blue.

Iodination mixture

The required quantity of radioactivity, 'carrier' free and with no reducing agent, is buffered by the addition of 1 ml of 9 : 1 alkaline glycine buffer. To this is added the quantity of iodine monochloride which will give the required degree of iodine substitution. The working solution contains 0·42 mg iodine per ml; 0·1 ml of this solution will give a mean of 1 atom of iodine per molecule for 20 mg albumin, assuming 100 per cent incorporation and a molecular weight for albumin of 60,000. For other proteins the volume of iodine monochloride solution required can be calculated from the expression:

$$\frac{\text{mg protein} \times 0.005 \times 60,000}{\text{M.W. of protein}}$$

$$= \frac{\text{mg protein} \times 300}{\text{M.W. of protein}} \text{ ml of working ICl solution to give 1 atom/mol.}$$

The iodination mixture (i.e. activity + 9 : 1 glycine buffer + ICl) is then mixed rapidly with the buffered protein solution. In theory the radioactivity should be added to the protein solution, otherwise all the activity might become attached to the first part of the added protein. However, less handling of activity is required if the protein solution is shot into the iodination mixture with a Pasteur pipette. No evidence of denaturation has been found after extensive biological testing of protein labelled in this way.

Non-protein-bound radioactivity is removed by passage through an anion-exchange column (prepared as above), and washed through with a few millilitres of saline (0·15 M). When small quantities of protein are being used, losses of protein can be reduced by washing the exchange column, prior to use, with dilute protein solution (e.g. 1 per cent albumin). Alternative methods for removing non-protein-bound activity are dialysis and gel filtration; these methods are also subject to protein loss due to unspecific adsorption, but this can be reduced by adding carrier protein in the same way.

Finally, when activities above 1 mC are being used, or when the labelled material is to be stored for more than a week, 'carrier' protein should be added (to a final concentration of 20 mg/ml) to minimize radiation damage.

Electrolytic iodination [7]

This method shares with the iodine monochloride method the advantage that no oxidizing agents are required to liberate iodine from iodide; thus one potential hazard to the protein molecule is avoided. However, in electrolytic iodination it is possible to use very little iodine so that tagging of small quantities of protein is easier than in the iodine monochloride technique.

The method given below is as described by Rosa *et al* [7], the only modifications being the omission of the reference electrode in the electrolytic chamber and the use of a platinum crucible as both anode and vessel. The electrolytic chamber consists of a platinum vessel the volume of which can be adjusted to suit individual requirements (6–10 ml has been found convenient). The cathode consists of a platinum wire contained in a tube, the bottom of which is sealed by a semi-permeable membrane; this is held so that the membrane dips into the protein solution and is roughly equidistant from all parts of the anode. A small inert magnetic stirrer is incorporated. The current to perform the electrolysis is supplied by a 6 V accumulator, and regulated to give a constant current between 50 and 500 μA.

Reagents required
1. Carrier-free radioactive iodine without reducing agent.
2. $2 \cdot 5 \times 10^{-4}$ M KI.

A known weight of protein in 0·15 M NaCl is placed in the electrode vessel, and the cathode tube is filled with NaCl of the same molarity. The radioactivity (a selected quantity) is put in the vessel together with sufficient KI to give the required level of iodine substitution. The working solution ($2 \cdot 5 \times 10^{-4}$ M KI) contains 0·032 mg I per ml; 1 ml of this is sufficient to give a mean substitution of 1 atom per molecule for 20 mg albumin assuming 100 per cent incorporation of iodine and a molecular weight for albumin of 68,000. For other proteins, the quantity to be added can be calculated from the expression:

$$\frac{\text{mg protein} \times 0 \cdot 05 \times 68,000}{\text{M.W. of protein}} \quad \text{ml KI required to give 1 atom/mol.}$$

$$= \frac{\text{mg of protein} \times 3400}{\text{M.W. of protein}}$$

As in the iodine monochloride method, the weight of iodine in the radioactivity is small enough to be ignored. One of the features of the electrolytic method is that stable iodine is not essential for the reaction; thus trace quantities of protein can be iodinated using only the isotopic iodine.

Electrolysis is carried out at a constant current for about half an hour. For albumin and γG globulin 300 μA for 25 minutes is sufficient. In the system described by Rosa *et al* [8] the potential can be measured between a third (calomel) electrode and the anode; as iodination nears completion a rise in potential will be observed.

After iodination has been completed, non-protein-bound activity is removed by the procedures described for method 1. The theoretical yield of this method is 100 per cent but, as with the previous technique, some of the iodine may be used to oxidize sulphydril groups; a preliminary preoxidation at pH 4·5, or electrolysis with stable iodine at this pH, should increase the yield. This is particularly important when very low substitutions are sought.

Chloramine-T. Hunter & Greenwood [9]

This is the most convenient of the methods employing oxidizing agents to liberate elemental iodine from iodide and, when using high levels of activity, there is minimal handling of radioactive material and little exposure to iodine vapour. Although very high specific activities can be obtained in this way, there is some evidence [12, 13] that minor alterations produced in the protein molecule are sufficient to cause more rapid catabolism of the labelled molecules during *in vivo* studies.

Reagents

1. Carrier-free radioiodine (e.g. IBS/3); this should be used shortly after delivery.
2. Chloramine T (BDH) 1·0 mg per ml in 0·15 M phosphate buffer pH 7·6.
3. Phosphate buffer 0·15 M pH 7·6.
4. Sodium metabisulphite. 1·25 mg/ml in phosphate buffer.
5. Sodium iodide 10 mg/ml in phosphate buffer.

The protein to be labelled is buffered to pH 7·6 with phosphate buffer and added to the radioactivity; this may be done through the rubber seal of the radioactivity bottle. The chloramine T is then added rapidly and the bottle shaken; the amount of chloramine T added is not critical but to reduce damage to the protein the quantity should be kept small. Loss of activity, due to reactions other than entry of iodine into the tyrosine ring, can be avoided by adding KI to protein samples. The amount of KI is equivalent to that used in the electrolytic method, and the total quantity of chloramine T should equal one part in two hundred (by weight) of protein. With smaller weights of protein (i.e. less than 1/mg) the proportion of chloramine T should be increased; Hunter and Greenwood recommend 88 μg of chloramine T to 5 μg of protein (growth hormone). After the addition of chloramine T the reaction is allowed to proceed at room temperature for about 30 minutes. 0·2 ml of sodium metabisulphite is then added to stop any further reaction, and excess iodide is removed as in the previous methods. More complete removal of the iodide can be effected if a small quantity of stable iodine (0·3 ml of 10 mg/ml) is added as 'carrier'. When trace quantities of protein are being iodinated, the loss of protein during this stage can be prevented by washing the ion-exchange column or gel bed with protein solution prior to passage of the active material. Carrier protein is necessary to prevent radiation damage with high specific activities.

Summary

Three methods for iodinating protein are available, none of them taking more than about 30 minutes; two of them require little in the way of apparatus. Although iodination may be simple, and need not cause damage to the protein, it will not restore an already denatured protein and so the protein for labelling must be carefully selected. It is always necessary to show that the results obtained from labelled-protein work truly reflect the behaviour of native protein.

References

[1] CAMPBELL R.M., CUTHBERTSON D.P., MATTHEWS C.M.E. & MCFARLANE A.S. (1956) Behaviour of ^{14}C and ^{131}I labelled plasma proteins in the rat. *Int. J. Appl. Radiation and Isotopes* 1, 66

[2] COHEN S., HOLLOWAY R.C., MATTHEWS C.M.E. & MCFARLANE A.S. (1956) Distribution and elimination of ^{131}I and ^{14}C labelled plasma proteins in the rabbit. *Biochem. J.* 62, 143

[3] FREEMAN T., MATTHEWS C.M.E., MCFARLANE A.S., BENHOLD H. & KALLEE E. (1959) Albumin labelled with ^{131}iodine in an analbuminaemic subject. *Nature, Lond.* 183, 606

[4] HUGHES W.L. (1966) The chemical requirements for a satisfactory label for proteins. *Symposium on Fundamental Aspects of Protein Labelling.* Pisa. In press

[5] MCFARLANE A.S. (1958) Efficient trace labelling of proteins with iodine. *Nature, Lond.* 182, 53

[6] HELMKAMP R.W., GOODLAND R.L., BALE W.F., SPAR I.L. & MUTSCHLER L.E. High specific activity iodination of γ-globulin with iodine^{131} monochloride. *Cancer Res.* 20, 1495

[7] ROSA U., SCASSELLATI G.A., PENNSIS F., RICCIONI N., GIAGNONI P. & GIORDANI R. (1964) Labelling of human fibrinogen with ^{131}I by electrolytic iodination. *Biochim. Biophys. Acta* 86, 519

[8] ROSA U., PENNISI G.F., DONATO L., BIANCHI R., FEDERIGHI G., ROSSI C.A., COZZANI I. & AMBROSINO C. (1966) Factors affecting protein iodination. *Symposium on Fundamental Aspects of Protein Labelling.* Pisa

[9] HUNTER W.M. & GREENWOOD F.C. (1962) Preparation of iodine^{131} labelled growth hormone of high specific activity. *Nature, Lond.* 194, 495

[10] FREEMAN T. (1959) The biological behaviour of normal and denatured human plasma albumin. *Clin. Chim. Acta* 4, 787

[11] BIANCHI R., FEDERIGHI G., DONATO L., ROSA U., PENNISI G.F. & SCASSELLATI G.A. (1966) Iodinated albumin for metabolic studies. *Symposium on Labelled Plasma Proteins for Metabolic Studies.* Pisa

[12] BOCCI V. (1964) Efficient labelling of serum proteins with I^{131} using chloramine T. *Int. J. Appl. Radiation and Isotopes* 15, 449

[13] BOCCI V. (1964) Efficient labelling of tissue-soluble proteins with I^{131} using chloramine T. *Nature, Lond.* 203, 985

CHAPTER 18

The Preparation of Radioiodinated Proteins of High Activity, Their Reaction with Antibody *in vitro:* The Radioimmunoassay

W. M. HUNTER

Introduction

The measurement of pico-grammes (10^{-12} g) of an antigen is relatively simple, precise and rapid if the antigen is radioactively labelled. The scope and precision obtained by the use of labelled antigens for the study of antigen–antibody reactions is considerable and their use has already facilitated the detection of non-precipitating antibodies to exogeneously administered insulin in man [1], of antibodies to a protein (glucagon) believed to be non-antigenic [2] and the investigation of primary interaction between antigen and antibody of non-precipitating [3] and precipitating systems [4].

When a labelled antigen is used it is only this label which is measured; thus, to obtain a precise measurement of the 'antibody-bound' labelled antigen as opposed to the unreacted or 'free' labelled antigen, a method for separating the 'free' from the 'bound' labelled antigen is necessary. This separation may be achieved in various ways and these make use of different physical or chemical properties of the substances, e.g. solubility, molecular size or charge. One of the limitations in the use of labelled antigen is that it is not possible to determine directly the quantity of antibody in the antigen–antibody complex. This can only be done if other measurements beside those of radio-activity are also made simultaneously.

The earliest applications of this method involved labelling well-characterized homogeneous antigens (insulin, bovine serum albumin, glucagon), but the system has also been used to examine the similarity or difference between the same antigen (insulin) derived from a large number of mammalian sources (beef, pork, sheep, horse, whale and man), to relate the structure and compo-sition of these related proteins by the use of immunological methods [5, 6] and to throw some light on the degree of heterogeneity of a given antigen [7]. However, the realization by Yalow & Berson in 1960 [8] that in a reaction with a fixed quantity of antibody, unlabelled antigen will compete with labelled antigen for the limited number of binding sites available, prompted them to use this system for the detection and assay of specific protein hormones in body fluids where these substances are present only in nano-gramme (10^{-9} g) quantities. This, the radioimmunoassay technique, has found widespread use in endocrinology, where the biological assay of specific protein hormones presented formidable problems of sensitivity (growth hormone and glucagon), specificity (insulin) or practicality (thyrotrophic hormone). Radioimmuno-assays for over a dozen protein hormones have been developed since the first brilliant papers of Bersen & Yalow in 1956–60 [1, 3, 5, 6, 8] and as almost another twelve highly purified protein and polypeptide hormones are now available, there is no doubt that this micro-method will be used more extensively in the future. It seems to the author that there must be proteins other than hormones whose assay is desirable and for which this method may be valuable. It is also hoped that the technique may be used more extensively by immunologists and other workers whose attention and scrutiny it may well merit.

Methods of labelling

The preparation of radioactively labelled proteins of high specific activity will be discussed here. Trace labelling is described in Chapter 17.

While labelling of proteins with tritium (by an exchange reaction) or with (^{14}C)-acetyl groups has been occasionally used [9] there has been widespread reliance on the use of radioiodine. Future development in chemistry will increasingly provide synthetic polypeptides as possible antigens and these may permit internal labelling with ^{14}C and so obviate the necessity for repeated labelling with nuclides* of short half-life. However, the shorter-lived radio-nuclides can provide higher specific activities than are possible with the slowly decaying nuclides. The relative advantage of radioiodine may be seen by a simple calculation that one atom of I-131 substituted into a molecule of insulin provides 200 times as many radioactive disintegrations per unit of time as would be produced if all 263 carbon atoms in the molecule were C-14; 586 atoms of tritium would be required to bring the same number of counts as one atom of I-131.

Although under some circumstances iodine may react with sulphydryl groups or with tryptophan, the chemistry of radioiodination is essentially the chemistry of substitution of iodine into tyrosine groups [10]. The reaction consists of substitution of iodine, produced by oxidation of iodide in the presence of protein. Various oxidizing agents including persulphate, iodate and nitrite have been used. In this method a maximum theoretical utilization of half of the available iodine can be expected:

---

* The use of the term 'nuclide' or 'radionuclide' is preferred to the more usual but erroneous use of 'isotope' or 'radioisotope'.

$$\text{(C}_6\text{H}_4\text{O}^-\text{R)} + I_2 \rightleftharpoons \text{(C}_6\text{H}_3\text{IO}^-\text{R)} + HI$$

Where small amounts of radioiodine are used this is unimportant but a reaction of higher efficiency is desirable when high specific activities are required as in this way a smaller quantity of radioactivity may be handled.

In 1958, McFarlane [11] introduced the use of iodine monochloride which facilitates a maximum possible iodine utilization of 100 per cent:

$$\text{(C}_6\text{H}_4\text{O}^-\text{R)} + ICl \rightleftharpoons \text{(C}_6\text{H}_3\text{IO}^-\text{R)} + HCl$$

Using this method [131]iodide is oxidized to [131]iodine which is equilibrated with [127]ICl and this is then reacted with the protein.

Preparations of ^{131}I-insulin of high specific activity (300–600 $\mu c/\mu g$) were made using 10–20 mc I-131 [12]. 20 μl of iodine monochloride was added to the thiosulphate-free Na[131]I and this was followed by 20 μg insulin in a borate buffer at pH 7·8 and the mixture shaken for 4 minutes and then dialysed.

Hales & Randle [13] have used iodine monochloride for the preparation of ^{131}I-insulin of 5–20 $\mu c/\mu g$ for the immunoassay of insulin. To obtain these moderately high specific activities relatively large quantities of [131]iodide (2–8 mC) were used. ^{131}I-insulin was separated from low molecular weight reactants by means of dialysis. In the calculations of specific activity by these authors no allowance was made for adsorption of protein to glassware or dialysis tubing, and the immunological behaviour of the preparations of ^{131}I-insulin was not discussed.

Chloramine-T method

Chloramine-T is the sodium salt of the N-monochloro-derivative of p-toluene sulphonanide:

$$[\text{Na}]^+ \left[CH_3\text{—C}_6\text{H}_4\text{—SO}_2\text{—N}\diagup^{Cl} \right]^-$$

In aqueous solution it slowly yields hypochlorous acid and hence is a mild oxidizing agent. It finds, or found, some use as an antiseptic. On addition of chloramine-T to a slightly alkaline aqueous solution of protein and iodide, a quantitative incorporation of iodine into the protein is obtained. The mechanism of this reaction is not fully described but presumably cationic iodine [I⁺] is formed in the presence of chloramine-T and the reaction then goes to completion. This reagent enables the iodination of proteins to be carried out in aqueous solution under very mild conditions (pH 7·5) and only very low concentrations of the reagent are required. Extraction and handling of radioiodine in volatile solvents is obviated and the quantity of radio-active material required is reduced to a minimum. Very small quantities of protein (5 μg) may be iodinated if necessary and separation of the iodinated protein from unreacted iodide and other low molecular weight reactants can be rapidly achieved and fully quantitated by means of gel filtration on the cross-linked dextrans (Sephadex). This method will be fully described and

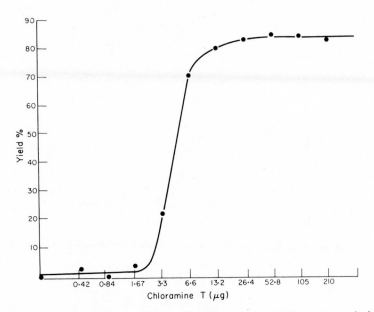

FIG. 18.1. Chloramine-T requirement for iodination. 100 μg of BSA was reacted with 100 μmg ^{127}iodide (as KI) plus a trace amount of Na^{131}I.

discussed since the author has been associated with its development and use [14, 15, 16]. The reaction has been widely used for the iodination of growth hormone [17, 18], insulin [19], and insulin subfractions [20], glucagon [21], parathormone [22], adrenocorticotrophic hormone (ACTH) [23], TSH [24] and vasopressin [25]. Most of the authors using this method for the iodination of protein hormones have used it for obtaining high specific activity prepara-tions but the procedure may be used and is one of the simplest available for preparations of low specific activity also (see Chapter 17 of this book). The reaction has a pH optimum of 7·5. The yield (per cent utilization of iodine) is dependent upon the concentration of the protein: being 100 per cent above 1 mg/ml, 80–90 per cent at 300 μg/ml and 60–70 per cent at 50 μg/ml.

Figure 18.1 shows the chloramine-T requirement for iodination of 100 μg of bovine serum albumin (BSA) with 100 μg of iodide ($K^{127}I$) and indicates

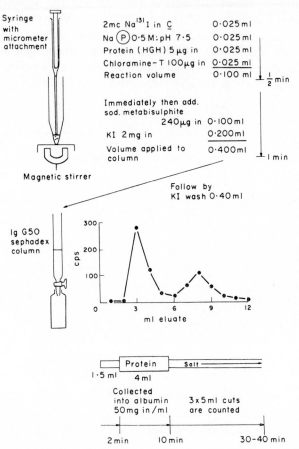

Fig. 18.2. Flow diagram for iodination using the chloramine-T method. Amounts and volumes are for reaction of 5 μg protein with 2 mc $Na^{131}I$ and volumes are kept to a minimum because of the low protein concentration. Specific activities 200–300 μc/μg with these quantities—which may, however, be varied according to requirements.

that a maximum yield can be achieved with only 25 μg of the reagent. For trace labelling without carrier very much lower concentrations of chloramine-T are required. If there is reason to believe that this reagent or the sodium metabisulphate used to reduce the excess chloramine-T may damage the protein being iodinated, then a trial experiment should be performed in which the chloramine-T requirement for the particular purpose is determined. Such an experiment may be readily monitored by determining the minimum amount of chloramine-T which in the presence of the protein will give maximum precipitation of I-131 by 10 per cent trichloracetic acid. It may be necessary to add carrier protein after the addition of metabisulphite to produce adequate precipitation. It may be expedient to use a suboptimal quantity of chloramine-T and to accept a slightly reduced yield if there is evidence that these reagents cause chemical damage to the protein.

Figure 18.2 is a flow diagram for the preparation of 2 to 3 μg of ^{131}I-HGH of 200–300 μc/μg using 5 μg of HGH and 2 mC of Na^{131}I. These quantities may be varied for any particular purpose and are merely used here to simplify description. The volumes of the reactant solutions are kept to a minimum because of the marked dependence of yield upon the protein concentration. After the iodination reaction has occurred, sodium metabisulphite is added in slight excess to reduce both the chloramine-T and also any unreacted iodine to iodide. Carrier iodide is then added and the reaction mixture is transferred to a small G50 Sephadex column which has been prepared earlier. This allows the rapid passage of the iodinated protein which appears immediately after the hold-up volume of the outside compartment of the gel. The first peak in the elution pattern represents ^{131}I-protein, this is followed by the second 'salt' peak which contains unreacted ^{131}iodine (now as ^{131}iodide) and other low molecular weight reagents used for the iodination reaction. In the example given, the column size is kept small to minimize loss due to adsorption which becomes important when only a few microgrammes of protein are being handled. In this interest also the column used here is presaturated by passing 20 mg of BSA through the gel and subsequently washing with buffer before the iodination mixture is applied. The protein fraction from the column is collected into 1 ml of 50 mg/ml BSA to minimize adsorption to glassware and to prevent significant radiation damage. Where quantities of protein of 1 mg and above are used larger column dimensions may be employed, the separation of protein from salt becomes complete and no presaturation is necessary.

The times marked in Fig. 18.2 indicate the approximate times required from the initial addition of protein to the radioiodine to completion of the various stages. These times illustrate the advantage of speed possessed by this method. This speed, though always convenient, becomes critical only when high concentrations of radioiodine solutions are used or when the protein being reacted is particularly unstable.

If the empty tube after transfer of the reactants, the pipette used to load the column and all the eluates are counted, then all of the initial radioiodide will be accounted for except any which may be adsorbed to the column.

Adsorption of [131]iodide is not significant and this can readily be demonstrated by omitting the protein in an iodination, when the initial [131]iodine is quantitatively recovered in the 'salt' eluates from the column. Any losses on the column during an actual iodination must therefore be due to adsorption of protein. (Such adsorption can be easily demonstrated by passing small quantities of iodinated protein through this manipulation in the absence of [131]iodide.) The yield of the reaction is therefore best calculated as 100 per cent minus percentage of initial [131]iodine recovered in the salt fractions. This form of calculation is essential where only a few microgrammes of protein are being iodinated. When the amount of protein used is 1 mg and above, adsorption is insignificant and the yield calculated by this method becomes virtually identical with the percentage of initial [131]iodine recovered in the protein portion of the column eluates.

Extent of iodine substitution into proteins using the chloramine-T method
The substitution of iodine into the tyrosine in proteins probably proceeds largely by a series of di-iodinations: since (1) the second reaction proceeds more rapidly than the first, and (2) little monoidotyrosine is recovered after hydrolysis of iodinated proteins and this small quantity is thought to be an artefact due to partial proteolysis [26]. The tyrosines present in a protein will not all iodinate equally readily; thus Springell [26], using the iodine mono-chloride method at pH 1·0, found that iodine atoms were incorporated in proportion to those reacted up to 4 atoms per molecule, after this the reaction proceeded more slowly up to 6 atoms per molecule, all of which were located in the A chain—the B chain being resistant perhaps because of intra-molecular hydrogen bonding. At pH 9, however, incorporation was proportional to iodine reacted up to 10 atoms iodine per molecule; the last pair of iodine atoms were more slowly incorporated. The C-terminal tyrosine group of α-chymotrypsin is more reactive towards iodine than the other tyrosines [27].

Figure 18.3 shows the extent of iodination with [127]iodine using the chloramine-T method of bovine serum albumin (mol. wt. 65,000), HGH (mol. wt. 21,450) and a polypeptide gastrin (mol. wt. 2114); the latter was supplied by Professor R.A.Gregory, Department of Physiology, University of Liverpool. Gastrin [28] which has one tyrosine only takes 2 atoms of [127]iodine but no more while substitution of [127]iodine into HGH proceeds lineally until 2 atoms are present for each of the seven tyrosines in the molecule. This linear substitution indicates that the tyrosine residues are all equally reactive towards iodine under the conditions of the reaction used. BSA takes the first 30 atoms of iodine equally readily but the remaining atoms up to the plateau of 56 atoms per molecule are more difficult to incorporate. This suggests that fifteen tyrosines are equally available for iodination but that thereafter a further thirteen are less readily iodinated.

The preparation of iodinated proteins of high specific activity

When attempts are made to achieve high specific activities, certain problems arise which are insignificant in trace-labelling experiments. The causes of these may be summarized as: (1) alteration due to substitution of iodine for hydrogen in the structure of the protein; (2) radiation damage to the protein; (3) chemical damage caused by more concentrated reagents required to oxidize iodide to iodine in solutions of high radioactivity; and (4) chemical damage caused by noxious substance(s) present fortuitously in the radiochemical reagent.

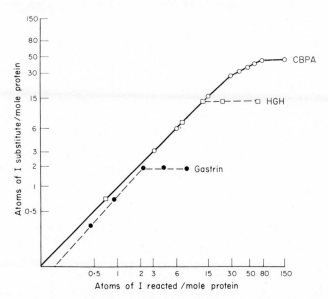

FIG. 18.3. Extent of substitution of three proteins (or peptides) with ^{127}I (using a trace amount of $Na^{131}I$) by means of the chloramine-T method. The experiments on gastrin are those of Dr P.C.Ganguli and those on CBPA were carried out by Dr P.M.Wilson, both in this laboratory.

1. *Alteration due to substitution of iodine for hydrogen in the structure of the protein*

It should be emphasized that even trace iodination may alter a protein significantly, thus if we consider gastrin 1 with a molecular weight of 2114, the disubstitution of its one tyrosine will increase the molecular weight by 12 per cent and will also alter the isoelectric point. However, all that need concern the user of an iodinated protein is whether labelling alters it with respect to the reaction or properties being studied. It is perhaps surprising, in view of the present widespread use of radioiodinated antigens, that there is only one study known to the author in which the effect of substitution of [127]I into a protein upon its immunological integrity has been investigated. Figure 18.4 shows a comparison of the ability of [127]I-HGH and unlabelled HGH to compete with ^{131}I-HGH for antibody binding sites. It will be seen that when the tyrosines of the protein are half-saturated with [127]iodine (7 atoms iodine per 21,450 mol. wt.) no alteration is detectable. However, at full saturation (14 atoms iodine per 21,450 mol. wt.), immunological integrity is grossly impaired and only when much larger quantities are used (Fig. 18.5) is there any effective competition with ^{131}I-HGH for antibody. It may be noted that even when large quantities of [127]I-HGH are used, the slope of

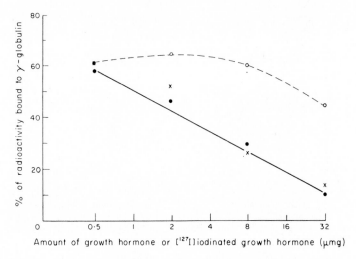

FIG. 18.4. Comparison of [127]I-HGH with unlabelled HGH in their ability to compete with a small amount of ^{131}I-HGH for antibody binding sites. The [127]I-HGH contained: ● 0·7 atoms [127]I/molecule; × 7 atoms of [127]I/molecule, ○ 14 atoms of [127]I/molecule. The full line represents unlabelled HGH (experimental points omitted).

the curve is less steep than that of HGH. Such a difference is indicative of a protein showing complete cross-reaction with the antigen; other examples of this will be cited below.

Preparations of Na[131]I and Na[125]I are available from suppliers of radio-chemicals and where these are prepared for high specific activity labelling, no carrier [127]iodide is added. However, considerable quantities of [127]iodide are present in the initial distillates from the target material and these form an irreducible contamination. The percentage of radioiodine in such a preparation is termed the *isotopic abundance*. The Na[131]I preparation, code number

IBS/3,* has an isotopic abundance (^{131}I) of 15–20 per cent on the day of preparation: (information made available by the Radiochemical Centre, Amersham) i.e. contains 5–7 atoms ^{127}I for each one of ^{131}I. Hence, though 1 mc of ^{131}I weighs 8 μmg the total iodine represented amounts to 40–60 μmg and from this the quantity of total iodine present in an iodinated protein of a given specific activity may be calculated.

No firm data is available for the isotopic abundance of the corresponding Na^{125}I preparation (IMS/3); however, what information is available suggests

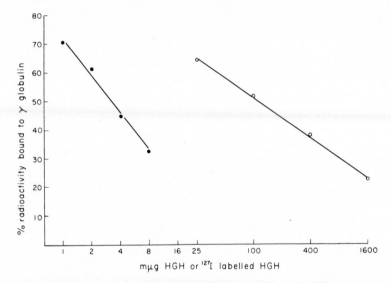

FIG. 18.5. Comparison of ^{127}I-HGH with unlabelled HGH in their ability to compete with a small amount of ^{131}I-HGH for antibody-binding sites. ● unlabelled HGH, ○ ^{127}I-HGH containing 14 atoms ^{127}I/molecule.

that it is approximately 25 per cent. Because of the difference in half-life of ^{125}I (60 days) and ^{131}I (8 days), the specific activity of ^{125}I is much lower, thus 1 g atom of ^{125}I produces only about one-seventh of the number of disintegrations given by ^{131}I. If the isotopic abundance of the ^{125}I preparation is in fact 25 per cent, then a ^{131}I preparation would yield five times as many disintegrations (per unit of time) per gramme of total iodine as would a ^{125}I preparation. If we consider that in the sodium iodide well-type scintillation counter ^{125}I is counted with about 80 per cent efficiency and ^{131}I with only 40 per cent efficiency we see that the ratio now moves to 2·5 : 1, i.e. with less

* The author has used only the Na^{131}I preparation (code No. IBS/3) and Na^{125}I preparation (code No. IMS/3), both of which are supplied by the Radiochemical Centre, Amersham, Bucks. Readers are referred to specific papers mentioned (notably ref. 19) for an indication of the suitability of preparations from other sources.

difference between the two radioisotopes. If 1 week elapses between preparation of iodinated proteins and their counting a further factor of 2 in favour of ^{125}I (because of its longer half-life) is entered and the two radioisotopes become equal. Thus, we see that there is nothing to choose between the ^{125}iodine and ^{131}iodine with respect to the number of iodine atoms required to yield the same number of counts. Naturally the relative merits would change if the isotopic abundance of the Na^{125}I preparations is later found to be markedly different from 25 per cent.

2. *Radiation damage*

The requirement in any laboratory from one batch of iodinated protein is probably for not more than 0·1 μg of the labelled protein which at 200 μc/μg

TABLE 18.1

Comparison of the amounts of I-131 used in different procedures

Method	Reference	Amount I-131 used initially (mc)	Amount I-131 reacted with protein (mc)	Amount of protein used (μg)	Specific activity of ^{131}I protein (μc/μg)
Oxidation of ^{131}iodide to ^{131}iodine and extraction into chloroform which is then shaken with protein solution	8	30–80	15–40	20	75–300
Iodine monochloride	12	10–20	10–20	20	300–600
Chloramine-T	14, 15	2	2	5	200–300

means 20 μc ^{131}I. The overall efficiency of a labelling process may be simply judged from the initial quantity of ^{131}I which must be handled in order to produce this requirement. The initial quantity of ^{131}I may be subjected first to an extraction process so that considerably less is actually reacted with, and hence can cause radiation damage to the protein. Table 18.1 summarizes the quantities of protein and Na^{131}I used in the preparation of ^{131}I proteins of high specific activity by various methods. It will be seen that considerably less starting radioactive material is required for the chloramine-T method than for the other methods.

In all preparations of high specific activity proteins, the volumes of the reagents are kept to the minimum which is consistent with accurate measurement because the reactions are favoured by high concentrations and because the use of minimum quantities of radioactivity is implicit. Therefore during the iodination reaction the protein may be subjected to a level of radiation which is many times higher than the self-irradiation which will occur later during storage and use. Thus after preparation the iodinated protein may be stored in dilute solution and it can be protected by the addition of carrier protein.

In a well-standardized procedure radiation damage may be distinguished from damage due to chemical onslaught in that it should be proportional to the amount of radioactivity reacted and should not vary with different batches of radioiodine. Specific activities of 600 $\mu c/\mu g$ for ^{131}I-HGH have been achieved using 4 mc of ^{131}I with the chloramine-T method without loss of immunological integrity [14] and it was concluded that radiation damage was not detectable at this level. It is doubtful whether iodination of any protein at the levels currently used with the chloramine-T method results in radiation damage.

3. Chemical damage due to reagents used

Iodination with elemental iodine may involve oxidation of sulphydryl groups, oxidative cleavage of disulphide bonds as well as denaturation of protein by the organic solvent (usually carbon tetrachloride) used for the extraction of the iodine. Iodine monochloride is a stronger oxidizing agent than elemental iodine and is also used in organic solvents.

Chloramine-T is an oxidizing agent and after iodination with this reagent a small excess of reducing agent (sodium metabisulphite) is added. Either or both of these reagents might impair the immunological integrity of an antigen.

In the preparation of the ^{127}I-HGH referred to above (Fig. 18.4) the quantities of chloramine-T and metabisulphite were the same as those used for high specific activity preparations. The data referred to (Fig. 18.4) therefore also shows that no detectable alteration in the HGH has resulted from exposure to these reagents. However, the quantity of chloramine-T (and therefore of metabisulphite) required may vary for different quantities of radioiodide, for solutions of radioiodide from different suppliers and also for different batches from one supplier. The effect of these reagents on any protein being studied should therefore be determined and the concentrations used should be kept below those known to cause detectable alterations.

4. Chemical damage due to noxious substances in the radiochemical reagent

Methods involving extraction of iodine (as such or as iodine monochloride) into organic solvents do not involve direct contact between protein and radiochemical reagent. Chemical damage, due to this, therefore does not occur with these methods. Such damage can occur—and indeed may be a major factor limiting the specific activities which can be achieved—when the chloramine-T method is employed.

The $Na^{131}I$ preparation IBS/3 is prepared by passing a stream of CO_2-free oxygen over the target material and into N/50 NaOH. The specification guarantees a pH of 8–10 and an ^{131}iodate content of <5 per cent of the total ^{131}I. Even at 300 $\mu c/ml$ the concentration of total iodide is only 18 $\mu mg/ml$ (assuming 15 per cent isotopic abundance for ^{131}I). Other non-radioactive substances may be present in considerably greater quantities than this and yet entirely escape detection by methods of chemical analysis. During 1963 some batches of IBS/3 could be used by reacting 4 mc with 5 μg HGH to achieve specific activities up to 600 $\mu c/\mu g$ without immunochemically detectable damage. However, most batches caused damage when 4 mc was used and none when only 2 mc was used [15]. Since early 1964, however, damage has frequently been encountered when 2 mc of IBS/3 was used. That this damage is due to the effects of noxious substances present in the radiochemical reagent is evidenced from its consistent occurrence or absence in all preparations from any one batch of $Na^{131}I$. The extent of damage varied considerably between different batches. Some workers [8, 18, 19, 29] have accepted damage during iodination at high specific activities and have relied on methods for removing damaged fractions after iodination. This approach is particularly well established for insulin [8, 19]. The immunologically intact ^{131}I-insulin is adsorbed strongly by cellulose powder whilst the damaged components pass through the column. The intact material is later eluted with plasma and is demonstrably free of discrete damaged components [19] and further can be shown to be indistinguishable from unlabelled insulin in its behaviour with antiserum. Insulin, however, may be regarded as a special case and indeed it is surprising that damage so slight as to require subtle testing procedures (see below) for its immunochemical detection can also be exploited for its separation from intact antigen. In general, the author believes that (except for insulin) labelling procedures should, where possible, be so used that the immunochemical integrity of the antigen is not impaired.

Separation of antibody-bound from free labelled antigen
In the systems under consideration only labelled antigen is determined and the reaction with antibody may be investigated if the labelled antigen bound to antibody can be separated from the unreacted 'free' antigen. This separation may be achieved either physiochemically (electrophoresis, chromatography, gel diffusion, etc.) or by means of a second immunological step. In this, the 'double-antibody' system, the antibody γ globulin complexed to the labelled antigen is precipitated by anti-γ globulin raised in a second species.

Methods of separation may be judged on their efficiency, i.e. separative ability—a perfect system would show no labelled antigen in the 'bound' fraction in the absence of antibody and 100 per cent of the labelled antigen in the 'bound' fraction after incubation with excess antibody. The practicality of rapidly handling several scores or even hundreds of samples must be considered in methods used for routine procedures such as radioimmuno-assays, whereas such considerations are less important if, for example, the detection of antibodies in relatively few sera is required. A further considera-tion is the volume of incubate which can be separated, since this will affect the specific activity required, counting time, precision and sensitivity of the system. Finally, an ideal system should separate 'bound' from 'free' rapidly because some dissociation of the complex may occur during a prolonged separation.

Physiochemical methods of separating 'bound' from 'free' labelled antigen
Since antibody γ globulins are larger proteins than many antigens (this happens to be particularly true of hormones as antigens) an antigen : antibody complex consisting of Ag : Ab will approximate to γ globulin in its physio-chemical behaviour. In some systems, notably those based upon salt fractiona-tion and electrophoresis, used to separate bound antigen both the nature of the antigen and the number of antigen molecules in the complex may be expected to affect the behaviour of the 'bound' moiety. However, if these possibilities are borne in mind it remains a matter of experience that the 'bound' component behaves similarly in most systems despite differences in the nature of the antigen. This being so, the establishment of a suitable separative system becomes essentially an investigation of the behaviour of free labelled antigen. For most applications antigen will be present in very low concentrations so that adsorption forces are an important consideration. Adsorption of the 'bound' component is much less intrusive because non-specific antibody γ globulin is always present and of course more non-immune γ globulin (or whole serum) may be added as carrier. The addition of non-radioactive antigen as carrier cannot be tolerated because the antigen–antibody reaction is reversible and even the late addition of suitable carrier quantities of non-radioactive antigen would seriously interfere with the system.

Any separative system must exert a force which tends to cause dissociation of the antigen : antibody complex. In antigen excess, mere removal of one of the reactants (the free antigen) from the system will of course favour dissocia-tion, but the rate of reaction in this direction does not, unless the energy of the reaction is very low and the separative process particularly protracted, result in appreciable release of free antigen. Further, any physical method which separates free antigen from the complex will tend also to leach antigen from the complex. Considerable dissociation causing a trail of free ^{131}I-insulin behind migrating antibody complexes of low energy was noted by Yalow & Berson [19] during 18 hours' paper electrophoresis in which free insulin was also being subjected to adsorptive forces by the paper. This trailing was absent, and a single radioactive peak appeared in the inter β-γ zone, when the same complexes were separated by rapid electrophoresis at high voltage.

Separation by electrophoresis
It may be counted a fortunate property of antibody γ globulin that it has a distinct and somewhat unusual electrophoretic mobility.

Hunter & Greenwood [17] used electrophoresis on cellulose acetate membranes for the separation of bound and free ^{131}I-HGH (Fig. 18.6). Certain theoretical considerations led to the selection of the conditions to be described. Since the spreading of zones is proportional to the distance travelled, the separation of two substances is most efficiently achieved by arranging the conditions so that both move an equal distance on either side of a central start-line. However, because of adsorptive forces (see above, page 621) it is much easier to move the 'bound' than the 'free' moiety and the best separation was achieved by causing the γ globulin to move from a central start-line towards the cathode under the influence of the exaggerated electro-endosmotic flow which can be induced by using a buffer of very low ionic strength. The free ^{131}I-HGH moves slightly towards the cathode but this process is restricted by adsorption. Some of the asymmetry of the 'free' HGH is due to electrophoretic heterogeneity of this protein as generally prepared. The best preparations, however, are immunochemically homogeneous [7]. Figure 18.6b shows that the separation of a mixture of 'bound' and 'free' ^{131}I-HGH is considerably less complete than would be expected from the behaviour of the 'free' and 'bound' fractions on separate strips. This arises for the following reason: Fig. 18.6a represents fully bound ^{131}I-HGH—a situation only achieved in antibody excess. In this region the complex consists of Ab_n Ag where n is perhaps 2–4 and the complex therefore moves with the γ globulins. In Fig. 18.6b, however, there is antigen excess and the complexes therefore consist largely of Ab Ag and hence the complex is more electronegative and moves only in the inter β-γ zone. Cellulose acetate electrophoresis has two further disadvantages: (i) the maximum quantity of incubation mixture which can be applied to one strip is 0·05 ml and this makes obligatory the use of high specific activity proteins for the assay of this hormone at the levels found in plasma; (ii) cellulose acetate membranes are expensive for routine use in large numbers.

Starch grain (block) electrophoresis was used [1] to achieve a separation of 'bound' and 'free' ^{131}I-insulin by means of an electric field in the absence of adsorption forces which are considerable on paper but minimal on starch [30].

The polyacrylamide gel electrophoresis method of Ornstein & Davies [31] was used [32] to separate bound and free ^{131}I-HGH. It was suggested that the concentration effect which occurs at the face of the small-pore gel would increase the concentration of antigen and antibody and that this would enable the highly diluted systems necessary for the assay of HGH in plasma to react

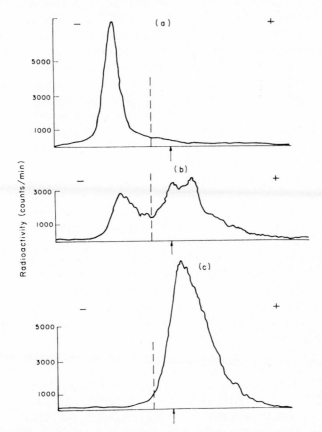

FIG. 18.6. Separation of free ^{131}I-labelled growth hormone from ^{131}I-labelled growth hormone bound to immune γ globulin. Samples from incubation mixtures of ^{131}I-labelled growth hormone and antiserum were applied to cellulose acetate strips at the points marked by arrows. After electrophoresis the strips were scanned for radioactivity from the anode (+) to the cathode (−). The broken line represents the cut taken as a routine to separate bound and free ^{131}I-labelled growth hormone. The final dilutions of antiserum in the incubation mixtures were 1 : 20, 1 : 20,000 and 1 : ∞ in (a), (b) and (c) respectively.

rapidly within the gel. It seems unlikely that the very short time (60 minutes) available during which concentration by passage through the gel occurs would be adequate materially to increase the rate of a reaction which, even with a very avid antiserum, takes 1–2 weeks to equilibrate. However, as a system for separating B and F polyacrylamide gel offers considerable advantages. It may be considered where the separation cannot be achieved on cellulose acetate electrophoresis because the mobility of the free iodinated protein is not sufficiently different from that of the 'bound' and where this cannot be accomplished on a routine basis by gel filtration because only G200 Sephadex or long columns of G100, both with very slow flow-rates, are required to effect a good separation. Provided the 'free' moves well in polyacrylamide an excellent separation may be expected since the 'bound' fraction will move slowly because of the combined effects of low electronegativity and large size. This method is rapid (20–30 minutes), can handle moderate volumes of the incubates, is inexpensive and practically, though not perhaps the most convenient of methods, may be adapted to handling moderately large numbers of samples.

Chromatography and chromatoelectrophoresis

The discovery that at low concentrations insulin adsorbs strongly to paper [1] during electrophoresis provided the starting-point for the development of a most efficient and expedient system for separating bound and free antigen [1, 8, 19]. Whatever variant is used this method is essentially adsorption chromatography. Some variation between batches of the usual electrophoresis grade of Whatman paper (3 MM) was encountered [19]: more recently a new designation (3 MC) has been given to paper selected on the basis of a low carboxyl content. This paper is recommended by the manufacturers for use in radioimmunoassays for insulin. Berson and Yalow favour its use in chromatoelectrophoresis in open tanks [19]. In this system (Fig. 18.7) free insulin is adsorbed at the start-line whilst that bound to antibody moves towards the centre of the paper strip with the (carrier) plasma proteins in the flow of buffer caused by evaporation from the centre of the strip. This separation takes about 20 minutes but must be carried out at 4° C since if run at room temperature the additional heat generated by the current may cause dissociation. Alternatively, these workers showed that the flow of buffer along a strip may be effected very simply by evaporation. A strip of 3 MC paper (46 × 5 cm) is wetted, blotted lightly and placed horizontally over nylon lines with one end folded to form a vertical wick dipping into a trough of barbitone buffer (pH 8·6 0·07 M in barbituric acid) with the buffer surface 4 cm below the plane of the paper. Free insulin is adsorbed at the start-line which is at the wick end of the horizontal portion of the strip. In about 30–45 minutes the (carrier) plasma proteins move some 8–10 cm. This system may be used at room temperature. The movement of 'bound' insulin on these systems can conveniently be followed by adding bromophenol blue which stains the albumin of the carrier plasma. This simple chromatographic technique was used to obtain the data shown in Figs. 18.8, 18.12 and 18.16. The following advantages can be claimed for these paper systems: the separation of B and F is complete and is not affected by wide differences in concentration of protein (an important point in assays of hormones or other proteins present in plasma); large numbers of samples can be handled (in this laboratory 100 strips are run by one technician in an ordinary working day). Volumes of up to 0·4 ml may be run on strips 5 cm wide but this is somewhat tedious because the solution flows over the outside of the paper unless the sample is applied slowly. Volumes up to 0·2 ml may be applied quite rapidly. These volumes

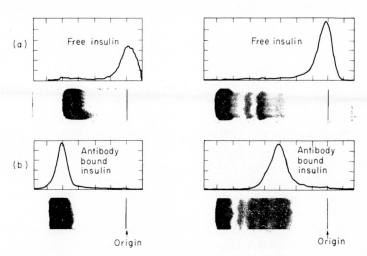

FIG. 18.7. Behaviour of free and antibody-bound ^{131}I-insulin in paper electrophoresis (right) and chromatoelectrophoresis (left): (a) non-immune plasma, (b) immune plasma. In the latter procedure strips are exposed to the open atmosphere during electrophoresis for 45–90 minutes so that the migration of plasma proteins (which may be followed by addition of bromophenol blue stain) results primarily from hydrodynamic flow chromatography. (From ref. 19.)

are intermediate between the very restrictive ones imposed by cellulose acetate and the virtually unlimited volume which can be handled by precipitation techniques (see below). Separation by means of 3 MC paper has been used, also for glucagon [2]. HGH [18], ACTH [23], parathormone [22], and TSH [34].

Ion-exchange paper chromatography

Bound ^{131}I-HGH has been separated from free by means of DEAE paper [18]. This exploits the difference in charge between the two components, the 'free' being held at the point of application while the bound migrates. DEAE paper is more delicate than 3 MC paper and (unlike the latter) crinkles on drying and tends to tear when fed into a chromatogram scanner. It cannot take the larger volumes possible with 3 MC paper. The separation should be good but the published details on this and on the conditions used are inadequate either for ensuring ready reproduction or for a proper assessment of the merits of the system.

Solvent precipitation systems

These systems have always attempted to precipitate the bound moiety whilst leaving the free in solution. Counting is performed on the whole of the precipitate (after washing it with the precipitating mixture if great precision is required), or on an aliquot of the supernatant. Early attempts were made with insulin using sodium sulphate and ether [1] or sodium sulphite [35]. The latter workers used 15 per cent urea to prevent serious co-precipitation of the free insulin. No concentration of ammonium sulphate could be used to precipitate bound HGH without very considerable contamination with free: urea improved this separation only slightly [17]. More recently, Odell *et al* [36] exploited the greater solubility of human TSH (a glycoprotein) and were able to precipitate the bound component fully. Under the conditions used (the addition of 4 ml of ethanol and 2·3 ml 16 per cent NaCl to 1 ml of incubation mixture) only a very small amount of the free ^{131}I-TSH was precipitated, and this could be removed by a single wash. This method has been used, with minor modifications in the volume of ethanol added, in this laboratory by Dr P.M.Wilson for the separation of bound from free ^{131}I-TSH and ^{131}I-luteinizing hormone (LH). The procedure is simple and large numbers of samples may be handled. Large volumes (1 ml or more) of incubate may be separated and hence very high specific activity iodinated proteins need not be used. The precipitation of the γ globulin (which is centrifuged down by 1800 g for 10 minutes at 4° C when flocculation appears after about 2–3 hours) exposes the Ag : Ab complex to a solvent which might cause dissociation, though no experimental evidence is yet available on this point. Another possible disadvantage is that the extent of co-precipitation of 'free' appears to be significantly dependent upon the dilution of plasma in the incubate. This difficulty might be overcome either by adding plasma immediately before the precipitation step to bring all solutions to the same concentration, or by washing the precipitates.

Methods depending upon molecular size

Ultracentrifugation has been used by Berson *et al* [1] to show the presence of antibody-bound ^{131}I-insulin which sedimented much more rapidly than free ^{131}I-insulin and was found only in serum from patients who had received beef–pork insulin. This provided a method based upon entirely different properties of the complex from those exploited in the paper-electrophoretic method used in the test of the studies by these workers, and hence provided independent evidence of the presence of antibodies.

Gel filtration on Sephadex columns can readily separate antigens of small molecular dimensions from their immune complexes. In practical terms the lowest numbered Sephadex grade which is capable of retarding the free antigen would be used since flow-rates diminish in sequence G25–G200. G75 columns have been used to separate 'bound' from 'free' ^{125}I-insulin [37]. An accurately measured volume of incubate was applied to the column and only the bound collected in a predetermined volume was counted. The columns were washed with buffer and could apparently be used repeatedly for periods up to 9 months. Gel filtration would seem to be most useful where the antigen is small—so that the faster G25 or G50 column may be used, and where the antigen shows little tendency to adsorb, since adsorption may preclude reuse of the columns and complicate quantitation. It certainly offers a useful and general method for detecting antibodies to small molecular-weight antigens.

Recently a method referred to as instant dialysis has been used to separate 'bound' and 'free' ^{131}I-insulin [38]. Charcoal which strongly adsorbs free insulin is coated with dextran which, acting as a molecular sieve, permits transit of 'free' but not of 'bound' insulin from the solution. The 'bound' fraction is merely decanted after centrifugation of the coated charcoal precipitate. This method should prove capable of rapidly separating large numbers of samples whose volume need not be small. If confirmed it may therefore become widely used.

The double-antibody system

This method depends upon the finding that the antigenic properties of γ globulin are retained when it complexes with an antigen. Consequently an antibody raised, for example in a rabbit, to a guinea pig γ globulin will still precipitate the guinea-pig anti-insulin γ globulin when the latter is bound to insulin. This method has certain advantages. It is the only really general method; it is gentle—i.e. exerts no strong force which might tend to dissociate the complex, and can handle large numbers of samples whose volume is not limited.

On the other hand the method is not rapid, and it requires considerable experimentation with the particular antisera used to determine optimum conditions. When the incubates contain appreciable concentrations of plasma (as in the radioimmunoassay of hormones in plasma) this method has proved seriously susceptible to non-specific interference. When used for radioimmunoassay of growth hormone [39] spuriously high results were obtained because damaged, immunologically inert components in the labelled growth hormone were held in solution (and hence appeared in the 'free' fraction) by interaction with plasma proteins but were precipitated (and hence read as 'bound') in their absence. A laborious extraction procedure, which separated an albumin fraction containing the growth hormone from the other plasma proteins, was used to avoid this effect [40]. More recently this non-specific effect has been avoided by using a better preparation of human growth hormone for iodination and by removing material which has been damaged during iodination [41]. Morgan and Lazarow have used the double-antibody system for radio-immunoassay of insulin [42]. This was excellent for standard solutions but inclusion of plasma in the incubates resulted in (i) inhibition of precipitation because of cross-reaction of rabbit anti-GP γ globulin with human γ globulin (this could be avoided by use of excess of rabbit anti-GP γ globulin) and (ii) interference by complement [43]—this could be prevented by addition of EDTA. Haemolysis may also affect this system. Hales and Randle have used two ingenious modifications to the double-antibody method for radio-immunoassay of insulin [13]. Firstly, the antibody to insulin was pre-precipitated with anti-γ globulin and this precipitate added as a suspension to react ^{131}I-insulin. This avoided problems of cross-reaction with human γ globulin. Secondly, separation of 'bound' insulin was accomplished by its retention on cellulose acetate ultrafiltration membranes, which allow free passage of the 'free' insulin. These membranes could be used to separate large volumes of incubate (e.g. 1 ml; though there is no limit with this method). The membranes were dried and mounted on planchettes for automatic handling on a β counter. Incubates may be handled at a rate of one per minute by one operator, and thus the method is suitable for handling large numbers of samples.

Summary and choice of method for separating bound and free iodinated antigens
Whilst the double-antibody system can in the hands of experienced and critical workers yield 'correct' answers it is suggested that its use should be limited to analysis carried out in pure solution (i.e. not involving addition of high concentrations of unextracted plasma) unless some other quite independent physical method is available for separating the bound and free fractions in the same incubate as a check on the specificity of the double-antibody method. Samols and Bilkus in a comparative study [44] showed that the percentage of ^{131}I-insulin bound to antibody always agreed to within ± 1 per cent when aliquots of the same incubate in pure solution were separated by chromatoelectrophoresis and by the double-antibody technique. No adequate comparison has been made where high concentrations of plasma have been included in the incubates.

The use of labelled antigen
In this chapter we are concerned with the *in vitro* reaction of antigen and antibody at concentrations which are so low that the solubility of the antigen–antibody complex is not exceeded. In many instances precipitation of the

immune complex does occur at higher concentration. This applies to so-called polyvalent antigens (antibody is presumed always to be polyvalent—even so a lattice cannot be built up and hence precipitation cannot occur if the antigen is univalent). In some instances (notably insulin) the antigen is usually univalent and the system is therefore non-precipitating even in high concentration. Glick *et al* [18] used papain digestion of antibody [45] to human growth hormone in order to make the system non-precipitating but this is not necessary at HGH concentrations below 10 μmg/ml.

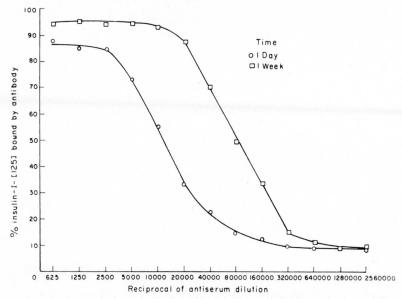

FIG. 18.8. Effect of time on binding of labelled insulin by antibody. ^{125}I-pork insulin 0·1 μmg/ml was incubated with antiserum in the dilutions shown. Aliquots (0·2 ml) were removed and applied to 3 MC paper strips, after addition of 0·05 ml dyed non-immune sheep serum as carrier, for chromatography at room temperature after incubation at 4° C for 1 day (○), and 7 days (□).

Detection of antibodies
The transfer of labelled antigen in an electrophoretic or other separative system, from its characteristic position in the free state to the position occupied by γ globulin after incubation with serum from an animal which has been injected with the antigen (and not in control serum) is evidence for the presence of specific antibodies. In order to avoid confusion due to possible artefacts of the separative system a second procedure based upon entirely different properties of the 'bound' and 'free' should be used.

The use of labelled antigen for the purpose of detecting antibodies is particularly valuable in non-precipitating systems, and during the last decade peptides of increasingly small size have been shown, by this method, to be antigenic [1, 2, 25]. Recently the octapeptide oxytocin, injected in adjuvant but without recourse to conjugation to a larger molecule, has been shown to be antigenic in the rabbit [25] (see Chapter 26).

The use of radioiodinated antigen provides the most sensitive system available for the detection of antibody. Assuming the (stringent) necessity for showing 50 per cent binding as evidence of the existence of antibody, this

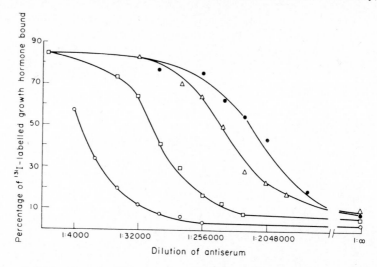

FIG. 18.9 Titration of rabbit antiserum to HGH with various concentrations of ^{131}I-HGH ∴ ○ 40 μmg/ml, □ 4 μmg/ml, △ 0·4 μmg/ml, ● 0·04 μmg/ml. Incubation 7 days at 4° C. Separation on cellulose acetate electrophoresis (see Fig. 18.6).

may be achieved with labelled antigen at 0·01 μmg/ml. If the antigen has a molecular weight of 30,000 we can therefore detect

$$\frac{50}{100} \times \frac{186,000}{30,000} \times 0{\cdot}01 = 0{\cdot}03 \ \mu\text{mg of antibody/ml.}$$

or 0·005 μmg of antibody N/ml.

Antiserum titration curves

Incubation of a constant amount of labelled antigen with serial dilutions of antiserum and subsequent separation of bound and free components will yield a plot of the form shown in Fig. 18.8. This shows the extent of binding of ^{125}I-insulin at 0·1 μmg/ml incubation mixture in 18 hours and 7 days. The system has equilibrated when each point on the curve reaches a percentage binding which shows no further increase with time. The equilibration time is a function of the concentration of antigen and antibody and upon the energy of the reaction. The energy of the reaction is related directly to association time and inversely to dissociation time. Antisera vary in their energy of reaction and this important quality of an antisera is termed its 'avidity' or average intrinsic association constant. Any given antiserum contains a mixture of antibodies of different avidities or association constants (see Chapter 14). Antigens also differ in their ability to elicit production of high avidity

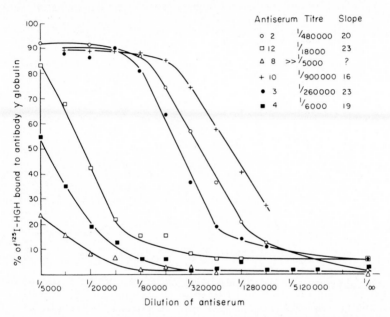

Fig. 18.10. Titration of different rabbit antisera to HGH with ^{131}I-HGH 1 μmg/ml. Incubation 7 days at 4° C and separation on cellulose acetate electrophoresis.

antisera. Figure 18.9 provides an illustration of the effect of concentration on equilibration time. At 40 μmg ^{131}I-HGH/ml (open circles) the system equilibrates overnight, at 4 μmg/ml (open squares) 2–3 days are required and at 0·4 μmg/ml (open triangles) 7–8 days. The mixtures used were in fact all separated on day 7 when the above three series had reached equilibrium, and these three curves are parallel lines spaced apart at ten-fold dilutions of antiserum. At 0·04 μmg/^{131}I-HGH/ml equilibration is not complete in 7 days (extrapolation suggested a requirement of 40–60 days for this system).

Figure 18.10 shows the curves for 6 rabbit anti-HGH sera after incubation with ^{125}I-HGH at 1 μmg/ml for 7 days. This illustrates two independent properties of antisera. Firstly 'titre', which is a purely quantitative factor, and may be defined as that concentration of antiserum which is necessary when the system has equilibrated to bind 50 per cent of labelled antigen at 1 μmg (labelled antigen) /ml incubation mixture. The titre of an antiserum increases following booster inoculation with antigen, plateaus at about 7–10 days, and then falls slowly. The second characteristic of an antiserum titration curve is the slope over the linear portion of the plot (from 20 and 80 per cent bound). The slope is conveniently defined as the fall in per cent bound per doubling dilution of antiserum and it is related to the avidity of the antiserum.* It will be seen that titre and avidity are independent properties since, for example,

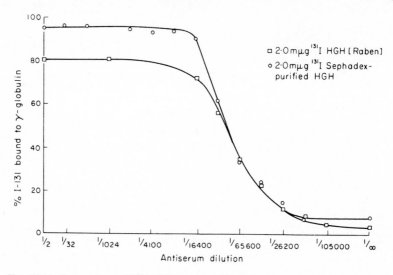

Fig. 18.11. Comparison of ^{131}I-HGH prepared by iodination of a crude preparation of HGH (□), and of a purified preparation ○. Incubation of ^{131}I-HGH at 0·2 μmg in 0·5 ml for 7 days at 4° C. Separation by cellulose acetate electrophoresis.

antiserum 12 (Fig. 18.10) has a relatively low titre but is of high avidity since it gives a steeper slope than the high titre antiserum 10. Avidity appears to increase with time following the primary injection of antigen, to reach a maximum after a certain time and to be unaffected by booster injections [47].

Antiserum titration curves may be used to gain information about the antigen. Figure 18.11 shows (open squares) that HGH prepared after an extraction procedure using hot acetic acid/acetone [48] contains some 20 per cent of material which does not react with antiserum. (The antiserum was raised against unpurified HGH.) After a further purification step using a Sephadex column [7] which removed most of this inert material the purified fraction

* For a discussion of the relationship of association constant to slope the reader is referred to Chapter 14 of this book and to the review [46] of Berson & Yalow.

was labelled and found to react almost quantitatively with the antiserum. This would seem to be the only method at present capable of detecting immunologically inert protein.

A steep slope which is linear over the whole range 20–80 per cent bound (Fig. 18.10) is consistent with the antigen being a homogeneous protein. Discontinuity in the curve would constitute evidence of a mixture of antigens since two proteins would be unlikely to elicit formation of antibodies of the same titre and avidity.

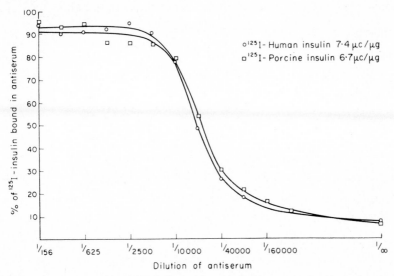

FIG. 18.12. Comparison of ^{125}I-human insulin and ^{125}I-porcine insulin in titration with a guinea-pig antiserum to porcine insulin. Concentration of labelled insulin 1·0 μmg/ml. Incubation 7 days, 4° C. Separation by paper chromatography.

Figure 18.12 shows the results of reaction of ^{125}I-human insulin and ^{125}I-porcine insulin with guinea-pig anti-pork insulin. The curves fall within the experimental error—indicating a reaction of identity. Antisera differ in their degree of cross-reaction with two closely related proteins—this question is best investigated by means of inhibition curves (see below) but differences in slope between cross-reacting proteins can be demonstrated by means of antiserum titration curves.

The above uses of antiserum titration curves require that the labelling procedure has not altered the antigen in respect to its reaction with the antibody being studied. The identical behaviour of iodinated preparations of widely different specific activities may be taken as evidence for their being unaltered but comparison of labelled and unlabelled antigen in inhibition studies (see below) provides superior evidence on this question. However, once the behaviour of immunologically unaltered labelled antigen with a given antiserum has been established the antiserum dilution curve may be used to test other iodinated preparations for damage caused during iodination. Figure 18.13 shows the behaviour of ^{125}I-HGH of very high specific activities, all of which have lost immunological activity during the over-labelling, in comparison with that of an undamaged preparation. In using the antiserum titration curve as a test for the integrity of the labelled antigen preparation it is clearly desirable that the results be available as soon after preparation of the iodinated material. Since the antigen : antibody system

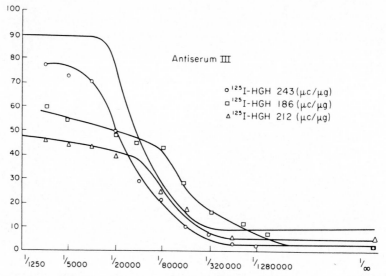

FIG. 18.13. Behaviour of undamaged ^{125}I-HGH (heavy line experimental points omitted) with three preparations showing gross loss of immunochemical integrity. Incubation 16 hours at 10 μmg labelled HGH/ml at 4° C. Separation on cellulose acetate electrophoresis.

equilibrates more rapidly at high concentration it is tempting to use, say, 10 μmg labelled antigen/ml incubate (this would equilibrate overnight at 4° C with a good antiserum). However, subtle damage can occur during iodination which merely reduces the rate of reaction with antibody. Such damage will escape detection in rapid testing at high concentration [16]. Testing should therefore be carried out at the lowest concentration at which it is intended to use the labelled preparation. It may be impractical to wait (7 days or more) for equilibration at this level but at a fixed shorter time (24 hours, say) undamaged labelled antigen will occupy a particular position (see Fig. 18.8) which can be established by experiment.

It is necessary to exercise some degree of caution in making quantitative deductions about fractions of iodinated antigens from curves of the form used in Fig. 18.11. Determinations of protein by both ultra-violet absorption (E_{280}) and by the Folin and Ciocaulteau colour reaction rely on the tyrosine content which may not be the same for each protein in a mixture. Biuret or total N determinations do not allow for carbohydrate or lipid contents of proteins. With iodination, however, it is necessary to consider not only relative tyrosine contents in a mixture but also the possibility of differential reactivity of different tyrosines within a given protein (see above). Further, dialysis or gel-filtration columns used to separate unreacted iodine from iodinated protein may also remove small molecular weight peptides present in the antigen or may show preferential adsorption of different fractions of a mixed antigen and hence the iodinated preparation may not faithfully represent the unlabelled material.

Antigen addition curves

If a mixture of labelled antigen and sufficient antibody to bind about 70 per cent of this label is incubated with serial additions of unlabelled antigen then labelled and unlabelled antigen will compete for the limited number of binding sites on the available antibody. There will consequently be a sequential fall in per cent bound through the series and a curve of the form shown in Fig. 18.14 is obtained. If unlabelled antigen is plotted on a log scale the regression becomes linear over a certain range. This forms the basis of the radioimmunoassay.

Before considering the most widely used form of this system—i.e. its use to assay antigen in unknown solutions—it may be valuable to consider how addition of unlabelled antigen and of related proteins may throw some light on the nature of the antigen itself. In making quantitative deductions from what follows, the same caution must be adopted as recommended above. Let us suppose that we are dealing with a protein of biological importance, which is not readily available in purified form. The actual preparation is an extract from the tissue of origin, but its purity is uncertain. Such a preparation might well be contaminated by plasma proteins. A mixture of labelled antigen and antiserum at a dilution just sufficient to bind 100 per cent of the label is incubated with plasma (say at one-tenth dilution to avoid incubation damage to the label—see below). If any plasma protein were present in the antigen and were represented in the label then inclusion of plasma in the incubation mixture would immediately provide a vast excess of this particular antigen and this would result in a corresponding depression of the per cent bound. The shape of an antigen dilution curve may also be used to provide evidence for the homogeneity of the antigen, a continuous curve being consistent with homogeneity and a discontinuous one suggestive of a mixture of proteins in the antigen.

x*

The radioimmunoassay

Standard curves: precision of assay in pure solution
A standard curve has certain characteristics which affect the precision, sensitivity and working range of the assay. These are best described by reference to Fig. 18.14 which shows an 'ideal' curve—that is, one which provides the highest precision and the widest working range with this particular antiserum.

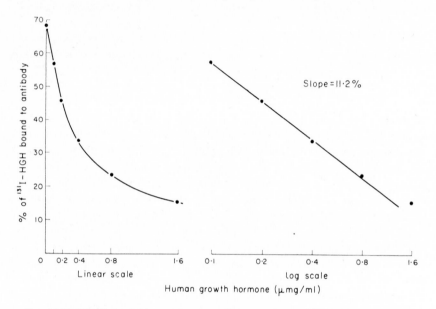

Fig. 18.14. 'Ideal' standard curve for the radioimmunoassay. ^{131}I-HGH 0·1 μmg/ml was incubated alone and with addition of unlabelled HGH as standard in the concentrations shown. All tubes contain the same amounts of ^{131}I-HGH and antiserum. An avid antiserum was used at a dilution sufficient to bind about 70 per cent of the ^{131}I-HGH in the absence of unlabelled HGH. Incubation 12–15 days at 4° C. Separation on cellulose acetate electrophoresis.

This system is not necessarily the most sensitive one but a higher sensitivity may be bought only at the cost of some loss in precision and working range—this subject will be discussed later.

In Fig. 18.14 which represents the mean values for twenty-seven standard curves run over a period of 3 months [17] the following factors emerge: the per cent of labelled HGH (used at 0·1 μmg/ml) bound to antibody in the absence of added unlabelled HGH (the '0' standard) is 68·2. Addition of an amount of unlabelled HGH (0·1 μmg/ml) equal to the concentration of labelled HGH results in a fall of 11·4 in the per cent bound. Such a fall can be measured with a high degree of accuracy. The per cent of label bound in the '0' standard can be increased by using a higher concentration of antiserum. However, this takes the system above the central linear part of the range and the fall in per cent bound for the first standard (0·1 μmg/ml) is reduced, so that the sensitivity of the assay is impaired. A reduction in the concentration of antiserum is less serious and merely results in lower per cent bound for the '0' standard and a shortening of the working range of the assay. The slope of the standard curve, defined as the fall in per cent bound per doubling dose of standard, is under these conditions (Fig. 18.14) approximately one-half of that of the antiserum dilution curve obtained with the same antiserum and using the same concentration of labelled antigen. The mean slope in the example given (Fig. 18.14) is steep enough to give a high order of precision but not so steep that the effective working range is restricted.

The assay of HGH in an unknown solution involves simply preparing dilutions such that their HGH content brings them within the range of the standard curve. In pure solution or using highly diluted pituitary gland extracts no problems need be considered other than those of statistical and manipulative precision. These are related to (a) the slope of the standard curve—the steeper the slope the greater the discrimination between two unknowns and hence the greater the precision; (b) the amount of radioactivity for counting after separation of bound and free labelled antigen. This is determined by the specific activity of the iodinated antigen, the volume of the aliquot which is taken for separation (of bound and free) and subsequent counting, the efficiency of the counting system and the counting time available. In a system in which only the bound or free component of an accurately measured volume of incubate is counted the precision is simply related to the number of counts recorded. The same relationship holds where bound and free are separately counted and plotted as a ratio, e.g. per cent bound, or B/F ratio. However, the actual precision obtained with these ratios is not so obviously clear from tables, and Fig. 18.15 gives some indication of what may be expected. This shows the standard deviation in per cent bound determined from repeated counting of a particular 'bound' and 'free' separation which gave a mean value of 20 per cent bound. A standard deviation of 0·5 in per cent bound with a slope of 11·2 per cent on the standard curve means a standard deviation of approximately ±5 per cent of the growth hormone in the unknown. This, of course, does not allow for manipulative errors. In 122 pairs of duplicate determinations [15] on two different dilutions of plasma the standard deviation of individual estimations from their means was ±10·8 per cent of the mean over the range 5–40 μmg/ml plasma; i.e. approximately twice the counting error. Similar results for precision were reported by Hales and Randle in the double-antibody method for insulin [13].

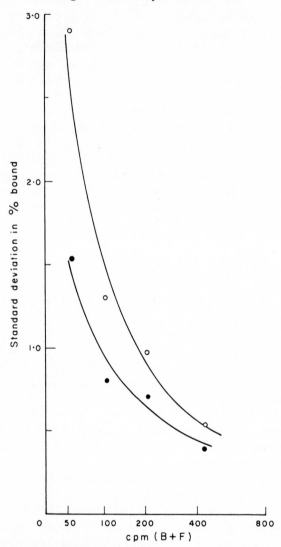

Fig. 18.15. Standard deviation in per cent of ^{131}I-HGH bound to antibody. The 'bound' and 'free' were separated on cellulose acetate electrophoresis and the strip cut into two parts (see Fig. 18.6), rolled into scrolls and counted in a sodium iodide well-type scintillation counter. Using a pulse height analyser with the 'window' set at 0·305–0·405 MeV the background was 20 count/min. The same pair of scrolls was counted thirty times for 10 minutes (each half of scroll) and the standard deviation in per cent bound calculated from these 10 minute determinations (○) and by treating the data as ten pairs of 30 minute determinations (●). The mean value was 19·8 per cent bound.

Assay of antigen in plasma

Duplicate estimations of growth hormone in plasma in the lowest range (1–5 μmg/ml) showed a standard deviation of ± 17 per cent of their means. The difference between this and the standard deviation in the higher range represents the small degree of non-specific interference due to incubation of labelled HGH with plasma dilution of one-fifth at 4° C for 15 days. This effect can be shown to be due to alteration in the physiochemical and immunological properties of the labelled antigen and has been discussed at length as 'incubation damage' by Yalow & Berson [8, 19] for insulin. Incubation of ^{131}I-HGH with plasma at one-fifth dilution produces only marginal changes, and provided no more concentrated solution is used these effects may be ignored [17]. If ^{131}I-HGH is incubated at 4° C with undiluted plasma there is increasing formation with time of a damaged fraction which is less electronegative, which interacts with denatured plasma proteins with which it tends to co-precipitate, and which is immunologically inert. ^{131}I-HGH which is bound to antibody is protected from this incubation damage. The damage is caused by the protein and not by the low molecular weight fraction of the plasma, and is not prevented by the enzyme inhibitor difluorophosphate. HGH provides difficulties for radioimmunoassay because damage, as shown by the appearance of immunologically inert material, may be caused by (i) the initial extraction procedure used to prepare the hormone from pituitary glands; (ii) iodination when high specific activities are attempted; and (iii) incubation with plasma. The effects of (i) and (ii) may not become apparent when assays are conducted in pure solution. However, when assays of plasma are attempted non-specific effects leading to grossly inaccurate estimates of the antigen may result from interaction of damaged labelled material with plasma proteins. Whether these effects result in over- or underestimation will depend upon the separative procedure used, but in most systems since the damaged fractions are immunologically inert they read as displacement of 'bound' labelled antigen into the 'free' compartment and hence appear as positive determinations of the antigen. This effect therefore generally results in overestimation. In assays which use the chromatographic or chromatoelectrophoretic separation of bound and free, however, damaged antigen loses its adsorption to paper and travels with the plasma proteins in the bound fraction. In this system damage results therefore in underestimation. These effects may be present in varying degrees with different proteins. The first effect raises problems of protein separation procedures which are not relevant to this chapter—but the radioimmunoassay technique can be most valuable in demonstrating the presence of damaged material. Iodination damage has been discussed above. Incubation damage to ACTH may be reduced by adding 2-mercaptoethanol 0·5 per cent and the trypsin inhibitor Trasylol 2 per cent to the incubates [29]. Alternatively, it may be necessary to extract the antigen from plasma so that it can be added to the incubates without also adding whole plasma. Extraction of HGH by means of a cold acid acetone procedure yielding essentially an albumin fraction has been used to concentrate the HGH in plasma and to give an approximately three-fold increase in the sensitivity of its assay (using the standard curve shown in Fig. 18.14) to 0·22 μmg/ml plasma [17]. However, the labour involved in extraction procedure is so considerable that other modifications in the procedure are preferable. These consist essentially of attempts to increase the sensitivity of the assay

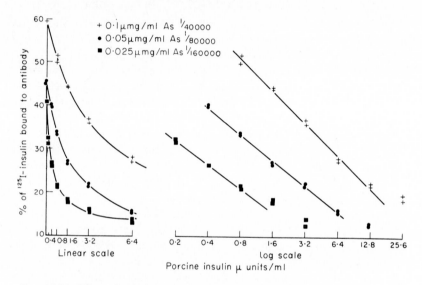

FIG. 18.16. Effect of dilution on the standard curve: attempt to obtain highest sensitivity in the assay of insulin with a given antiserum. The ratio of ^{125}I-insulin : antiserum is the same in each of the three curves. The working range and slope diminish as the system becomes attenuated.

so that unextracted plasma may be diluted to a sufficient degree to obviate significant incubation damage.

Sensitivity of the radioimmunoassay

At first sight it would seem that the only necessity for increasing the sensitivity of an assay is to reduce the concentration of labelled antigen, antiserum and consequently of standards. However, as a system is diluted the equilibration time increases: in practice an assay involving incubation of more than about 7 days is most inconvenient. Figure 18.16 shows the effect of dilution of the pork insulin, guinea-pig anti-pork insulin system. The three curves are identical in the ratio of antiserum : ^{125}I-insulin used and were all from mixtures incubated for 7 days. The per cent bound in the absence of unlabelled insulin shows a progressive reduction with dilution. This results also in a progressive reduction in both the slope of the standard curve (and hence in its precision) and also in the working range (linear portion) of the curve. The greatest absolute sensitivity, however, is found in the system giving the largest fall in per cent bound for a given standard. Thus the curve using the lowest concentration of ^{125}I-insulin (0·025 μmg/ml) is the most sensitive one, but the precision is lower and the working range smaller than with either of the other two

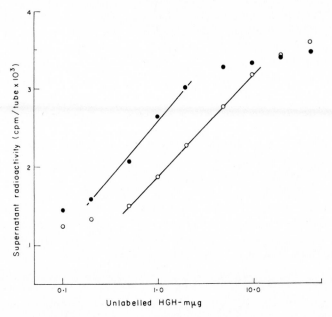

FIG. 18.17. Standard curves showing increased sensitivity of the assay when unlabelled HGH and antiserum were allowed to react for 24 hours (●) before addition of ^{131}I-HGH compared to when ^{131}I-HGH was added immediately (○). (From ref. 40.)

curves. A further reduction in concentration of label and antisera results in a further fall in per cent bound in the absence of unlabelled insulin and a diminished fall for the first standard. The actual sensitivity of the system is a function of the avidity of the antiserum used. In general the search for an avid antiserum is a haphazard process but if success is finally achieved the antiserum being very stable and being used in high dilution may last almost indefinitely.

For the above assays of insulin ^{125}I-pork insulin of 150 μc/μg was prepared by reaction of 1·5 mc of Na^{125}I with 5 μg insulin and damaged fractions removed by means of a small cellulose column [19]. With this specific activity and using the paper chromatographic separation which can take 0·2 ml of the incubate the amount of radioactivity is not a limiting factor in the sensitivity of the assay. However, specific activity can be the limiting factor in an assay and this is in fact so for ACTH assays which at present are limited by this to a sensitivity of 3–5 $\mu\mu$g/ml in pure solution [49].

Hales & Randle [13] showed that if the addition of the labelled antigen is delayed until the antiserum and standards have been allowed to react for some time, the standard curve is shifted to the left with a consequent increase in sensitivity. Figure 18.17 illustrates this point. The use of delayed addition of labelled antigen offers two further clear advantages: (i) it may be used to provide twice the quantity of radioactivity without loss of sensitivity—this may be used to reduce the counting time or to increase the precision; (ii) it reduces the exposure of labelled antigen to incubation damage and so may improve sensitivity by permitting the assay of less diluted plasma.

Methods of treating the data

In the above description the data has been treated in terms of the variation in per cent of labelled antigen bound to antibody. Other methods may be used and each system has certain advantages. The use of 'per cent of labelled antigen bound' enables the radioactive material to retain some chemical identity and facilitates the consideration of its homogeneity. (For example, using this form it is easy to think in terms of, say, 5 per cent of the label representing a contaminant, or of 15 per cent being immunologically inert.) Also linear regression lines are found for antiserum titration curves (essentially a plot of per cent B against log antiserum concentration) and for antigen addition curves (per cent B vs. log antigen concentration). The slopes of each of these can be expressed quantitatively and hence may be compared—even between systems for quite different antigens and in different laboratories. Hales & Randle [13] use (Fig. 18.18) a plot of radioactivity in the bound fraction in the absence of added standard ÷ radioactivity in the bound fraction with added standard. This uses the general principle of isotope dilution and takes the form:

$$\frac{C_0}{C_i} = i \cdot \frac{1}{i_0} + 1$$

in which

C_0 = bound radioactivity when concentration of unlabelled insulin = 0.
C_i = bound radioactivity when concentration of unlabelled insulin = i.
2i = concentration of unlabelled insulin.
$2i_0$ = concentration of ^{131}I-insulin.

In this equation C_0/C_i is linearly related to the concentration of unlabelled insulin. The authors point out, however, that this holds only if the affinity of antibody for labelled and unlabelled insulin is the same and if the amount of insulin bound by antibody is independent of the concentration of insulin. The latter condition may not in fact obtain in the radioimmunoassay—it is not fulfilled with the data from Fig. 18.14. However, as the authors point out, the data may still be treated in this way if standards are always run with

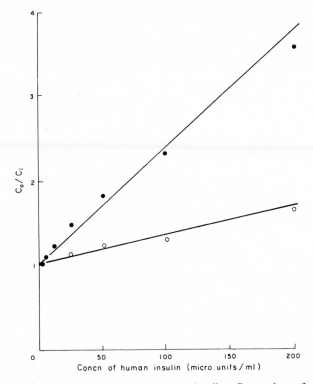

FIG. 18.18. Cross-reaction of human and bovine insulins. Comparison of antiserum to human (●) and bovine (○) insulins in the assay of human insulin. ^{131}I-bovine insulin was used. The plot of C_0/C_i against added unlabelled insulin is linear for both, but the slopes are different. (From ref. 13.)

unknowns. Using this method of plotting, the final standard curves do not contain an indication of how much of the label is bound to antiserum.

Yalow and Berson use the ratio Bound/Free (B/F). This is based firmly upon the treatment of the system in terms of mass action equations thus:

$$[Ag]+[Ab] \underset{k_2}{\overset{k_1}{\rightleftharpoons}} [Ag\,Ab]$$

$$K = \frac{k_1}{k_2} = \frac{[Ag\ Ab]}{[Ab]\ [Ag]}$$

then the molar concentration (molar concentration of antibody × valency of antibody) is $[Ab^0]$

$$[Ab^0] = [Ab] + [Ag\ Ab]$$

hence

$$K([Ab^0] - [Ag\ Ab]) = \frac{[Ag\ Ab]}{[Ag]}$$

let

$$B\ (\text{`Bound'}) = [Ag\ Ab]$$

and

$$F\ (\text{`Free'}) = [Ag]$$

thus

$$B/F = K([Ab^0] - B).$$

The reader is referred to papers by these authors for a very full treatment of the system in this form [5, 46]. The B/F ratio does not give a linear regression in antiserum titration curves or in the assay curves and hence these cannot be so readily compared with one another.

Specificity

The specificity of the radioimmunoassay depends upon: (i) the identity and homogeneity of the labelled antigen: (ii) the specificity of the immune reaction which requires that only protein(s) which are identical or closely similar (cross-reacting) to the protein represented in the label shall compete with the labelled antigen for binding sites on the antibody.

The identity and homogeneity of the labelled antigen may be considered first with respect to the protein available for labelling; this is essentially a problem of protein chemistry though immunochemical methods, including the radioimmunoassay technique, may assist in monitoring the process of purification. It is of interest that Berson and Yalow were able to prepare immunochemically homogeneous ^{131}I-human insulin by iodinating crude human insulin which contained only 25 per cent of insulin and then removing the contaminants [50]. Such an approach was of marginal value for insulin since these workers had already established an immunoassay for human insulin by using purified pork insulin for labelling and antiserum (to pork insulin) which reacted identically with pork and human insulin. However, it may be possible to approach the problem of the immunoassay of other proteins of biological importance which have not been isolated by effecting the final stages of purification *after* iodination.

The specificity of the immune reaction is not absolute. Antisera to bovine insulin react with pork or human insulin—proteins which though not identical are biologically related and also differ chemically by only one or two specific amino acids. Human pituitary luteinizing hormone cross-reacts immunologically with human chorionic gonadotrophin and more recently a placental protein has been prepared whose biological activity is uncertain but which is believed to be a new hormone because it is immunochemically related to pituitary growth hormone [51]. This placental hormone has more recently been shown to have the same amino-acid analysis as growth hormone [52]. Thus, although not absolute, immunological cross-reaction appears generally to be limited to proteins which are closely related biologically. In assessing the specificity of a radioimmunoassay for a protein in physiological fluids the behaviour of such cross-reacting proteins will generally not be relevant; for example, animal insulins will not be found in humans unless they have been administered. Placental hormones will interfere in the assay of their related pituitary principals only in pregnant women and patients with certain hormone-secreting tumours. Further, the assay procedure involves a graded response and related (cross-reacting) proteins will frequently give a different slope from that of the homologous antigen in the standard curve (see below). These considerations with the addition of those due to artefacts of the system which can arise as a result of the presence of immunochemically altered antigen, or of inhomogeneity, in the label (see above) provide the only limitations to the specificity of the radioimmunoassay method.

Effect of addition of modified antigen on the reaction of labelled antigen with antibody

The effect of substitution of HGH with ^{127}iodine has been discussed above (Fig. 18.5). Recent work on ACTH by Imura *et al* [53] provides an excellent example of the effect of related proteins and modified antigen in antigen addition curves. Figure 18.19 shows that with two different antisera raised to injected intact natural α^{1-39}ACTH from sheep, whole human, pig and sheep ACTH behaved as expected giving a significant fall in per cent bound with addition of an amount equal to that of the ^{125}I-ACTH and thereafter gave a slope of approximately 10 per cent per doubling dose. Polypeptides consisting of the twenty-four or twenty-six amino acids comprising the N-terminal portion of the molecule, α^{1-24}ACTH and α^{1-26}ACTH, were present in approximately ten times that required for the α^{1-39}ACTH before a significant fall in per cent ^{125}I-ACTH occurred. The slope of the curve was diminished. α^{1-17}ACTH and α^{1-19} failed to compete with the label even when added at one hundred times the concentration of ^{125}I-ACTH. These findings indicate that the immunologically reactive sites reside in the 19–39 end (i.e. the C-terminal half) of the peptide chain. Figure 18.19 shows the effect of the 22–39 peptide which is seen to show a fall in per cent bound with smaller amounts but to show the same slope that is found with $^{1-39}$ACTH. Thus $^{22-39}$ACTH was calculated to be six times more active than $^{1-39}$ACTH on a weight basis and three times more active on a molar basis. It is of interest that these highly active subfractions showed a slope identical to that of α^{1-39}ACTH; none showed a steeper slope.

Studies of this kind have important implications for the use of radio-immunoassays for the determination of hormones (or other biologically active proteins) in physiological fluids, for the object clearly is to obtain data which is of physiological significance. The biologically active sites of ACTH are confined to the N-terminal end of the molecule—that is, to the immuno-logically inactive portion. The C-terminal half ($^{22-39}$ACTH) which shows

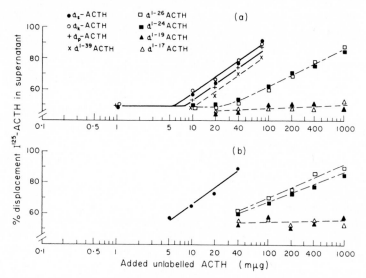

FIG. 18.19. Comparison of the ability of three natural preparations: α_s-ACTH (sheep), α_h-ACTH (human), α_p-ACTH (pig) and synthetic $\alpha_p{}^{1-39}$ACTH and fractions thereof to compete with ^{131}I-ACTH (natural human) for antibodies to natural sheep ACTH. (a) antiserum 28, (b) antiserum 26. (From ref. 53.)

substantially all of the immunological activity is inactive biologically. Similarly, oxidation of ACTH with periodate or incubation with fibrinolysin completely destroyed its biological activity but left unaltered or increased the immunological activity [53]. The question must inevitably be asked whether a protein might become altered (perhaps during interaction with its specific target tissue or during passage through the liver) in such a way that biological activity was lost whilst it still remained in the circulation and retained its immunochemical activity. Such altered material would be detected by immunoassays and this might lead to an entirely false estimate of the biological situation.

The acceptability of immunochemical methods, like other chemical methods for the assay of biologically active substances, must be questioned. The council of perfection would certainly suggest that immunochemical methods be compared with suitable biological assays on the same samples. Unfortunately, bioassays for HGH are 10,000–100,000 times less sensitive, and many times less precise than the radioimmunoassay, so that such checks would require the concentration of many litres of plasma even with the high concentrations found in acromegaly. Biological methods for the microassay of insulin in plasma have been based upon various minute changes in glucose uptake or gas exchange of preparations of rat diaphragm or epididimal fat pad and are of such doubtful specificity that the term 'insulin-like activity' is generally used. More recently those assays which give results of the same order as those found by radioimmunoassay have been regarded as the most specific. Alternatively, the bioassay has been conducted first with whole plasma and then again on the same plasma in the presence of antisera to insulin. The difference, the 'immunologically suppressible insulin' has been regarded as nearest to the true insulin value. Such thoughts, whilst perhaps flattering to the immunoassayist, are of little help in assessing the biological validity of immunochemical assays!

TSH provides the only example at present of a protein which has been estimated in physiological fluids by radioimmunoassay [34, 36] and also by bioassay [54] using a method whose specificity is not seriously in question. Comparisons of these two assays have not been carried out *on the same sample* and this is anticipated as an interesting development to be expected in the near future.

The behaviour of immunologically related (cross-reacting) proteins in antigen addition curves

These may be classified as: (i) reactions of identity; (ii) complete cross-reactions; (iii) incomplete cross-reactions.

(i) A protein showing a reaction of identity behaves in a manner indistinguishable from that of the antigen itself; the curve given by addition of increasing increments of such a protein will have the same slope throughout the entire range as that of the antigen. Some antisera may fail to distinguish between two slightly different proteins (i.e. the two proteins show reactions of identity), e.g. Fig. 18.20, whilst others from the same species of animal may distinguish between the same two proteins (i.e. the two proteins show complete cross-reaction).

(ii) Complete cross-reactions. A completely cross-reacting protein is capable of competing with the antigen for all of the binding sites on the antibody, but its affinity for antibody is diminished and hence more of the cross-reacting protein than of the antigen itself is required to effect an equal fall in per cent bound of labelled antigen. The slope of the curve is shallower than that given by the antigen. Figure 20 illustrates the differences between guinea-pig anti-pork insulin in their ability to distinguish between pork, human and ox insulins. It will be seen that antiserum GP.56.228 does not distinguish between insulins from these two species, but GP.75.228 antiserum does detect this difference.

It is of interest that the first use of the radioimmunoassay system—that developed by Yalow & Berson [8] for measuring endogenous insulin in human plasma made use of the reaction of identity shown by human and pork insulin (which differ only in the C-terminal amino acid of the B chain) with some guinea-pig anti-pork insulin sera. Purified human insulin was not available to these workers for the purpose of raising antisera or for labelling. Impure human preparations containing respectively 1·8 and 6·8 units/mg (i.e.

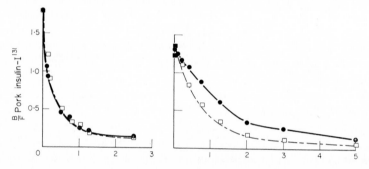

FIG. 18.20. Ability of one guinea-pig anti-pork insulin serum (GP. 75. 228) (right) to distinguish between human ●—● and pork insulin □ - - □ (added as standards in the amounts shown on the abscissa [μmg/ml]), and reaction of identity shown with another antiserum (GP. 56. 228) (left). (From ref. 56.)

6·45 per cent and 28·2 per cent pure insulin by weight by bioassay) were compared with purified pork insulin (27–29 units/mg) until an antiserum was found with which the insulins from the two species showed reaction of identity —i.e. had identical slopes. Radioimmunoassay of the human insulin preparations was therefore possible using pure pork insulin as standard. The ratio of potencies of these two human preparations to each other and to the pork standard was in excellent agreement with the potency ratios found by bioassay. It was therefore possible (provided this antiserum was used) to assay endogenous insulin in human plasma using pork insulin for labelling and as the standard. These workers later prepared pure radioiodinated human insulin by removal of the contaminants after labelling of a crude preparation. Using this material the validity of the earlier use of pork insulin has been fully justified [55].

Figure 21 shows curves for the addition of standards (of HGH which was the antigen), of serial dilutions of plasma from an acromegalic patient and of plasma from an adolescent. Curves for these materials are parallel, indicating the presence of a protein showing identity of immunological behaviour. The open squares represent the curve for plasma from a pregnant woman. This plasma contains the human placental lactogen which shows a complete cross-reaction with HGH. The plot of per cent bound against log added protein gives a linear regression and enables the cross-reaction to be quantitated by comparison of these slopes.

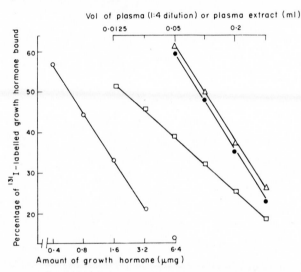

FIG. 18.21. Assay of a protein believed to be identical with the antigen and detection of a completely cross-reacting protein. Parallelism between curves for HGH standards (○) and dilutions of plasma from non-pregnant subjects (●, △) is evidence of identity of active substance in plasma and HGH. Lack of parallelism for dilutions of plasma from a pregnant woman (□) is indicative of the presence of a protein showing a complete cross-reaction with HGH.

It is possible to assay one protein using a standard which shows a different slope to that of the unknown, though the unknown (as well as the standard) must be assayed at several dilutions so that a full slope study can be made. The calculations then involve a correction factor which allows for this slope difference. However, such a method involves some loss of sensitivity and precision in comparison with one in which antigen, label, standards and unknown are immunologically identical.

(iii) Incomplete cross-reactions. A protein showing incomplete cross-reaction with the antigen is one which will react with some but not all of the antibodies directed against the specific antigen. In the radioimmunoassay the cross-reacting protein will compete with labelled antigen only over a certain range—an example is shown in Fig. 18.22 [36]. Human TSH in increasing amounts progressively decreases the per cent of ^{131}I-HTSH until none of the label is bound. Serum from pregnant women and from patients with hydatid mole depressed the binding of labelled TSH with a diminished slope (as for completely cross-reacting proteins) but this process stopped when some 50 per cent of the label was still bound to antibody. This must mean that the remaining ^{131}I-TSH was bound to antibodies which do not react

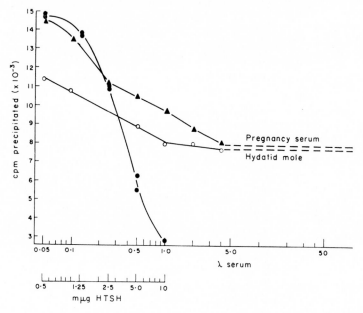

Fig. 18.22. Detection of a protein showing an incomplete cross-reaction. TSH (●) competes with ^{131}I-TSH for antibody over the whole range of binding. Plasma from normal and mole pregnancy contains a substance (which may be HCG) which competes for only some of the antibody sites which bind ^{131}I-TSH. (From ref. 36.)

with the cross-reacting protein, i.e. the two proteins show an incomplete cross-reaction. Though human chorionic gonadotrophin (HCG) has not been isolated the authors considered that this was the cross-reacting substance since partially purified preparations of HCG of 12,000 i.u./mg and a human luteinizing hormone (LH) preparation from post-menopausal urine (which resembles HCG in its biological and immunological activity) showed the same effect. The radioimmunoassay of TSH was therefore conducted with anti-TSH serum which had been absorbed with HCG and no interference was then found when plasma from pregnant women was assayed [36]. TSH and HCG (or LH) are not known to be related in their biological activity so their cross-reaction is surprising.

Specificity when assaying in unknown solutions
The above treatment has been concerned with the limitations of specificity with respect to the effects of immunochemically related proteins. In the section dealing with iodination the other source of non-specificity has been discussed —i.e. that due to alteration in the behaviour of the labelled antigen resulting from its incubation (particularly with undiluted plasma) in the assay. In assessing the specificity of an assay use may (as mentioned earlier) be made of the fact that we are dealing with a graded response. Thus, if an unknown solution gives a regression of per cent bound against dilution which parallels that of the antigen this is good evidence for identity. Duplicate determinations at the same dilution are no easier to carry out and they provide less information than the use of two different dilutions of unknown. This use of two different dilutions provides useful evidence of specificity at the threshold of sensitivity of the assay, i.e. in the range in which non-specific effects are (proportionately) more important. A response which parallels that of the standard at two dilutions in the logarithmic part of the standard curve is most likely to be due to the specific protein being assayed. Such parallelism is assessed more accurately and deviations more readily detected if the slope of the standard curve is steep. This again emphasizes the importance of an avid dilution.

It will be noticed that in the consideration of specificity no mention has been made of homogeneity of the antiserum. The concept of antiserum homogeneity is a dangerous illusion which runs menacingly through the literature of applied immunology. Such a reagent probably does not exist and if it did it would go unrecognized. The ability of an immunized animal to 'amplify' the presence of minute quantities of a contaminant protein is well illustrated by a rabbit antiserum to an HGH preparation which contained no detectable (<2 per cent) plasma albumin. This antiserum had a higher titre and avidity to albumin that it had to HGH. It is one of the strengths of the radioimmunoassay that the use of heterogenous antisera is quite irrelevant since only those antibodies directed towards protein represented in the label affect the system.

Conclusion
The use of labelled antigens permits the investigation of the primary reaction between antigen and antibody, whereas many other methods used in immunology require the development of a secondary effect (precipitation, agglutination, complement fixation, etc.). This consideration—as well as those of sensitivity and precision which have been mentioned—recommends this system to the attention of immunologists.

Acknowledgment

I am most grateful to Dr P.C.Ganguli for help with the manuscript and to the author and publishers for permission to reproduce Figs. 18.7, 18.17, 18.18, 18.19, 18.20 and 18.21.

References

[1] BERSON S.A., YALOW R.S., BAUMAN A., ROTHSCHILD M.A. & NEWERBY K. (1956) Insulin-I^{131} metabolism in human subjects: Demonstration of insulin binding globulin in the circulation of insulin treated subjects. *J. clin. Invest.* **35,** 170

[2] UNGER R.H., EISENTRAUT, A.M., McCALL, M.S., KELLER, S., LANZ, H.C. & MADISON, L.L. (1959) Glucagon antibodies and their use for immunoassay for glucagon. *Proc. Soc. exp. Biol., N.Y.* **102,** 621.

[3] BERSON, S.A. & YALOW R.S. (1959) Quantitative aspects of the reaction between insulin and insulin-binding antibody. *J. clin. Invest.* **38,** 1996

[4] FARR R.S. (1958) A quantitative immunochemical measure of the primary interaction between I*BSA and antibody. *J. infect. Dis.* **103,** 239.

[5] BERSON S.A. & YALOW R.S. (1959) Species-specificity of human anti-beef pork insulin serum. *J. clin. Invest.* **38,** 2017

[6] BERSON S.A. & YALOW R.S. (1959) Cross reactions of human anti-beef pork insulin with beef, pork, sheep, horse and human insulins. *Fed. Proc.* **18,** 11

[7] HUNTER W.M. (1965) Homogeneity studies on human growth hormone. *Biochem. J.* **97,** 199

[8] YALOW R.S. & BERSON S.A. (1960) Immunoassay of endogenous plasma insulin in man. *J. clin. Invest*, **39,** 1157

[9] COLLIPP P.J., KAPLAN S.A., BOYLE D.C. & SHIMIZU C.S.N. (1965) ^{14}C-acetyl BGH. *J. biol. Chem.* **240,** 143

[10] HUGHES W.L. (1957) The chemistry of iodination. *Ann. N.Y. Acad. Sci.* **70(1),** 3

[11] McFARLANE A.S. (1958) Efficient trace-labelling of proteins with iodine. *Nature, Lond.* **182,** 53

[12] SAMOLS E. & WILLIAMS H.S. (1961) Trace-labelling of insulin with iodine. *Nature, Lond.* **190,** 1211

[13] HALES C.N. & RANDLE P.J. (1963) Immunoassay of insulin with insulin-antibody precipitate. *Biochem. J.* **88,** 137

[14] HUNTER W.M. & GREENWOOD F.C. (1962) Preparation of iodine-131 labelled human growth hormone of high specific activity. *Nature, Lond.* **194,** 495

[15] GREENWOOD F.C., HUNTER W.M. & GLOVER J.S. (1963) The preparation of ^{131}I-labelled human growth hormone of high specific radioactivity. *Biochem. J.* **89,** 114

[16] HUNTER W.M. (1966) Iodination of protein compounds. Atomic Energy Commission Symposium Series. *Radioactive Pharmaceuticals,* ed. ANDREWS, KNISELEY & WAGNER, U.S. Atomic Energy Commission, Oak Ridge, Tennessee

[17] HUNTER W.M. & GREENWOOD F.C. (1964) A radio-immunoelectrophoretic assay for human growth hormone. *Biochem. J.* **91,** 43

[18] GLICK S.M., ROTH J., YALOW R.S. & BERSON S.A. (1963) Immunoassay of human growth hormone in plasma. *Nature, Lond.* **199,** 784

[19] YALOW R.S. & BERSON S.A. (1964) Immunoassay of plasma insulin. *Meth. biochem. Anal.* **12,** 69

[20] YAGI Y., MAIER P. & PRESSMAN D. (1965) Antibodies against the component poly-peptide chains of bovine insulin. *Science* **147**, 617.

[21] SAMOLS E., TYLER J. & MARRI G. (1965) Stimulation of glucagon secretion by oral glucose. *Lancet* **ii,** 1257

[22] SHERWOOD L.M., POTTS J.T., CARE A.D., MEYER G.P. & AURBACH G.D. (1966) Evaluation by radioimmunoassay of factors controlling the secretion of parathyroid hormone. *Nature, Lond.* **209**, 52

[23] YALOW R.S., GLICK S.M., ROTH J. & BERSON S.A. (1964) Radioimmunoassay of human plasma ACTH. *J. clin. Endocrin.* **24**, 1219

[24] UTIGER R.D., ODELL S.D. & CONDLIFFE P.G. (1963) Immunologic studies of purified human and bovine thyrotropin. *Endocrinology* **73**, 359

[25] GALLILAND P.F. & PROUT T.E. (1965) Immunologic studies of octapeptides. 1. Radioiodination of oxytocin. *Metabolism* **14**, 912

[26] SPRINGELL P.H. (1961) An unreactive tyrosine residue in insulin and the exclusive iodination of the A chain. *Nature, Lond.* **191**, 1372

[27] DUBE S.K. ROHOLT O.A. & PRESSMAN D. (1964) Identification of the most rapidly iodinating tyrosine residue in a chymotrypsin. *J. biol. Chem.* **239**, 3347

[28] GREGORY H., HARDY P.M., JONES D.S., KENNER G.W. & SHEPPARD R.C. (1964) The antral hormone gastrin. *Nature, Lond.* **204**, 931

[29] YALOW R.S. (1966) Preparation and purification of high specific activity labelled hormones. Atomic Energy Commission Symposium Series. *Radioactive Pharmaceuticals*, ed. ANDREWS, KNISELEY & WAGNER U.S. Atomic Energy Commission, Oak Ridge, Tennessee

[30] KUNKEL H.G. & SLATER R.J. (1952) Zone electrophoresis in a starch supporting medium. *Proc. Soc. exp. Biol., N.Y.* **80**, 42

[31] ORNSTEIN L. & DAVIES B.J. (1962) *Disc Electrophoresis.* Reprinted by Distillation Products Industries, Rochester, New York.

[32] FITSCHEN W. (1964) A quantitative study of antigen–antibody composition during disc electrophoresis in acrylamide gel using iodine-131 labelled human growth hormone. *Immunology, Lond.* **7**, 307

[33] UNGER R.H., EISENTRAUT A.M., MCCALL, M.S. & MADISON L.L. (1961) Glucagon antibodies and an immunoassay for glucagon. *J. clin. Invest.* **40**, 1280

[34] UTIGER H.D. (1965) Radioimmunoassay of plasma thyrotropin. *J. clin. Invest.* **44**, 1277

[35] GRODSKY G.M. & FORSHAM P.H. (1960) An immunochemical assay for total extract-able insulin in man. *J. clin. Invest.* **39**, 1070

[36] ODELL W.D., WILBER J.F. & PAUL W.E. (1965) Radioimmunoassay of thyrotropin in human serum. *J. clin. Endocrin.* **25**, 1179

[37] GENUTH S., FROHMAN L.A. & LEBOVITZ H.E. (1965) A radioimmunological assay method for insulin using insulin-^{125}I gel filtration. *J. clin. Endocrin.* **25**, 1043

[38] HERBERT V., LACE K.S., GOTTLIEB C.W. & BLEICHER S.J. (1965) Coated charcoal immunoassay of insulin. *J. clin. Endocrin.* **25**, 1375

[39] UTIGER R.D., PARKER M.L. & DAUGHADAY W.H. (1962) Studies on human growth hormone. 1. A radioimmunoassay for human growth hormone. *J. clin. Invest.* **41**, 254

[40] UTIGER R.D. (1964) Extraction and radioimmunoassay of growth hormone in human serum. *J. clin. Endocrin.* **24**, 60

[41] SCHALCH D.S. & PARKER M.L. (1964) A sensitive double-antibody immunoassay for human growth hormone in plasma. *Nature, Lond.* **203**, 1141

[42] MORGAN C.R. & LAZAROW A. (1963) Immunoassay of insulin: Two antibody system. Plasma insulin levels of normal, subdiabetic and diabetic rats. *Diabetes,* **12**, 115

[43] Morgan C.R., Sorenson R.L. & Lazarow H. (1964) Further studies of an inhibitor of the 2 antibody immunoassay system (for insulin). *Diabetes* **13**, 579.

[44] Samols, E. & Bilkus D. (1964) A comparison of insulin immunoassays. *Proc. Soc. exp. Biol. Med.* **115,** 79

[45] Porter R.R. (1959) Hydrolysis of rabbit-globulin and antibodies with crystalline papain. *Biochem. J.* **73,** 119

[46] Berson S.A. & Yalow R.S. (1964) Immunoassay of protein hormones. *The Hormones,* Vol. 4, Ch. 11, ed. Pincus, Thimann & Astwood. New York and London: Academic Press

[47] Gray H.M. (1964) Studies on changes in the quality of rabbit-bovine serum albumin antibody following immunization. *Immunology, Lond.* **7,** 82

[48] Raben M.S. (1959) Human growth hormone. *Recent Progr. Hormone Res.* **15,** 71

[49] Landon J., Livanou D. & Greenwood F.C. (1966) Problems in the radioimmuno-assay of human ACTH. *J. Endocrin.* **35,** P.1

[50] Berson S.A. & Yalow R.S. (1961) Preparation and purification of human insulin-I^{131} binding to human insulin-binding antibodies. *J. clin. Invest.* **40,** 1803.

[51] Josimovitch J.B. & MacLaren J.A. (1962) Presence in the human placenta and term serum of a highly lactogenic substance immunologically related to pituitary growth hormone. *Endocrinology* **71,** 209

[52] Friesen H (1965) Purification of a placental factor with immunochemical and chemical similarity to human growth hormone. *Endocrinology* **76,** 369

[53] Imura H., Sparke L.L., Grodsky G.M. & Forsham P.H. (1965) Immunologic studies of adrenocorticotrophic hormone (ACTH) dissociation of biologic and immunologic activities. *J. clin. Endocrin.* **25,** 1361–1369

[54] Kirkham K.E. (1962) A new bioassay technique for the measurement *in vitro* of thyrotrophic hormone in serum and in pituitary extracts. *J. Endocrin.* **25,** 259

[55] Yalow R.S. & Berson S.A. (1961) Immunological specificity of human insulin: application to immunoassay of insulin. *J. clin. Invest.* **40,** 2190

CHAPTER 19

Immunodiffusion and Immunoelectrophoresis

Ö.OUCHTERLONY

Introduction

Gel-diffusion techniques for immunoprecipitation analysis have a history of about 60 years. Back in 1897 Rudolf Kraus in Vienna gave the first report on precipitation caused by interaction of soluble antigens and corresponding antisera, and in 1905 Bechhold [2] in Germany reported on experiments concerning immunoprecipitates established in a gel medium. However, Bechhold's experiments were carried out as part of a study on Liesegang effects, and the phenomenon observed treated from the physicist's point of view. His reports obviously did not catch the eyes of the serologists and the diffusion-in-gel principle for immunological analyses was overlooked for a considerable period of time. In the 'thirties some bacteriologists made attempts to apply the diffusion principle for serological typing of various bacterial species but well-standardized techniques for immunodiffusion (ID) were not established until the middle of the 'forties. In 1946 Oudin in France gave his first report on the principles and application of the simple diffusion technique in tubes [31]. Somewhat later double diffusion methods were introduced in 1947 in Sweden by Ouchterlony [27] and in 1948 in England by Elek [8] and Oakley & Fulthorpe [26] in 1953. Since then the basic techniques have been further developed and several new ID methods based on the original principles have been reported. One of the most useful technical developments in this field is the method of immunoelectrophoresis (IE). An early attempt to combine paper electrophoresis with ID analysis was reported in 1952 by Poulik [34]. However, an IE technique, where the electrophoresis as well as the ID analysis is performed in the gel medium, was first described in 1953 by Grabar & Williams [10]. A great variety of ID and IE methods are nowadays commonly used for qualitative as well as quantitative analysis of immunoprecipitating materials, and they have been applied to many problems in research even outside the field of serology and immunology. Several extensive reviews on this topic have been published by, e.g. Crowle [6], Grabar & Burtin [11, 12], Ouchterlony [28, 29] and Oudin [32].

Diffusion and electrophoresis in fluid and gelified media

Diffusion of a dissolved substance in a fluid medium is a process by which the substance is transported from one part of the fluid to another as a result of random molecular motion. By this process a tendency towards an equalization of concentrations of the substance in the medium is induced. The following formula for free diffusion in one dimension in a fluid medium was presented by Fick in 1885

$$\frac{dQ}{dt} = -DA\frac{dC}{dx},$$

where Q is the amount of diffusing substance which at a time t passes an area A, where the concentration gradient is dC/dx and D is a constant of proportionality called the diffusion coefficient. In the CGS system D is expressed as cm^2/sec. The following characteristics of the diffusion process should be noted: (a) An increase of the initial concentration of the diffusing matter has an incremental influence on the rate of diffusion. (b) An increase in temperature increases the value of D. (c) D varies inversely with the cube root of the volume of the molecule in solution corrected for eventual hydration and deviation from spherical shape. (d) The distance travelled by any given concentration of the solute varies directly as the square root of the time of diffusion.

When studying diffusion in fluid media it is often difficult to avoid disturbances induced by currents caused for example by temperature differences. One way to overcome this obstacle is to employ a gelified medium, e.g. an agar or gelatin gel. The gel forms a mesh-like structure stabilizing the liquid and preventing convective currents. If the pores of the gel network are considerably greater than the particle size of the diffusing substance and provided that the substance does not react chemically or physically with the gelifying agent, it may be assumed that the laws of free diffusion should apply. It has been found that if the concentration of the gelling agent is sufficiently low the rate of diffusion for many substances of small particle size is about the same in a fluid as in a corresponding gelified medium. However, the diffusion of larger molecules can be impeded or prevented particularly if the concentration of the gelling agent is increased. The decreased pore size of the gel thus obtained gives a so-called sieve effect. It can be mentioned as an example that the average pore diameter of a 2 per cent agar gel has been estimated at about 3 mμ. A 0·3–1·5 per cent agar gel does not usually interfere with free diffusion of most immunoreactants (antibodies and antigens) of a moderate molecular size and a regular shape. It may be mentioned that when immunoprecipitates are formed in an agar gel of the aforementioned concentration range, the size of the aggregates rapidly exceeds the diameters of the pores and thus the diffusion of the antigen–antibody complexes is prevented.

Electrophoresis is the migration of charged particles in a conductive solvent under the influence of an electric field. Among the factors governing the migration may be mentioned the charge, size and shape of the particles, the concentration, ionic strength and pH of the solvent, the temperature and viscosity of the medium and the character and intensity of the electric field. In Tiselius's original method for free electrophoresis of proteins, the sample to be analysed is dissolved in an appropriate buffer solution and poured into a U-shaped tube with an electrode in each arm. A barbiturate buffer of pH 8·2 used for samples of blood serum or plasma gives most of the protein particles a net negative charge. When the electric field is established the particles move towards the anode. Differences in migration rate, governed by the amount of the charge of the particles, lead to a separation of the material, and several fractions of the blood proteins, e.g. albumin, α, β and γ globulins and subgroups thereof, are accordingly registrable.

Various methods have been developed where the conductive solvent in the electrophoresis is stabilized by a porous material, e.g. glass spheres, foam rubber, paper, starch, cross-linked dextrans, polyvinyl chloride, pectin, gelatin and agar. The electrophoretic migration of the solute in a gelified medium corresponds to that in the liquid solvent provided that the size of the pores is sufficiently large and that the gel is electrically neutral. The network of the gel prevents disturbing convection currents in the fluid and stabilizes the location of the electrophoresed material immediately after the run. If after the electrophoresis the gel is kept wet and no fixatives are applied, free diffusion of the fractionated material takes place. By employment of a translucent gel such as agar, conditions can be established for a direct analysis by immunodiffusion, where the precipitates become clearly visible in the gel. Some peculiarities of gel electrophoresis deserve mention as they represent technical obstacles which are usually not encountered in free electrophoresis. The voltage of the current used in electrophoresis—usually denoted as field strength or gradient of volt/cm—has an influence on the migration rate and the separation of different components. A more rapid separation is obtained if the voltage is increased. Under such circumstances the resistance of the gelified medium, including its connections with the buffer solution in the electrode vessels by means of, e.g. wicks of filter paper, foam rubber or cellulose sponge, causes excessive heat and can lead to dehydration and deformation of the gel and induce a heterogeneity or break of the electrical field. This undesirable heat production can be reduced, but only to a certain degree, by lowering the ionic strength of the buffer in the gel. Removal of excessive heat may be obtained if a cooling system is used. An effective cooling system is not always easy to construct. Another factor to be considered in gel electrophoresis is the electroendosmosis. The correspondence of electrophoretic migration of particles in a fluid medium and a neutral gel was mentioned earlier. Commercially available agar, even if purified, forms a gel with a negative electrical charge. When this type of gel is used for electrophoresis, water is transported by the electroendosmosis through the gel towards the cathode. This flow slows down the electrophoretic migration of particles moving towards the anode. If agar is substituted by, e.g. agarose obtained from agaropectin, the electroendosmotic effect can be reduced as this substance forms a gel devoid of polar groups.

Precipitation and flocculation reactions

When a solution of precipitinogen is mixed with its corresponding antiserum, the antigen very rapidly combines with the antibody, and if the conditions are suitable the reactants then form precipitating or flocculating aggregates. Like serological reactions in general the precipitation is a characteristic of the immunospecificity of the reactants. The rate of the reaction is influenced by a number of physico-chemical as well as immunological factors. For example, the velocity of formation of aggregates is, up to a certain limit, increased with increased temperature. The amount of precipitate, however, may be less at a higher temperature. The temperature commonly used for precipitin reactions varies from 0–56° C. It should be mentioned that for certain precipitating systems the optimal temperature is in the lower part of the range and that the aggregation takes place only in the cold. An increase of the velocity of precipitation is observed as a result of agitation of the antigen–antibody mixture. An increase of the viscosity has a retarding effect on the precipitation. The content of electrolytes in the system and the pH have also proved to be of importance. The presence of a certain amount of electrolyte is considered necessary for the formation of precipitates, but the optimal concentration range varies for different immunoprecipitating systems. The employment of a pH outside the range of 6·5–8·2 may retard the immunoprecipitation and induce a non-specific precipitation. A factor of great importance for the rate and extent of immunoprecipitation is the proportion of antigen and antibody in the mixture. The ratio of the reactants at the shortest time of precipitation or flocculation is denoted OR (optimal ratio), which usually corresponds to approximately equivalent amounts of antigen and antibody. At an excess of the antigen the reaction time is increased and the formation of the precipitate is partially or totally inhibited. An excess of the antibody may have a similar effect on the precipitation as observed for certain immunosystems, e.g. flocculating antibodies in horse sera against protein antigens. It should be noted that the above-mentioned influence of antigen and antibody excess is not limited to the formation of precipitates but also includes the possibility of changes in precipitates already formed. This reversibility of antigen–antibody binding may lead to a partial or total dissolution of established precipitates when exposed to an excess of one of the reactants. Newly formed aggregates are more sensitive to this dissolving effect than well-established precipitates, where the antigen–antibody binding is more firm.

A technique for quantitation of immunoflocculating reactants was developed in 1922 by Ramon [35]. In this method, also called the β technique,

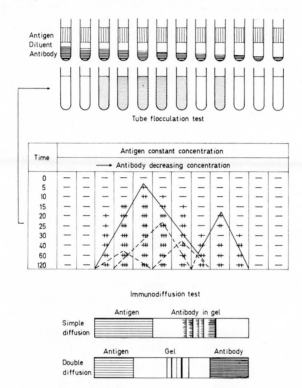

FIG. 19.1. A serological system containing five separate antigen–antibody systems analysed by a serial dilution test in tubes, β technique, and by immunodiffusion tests (concentration gradients in gel). Note that in the serial dilution test three pairs of antigen–antibody are 'hidden' within the flocculation zone of the dominant system.

the time is registered for the formation of floccules in a series of tubes containing a constant amount of antigen mixed with varying quantities of antibody. For the precipitin test a similar method, called the α technique was introduced in 1926 by Dean & Webb [7]. In this test a constant quantity of antibody is tested with varying quantities of antigen. In both methods quantitation is obtained by determining the antigen–antibody OR, as indicated by the tube where the mixture of reactions shows the shortest time for the formation of visible aggregates. In these two serial dilution methods, the varying

Y

solubility of antigen–antibody complexes, as related to differences in the ratio of the reactants, is indicated by the appearance of pre- and/or post-zones of inhibition and by differences in quantity of precipitated material within the precipitation or flocculation zone. Figure 19.1 illustrates a flocculation

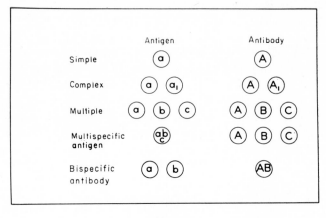

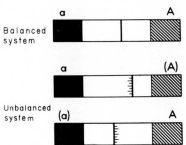

Precipitate soluble in excess of antigen only, or in antigen as well as antibody excess

Fig. 19.2. Nomenclature and symbols used in the text for the classification of immunoprecipitation systems and reactants and some of the subsequent figures. **a, b, c** serologically non-related antigens and **A, B, C** corresponding non-related antibodies: **a, a₁** serologically related antigens, **a** having induced the formation of **A** as well as **A₁** antibodies: **(a)** and **(A)** concentration of reactant less than **a** and **A**, **a̲** and **A̲** concentration of reactant greater than **a** and **A**. The lower part of the figure shows balanced and unbalanced ID systems. Antigen, black; antibody, shaded; diffusion area, white.

test by means of the β technique and it may be noted that in the example given two separate flocculation systems are observable.

For the classification of immunoprecipitation systems and reactants the following nomenclature can be used (see Fig. 19.2). A serological system is referred to as: (a) simple if only one antigen is combining with its corresponding antibody, (b) complex when the reaction involves serologically related but not identical reactants and (c) multiple when several serologically unrelated reactants are involved. It should be remembered that the antigen particle is polyvalent carrying a multitude of reactive sites. The particle may be monospecific carrying determinants of the same specificity, or multispecific carrying determinants of different specificities. Precipitating antibodies are bivalent and the particle usually carries reactive groups of the same specificity. However, the existence of antibody particles where the two reactive sites represent different specificities cannot be excluded. As previously mentioned a differentiation of precipitation systems can also be based on the variation in solubility of the antigen–antibody complex in excess of a reactant. For the understanding of reactions obtained by means of ID techniques this differentiation is important to keep in mind. Of the nomenclature used in connection with these techniques the expressions balanced and unbalanced serological systems may need an explanation. In double diffusion with the reactants at equivalent concentrations at the sources of diffusion, the term balanced system is employed. If the concentrations of the reactants are not equivalent, the expression unbalanced system is used. As will be seen later an unbalanced system is a prerequisite for the simple diffusion techniques.

Immunoprecipitation in gelified media
As has been mentioned the formation of immunoprecipitates very much depends on the antigen–antibody ratio in the medium where the reactants combine. In the classical techniques suitable ratios are found by testing serial dilutions of one of the reactants with a constant amount of the other. In the ID methods the stepwise dilutions are replaced by a dilution obtained by diffusion in a gel medium. Concentration gradients of one or both of the reactants are established in an aqueous transparent gel in such a way that somewhere in the medium antigen as well as antibody are present at concentrations suitable for immunoprecipitation. This latter procedure is advantageous as the gradient represents a continuous variation of the amount of reactant from a maximum at the source of diffusion to zero somewhere in the diffusion medium. The employment of concentration gradients permits the establishment of more or less narrow zones in the medium where the ratio of the reactants is favourable for precipitation, outside of which, aggregation does not take place due to either excess or lack of reacting material. Test material containing two or more precipitating systems thus induces the formation of a precipitation spectrum where each line corresponds to each pair of antigen and antibody. The difference in resolving power between the application of concentration gradients and serial dilutions, when testing a multiple system, is illustrated in Fig. 19.1.

According to the type of diffusion arrangement used for the analysis of immunoprecipitation in gels the following classification of methods is applicable (see Fig. 19.3). Simple diffusion is the expression used when a concentration gradient is established for only one of the reactants. The gelified diffusion medium contains antigen or antibody at a comparatively low concentration, and the corresponding reactant at a definitely higher

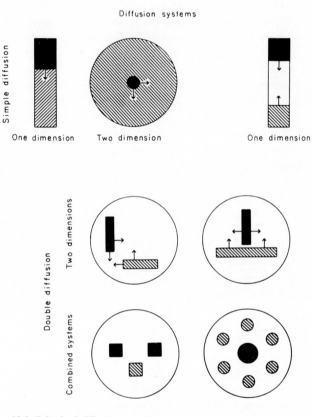

FIG. 19.3. Principal diffusion systems. Antigen, black; antibody, shaded.

concentration diffuses from an external source into the gel. Double diffusion is the expression used when concentration gradients are established for both reactants. The antigen and antibody diffuse from external, separate sources into an initially, serologically neutral gel. Simple as well as double diffusion methods can be further characterized by the dimension employed—techniques of one-, two- or three-dimensional diffusion. The three-dimensional technique, however, is seldom used. For techniques where several sources of diffusion are employed and reactants analysed under conditions rendering interaction between precipitation systems possible, the name combined systems has been proposed. It may be mentioned, however, that when ID methods are referred to, expressions like tube, plate, slide, cell, or chamber techniques are often employed, sometimes with the addition of the name of the originator of the method—Oudin tubes or Ouchterlony plates, etc. The nomenclature

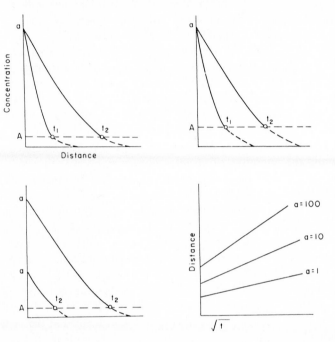

FIG. 19.4. Diagrams of one-dimensional simple diffusion applied to an immuno-system a–A. In the upper figures and the lower left figure the ordinates represent concentrations of antigen and antibody expressed in equivalent units. Abscissae represent distances from the initial boundary. Curves indicate varying concentrations of antigen in the gel, straight dotted lines the uniform antibody concentration in the gel. Time of diffusion, $t_1 < t_2$. Intersection of curve and straight dotted line indicates the site of the leading edge of the precipitate at the time noted. In the lower right figure the ordinate represents distances of precipitate from the interface and the abscissa the square root of the time of diffusion. In the three illustrated experiments the same antibody concentration was present in the gel; the concentration of antigen, the external reactant, varied.

indicating the type of diffusion employed seems more informative and in my opinion it is to be preferred.

In order to illustrate some of the basic factors which influence the formation and changes of immunoprecipitates in diffusion-in-gel tests the following examples may be given. A simple, one-dimensional ID system can be established as follows. A fluid, agar-mixed antibody solution is poured into a glass tube. After congelation, a solution of the antigen, serologically corresponding to the antibody in the gel, is poured on top of the gel column and the tube is incubated at a suitable temperature. As the antigen, external reactant, diffuses into the column, antigen–antibody aggregates are formed just below the solution-to-gel interface. A precipitation band or line will be observed provided that the concentration of antibody, internal reactant, is above the threshold value for the formation of a visible precipitate. At the site of the precipitation the reactants are present at equivalent concentrations. As the diffusion continues, more and more antigen material comes into the gel, and the excess of antigen thus created gradually dissolves the initial precipitate. However, new precipitating aggregates are formed in the adjacent part further down in the gel column. The continuation of this process of precipitation, dissolution and reprecipitation creates the image of a slowly migrating precipitate with a sharp leading edge and a more or less extended tail. How the site and the migration of an immunoprecipitate are affected by the concentrations of antigen and antibody and by the time of diffusion is exemplified by the diagrams in Fig. 19.4. The influence of these variables may be summarized as follows. A prerequisite for obtaining migrating precipitates is that the initial concentration of the external reactant exceeds that of the internal reactant. The distance from the interface to the leading edge of the precipitate is proportional to the square root of the time of diffusion. An increase of the initial concentration of the external reactant increases the rate of migration of the precipitate while an increase of the concentration of the internal reactant has a retarding effect. If equivalent concentrations of the external and internal reactants are employed the precipitate is formed at the interface and remains stationary.

A double, one-dimensional ID system can be established as follows. A fluid, agar-mixed antibody solution is poured into a glass tube and after congelation a layer of neutral agar is established on top of the gel containing the antibody. On top of this two-layer gel column a solution of the antigen corresponding to the antibody is poured. Thus two interfaces are created, antigen to neutral gel to antibody. The tube is then incubated at a suitable temperature. When the reactants diffuse towards each other into the neutral gel, antigen and antibody will at some time and at some site meet at equivalent concentrations (see Fig. 19.5). Provided that the concentration exceeds the threshold value for visible aggregation, a precipitation line or band can be registered. If the serological system is balanced, the line remains stationary, and its density gradually increases. If the system is considerably unbalanced, the initial precipitate will gradually grow in the direction of the diffusion of the reactant present in excess. If the precipitate is completely soluble in this excess of reactant, the primary precipitate will gradually dissolve and a migrating band with a leading edge and a more diffuse tail will be formed. If the precipitate is insoluble or only partially soluble in the excess reactant, a broadening of the band in the direction of the diffusion of the more concentrated reactant will take place, but little or no dissolution of the primary precipitate will occur. In the double diffusion system the site of the primary

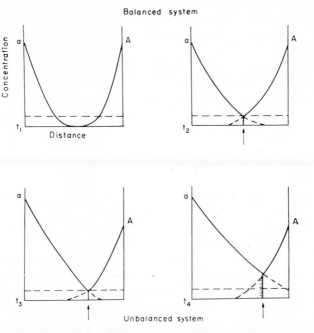

FIG. 19.5. Diagrams of one-dimensional double diffusion applied to an immunosystem a–A. The ordinates represent concentrations of antigen and antibody expressed in equivalent units. The abscissae represent the distance between the antigen–neutral gel and antibody–neutral gel interfaces. The straight dotted lines indicate the minimal concentration of reactants necessary for the formation of a visible precipitate. Curves indicate concentration gradients of reactants after diffusion times $t_1 < t_2$ and $t_3 < t_4$. Arrow indicates site of precipitate.

precipitate is influenced mainly by two factors, the diffusibility of the reactants and their initial concentrations at the sources of diffusion. For balanced systems this relation can be expressed as

$$\left(\frac{X_{Ab}}{X_{Ag}}\right)^2 = \frac{D_{Ab}}{D_{Ag}},$$

where X_{Ag} and X_{Ab} are the distances of the precipitate to the respective interfaces between the middle layer and the antigen and antibody depots. D_{Ag} and D_{Ab} are the diffusion coefficients of the reactants.

The number of precipitation bands created in simple as well as double diffusion systems is related to the number of precipitating systems present. When a simple serological system is tested only one precipitation line or band is formed. When a multiple serological system is tested one precipitation band is formed for each pair of antigen and antibody. The site, density and migration of the precipitates are as if the individual serological systems were tested separately and the precipitation patterns placed together. For a complex serological system where antibodies of varying degrees of specificity are tested against a mixture of related antigens the pattern does not develop as if separate simple systems were just superimposed. The interaction of the related reactants has to be taken into consideration. In a simple diffusion system with the antigen as the external reactant the number of lines depends on which antigen, the more or the less specific, which has the leading edge during diffusion. In a double diffusion system the number of lines depends not only on which antigen but also on which antibody, the more or the less specific, which has the leading edge during diffusion. The rule is that the number of lines formed by a complex system is equal to or less than the number of serological systems present. A more detailed treatment of pattern formation is given later (see Figs. 19.6 and 19.9).

Immunodiffusion techniques

The gelifying agent most often used in ID methods is agar. The commercially available product comes from various sources and its grade of purity differs to a wide extent. Some brands may be used for immunodiffusion without further purification, e.g. Difco Bacto Agar, Difco Special Agar (Noble), Oxoid Ion Agar and Behringwerke Rein Agar. Purification of raw agar products, named only as of Mexican, Korean, Japanese or New Zealand origin, may be performed as follows. The agar is dissolved at a concentration of 6 per cent in boiling water, clarified by precipitation with calcium chloride and the hot solution filtered through glass wool. After solidification the bottom layer is removed and the rest cut into small cubes which are washed for 3 days against running tap water and for another 3 days against distilled water. The agar cubes are then melted and after estimation of the dry weight, hot distilled water is added corresponding to a 3 per cent agar concentration. The agar is dispensed in bottles or tubes and kept as a stock solution in the cold. When the agar is to be used as a diffusion medium for ID analysis the stock solution is melted and diluted to a suitable concentration varying from 0·3 to 1·5 per cent depending on the ID technique to be used. Usually electrolytes are added, for example, sodium chloride to a final concentration of 0·85 per cent or a buffer solution, e.g. a veronal buffer of pH 7·4. In order to avoid growth of contaminating micro-organisms in the gel or on its surface 0·01–0·05 per cent sodium azide, 0·10–0·12 per cent merthiolate or 0·1 per cent phenol can be added. In ID and IE methods, glass apparatus is most often used to support the gel. Since leaks between the glass and the gel must be avoided the technique of agar precoating is necessary. The glass is heated to 70–80° C and covered with a thin layer of a diluted agar solution of the same temperature. It is then placed for drying in the open air or in a desiccator. When the glass is used later as a support for the diffusion medium the precoating usually permits good adherence of the agar gel.

Simple diffusion in one dimension
Oudin's method for qualitative and quantitative analysis of immuno-precipitating systems is based on this type of diffusion arrangement.

Tube technique (see, e.g. Oudin [32])
In this technique agar-precoated glass tubes of 3 mm inner diameter were originally recommended. However, it is often more convenient to use slightly wider tubes. The internal reactant, usually the antiserum, is incorporated in a melted 0·3 per cent agar solution cooled at 46° C. The mixture is poured by means of a Pasteur pipette into a tube at the same temperature. The agar column formed should be 35–45 mm high. After congelation the tubes are placed at the temperature of the experiment and the external reactant is added, also by means of a Pasteur pipette, on to the top of the gel column. The height of the fluid column should be about 30 mm. If desired, a 0·3 per cent agar mixture of the external reactant can be employed instead of the fluid. The tubes are sealed in order to avoid evaporation. It is essential to keep the tubes at a constant temperature during the experiment in order to avoid precipitation artefacts caused by temperature changes. With a scattered-light arrangement—black background and oblique lighting—the formation and sites of immunoprecipitates in the gel column of internal reactant can be observed with the naked eye or with slight magnification. For a permanent registration of patterns, photographs are taken. The distance from the interface to the leading edge of each precipitation band can thus be determined with great accuracy. A one-week observation period with successive readings is the usual procedure. It should be remembered that a concentration of the external reactant definitely higher than that of the internal has to be used in order to induce diffusion of the former reactant into the gel. This condition is essential for the establishment of migrating precipitates. Since it is desirable that these precipitates appear as narrow bands with a sharp leading edge and a minimum of trailing, antiserum is preferable as the internal reactant. Advantage is thereby taken of the more general solubility of newly formed antigen–antibody aggregates in an excess of antigen.

Precipitation patterns obtained by simple, multiple and complex serological

Y*

systems are exemplified in Fig. 19.6. The example of the simple system—the antigenic factor **a** as the external reactant and the corresponding antibody component **A** in the gel—illustrates the formation, site and migration of the precipitate **aA** in relation to the time of diffusion and the concentration of

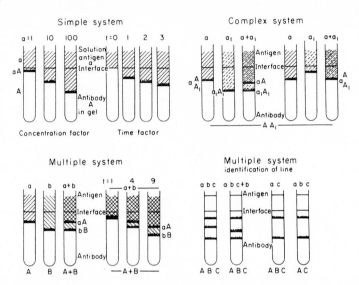

FIG. 19.6. Precipitation patterns of simple, multiple and complex serological systems tested with one-dimensional simple diffusion (Oudin tube technique).

the external reactant (Figs. 19.6 and 19.4). The formulae for the influence of the concentration of the reactants has been given by Oudin as

$$\frac{X}{\sqrt{t}} = \gamma \log \frac{Ag}{Ag_0}$$

and

$$\frac{X}{\sqrt{t}} = \alpha \log \frac{Ab}{Ab_0}$$

where X is the distance of displacement from the interface to the leading edge, t is the time of diffusion, Ag and Ab the initial concentrations of the reactants, Ag_0 and Ab_0 the extrapolated value for $X/\sqrt{t} = 0$. γ is a coefficient > 0 and α is a coefficient < 0. Both formulae apply to each given value of Ag and Ab, respectively, provided the value of $X/\sqrt{t}$ is low. It should be mentioned that it has been observed that low values of $X/\sqrt{t}$ approach a linear relationship to log C, while for high values of $X/\sqrt{t}$, X^2/t becomes a linear function of log C (C = initial concentration of the external reactant). For example, a quantitative analysis of antigen solutions can be made by testing them as external reactants using the corresponding antibody at a constant low concentration as the internal reactant. As a reference an antigen standard should be tested simultaneously.

The development of a precipitation pattern representing a multiple system —antigen factors **a** and **b** and corresponding antibodies **A** and **B**—is given in Fig. 19.6. Two precipitation bands, **aA** and **bB** are formed corresponding to the paired reactants. The two precipitates migrate independently. It might happen that the site of the initial precipitation of one system coincides with or comes very close to that of another, but as the precipitates usually migrate downwards at a different rate the presence of separate bands is soon revealed. Two ways of identifying precipitation bands in a multiple system are exemplified in Fig. 19.6. The multiple system, **abc–ABC**, gives a three-band pattern **aA**, **bB** and **cC**. Retesting after specific absorption of one of the antigens or antibodies gives a two-band pattern and comparison of this pattern with the original pattern permits identification of the third line. Another way of line-identification is to compare two tubes with multiple systems identical except for a difference in concentration of the antigen factor the band of which is to be identified. The patterns should be the same except for the location and migration of the band in question.

The development of precipitation patterns of complex systems is illustrated in Fig. 19.6. In the example given, a mixture of the serologically related antigens, **a** and $\mathbf{a_1}$ is tested by an antiserum obtained after hyperimmunization with the antigen **a**. The serum contains antibodies of varying specificity, **A** reacting only with the corresponding antigen **a**, and the less specific $\mathbf{A_1}$ reacting with **a** as well as $\mathbf{a_1}$. As may be seen in the figure there are two alternatives of precipitation pattern depending on which of the antigens has the leading edge during diffusion. If **a** diffuses ahead of $\mathbf{a_1}$ only one precipitation band $\mathbf{a_{A_1}^A}$ will appear caused by the homologous reaction. If $\mathbf{a_1}$ diffuses ahead of **a**, two bands will be formed, $\mathbf{a_1 A_1}$ caused by the heterologous reaction and one, higher up in the column, caused by the homologus reaction between **a** and the antibodies of higher specificity **A** not reacting with $\mathbf{a_1}$.

Provided that antigen–antibody systems present at a concentration of the reactants too low to form visible precipitates are ignored, the number of bands is equal to the number of immunosystems (simple, multiple and complex systems with an $\mathbf{a}/\mathbf{a_1}$ ratio <1) or is less than the number of immunosystems (complex systems with an $\mathbf{a}/\mathbf{a_1}$ ratio >1). Under certain circumstances deviation from these rules may be observed. For example, if the regularity of the diffusion of the external reactant is disturbed by, e.g. abrupt changes of the temperature during the experiment, the formation of additional, artefact precipitation bands may be induced. Such bands, however, usually remain stationary. An artificial duplication of bands may also occur if, during the experiment, the external reactant is replaced by a solution of a markedly higher concentration.

Simple diffusion in two dimensions

Plate technique (*halo formation*) (see, e.g. Petrie [33], and Ouchterlony [28])

In this technique a 2–3 mm thick layer of 0·8–1·5 per cent agar mixed with an appropriate amount of internal reactant, usually antiserum, is poured into a glass dish with a flat bottom. It is essential to have the dish on a horizontal surface in order to produce a uniform agar layer. After congelation sources of diffusion for the external reactant are prepared by punching holes of a suitable size and shape in the agar layer. If in the test larger amounts of the external reactant than such basins would supply are desired, cups placed on the surface of the agar layer can be used as receptacles for the reactant. Cups used for antibiotic testing are suitable for this purpose. In order to get a tight seal between cup and agar, the cups should be heated slightly before they are placed on the agar surface. Filter paper discs saturated with the external reactant have also been used as sources of diffusion. After filling the basins or cups with the external reactant (in solution or gelified) the plate is placed horizontally in a humid atmosphere and at constant temperature. If the source of diffusion is circular and a suitable concentration ratio of matching reactants is attained, ring-shaped bands of precipitate, haloes, will form concentrically around the source of the diffusing reactant. As the diffusion process goes on the diameter of the rings will gradually increase. The development of precipitation patterns is governed by the same factors as those mentioned for the tube technique, for example the type of serological systems present, the diffusibility of the external reactant, the concentration of the external as well as the internal reactant, etc. However, for quantitation by means of precipitation site and rate of migration, a formula for radial diffusion should be applied.

In the plate technique, as distinguished from the aforementioned tube technique, the migration of the precipitates ceases comparatively soon. The reason is that the amount of the external reactant is usually relatively small compared to that of the internal reactant. This observation has led to a more convenient method for quantitation by means of the halo plate technique. In this method, originally described by Mancini *et al* [23, 24], the determination of the rate of migration of the leading edge of precipitate has been substituted by the measurement of the area of the halo after the diffusion of the external reactant has ceased. A warm fluid 3 per cent agar gel buffered at pH 8·6 is mixed with an appropriate amount of antiserum and poured as a 1 mm thick layer on a Perspex plate. After congelation circular wells of the desired diameter, usually 1–2 mm, are punched out. An accurately measured volume of antigen solution is introduced into each of the wells by means of a micropipette.

The plate is then incubated in a humid atmosphere. When the diffusion of the external reactant has ceased, as indicated by the change from a migrating to a stationary precipitate, the area of the halo is determined. This can be done either directly by diameter measurements under slight magnification and a scattered light arrangement or after washing, drying and staining the plate. Quantitation is based on the observation that for a given concentration of the internal reactant the ring diameter or the area of the halo shows a linear relationship to the initial concentration of the external reactant. It is advisable to employ a series of dilutions of a standard antigen as a reference in the test plate.

The halo plate technique can be used for qualitative comparative analyses, by means of combined systems. If sources of diffusion are placed in such a pattern that the haloes developed around each centre grow into a common area the presence or absence of interactions of precipitates makes serological comparisons possible. Such comparative analyses are exemplified in Fig. 19.7. An absence of interaction indicates a serological non-identity of the compared external reactants while a coalescence of the rings with a dissolution of the precipitate in the region between the two sources of diffusion indicates a serological similarity or identity. The principles for the interpretation of patterns established by combined systems will be further discussed in connection with the double diffusion techniques. The halo plate technique can also be utilized for the analysis of soluble antigens from growing colonies of micro-organisms. In such tests the antiserum is incorporated in a nutrient agar medium, and after congelation the organisms are inoculated on the surface of the plate. The plates are then incubated at a temperature suitable for the growth of the organism. When streaks or single colonies of bacterial growth develop, halo precipitates are formed, provided that the amount of antigen produced gives a concentration higher than that of the matching antibody in the medium.

Double diffusion in one dimension
Tube technique (see, e.g. Oakley and Fulthorpe [26])
The originators' recommendation is to use glass tubes 8 mm in diameter. Narrower tubes might be difficult to fill without touching the walls of the upper part of the tube. The immune serum or dilutions thereof is mixed at 54°C with an equal amount of a melted 2 per cent agar solution containing 1 per cent NaCl. The mixture is poured into the tube to form a column of suitable height. After congelation a second layer of a 1 per cent agar solution containing 1 per cent NaCl is poured on top of the primary column. The height of the second column is varied to suit the analysis in question but usually an 8 mm layer is employed. After congelation the antigen solution, as a fluid or as an agar mix, is poured on top and the tube is sealed and incubated at a suitable, constant temperature. The precipitates formed by the

reactants diffusing from opposite directions into the middle layer are usually recorded after 24 and 48 hours. An extension of the time is advisable if a greater height of the middle layer is used or when the initial concentration of the reactants is comparatively low. The influence of the type of serological

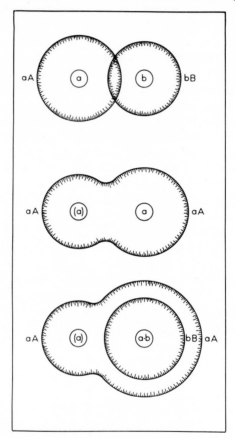

Fɪɢ. 19.7. Schematic representation of interacting and non-interacting halo reactions in the simple diffusion plate technique. An immune serum containing the antibody components **A** and **B** incorporated in the diffusion medium.

system and the diffusibility and concentration of the reactants on the formation of precipitation patterns is essentially the same as that described later under plate technique.

Gradient tube technique (see, e.g. Hayward & Augustin [14])
This technique was developed for quantitative analysis. It is similar to the standard double diffusion tube technique, but the reactant in the layer

is permitted to prediffuse into the middle layer (see Fig. 19.8). The standard procedure recommended is to use glass tubes of 8 mm diameter, a lower gel layer of 6 mm in height, a middle layer of 4–8 mm and about 0·25 ml of the test solution. This reactant is poured into the tubes after they have been preincubated for 15 hours. The tubes are kept at 37° C and precipitation recorded after 48 hours. For the quantitation of antigens the immune serum is placed as the lower reactant and serial dilutions of the antigen tested using the tube with the precipitation line formed tangentially at the upper meniscus (interface) as the end-point of the titration.

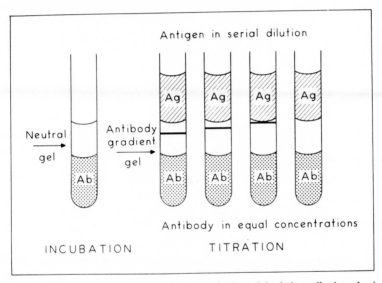

FIG. 19.8. Gradient tube technique for quantitation. Stippled, antibody gel-mix; shaded, antigen solution; white, neutral gel and after incubation, antibody gradient gel.

Plate technique (see, e.g. Ouchterlony [28])
A 0·8–1·5 per cent agar solution containing 0·8 per cent NaCl is poured hot into a glass dish, e.g. Petri dish, in order to form a thin, sealing, bottom layer. Instead of Petri dishes, which often show irregularities in the glass, a suitable plate with an even bottom can be prepared by attaching a metal or plexiglass ring of a suitable height and diameter to a glass plate. After congelation of the primary agar layer a two-matrix template is placed on the surface of the thin agar layer. A second agar layer of about 2–3 mm thickness is then poured into the dish. After congelation the template is removed leaving basins corresponding to the matrices in the top layer (see Fig. 19.9). In order to prevent the agar from sticking to the matrices it is advantageous to

have the matrices coated with a thin paraffin film. A convenient and more rapid way to obtain basins in the gel is to punch holes by means of a cutter and aspirate the agar from each well with a pipette attached to a vacuum system. When the punch method is employed no primary bottom layer of agar is needed but it is advisable to seal the bottom of the basins with a minute amount of hot agar in order to avoid leakage between the gel and the glass bottom. The form and size of the basins and distance between the depots should be chosen to fit the serological system to be analysed. In the examples comprising Fig. 19.9 two parallel rectangular basins are used. It is preferable to employ basins large in relation to the gel volume in order to maintain a comparatively stable concentration of reactants in the depots as long as possible. The distance employed between the adjacent margins of the two basins is usually 6–20 mm. For the ID test the two basins are filled with antigen and antibody solutions, respectively, and the plate is sealed or covered and placed in a humid atmosphere at a convenient, constant temperature.

The basic precipitation patterns formed by simple, multiple and complex serological systems with the one-dimensional double diffusion techniques are illustrated in Fig. 19.9. Each line in a precipitation spectrum corresponds to each matching pair of antigen–antibody. The absence of an antigenic factor or an antibody component is indicated by the absence of the corresponding line of the spectrum. This principle can be used for the identification of lines in precipitation spectra. Each precipitate functions as a barrier for the reactants forming the precipitate in question and prevents their diffusion beyond the site of precipitation. However, the barrier effect is immunospecific and the diffusion of other reactants is not hindered unless the density of the aggregates causes a mechanical obstacle. The specific barrier effect is a characteristic for the balanced system where the precipitate grows in density but remains stationary. In unbalanced systems, however, the barrier effect of a precipitate is influenced by the reactant in excess, which might induce a process of gradual dissolution and reprecipitation, giving the impression of a migrating precipitate. The similarity to the pattern in a simple diffusion test is obvious. The basic alternative patterns for complex systems given in the figure illustrate how the number of lines and the composition of the precipitates are influenced by the reactants having the leading edge during diffusion. Under certain conditions artificial duplications of lines may occur in double diffusion tests. For example, if high concentrations of reactants are used in the test a splitting of lines can be caused by the mass of aggregates formed in a narrow zone. In greatly unbalanced systems there is sometimes a tendency to duplication of lines within the zone of the migrating precipitate. If, at the sources of diffusion, the concentration of one or both reactants is abruptly changed, e.g. by refilling of depots during the experiment, line duplications are likely to occur as artefacts.

The one-dimensional double diffusion technique offers possibilities for quantitative analyses although with less accuracy than with the simple diffusion technique. A known simple serological system, where the specific precipitation band is established at some predetermined site, is used as a reference. Serial dilutions of the test sample, antigen or antibody, are analysed by means of the corresponding reactant at the same concentration as in the reference system. The concentration of the test dilution giving a precipitate

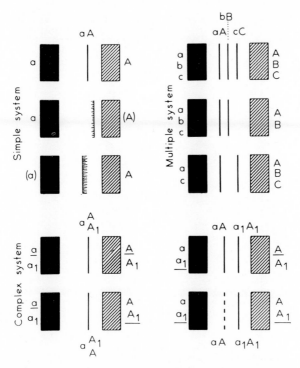

Fig. 19.9. Principles of the formation of immunoprecipitation patterns of simple, multiple and complex serological systems tested with one-dimensional double diffusion. Dotted line indicates an eventual precipitate. Antigen, black; antibody, shaded.

at a site corresponding to the reference precipitate is accordant with the concentration of the reference reactant.

Gradient plate technique (see, e.g. Feinberg [9])
This technique was elaborated for quantitative analysis and its similarity to the gradient tube technique is obvious. In a standard agar diffusion plate small circular wells are placed circumferentially around a larger circular

well (see Fig. 19.10). This pattern of wells is obtained by means of a special cutter. The antiserum is poured into the central well and the plate is pre-incubated, usually for 1–3 days, a time calibrated for the establishment of an antibody gradient extending beyond the circumferential wells. Serial dilutions of the antigen are then poured into the peripheral wells and the plates are incubated for 24 hours. The highest antigenic concentration giving a complete ring around the well is noted as the end-point of the titration.

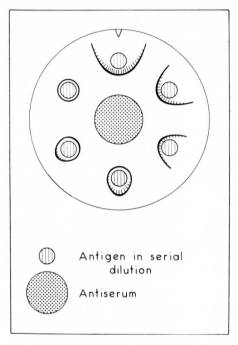

Antigen in serial dilution

Antiserum

Fig. 19.10. Gradient plate technique for quantitation. Two-dimensional double diffusion plate technique. Antigen, shaded; antibody, stippled.

Double diffusion in two dimensions

Plate technique (see, e.g. Ouchterlony [28])

The diffusion plate is prepared in the same way as described previously. However, the rectangular basins are placed at right-angles as shown in Fig. 19.11. A suitable distance between the nearest corners of the two basins is 5–7 mm. In the experiment one basin is filled with the antigen solution and the other with the antiserum. Incubation, recording of precipitates, etc., is performed as described above. The principles for formation of the basic pattern in relation to the type of serological systems and concentrations of the reactants are in accordance with those given for the one-dimensional double diffusion technique. With the right-angled arrangement of the basins, the initial precipitation will take place in the region between the nearest corners. From this site the precipitates will gradually grow peripherally forming straight lines at constant angles to the basins. At equivalent concentrations of the reactants the angle of the line is determined by the ratio of the diffusion coefficients of the reactants according to the formula

$$\frac{D_{Ab}}{D_{Ag}} = \left(\frac{X_{Ab}}{X_{Ag}}\right)^2$$

and

$$tg\ \alpha = \frac{X_{Ab}}{X_{Ag}},$$

where α is the angle between the line and the margin of the basin containing the antibody. The rate of extension of the precipitation line will be inversely proportional to the square root of the time of diffusion.

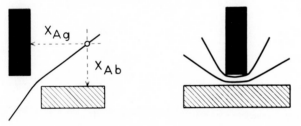

Fig. 19.11. Diagrammatic illustration of two-dimensional double diffusion plate technique with rectangular basins at right angles. Antigen, black; antibody, shaded.

A slightly different arrangement of basins for two-dimensional double diffusion is illustrated in Fig. 19.11. As will be seen later this pattern of depots for reactants comes close to the double diffusion arrangement used in the IE technique. The right-angle technique can also be employed for the direct analysis of soluble antigens from bacteria growing on a solid medium in a plate. In such tests a trench is cut in the nutrient agar and is filled with an antiserum agar mix. The bacterial inoculum is streaked across the trench at right-angles and the plate is incubated at a temperature suitable for growth. Soluble antigens produced from the growing micro-organisms diffuse into the medium and meet antibodies diffusing from the trench. Matching pairs of reactants will under such circumstances form precipitates and the pattern formation follows the same principles as illustrated in Figs. 19.9 and 10.

Comparative double diffusion

The principles of this type of analysis were independently introduced by Ouchterlony [27] and Elek [8].

Comparative three-basin plate technique (see, e.g. Ouchterlony [28, 30])
Standard agar diffusion plates as described above are used in this technique. With a three-matrix template corresponding basins are formed in the gel. The shape of the basins is square or rectangular and the wells are placed in such a way that two right-angle basin systems with one well in common are

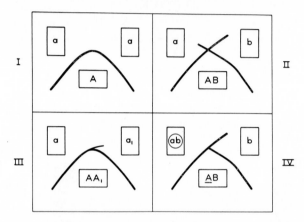

Reaction Type	Interference	Inhibition	Deviation	Fusion
I	Yes	No	Yes	Complete
II	No	No	No	No
III	Yes	No	Yes	Partial
IV	Yes	Yes	No	No

Fig. 19.12. Basic comparative precipitation patterns in combined systems (Ouchterlony plate technique).

established (see Fig. 19.12 and Plate 19.1). In the original technique the size of each basin was 10×10 mm with a depth of 2–3 mm. The upper basins were placed 20 mm apart and the third basin was placed between and 5 mm below them at a distance of 7·1 mm between adjacent corners. A similar pattern of smaller, rectangular basins placed more closely has been found suitable (see Fig. 19.18). For the experiment, the reactants, as agar-mixtures if so desired, are poured into the basins; the plates are closed and then incubated at a constant temperature in a humid atmosphere. The two upper basins are used for the reactants to be compared, e.g. two antigen solutions tested versus a suitable immune serum in the lower basin. Repeated readings and recordings of appearances and changes of lines, are made for up to one week. If refilling of the basins is done, which may be advantageous if the concentrations of antigen and antibody are low, care should be taken to empty the basins before each refilling. The possibility, that refilling might induce artefacets, i.e. duplication of lines, particularly in unbalanced systems, should be kept in mind.

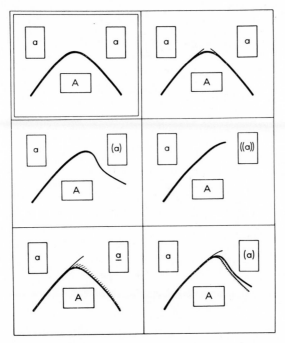

FIG. 19.13. Reaction type I and variations when identical antigens at varying concentrations are compared. (For symbols, see Fig. 19.2.)

The precipitation line or lines, which appear at each side of the central basin if the experimental conditions are suitable, will initially have the same patterns as those which would be created by the two right-angle basin systems considered separately. However, as the lines of precipitation gradually extend into the central area, changes in the regularity of the extension of the lines may or may not occur. The basic precipitation patterns for combined, balanced systems are given in Fig. 19.12. The comparison is primarily based on the recording of the presence or absence of interaction between the two precipitation patterns. If interference is present this phenomenon can be further characterized by the presence or absence of three characteristics:

inhibition, deviation, and fusion (coalescence) of lines. The fusion of lines can be complete or partial. The development of patterns and the interpretation of the four types of reaction which can be differentiated as described above may be summarized as follows. Reaction type II is most clear-cut, no interaction is recorded. The absence of interference is most evident, when the precipitation lines from each side extend so far into the central area that a crossing of the lines occurs. This type of reaction indicates that there is no

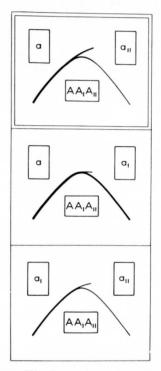

Fig. 19.14. Reaction type III. Comparison of serologically related antigens, a—a_1—a_{11}, a having induced the formation of antibodies A—A_1—A_{11} of varying specificity.

serological relationship between the reactants compared. In reaction type I the precipitation lines from each side deviate and make a complete fusion in the central area. For balanced systems this arc formed by the fusing lines is symmetrical. The reaction indicates the presence of identical antigenic determinants in the compared reactants. Reaction type III is very similar to type I with the exception that the fusion of lines is incomplete, a so-called true spur on the arc of interference is formed. This reaction indicates a serological relationship but no identity of the compared antigens. In reaction type IV the interference appears as a one-sided inhibition without deviation. This pattern might indicate the presence of multispecific antigen particles in one of the reactants compared.

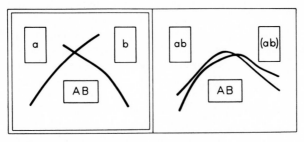

FIG. 19.15. Reaction type II. Comparison of serologically unrelated antigens.

Variations of the types of pattern may be observed when for instance unbalanced systems are tested. Examples of these are illustrated for the type I reaction in Fig. 19.13. For instance an asymmetric arc of fusion is seen when the compared reactants are present at distinctly different concentrations in

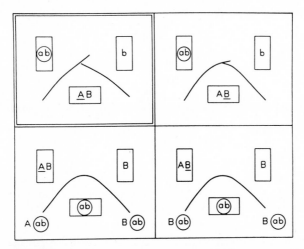

FIG. 19.16. Reaction type IV and its relation to types I and III. Comparative patterns involving multispecific antigens.

the two depots. When the concentration of one of the compared reactants is below the threshold value for the formation of a visible precipitate, its presence might be revealed by the deviation induced in the pattern on the opposite side. Highly unbalanced systems not only induce migrating bands but also eventually cause duplication of lines and the formation of so-called false spurs. Such spurs, however, are gradually dissolved while true spurs grow in length. Variations in the formation of true spurs in the type III reaction can give information of interest concerning serological relationships as exemplified in Fig. 19.14. When closely related antigens, **a** and **a₁**, are compared the spur is small and shows a marked deviation. For less related antigens, **a** and **a₁₁** the spur is more pronounced and shows less deviation. When two heterologous systems are compared by means of the same antiserum the spur extends in the direction towards the source of the less closely

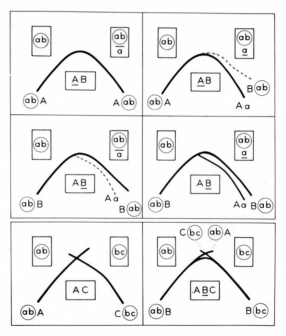

Fig. 19.17. Variations of comparative patterns with different ratios of antigenic factors or antibody components. Note that the reactant forming the leading edge at the diffusion is underlined. Dotted lines indicate eventual precipitates.

related antigen. The interpretation of variations of the type II pattern usually does not give rise to any particular difficulty. It should be mentioned, however, that the principal characteristic is the absence of interference and that the undisturbed crossing of lines is a verification of the non-interference. This verification might be missing if the lines have a limited extension or grow in directions which make a crossing unlikely in the plate. A mixture of antigens containing two or more factors does not always induce precipitation lines of the same individual order although tested by the same antiserum.

This is illustrated by the crossing of lines in the example in Fig. 19.15 where two different concentrations of the same antigen solution are compared. The pattern is explained by the fact that the displacement of a line is more pronounced if the reactant at the source of diffusion has been diluted to a concentration level close to the value for the formation of a visible precipitate. In the type IV reaction, exemplified in the upper left part of Fig. 19.16, the inhibition of one line without deviation is explained by the difference in composition of the two precipitation lines. However, with a change of the

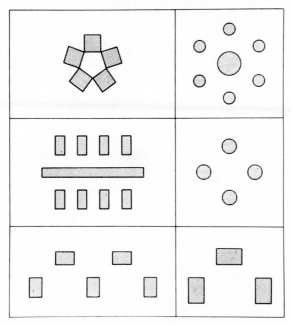

FIG. 19.18. Some arrangements of depots for reactants in comparative double diffusion plates.

ratio of the two antibody components in the serum a type III reaction is formed at the comparison of the same antigenic reactants—see upper right part of Fig. 19.16. This change of pattern is explained by the fact that the antibody component forming the leading edge during diffusion is not the same in the two examples. Figure 19.17 illustrates some pattern variations obtained by mono- and multispecific antigens and suitable immune sera. The influence on the pattern formation of the reactant forming the leading edge during diffusion is obvious. It should be mentioned that, although only comparisons of antigens have been exemplified here, comparative analyses of antisera can be made by the combined system technique and that the aforementioned principles are applicable to the interpretation of the pattern thus obtained.

Many modifications of the combined system technique have been developed and the number, size, shape and individual sites of the depots have been varied according to the problems to be investigated. Examples of some of the more commonly used arrangements of patterns of wells are illustrated in Fig. 19.18. The interpretation of comparative patterns obtained by these variants follows the aforementioned basic principles for the three-basin plate technique patterns. An example of comparative patterns formed with the five-basin technique is given in Fig. 19.19.

Plate chamber techniques (see, e.g. Holm [17] and Wadsworth [39, 40])
In these techniques the gelified diffusion medium is enclosed and the depots for the reactants are in a translucent material covering the gel layer. An

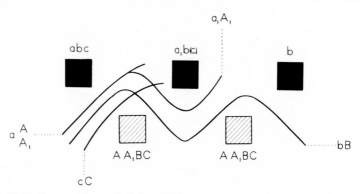

Fig. 19.19. Comparative analysis in a five-basin comparative double diffusion plate.

advantage of this technique as compared with the regular open-plate technique is that for example the evaporation from the gel surface is eliminated and that a thinner gel layer can be used in combination with increased volumes of the depots. Disturbances of the diffusion process are less likely to occur and considerable amounts of reacting material can be diffused into the thin gel layer without refilling of the wells. A convenient macroplate chamber technique has been elaborated by Holm and is schematically illustrated in Fig. 19.20. In a plexiglass cover depots of desired size, shape and arrangement are cut out. The cover is placed on an agar-precoated glass slide. By means of small pieces of waterproof tape previously attached at each corner of the lower surface of the cover, a 0·6 mm slit between the cover and the bottom glass is obtained. A hot agar solution (1 per cent agar and 0·85 per cent NaCl) is poured into the plate and by capillary force the space between the glass and the cover is filled by the fluid agar. After gelification the agar in the basins is removed by a capillary tube attached to a water vacuum pump after cutting along the sides of the basins. The maximum basin capacity in the example illustrated is 0·185 ml. The reactants are pipetted into the basins and the plate is placed horizontally in a humid chamber at a constant temperature. A useful microplate chamber technique has been elaborated by Wadsworth and is schematically illustrated in Fig. 19.21. A suitable pattern of depots in the plexiglass cover is obtained by drilling holes of 3 mm diameter with an aperture at the lower surface of 2 mm. Finely drawn capillary

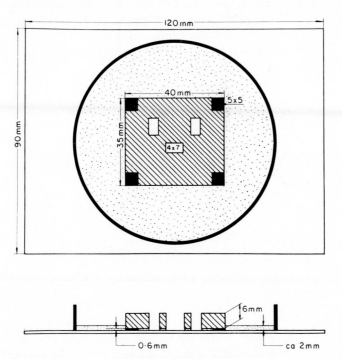

FIG. 19.20. Schematic illustration of a diffusion chamber used for comparative double diffusion analysis, macrotechnique.

pipettes are used for filling the basins with the reactants and particular care should be taken to avoid bubbles at the lower aperture of the depots. The maximum capacity of a depot in the example given is 0·023 ml. In the two gel chamber methods just described the plexiglass cover may, in order to facilitate a final recording of patterns, be slid off, when the development of precipitates in the gel is judged complete. However, the depots should be emptied and thoroughly rinsed with physiological saline before the cover is removed.

Objective double diffusion plate technique (see, e.g. Jennings & Malone [18, 19]; Jennings [20])

This technique was established to serve a dual purpose, quantitation and a qualitative, comparative analysis of immunoprecipitating reactants. The diffusion plate as well as the reaction area and the three depots are triangular in shape. The reactants are mixed with melted agar and poured into the depots as indicated in Fig. 19.22. After congelation the plate is incubated at a suitable, constant temperature. The site and extension of the precipitation lines formed when the reactants diffuse from the gel-to-gel interface into the reaction area are recorded. In the example given an antigen of an unknown concentration is analysed by means of an antibody indicator and a corresponding reference antigen. The concentration of the reference antigen is calibrated so that the

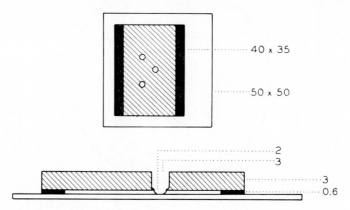

Fig. 19.21. Schematic illustration of a diffusion chamber used for comparative double diffusion analysis, microtechnique.

precipitation line in question bisects the angle RSI. After 4–24 hours of incubation the threshold isobars of the indicator and the unknown antigen are determined. The threshold isobar is a line marking the momentary site of the concentration of the reactant just sufficient to produce a visible precipitate and it is indicated by the most advanced tip of the extending precipitation line. The site, T, of the intersection of the presumptive precipitation lines is calculated and the distances TU and TS are measured. By means of these values the diffusivity ratio of the unknown antigen solution is determined according to 2 TU/TS. The diffusivity ratio is defined as the quotient of the distance travelled by the isobar of the unknown reactant and the isobar of the standard indicator. Knowing the diffusivity ratio the concentration of the unknown antigen can be calculated as there is a straight-line relationship between the diffusivity ratio and the log of the concentration. As has been described the measurements for quantitation are made before the precipitation lines have developed to a point where interference sets in. However, by further incubation of the plate the comparative pattern can be developed and used for a qualitative analysis.

Inhibition plate technique (see, e.g. Björklund [3, 5]; Nilsson [25])
This technique introduced by Björklund is schematically illustrated in Fig. 19.23. Its employment can be advantageous for the identification of lines in

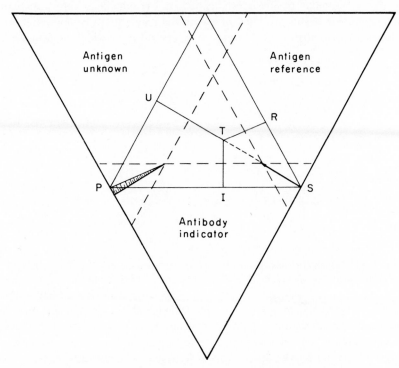

Fig. 19.22. Schematic illustration of the objective double diffusion technique (Jennings and Malone). For explanation see text.

multilinear precipitation spectra. As depots three triangular basins are used and arranged as given in the figure. The antigen mixture to be tested is poured into one of the upper basins and the corresponding immune serum in the other. The lower basin is used as a depot for the same immune serum to which an excess of some of the antigens present in the aforementioned mixture have been added. The total precipitation spectrum of the complete serological system develops between the upper basins. Its development towards the lower basin is however influenced in such a way that the spectrum splits in two parts with a deviation of the gradually extending lines to the lower left or right. This deviation in separate directions is explained by the influence of the antigenic factors and antibodies free to diffuse from the lower basin into the gel. The advantage of this technique for identification purposes is obvious. Another useful comparative inhibition plate technique has been developed by Nilsson. It is particularly suited for the comparison of systems involving solutions containing multispecific antigen particles and corresponding immune sera. By means of proper matrices a circular well surrounded by three rectangular basins is established in a regular agar diffusion plate. The rectangular basins are filled first with the reactants to be compared and the plate is incubated for 7–8 hours. The central well, which is situated in

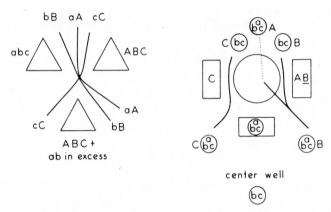

Fig. 19.23. Schematic illustration of precipitation patterns obtained by inhibition plate techniques, to the left Björklund's method and to the right Nilsson's technique.

the area of expected interaction is then filled with an agar-mixed reactant suitable for the differentiation. After congelation the plate is further incubated and the development of the comparative pattern followed. An example of the differentiating possibilities of this technique is schematically illustrated in Fig. 19.23.

Immunoelectrophoretic techniques

In immunoelectrophoresis two methods are combined, gel electrophoresis followed by immunodiffusion. A suitably buffered agar gel is used as the medium and the two steps of the analysis are performed in the same plate. The procedure is schematically illustrated in Fig. 19.24.

The gel is prepared in the same way as for the regular diffusion plates except for the addition of a suitable buffer salt solution instead of sodium chloride. A high quality of agar is recommended, e.g. Difco Bacto Agar,

Difco Noble Agar Special, Behringwerke Rein Agar and Oxoid Ion Agar can be used without previous purification. The use of agarose instead of agar is recommended if at the electrophoresis stage electroendosmosis is to be avoided. The agar concentration generally used is 1–2 per cent. Buffers between pH 6 and 9 may be used and veronal or borate buffers are commonly employed. For example, in serum analysis a veronal buffer pH 8·2 at an ionic strength

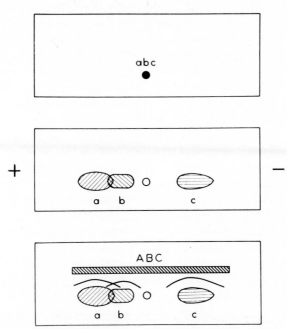

FIG. 19.24. Schematic representation of immunoelectrophoresis. First step, agar-gel electrophoresis of material containing a mixture of antigens, **a**—**c**—**b**. Buffered gel, white; antigen basin, black; separated fractions, shaded. Second step, double diffusion analysis by means of a corresponding immune serum, **A**—**B**—**C**, in longitudinal basin.

of 0·025 and with the addition of merthiolate 1:10,000 has been recommended. The choice of the concentration of the buffer is guided, e.g. by the desirability to escape variations in pH which may occur if too low buffer concentrations are utilized and by the need to avoid heating of the gel, during electrophoresis, which may take place if too high concentrations of buffer are incorporated.

Macrotechnique (see, e.g. Grabar & Williams [10]; Grabar & Burtin [11–12]) The melted buffered agar is poured on to a horizontal 13 × 18 cm glass plate. Before pouring the plate, strips of chromatograph filter paper are placed on the plate at both ends projecting about 3 cm. The congealed gel layer should be of uniform thickness (2–4 mm). Transverse and longitudinal trenches for the application of the test material and for the precipitating reactants are cut out or formed by matrices placed in position before pouring the plate. The transverse basins are filled with the material to be analysed, mixed with melted buffered agar at 45° C. For electrophoresis the plate is placed as a bridge between the anode and cathode reservoirs allowing the paper strips to dip down into the buffer solution of the reservoirs. Any cracks caused by the folding of the filter papers are filled in with melted agar. The buffer solution of the reservoirs corresponds to that used for the gel but a double ionic strength is recommended. The electrodes are connected with a transformer–rectifier and the gel electrophoresis is performed at a suitable voltage. A gradient of 3–6 V/cm can be used without damaging heat-effects, provided that a comparatively low concentration of buffering salts is employed. It is advisable to measure the potential drop between the ends of the gel plate and not only between the electrodes. If higher voltage is used to get an increase of the electrophoretic migration, a cooling system is recommended. The time of the electrophoresis has to be empirically determined. For example, an adequate separation of serum components will take place in about 4–6 hours under the described conditions. After the electrophoretic run serological reactants corresponding to the test material are pipetted into the longitudinal basins and the plate is placed horizontally at a convenient, constant temperature in a humid atmosphere. The immunodiffusion systems thus established will approximate a two-dimensional double diffusion arrangement and the precipitation patterns obtained can be interpreted according to the basic principles previously mentioned under double diffusion techniques. If the effect of electroendosmosis on the electrophoretic migration of the material has to be determined more accurately a substance lacking electromobility, e.g. dextrans, levans and glucose, is incorporated at a convenient spot in the gel layer before the electrophoresis. After the run the migration of this substance, a migration caused only by the electroendosmosis, is determined and a reference-point of zero-migration can be obtained.

The following modification of the standard macrotechnique has been introduced by Wadsworth & Hanson [42] (see Fig. 19.25). The gel-supporting glass plate consists of three pieces ($2 \times 8 \cdot 2$, $8 \cdot 2 \times 8 \cdot 2$ and $2 \times 2 \cdot 8$ cm). Before pouring the agar, the two smaller pieces are attached at the opposite ends of the third piece by employing a hinge of tape at the lower surface of the junctions. An agar layer of about $1 \cdot 5$ mm thickness and covering all three pieces is used. After congelation the desired number and pattern of circular basins of a suitable diameter, generally 2–3 mm wide, are cut out. The liquid or agar-mixed test material is pipetted into the basins. Before the plate is placed on the electrode vessels the agar is cut directly above the hinges so that the end pieces may hang down into the buffer solution in the reservoirs. The discontinuity of the gel layer just created is filled in with melted buffered agar. Thus the current flows through a continuous slab of agar between the vessels. It is preferable to perform the electrophoresis in a closed box in order to maintain a constant humid atmosphere during the run. At the

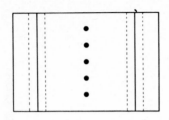

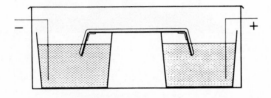

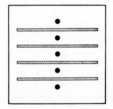

Fig. 19.25. Schematic representation of the hinged-plate immunoelectrophoretic technique. Top, plate with centre basins filled with immunoreactant to be separated; centre, arrangement for the electrophoretic run; bottom, plate with longitudinal basins filled with corresponding immunoreactant for double diffusion analysis.

completion of the run the hinged glass pieces are removed by cutting through the tape hinges. It can be mentioned that by means of this technique using 0·05 molar sodium veronal buffer, pH 8·4 and a potential drop of 5 V/cm in the agar an adequate separation of blood serum proteins is obtained within

z

approximately 1 hour. For the precipitation analysis longitudinal basins usually 70 × 2 mm in size are cut 2–8 mm from the original circular wells and parallel to the direction of the electrical flow. The immunodiffusion analysis is performed as in the regular macroplate technique. A diagrammatic representation of an IE pattern of human plasma is shown in Fig. 19.26.

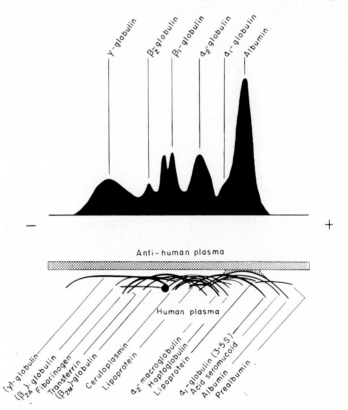

FIG. 19.26. (a) Photometric curve of fractions of human plasma after agar-gel electrophoresis. (b) Corresponding immunoelectrophoretic pattern of human plasma.

Microtechnique (see, e.g. Scheidegger [36])

Several micromethods of the regular immunoelectrophoretic technique have been developed. Scheidegger was the first to devise a technique of this type. It is simple, rapid, saving in material and commonly used, particularly for screening purposes. As a support for the gel layer a microscope slide of standard size (25 × 75 mm) is used. Two millilitres of buffered agar are poured on top giving a gel layer of about 1 mm thickness. The test material is poured into small circular basins, diameter 1·2 mm, punched out by means of a capillary pipette or preferably a steel cutter. One or two longitudinal basins or trenches 40 × 2 mm are cut parallel to the electrical flow and at a suitable distance, 3 or 4 mm, from the circular well or wells. Filter paper is used for the connection to the electrode vessels. For the electrophoresis of a serum sample— type and concentration of buffer in the gel and vessels the same as in the regular macrotechnique—an adequate separation of fractions is obtained within 45 minutes using a potential drop of 6 V/cm in the gel. After the run of the electrophoresis the immunodiffusion analysis is performed according to the same principles as in the macrotechnique. The complete pattern is usually

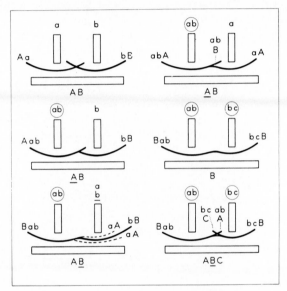

FIG. 19.27. Comparative patterns formed by various serological systems with a double diffusion arrangement similar to that used for the ID analysis in immuno-electrophoresis.

developed within 12–24 hours. The amount of test material in the circular well is about 0·001 ml and the amount of reactant used in the trench about 0·05 ml.

Precipitation patterns in immunoelectrophoresis
As has been mentioned the diffusion arrangement in the regular IE technique is approximately the same as in the regular plate technique using double diffusion from troughs at right-angles. There is, however, an important difference. In the IE analysis the test material or its separated fractions do not represent well-defined sources of diffusion with uniform concentrations of the reactant. The precipitation lines in an IE pattern are therefore formed

as more or less elongated symmetrical or asymmetrical arcs. The serological identification of the precipitation arcs is achieved by the employment of reactants of suitable composition in the longitudinal trough. The configuration of the arcs often makes it possible to locate the centre of concentration of the individual substances after the electrophoretic migration. Elongated precipitation lines instead of the usual characteristic arc-formation may be observed if the test material or fractions thereof are retained by the gel. Elongated lines may also be seen if the migrating material contains substances of the same serological specificity but with different mobilities and no marked centre of concentration is created. When arcs in the ID pattern

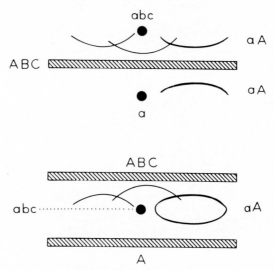

Fig. 19.28. Schematic illustration of ways to locate and serologically identify a constituent in a mixture after agar electrophoresis. Top, with the pure constituent: bottom, with a factor-specific antiserum.

develop in areas where they may interact, a comparative analysis can be made. This is exemplified in Fig. 19.27 where a standard double diffusion arrangement has been chosen, closely resembling the experimental conditions of the ID analysis in the IE technique. It is obvious that the patterns exemplified here can be interpreted as previously described according to the principles for the basic type reactions in standard combined systems. The number of precipitation arcs or lines in an IE pattern is an indicator of the number of immunoreacting constituents in the test material. This is in accord with the results obtained with the same reactants tested by standard double diffusion. However, an advantage of the IE technique is the increased resolving power due to the electrophoretic separation of the test material before the ID analysis is performed. This advantage is pronounced when immuno-systems forming multilinear spectra are analysed. The sensitivity of the IE method is however somewhat less because during the electrophoretic migra-tion of a substance dilution takes place due to the spreading of the material into a greater area. Therefore the concentration of a reactant at the source of the diffusion after the electrophoretic run is always lower than in the original solution.

A direct and reliable way of locating and serologically identifying a consti-tuent in a mixture, after the electrophoresis in the gel, is to employ a corres-ponding monospecific reactant for the ID analysis (see Fig. 19.28). A parti-cular line in a multilinear IE pattern obtained by the complete antiserum to a heterogeneous test material can be identified by employing a suitable monospecific antiserum in the same plate but in a separate longitudinal basin. The two basins are placed on opposite sides of the circular well and the re-lative position of the arc formed by the monospecific serum may be used for the recognition of the arc in question in the multilinear pattern. For serologi-cal verification, however, one must let the two precipitates grow and extend in order to get a fusion of the lines. It is also possible to identify an arc of precipitation by placing an additional square or circular basin in the area into which the line in question is calculated to extend. The observation if and how the diffusion of a suitable reactant poured in the latter basin in-fluences the further development of the line may give the desired information. In standard immunoelectrophoresis the identification of lines in a multi-linear pattern can also be obtained by using the polyvalent serum after absorp-tion with a pure antigen. The complete and the absorbed antiserum are placed in the longitudinal basins on opposite sides of the circular well. The absence of a line in the pattern formed by the absorbed serum as compared to the complete pattern is used for the identification.

Comparative immunoelectrophoresis (see, e.g. Heremans [15, 16]; Wadsworth & Hanson [42])
A series of modifications of the standard IE technique particularly suitable for identification purposes have been elaborated. The principle is to utilize sup-plementary sources of diffusion. By suitable arrangements of such basins and by employment of appropriate reactants a supplementary precipitation pattern is established at a location permitting interaction with the develop-ment of the normal IE pattern. Some examples of such comparative patterns are given in Fig. 19.29. As may be seen the straight-line development of a precipitate in the supplementary pattern is influenced by the arc formation of the IE pattern giving a fusion of lines provided that there is a serological identity of the reactants in question. This type of comparative IE technique may permit the demonstration of material not demonstrable in the standard

technique due to too low concentration of the reactant in question. The example in Fig. 19.29 shows that the straight-line development of the precipitate induced by the reactant in the supplementary basin is influenced by the same reactant present in the original material but at a concentration too low for the formation of a precipitate in the normal IE analysis.

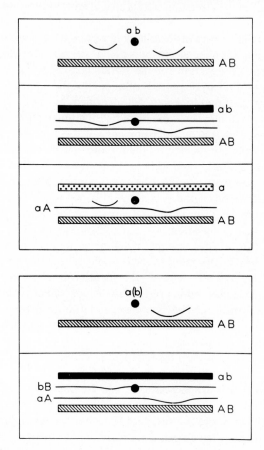

Fig. 19.29. Schematic representation of the principle of comparative immunoelectrophoresis. For interpretation see text.

Quantitative immunoelectrophoresis (see, e.g. Backhausz *et al* [1], Ouchterlony [32])

In the standard IE technique double diffusion is used for the formation of the precipitation patterns. If an antiserum is employed where the concentrations of the antibody components are known, the shape and site of the arcs may give some information regarding the concentration of the antigens separated by the electrophoresis. The principle for this type of quantitation is the same as for the one-dimensional double diffusion plate technique and the results thus obtained are only semiquantitative at best. As has been mentioned earlier simple diffusion methods are better suited for quantitative analysis. By combining the gel electrophoresis with the last-mentioned type of immunodiffusion analysis quantitation with higher accuracy can be obtained. The agar plate electrophoresis and the double diffusion analysis is performed as in the normal IE technique. However, a simple diffusion arrangement is added by cutting out a broader longitudinal trough parallel to the narrow longitudinal basin but at the opposite side of and adjacent to the transverse depot (see Fig. 19.30). Normal diffusion agar containing a comparatively low concentration of antiserum is poured into the larger basin thus establishing conditions for simple diffusion into the antibody-containing gel. In this area, arc-shaped migrating zones of precipitates are formed and the displacements (X) of the leading edges of the precipitates in relation to time can be determined. In the calculation for quantitation the formula for simple diffusion mentioned earlier is employed,

$$\frac{X}{\sqrt{t}} = K = \gamma \log \frac{Ag}{Ag_0}.$$

A series of troughs arranged as in Fig. 19.30 and containing known concentrations of the reactant to be quantitatively determined can be used as reference sources of diffusion. This procedure eliminates the trouble of repeated measurements.

Antigen–antibody crossed electrophoresis (see, e.g. Laurell [21, 22])
An interesting modification of the regular IE technique suitable for qualitative and quantitative analysis has recently been described by Laurell. The method has been named antigen–antibody crossed electrophoresis and offers not only higher resolution and simpler identification than the standard IE technique but it can also be standardized for quantitative work. So far its application seems to have been limited to the analysis of serum proteins but the principle could obviously be of advantage for the analysis of other materials. The first part of the procedure, see Fig. 19.31, is a regular agarose gel plate electrophoresis (barbital buffer pH 8·6 ionic strength 0·05 and calcium lactate 1 mM with 1 per cent agarose). The test material (serum) is poured into a transverse slit in the gel layer (thickness 1·5 mm) and the plate is placed on a cooled surface. The electrophoresis is performed for about 3 hours with a potential drop of 10 V/cm. Afterwards a narrow longitudinal strip containing the separated fractions is cut out along the middle of the

gel. The next part of the electrophoresis is carried out in a gel plate (agarose buffer solution as described above, thickness of layer 1·5 mm) containing a comparatively low concentration of an antiserum corresponding to the test material. The aforementioned gel strip is placed on the plate and a potential gradient of 10 V/cm is applied over the plate at an angle of 90° to the previous direction of the electrophoretic separation. The time of the second run is 30–90 minutes depending on the relative proportions of antigens and antibodies. In this second run the antigens in the gel strip as well as the antibodies incorporated uniformly in the gel plate migrate according to their electrophoretic mobility slightly counteracted by the slow electroendosmotic flow in the agarose gel. Precipitation zones for each antigen–antibody system

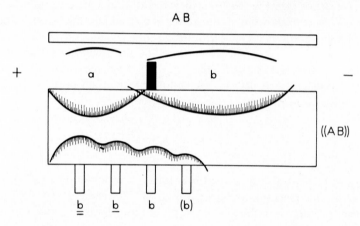

FIG. 19.30. Schematic illustration of precipitation patterns in quantitative immunoelectrophoresis. **A** and **B**, antibodies to separated constitutent **a** and **b**, the latter quantitated by means of simple diffusion technique.

present are rapidly formed and these zones 'migrate' under the influence of antigen excess primarily caused by the electrophoretic migration of the antigens. The precipitation patterns obtained by this antigen–antibody crossed ID technique differs from those formed in the standard IE technique. The span of the arc is shorter in proportion to the height and the differentiation between the individual precipitation lines is thereby facilitated. An interesting additional observation is that for a given concentration of an antibody component the height of the peak is roughly proportional to the concentration of the corresponding antigen provided that the time of the second run is sufficiently extended.

    This observation has led to the development of a rapid and accurate quantitative IE method for estimation of proteins with a charge differing from that of antibody proteins. An oblong glass plate with a gel layer of uniform thickness (1·5 mm) is used. For the analysis of serum components the agarose buffered gel, pH 8·6 is used, mixed with an appropriate amount of a suitable antiserum as mentioned earlier. Holes (3 mm diameter and at least 8 mm apart) are cut out along a line parallel with one of the long edges of the plate. The test material and dilutions of a standard antigen used for calibration are poured into the wells. The electrophoresis is performed as described

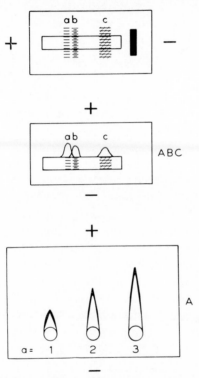

Fig. 19.31. Schematic illustration of the principle of antigen–antibody crossed electrophoresis. Top, gel-layer electrophoresis in agarose gel of mixture containing three constituents with different mobilities. After first run longitudinal strip removed. Middle, second run, strip laid on antibody-containing gel. Bottom, quantitation of antigen **a** by means of electrophoresis in gel containing antibody **A**.

and the time of the run is about 2–10 hours depending on the charge and amount of antigen in relation to the concentration of antibody in the gel. Migrating peak-formed precipitation zones originating from the circular wells, are developed (see Fig. 19.31). The leading edge of the precipitate is displaced at a decreasing rate towards one of the electrodes. The edge becomes stationary when an antigen excess can no longer be induced. For a given antibody concentration the relationship between the distance travelled by a

z*

precipitate and the antigen concentration is linear. Thus the test material can be quantitated using the peaks of two antigen solutions of known but different concentrations as a reference.

Immune gel filtration (see, e.g. Hanson *et al* [13])
A technique involving the combination of thin-layer Sephadex gel filtration and immunodiffusion has recently been described. Its application to the analysis of, e.g. human serum, fractions thereof and cerebrospinal fluid

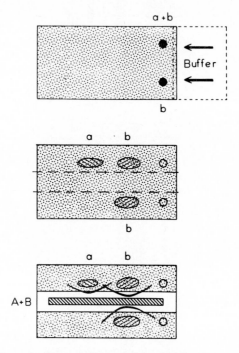

Fig. 19.32. Schematic representation of the principle of immune gel filtration. Application site of test material, black; Sephadex gel layer, stippled; buffered diffusion agar, white; antiserum in longitudinal basin.

has been reported. The principle of the technique is schematically illustrated in Fig. 19.32. The procedure for analysis of serum proteins by means of this technique is briefly as follows. An 8×20 cm glass plate is prepared with a 0·5 mm thick layer of gel, Sephadex G100 or 200 (sodium barbital buffer 0·05 M pH 8·4). The plate is tilted at a suitable angle and its upper part connected with a buffer reservoir (0·02 M tris-HCl, 0·2 M NaCl pH 8·0) by means of a filter paper wick. The gel is equilibrated by allowing this buffer to flow through the gel before applying the test samples. Samples of 1–2 μl and a reference, e.g. dyed albumin, are put into the gel at intervals of 1 cm. The gel filtration is continued until the albumin has migrated 5 cm, then it is interrupted and the plate is placed horizontally. The parts of the Sephadex gel not containing the migrating material are removed (longitudinal strips between the places of the original application of the samples, see Fig. 19.32). The whole plate is flooded with a fluid buffered agar gel (1 per cent) filling the trenches, overflowing the remaining Sephadex strips, and creating an even gel layer about 1 mm thick. After congelation longitudinal basins parallel to the Sephadex strips are cut out of the agar gel and used as depots for suitable immune sera. The double diffusion analysis is performed as described for the standard IE technique. The advantage of this combined technique is

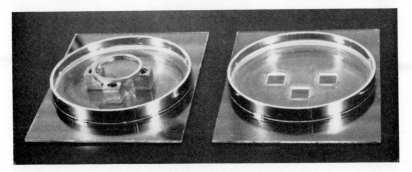

Fig. 19.33. Comparative double diffusion plate. Three-matrix template in place for pouring of agar and plate ready for filling with reactants.

that in the same plate material characterized by migration in a well-defined Sephadex gel (molecular size) can be classified according to its serological properties.

Permanent records of precipitation plates
As has been mentioned earlier the recording of precipitation patterns in the translucent gel can be done by employing transmitted or scattered light arrangements. With the former the precipitates are visualized as more or less dark bands against a light background. The latter arrangement, which gives a definitely better recording, illuminates the precipitates which are pictured against a dark background (see Figs. 19.34 and 19.35). For this dark-field illumination the oblique light from a circular source is directed through the gel plate from below and transmitted at an angle of about 20–25°. For permanent records photographs which also facilitate accurate analyses can easily be made with this type of illumination. Photographic plates and films of various trademarks have been recommended, e.g. Ilford Thin-film half-tone plate No. 50 (blue sensitive, high contrast), Ilford Film

N5 30 (blue sensitive), Kodak Panatomic X film and Contrast process pan film. Accurate recordings can be obtained more rapidly by utilizing the Polaroid procedure, Polaroid Land Film Type 55 N/P or Type 42 [41].

For the preservation of completed precipitation-in-agar plates various methods can be employed. The first step, common to most of these methods, is to elute unprecipitated material by washing the plates in physiological saline. Before placing the plates in the saline solution, basins or troughs still containing fluid reactants should be emptied. The time necessary for the elution depends on the thickness of the agar layer. For standard plates 1–3

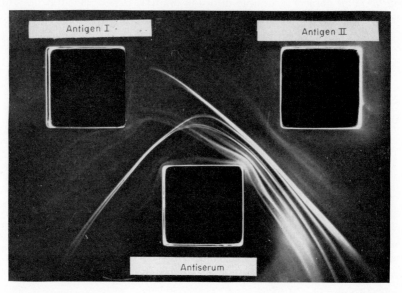

FIG. 19.34. Photograph of a comparative precipitation pattern obtained with double diffusion plate technique.

days is usually sufficient. After washing the precipitation plates can be preserved by sealing and storage in the cold. In order to prevent crack formation in the gel it is advisable to pour a thick layer of hot standard diffusion agar over the surface before the sealing, thus also filling the emptied basins with gel. By this simple procedure the original plate can be kept for a considerable time. If a permanent record is wanted the precipitation plate, after washing, can be dried in a dry-air incubator at a moderate temperature, e.g. 37° C. It is advisable to cover the moist plate with filter paper during the dehydration in order to remove salts and avoid cracks in the agar film formed. The thin translucent agar film usually sticks well to the glass and the precipitation lines are easily observed by means of a transmitted light arrangement.

Staining of immunoprecipitates has been introduced as an improvement for the preparation of permanent records as well as a technique for biochemical characterization of precipitates. Stains for proteins are usually employed for non-selective staining because the precipitates always contain antibody protein. Staining of either the washed moist plate or of the dried agar film can be performed. Protein stains commonly used are, e.g. Amido black, Bromphenol blue, Azocarmine, Nigrosin and Light green. The staining time is short for dried plates, e.g. 15–180 minutes, but considerably longer when moist plates are stained, particularly if the agar layer is thick. After staining, excess stain is washed out with a suitable solvent, thereafter the plate is dried and can be kept as a permanent record. The following is an example of a suitable procedure. The plate is washed and dried as previously

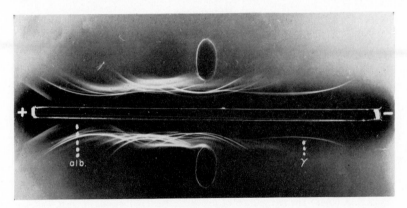

FIG. 19.35. Photograph of immunoelectrophoretic precipitation patterns of two human sera.

described. A staining solution of Amido black (1 g dissolved in 450 ml 12 per cent acetic acid, 1·6 per cent sodium acetate and 100 ml glycerol) is applied to the plate for 3 hours. The staining is followed by washing out excess stain by repeated washing for 1–2 hours using 2 per cent acetic acid solution containing 10–15 per cent glycerol. After washing the plate is dried at 37° C in a dry-air incubator. It should be mentioned that glycerol in the staining and washing solutions makes it possible to strip the dry agar film from the supporting glass and to preserve the film as a permanent record. In order to prevent the agar film from getting brittle a soaking in 1–2 per cent glycerol before the final drying is advisable. If the agar film is to be preserved adhering to the glass plate the glycerol should be omitted at all stages.

Staining procedures have also been employed for differentiation and identification of immunoprecipitates in agar gel. This technique was introduced by Björklund (1954) who reported on colour reactions of precipitates using basic fuchsin and Mayer's mucicarmine. A series of suitable selective staining methods have since been elaborated [37, 38]. As has been mentioned stains like Amido black will mark all immunoprecipitates due to their antibody content. The selective staining methods, however, are mostly used for the characterization of the precipitation lines due to their content of substances other than proteins. For instance Oil red, Sudan IV and Sudan black have been employed for the identification of lipoids and lipoproteins and periodic acid, Schiff's or Nada's reagent, for polysaccharides and glycoproteins. It should be mentioned that selective staining as well as the normal protein staining may be performed in the same plate.

References

[1] BACKHAUSZ R., VERES G. & VETÖ I. (1960) Recherches immunologiques sur des gamma-globulines. *Ann. Immunol. Hungaricae* **3**, 116
[2] BECHHOLD H. (1905) Strukturbildung in Gallerten. *Z. phys. Chem.* **52**, 185
[3] BJÖRKLUND B. (1952) Specific inhibition of precipitation as an aid in antigen analysis with gel diffusion method. *Proc. Soc. exp. Biol..* **79**, 319
[4] BJÖRKLUND B. (1954) Qualitative analysis of gel precipitates with the aid of chemical colour reactions. *Int. Arch. Allergy* **5**, 293
[5] BJÖRKLUND B. (1956) Antigenicity of malignant and normal tissues by gel diffusion techniques. *Int. Arch. Allergy* **8**, 179
[6] CROWLE A.J. (1961) *Immunodiffusion.* New York and London: Academic Press Inc.
[7] DEAN H.R. & WEBB R.A. (1926) The influence of optimal proportions of antigen and antibody in the serum precipitation reaction. *J. Path. Bact.* **29**, 473
[8] ELEK S.D. (1948) The recognition of toxogenic bacterial strains in vitro. *Brit. med. J.* **i**, 483
[9] FEINBERG J.G. (1957) Identification, discrimination and quantification in Ouchterlony gel plates. *Int. Arch. Allergy* **11**, 129
[10] GRABAR P. & WILLIAMS C.A. (1953) Méthode permettant l'étude conjuguée des propriétés électrophorétiques et immunochimiques d'un mélange de protéines. Application au sérum sanguin. *Biochim. biophys. Acta* **10**, 193
[11] GRABAR P. & BURTIN P. (1960) *Analyse immuno-électrophorétique.* Paris: Masson et Cie Editeurs.
[12] GRABAR P. & BURTIN P. (1964) *Immuno-electrophoretic Analysis.* Amsterdam, London, New York: Elsevier Publishing Company
[13] HANSON L.Å., JOHANSSON B.G. & RYMO L. (1966) Further applications of thin-layer gel filtration: Two-dimensional gel filtration-electrophoresis and immuno-gel filtration. *Clin. chim. Acta.* **14**, 391
[14] HAYWARD B.J. & AUGUSTIN R. (1957) Quantitative gel diffusion methods for assay of antigens and antibodies. *Int. Arch. Allergy* **11**, 192
[15] HEREMANS J.F. (1960) Les globulines sériques du système gamma. *Thesis*, pp. 38–42. Bruxelles: Editions Arscia S.A.
[16] HEREMANS J.F. (1963) *Die Immunoelektrophorese und ihre klinische Bedeutung, in Ergebnisse der inneren Medizin und Kinderheilkunde.* 20, pp. 196–199. Berlin, Göttingen, Heidelberg: Springer-Verlag

[17] HOLM S.E. (1965) A modified gel chamber technique for immunodiffusion analysis. *Int. Arch. Allergy* **26**, 34

[18] JENNINGS R.K. & MALONE F. (1954) Rapid double diffusion precipitin analysis. *J. Immunol.* **72**, 411

[19] JENNINGS R.K. & MALONE F. (1957) Objective double diffusion precipitin analysis. *J. Path. Bact.* **74**, 81

[20] JENNINGS R.K. (1958) Objective interpretation of precipitate patterns in agar diffusion precipitin plates. *J. Lab. clin. Med.* **51**, 152

[21] LAURELL C.B. (1965) Antigen–antibody crossed electrophoresis. *Analyt. Biochem.* **10**, 358

[22] LAURELL C.B. (1966) Quantitative estimation of proteins by electrophoresis in agarose gel containing antibodies. *Analyt. Biochem.* (in press)

[23] MANCINI G., VAERMAN J.P., CARBONARA A.O. & HEREMANS J.F. (1964) A single-radial-diffusion method for the immunological quantitation of proteins. In *Prot. biol. Fluids 11th Colloqu. Bruges*, pp. 370–373, ed. PEETERS H.

[24] MANCINI G., CARBONARA C.O. & HEREMANS J.F. (1965) Immunochemical quantitation of antigens by single radial immunodiffusion. *Immunochemistry* **2**, 235

[25] NILSSON L.Å. (1966) Diffusion-in-gel analyses of acute phase protein antisera by means of a comparative inhibition technique. *Int. Arch. Allergy* (in press)

[26] OAKLEY C.L. & FULTHORPE A.J. (1953) Antigenic analysis by diffusion. *J. Path. Bact.* **65**, 49

[27] OUCHTERLONY Ö. (1948) In vitro method for testing the toxic-producing capacity of diphtheria bacteria. 8th Scandinavian Pathological Congress 1947. *Acta path. microbiol. scand.* **25**, 186

[28] OUCHTERLONY Ö. (1958) Diffusion-in-gel methods for immunological analysis. In *Progress in Allergy*, Vol. V, pp. 1–78, ed. KALLÓS P. Basel and New York: Karger

[29] OUCHTERLONY Ö. (1962) Diffusion-in-gel methods for immunological analysis. II. In *Progress in Allergy*, Vol. VI, pp. 30–154, ed. KALLÓS P. & WAKSMAN B.H. Basel and New York: Karger

[30] OUCHTERLONY Ö. (1962) Quantitative immunoelectrophoresis. *Acta path. microbiol. scand.* **Suppl. 154**, 252

[31] OUDIN J. (1946) Méthode d'analyse immunochimique par précipitation spécifique en milieu gélifié. *C.R. Acad. Sci.* **222**, 115

[32] OUDIN J. (1952) Specific precipitation in gels and its application to immunological analysis. In *Methods in Medical Research*, Vol. V, pp. 335–378, ed. CORCORAN A.C. Chicago, Ill.: Year Book Publishers Inc.

[33] PETRIE G.F. (1932) A specific precipitin reaction associated with the growth on agar plates of meningococcus, pneumococcus and B. dysenteriae (Shiga). *Brit. J. exp. Path.* **13**, 380

[34] POULIK M.D. (1952) Filter paper electrophoresis of purified diphtheria toxoid. *Canad. J. med. Sci.* **30**, 417

[35] RAMON G. (1922) Flocculation dans un mélange neutre de toxine–antitoxine diphtériques. *C.R. Soc. Biol.* (*Paris*) **86**, 661

[36] SCHEIDEGGER J.J. (1955) Une micro-méthode de l'immune-électrophorèse. *Int. Arch. Allergy* **7**, 103

[37] URIEL J. & GRABAR P. (1956) Étude des lipoprotéins sériques par l'électrophorèse en gélose et l'analyse immunoélectrophorétique. *Bull. Soc. Chim. biol.* (*Paris*) **38**, 431

[38] URIEL J. (1960) Les réactions de caractérization des constituants protéiques après électrophorèse ou immuno-électrophorèse en gélose. In *Analyse immuno-électrophorétique*, pp. 32–56, ed. GRABAR P. & BURTIN P. Paris: Masson et Cᶦᵉ

[39] WADSWORTH C. (1957) A slide microtechnique for the analysis of immune precipitates in gel. *Int. Arch. Allergy* **10,** 355

[40] WADSWORTH C. (1962) A microplate technique employing a gel chamber compared with other micro- and macroplate techniques for immune diffusion. *Int. Arch. Allergy* **21,** 131

[41] WADSWORTH C. (1963) Comparative testing of a new photographic material for rapid registration of immunoprecipitates. *Int. Arch. Allergy* **23,** 103

[42] WADSWORTH C. & HANSON L.Å. (1960) Comparative analysis of immune electrophoresis precipitates employing a modified immune electrophoretic technique. *Int. Arch. Allergy* **17,** 165

CHAPTER 20

Micro-complement Fixation

LAWRENCE LEVINE

Since the first demonstration of the complement (C′) fixation reaction in 1901 [1], there have been a number of techniques developed for measurement of C′ fixation. A description and critique of many of these procedures have been reviewed by Osler [2]. In all of these procedures, C′ fixation is measured by the capacity of C′, after incubation with antigen–antibody complexes to haemolyse sensitized sheep red blood cells. Thus, it is apparent that fixation of C′ by antigen–antibody complexes and lysis by C′ of sensitized sheep red blood cells involve some, if not all, of the same components that comprise the C′ system. The sequence of C′ component reactions and some of the molecular changes accompanying these reactions in immune haemolysis have been studied intensively [3]. The sequence of C′ component fixation to antigen–antibody complexes has also been studied [4] and it is generally assumed that the initial sequence of events following C′ fixation by antigen–antibody complexes or sensitized sheep red blood cells is the same. This sequence can be schematically represented as follows:

$$(Ag\text{–}Ab)_i + C'1 \xrightarrow{\ Ca^{++}\ } (Ag\text{–}Ab)_i C'1a \tag{1}$$

$$(Ag\text{–}Ab)_i C'1a + C'4 \longrightarrow (Ag\text{–}Ab)_i C'1a,4 \tag{2}$$

$$(Ag\text{–}Ab)_i C'1a,4 + C'2 \xrightarrow{\ Mg^{++}\ } (Ag\text{–}Ab)_i C'1a,4,2a \tag{3}$$

(Ag = antigen; Ab = antibody; $(Ag\text{–}Ab)_i$ = antigen–antibody complex; C′1, C′2, C′4 = components of C′ and C′1a; and C′2a = C′ component reaction products.)

While C′3 can be fixed under certain experimental conditions, C′3 is not fixed either at 0° or at 37°C with the concentrations of antigen, antibody and C′ used in most C′ fixation procedures [5]. This schematic representation does not signify which component, depleted from the C′ system by the antigen–antibody complexes, is responsible for the loss of C′ activity towards the sensitized sheep red blood cells. It is likely that a decrease in all three components of (C′1, C′4 and C′2) affects the residual haemolytic activity of the C′ system.

707

In our laboratory analyses of antigen–antibody reactions by C' fixation [6] are done in the presence of sufficient C' for quantitative estimation of residual haemolytic activity. Since dilute solutions of C' are used in the reaction mixtures, small amounts of antibody and consequently small quantities of antigen are required to obtain a complete antigen–antibody curve.

Principle

The complement system of fresh guinea-pig serum has the capacity to combine irreversibly with antigen–antibody complexes. If the antigen is associated with the sheep erythrocyte cell surface, such a combination may result in lysis of the erythrocyte and, thus offers an excellent indicator system for C' activity. If two different antigen–antibody systems are added to guinea-pig serum, a competition for the C' components would result. If, however, C' is allowed to incubate with the antigen–antibody system under study, then its combination can be estimated by the residual haemolytic activity it possesses when a known quantity of antibody-coated, i.e. sensitized erythrocytes, is added at a later time.

Reagents

Diluent

In a 1 litre volumetric flask, dissolve 81·6 g NaCl and 12·1 g tris(hydroxymethyl)aminomethane in about 800 ml distilled water. Add 6·6 ml concentrated HCl, mix and add 33 ml 0·15 M $MgSO_4$ and 15 ml 0·1 M $CaCl_2$. Adjust volume to 1 litre with distilled water. The pH should be 7·4. This buffer stock is ten times more concentrated than that used in the assay. Therefore, for use, make precise tenfold dilutions with distilled water. Bovine serum albumin, 0·1 per cent, should be added to protect the dilute solutions of proteins used in the assay. The dry bovine serum albumin can be added to the NaCl-tris buffer after it is brought to isotonicity.

Sheep erythrocytes

Sheep blood, in an equal volume of Alsever's solution, can be obtained commercially. The sterile blood is kept at 2–4° C for at least a week after bleeding, at which time the red blood cells are uniformly susceptible to immune haemolysis and remain so for a period of about 2 months. To prepare the standardized red blood cells, an aliquot (about 8 ml is sufficient for the day's experiments) of the sheep blood is centrifuged and the plasma removed by aspiration. The packed cells are resuspended in about 10 ml diluent and the washing procedure repeated three times. The second and third washes should be colourless. After the last cycle of washing, 1·0 ml of the packed cells are evenly suspended in 19·0 ml diluent. The erythrocyte suspension is standardized by lysing 1·0 ml with 14·0 ml of 0·1 per cent Na_2CO_3. A cell suspension containing 1×10^9 erythrocytes/ml will have an optical density (OD) of 0·680 at 541 mμ in a cuvette having a path length of 1 cm. Usually, the 5 per cent lysed cell suspension will give a higher reading and should be adjusted to a final OD of 0·680 by appropriate dilution.

Sensitization of the sheep erythrocytes

The haemolytic rabbit antibody is available commercially. With the several lots of commercial haemolytic antibody used in our laboratory during the past several years, a dilution of 1/1000 has been suitable. If, however, the haemolytic antibody is to be titred for optimum sensitization of cells, the method of Osler *et al* [2] should be used. A stock haemolytic antiserum dilution of 1/50 in diluent is stored at $-20°$ C.

For sensitization of the cells, 10·0 ml of the haemolytic antibody, diluted 1/1000, is added slowly to 10·0 ml of the standardized cell suspension in a 500 ml Erlenmeyer flask with constant swirling of the contents. After incubation of 37° C for 15 minutes to allow maximum sensitization, 180 ml of diluent is added and the cell suspension which now contains 5×10^7 sensitized cells (EA) per ml, is kept at 0° C until used.

Complement (C')

Lyophilized guinea-pig serum, obtained commercially, is reconstituted with the supplied diluent. This reconstituted guinea-pig C' has haemolytic activity equal to that of the commercially available frozen C'. C' pools can be prepared in lots of 40 ml and should be stored in 2 ml quantities in screw-capped tubes at $-20°$ C to minimize the loss of C' activity which may occur following repeated freezings and thawings. The C' is titred as follows: to a series of 40 ml centrifuge tubes in an ice-bath are added, in order, 5·0 ml diluent and 1·0 ml C', diluted 1/150, 1/175, 1/200, 1/250, 1/275, 1/300. After incubation at 16–18 hours at 2–4° C, 1·0 ml of EA is added and haemolysis allowed to proceed at 35–37° C with occasional swirling for 60 minutes. The reaction mixtures are centrifuged to sediment the unlysed cells, and the supernatant fluid is read at 413 mμ. That dilution of C' which gives 90 per cent haemolysis is used in the C' fixation test and has been found to vary from 1/225 to 1/275 in our laboratory.

C' fixation procedure

To a series of 40 ml centrifuge tubes in an ice-bath is added, in order, 1·0 ml diluted antiserum, 3·0 ml diluent, 1·0 ml diluted C' (previously titred), and finally 1·0 ml antigen solution serially diluted twofold. Appropriate dilutions of antigen (usually the highest concentration) and C', antibody and C', diluent and C', and diluent in a total volume of 6·0 ml serve as controls and

TABLE 20.1

Micro-C′ fixation protocol and results

Reaction Mixture	1	2	3	4	5	6	7	8	9	10	11
Ra–anti-pork haemoglobin (1 : 200), ml	1·0	1·0	1·0	1·0	1·0	1·0	1·0	—	—	—	—
Diluent, ml	3·0	3·0	3·0	3·0	3·0	3·0	4·0	4·0	5·0	4·0	6·0
C′ (1 : 260)	1·0	1·0	1·0	1·0	1·0	1·0	1·0	1·0	1·0	2·0	—
Antigen (pork haemoglobin), ml	1·0	1·0	1·0	1·0	1·0	1·0	—	1·0	—	—	—
μg antigen/ml (pork haemoglobin/ml)	0·5	0·25	0·12	0·06	0·03	0·015	—	0·5	—	—	—
						16–18 hours, 2–4°C					
EA (5 × 10^7/ml), ml	1·0	1·0	1·0	1·0	1·0	1·0	1·0	1·0	1·0	1·0	1·0
						1 hour, 37°C					
Haemolysis, OD 413 mμ	0·489	0·253	0·114	0·199	0·341	0·459	0·489	0·502	0·511	0·631	0·002
C′ fixation, Δ OD, Control OD (average) minus reaction OD	0·012	0·248	0·387	0·302	0·160	0·042					
Per cent C′ fixation (Δ OD/control OD) × 100	2	49	77	60	32	8					

are included in every experiment. After incubation at 2–4° C for 16–18 hours, 1·0 ml of EA is added and haemolysis allowed to proceed, with occasional swirling, in a water-bath at 35–37° C until controls are visually estimated to be 80–90 per cent haemolysed, about 40–60 minutes. After immersion in an ice-bath to stop the haemolytic reaction, the mixtures are centrifuged for 10 minutes to sediment the unlysed EA, and the optical density of the supernatant fluid is determined at 413 mμ. Providing that the antigen and antibody controls do not give evidence of independent pro- or anti-C′ activity, the

TABLE 20.2

The relationship of antigen concentration to maximum C′ fixation

Immune system	Approximate molecular weight of antigen	Amount of antigen added to give maximum C′ fixation (μg/6 ml)[a]
Bovine pancreatic ribonuclease	13,500	0·01
Human growth hormone	27,000	0·05
Swine pepsinogen	42,000	0·01
Egg albumin	46,000	0·05
Swine haemoglobin	66,000	0·1
Human haemoglobin	66,000	0·05
Bovine serum albumin	68,000	0·04
Calf skin tropocollagen	130,000	0·1
Lactic dehydrogenase	150,000	0·05
Horse spleen ferritin	460,000	0·03
Bacteriophage T$_4$ DNA	$1·2 \times 10^8$	0·01
Bacteriophage T$_4$	$2·4 \times 10^8$	0·12
Pneumococcus polysaccharide	[b]	0·01
Colicine K	[b]	0·3
Dogfish pepsinogen	[b]	0·1

[a] These values are given for a dilution of antibody which will give 70–80 per cent maximum C′ fixation.

[b] Molecular weight unknown.

results may be expressed in either one of two ways: (i) as the difference between the OD of the controls (antigen, antibody and C′) and the OD of the experimental tubes (Δ OD); or (ii) as the percentage of C′ fixed, calculated as (Reaction Δ OD/Control OD) × 100. A typical protocol and results of a C′ fixation experiment using a porcine haemoglobin–anti-porcine haemoglobin immune system is shown in Table 20.1.

The dilution of antiserum to be used in the micro-C′ fixation procedure is found empirically. The undiluted rabbit antiserum is first heated to 60° C for 20 minutes to destroy endogenous C′ activity. C′ fixation is then performed with varying dilutions of the antiserum (1/200, 1/400, 1/800, 1/1600, etc.)

using antigen concentrations varying from 0·001 to 1·0 μg. The dilution of antiserum which gives a complete C' fixation curve with maximum fixation around 70 per cent should then be used for subsequent studies. As shown in Table 20.2, with most immune systems studied, the antigen concentrations required for maximum C' fixation with the antibody dilution giving a complete fixation curve varies from 0·01 to 0·1 μg.

C' fixation inhibition procedure

Hapten inhibition of antigen–antibody interaction as measured by C' fixation is performed in the same manner as micro-C' fixation, except that the antigen is kept constant and the diluent now contains various quantities of inhibitor. The constant quantity of antigen to be used in the assay is the amount that gives maximum C' fixation in a previously characterized immune system.

To a series of 40 ml centrifuge tubes in an ice-bath is added, in order, 1·0 ml diluted antiserum, 2·0 ml diluent, 1·0 diluted C',1·0 ml hapten solution serially diluted twofold, and finally 1·0 ml of solution containing the constant amount of antigen. Appropriate dilutions of the C', hapten solutions (usually the highest concentration) and C', antibody and C', antigen and C', diluent and C', and diluent in a total volume of 6·0 ml—serve as controls and are included in every experiment. After incubation at 2–4° C for 16–18 hours, 1·0 ml EA is added and haemolysis allowed to proceed, with occasional swirling, in a water-bath at 35–37° C until controls are visibly estimated to be 80–90 per cent haemolysed. After immersion in an ice-bath to stop the haemolytic reaction, the mixtures are centrifuged for 10 minutes to sediment the unlysed EA, and the optical density of the supernatant fluid is determined at 413 mμ. Providing the inhibitor, antigen and antibody controls do not give evidence of independent pro- or anti-C' activity, the inhibition may be expressed as the percentage of C' fixed in presence of hapten divided by the C' fixed in absence of hapten × 100. A typical protocol and results of a C' fixation inhibition by tetra-D-lysine of a poly-D-lysine immune system [3] is shown in Table 20.3.

Quantitative estimation of antigen concentration

Estimation of antigens by immunological techniques is dependent upon the rigorous demonstration of the immunochemical homogeneity of the immune system. The C' fixation curve with the purified antigen can then be used as a calibration curve to estimate the quantity of antigen in crude material or antigen unmasked as a result of some physical or chemical treatment. The quantitative appearance of the single strand DNA when native double strand DNA is exposed to different temperatures for 10 minutes and quickly chilled is represented by the C' fixation curves shown in Fig. 20.1 [4]. The ratio of the extent of reaction at a specific temperature

TABLE 20.3

Inhibition of poly-D-lysine-anti-poly-D-lysine by tetra-D-lysine

Reaction mixture	1	2	3	4	5	6	7	8	9	10	11	12
Ml antiserum (1 : 1500)	1·0	1·0	1·0	1·0	1·0	1·0	1·0	—	—	—	—	—
Ml Tris buffer	2·0	2·0	2·0	2·0	2·0	3·0	4·0	4·0	4·0	5·0	4·0	6·0
Ml C' (1/251)	1·0	1·0	1·0	1·0	1·0	1·0	1·0	1·0	1·0	1·0	2·0	—
Ml tetralysine dilution	1·0	1·0	1·0	1·0	1·0	—	—	—	1·0	—	—	—
Tetralysine, mμM added	69·0	23·0	7·7	2·6	0·9	—	—	—	69·0	—	—	—
Ml poly-D-lysine (0·06 μg/ml)	1·0	1·0	1·0	1·0	1·0	1·0	—	1·0	—	—	—	—
						2·4°C—20 hours						
Ml EA, 5×10^7/ml	1·0	1·0	1·0	1·0	1·0	1·0	1·0	1·0	1·0	1·0	1·0	1·0
						Haemolysis, 37°C—45 minutes						
OD 413 mμ	0·485	0·390	0·242	0·146	0·071	0·050	0·510	0·550	0·530	0·579	0·650	0·021
C' fixation : average of the OD values of C' Ab, Ag, and I controls minus reaction OD	0·057	0·152	0·300	0·396	0·471	0·492	—	—	—	—	—	—
Per cent inhibition	88%	69%	39%	20%	4%	0%	—	—	—	—	—	—

to the extent of reaction of DNA which had been heated at 100° C to denature all the molecules (the C′ fixation calibration curve) can then be used to calculate the amount of denatured DNA in any sample.

Antigen structure

As shown by Osler & Hill [5, 6], the C′ fixing capacity of rabbit immune systems depends on the affinity of antibody for its antigen and their subsequent aggregation. Since the micro-C′ fixation assay employs antiserum at very low concentrations, it is likely that only the antibodies of highest affinity are being measured. A change which alters the complementarity

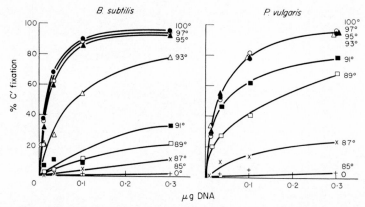

FIG. 20.1. Fixation of C′ in a rabbit by increments of *B. subtilis* and *P. vulgaris* DNA after incubation of the samples (3 μg/ml) for 10 minutes at the designated temperature in 0·15 M NaCl-tris buffer (pH 7·4) followed by fast cooling and appropriate dilution. Antiserum was anti photo-oxidized T4 DNA. (From Seaman *et al.* [4].)

between one of the antigenic determinants on the protein and its specific antibody may also decrease the affinity between them. Thus, even a local conformational change in only one of several antigenic determinants may be magnified during the process of antigen–antibody aggregation and be sufficient to alter the C′ fixation curve.

The changes in the C′ fixation curve which presumably reflect these changed states of aggregation have been found to be the following: (i) a decrease in C′ fixation at the same antigen concentration originally required for maximum fixation (vertical shift), and (ii) an increase in antigen concentration required to reach maximum fixation with or without a decrease in the maximum fixation (lateral shift).

Such changes in C′ fixation curves are illustrated in the following immune systems:

(a) *Vertical shift*

Hydrolysis by carboxypeptidase A of the two C-terminal amino acids from the β chains of haemoglobin (α_2^A, α_2^A) results in a conformational change of the molecule as judged by the loss of its characteristic oxygenation properties [7]. On the other hand, removal of the C-terminal amino acids of the α chains by carboxypeptidase B does not affect the heme–heme interaction exhibited by haemoglobin. The C′ fixing properties of these molecules [8] are shown in Fig. 20.2. Where a conformational change occurred, as judged by oxygenation

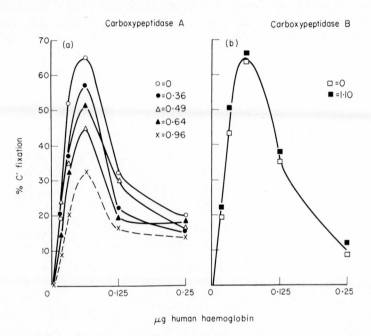

FIG. 20.2. Effect of carboxypeptidase hydrolysis on the C′ fixing activity of A_1 haemoglobin: (a) μmole *his* released per $\alpha\beta$ unit, (b) μmole *arg* released per $\alpha\beta$ unit. (From Reichlin *et al.* [8])

properties, a decrease in C′ fixation is observed. Removal of the C-terminal amino acids by carboxypeptidase A does not affect the C′ fixing capacity of haemoglobin H (β_4^A), a molecule which exhibits no heme–heme interaction. A decrease in serologic activity has also been observed by Reichlin *et al* [9] when comparing oxygenated and deoxygenated haemoglobins, molecules differing only in the distance between their β chains [10].

A decrease in C′ fixation accompanied by a vertical shift is most easily interpreted as decreased antigen–antibody aggregate formation due to altered complementarity of one or a minority of antigenic determinants; i.e. while the altered antigenic determinant will not react or will have a lowered affinity for its antibody, most of the other antigenic determinants will remain unchanged.

(b) *Lateral shift*

When pepsinogen (1 mg/ml) is exposed to varying concentrations of urea for 1 hour at 25° C then rapidly diluted into cold diluent and assayed with anti-pepsinogen by C′ fixation, the data shown in Fig. 20.3 are obtained. Two molar urea produces a lateral shift of the curve, while 4–6 M urea causes a further shift and slight decrease in maximum fixation. If these same samples are diluted so as to diminish the urea concentration below 0·8 M and then

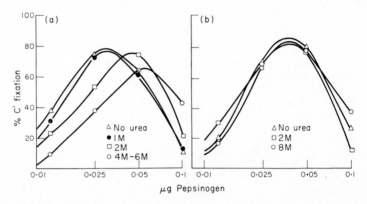

FIG. 20.3. The C′ fixation curves of pepsinogen (1 mg/ml) exposed to various concentrations of urea (pH 7·6) for 1 hour at 25° C and (a) diluted into veronal buffer and reacted rapidly with antipepsinogen; or (b) diluted in 1 : 10 in buffer and allowed to stand for 1 hour prior to assay with antipepsinogen. (From Gerstein *et al.* [11])

allowed to stand for 1 hour at 25° C before further dilution and contact with the antibody, the curves shown in Fig. 20.3b are obtained. By C′ fixation, renaturation is complete from all concentrations of urea. The conformational change in pepsinogen induced by urea was measured concomitantly by potential peptic activity and relative fluorescence intensity [11]. The lateral shift was also observed when pepsinogen was exposed to temperatures between 45 and 65° C.

The reduced affinity of a majority of the antigenic determinants requires a higher concentration of antigen for maximum fixation. The lateral shift then indicates a more general conformational change than the vertical shift. In certain cases, both a vertical and lateral shift is observed as when pepsinogen is heated to temperatures above 65° C [12].

Advantages

A comparison of three different quantitative immunochemical techniques (precipitation, the C′ fixation method of Mayer *et al* [13], and micro-C′ fixation) for distinguishing structural differences in proteins is given in Table 20.4.

The effect of chemical, physical or enzymatic treatment in altering the immunochemical properties of proteins can be determined by the changes in direct C′ fixation. This technique can profitably be used in conjunction with some of the other techniques presently utilized to investigate conformational changes in proteins. Indeed, the C′ fixation assay has proven to be

TABLE 20.4

Comparison of sensitivity of immunological methods

Antiserum	Heterologous antigen	Quantitative precipitin reaction	Cross-reaction[a]	
			Macro-complement fixation	Micro-complement fixation
Anti-human haemoglobin A	Human haemoglobin S	100[b]	86[b]	41[b]
Anti-human serum albumin	Chimpanzee serum albumin	97	89	46
Anti-chicken ovalbumin	Turkey ovalbumin	96	89	3
Anti-chicken H_4 LDH	Turkey H_4 LDH	91	90	32

[a] The heterologous reaction is expressed as a percentage of the homologous reaction.
[b] From unpublished data of M.Reichlin, A.Wilson and L.Levine.

more informative in some cases. For example, exposure of lactic dehydrogenase to urea, followed by dialysis, yields a protein that has regained its original polarization of fluorescence properties. It has, however, refolded to a conformation that differs from the native molecule as revealed by its C′ fixation [14]. With proteins possessing no biological activity, the micro-C′ fixation assay offers, perhaps, the simplest and most sensitive tool for determining whether renaturation has yielded the original molecule. The advantage it has over the other quantitative immunochemical techniques which are commonly used to detect conformational changes is best illustrated in Table 20.4. The ability to detect similarities in the same protein from different tissues or different species is, of course, an obvious use for the assay. The requirement for extremely small amounts of reactants and the ease of performing the analyses, once the system has been standardized, have already been mentioned. Since the antibody is highly specific for the protein antigen, it is possible to study the conformational changes which the antigen undergoes in the presence of other proteins, provided the latter do not cross-react with the antibody.

Disadvantages

Because of the complex interrelationships of the C′ system, the C′ fixation procedure does not permit any marked fluctuation of environmental conditions. For example, the assay cannot be performed at ambient temperatures or in 8 M urea. In addition, metals, amines, chelating agents, enzymes, organic solvents, etc., can destroy the haemolytic activity of C′ if present at certain concentrations. Appropriate dilution from the reaction mixture into buffer, prior to addition to the C′ fixation reaction mixtures, can usually circumvent these difficulties. The antigen controls serve to detect such interference if it exists at the dilution of antigen being used for the C′ fixation assay. The changes measurable by the C′ fixation procedure in proteins that are reversibly denatured are probably not maximum. The time between treatment of the antigen and its dilution and addition to the antibody-containing reaction mixture, therefore, may be critical.

References

[1] WASSERMAN E. & LEVINE L. (1960) Quantitative micro-complement fixation and its use in the study of antigenic structure by specific antigen–antibody inhibition. *J. Immunol.* **87,** 290

[2] OSLER A.G., STRAUSS J.H. & MAYER M.M. (1952) Diagnostic complement fixation method. *Am. J. Syph. Gonor. and Ven. Dis.* **36,** 140

[3] VAN VUNAKIS H., KAPLAN J., LEHRER H. & LEVINE L. (1966) Immunogenicity of polylysine and polyornithine when complexed to phosphorylated bovine serum albumin. *Immunochemistry* **3,** 393

[4] SEAMAN E., LEVINE L. & VAN VUNAKIS H. (1965) Immunochemical studies on bacteriophage deoxyribonucleic acid. V. Specificity of antibodies to deoxyribonucleic acid after immunization with methylated bovine serum albumin deoxyribonucleic acid complexes. *Biochemistry* **4,** 2091

[5] OSLER A.G. & HILL B.M. (1955) Kinetic studies of complement fixation. I. A method. *J. Immunol.* **75,** 137

[6] HILL B.M. & OSLER A.G. (1955) Kinetic studies of complement fixation. II. The role of the aggregating capacity of antibody and its heterogeneity. *J. Immunol.* **75,** 146

[7] ANTONINI E., WYMAN J., ZITO R., ROSSI-FANELLI A. & CAPUTO A. (1961) Studies on carboxypeptidase digests of human haemoglobin. *J. biol. Chem.* **236**

[8] REICHLIN M., HAMMERSHLAG R. & LEVINE L. Effect of carboxypeptidase hydrolysis on the serologic activity of A_1 haemoglobin. Unpublished data

[9] REICHLIN M., BUCCI E., WYMAN J., ANTONINI E. & ROSSI-FANELLI A. (1965) The role of α and β chains in the immunochemical difference between oxy and deoxy human haemoglobin. *J. molec. Biol.* **11,** 775

[10] MUIRHEAD H. & PERUTZ M.F. (1963) Structure of haemoglobin. A three dimensional fourier synthesis of reduced human haemoglobin at 5·5 Å resolution. *Nature* **199,** 633

[11] GERSTEIN J.F., LEVINE L. & VAN VUNAKIS H. (1964) Altered antigeneity of pepsinogen and pepsin as an index of conformational change: Effect of urea and reducing reagents. *Immunochemistry* **1,** 3

[12] GERSTEIN J.F., VAN VUNAKIS H. & LEVINE L. (1963) Heat and alkali-induced changes in the conformation of pepsinogen and pepsin. *Biochemistry* **2,** 964

[13] MAYER M.M., OSLER A.G., BIER O.G. & HEIDELBERGER M. (1948) Quantitative studies of complement fixation; method. *J. Immunol.* **59,** 195

[14] LEVINE L. (1962) Determinants of specificity of proteins, nucleic acids, and polypeptides. *Fed. Proc.* **21,** 711

CHAPTER 21

Passive Haemagglutination

W.J.HERBERT*

Introduction

The agglutination of a particulate antigen by its specific antibody is classically the simplest way of estimating the quantity of that antibody in a serum. Some soluble antigens can be coated on inert materials such as bentonite or latex which are then found to react as if they were themselves particles with the antigenic specificity of the antigen. These can then similarly be used for agglutination tests. However, such particles are difficult to coat, preserve, and standardize, and they have not shown the wide range of usefulness that was at first expected of them.

Red blood cells, on the other hand, have been found to be extremely convenient passive carriers of antigen. Not only is it possible to coat almost any antigen on their complex surfaces, but the coated cells have been found to be amongst the most sensitive available indicators of antibody. The convenience with which agglutination tests may be carried out is also greatly increased by the fact that the cells lend themselves to the observation of settling patterns in the wells of perspex trays for end-point determinations, rather than of gross agglutination in separate tubes.

Red blood cells have an elaborate antigenic surface. Though this may facilitate the attachment of many antigens it entails a complication in the test due to the frequent presence of natural heterophile antibodies to the cells in the sera of most animals and which must be removed before the test proper is carried out. The antigenic surface has, however, also been used to facilitate the firm attachment of antigen to a cell by coupling it first to an anti-red cell antibody [15].

With some antigens, particularly the polysaccharides, red cells may be effectively coated by merely exposing them to the antigen for a short time. With most proteins this type of direct coating can also take place, but the sensitivity of the resultant cells is greatly improved if their agglutinability has been increased by previous tanning [7]. A more sure coating of the cells can

* The studies carried out by the author were made in the Immunology Unit, Bacteriology Department, University of Edinburgh, and were supported by a grant from the Animal Health Trust.

be accomplished by attaching the antigen to them through a chemical bond.

Three types of coating may therefore be distinguished: direct adsorption of the antigen by the cells, the tanned cell technique, and the firm bonding of antigen to the cells by various, usually chemical, means. The reagent produced is, however, much the same however prepared and will give very similar results in the agglutination test.

It must also be noted that it is possible to reverse tests of this type by coating the cells with antibody and using them thereafter to test for the presence of antigen [19, 72]. Though difficulties may be encountered in obtaining antibody of sufficient purity, this reversed technique would appear to have a useful future, particularly in the diagnosis of viral diseases.

The choice and preservation of cells

To avoid difficulties caused by the presence in the sera being examined of agglutinins against non-homologous red cells, it would seem logical to use cells of the same species whenever possible. However, most reports are of the use of either sheep or human group O cells, both being fairly easy to obtain in quantity. It is usual to absorb out non-specific agglutinins against these cells in an initial dilution stage before the titration proper. In most respects sheep cells have proved satisfactory in practice, though human cells are said to make more sensitive cells for the tanned cell technique [81]. Difficulties have been experienced with rabbit, mouse and chicken cells in some systems [26, 42] though found adequate in others [61, 90]. Pig cells have been found to be very suitable as carriers in a completely homologous system [49] and horse, monkey, and guinea-pig cells have also been successfully used [26, 61, 90].

Sheep blood may be collected from an abattoir and defibrinated by shaking in a bottle with a wire spiral. If gross contamination is avoided, and the blood kept at 4° C, the cells may be used for a period of 3–4 days after collection. Thereafter the sensitized cells may be useful for a further 3–4 days [42]. By aseptically collecting sheep blood into an equal volume of Alsever's solution:

Dextrose	2·05 g
Sodium citrate	0·80 g
Sodium chloride	0·42 g
Distilled water	100 ml

(adjusted to pH 6·1 with 10 per cent citric acid before autoclaving at 10 pounds for 15 minutes) and adding an antibiotic (say, Aureomycin at 5 mg per 100 ml), it may be preserved for use for at least 2 weeks [39, 74]. Heparinized blood has also been found to be satisfactory [79].

For the long-term preservation of cells, either before or after coating, they must be formalinized. This may lead to additional difficulties due to the effect of the formalin on the coating antigen [30, 41] and the preserved cells are somewhat less sensitive than the fresh ones [41]. Many methods for formalinization have been described but some of them take a long time to carry out and produce agglutinated or clumped cells which have to be broken up by heroic means [45, 55, 77].

A simple method of formalinizing cells in quantity for subsequent coating is that of Csizmas [18]. The conditions under which this is carried out have not been found to be critical and a suitable technique is as follows:

1. Freshly collected red blood cells are washed five times with physiological saline and packed after the final wash (750 *g* for 15 minutes). There should be no haemolysis.

2. Twenty-five millilitres of the packed cells are resuspended to 200 ml in phosphate buffered saline pH 7·2 and placed in a 500 ml conical flask.

3. Fifty millilitres of commercial formalin (40 per cent formaldehyde) are introduced into a length of dialysis tubing which is then tied off so that, though air is excluded, the tube is only two-thirds full. This allows for the expansion in volume, due to osmotic effect, which occurs during the next stage.

4. The filled dialysis tube is submerged in the red cell suspension and the whole gently agitated at room temperature. The flask may be placed in a reciprocating shaker or a magnetic stirrer may be used [73] but care should be taken to avoid the production of much foam. Gentle rotation such as that provided by a Matburn* blood cell suspension mixer has been found ideal and a wire mesh glassware crate can easily be attached to this machine to hold the flask.

5. After about 3 hours the swollen dialysis sac is punctured, to allow the formalin to escape, and removed. Gentle mixing is then continued for about 12 hours or overnight.

6. The dark brown suspension produced is filtered through muslin to remove scum and debris. It is then washed five times with physiological saline or distilled water to remove the formalin. Once formalinized, the cells are difficult to resuspend after each centrifugation and gentle stirring with a glass rod is of assistance. Care should be taken to ensure that resuspension is complete before centrifugation after each washing.

7. Finally the cells are made up to about a 25 or 50 per cent suspension in physiological saline. A little formalin or thiomersal (see below) may be added as preservative and they are stored at 4° C. The exact concentration of the suspension should be determined in a haematocrit tube as from this must be

* Matburn Ltd, 20–24 Emerald Street, London, W.C.1.

calculated the volume of suspension which will contain the quantity of packed cells wanted for subsequent procedures.

Cells prepared in this manner are of normal shape, are not clumped, and are resistant to damage by distilled water or even ultrasonication. They do, however, retain most of the surface properties of the fresh cells and have been found to be suitable replacements for them in the tests to be described. A modification of the method which may be valuable is to adjust the pH of the formalin to about pH 5·5–6·0 with 1 N NaOH before use [1].

Other formalinization techniques which have been described are particularly useful if preservation is undertaken *after* a tanning or coating stage.

A. An 8 per cent suspension of cells in phosphate buffered saline at pH 7·2 is added to an equal volume of 3 per cent formaldehyde, well mixed and then gently agitated at 37° C for 18 hours. The preserved cells are washed five times and preserved as a 10 per cent suspension with thiomersal [12].

B. Formalin, previously neutralized with NaOH using phenolphthalein as indicator, is added to the cell suspension so as to give a final concentration of 3 per cent for sheep cells or 1 per cent for human cells. After gentle agitation for 20 hours at 37° C the cells are washed four times with distilled water before storage [87].

C. Merely pouring a 2 per cent suspension of the coated cells into buffered saline containing 20 per cent formalin may be adequate [29]. A better technique is very slowly to add 50 ml of formalin, over a period of 30 minutes or longer, from a burette to a suspension of 10 ml of packed cells in 500 ml of borate–succinate buffer, stirring being carried out continuously. The mixture is then left overnight at 4° C before another 50 ml of formalin is added in one lot. Twenty-four hours later the preserved cells are washed several times before being stored at 4° C in the presence of 0·2 per cent of formalin [32, 88].

Some authors have taken great care to eliminate all traces of formalin by extensive washing and chemical treatment [55]. If it is considered that this is necessary, residual formaldehyde may be tested for by adding 1·5 ml of concentrated sulphuric acid to 1·0 ml of the washing water and then a few crystals of chromotrophic acid. The development of a violet-pink colour indicates the presence of formaldehyde [77].

Formalinized cells may be kept for some weeks or months at 4° C before use without deterioration even if they have been very well washed [91]. The development of slight distortion and crenellation has been found to have no deleterious effect on sensitization [12]. However, bacterial action develops sooner or later, leading to clumping or destruction of the cells [73]. It is therefore preferable either to keep them deep frozen in volumes suitable for subsequent use [33] or to add 0·2 per cent formalin [30] or 1 : 10,000 thiomersal [12, 77] as a preservative.

AA

Packed fresh cells can readily be drawn up into a pipette for measurement, but a different technique must be employed with formalinized cells as they settle to a very compact mass. A suspension of known concentration, as determined by haematocrit, is therefore prepared and quantities sufficient to give the required volume of packed cells withdrawn from it. It is of course essential to ensure that a complete resuspension of the cells has been made before the sample is removed.

Final storage after coating may be at 4° C, deep frozen at −20° C, or in the freeze-dried state, though the first may safely be used for short periods only, unless a preservative is added. If the cells are to be frozen, this is best done by quick freezing small vials of them in a dry-ice and acetone bath. The vials should not be placed directly in a deep-freeze cabinet because the gradual development of ice crystals combined with sedimentation leads to gross clumping of the cells along the crystal planes. On thawing, such cells have to be very violently agitated or even subjected to a short period of ultrasonication before an even suspension for use can be obtained [41].

Though it is unnecessary to have any freezing protectant, such as glycerol [24], present; the final storage temperature may be important. Some highly purified protein coatings such as chromatographically prepared ovalbumin are stable for years at ordinary deep-freeze temperatures (−20° C). Other substances such as human γ globulin lose their activity in 6–9 months at this temperature [42]. When a serum stabilizer is present in the final suspension, it is important to realize that the material will not be completely frozen at −20° C [37]. It is therefore preferable to preserve the cells at a lower temperature such as −30° C or by storage in a dry ice cabinet. The dehydrating effect of complete freezing can be observed with formalinized cells which are of a salmon-pink colour at −70° C or when dried on filter paper, but at −20° C retain their normal dull brown colour as at room temperature.

To enhance stability and portability the coated cells may also be lyophillized in their ready-to-use state, being reconstituted with distilled water for use. The settling patterns produced by dried cells are, however, not always as satisfactory as those obtained with frozen cells.

Simple adsorption of antigen by red cells

Many polysaccharides will coat cells in a simple fashion so that they are immediately reactive to antibody. However, it is thought that the presence of a fatty acid portion is necessary for this to occur [86] and there may be some evidence for this in the effective way in which the lipopolysaccharides of Gram-negative bacteria are able to coat cells.

Very simple methods are usually satisfactory for the coating procedure, the antigen being merely incubated with washed fresh or formalinized cells. There is often a direct relationship between the sensitivity of the resultant cells to antibody, the concentration of antigen used, and the time of exposure of the cells to it [51], but the temperature at which the reaction is carried out does not appear to be critical [51].

In the case of the bacteria, Neter [59] gives a useful list of those species from which coating antigens have been extracted. In some cases it has been possible to differentiate between antibodies raised against a number of different antigens of a micro-organism (e.g. *Coxiella burnetii*) in that some of the antigens can be coated directly on cells whilst others are nonreactive unless the cells have first been tanned [3].

Methods

A. *Bacterial antigens*

The overnight growth from three plates inoculated with *Escherichia coli* is suspended in 10 ml of physiological saline. The antigens are then extracted by steaming the mixture for 1 hour. To the supernate after centrifugation are added fresh red cells so as to give a 2·5 per cent suspension. The mixture is then incubated at 37° C for 1 hour before the cells are washed three times and made up for use as a 1 per cent suspension [33, 60, 61, 89]. Both fresh and formalinized cells can be coated simultaneously or sequentially with up to ten separate antigens of this type, and they are found to react specifically with antibodies raised against each of them [33]. The test is carried out in perspex agglutination plates, the antiserum being diluted by twofold steps in 0·1 ml volumes of physiological saline. To each well is added 0·1 ml of the cell suspension, the plate is then left undisturbed for 2 hours, after which the end-point of the titration is determined by inspection of the settling patterns of the cells (for details of these see the tanned cell technique, below).

Fresh cells may similarly be coated with phenol extracts of *Pasteurella* spp. by incubating the mixture for 18 hours at 4° C [90]. Formalinized cells preserved by freezing can be used for this purpose and are particularly useful for the identification of the many serotypes [13].

'Old tuberculin' or extracts of tubercle bacilli are coated on cells by incubation with them at 37°C and pH 7·2 for 2 hours with agitation; 10 ml of the extract being mixed with 0·5 ml of packed cells [57].

The endotoxin (galactan) of *Mycoplasma mycoides* has been coated on formalinized cells by exposing a 5 per cent suspension of them to it at a concentration of 50 μg/ml for 3 hours at 4° C with continual agitation. A single following wash was then found to be sufficient to remove the excess antigen. The product was subsequently lyophilized [62].

B. *Viruses*

As with bacterial extracts, non-haemagglutinating viruses may become attached to red blood cells and they are then subject to agglutination by the appropriate antibody. Similar effects may also be seen with the residual particles of a haemagglutinating virus after it has eluted, or if it is used to coat the cells in sub-haemagglutinating doses [10, 11].

C. *Antibiotics*

Penicillin may be coated on cells by adding 8 ml of whole blood in Alsever's solution to a bottle containing 200,000 units of crystalline penicillin G. The mixture is then incubated at 37° C for 1 hour and washed three times with physiological saline before being used in the test [51]. It may perhaps be noted that, as with the antigens of *C. burnetii*, there appears to be a difference between the antibodies detected by cells to which penicillin is merely adsorbed and those to which it is firmly linked by a chemical bond [21].

D. *Proteins*

At least some proteins are directly adsorbed by fresh or formalinized cells.

Ovalbumin as a 0·25–1·0 per cent solution is incubated with a 1 in 6 suspension of sheep cells for 2 hours at 37° C. The coated cells may then be washed three times but remain fully sensitized [75]. Such cells may be used in both haemagglutination tests and, if complement is present, haemolysis tests for anti-ovalbumin antibody.

Formalinized chicken cells may be coated with either bovine serum albumin or ovalbumin by mixing 5 ml of a 2 per cent suspension of the cells with 5 ml of buffer containing 1 mg of the antigen. This is followed by constant mixing at room temperature for 4 hours. The cells are then washed three times and resuspended for use as a 1 per cent suspension in phosphate buffer at pH 7·2. To obtain the optimum results it is necessary, at the coating stage, to use an acetate buffer at pH 5·0 for the bovine serum albumin, and at pH 4·0 for the ovalbumin [43].

E. *Haptens*

Chemical groupings suitable for the detection of anti-dinitrophenyl antibodies and cross-reacting anti-picryl antibodies have been found to become directly attached to red cells without the necessity for a protein carrier of the hapten. Treatment of a 10 per cent suspension of the cells was carried out in an EDTA buffer pH 8·4 with 3 per cent 1,3-difluoro-2,4-dinitrobenzene. Haemagglutination tests carried out with such cells were found to equal passive cutaneous anaphylaxis in sensitivity [9]. The preparation of cells which will react with anti-phenylarsonic acid azo sheep serum has also been described, the cells being exposed for a few minutes to neutral diazotized arsanilic acid solution and subsequently well washed [44, 65].

The tanned cell technique

Though it is generally assumed that tannic acid acts on red cells in such a way as to cause them to take up protein antigens, this may not be its main function. Cells have been shown to adsorb such antigens and become agglutinable without the aid of tannic acid [43, 75] though the sensitivity of such preparations is usually low [42]. The quantity of protein antigen becoming attached to the cells is increased after they have been treated with tannic acid [74] but its chief function is, almost certainly, to increase the instability of the cells so making a normally non-agglutinating reaction result in agglutination [63]. The role of tannic acid may be analogous to that of some enzymes, for it has been observed that the red blood cells of cold-blooded animals may adsorb bacterial antigens but are not agglutinated by the homologous antibody unless they have been altered in some way by the action of proteolytic enzymes [60]. Such treatment may be carried out before or after coating whereas tanning is usually ineffective unless done before the coating stage [41]. Once treated with tannic acid at the right concentration, the red cells will show agglutination settling patterns. However, this tendency to agglutinate may be balanced by adding normal serum as a stabilizer [2] so that it is just cancelled out. The coated cells are thus in a very sensitive state ready to agglutinate in the presence of a very small quantity of antibody, hence the great sensitivity of the test.

Materials for the tanned cell test
Tannic acid
A good reagent grade of tannic acid should be used but there is little difference in effectiveness between the products of different manufacturers [6, 35, 74, 79, 84]. Even quite crude preparations may be found to be effective [91]. Though stock solutions for subsequent dilution can be prepared this is not recommended; it is preferable to make up the solution freshly each time that a batch of cells is to be prepared [6].

Buffers
The phosphate buffered saline described in the original paper of Boyden is a mixture of equal parts of 0·15 M buffer and physiological saline [7, 40]. This is usually satisfactory but occasionally difficulties have been traced to its use [41]. A reduction of the proportion of the buffer component to one part in ten of saline is preferable. Otherwise, a buffered saline (pH 7·2) may be prepared directly, thus:

NaCl	36·0 g
Na_2HPO_4 (anhydrous)	7·4 g
KH_2PO_4 (anhydrous)	2·15 g

These salts may be dissolved either in 5 litres of distilled water for immediate use or in 1 litre to make a stock solution of which portions are diluted down when required. The latter is easier to keep free of fungal and algal contamination without the necessity of adding a preservative. It is best stored at 4° C, or may be autoclaved, or kept frozen as aliquots.

With formalinized cells, a plain buffer of any reasonable molarity may be used as the cells are not susceptible to lysis. There would also appear to be scope here for experiment to determine the best conditions for coating such cells as they may have ion-exchange properties for which the usual physiological conditions may not be ideal.

Antigen

An important problem concerns the influence of mixed antigens in the coatings of tanned cells and the possibility that one antigen may mask another. Evidence from simple coating without tanning seems to indicate that many different antigens can be coated on a single cell and that it will react equally to each of them [34]. Mixed antigens have also been found to coat tanned cells which subsequently can be shown to be sensitive to each of them [41]. In some cases, however, the masking of a 'weak' antigen (bovine serum albumin or bovine γ globulin) by a 'strong' one such as a whole serum has been reported [50, 53]. This might perhaps be expected when the cell is exposed to such a great range of antigens as is contained in whole serum. However, when serum is used for stabilization it does not appear to mask the reactions of the cells.

A difficulty of this type of considerable practical importance is the suggestion that the slight contamination of ovalbumin by conalbumin, which usually occurs when the protein is prepared by the crystallization process, may lead to cells coated with the material being chiefly sensitized to the conalbumin rather than to the ovalbumin [6]. By using very highly purified materials it is, however, possible to show that cells so coated will respond in proportion as the two antibodies are present in the serum with which they are tested [92]. Conalbumin is a good antigen in the rabbit so that sera raised against crystalline ovalbumin may well contain an unexpectedly large component of anti-conalbumin as well as anti-ovalbumin and this may lead to anomalous results in the tests. Effects of this type are of great importance with a test having the sensitivity of the tanned cell technique. Every possible precaution must be taken as it could be all too easy to measure an antibody–antigen system other than that intended [70].

The preparation of antigens of very high purity is often laborious and difficult, but the test often shows a much greater sensitivity with highly purified than with crude materials [84, 85]. This may be only a concentration effect but in some cases the test has only been found to work at all if an adequately purified antigen is used [27]. Where the antigen has been obtained commercially, marked differences in sensitizing ability have sometimes been found between the products of different manufacturers [48].

The physical state of the antigen appears to have an influence on its ability to coat cells. A solution of ovalbumin from which all aggregated particles had been removed by centrifugation was found not to coat cells until it had been denatured with urea [34]. Very pure preparations of ovalbumin have also been found to have a poor coating ability which may be related to their freedom from denatured material [75]. Even in simple coating procedures, good sensitivity may only be obtained if the antigen is in an aggregated or partially denatured form [14, 23] and the same appears to apply to the tanned cell technique [76]. It has been suggested that positively charged groups on the antigen are necessary to enable it to coat the cells, and that denatured materials have more such groups [56]. When an antigen appears to be non-reactive in the test it may therefore be worth while to consider gentle denaturation with urea [34], or heat, or even freezing and thawing [22]. Excessive measures to remove turbidity in an antigen solution may also be inappropriate.

Finally it must be remembered that some antigens may themselves contain agglutinins for the cells being coated and it is necessary to remove these before the coating procedure is carried out [40]. An absorption stage employing 1 volume of packed cells to 4 volumes of antigen solution, leaving the mixture at room temperature for 1 hour, may be sufficient for this. With some materials, particularly toxins and toxoids, it has been found that non-specific agglutinins can be removed by simple dialysis [29].

Stabilizer

To balance out the agglutinating effect of the tannic acid, the stabilizer commonly used in the final washes and suspending fluid is normal rabbit serum [7, 26, 34]. This is inactivated and well absorbed with the cells being used and is employed as a 1 per cent addition to phosphate buffered saline; lower concentrations may, however, be effective [35]. Other sera used for the purpose have been: that from the same species of animal as the cells used [54], 1 per cent horse serum [29], 0·2 per cent human serum [39], and 0·4 per cent guinea-pig serum [78]. Derivatives of serum such as bovine serum albumin at a concentration of 0·125 per cent [83], and bovine γ globulin [79], have also been used, as have also other protein solutions such as gelatin [79]. Polyvinylpyrrolidone is also an effective stabilizer used at a dilution of 0·35 per cent [6]. It is evident that the protein stabilizers themselves become attached to the cells, the amount adsorbed being directly related to the concentration used. This is not affected by the quantity of protein in the active coating [74], and is presumed not to affect its activity.

Methods of preparing cells for the tanned cell test

Despite the difficulties which some experimenters have found, the technique of preparing tanned cells is simple and the conditions can be varied within quite wide limits whilst still obtaining a product which is sensitive to antibody. For the maximum sensitivity it is, however, sometimes necessary to test out all the possible variations that can be introduced at each stage of the test. When it is intended to use the test to detect antibodies to complex or unusual antigens, those unfamiliar with it would be well advised to try out the technique first with some simple antigen such as ovalbumin or bovine serum albumin and the appropriate antiserum.

Before discussing each step in the technique, a suggested method will be detailed. This has been designed for use with 1 oz (28 ml) screw-cap 'McCartney' bottles [17] and a bench centrifuge. Bottles are particularly convenient containers as they can be stood on the bench during the many manipulations rather than having to be held in a rack, and the caps make a safe seal. The method below gives a yield of 50 ml of cell suspension ready for use in the test. Larger bottles are therefore needed for the final suspension, but if a small quantity will suffice, the quantities can be halved and the final suspension made up to fill the bottles which have been used throughout.

Materials required:

Sheep blood in Alsever's solution or defibrinated, or formalinized cells in suspension.

Physiological saline.

Phosphate buffered saline, pH 7·2 (PBS).

Tannic acid solution, 5 mg in 50 ml PBS.

Antigen solution.

Normal rabbit serum, inactivated and absorbed twice with a quarter of its volume of packed cells from the same batch as those being coated.

Two 1 oz screw-cap bottles, two 50 or 100 ml bottles.

Graduated 1 and 10 ml pipettes, Pasteur pipettes, and a 100 ml cylindrical measure.

Method employed:

1. (a) Fresh cells are washed* three times with physiological saline or PBS and then packed at 750 g for 15 minutes; 0·6 ml of the packed cells are pipetted into each of two 1 oz bottles and suspended in 10 ml of PBS. (b) If formalinized cells are to be used, the calculated volume of the stock suspension

---

* 'Washing' is carried out by sedimenting the cells by centrifugation at about 750 g for 5–10 minutes preferably at 4° C, removing the supernate and resuspending in fresh saline. It will be found convenient to have a Pasteur pipette attached to a filter pump for the removal of supernate from the fresh cells. Formalinized cells usually sediment to a pellet so firm that the supernate can safely be poured off.

which will contain 0·6 ml of packed cells is measured into each of two 1 oz bottles. If no preservative is present the bottles are centrifuged once, the supernate removed, and cells in each resuspended to 10 ml with PBS. Otherwise the cells are washed twice with PBS before being made up to 10 ml.

(Note: A starting volume of 0·6 ml rather than 0·5 ml of packed cells is used to allow for loss of cells during the many washing processes necessary during the preparation of the sensitized cells.)

2. Ten millilitres of the tannic acid solution are added to the cell suspension in each bottle and the contents of each is well mixed. The bottles are then incubated for 15 minutes at 37° C in a water-bath.

3. Both bottles are centrifuged for 5 minutes at 750 *g* to bring down the cells, the supernate is removed and the cells resuspended and washed once with about 20 ml of PBS. Finally they are resuspended* in 10 ml of PBS in each bottle. (With some antigens it may be necessary at this stage to resuspend the cells in buffered saline of pH other than 7·2 but this will be found satisfactory for most simple proteins.)

4. One bottle is set aside; this will provide uncoated cells for controls and absorptions. To the other is added 10 ml of PBS containing the antigen (say 20 mg of ovalbumin or bovine serum albumin). After gentle mixing, this bottle is incubated at 37° C for 30 minutes in a water-bath. The bottle should be shaken gently once or twice during this period.

5. The cells in both bottles are spun down, the volume in the bottle of control cells having been made up to 20 ml with PBS in order to balance the centrifuge. After removal of the supernate, the content of each bottle is resuspended in 20 ml of PBS containing 1 per cent of inactivated and absorbed normal rabbit serum. The cells are washed three times with this serum-saline before the content of each bottle is resuspended to 50 ml with the same serum-saline to give a 1 per cent suspension ready for use in the test. If formalinized cells have been used, it is possible to carry out the washes and make up the final 1 per cent suspension with PBS alone. The correct quantity of normal rabbit serum for adequate stabilization is then determined by titration and added to the bulk suspension.

Many variations of the technique are reported in the literature, some of which are supported by comparative experimental data.

Tanning

The concentration of the tannic acid used is of the first importance; other things being equal, the greater the quantity of tannic acid used (within limits) the greater the sensitivity of the cells produced [91]. However, the cells must

---

* It will be found much easier to resuspend the fresh cells evenly after centrifugation and removal of the supernate if only 1–2 ml of PBS is introduced into the bottle at first and the cells are gently resuspended in this. The volume is then made up as required.

AA*

not be made so agglutinable that they cannot be stabilized. It is normal to arrange that the cells as a 1·0 or 1·5 per cent suspension are exposed to a 1 : 40,000 dilution of the tannic acid [1, 6, 32, 34, 79], though lower concentrations have sometimes been found to be effective [8, 39]. Some batches of cells are abnormally sensitive to the action of tannic acid. If difficulty is found with panagglutination it may therefore be advisable to carry out tests with several different concentrations of tannic acid, changing only this item in the method described [73]. If a 10 per cent cell suspension is to be tanned, tannic acid at a concentration of 1 : 5000 may be required [77], whilst to obtain adequate tanning of a 50 per cent suspension the author found it necessary to employ an equal volume of 1 : 300 tannic acid [91].

There appears to be universal agreement that the reaction should be carried out at pH 7·2, the only modification proposed being that the pH of the tannic acid solution itself be adjusted to that figure with 1 N sodium carbonate [39].

Tanning is usually carried out at 37° C [34, 39, 79] but appears to be effective in the cold [74] or at room temperature [8].

A period of about 10 minutes has been considered sufficient for the reaction and there is evidence that it is completed very rapidly, increased time of exposure having no effect on the sensitivity of the cells produced [91].

After tanning, a single wash has been found by all workers to be sufficient to remove any excess reagent. The tanned cells may be kept for several days before being coated if this is necessary [54, 79] and formalinized tanned cells can be preserved for months without deterioration [41].

Coating

There is good evidence that only a very small proportion, less than 1 per cent, of the antigen available is taken up by the cells [54, 70], however, the quantity adsorbed appears to be dependent on the amount present. It is known that a single antigen solution may sometimes be repeatedly used to coat batches of cells without losing its activity.

A series of tanned cell suspensions (2 per cent) exposed to ovalbumin in solutions containing from 0·2 to 8·0 mg/ml of antigen have been found to be equally sensitive to antibody [91], and it is commonly found that satisfactory sensitization is obtained over a wide range of antigen concentrations. On the other hand, an excess of antigen has been reported to cause non-specific panagglutination [39, 79, 83]. It may therefore be necessary to test dilutions of antigen if this trouble is encountered, and in many cases it will be found necessary specifically to determine the optimum concentration of antigen to be used in the system being examined. The following figures may be of assistance as base lines. They are for final cell suspensions (i.e. after addition of the antigen solution) of 1–2 per cent.

Ovalbumin	0·0125–5·0 mg/ml	[79, 82]
Bovine serum albumin	0·04–25·0 mg/ml	[4, 54]
Thyroglobulin	2·0 mg/ml	[32]
Bence-Jones proteins and antibody fragments	1·0 mg/ml	[23]
Tissue antigens	20 μg protein N/ml	[5]
Helminth antigens	0·6–9·0 μg protein N/ml	[47]

In many cases, particularly where complex antigens such as those extracted from *Toxoplasma* or trypanosomes have been used [77], no attempt to quantitate the antigen has been made. However, from general experience and from the figures given above it appears that as long as a reasonable amount of antigen is available the failure of the reaction is unlikely to be traced to this part of the process.

Following Boyden's original recommendation it has been usual to carry out the coating process at pH 6·4 whereas the other processes are carried out at pH 7·2 [7]. Tests have shown that no sensitization is obtained with herpes simplex virus if coating is carried out above pH 6·4 [26], but in the case of antigens extracted from tissues there was a great increase in sensitivity as the pH was raised from 5 to 8 [5]. With certain plant viruses the optimum pH was found to be 5·0 [68]. However, simple proteins such as ovalbumin, human γ globulin, and human serum albumin, appear to be effectively coated on the cells over the whole pH range 4·8–8·0 [91, 74].

It is usual to coat the cells at room temperature [6, 34, 79] but coating at 4° C is also effective [1] and batches of cells coated with ovalbumin at 20°, 37°, or 56° C have been found to have identical sensitivities [91].

Most of the antigen appears to be adsorbed by the cells as soon as they are exposed to it and only a further 25 per cent is adsorbed if the time of exposure is prolonged to 30 minutes [74]. Cells coated with ovalbumin over a period of 64 minutes were found to be only very slightly more sensitive to antibody than those exposed for 1 minute [91]. Herpes simplex virus, however, was found to require an exposure of at least 10 minutes for effective coating [26]. The usual practice of incubating the mixture of tanned cells and antigen for between 10 and 30 minutes seems, therefore, to be fully adequate [6, 34, 77, 79].

Though some workers have washed the cells only once after coating [77, 79], most have found it necessary to do this at least three times completely to eliminate free antigen [4]. Elution of antigen from the washed tanned cells may occur and this may increase with time if the cells are stored [25]. One worker has overcome the problem by storing formalinized, tanned, and *Echinococcus*-antigen coated cells in the antigen solution itself. They are washed several times immediately before use [1]. The pH of the washing and suspending saline is usually 7·2, but on occasion it may be more satisfactory to use a lower value than this; pH 5·7–6·0 has been found optimal for diphtheria-antigen coated cells [27].

The preparation of large quantities of cells

In many experiments it is convenient to prepare a single large batch of cells at one time. These are then preserved in aliquots so that cells of a standard sensitivity are available when required. To overcome the difficulty of manipulating large volumes, the following method may be found useful. This is for the preparation of 500 ml of a 1 per cent suspension of formalinized sheep cells, tanned and coated with ovalbumin, and is carried out in 1 oz (28 ml) glass bottles with screw caps.

1. A 1 oz bottle is marked at the 12 ml level. Formalinized cell suspension equivalent to 6 ml of packed cells is then measured into it and centrifuged down to form a thick pellet (5 minutes at 750 *g*). In subsequent washes it is necessary to stir this pellet gently with a thin glass rod to ensure adequate resuspension. If a preservative has been used with the cells, they should be washed three times before use. When ready, sufficient phosphate buffered saline at pH 7·2 (PBS) is added to the pellet to fill the bottle to the 12 ml mark and the cells are very carefully and fully resuspended in this.

2. Forty milligrammes of tannic acid are dissolved in 12 ml of PBS and the solution added to the cell suspension. As the tanning action takes place almost instantaneously it is most important that this addition be done very quickly and the whole bottle be vigorously shaken at once, stoppered only by a finger. Any delay will result in uneven tanning and failure of the method. The bottle is then incubated at room temperature for 15 minutes with frequent agitation. This is best carried out by clipping it to a Matburn blood cell suspension mixer.

3. After tanning, the cells are sedimented by centrifugation and washed once with enough PBS to fill the bottle. They are then resuspended again to the 12 ml mark with PBS.

4. Twenty milligrames of ovalbumin are dissolved in 12 ml of PBS, the solution added to the cell suspension and the whole well mixed. The bottle is then gently agitated (on the Matburn mixer) for 45 minutes at room temperature.

5. After centrifugation and removal of the antigen solution, the coated cells are washed three times with PBS. They are then made up to 500 ml of 1 per cent suspension in plain PBS and stored at 4° C whilst the following two tests are carried out.

(a) A doubling dilution series of inactivated and absorbed normal rabbit serum is made in 0·1 ml volumes in the wells of a perspex agglutination plate: 0·1 ml portions of the cell suspension are added to each well and, after mixing, the plate is left undisturbed at room temperature overnight. The highest dilution of serum which has brought the cells in the suspension down to a good negative button is noted. Sufficient serum to bring the whole 500 ml batch of cells to this dilution is then added to the suspension.

(b) To 10 ml of the suspension is added 0·1 ml of inactivated and absorbed normal rabbit serum. This stabilized suspension is then tested against a suitable anti-ovalbumin serum to check the activity and sensitivity of the cells.

6. On satisfactory completion of the tests the cells are evenly resuspended, distributed into suitable bottles, frozen by immersion in solid CO_2 and acetone, and stored at $-20°$ C.

The titration of antibody with tanned and coated cells

If high titred sera and tanned cells are mixed in test tubes, gross agglutination may be seen similar to that of a bacterial suspension in the Widal and similar tests. A test employing tanned cells has been described in which three drops of diluted serum are mixed with three drops of sensitized cells on a glass plate, the agglutination being read on gentle agitation after 10 minutes [82]. Observations of this type do not, however, exploit the sensitivity of the test to the full. If the cells are allowed to settle to the bottoms of test tubes or the wells of a plastic agglutination plate they exhibit agglutination patterns similar to those described for viral haemagglutination [69]. Agglutination is indicated by a complete carpet of cells covering the bottom of the tubes whereas non-agglutinated cells slide down to form a compact button or small ring at the centre of the curved tube bottom. In a doubling dilution series, a gradation between these two appearances usually occurs over three to four tubes. This is usually graded as $+++$ (an even carpet of cells) $++$, $+$, $\pm$, and $-$ (a negative button). The most consistent end-point $+$ being taken as an even carpet of cells with a slight ring at the edge [30]. Some experience is necessary to choose an unambiguous end-point appearance. It is helpful when carrying out a number of titrations simultaneously to inspect a number of the dilution rows for pattern effects before picking the end-point to be used and starting to record the results. It may be noted here that agglutinated cells can be completely and evenly resuspended after settling but show no agglomeration except where the antibody is highly concentrated [45]. The resuspended cells will settle again to patterns showing the same end-points.

The test is most conveniently carried out in the wells of plastic agglutination plates by adding 0·1 ml volumes of a 1 per cent suspension of sensitized cells to a doubling dilution series of the serum to be examined in 0·1 ml volumes of physiological saline. Sometimes, better results are obtained if the serum is diluted in a saline containing 1 per cent rabbit serum [6]. This is particularly necessary if the test is to be carried out in tubes and the dilutions are made in larger volumes, say 0·5 ml. In this case the sensitized cells are made up as a 2·5 per cent suspension and 0·05 ml of this is added to each serum dilution [79].

Heterophile agglutinins for the red cells must be removed from the sera being examined. This is conveniently done by making an initial 1 : 10 dropwise dilution of the serum with a 1 per cent suspension of uncoated tanned cells. The mixture is left on the bench for half an hour before the cells are removed by centrifugation and the dilution series made from the supernate. In some cases, it may be necessary to absorb a serum with a more concentrated cell suspension completely to remove these non-specific agglutinins. To confirm their removal a control consisting of serum at the initial dilution and tanned, but uncoated, cells is set up for each titration. Controls with coated and uncoated cells in saline alone are also prepared for each group of tests.

When fresh cells are used the test may be read after 2 hours, but it is usually necessary to allow formalinized cells to settle overnight. The plates may be left on the bench as other temperatures have not been found to affect the end-points [12, 73, 79]. The plates or tubes must, however, be carefully protected from disturbance or vibration such as that caused by a near-by centrifuge.

With some very high titred sera, as from hyperimmunized horses, prozones may be seen. Such antibodies may also be inefficient agglutinators showing much higher titres in the inhibition type of test than in straightforward agglutination [29, 70]. There have been suggestions that the patterns shown by the sedimented cells can be related to the presence of antibodies of different molecular size, IgG giving the normal even carpet of cells and IgM a collapsed appearance [4, 64]. It may also be noted that IgM has been shown to be about 750 times more efficient at agglutinating cells than IgG [38]. This may explain some of the reports of inconsistency between tanned cell titres and antibody estimations made by other methods, viz. complement fixation tests for *Haemonchus contortus* antigens [78], quantitative precipitation for anti-bovine γ globulin in early sera [67], co-precipitation for human thyroglobulin antibodies [32], and the neutralization of diphtheria antitoxin [71]. However, it is probable that many of these ambiguities arise because antibodies to different antigens are being measured [66].

Panagglutination

A common difficulty found with the tanned cell test is that the coated cells panagglutinate. The following suggestions may be considered if this occurs.

Use freshly diluted sera both in the test and as the stabilizer, and not sera which have been left standing without preservative even if at 4° C [45].

Ensure that the stabilizer used is completely free from agglutinins for the cells employed, as slight traces of these may build up on the cells during the repeated washing processes. Check that the cells are not abnormally sensitive to tannic acid or that the tannic acid used is not of a batch showing unusually strong agglutinating properties [73].

Ensure that the antigen is not present in excess [39, 79, 83] and does not contain agglutinins for the cells being coated. Check the pH of the final stabilizing solution and if necessary try other pH values for this [27, 35].

Finally, there is the suggestion that washing the cells, after tanning, with 0·1–1·0 per cent bovine serum albumin, and thereafter carrying on with the usual coating procedure, may be useful, particularly with antigens extracted from tissues [20].

The attachment of antigen to red cells by the agency of an intermediate compound

Bis-diazotized benzidine
This is a simple and effective way of attaching antigen to red cells by means of chemically stable covalent azo bonds which was originally devised by Pressman, Campbell & Pauling [65]. Fresh cells may be used but they are rather susceptible to haemolysis after treatment; it is therefore preferable to use formalinized material. The method is to prepare the benzidine compound (BDB) first and store it at $-20°$ to $-40°$ C for use as required. Coupling the antigen to the cells is then a simple matter of incubating cells, BDB, and antigen together for a short while and then washing the sensitized cells [12, 36, 65, 80].

Method: 1. *Preparation of BDB.* Dissolve 0·23 g of benzidine in 45 ml of 0·2 N HCl. Cool the mixture in an ice-bath. Dissolve 0·175 g of $NaNO_2$ in 5 ml of distilled water and cool similarly before adding this to the benzidine solution. This addition should be carried out over a period of about 1 minute with constant stirring.

Allow the reaction to proceed for 30 minutes in the ice-bath stirring every 5 minutes. The reagent is then pipetted, in 2 ml volumes, into clean ampoules. These are sealed whilst still immersed in the ice-bath and deep frozen in a bath of acetone and solid CO_2. The frozen material is stored at $-20°$ C.

2. *Sensitization of the cells.* To 3 ml of a solution of the antigen in phosphate buffered saline is added 0·1 ml of a 50 per cent suspension of washed fresh or formalinized cells. An ampoule of BDB is thawed out and immediately diluted as required in phosphate buffered saline pH 7·2 (see below). One millilitre of the diluted BDB is added to the antigen and cell suspension and the whole incubated at room temperature for 15 minutes. The mixture is

then centrifuged at 4° C, the supernate removed and the cells washed twice. Finally, they are made up to 5 ml of a 1 per cent suspension in saline containing 1 per cent of normal rabbit serum which has been inactivated and absorbed with the cells being sensitized.

It is necessary to carry out tests to determine the optimal ratio of BDB to antigen. Where the antigen solution contained 0·75 mg of ovalbumin, 0·03 ml of BDB (i.e. 1 ml of a 1 : 30 dilution of the ampouled solution) was found suitable [12]. A similar quantity effectively coupled 2·25 mg of pollen antigen [36].

Though the test may be carried out, as with the tanned cell technique, using 0·1 ml volumes of serum in the wells of a plastic plate to which 0·1 ml volumes of a 1 per cent suspension of sensitized cells is added, some authors have used other proportions. The serum is diluted in tubes in either 0·5 or 0·8 ml volumes of saline containing 1 per cent of normal rabbit serum, and 0·05 ml volumes of a 2 per cent sensitized cell suspension added. In all cases the end-point is determined by inspection of the settling patterns of the cells.

Fresh cells sensitized in this manner do not keep long and it is necessary to use them within a few hours of preparation [21], the test itself being read 6–12 hours later.

Sera to be tested should be absorbed with uncoated cells to remove nonspecific agglutinins. Controls are set up with sensitized and unsensitized cells in saline, and with unsensitized cells in serum at the starting dilution.

Formalinized cells appear to be most useful for this technique as they can be preserved after coating and can be coated more effectively with antigen. This is because relatively more BDB can be used without making the cells too fragile and the sensitivity of the test appears to be in part related to the quantity of antigen that can be attached to the cells. This in turn is related to the quantity of BDB employed rather than to the antigen concentration [12] in contrast to the tanned cell technique where the amount of antigen adsorbed is related to the quantity of antigen present [58].

Chromic chloride

Jandl & Simmons [46] have reported a method of coupling proteins to red cells by the use of metallic cations. They found the most useful of these to be chromium, and tests based on their method have been used to measure antibodies to several of the commonly used protein antigens [28].

Method. To 0·5 ml of a 50 per cent suspension of chicken or human red cells is added 1 ml of a 2·5 μM solution of $CrCl_3$ and 2·5 ml of a 1 per cent solution of bovine γ globulin. The solutions are mixed rapidly and allowed to stand at room temperature for 1 hour. The cells are then washed six times with physiological saline before finally being made up to 20 ml of a 1 per cent suspension with saline. Tube, rather than settling pattern agglutination tests are carried out with this reagent.

Ovalbumin can similarly be coated on cells using a 10 per cent ovalbumin solution and 15 μM $CrCl_3$. Physiological saline is used as the vehicle for all the reagents and defibrinated blood is employed [46].

Difluorodinitrobenzene

Ling [52] has used difluorodinitrobenzene (DFDNB) as a coupling agent.

Method. Two grammes of 1,3-difluoro-4,6-dinitrobenzene are dissolved in 100 ml of acetone. The solution is stored in a glass-stoppered bottle at 4° C and renewed weekly.

All other manipulations are carried out in an EDTA buffer. This is prepared by dissolving 17 g of EDTA in distilled water, bringing the pH to 8·4 or 7·5 with 2 N NaOH and making the whole up to 1 litre. An equal volume of physiological saline is then added.

To 1 ml of the buffer at pH 8·4 containing 0·015 ml of the DFDNB solution is added 0·5 ml of a 10 per cent suspension of human red cells. This mixture is incubated for 30 minutes at room temperature after which the cells are centrifuged down and the supernate discarded. The cells are then resuspended in 1 ml of buffer at pH 8·4 and 10 mg of purified protein antigen added. The mixture is incubated at 37° C for 1 hour, before the cells are washed three times with pH 7·5 buffer and finally resuspended to 20 ml in the same buffer. Sera to be tested are first absorbed with cells which have been treated with DFDNB but not coated. They are then diluted in 0·25 ml volumes in the wells of a perspex plate and an equal volume of the cell suspension added to each dilution. The end-points are read by the pattern method.

Fulthorpe, Parke, Tovey & Monckton [31] have used this method to coat formalinized cells with human chorionic gonadotrophin.

One litre of a 1 per cent suspension of formalinized cells in EDTA buffer is warmed to 37° C before the addition of 5 ml of 2 per cent DFDNB in dioxane. The mixture is incubated at 37° C for 30 minutes with stirring before the cells are brought down by centrifugation and the supernate removed. The cells are then resuspended in 200 ml of the EDTA buffer (giving a 5 per cent suspension) and to this is added 3500 units of human chorionic gonadotrophin in 3 ml of the buffer. After further incubation at 37° C for 90 minutes the cells are washed three times with a borate succinate buffer and stored as a 10 per cent suspension with 5 g of sucrose and 10 ml of normal rabit serum.

The sensitized cells were used by Fulthorpe *et al* in an inhibition test to detect the presence of the hormone. To this end they were diluted to 1 per cent, agglutinated with the appropriate antiserum, and then freeze dried. A modification of the method involved the formalinization of the cells in the presence of 0·15 per cent hydroquinone. The cells then appear to have been able to adsorb the hormone without further treatment [31].

Antibody

Coombs & Fiset [15] have described a method of coupling antigen (ovalbumin) to sheep red cells by means of antibody to the Forssman antigen. An anti-Forssman serum was prepared by inoculating rabbits with fowl red cells. The globulins were separated from the serum by half saturation with ammonium sulphate. This antibody was then photo-oxidized by the agency of eosin Y in an atmosphere of oxygen and very strong lighting, so making it non-agglutinating but still capable of attachment to sheep red cells. The product was coupled to ovalbumin by means of bis-diazotized benzidine. The resultant 'photo-oxidized globulin sheep cell antibody azo-benzidine-azo ovalbumin' could be stored for long periods at $-20°$ C and be used to sensitize sheep cells at will. This was carried out by mixing the reagent with them, incubating at $37°$ C and subsequently washing twice. The sensitized cells could be directly agglutinated by the anti-ovalbumin in some human sera, whilst the further addition of Coombs' anti-globulin serum showed the presence of 'incomplete' antibodies in others.

Steele & Coombs [81] later modified the method. They tested various dyes in the photo-oxidation process, finding that 0·1 per cent rose bengal was the most suitable, and they simplified the method, carrying it out by exposure to a good north light. An anti-whole red cell serum was used in place of the anti-Forssman antibody. It was also found that the antigen would quite simply become attached to the antibody during the photo-oxidation process, thus cutting out a step and so making the whole technique very simple. Coombs, Howard & Wild [16] have also described a method by which antigen may be attached to human Rh + cells by the agency of incomplete Rh antibody.

References

[1] ALLAIN, DOROTHY S. & KAGAN I.G. (1961) The use of formalinized red cells in the serology of hydatid disease. *J. Parasit.* **47,** 61

[2] ATKIN E.E. (1909) Spontaneous agglutination of horse erythrocytes suspended in sodium chloride solution. *Z. ImmunForsch.* **1,** 387

[3] BAKEMEIER R.F. (1965) A study of phase variation in *Coxiella burnetii* employing hemagglutination tests. *J. Immunol.* **95,** 880

[4] BENEDICT A.A., BROWN R.J. & AYENGAR R. (1962) Physical properties of antibody to bovine serum albumin as demonstrated by hemagglutination. *J. exp. Med.* **115,** 195

[5] BJÖRKLUND B. & PAULSSON J.E. (1962) Studies of hemagglutination as a means for assay of malignant and normal human tissue antigens. *J. Immunol.* **89,** 759

[6] BORDUAS A.G. & GRABAR P. (1953) L'hemagglutination passive dans la recherché des anticorps antiprotéiniques. *Ann. Inst. Pasteur* **84,** 903

[7] BOYDEN S.V. (1951) The adsorption of proteins on erythrocytes treated with tannic acid, and subsequent hemagglutination with antiprotein sera. *J. exp. Med.* **93,** 107

[8] BOYDEN S.V. & SORKIN E. (1955) A study of antigens active in the tannic acid hemagglutination test present in filtrates of culture of *Mycobacterium tuberculosis. J. Immunol.* **75,** 15

[9] BULLOCK W.E. & KANTOR F.S. (1965) Hemagglutination reactions of human erythrocytes conjugated covalently with dinitrophenyl groups. *J. Immunol.* **94,** 317

[10] BURNET F.M. (1946) Modification of human red cells by virus action. III. A sensitive test for mumps antibody in human serum by the agglutination of human red cells coated with a virus antigen. *Brit. J. exp. Path.* **27,** 244

[11] BURNET F.M. & ANDERSON S.G. (1946) Modification of human red cells by virus action. II. Agglutination of modified human red cells by sera from cases of infectious mononucleosis. *Brit. J. exp. Path.* **27,** 236

[12] BUTLER W.T. (1963) Hemagglutination studies with formalinized erythrocytes. Effect of bis-diazo-benzidine and tannic acid treatment on sensitization by soluble antigen. *J. Immunol.* **90,** 663

[13] CARTER G.R. & RAPPAY D.E. (1962) Formalinized erythrocytes in the haemagglutination test for typing *Pasteurella multocida. Brit. vet. J.* **118,** 289

[14] CHRISTIAN C.L. (1958) Characterization of the 'reactant' (gamma globulin factor) in the F II precipitin reaction and the F II tanned sheep cell agglutination test. *J. exp. Med.* **108,** 139

[15] COOMBS R.R.A. & FISET M.L. (1954) Detection of complete and incomplete antibodies to egg albumin by means of a sheep red cell-egg albumin antigen unit. *Brit. J. exp. Path.* **35,** 472

[16] COOMBS R.R.A., HOWARD A.N. & WILD F. (1952) Titration of antisera to soluble proteins on the basis of an agglutination reaction: Conjugation of egg albumin and chicken serum globulin to the incomplete Rh antibody and the subsequent use of Rh-positive cells, sensitized by such conjugated incomplete antibodies, to titrate antisera against egg albumin and chicken globulin. *Brit. J. exp. Path.* **33,** 390

[17] CRUICKSHANK R. (1965) *Medical Microbiology,* 11th ed., p. 723. Edinburgh: Livingstone

[18] CSIZMAS L. (1960) Preparation of formalinized erythrocytes. *Proc. Soc. exp. Biol., N.Y.* **103,** 157

[19] CUA-LIM F., RICHTER M. & ROSE B. (1963) The reversed BDB technique. The agglutination of antibody coated red cells by homologous antigen. *J. Allergy* **34,** 142

[20] EIDINGER D. (1964) A modified tanned cell haemagglutination procedure for the study of organ antigen–antibody systems. *Nature, Lond.* **201,** 1046

[21] EPP M. (1962) Penicillin antibody in maternal and cord bloods and its possible relationship to hypersensitivity. *Immunology* **5,** 287

[22] EPSTEIN W.V. (1961) Demonstration of serological specificity in the reaction of individual gamma globulins with rheumatoid factors by hemagglutination. *Proc. Soc. exp. Biol., N.Y.* **108,** 744

[23] EPSTEIN W.V. & GROSS D. (1964) Naturally occurring human antibody reacting with Bence Jones proteins. *J. exp. Med.* **120,** 733

[24] FAHEY J.L. & HUMPHREY J.H. (1962) Antibodies with differing molecular sizes in mice. *Immunology* **5,** 104

[25] FEINBERG R.J. & FLICK J.A. (1957) Elution of pollen antigens from tannic acid treated erythrocytes. *Proc. Soc. exp. Biol., N.Y.* **96,** 71

[26] FELTON, FRANCES G. & SCOTT L.V. (1961) Studies on hemagglutination with herpes simplex virus. II. The factors involved in the technique. *J. Immunol.* **86,** 42

[27] FISHER S. (1952) The estimation *in vitro* of small amounts of diphtheria antitoxin by means of a haemagglutination technique. *J. Hyg. Camb.* **50,** 445

[28] FUDENBERG H.H., DREWS, GENEVIEVE & NISONOFF A. (1964) Serologic demonstration of dual specificity of rabbit bivalent hybrid antibody. *J. exp. Med.* **119,** 151

[29] FULTHORPE A.J. (1957) Tetanus antitoxin titration by haemagglutination. *J. Hyg. Camb.* **55,** 382

[30] FULTHORPE A.J. (1962) Multiple diphtheria antigen–antibody systems investigated by passive haemagglutination techniques and other methods. *Immunology* **5,** 30

[31] FULTHORPE A.J., PARKE J.A.C., TOVY J.E. & MONCKTON J.C. (1963) Pregnancy diagnosis by a one-stage haemagglutination inhibition method. *Brit. med. J.* **i,** 1049

[32] FULTHORPE A.J., ROITT I.M., DONIACH D. & COUCHMAN K. (1961) A stable sheep cell preparation for detecting thyroglobulin auto-antibodies and its clinical applications. *J. clin. Path.* **14,** 654

[33] GANGULI L. (1966) Personal communication

[34] GEORGE, MARIAM & VAUGHAN J.H. (1962) Observations on the nature of the antigen in tanned red-cell hemagglutination. *J. Immunol.* **88,** 191

[35] GILL B.S. (1964) A procedure for the indirect haemagglutination test for the study of experimental *Trypanosoma evansi* infections. *Ann. trop. Med. Parasit.* **58,** 473

[36] GORDON J., ROSE B. & SEHON A.H. (1958) Detection of 'non precipitating' antibodies in sera of individuals allergic to ragweed pollen by an *in vitro* method. *J. exp. Med.* **108,** 37

[37] GREAVES R.I.N. (1965) Preservation of antigens and antibodies. *Fed. Proc.* **24,** S–253

[38] GREENBURY C.L., MOORE D.H. & NUNN L.A.C. (1963) Reaction of 7S and 19S components of immune rabbit antisera with human group A and AB red cells. *Immunology* **6,** 421

[39] HELLER G., JACOBSON A.S., KOLODNY M.H. & KAMMERER W.H. (1954) The hemagglutination test for rheumatoid arthritis. II. The influence of human plasma fraction II (gamma globulin) on the reaction. *J. Immunol.* **72,** 66

[40] HELLER G., JACOBSON A.S., KOLODNY M.H. & SCHUMAN R.L. (1952) The hemagglutination test for rheumatoid arthritis. I. An immunological analysis of the factors involved in the reaction. *J. Immunol.* **69,** 27

[41] HERBERT W.J. (1964) Studies on mineral oil antigen adjuvants. Thesis, University of Edinburgh

[42] HERBERT W.J. Unpublished observations

[43] HIRATA A.A. & STASHAK P.W. (1965) Simplified procedure for passive haemagglutination tests with protein antigens. *Nature, Lond.* **205,** 1233

[44] INGRAHAM J.S. (1952) Specific, complement-dependent hemolysis of sheep erythrocytes by antiserum to azo hapten groups. *J. infect. Dis.* **91,** 268

[45] INGRAHAM J.S. (1958) The preparation and use of formalinized erythrocytes with attached antigens or haptens to titrate antibodies. *Proc. Soc. exp. Biol., N.Y.* **99,** 452

[46] JANDL J.H. & SIMMONS R.L. (1957) The agglutination and sensitization of red cells by metallic cations: Interactions between multivalent metals and the red-cell membrane. *Brit. J. Haemat.* **3,** 19

[47] JUNG R.C. & PACHECO G. (1960) Use of a hemagglutination test in *visceral larva migrans. Amer. J. trop. Med.* **9,** 185

[48] LANDY M., TRAPANI R.J., FORMAL R. & KLUGLER I. (1955) Comparison of a haemagglutination procedure and the rabbit intradermal neutralization test for the assay of diphtheria anti-toxin in human sera. *Amer. J. Hyg.* **61,** 143

[49] LANG B.G. (1965) Personal communication

[50] LECOCQ E. & LINZ R. (1962) Agglutination d'hématies tannées traitées par deux antigènes. II. Traitements successifs par deux antigènes. *Ann. Inst. Pasteur* **102**, 437

[51] LEY A. B., HARRIS J.P., BRINKLEY M., LILES B., JACK J.A. & CAHAN A. (1958) Circulating antibody directed against penicillin. *Science* **127**, 1118

[52] LING N.R. (1961) The coupling of protein antigens to erythrocytes with difluorodinitrobenzene. *Immunology* **4**, 49

[53] LINZ R. & LECOCQ E. (1962) Agglutination d'hématies tannées traitées par deux antigènes. I. Hématies traitées par un mélange de deux antigènes. *Ann. Inst. Pasteur* **102**, 92

[54] LINZ R., LECOCQ E. & MANDELBAUM E. (1961) L'adsorption d'antigènes par des hématies tannées. *Ann. Inst. Pasteur* **101**, 367

[55] McKENNA J. (1957) A stable preparation of antigen sensitized erythrocytes. *Proc. Soc. exp. Biol., N.Y.* **95**, 591

[56] MAURER P.H., GERULAT B.F. & PINCHUCK P. (1963) Antigenicity of polypeptides (poly-α-amino acids). V. Studies in rabbits. *J. Immunol.* **90**, 381

[57] MIDDLEBROOK G. & DUBOS R.J. (1948) Specific serum agglutination of erythrocytes sensitized with extracts of tubercle bacilli. *J. exp. Med.* **88**, 521

[58] MÜLLER H.E. & GRAMLICH F. (1963) Über das Antigen-AntiKörper-Verhältnis bei der indirekten Hamagglutination mit Benzidintetrazotat behandelten und tannisierten Erythrozyten. *Z. ImmunForsch.* **125**, 199

[59] NETER E. (1956) Bacterial hemagglutination and hemolysis. *Bact. Rev.* **20**, 166

[60] NETER E., COHEN E., WESTPHAL O. & LÜDERITZ O. (1959) The effects of proteolytic enzymes on agglutination by bacterial antibodies of lipopolysaccharide modified erythrocytes. *J. Immunol.* **82**, 85

[61] NETER E., LEE F.B., ZAK D.A., MURDOCK M.R. & ARBESMAN C.E. (1952) Studies on hemagglutination and hemolysis by *Escherichia coli* antisera. *J. exp. Med.* **96**, 1

[62] PERREAU P., PROVOST A., REGNOULT R. & ORUE J. (1964) Valeur de la réaction d'hémagglutination indirecte dans la péripneumonie bovine. Emploi d'hématies formolees, sensibilisees et lyophilisees. *Rev. Elev.* **17**, 5

[63] PIROFSKY B., CORDOVA, MARIA & IMEL T.L. (1962) The function of proteolytic enzymes and tannic acid in inducing erythrocyte agglutination. *J. Immunol.* **89**, 767

[64] PORTER R.J. (1960) Studies on antibody formation. Effects of X-irradiation on adaptation for the secondary response of rabbits to bovine γ-globulin. *J. Immunol.* **84**, 485

[65] PRESSMAN D., CAMPBELL D.H. & PAULING L. (1942) The agglutination of intact azoerythrocytes by antisera homologous to the attached groups. *J. Immunol.* **44**, 101

[66] RICHTER M. (1964) Lack of correlation of antibody titres as determined by the precipitin and hemagglutination technique. *Acta allerg., Kbh.* **19**, 1

[67] ROSENBLATT E. & JOHNSON A.G. (1963) Size of antibody and role of autonomic nervous system in the adjuvant action of endotoxin. *Proc. Soc. exp. Biol., N.Y.* **113**, 156

[68] SAITO Y. & IWATA Y. (1964) Hemagglutination test for titration of a plant virus. *Virology* **22**, 426

[69] SALK J.E. (1944) A simplified procedure for titrating hemagglutinating capacity of influenza-virus and the corresponding antibody. *J. Immunol.* **49**, 87

[70] SCHEIBEL I. (1956) A comparative study on intracutaneous and haemagglutination procedures for assaying diphtheria antitoxin, with special reference to the avidity of the antitoxin. *Acta path. microbiol. scand.* **39**, 455

[71] SCHEIBEL I., BENTZON M.W., TULINIUS S. & BOJLEN K. (1962) Duration of immunity to diphtheria and tetanus after active immunization with mention of non-conformity between haemagglutinating and neutralizing diphtheria antitoxin titres in some human sera. *Acta path. microiol. scand.* **55**, 483

[72] SEGRE D. (1962) Detection of hog cholera virus by a hemagglutination test. *Amer. J. vet Res.* **23**, 748

[73] SEWELL M.M.H. (1966) Personal communication

[74] SHIOIRI K. (1964) The observation of proteins adsorbed on erythrocytes treated with tannic acid in passive hemagglutination tests (Boyden's method). *Jap. J. exp. Med.* **34**, 345

[75] SINDO T. & WAKAKURA K. (1952) Studies on the antigen–antibody reactions using crystalline ovalbumin as an antigen. With special reference to the possibility of hemagglutination, hemolysis tests without preliminary treatment of erythrocytes. *Jap. J. exp. Med.* **22**, 285

[76] SINGER J.M., ORESKES I. & ALTMANN G. (1962) The mechanism of particulate carrier reactions. IV. Adsorption of human γ globulin to tanned sheep erythrocytes and their sensitization for agglutination with rheumatoid arthritis serum *J. Immunol.* **89**, 227

[77] SMIT G.L. (1964) The use of formalin-preserved human erythrocytes in the toxoplasma haemagglutination test. *Trop. geogr. Med.* **16**, 152

[78] SOULSBY E.J.L. (1960) The use of the haemagglutination technique for the detection of antibodies in gastro-intestinal nematode infections of sheep. *Brit. vet. J.* **116**, 302

[79] STAVITSKY A.B. (1954) Micromethods for the study of proteins and antibodies. I. Procedure and general application of hemagglutination and hemagglutination inhibition reactions with tannic acid and protein treated red blood cells. *J. Immunol.* **72**, 360

[80] STAVITSKY A.B. & ARQUILLA E.R. (1955) Procedure and applications of hemagglutination inhibition reactions with bis-diazotized benzidine and protein-conjugated red blood cells. *J. Immunol.* **74**, 306

[81] STEELE A.S.V. & COOMBS R.R.A. (1964) The red cell linked antigen test for incomplete antibodies to soluble proteins. *Int. Arch. Allergy* **25**, 11

[82] STEFFEN C. & ROSAK M. (1963) *In vitro* demonstration of anti-ovalbumin specificity of lymph node cells in delayed type sensitivity. *J. Immunol.* **90**, 337

[83] STEIN B. & DESOWITZ R.S. (1964) The measurement of antibody in human malaria by a formolized tanned sheep cell haemagglutination test. *Bull. World Hlth. Org.* **30**, 45

[84] SURJÁN, MARGARET & NYERGES, GEORGETTE (1962) Haemagglutination procedure for the assay of tetanus antitoxin of children's sera. *Z. ImmunForsch.* **124**, 390

[85] SURJÁN, MARGARET & NYERGES, GEORGETTE (1962) Diphtheria antitoxin titration of human sera by haemagglutination. *Z. ImmunForsch.* **124**, 401

[86] TSUMITA T. & OHASHI M. (1964) A synthetic acyl polysaccharide and the hemagglutination activity. *J. exp. Med.* **119**, 1017

[87] WEINBACH R. (1958) Die verwendbarkeit formolbehandelter Erythrocyten als Antigenträger in der indirekten Haemagglutination. *Schweiz. Z. Path.* **21**, 1043

[88] WEIR D.M. (1962) Personal communication

[89] WHANG H.Y. & NETER E. (1963) Comparative study of latex agglutination and hemagglutination tests for demonstration of enterobacterial antibodies. *Amer. J. clin. Path.* **40**, 136

[90] WRIGHT G.G. & FEINBERG R.J. (1952) Hemagglutination by tularemia antisera: Further observations on agglutination of polysaccharide-treated erythrocytes and its inhibition by polysaccharide. *J. Immunol.* **68**, 65

[91] HERBERT, W.J. (1967) A study of factors influencing the sensitivity to antibody of tanned, ovalbumin coated, formalinized sheep red-cells. *Immunology* (in press)

[92] HERBERT, W.J. (1967) Ovalbumin, conalbumin, and the tanned red-cell agglutination test. *Immunology* (in press)

CHAPTER 22

Passive Cutaneous Anaphylaxis (PCA)

W.E.BROCKLEHURST

Introduction

This name and the prototype experimental procedure were introduced by Ovary in 1952 [1]. PCA is closely related to the P–K reaction of man, but as usually carried out may involve antibodies of both reaginic and other types. In the P–K test, both sensitizing and challenging substances are given intradermally at the same site. In PCA sensitization is produced by intradermal injection of antibody, but the antigen is given intravenously, so that it is presented simultaneously and uniformly to the whole sensitized area. The 'response' is the rapid occurrence of a marked increase in the permeability of capillaries to large molecules. This is demonstrated by the leakage of a blue dye into the tissue-space, which permits reproducible evaluation of the area and intensity of the reaction.

Dye is given at the same time as the antigen (or shortly before the intradermal injection of known permeability factors which may be used to establish a standard reponse in different animals). The dye must be of large molecular size, such as Evans blue, or have strong affinity for the plasma proteins so that it will be largely retained in the bloodstream except where the vessels are abnormally permeable. Protein markers include Coumassie blue, which gives very clear differentiation of the reaction because the normal skin is barely coloured, Pontamine sky blue (Chicago blue), which has been very widely used, but must be tested because some batches are not satisfactory, and Trypan blue, which is strongly electronegative and has some anti-inflammatory actions which may be undesirable.

Most work has been done in male albino guinea-pigs which react to very low doses of antibody, but rats have been extensively used, especially where the study has involved reactions initiated by drugs. Rabbits, mice and hamsters have also been employed. Monkeys have come into favour more recently because they can be sensitized with human IgA, and they can sometimes be used more than once, thus reducing the cost, provided that the skin is light-coloured and the PCA responses can be 'read' from the exterior.

Usually homologous antibody is the most active, and of course some heterologous antibodies are not compatible with the test species and do not cause sensitization.

Complications arise from the use of different classes of antibody globulin. For example, human reaginic antibody will sensitize the skin of primates but not that of the guinea-pig, whereas human γG is effective in both species. Furthermore, homologous γA is many times more active than homologous γG in the guinea-pig's skin. Much of the published work employed whole γ globulin, therefore any quantitative data reported (e.g. minimum amount of antibody-N to produce a response) is likely to be a gross overestimate. It is now evident that one cannot predict, from considerations of the amount of precipitable antibody present, what the sensitizing potency of a serum will be. The use of whole γ globulin has also resulted in disagreement about the pharmacology underlying the 'blueing' response, which may be expected to differ with antibody which activates complement, compared with that which does not.

The test

The following is a typical procedure. Purified antibody or serum containing antibody is diluted with Tyrode or mammalian Ringer solution so that the dose is contained in 0·05 ml or 0·1 ml. Doses are usually in the ratio 1 : 3 : 9 or 1 : 2 : 4 : (8), to give diameters of lesion which approximate a linear relationship. The doses are injected using a tuberculin syringe and a small needle at a site on the shaved abdomen previously marked indelibly, e.g. with a laundry-marking pencil. After 4 hours, antigen and dye are given together intravenously in the smallest practicable volume. Exactly 20 minutes later the animals are killed, and the skin opened, freed from the subcutaneous attachments and reflected so that the lesions can be evaluated. Measurements of both diameters and an assessment of intensity are usually made. This can be postponed until all the animals have been killed, but the delay is not advised and should not exceed 2 hours. The skin must not be allowed to dry; indeed, it is better to decapitate the animal and delay the dissection until quite ready to evaluate the lesions.

Since the reaction depends upon a good blood-flow in the skin it is most satisfactory in animals which are not anaesthetized and are not frightened or excited [2]. It is therefore essential that the intravenous injection should be performed quickly and skilfully without excessive restraint of the animal, and in monkeys it would seem reasonable to use animals under sedation. Warmth is obviously important; it will influence both the washing away of unbound antibody from the injection site, and the intensity of blue resulting from extravasation of plasma proteins during the anaphylactic reaction. Ideally the whole test should be conducted in a draught-free room, evenly heated to about 24° C.

Details of the test will depend on the nature of the experiment, the accuracy necessary, and the species used (see Appendix 1 for statistical methods applicable to skin-test data).

The syringes used for the intradermal injection must not leak even under heavy injection pressure. Plastic disposable tuberculin syringes are excellent in this respect, but the calibration at 0·05 ml must be checked. Glass tuberculin syringes must be tested for leaks both at the needle butt and past the piston. Needles with 'short bevel' points are made specially for intradermal injections, and are usually $\frac{1}{2}$ in. × 26 gauge. Normal or long bevel needles are more likely to lead to subcutaneous injections by puncturing the dermis. Miles has illustrated the correct depth of intradermal injection [2] and a useful criterion is that real pressure is needed to inject, and the bleb is clearly visible for at least 5 minutes. For the intravenous injection a 2 or 5 ml all-glass syringe is needed, depending on the size of the animal. The piston must be easy-moving so that there is no doubt that the needle is in the vein when the smallest pressure is applied. The needle must be very sharp and as large as is reasonable for each species. For guinea-pigs about $\frac{3}{4}$ in. × 22 gauge is satisfactory for the dorsal veins of the penis or the vein which runs on the dorsal surface of the hind foot between the metatarsals of the outer and middle toes. For injection into the ear an 'intradermal' needle is used, but this route is not recommended for doses of 1 ml or greater. The intracardiac route is difficult and uncertain quite apart from the effect on the animal.

For rats, a tail vein is the obvious choice, but it is easy to get into the sheath rather than the lumen of the vein unless it is distended by warming the tail under an infra-red lamp or in water at about 44° C for 1 or 2 minutes. An alternative site is a vein which runs diagonally across the thigh towards the base of the tail. In the mouse the tail is the best site. In rabbits the vein running along the rear margin of the outer skin of the ear is by far the most useful site, but as in all the larger animals there are plenty of veins more or less easily accessible.

The site and pattern of the antibody injections must take account of the thickness of the skin and its vascularity. The abdomen is the most satisfactory site in guinea-pigs because males fight and often have scarred backs, and because the skin of the abdomen is thinner, thus being easier to inject. The usual pattern is three injections equally spaced between the nipple and the costal margin on either side of the midline. If 'check' responses to histamine or bradykinin are needed, these can be placed more laterally or even above the costal margin. If eight or nine test reactions are needed, two or three doses may be placed in the midline with three doses either side, arranged to give the maximum available separation without spreading too far laterally on to the sides of the animal. Provided that enough material and animals are available, the site used for each dose should be randomized throughout the group of animals, e.g. six doses, six animals, each dose being located at a different site on each animal of the group.

When the potency of a sensitizing antibody is unknown a wider range of doses may seem useful, but the results are often misleading if the top dose is too large because this sometimes causes obvious symptoms of systemic anaphylaxis, resulting in reduced cutaneous blood-flow, and in any case tends to obscure and to diminish adjacent skin reactions. The highest dose should give lesions of 15 to 20 mm diameter, and the smallest about 5 mm diameter (i.e. about the size of the initial bleb caused by the injection). This difference is usually achieved with doses varying less than 10 : 1.

The delay of 4 hours between intradermal injection of antibody and intravenous antigen was originally chosen because at this time the lesion produced using rabbit antibody in guinea-pigs or rats was approaching maximum yet still retained clearly defined edges, and a relatively regular shape [1, 3]. Recently it has been found that at this time the response to IgA (guinea-pig antibody in guinea-pig) is not maximum although that to IgG is. Furthermore, the effect of IgG has disappeared at 24–36 hours when that of IgA is about maximum, and it is thus practicable to differentiate between the responses due to IgA and those due to IgG, by delaying the challenge [4]. This can of course be done in the same animal by giving the intradermal doses of antigen on two occasions at 24 hours interval so that challenge is at 28 and 4 hours respectively. Antibody is rapidly lost from the site in the rabbit, and it is usual to challenge only 30 minutes after injection in this species.

The dose of antigen for optimum reaction in PCA is much less critical [2, 4] than that for systemic anaphylaxis as established by Liacopoulos *et al* [5]. One may speculate that since the antigen must leave the bloodstream before it reacts with antibody on the cells, the concentration in the tissue spaces is unlikely to pass through the range of optimum proportions so quickly that it will fail to trigger the tissue reactions leading to the observed lesion. Whatever the reasons, the wide limits are fortunate for those who wish to use mixed antibodies, some of which may diminish the local concentration of antigen although they do not sensitize the skin, e.g. 19S antibody. The usual amount of antigen given has been about 10–20 mg/kg body weight for proteins of molecular weight about 10^5 (i.e. about 1 ml of 0·1 mM per kg) but if the antigen is in short supply, as little as 100 μg gives a satisfactory graded response [4]. It may be given as 1–10 per cent solution in 0·9 per cent sodium chloride.

Monovalent antigen (hapten) is ineffective in producing PCA, but if present at the time of challenge by the complete antigen, causes inhibition, presumably by continuing to occupy the antigen-combining sites of the antibody although the union is weak and impermanent.

The dose of dye must be chosen so that it gives strong coloration within the lesion but negligible colour elsewhere. Pontamine blue has been used in doses of 20–100 mg/kg body weight and is generally given as 2 or 5 per cent aqueous solution [1, 2, 3]. Coumassie blue is available (I.C.I.) as 2 per cent solution in ampoules for the determination of the circulation time in man, 10–20 mg/kg is suitable for PCA. Evans blue is used as a 2 per cent solution and the dose is 20–100 mg/kg [6]. Trypan blue 40 mg/kg as 1 per cent solution has been used mainly in experiments involving chemically induced lesions [7]. It has been extracted from the comminuted tissue with 25 per cent aqueous pyridine after defatting with ethanol. The amount of dye, determined in an absorptiometer, is taken as a measure of the reaction [8]. Although this procedure has the ring of scientific accuracy, it is time-consuming if properly done, and will lose information by giving equal values to a small but intense reaction and a large more diffuse one. A method for the extraction and evaluation of Evans blue has also been described [10].

Evaluation of the size of lesions is usually done with a transparent ruler against the trans-illuminated skin. Errors due to distortion (stretching) of the skin can be minimized if the site of the reaction is marked by a ring of known size at the time of the sensitizing injection. This can be done with the end of a piece of brass tube covered with quick-drying green stain (from a pad), applied to the unstretched skin and gently rotated to give a firm line.

Intensity of blueing is often expressed arbitrarily as + to + + +, but it is usually possible to match the intensity of blue with a tint scale made of celluloid or glass, giving a five or six point range. Most lesions are of rather uniform intensity throughout, those with 'pale centres' cannot be assessed because this area of powerful vasoconstriction is probably due to release of large amounts of histamine possibly together with 5-hydroxytryptamine, and is the result of using an unduly large dose of antibody.

Usually either area *or* intensity will be of major interest depending on whether sensitization or inhibition is the most important consideration. Only occasionally will the product of area and intensity be useful, and a table showing both would usually be preferable.

Since the relationship between area of response and the dose is roughly linear, the plot of mean diameter upon log dose will also be linear [2] and it is possible to read off equiactive doses of different antibody samples direct from such a plot of their regression lines. The effectiveness of inhibitors can also be readily seen on the graph of log dose/mean diameter and the pA_2 value [9] calculated.

Modifications of the test have been used, especially where the antigen is being investigated. If only minute amounts of antigen are available it may be injected directly into the sensitized site, as in the P–K reaction. The animal should be 'blued' 10–15 minutes previously by intraveneous injection. It is vital to show that the antigen alone does not cause a blue area.

A similar technique may be employed to show that an impure material does or does not contain a given antigenic substance. If this is a quantitative study to compare the content of several samples, it may be preferable to sensitize the whole animal by the intravenous route 12–36 hours previously, then to give blue dye, and finally inject the various samples of antigen intradermally in graded doses.

The local injection of antigen loses the great advantage of uniform, simultaneous challenge, which is a feature of intravenous administration. Quite apart from the chance that the antigen may not entirely overlap the sensitized area, there must be a very wide range of relative concentrations of antigen and antibody in different parts of the site. But above all, the release of active agents in the first few minutes after injection will inevitably modify blood and lymph flow so that the full blue reaction may not develop. The choice of doses of antigen should therefore be fairly near threshold, which must be determined by preliminary trial over a range of say 10–200 ng. Similar considerations apply to active sensitization, and serve to show up the advantages of the usual PCA technique.

A sensitive method for the detection and characterization of antigenic material in an impure state has been described by Janoff *et al* [11]. This utilizes the PCA reaction as an indication of the neutralization of sensitizing antibody by prior contact with antigen. The antibody and the material to be tested for the presence of antigen are mixed prior to intradermal injection, but in all other respects the test is the same as the usual PCA—with challenge after 4 hours. The neutralized antibody fails to give a reaction, or gives a response smaller than that produced by untreated antibody injected in an adjacent site on the same animal. If necessary, the amount of antigen can be roughly estimated by plotting data showing the change in PCA response resulting from the addition of graded amounts of authentic antigen to the sensitizing antibody. This method is used to identify traces of antigenic material in samples of biological fluid such as serum, provided that the sample itself does not cause a severe reaction when injected, and might thus interfere with the process of sensitization or the ability of the tissue to give a PCA reaction later. The antigen used for challenge must be pure, and the amount needed is comparatively large, e.g. 2 –5 mg for a small guinea-pig.

Passive cutaneous anaphylaxis is said to be 'reversed' when the antigen is given before the antibody. 'Reversed PCA' has been used to demonstrate that certain antigenic substances such as γ globulins, γ globulin–hapten conjugates, and γ globulin fragments produced by partial proteolysis, are retained in the skin. 'Fixation' in the injection site is shown by a PCA response to the injection of antibody after 3 or 4 hours. Albumin and practically all non-globulin proteins and macromolecules are quickly dispersed after intradermal injection, and consequently give no local reaction. A comparatively large amount of antibody is necessary to give a satisfactory reversed PCA reaction. One must assume that both IgA and IgG will contribute to this reaction, and the optimum amount of a particular antiserum can only be established by trial. The amount is of the order of 200 times that which gives a good positive response in the ordinary PCA test.

A more exhaustive survey of the experimental potentialities of cutaneous anaphylactic reactions is to be found in the review by Ovary [12].

References

[1] OVARY Z. (1952) Cutaneous anaphylaxis in the albino rat. *Int. Archs. Allergy appl. Immun.* **3**, 293

[2] MILES A.A. & MILES E.M. (1952) Vascular reactions to histamine, histamine-liberator and leukotaxine in the skin of guinea pigs. *J. Physiol. (London)*, **118**, 228

[3] BROCKLEHURST W.E., HUMPHREY J.H. & PERRY W.L.M. (1955) The role of histamine in cutaneous antigen–antibody reactions in the rat. *J. Physiol. (London)* **129**, 305

[4] COLQUHOUN D. & BROCKLEHURST W.E. (1965) Passive sensitization of skin and lung by guineapig immunoglobulins. *Immunology* **9**, 591

[5] LIACOPOULOS P., HALPERN B.N. & FRICK O.L. (1963) The effect of antigen excess on the anaphylactic reaction. *J. Immun.* **90**, 165

[6] SEVITT S. (1958) Early and late odema and increase in capillary permeability after burns in the skin. *J. Path. Bact.* **75**, 27

[7] SPECTOR W.G. (1958) Substances which affect capillary permeability. *Pharmac. Rev.* **10**, 475

[8] JUDAH J.D. & WILLOUGHBY D.A. (1962) A quantitative method for the study of capillary permeability: Extraction and determination of trypan blue in tissues. *J. Path. Bact.* **83**, 567

[9] SCHILD H.O. (1947) pA—a new scale of drug antagonism. *Brit. J. Pharmacol.* **2**, 189

[10] FRIMMER M. & MÜLLER F.W. (1962) Usefulness and limitations of dye methods in the determination of increased permeability in the skin capillaries. *Med. exp. (Basel)* **6**, 327

[11] JANOFF A., ZWEIFACH B., NAGLER A.L. & OVARY Z. (1961) Detection of ferritin in the plasma of guinea-pigs in experimental shock. *Circulat. Res.* **6**, 407

[12] OVARY Z. (1964) Passive cutaneous anaphylaxis. *Immunological Methods*, pp. 259–283, ed. ACKROYD J.F. Oxford: Blackwell

CHAPTER 23

Histochemistry in Experimental Immunology

LUCILLE BITENSKY

Introduction

The meaning of histochemistry

The term 'histochemistry' has come to refer to two types of study or discipline. One, which is well exemplified in the recent books of Burstone [1] and of Barka and Anderson [2], is more a branch of histology than of chemistry; it justifies its claim to being histochemistry because it lays emphasis on the chemistry underlying the staining reactions of tissues. This form of the subject will not be discussed further in the present chapter since for an immunologist, the mere effect of colouring his material is of little value, however exquisitely and rationally it is achieved; it is not the staining but the cellular chemistry or physiology that concerns him. Moreover, this form of histochemistry has been severely attacked, particularly by Chayen [3], on scientific grounds.

The form of histochemistry that will be considered in this chapter is that which aims at disclosing the chemical behaviour of the tissue, and the metabolic changes induced in it by external agents or conditions. It resembles the first type of histochemistry in that the metabolic reaction which is tested is made to yield a coloured end-product which can be seen at, or very close to, the site of the enzymes or other active groups responsible for the function studied. On the other hand it is concerned with the function rather than the stain. It is believed that this form of histochemistry can yield information which is of direct, and of fundamental, interest to the immunologist in that it informs him of the cellular biochemistry which is responsible for the gross changes to which his observation is so often limited. However, while the approach, and the critical criteria, may be those of biochemistry, this form of histochemistry can be of more use, in this context, than can more conventional biochemistry. This follows from two factors: the first is that it can be done on minute pieces of tissue; indeed, since the sites of active groups are rendered visible, it is possible to observe a reaction which occurs at a single locus in one cell of a tissue section. Even when not pressed to such extreme lengths, this form of cellular chemistry does avoid the tissue dilution artefact of more conventional biochemistry [4, 5] in that the activity of particular cells, within a heterogeneous population, can be assessed by direct microscopic

752

examination. The second factor is that unlike conventional biochemistry, histochemistry does not involve the disruption of the tissue. Because of this it can disclose the spatial relationships that may exist between related metabolic systems, not only in their structural topography within the cell but also in their chemical linkage one to the other. At present this is a relatively new concept of the role of histochemistry which was defined by Chayen [3] as ' . . . histochemistry is concerned with visualizing cellular chemistry . . . it is an extension of biochemistry which can be performed on histologically acceptable sections; and . . . it has already a certain amount of scientific information which is related to the special conditions concerned with the chemistry of intact sections'. As yet, this form of histochemistry has been applied only to a few problems in immunology. However, since it is likely to be the more fruitful concept of histochemistry, it is this form of the subject that will be considered in the present chapter.

The function of histochemistry in immunological studies
The immunologist is well aware of the gross effects of immune reactions within an organism, yet even with these he may be concerned to know the actual mechanism by which the recognition of foreign matter becomes translated into the death of the foreign tissue. For example, it is likely that the primary effect of the rejection mechanism may be related to fluctuation in the concentration of histamine-like substances in the region of the graft. Histochemistry has already proved useful in suggesting a rather novel role for the mast cell in controlling the concentration of histamine in tissue [6], extension of such studies and of the direct investigation of the histochemistry of such compounds as histamine [7, 8], 5-hydroxytryptamine [9, 10, 11], dopamine [12], and catecholamines [13, 14], may be helpful in elucidating the mechanism of graft rejection, or tissue damage in the 'delayed' type of hypersensitivity.

At the less gross level, the study of immune cytolysis may be taken as a clear example of how histochemistry can extend immunological knowledge [15]. It is well known that when ascites cells are exposed to specific antibody in the presence of complement, they undergo cytolysis. Histochemistry is not required to show this, but it has indicated the mechanism by which such an immunological reaction may cause cell death [15, 16]. Moreover, histochemistry has been able to disclose more than this: it has shown that if cell death is the only response recorded, the observer misses many of the responses of the cells to the interaction of antibody and antigen. Thus by the application of histochemistry, Dumonde *et al* [17, 15] were able to show chemical changes induced by a soluble antibody which was reacting in the absence of added complement, with a cellular antigen located at the cell surface. No structural alteration, and no lysis, were seen even though marked functional changes could be detected histochemically. Moreover, Dumonde, Bitensky and Chayen were able to show that the behaviour of ascites cells which suffered immune cytolysis depended on the nature of the experimental system [18, 15, also see below]. These differences were best seen by the use of interference microscopy. Thus histochemistry, in the sense used by the present author and her associates, includes not only the metabolic biochemistry of cells, but also their physical biochemistry, for which biophysical methods may be more appropriate than more conventional microbiochemistry.

The value of histochemistry becomes even more marked at the subcellular and functional level. It is obvious that the problem of sensitization is not one of morphology but must depend on metabolic changes. Similarly, it is suggested that the question of auto-immunity may depend on subtle configurational changes within macro-molecules; structural alterations in the binding between lipid and protein, which may be related to auto-immunity, have been detected histochemically [19]. But although the fact of auto-immunity is important in itself, the mechanism by which it causes disease may be of greater concern. This certainly is the province of histochemistry. For example, there is some evidence that auto-immunological reactions may disturb lysosomes and so allow their lytic enzymes to leak out of the affected cells into the surrounding connective tissue. A comparable situation was disclosed biochemically by Fell and her co-workers who showed that excess vitamin A induced the lysis of cartilage matrix by damaging the lysosomes of the chondrocytes [20, 21, 22, 23].

The type of immunological problem which might be investigated histochemically

Respiration as an indicator of the ultimate rejection of a tissue graft

If a tissue is under such deleterious environmental circumstances that it will ultimately be killed and so rejected by the host organism, this may be disclosed by changes in respiratory activity. For example, it may be that the normal energy supply of that tissue will be reduced, owing to interference with the entry of substrate by the host reaction; in this case, it might be supposed that the Krebs' cycle will show impaired activity. Equally there might be some attempt by the graft to grow, as a regenerative effect to counteract the host reaction; in this case, some evidence of enhanced pentose-shunt activity might be expected, however slight and ineffectual it might be. Both these responses have been observed by various workers. For example, depression of succinic and malic dehydrogenase activity was reported by Williams *et al* [24] in homotransplants of dog kidney biopsied 6 days after insertion of the graft. These histochemical observations were confirmed, by the same authors, by quantitative biochemical studies on homogenates of the renal cortex from the same kidneys. At this time, there was little or no histological evidence of damage. Chiba *et al* [25] found that the activity of malic dehydrogenase was depressed in specimens from homografted dog hearts. Alteration in the activity of a number of dehydrogenases was reported by Lindquist & Hager [26] to occur as early as two days after the insertion of renal homografts in dogs, at a time when no histological abnormalities could be detected. Thus, in the convoluted tubular epithelium, the following dehydrogenases showed reduced activity—β-hydroxybutyric, glutamic, α-glycerophosphate, lactic, isocitric, succinic and malic; diphosphopyridine and triphosphopyridine nucleotide (DPNH and TPNH) diaphorase activity was also depressed. These changes were believed to be due to the process of homograft rejection, since they were not observed in the autograft controls. Similar results were obtained by Lindquist & Hager [26] in experiments on mouse skin grafts, and by Ballantyne *et al* [27] on skin grafts in rats.

Only the enzymes of the pentose–shunt failed to show this reduced activity. Thus Lindquist & Hager [26] found even a slight to moderate increase in the activity of glucose-6-phosphate and 6-phosphogluconate dehydrogenases in both the 2-day-old renal homografts and the skin homografts.

Other changes associated with graft rejection

Williams *et al* [24] reported depression of cytochrome oxidase activity in canine renal homografts 6 days after the operation; this, assumably, correlated with the reduction in the associated dehydrogenases since both succinic dehydrogenase and probably DPNH diaphorase are linked to this enzyme. Their evidence that β-glucosaminidase activity was also reduced is less easily fitted into a cellular metabolic pattern. They also reported changes in the intracellular distribution of acid phosphatase; the fact that the localization of this enzyme was different in the homograft and in the autograft must be considered significant, but their precise findings are not so significant owing to the histochemical procedure used.

It may be emphasized that merely to provide evidence that a histochemical reaction gives enhanced, depressed or unaltered results may even be unhelpful to the immunologist who is concerned, not with the staining properties, but with cellular or physiological responses. The aim of histochemistry should be to elucidate the mechanism of these responses. Hence it is not very surprising that Scothorne & Tough [28] failed to demonstrate any differences in the glycogen and ribose nucleic acid content of human skin autografts and homografts from the time of transplantation even up to their rejection. From what is known of the metabolism of these substances, it would have been rather surprising if these had been affected early in the process of graft rejection.

Protein synthesis and the production of antibodies

The production of antibodies is likely to be associated with actual synthesis of protein as well as with changes which render non-specific protein immunologically specific. Evidence that certain cells are involved in protein synthesis can be found readily by histochemical methods. The extensive researches of Brachet [29], of Caspersson [30] and of their colleagues had established that high cellular concentrations of ribose nucleic acid (RNA) were associated with the biosynthesis of protein; the biochemical mechanisms involved have been established rather more recently [31, 32]. Thus cells which synthesize protein are likely to stain intensely for RNA; either methyl green–pyronin [33], or acridine orange [34], or even toluidine blue [35, 36] can be used for this purpose. However, there is considerable evidence that pentose-shunt activity [37, 38] may be involved in the synthesis of the ribose moiety of the nucleic acid which eventually is used in the biosynthesis of protein. Consequently the earliest indication that protein, such as antibody, is being synthesized by antibody-making cells, may be an increase in the activity of enzymes of the pentose-shunt which oxidize glucose-6-phosphate and 6-phosphogluconate. Excellent histochemical procedures for these enzymes have been developed recently (see below).

The binding of antibody and the resultant alterations to the surface membrane of affected cells

The fact that antibody becomes attached to the cell surface can be demonstrated by suitable histochemical immunofluorescence techniques (see Holborow & Johnson, Chapter 16; also Dumonde *et al* [16]). Yet while these and the ferritin techniques (see Andres, Hsu & Seegal, Chapter 15) may show the actual localization of the antibody, they tell nothing of the functional disorders which are caused by this attachment of antibody and which in the presence of complement lead finally to cytolysis. Cell death under these circumstances would be due primarily to changes in the cell membrane, as indicated by Easty & Ambrose [39] and by Easton *et al* [40].

Thus it may be of particular advantage to be able to study the integrity of the cell membrane. This can be done histochemically in two ways. The first depends on the fact that the structural integrity of the cell surface is maintained by a particular lipid-protein configuration (e.g. see Davson & Danielli [41]). In the normal membrane, the lipid molecules are linked to protein and are maintained in a special orientation sandwiched within outer layers of protein. Consequently they will not stain appreciably with reactions for phospholipids, nor will they show a strong affinity for dyes or fluorochromes which are normally used for colouring lipids. However, if the structure is sufficiently deformed, the phospholipids become 'unmasked' [42, 43] to a lesser or greater extent, depending on the degree of damage done to the membrane. They will then stain with histochemical methods for phospholipids. Moreover, the unmasked phospholipids will disclose fatty properties in the membrane, which previously were concealed by the outer shell of protein, so that the membrane will concentrate lipid dyes or fluorochromes into it from an aqueous dispersion. These principles were used by Dumonde *et al* [16] (also see Bitensky [15]) in studying the cytotoxic effect of antibody and complement on EL_4 mouse ascites cells. They used the acid haematein method (see below) for demonstrating the unmasked or freely available phospholipid, and the fluorescent dye, 3 : 4-benzpyrene in aqueous dispersion, for testing the fattiness of the membrane. Air-dried smears of untreated cells gave almost no reaction with the acid haematein method; suspensions of these cells showed only general fluorescence in the cytoplasm when studied with benzpyrene; both results demonstrated that the lipids of the membranes were well masked against these procedures. In contrast, similar preparations of cells which had been treated with antibody and complement showed strong staining of the membrane by both techniques. Hence it followed that one effect of treatment with antibody and complement was to disturb the integrity of the membrane sufficiently to unmask the lipids of the membrane and so make them available to these histochemical reactions.

However, the histochemical methods were sufficiently delicate to disclose similar, albeit lesser, changes in the surface membrane when antibody was used even in the absence of added complement, when no gross cytotoxic effects were observed. In cells treated with antibody alone, the acid haematein reaction demonstrated some unmasking of membrane lipids and also of cytoplasmic lipids. These changes were also associated with alteration of intracellular metabolic activity, as will be discussed later.

The second way of studying changes in the integrity of the cell membrane is indirect, but more functional in that it tests the ability of the membrane to maintain the osmotic balance of the cells. If the cell membrane allows excess water to enter the cell, the cytoplasm may either become diluted, or watery vesicles will form. The latter can be observed very readily, even with phase-contrast illumination, but proof of either effect depends on being able to measure the concentration of dry matter in the protoplasm. This can be done directly by phase contrast refractometry [44] but this involves immersing the cells in various solutions which may not be suitable, or convenient. The indirect method is to measure the actual dry mass of the protoplasm, or the vesicle, and relate this value to its projected area. The dry mass of the protoplasm in a cell, or in a selected part of a cell, can be measured with remarkable accuracy by interference microscopy [44–47]. This procedure was used by Dumonde *et al* [18] and by Easty & Ambrose [39] in studies on mouse ascites cells exposed to antibody and complement. Dumonde *et al* [18] were able to show that when the antibody was presented as whole immune serum, the cytoplasm coagulated around the nucleus and the cell membrane swelled away from the congealed protoplasm, forming a huge watery vesicle. On the other hand, when it was presented as a relatively purified γ globulin fraction, the swelling of the membrane was accompanied by dilution of the cytoplasm which filled the whole swollen space (see Bitensky [15]).

It should be emphasized that this indirect method may indicate the reduced ability of the cytoplasm to do osmotic work rather than simple changes in the integrity of the surface membrane. This is likely because there is no evidence that the swollen membrane allows large molecules to leak out until true lysis occurs [39, 48, 18]. This gives special relevance to the demonstration of changes in intracellular organelles, produced by the action of a membrane-located antibody, acting even in the absence of added complement (see below).

The effects of immune reactions on intracellular organelles
The work of Dumonde *et al* [17] (also considered above) has shown that an antibody, acting at the surface of ascites cells in the absence of added complement, may change the membrane fragility of intracellular lysosomes. As has just been discussed, the swelling of cell membranes in immune cytolysis may also represent an inability of intracellular enzyme systems to do enough osmotic work to maintain the osmotic balance of the cells. Furthermore, if the effect of interaction between antibody, antigen and possibly complement, in the vicinity of a target tissue, were to cause the liberation of histamine, this too could produce profound changes in the permeability of intracellular metabolic barriers [49, 50]. Thus the first stage of graft rejection could involve increased local concentrations of amines like histamine which, only in later stages, would produce the dilatation of vessels and cessation of blood flow which is a regular feature of graft rejection [51]. Local increases in the concentration of such amines can be detected histochemically by the changes they induce in the permeability of intracellular organelles, such as mitochondria. The enhanced permeability thus produced results in increased enzymatic response to histochemical reactions for many enzymes, but notably glutamic dehydrogenase [52, 53], and monoamine oxidase [49, 50, 54]. Some of the more obviously significant enzymes will be considered briefly.

(a) *Acid phosphatase*
This enzyme is very useful as a marker for the activity of the lysosomes, since, in most tissues, it occurs solely within these organelles. Moreover, when studied by suitable histochemical methods, its activity can be used as a measure of the integrity and permeability of the lysosomal membrane. The lysosome was defined by de Duve [55, 56, 57] as a cellular organelle, of about the size of a small mitochondrion, within which were located many of the hydrolytic enzymes of the cell; these were maintained in an inert or latent

state, separated from the rest of the cell by an impermeable bounding membrane. With such latent enzymes generally, their total cellular content is of little significance; the point of interest is whether the condition of the membrane has allowed their activity to become manifest in the cell. Consequently Bitensky [58] devised a fragility test for assessing the condition of the membrane. It will be obvious that such a test cannot be performed on fixed tissues since the object of fixation is to impose some degree of denaturation on the protoplasm; a consequence of this is that all membranes become totally permeable, so rendering such a fragility test impossible. The mechanism of the test depends on the fact that the permeability of the lysosomal membrane increases with prolonged exposure to acid conditions, including those in which the acid phosphatase reaction is performed. It follows, therefore, that the fragility of the membrane can be assessed by estimating the shortest time required to produce a reaction in the normal tissue and observing the effect produced by this treatment on the abnormal lysosomes.

By the use of this fragility test, Dumonde *et al* [17, 16, 15] were able to show that antibody to mouse ascites tumour cells altered the nature of the intracellular lysosomal membranes even when, in the absence of added complement, the antibody was restricted to the cell surface. In this way, histochemistry was able to disclose metabolic changes deep within the cell even where these were reversible [57, 17], and where no structural changes had been demonstrated, inside the cell, by either light or electron microscopy [60].

(b) *Aminopeptidase*

It has been shown recently by Sylvén & Bois-Svensson [61], and by McCabe & Chayen [62] that aminopeptidase activity occurs in lysosome-like particles and is probably an indication of lysosomal proteolytic potentiality [62]. It is possible, therefore, that the changes in lysosomal acid phosphatase activity found by Dumonde *et al* [17] would be correlated with unmasking of aminopeptidase activity. Release of this activity could be connected with either autolysis or, more likely, death of near-by cells. Consequently histochemical studies of aminopeptidase may be valuable for providing information concerning the mechanism of graft rejection or of cell damage following various immune reactions.

(c) *Mitochondrial glutamic dehydrogenase*

There is considerable evidence [63, 52] that the degree of activity shown by this enzyme is related to the integrity of the mitochondrial membrane. Since damage to the tissue can alter this drastically, it is likely that the severity of damage caused by immune reactions can be assessed by measuring the activity of the glutamic dehydrogenase system. This can be done by quantitative histochemistry [52] although qualitative results may suffice for most purposes [64].

It is possible that drastic alterations in glutamic dehydrogenase activity may, in certain circumstances, be indicative of a general metabolic change to one of katabolism, presaging severe cell disturbance and even death. This follows from the association between this dehydrogenase and the transaminases, which are known to leak into the serum, in elevated amounts when tissues are damaged or develop foci of necrosis [65]. Simply, the association between these enzymes can be shown as follows (after Baldwin [66]):

It will be appreciated that increased activity of the glutamic dehydrogenase might be expected to shift the transamination equilibrium from the left to the right, causing a need for more free amino acid which can be supplied by further breakdown of protein. Consequently, under some circumstances, the increased activity of the glutamic dehydrogenase will be reflected in enhanced transaminase activity and a tendency towards katabolic metabolism in the affected cells.

(d) *Monoamine oxidase*

It is likely (for example, see Humphrey [67], Osler [68] and Dixon [69]) that many of the gross effects which concern immunologists derive immediately from an increase in local concentration of amines like catecholamines or histamine. The most striking example is the phenomenon of anaphylaxis in which mast cells and histamine have been implicated [70, 71]. It has been suggested that these amines can be detected by direct histochemical procedures [7–14] although it is not certain that the methods are sufficiently sensitive for most immunological problems. However, the indirect demonstration of the presence of these amines, namely by enhanced monoamine oxidase activity, does appear to be very sensitive. It follows from the fact that all these compounds greatly increase the permeability of the membrane which surrounds this enzyme. Consequently, when tested histochemically, the substrate penetrates into the organelle in greater concentration than normally, and so produces a strikingly enhanced stain [49, 50].

Methods

The preparation of tissue sections

It has been emphasized (above) that the type of histochemistry favoured by the present author is a histological form of biochemistry which benefits from the fact that the tissue is not disrupted or homogenized. It is because of this that this form of inquiry can disclose the spatial relationships and binding that may exist between metabolically related systems and substances. For example, the degree of binding between phospholipids and proteins would seem to be a delicate marker of the normality of cells, and this can be assessed by the acid haematein procedure. Similarly, the extent of the manifest activity of otherwise latent lysosomal enzymes depends on the state of the lysosomal membrane. Another example, at a more complex level of chemical organization, would be the activity of monoamine oxidase, which seems to depend not only on the condition of the membrane surrounding the particle which contains the enzyme, but also on the presence of related enzymes (see below; also Cohen *et al* [54]).

It will be obvious, therefore, that the method of preparing the tissues will be of critical importance. For example, the use of fat-solvents may so split lipid–protein associations that their effect would obliterate that of an immune response in unmasking some of the phospholipid. Similarly ice damage, which may occur during some types of freeze-sectioning, might be expected to cause as much disruption as biochemical homogenization.

The method recommended for these studies depends apparently on super-cooling the water-phase of the tissues so that no ice damage can occur [72]. The tissue is then sectioned under conditions which do not seem to disturb this super-cooled state [73]. The procedure is as follows: pieces of tissue, up to about 0·5 cm cubed, are plunged into hexane (BDH, 'free from aromatic hydrocarbons' grade) which has been cooled previously to $-70°$ C by means of an outer bath of solid carbon dioxide and alcohol. Such pieces of rat liver were found to reach $-40°$ C in about 9 seconds [72]. They are left for about 1 minute and are then transferred, with chilled forceps, to empty corked glass tubes which had been equilibrated against solid carbon dioxide.

A microtome chuck is cooled with the CO_2–alcohol mixture and a small drop of water, placed on top of it, is allowed to freeze. When only a last film of moisture remains, the tissue is rapidly transferred from the tube to it, so as to become sealed on to the chuck. This is the most critical part of the procedure since the tissue must not be allowed to become appreciably warmed. It may be preferable to do this transfer in a refrigerated cabinet, e.g. in the cryostat itself.

The tissue is then sectioned, usually at 8 μ, at an ambient temperature of about -25 to $-30°$ C. The knife is cooled still lower by having solid carbon dioxide packed around its handle [73]. The sections are picked up, off the knife, with a glass slide taken from the temperature of the laboratory; the warmth of the slide probably aids in removing much water from the section. In this way, true freezing of the water of the sectioned tissue in the cryostat is avoided; moreover, this rapid 'thawing' would appear to be beneficial. These sections, apparently because they have lost so much moisture, can be stored for a few hours in the cryostat until they are used. They are then plunged into the relevant histochemical incubation media, at 37° C if required, or they can be labelled, etc., on the bench for as long as 5–15 minutes before beginning the reaction.

One difficulty which is often met in working with cryostat sections, is that routine staining with haematoxylin and eosin frequently yields histo-logical pictures which are difficult to relate to those seen after conventional histological procedures. This may be overcome, to a large extent, by allowing the sections to dry, preferably by warming them gently, and then using Roberts's modified celestin blue eosin procedure (personal communication). This depends firstly on the use of the complex picric fixative, devised and studied by Bitensky *et al* [74], to which is added 5 per cent acetic acid, and then on the use of a mixture of celestin blue iron alum and Mayer's haemalum (as suggested by Lendrum [75]).

Staining procedure
Fresh frozen sections are dried and then fixed for 3 minutes in the picric

acid fixative which consists of 10 ml of formalin, 56 ml of absolute alcohol, 5 ml of glacial acetic acid, 0·18 g sodium chloride, 0·15 g picric acid and 30 ml of distilled water. The sections are rinsed in 70 per cent alcohol and then stained in the celestin blue iron alum mixture for 3 minutes. (This mixture is prepared by dissolving 2·5 g of iron alum in 50 ml of distilled water; to this solution is added 0·25 g of celestin blue; the solution is boiled for 3 minutes and filtered when it is cool.) The sections are then rinsed in water and stained in Mayer's haemalum for 3 minutes. After this, the sections are again rinsed in water, differentiated briefly in 1 per cent acid alcohol, and 'blued' in water containing a few drops of a saturated solution of lithium carbonate. They are counterstained in 0·5 per cent aqueous eosin for 5 seconds, dehydrated and mounted in DPX.

Methyl green–pyronin method for nucleic acids [76, 33, 77]
The basis of this technique is the competitive action of two basic dyes [76], one of which can bind through a single charged group while the other can combine with two charged groups. Although both will stain both types of nucleic acid, pyronin will stain more actively than will methyl green, and will drive it out of all dye-substrate combinations where the dye is held by a single electrostatic bond. However, where the methyl green can bind to substrate by two bonds, as it can when it links to highly polymerized and orientated DNA [78, 79, 80], it is not displaced by the highly competitive pyronin. Thus in correctly prepared sections, where the orientation and polymerization of the DNA has been preserved, pyronin stains all nucleic acid-containing structures other than the DNA of the chromatin which combines with and retains the doubly charged methyl green (also see Vercauteren [81]). Some nuclei stain reddish-green or blue, apparently owing to some RNA or possibly to some other acidic matter [76]. Occasionally polymerized phospholipids may also bind the methyl green, although this is rather rare [82]. Rigorous specificity can be obtained by the use of nucleases, to remove the specific nucleic acid whose presence is suspected (see Jacobson & Webb [83]).

Method. A 0·25 per cent solution of 'Revector' brand (Hopkin and Williams) methyl green in 0·2 M acetate buffer at pH 4·2 is first cleansed of methyl violet by repeated extraction with chloroform. After leaving to stand, to allow the chloroform to evaporate, this solution is added to an equal volume of a 0·5 per cent solution of pyronin G in similar buffer. Fresh frozen sections are immersed in this solution for half an hour. No fixation is required since this is effected by the acetate buffer at the pH used in the dye mixture. More intense reactions, i.e. to disclose the maximum amount of nucleic acids present in the section, can be obtained if the sections are fixed in an acetic–alcohol mixture (e.g. 5 : 95 v/v or even 1 : 3 v/v). After staining, the sections are

BB*

rinsed very briefly in distilled water, blotted dry very carefully, dehydrated in N-butyl alcohol, and mounted in Euparal.

Acridine orange method for nucleic acids [34, 84]
Like the methyl green–pyronin procedure, this technique differentiates between highly polymerized and less highly polymerized nucleic acids; in general, the former represents DNA and the latter RNA. In this case, however, only one dye, acridine orange, is used to effect this. It seems possible that the difference in fluorescence shown by this fluorochrome when linked to acidic molecules of different molecular weights and configurations may be a form of metachromasia [85, 86]. This would be comparable to that of toluidine blue when it stains red with acidic polysaccharides instead of its more usual blue with other acidic substances (the mechanism of this is described by Sylvén [87], and by R. Chayen & Roberts [88]). Diengdoh [84] has shown that, at least in fresh cryostat sections, the nature of the buffer may have profound effects on the reaction.

Method. Fresh frozen sections are treated for a few minutes with Walpole's acetate–HCl buffer at pH 4·2 [89] and then immersed for 30 minutes in a 1 : 2000 solution of acridine orange in the buffer. They are rinsed for 15 minutes in the buffer, mounted in buffered glycerine (4 volumes glycerine, 1 volume of the buffer) and examined by fluorescence microscopy using blue light. A strong barrier filter in the eyepiece is necessary to remove all the blue light used in exciting the fluorochrome.

Results. The colours seen will depend on the light used for evoking the fluorescence. With visible blue light, DNA appears to be coloured yellow while RNA is flame-red (see Armstrong [34], who also describes the effects seen with ultra-violet light). Other polymers may also fluoresce with this method, particularly keratin (usually darker green).

Methods for dehydrogenases acting on glucose-6-phosphate and on 6-phosphogluconate [90]
These enzymes are of interest in that exceptional increases in their activity may be indicative of enhanced ribose synthesis and thus of potential increases in the nucleic-acid content of cells [38, 91, 37]. Increases in concentration of RNA have been correlated with protein synthesis [29, 30, 92]. Enhanced activity of these dehydrogenases, which form part of the hexose monophosphate pathway or pentose-shunt [93] has been found histochemically in proliferating tissues [94] and may be expected in cells which begin to synthesize protein, e.g. during the production of antibody.

Both of these pentose-shunt dehydrogenases are considered biochemically to be soluble enzymes [95] and consequently, some histochemists seem to have despaired of being able to demonstrate them adequately in unfixed sections.

However, Altmann [96] and Altmann & Chayen [97, 90] have shown that these enzymes can be demonstrated, and even measured quantitatively, without their becoming lost from the section during the incubation, provided that an inert colloid-stabilizer, polyvinyl alcohol, is added to the medium.

The histochemical method depends on the removal of hydrogen from glucose-6-phosphate, or from 6-phosphogluconate, by the relevant enzyme; this occurs only in the presence of the coenzyme triphosphopyridine nucleotide (TPN; now renamed NADP) which accepts the hydrogen. The reduced coenzyme, TPNH or NADPH, is then oxidized by the diaphorase which, either directly or by some intermediate, passes the hydrogen to the almost colourless tetrazolium salt which, becoming reduced, is precipitated as the coloured formazan. Neotetrazolium chloride has been used because it is effective, cheap, and can be eluted for quantitative study [90, 98]. It precipitates crudely and does not give as precise a localization as can be obtained with nitroblue tetrazolium (NBT) which can be substituted for it, especially in cells which give only weak reactions for these enzymes. However, the intracellular localization of either formazan is not significant for an enzyme system which appears to be distributed throughout the cytoplasm.

Method. Fresh frozen sections are incubated at 37° C in a medium consisting of 0·05 M glycyl glycine buffer, 0·15 per cent neotetrazolium chloride (Sigma Chemical Company, U.S.A.), NADP (2·5 mg/ml obtained from Boehringer GmbH, Germany), 0·01 M potassium cyanide, 0·08 M calcium chloride and 20 per cent polyvinyl alcohol (Polyviol MO5/140 obtained from Bush, Beach & Segner Bayley Ltd, London). The relevant substrates glucose-6-phosphate (sodium salt; Boehringer) or 6-phosphogluconate (tri-sodium salt; Wessex), are added at a concentration of 1·5 mg/ml and the pH of the medium is adjusted to pH 8·5 for glucose-6-phosphate dehydrogenase and pH 8·0 for 6-phosphogluconate dehydrogenase.

The time of incubation depends on the activity of these dehydrogenases in the tissue to be studied, but under these conditions, 20 μ sections of normal rat liver give a moderately intense reaction after 20 minutes. At the end of the incubation, the sections are rinsed in distilled water and mounted in Farrants' medium.

Method for mitochondrial glutamic dehydrogenase activity

Although biochemical studies may be used to show the total potential glutamic dehydrogenase activity present in a tissue, the especial advantage of histochemistry is that it discloses the degree of activity actually present [52, 53]. It does this by virtue of retaining the mitochondrial system intact, so that the activity recorded is controlled by the state of the membrane bounding the mitochondria. Thus the activity is a measure of the rate of penetration of glutamate and coenzyme through the mitochondrial membrane to the site of the enzyme complex.

As in all histochemical demonstrations of dehydrogenases, the method requires that the unfixed sections are incubated in the presence of the substrate, coenzyme and activators, if required, and a suitable hydrogen acceptor which takes the place of oxygen in normal respiration. It is not certain that the whole cellular complement of glutamic dehydrogenase is located solely in the mitochondria and some cytoplasmic activity might be detected by using a hydrogen acceptor, like NBT, which can accept hydrogen avidly, even possibly from the relevant diaphorase [99]. In the present technique neotetrazolium is used since, with enzymes which are dependent on the coenzyme DPN (or NAD), this can accept hydrogen only from the intact hydrogen transport system [99] that occurs within the mitochondrion [100]. Consequently, this method is limited to the mitochondrial glutamic dehydrogenase. Moreover, the formazan of neotetrazolium can be estimated quantitatively (see below).

Method. Fresh frozen sections are incubated for 1 hour at 37° C in a medium consisting of 0·05 M phosphate buffer, pH 7·8, containing neotetrazolium (1 mg/ml), NAD (5 mg/ml) and sodium glutamate (17 mg/ml). The sections are rinsed in distilled water and mounted in Farrants' medium.

Quantitative estimation of dehydrogenase activity

Provided that neotetrazolium is used, the quantitative activity of any dehydrogenase may be assessed. Ideally the correct conditions for the incubation should be established for each enzyme, and possibly for each tissue. This has been done for succinic dehydrogenase in rat liver [98] and for pentose-shunt dehydrogenases in rat liver [96]; however, the quantitative estimation of the formazan produced is recommended in place of more subjective criteria even if the optimal conditions have not been established. The formazans which are more substantive for protein, i.e. those which bind to protein and so yield a more precise localization of the site from which the tetrazolium salt has accepted the hydrogen, are unsuitable since their binding to the section resists extraction for quantitative study.

Method. The sections are incubated in the same media for quantitative as for qualitative study, except that the media are placed in microcells [101] on the section instead of lying free, in drops; this ensures a known and constant volume of incubation medium. The formazan is eluted from the dried, stained section in 10 per cent hapten-1-ol in tetrachlorethane and the colour is measured at 550 mμ in a spectrophotometer. The activity can be related to the area of the section (e.g. see Altmann & Chayen [90]) to the nucleic acid content (Butcher & Chayen [102]) or to the nitrogen content of the section (Sloane-Stanley & Jones [103]).

Monoamine oxidase

This enzyme oxidizes and deaminates simple amines like adrenalin, hydroxy-tryptamine and tyramine; it probably is concerned in much of the physio-logical deactivation of catecholamines. It seems unable to affect histamine. Histochemical studies have shown it to occur in discrete particles, of the size of mitochondria [54]; this agrees with biochemical investigation [104]. Histochemistry has shown, moreover, that the membrane around these par-ticles is made more permeable by histamine and by substances like adrenalin, which thereby enhance the histochemical reaction. Thus a strong reaction may indicate that pharmacologically active amines have been acting on the tissue prior to biopsy. Furthermore, Cohen *et al* [54] have suggested that disruption of the particles, with freeing of the enzyme diffusely into the cyto-plasm, may indicate that it is no longer functional. If this is correct, such diffuse staining may precede cell death.

Method. Fresh frozen sections are incubated for 1 hour at 37° C in a med-ium consisting of tryptamine hydrochloride (25 mg), nitroblue tetrazolium (5 mg), 0·1 M phosphate buffer at pH 7·6 (5 ml) and distilled water (15 ml). The sections are rinsed in distilled water and mounted in Farrants' medium.

Acid phosphatase

Lysosomes were defined by de Duve [55, 56, 57] as intracellular organelles which contain a number of hydrolytic enzymes, including acid phosphatase, within an impermeable bounding membrane. The activity of these enzymes remains latent until the membrane has been altered by such conditions as exposure to acidic or hypertonic solutions. It has been shown that, provided the tissue is suitably prepared and stained, particles which conform to these biochemical criteria can be demonstrated histochemically in many tissues, including rat liver [105], mouse skin [106] and human endometrium [107]. These particles appear to respond to a wide variety of conditions, and their increased fragility is a very sensitive indication of cell damage, or even the response of cells to potentially damaging agents, for example, the response of ascites tumour cells to the action of an antibody acting on their surface [17, 59, 15, 58]. It follows that there is a special advantage in retaining these organelles unchanged in tissue sections. The fragility of lysosomes in sections of normal tissue is measured by the time of incubation in the acidic medium necessary to produce only just visible particulate staining. The ability of the sections from the treated tissue to withstand this time is tested and an assess-ment of whether the lysosomal membranes are as fragile, more fragile or less fragile than the normal can be made from the intensity of the staining reaction [58].

Method. The preparation of the incubation medium is as described by Holt [108] for the Gomori acid phosphatase procedure [109]. The medium which consists of 0·05 M acetate buffer at pH 5, containing 0·004 M lead nitrate and 0·01 M sodium β-glycerophosphate (BDH), is incubated for 24 hours at 37° C and then filtered. Fresh frozen sections are incubated at 37° C in the filtered medium; they are rinsed in distilled water, before immersion for 2 minutes in distilled water which has been saturated with hydrogen sulphide gas; finally they are rinsed again in distilled water and mounted in Farrants' medium. The solution of hydrogen sulphide is prepared by bubbling the gas, made from zinc sulphide and hydrochloric acid in a Kipp's apparatus, for 5 minutes through distilled water immediately before use [110]. As controls, serial sections are treated in the same way, but with 0·01 M fluoride in the incubation medium.

Demonstration of aminopeptidase activity

Although there has been a great deal of detailed research on the chemistry of these enzymes [61, 111, 112, 113] it is probably best to regard this histochemical reaction as due to proteolytic activity which, in normal cells, is mainly lysosomal [62], but which may leak out harmfully into surrounding tissue. In the histochemical method, leucylnaphthylamide is split enzymatically to liberate naphthylamine which must be immediately trapped and precipitated by a coupler to produce a coloured azo-dye at the site of the enzymic activity. Thus the speed of coupling is critical; of the substances in common use, Fast blue B has been shown to be the most effective [62].

Method [114]. The incubation medium, which is made up immediately before use, consists of the following: 8 mg leucyl-β-naphthylamide dissolved in 1 ml distilled water, 8 ml of 0·85 per cent sodium chloride, 10 ml of 0·1 M acetate buffer at pH 6·5–6·8, 1 ml of 0·02 M potassium cyanide and 10 mg of Fast blue B salt. Fresh frozen sections are incubated at 37° C in this medium. The incubation time varies with the enzyme activity of the tissue; for example, rat liver gives a moderate reaction after 2 hours' incubation, whereas rat kidney sections are strongly coloured after only half an hour. At the end of the incubation, the sections are washed in 0·85 per cent sodium chloride, and then transferred to a solution containing 0·1 M copper sulphate for 2 minutes. The sections are rinsed again in 0·85 per cent sodium chloride and mounted in Farrants' medium.

The staining of phospholipids

The evidence that phospholipids occur at a particular site in a cell depends on two properties: firstly the physical proof of 'fattiness' and secondly the more chemical evidence of unsaturation of the type associated with fatty acids in a polar environment. The lipid nature of a structure is demonstrated by the ability of a fat-soluble dye to be concentrated by that structure from out of a solution in which the dye is barely soluble. The Sudan dyes and oil red O are often used for this purpose: a structure which can absorb these preferentially out of an alcoholic solution must be very fatty. Consequently these dyes are excellent for staining relatively gross accumulations of lipids, such as fat droplets. However, phospholipids may occur in less fatty conditions, as in association with proteins in membranous structures. For these conditions, the uptake of benzpyrene from a hydrotropic dispersion in water is a far more delicate test both because benzpyrene is hydrophobic and because it is a fluorescent dye.

The second type of evidence is obtained by the use of the acid haematein test. In essence, this began as an empirically derived staining method. The studies of Baker [115, 116], whose name is usually coupled with the procedure, produced a specific histochemical test for phospholipids. It would appear that the method depends on the presence of unsaturated groups in the fatty acid moieties of the phospholipid; these groups react with the chromium in the mordant and bind it. (It is probable that the polar groups, i.e. phosphate, choline, etc., help the hydrophilic dichromate to penetrate to the fatty acids.) Thus at present the control for the specificity of this reaction is to saturate the fatty acids by treating them with bromine [117]; this should abolish the true acid haematein reaction.

3 : 4-*benzpyrene method* [118]
Preparation of the aqueous dispersion of benzpyrene
A saturated solution of caffeine is prepared by allowing a solution containing about 1·5 per cent caffeine to stand at room temperature for 2 days. A few crystals of benzpyrene (about 2 mg) are added to 100 ml of filtered caffeine solution, and the solution is then incubated at 35° C for 2 days. After this, the excess benzpyrene is filtered off, and the solution is then diluted with an equal volume of water to prevent crystallization of the caffeine; the solution is filtered again after it has been allowed to stand for 2 hours. This reagent should contain about 0·75 mg benzpyrene/100 ml and it will keep for some months in a dark bottle.

Staining method
Sections are stained with the benzpyrene reagent for about 20 minutes. They are then rinsed and mounted in water and are examined in ultra-violet light (365 mμ) by fluorescence microscopy. Wet preparations of cell suspensions can be examined directly by adding about 0·6 ml of the benzpyrene solution to about 1 ml of cell suspension in Ringer's solution.

The acid haematein method (Bitensky *et al* [119] after Baker [115])
Fresh frozen sections are fixed in Baker's dichromate mordant (an aqueous solution of 5 per cent potassium dichromate and 1 per cent calcium chloride)

and left for 1 day, followed by another day at 60° C. They are washed well in distilled water and then immersed in the acid haematein solution for 5 hours at 37° C. This solution is prepared by warming a mixture of 0·05 g haematoxylin (BDH reagent grade), 48 ml of distilled water and 1 ml of 1 per cent sodium iodide; the solution is warmed until it just begins to boil, after which it is cooled and then 1 ml of glacial acetic acid is added. The sections are rinsed again in distilled water, and then are differentiated in the borax–ferricyanide solution (an aqueous solution of 0·25 per cent potassium ferricyanide and 0·25 per cent sodium tetraborate) for 18 hours at 37° C. They are then washed again in water, dehydrated in tertiary butanol and mounted in Euparal.

Acknowledgment

It is a privilege to acknowledge the help and guidance given to me by Dr J.Chayen.

References

[1] BURSTONE M.S. (1962) *Enzyme Histochemistry*. New York: Academic Press
[2] BARKA T. & ANDERSON P.J. (1963) *Histochemistry*. New York: Harper & Row
[3] CHAYEN J. (1963) The development of histochemistry. *Nature, Lond.* **200,** 1249
[4] CHAYEN J., JONES G.R.N., BITENSKY L. & CUNNINGHAM G.J. (1961) Histological variation as a source of biochemical error. *Biochem. J.* **79,** 34P
[5] JONES G.R.N., BITENSKY L., CHAYEN J. & CUNNINGHAM G.J. (1961) Tissue dilution artefact; a re-interpretation of variations in levels of succinic dehydrogenase during chemical carcinogenesis. *Nature, Lond.* **191,** 1203
[6] CHAYEN J., DARRACOTT S. & KIRKBY W.W. (1965) A re-interpretation of the role of the mast cell. *Nature, Lond.* **209,** 887
[7] SCHAUER A. & WERLE E. (1959) Zur histochemischen Derstellung des Histamins der Mastzellen. *Z. ges. exptl. Med.* **131,** 100
[8] LAGUNOFF D., PHILLIPS M. & BENDITT E.P. (1961) The histochemical demonstration of histamine in mast cells. *J. Histochem. Cytochem.* **9,** 534
[9] RILEY J.F. (1958) Fluorescent mast cells in precancerous mouse skin. *Experientia* **14,** 141
[10] COUPLAND R.E. & RILEY J.F. (1960) Mast cells and 5-hydroxytryptamine in precancerous mouse skin. *Nature, Lond.* **187,** 1128
[11] FIORE-DONATI L., DE BENEDICTIS G. & CHIECO-BIANCHI L. (1962) Development of mast cell reaction during chemical skin carcinogenesis of mouse. *Nature, Lond.* **193,** 287
[12] COUPLAND R.E. & HEATH I.D. (1961) Chromaffin cells, mast cells and melanin. II. The chromaffin cells of the liver capsule and gut of ungulates. *J. Endocrinol.* **22,** 71
[13] FALCK B. (1962) Observations on the possibilities of the cellular localization of monoamines by a fluorescence method. *Acta physiol. scand.* **56, Suppl. 197**

[14] CARLSSON A., FALCK B. & HILLARP N-A. (1962) Cellular localization of brain monoamines. *Acta physiol. scand.* **56, Suppl. 196**

[15] BITENSKY L. (1963) Cytotoxic action of antibodies. *Brit. med. Bull.* **10**, 241

[16] DUMONDE D.C., BITENSKY L., CUNNINGHAM G.J. & CHAYEN J. (1965) The effects of antibodies on cells. 1. Biochemical and histochemical effects of antibodies and complement on ascites tumour cells. *Immunology* **8**, 25

[17] DUMONDE D.C., WALTER C.M., BITENSKY L., CUNNINGHAM G.J. & CHAYEN J. (1961) Intracellular response to an iso-immune reaction at the surface of ascites tumour cells. *Nature, Lond.,* **192**, 1302

[18] DUMONDE D.C., BITENSKY L. & CHAYEN J. In preparation

[19] CHAYEN J., BALDWIN R.W., BITENSKY L. & DUMONDE D.C. In preparation

[20] FELL H.B. & MELLANBY E. (1952) The effect of hypervitaminosis A on embryonic limb-bones cultivated *in vitro. J. Physiol.* **116**, 320

[21] DINGLE J.T., LUCY J.A. & FELL H.B. (1961) Studies on the mode of action of excess of vitamin A. 1. Effect of excess of vitamin A on the metabolism and composition of embryonic chick-limb cartilage grown in organ culture. *Biochem. J.* **79**, 497

[22] LUCY J.A., DINGLE J.T. & FELL H.B. (1961) Studies on the mode of action of excess of vitamin A. 2. A possible role of intracellular proteases in the degradation of cartilage matrix. *Biochem. J.* **79**, 500

[23] DINGLE J.T. (1961) Studies on the mode of action of excess of vitamin A. 3. Release of a bound protease by the action of vitamin A. *Biochem. J.* **79**, 509

[24] WILLIAMS M.A., TYLER H.M., MORTON M., NEMETH A. & DEMPSTER W.J. (1962) Some biochemical changes in the transplanted kidney. *Brit. med. J.* **2**, 1215

[25] CHIBA C., WOLF P.L., GUDBJARNESON S., CHRYSOHOV A., RAMOS H., PEARSON B. & BING R.J. (1962) Studies on the transplanted heart. *J. exp. Med.* **115**, 853

[26] LINDQUIST R.R. & HAGER E.B. (1964) Histochemical studies of renal grafts. *Ann. N.Y. Acad. Sci.* **120**, 52

[27] BALLANTYNE D.L., CASCARANO J. & CONVERSE J.M. (1964) Histochemical diagnosis of homograft rejection. *Ann. N.Y. Acad. Sci.* **120**, 46

[28] SCOTHORNE R.J. & TOUGH J.S. (1952) Histochemical studies of human skin autografts and homografts. *Brit. J. Plast. Surg.* **5**, 161

[29] BRACHET J. (1950) *Chemical Embryology,* transl. BARTH L. New York: Interscience

[30] CASPERSSON T. (1950) *Cell Growth and Cell Function.* New York: Norton

[31] HOAGLAND M.B. (1958) Enzymatic reactions between amino acids and ribonucleic acids as intermediate steps in protein synthesis. *Symp. VIII, 4th Int. Congr. Biochem.,* Vienna, pp. 199

[32] ASKONAS B.A., SIMKIN J.L. & WORK T.S. (1958) Protein synthesis in cell free systems. *Symp. VIII, 4th Int. Congr. Biochem., Vienna,* pp. 181

[33] KURNICK N.B. (1955) Histochemistry of nucleic acids. *Int. Rev. Cytol.* **4**, 221

[34] ARMSTRONG J.A. (1956) Histochemical differentiation of nucleic acids by means of induced fluorescence. *Exp. Cell. Res.* **11**, 640

[35] SINGER M. (1954) The staining of basophilic components. *J. Histochem. Cytochem.* **2**, 322

[36] SWIFT H. (1955) Cytochemical techniques for nucleic acids. In *The Nucleic Acids,* Vol. II, pp. 51–92, ed. CHARGAFF E. & DAVIDSON J.N. New York: Academic Press

[37] HORECKER B.L. & MEHLER A.H. (1955) Carbohydrate metabolism. *Ann. Rev. Biochem.* **24**, 207

[38] KORNBERG A. (1957) Pathways of enzymatic synthesis of nucleotides and polynucleotides. In *The Chemical Basis of Heredity,* pp. 579–608, ed. McELROY W.D. & GLASS B. Baltimore: Johns Hopkins Press

[39] Easty G.C. & Ambrose E.J. (1957) The antigenic composition of mouse ascites tumour cells using *in vitro* and gel-diffusion techniques. *Brit. J. Canc.* **11**, 287

[40] Easton J.M., Goldberg B. & Green H. (1962) Immune cytolysis: Electron microscopic localization of cellular antigens with ferritin–antibody conjugates. *J. exp. Med.* **115**, 275

[41] Davson H. & Danielli J.F. (1943) *The Permeability of Natural Membranes.* London: Cambridge University Press

[42] Chayen J., Gahan P.B. & La Cour L.F. (1959) The masked lipids of nuclei. *Quart. J. micr. Sci.* **100**, 325

[43] Chayen J., Chayen R., Cunningham G.J. & Bitensky L. (1961) Bound lipids, and their significance in cell biology. *Path. et Biol.* **9**, 925

[44] Barer R. (1959) Weighing cells with the microscope; some aspects of phase contrast and interference microscopy. In *Tools of Biological Research*, pp. 122–143, ed. Atkins H.J.B. Oxford: Blackwell Scientific Publications

[45] Davies H.G., Wilkins M.H.F., Chayen J. & La Cour L.F. (1954) The use of the interference microscope to determine dry mass in living cells and as a quantitative cytochemical method. *Quart. J. micr. Sci.* **95**, 271

[46] Hale A.J. (1958) *The Interference Microscope in Biological Research.* Edinburgh: Livingstone

[47] Barer R. (1956) Phase contrast and interference microscopy in cytology. In *Physical Techniques in Biological Research*, Vol. III, pp. 29–90, ed. Oster G. & Pollister A.W. New York: Academic Press

[48] Green H., Fleischer R.A., Barrow P. & Goldberg B. (1959) The cytotoxic action of immune gamma globulin and complement on Krebs ascites tumour cells. II. Chemical studies. *J. exp. Med.* **109**, 511

[49] Kirkby W.W. (1964) The effect of histamine on monoamine oxidase in rat liver cultured *in vitro*. *Biochem. J.* **93**, 7P

[50] Diengdoh J.V. (1964) Experimentally induced activation of monoamine oxidase in mouse skin. *Biochem. J.* **93**, 6P

[51] Converse J.M. & Rapaport F.T. (1956) The vascularization of skin autografts and homografts. *Ann. Surg.* **143**, 306

[52] Wells P.J., Bitensky L., Altmann F.P. & Chayen J. (1965) The effect of mechanical damage on the latency of glutamic dehydrogenase. *Biochem. J.* **96**, 36P

[53] Chayen J., Wells P.J. & Bitensky L. (1965) The meaning of a 'good' histochemical reaction in relation to the problem of latent enzyme activity. *J. Roy. Micr. Soc.* **84**, 400

[54] Cohen S., Bitensky L. & Chayen J. (1965) The study of monoamine oxidase activity by histochemical procedures. *Biochem. pharmacol.* **14**, 223

[55] Gianetto R. & Duve C.de (1955) Tissue fractionation studies. 4. Comparative study of the binding of acid phosphatase, β-glucuronidase and cathepsin by rat liver particles *Biochem. J.* **59**, 433

[56] Duve C.de (1959) Lysosomes, a new group of cytoplasmic particles. In *Subcellular Particles*, pp. 128–159, ed. Hayashi T. New York: Ronald Press

[57] Duve C.de (1963) The lysosome concept. In *Ciba Foundation Symp. on Lysosomes*, pp. 1–31, ed. de Reuck A.V.S. & Cameron M.P. London: Churchill

[58] Bitensky L. (1963) The reversible activation of lysosomes in normal cells and the effects of pathological conditions. In *Ciba Foundation Symp. on Lysosomes*, pp. 362–375, ed. de Reuck A.V.S. & Cameron M.P. London: Churchill

[59] Bitensky L. & Gahan P.B. (1962) The reversible activation of lysosomes in normal cells. *Biochem. J.* **84**, 13–14P

[60] GOLDBERG B. & GREEN H. (1959) The cytotoxic action of immune gamma globulin and complement on Krebs ascites tumour cells. I. Ultrastructural studies. *J. exp. Med.* **109,** 505

[61] SYLVÉN B. & BOIS-SVENSSON I. (1964) Studies on the histochemical 'leucine aminopeptidase' reaction. IV. Chemical and histochemical characterization of the intracellular and stromal LNA reactions in solid tumor transplants. *Histochemie* **4,** 135

[62] MCCABE M. & CHAYEN J. (1965) The demonstration of latent particulate aminopeptidase activity. *J. Roy. Micr. Soc.* **84,** 361

[63] BENDALL D.S. & DUVE C.DE (1960) Tissue fractionation studies. 14. The activation of latent dehydrogenases in mitochondria from rat liver. *Biochem J.* **74,** 444

[64] KIRKBY W.W. (1965) The use of histochemical examination of maintenance-cultured tissue in assessing potential cytotoxic substances. *Biochem. J.* **94,** 24–25P

[65] MACLAGAN N.F. (1964) Diseases of the liver and biliary tract. In *Biochemical Disorders in Human Disease.* pp. 122–125, ed. THOMPSON R.H.S. & KING E.J. London: Churchill

[66] BALDWIN E. (1959) *Dynamic Aspects of Biochemistry,* 3rd ed., p. 262. London: Cambridge University Press

[67] HUMPHREY J.H. (1959) Cellular components involved in the immediate allergic reactions. *1st Int. Symp. on Immunopathology.* pp. 215–221, ed. GRABER P. & MIESCHER P. Basel: Benno Schwabe.

[68] OSLER A.G. (1959) The role of complement in the mediation of tissue injury induced by allergic reactions of the immediate type. In *1st Int. Symp. on Immunopathology,* pp. 227–236, ed. GRABAR P. & MIESCHER P. Basel: Benno Schwabe

[69] DIXON F.J. (1962) Tissue injury produced by antigen–antibody complexes. In *2nd Int. Symp. on Immunopathology,* pp. 71–86, ed. GRABAR P. & MIESCHER P. Basel: Benno Schwabe

[70] RILEY J.F. (1959) *The Mast Cells.* Edinburgh: Livingstone

[71] MOTA I. (1963) The behaviour of mast cells in anaphylaxis. *Int. Rev. Cytol.* **15,** 363

[72] BITENSKY L., LYNCH R., SILCOX A.A. & CHAYEN J. (1965) Studies on chilling and sectioning tissue for histochemistry. *J. Roy. Micr. Soc.* **84,** 397

[73] SILCOX A.A., POULTER L.W., BITENSKY L. & CHAYEN J. (1965) An examination of some factors affecting histological preservation in frozen sections of unfixed tissue. *J. Roy. Micr. Soc.* **84,** 559

[74] BITENSKY L., ELLIS R., SILCOX A.A. & CHAYEN J. (1962) Histochemical studies on carbohydrate material in liver. *Ann. Histochim.* **7,** 7

[75] LENDRUM A.C. (1949) The staining of erythrocytes in tissue sections. *J. Path. Bact.* **61,** 443

[76] CHAYEN J. (1952) The methyl green–pyronin method. *Exp. Cell Res.* **3,** 652

[77] BITENSKY L. (1962) Histochemical studies on experimentally induced liver tumours in rats. Ph.D. thesis. University of London.

[78] KURNICK N.R. & MIRSKY A.E. (1950) Methyl green-pyronin. II. Stoichiometry of reaction with nucleic acids. *J. gen. Physiol.* **33,** 265

[79] KURNICK N.R. (1950) The quantitative estimation of desoxyribosenucleic acid based on methyl green staining. *Exp. Cell Res.* **1,** 151

[80] KURNICK N.R. (1952) The basis for the specificity of methyl green stain. *Exp. Cell Res.* **3,** 649

[81] VERCAUTEREN R. (1950) The structure of desoxyribose nucleic acid in relation to the cytochemical significance of the methyl green–pyronin staining. *Enzymologia* **14,** 134

[82] CHAYEN J. & NORRIS K.P. (1953) Cytoplasmic localization of nucleic acids in plant cells. *Nature, Lond.* **171,** 472

[83] JACOBSON W. & WEBB M. (1952) The two types of nucleoproteins during mitosis. *Exp. Cell Res.* **3,** 163

[84] DIENGDOH J.V. (1965) Ph.D. thesis, in preparation. Also personal communication.

[85] HÖFLER K. (1949) Fluorochromierungstudien an Pflanzanzellen. In *Fluoreszenzmikroskopie,* pp. 46–70, ed. BRÄUTIGAM F. & GRABNER A. Vienna: George Fromme

[86] MESSART L., PEETERS G., DE LEY J., VERCAUTEREN R. & VON HONCKE A. (1947) The mechanism of the biochemical activity of acridines. *Experientia* **3,** 288

[87] SYLVÉN B. (1954) Metachromatic dye-substrate interactions. *Quart. J. micr. Sci.* **95,** 327

[88] CHAYEN R. & ROBERTS E.R. (1955) Some observations on the metachromatic reaction. *Sc. J. Roy. Coll. Sci.* **25,** 50

[89] PEARSE A.G.E. (1960) *Histochemistry,* 2nd ed., p. 779. London: Churchill

[90] ALTMANN F.P. & CHAYEN J. (1965) The significance of a functioning hydrogen-transport system for the retention of 'soluble' dehydrogenases in unfixed sections. *J. Roy. Micro. Soc.* **85,** 175

[91] CHAIN E.B. (1959) Recent studies on carbohydrate metabolism. *Brit. med. J.* **2,** 707

[92] CASPERSSON T. (1947) The relations between nucleic acid and protein synthesis. *Soc. Exp. Biol. Symp.* **1,** 127

[93] DICKENS F., GLOCK G.E. & McLEAN P. (1959) Some problems in the choice of oxidative pathways of carbohydrate metabolism. In *Ciba Found. Symp. on Regulation of Cell Metabolism,* pp. 150–182, ed. WOLSTENHOLME G.E.W. & O'CONNOR C.M. London: Churchill

[94] CHAYEN J., BITENSKY L., AVES E.K., JONES G.R.N., SILCOX A.A. & CUNNINGHAM G.J. (1962) Histochemical demonstration of 6-phosphogluconate dehydrogenase in proliferating and malignant cells. *Nature, Lond.* **195,** 714

[95] GLOCK G.E. (1961) In *Biochemists' Handbook,* pp. 343–346, ed. LONG C. London: Spon

[96] ALTMANN F.P. (1965) The retention and estimation of 'soluble' dehydrogenases in unfixed tissue sections. *Biochem. J.* **96,** 53–54P

[97] ALTMANN F.P. & CHAYEN J. (1965) The retention of nitrogenous material in unfixed sections during incubation for histochemical demonstration of enzymes. *Nature, Lond.* **207,** 1205

[98] JONES G.R.N., MAPLE A.J., AVES E.K., CHAYEN J. & CUNNINGHAM G.J. (1963) Quantitative histochemistry of succinate dehydrogenase in tissue sections. *Nature, Lond.* **197,** 568

[99] NACHLAS M.M., MARGULIES S.I. & SELIGMAN A.M. (1960) Sites of electron transfer to tetrazolium salts in the succinoxidase system. *J. biol. Chem.* **235,** 2739

[100] GREEN D.E. (1959) Structure-function interrelationships in mitochondrial electron transport and oxidative phosphorylation. *Disc. Faraday Soc.* **27,** 206

[101] JONES G.R.N. (1964) Quantitative histochemistry: Design and use of a simple microcell for standardized incubation on the slide. *Stain Technol.* **39,** 155

[102] BUTCHER R. & CHAYEN J. In preparation

[103] SLOANE-STANLEY G.H. & JONES G.R.N. (1963) Simple methods for the determination of very small amounts of nitrogen in organic matter. *Biochem. J.* **86,** 16P

[104] BAUDHUIN P., BEAUFAY H., RAHMAN-LI Y., SELLINGER O.Z., WATTIAUX R., JACQUES P. & DUVE C.DE (1964) Tissue fractionation studies. 17. Intracellular distribution of monoamine oxidase, aspartate aminotransferase, alanine aminotransferase, D-amino acid oxidase and catalase in rat-liver tissue. *Biochem. J.* **92,** 179

[105] BITENSKY L. (1962) The demonstration of lysosomes by the controlled temperature freezing-sectioning method. *Quart. J. micr. Sci.* **103,** 205

[106] DIENGDOH J.V. (1964) The demonstration of lysosomes in mouse skin. *Quart. J. micr. Sci.* **105,** 73

[107] BITENSKY L. & COHEN S. (1965) The variation of endometrial acid phosphatase activity with the menstrual cycle. *J. Obstet. Gynaec. Brit. Comm.* **LXXII,** 769

[108] HOLT S.J. (1959) Factors governing the validity of staining methods for enzymes, and their bearing upon the Gomori acid phosphatase technique. *Exp. Cell Res.* **Suppl. 7,** 1

[109] GOMORI G. (1941) Distribution of acid phosphatase in the tissues under normal and under pathologic conditions. *Arch. Path.* **32,** 189

[110] BITENSKY L. (1963) Modifications to the Gomori acid phosphatase technique for controlled-temperature frozen sections. *Quart. J. micr. Sci.* **104,** 193

[111] SYLVÉN B. & BOIS I. (1963) Studies on the histochemical 'leucine amino-peptidase' reaction. II. Chemical and histochemical comparison of the enzymatic and environmental factors involved. *Histochemie* **3,** 341

[112] SYLVÉN B. & SNELLMAN O. (1962) A new metal-dependant enzyme present in cathepsin C preparations. *Biochim. Biophys. Acta* **65,** 350

[113] SYLVÉN B. & SNELLMAN O. (1964) Studies on the histochemical 'leucine amino-peptidase' reaction. III. On the different LNA-splitting enzymes from spleen. *Histochemie* **3,** 484

[114] NACHLAS M.M., CRAWFORD D.T. & SELIGMAN A.M. (1957) The histochemical demonstration of leucine aminopeptidase. *J. Histochem. Cytochem.* **5,** 264

[115] BAKER J.R. (1946) The histochemical recognition of lipine. *Quart. J. micr. Sci.* **87,** 441

[116] BAKER J.R. (1947) Further remarks on the histochemical recognition of lipine. *Quart. J. micr. Sci.* **88,** 463

[117] MAGGI V., CHAYEN J., GAHAN P.B. & BRANDER W. (1964) A histochemical study of the bound lipids of arteries: Their possible role in arteriosclerosis. *Exper. Mol. Path.* **3,** 413

[118] BERG N.O. (1951) A histological study of masked lipids. Stainability, distribution and functional variations. *Acta Pathol. Microbiol. Scand.* **Suppl. XC,** 1-192

[119] BITENSKY L., BALDWIN R.W. & CHAYEN J. (1960) A histochemical study of the early stages of carcinogenesis in rat liver: Changes in cellular lipids and mitochondria. *Brit. J. Canc.* **14,** 696

PART C

APPLIED METHODS

CHAPTER 24

Immunological Methods in Virology

D.A.J.TYRRELL

Introduction

This chapter deals with immunological methods used in virology and because of the limitations of the author mainly with the virology of man and animals; there are certain other limitations which should also be stated in order that it may be used as effectively as possible. In the first place, it does not pretend to be a complete catalogue of all the methods which have been used in virology; those of historical interest only have been ignored, those which represent minor variations of other tests have been either omitted or merely referred to, and methods which are likely to be of interest to only a limited number of readers have been outlined, but not described in detail. Methods which are described elsewhere in this book—complement fixation or gel diffusion, for example—are not described in full here, but modifications which are important in virology are given in a certain amount of detail. Finally, although this is intended to be a practical book an attempt has been made throughout to stress principles rather than small details, because in fact it is possible to vary the details of most of the technical procedures to be described without detriment to the results, provided the important principles of the test are not violated; in fact, some variations in detail may be advantageous if they are made with a clear understanding of the basic requirements of the test. The methods given therefore serve as models which an individual worker can modify to suit his own needs. Nevertheless, because all but one of the methods described in detail are based on personal experience, it should be possible to set up a working test without difficulty if the procedures are carried out exactly as described.

776

The place of immunological methods in virology

All viruses contain at least one protein differing from that of the animal they parasitize and many virus proteins are very potent antigens. Therefore, antibodies are often formed by the host following non-fatal virus infections and may also be induced in any one of a variety of animal species by injections of killed virus or of virus which cannot multiply.

If a rising titre of antibody is detected in the serum of a patient this suggests that his illness was caused by a virus related to the one used to detect the antibody. This is the basis of a great many serological diagnostic tests. Similarly, the presence of antibody in a healthy person suggests that he has previously been infected with the virus used in the test or with one related to it. This test may also be useful for the retrospective diagnosis of an infection and serological surveys may be carried out; that is, it may be possible to show the presence of viruses in a certain population by testing the sera of representative individuals for the presence of specific antibodies.

Sera from animals given experimental infections or injections of killed virus can be used as specific reagents for identifying the antigenic type of virus. Unidentified viruses are usually put into their biological group by properties such as the type of cells they attack, or whether they produce haemagglutinins. They are then allowed to react with a series of sera prepared against viruses of that group. If a reaction occurs with a serum the virus can be assigned to the corresponding serotype. Immunological methods may thus be used for the serotyping and identification of viruses.

Finally, since many virus proteins are specific antigens they may be recognized by immunological methods after a virus particle has been broken up or become non-infectious. Thus the antigenic structure of a virus particle may be studied, and small amounts of virus protein may be detected in the presence of large amounts of contaminating material. Furthermore, virus antigens may be detected within the cells in which they are synthesized and before any infectious virus is produced; by staining with fluorescent antibody individual infected cells may be identified and also the part of the cell in which the specific antigen is present.

Specific tests are mentioned in subsequent sections and also outlines of the ways in which each may be used. However, a reader wishing to find the methods which are applicable to a certain virus or group of viruses should also read a systematic textbook of virology or virological techniques [1] or [2].

The preparation of antibodies against virus antigens

The infection of a susceptible animal or the injection of an insusceptible one may be used. These methods may be illustrated by one which is widely used for the preparation of antiserum against influenza A virus in the ferret

[3]; a procedure similar to this can be used for immunizing ferrets, guinea-pigs and hamsters against influenza, parainfluenza and respiratory syncytial viruses [4, 5]. Certain viruses such as arboviruses and coxsackieviruses kill new-born mice, but not adults. Potent antisera may be obtained against these by inoculation of adults with tissue extracts from infected infant mice; in these animals it is probable that a limited degree of virus multiplication takes place. Another method is used to prepare antisera in the rabbit [6]—procedures similar to this have been used to prepare sera against enteroviruses, adenoviruses and reoviruses [7, 8, 9].

1. *Infection of a ferret with influenza A virus*
Egg-adapted influenza A virus diluted 10^{-3} in buffered saline containing antibiotics is inoculated into five 10-day-old chicks embryos by the allantoic route. The eggs are incubated at 35° C for 2 days. The eggs are chilled and harvested; the allantoic fluids are pooled and stored at $-70°$ C if there is to be a delay before the animal is inoculated.

The ferret, half- to full-grown, is anaesthetized with ether and 5-10 ml of blood is removed by cardiac puncture. While still anaesthetized and lying on its back 0·5 ml of allantoic fluid is instilled into each nostril. The rectal temperature of the animal may be taken daily before and after inoculation if desired, as a febrile response indicates that an infection has been successfully induced. Two to three weeks later the animal is bled again. The blood samples are all processed immediately after collection by sterile techniques and serum is separated and stored at $-20°$ C until needed.

2. *Preparation of antiserum against influenza A virus in a rabbit*
A pool of allantoic fluid prepared as described above is clarified by centrifugation, if necessary. A young rabbit, about 2 kg in weight, is bled from the marginal ear vein. Then 10 ml of allantoic fluid, which should have a haemagglutinin titre of at least several hundred is slowly injected intravenously. Two weeks later the rabbit is bled again.

If desired the antibody titre of both rabbit and ferret can be raised by further injections of up to 10 ml of antigen given intraperitoneally or intravenously.

These methods produced 'impure' sera which contain antibodies against both the surface or V antigen of the virus and also the internal, S or g antigen. Antisera reacting against only the S antigen may be obtained by immunizing a rabbit from the beginning with a purified virus fraction [10] or by waiting till the primary antibody response of an infected guinea-pig declines and then stimulating it by intraperitoneal injection of purified S antigen [11]. Similarly, anti-V antiserum may be obtained by immunizing with purified V antigen or by stimulating a previously infected guinea-pig with purified V antigen.

If complement fixation, precipitation or similar tests are to be used it is essential to remember that, except in the sera of animals convalescent from infection, there is likely to be antibody against not only the virus but also against the proteins of the host in which the virus was prepared—chick proteins in the case of example 2 above. In the case of myxoviruses in general it is impossible to remove these host antigens by purification for they are incorporated into the particle itself. However, even impure antigens may induce only antiviral antibodies if the virus is grown in cells of the animals of the species to be immunized—for example, respiratory syncytial virus may be grown in tissue cultures of ferret kidney cells maintained with ferret serum and this may be used to stimulate antibody production in previously infected ferrets [12, 13].

Preparation of antisera against 'poor' antigens

It is difficult to make antisera against some viruses and this is often because very little virus is produced during an infection, and also because this little is heavily contaminated by host protein, which comprises more than 99 per cent of the average virus preparation.

Adjuvants may be used with viruses as with other antigens. Aluminium phosphate is not necessarily a useful adjuvant, but virus adsorbed to it is also concentrated and purified to some extent and can be further incorporated into Freund-type adjuvant, preferably including tubercle bacilli to give a maximal antigenic stimulus. Aluminium hydroxide may also be an efficient adjuvant, but the optimal effect may be obtained only if exactly the right amount is added to, for example, a preparation of NDV virus [15]. The Freund adjuvant may greatly enhance the antigenicity of some myxoviruses [16, 17], but does not have a regular effect on picornaviruses or adenoviruses [18, 19, 20]; the effect may also vary from species to species [20].

The author has found on several occasions that it may also be helpful in these cases to prepare the animal by frequent subcutaneous or intravenous injections of virus or by an intramuscular injection of virus in adjuvant; the animal may then be left for at least 6 weeks and sometimes 6 months, and then given an intravenous injection of as much virus as possible. One week to 10 days after inoculation good titres of antibody are usually present.

3. *The preparation of antisera against rhinoviruses in goats*

Virus is prepared by infection of tissue cultures of human diploid fibroblast cell strains or malignant cells maintained in a medium containing 1 or 2 per cent normal goat serum and Eagle's medium. About 500 ml of culture fluid of a titre of at least $10^{4.5}$ TCD_{50}/ml is mixed with a final concentration of 1–2 mg/ml of sterile aluminium phosphate gel, mixed thoroughly at 0° C for 60 minutes and the gel and adsorbed virus are then centrifuged off at low speed. It is necessary to ensure that the batch of gel will adsorb virus efficiently under the conditions used. The gel is resuspended in saline or Eagle's basal medium and mixed with an equal volume of complete Freund adjuvant and emulsified by means of a blender. One millilitre of the mixture is inoculated intramuscularly into each of the four quarters of a goat, and the injections are repeated 1 week later. The goat is given a further intravenous dose of 100 ml or more of virus adsorbed on to aluminium phosphate or as plain culture fluid about 6 months later. A test bleed is taken 10 days later and if a high titre of antibody is present the animal is exsanguinated under anaesthesia and 1–2 litres of serum are obtained. If a high titre of virus is obtained tissue culture fluid incorporated into adjuvant may induce antibodies without the use of aluminium phosphate or a 'rest' period followed by reinoculation [21].

Adsorption of sera

Antibodies against host cells may interfere with serological tests in various ways, such as fixing complement with host antigens, agglutinating red cells or damaging culture cells or making them virus-resistant [22]. It is therefore necessary at times to absorb these sera, and the usual method is to obtain a sedimentable preparation of cellular antigens, mix it with the serum, and hold them together with shaking for some time, usually for several hours, and then centrifuge the mixture. The supernatant is the absorbed serum. Liver may be blended in saline and the sediment obtained and washed with saline; when precipitated and dried with acetone it can be stored until needed [23]. We have also used trypsinized tissue or culture cells, sometimes stored at $-20°$ C in 50 per cent glycerol, to remove anti-tissue antibodies which were interfering with the fluorescent antibody staining of virus [24].

It is also possible to absorb antiviral antibodies from sera. However, it may be difficult to obtain enough virus to absorb a detectable amount of antibody and it is usually necessary to use an ultracentrifuge to separate the virus–antibody complexes. The following is a simple method for the absorption of sera with influenza virus.

4. Absorption of virus antibodies from serum

Ten millilitres of allantoic fluid containing influenza A virus of a haemagglutinin titre of 1000 or greater are centrifuged at 3000 rev/min for half an hour and placed in an ultracentrifuge tube. The tube is centrifuged at 30000 rev/min for half an hour to deposit the virus and subcellular particles; the supernatant is poured off and the deposit resuspended in 1 ml of saline by grinding with a glass rod and by repeated pipetting. Three millilitres of rabbit antiserum diluted 1/5 in saline are added and the mixture held at $4°$ C overnight. Next morning the mixture is centrifuged again at 30000 rev/min for half an hour and the supernatant is the absorbed serum.

To simplify this procedure, stocks of influenza virus irreversibly adsorbed on to formalin-treated red cells can be prepared and kept in the refrigerator [25]. In order to absorb any serum it is then only necessary to take a standard aliquot of red cells and mix it with a portion of serum, allow the mixture to react and then centrifuge it at low speed to remove the red cells with the attached virus and antibody. Antibodies against homologous virus are absorbed by this technique. Some sera contain antibodies against the immunizing virus and also other viruses related to it. If the serum is absorbed with the immunizing virus all the antibodies may be absorbed; if it is absorbed with a related virus then only antibodies against the related virus used may be absorbed [25, 26].

Methods based on the inactivation of the specific biological activity of viruses

Haemagglutination inhibition
In recent years it has become clear that many viruses agglutinate red cells of certain species. For instance, the influenza, mumps and parainfluenza viruses agglutinate chicken, human and guinea-pig cells, measles virus agglutinates monkey cells, all the adenoviruses agglutinate rat or monkey cells or both, the reoviruses and many enteroviruses agglutinate human cells, and the majority of the arboviruses day-old-chick or goose cells. Many agglutination reactions have optimal temperatures at some point between refrigerator temperature and 37° C, and many can be readily performed at room temperature. Of the order of a million virus particles may be needed to produce demonstrable haemagglutination [27] so the test is usually a much less sensitive test for the presence of virus than is infectivity, but noninfectious virus often haemagglutinates, and this may be an advantage. Haemagglutination is generally mediated by the same areas on the surface of the virus particle as are concerned in the early stages of virus infection and they can be inactivated by combination with specific antiviral antibody. Therefore virus-neutralizing antibodies are often also haemagglutination-inhibiting antibodies, and although the tests are not exactly equivalent it is often possible to use simple haemagglutination tests instead of neutralization tests in the study of the composition of virus antigens and of the titres of antiviral antibodies in sera.

The haemagglutinins of many viruses are inhibited by substances other than antibodies which are present in tissue extracts and in sera and these must be removed in order to obtain accurate measurements of antibody concentrations. Although called 'non-specific' inhibitors they would be better called 'non-antibody' inhibitors since different substances such as lipoproteins, glycoproteins inhibit specifically agglutination by viruses of different groups. Some methods of removing these inhibitors are listed in Table 24.1. There follows now a description of a typical haemagglutination inhibition test using the influenza virus as a model once again.

5. *Haemagglutination inhibition test*

Chicken red cells are collected aseptically from the wing vein of a cock, suspended in sterile saline in a graduated tube and centrifuged at 3000 rev/min for 5 minutes in a bench centrifuge. The supernatant is discarded. The cells are washed three times in this way. From the packed-cell volume the calculated amount of dextrose–gelatin–veronal (DGV) solution is added to form a 10 per cent suspension which is stored at 4° C. A suspension of 0·5 per cent cells is made by making a 1/20 dilution of the DGV suspension in saline. Allantoic fluid containing influenza virus is diluted 1/10 in broth and from this solution serial twofold dilutions are made in a plastic tray in the following way. Volumes of 0·25 ml of saline (buffered at pH 7·1 with 0·01 M sodium phosphate buffer) are added to the cups in a WHO pattern plastic agglutination tray using an automatic dispenser or pipetting machine. A pasteur pipette has been previously constricted and calibrated with a weighed drop of mercury to contain 0·25 ml. This is used to make serial dilutions of virus; each mixture is made by pipetting up and down five or six times and after the last volume is discarded the pipette is cleaned by rinsing in cold saline, boiling water and clean sterile saline. Alternatively a fresh pipette may be used. Two series of dilutions are made and then 0·25 ml of 0·5 per cent red cell suspension is added to each cup. The cells and virus are mixed by adding the suspension vigorously and if necessary shaking the plate. The plate is then allowed to stand on the bench, protected from draughts and air currents either by stacking the plates or putting them in plastic bags. After $1-1\frac{1}{4}$ hours the plates are inspected. Agglutinated red cells form an even carpet on the bottom of the cup, or in high concentrations rather granular clumps near the centre. Unagglutinated cells form a smooth button at the centre. Partial agglutination is taken as the end-point. If the two titrations agree within one dilution the final end-point is taken as the average of the two; if they do not agree the test is repeated.

Serum dilutions have usually been prepared earlier. Volumes of 0·2 ml of serum are mixed aseptically with 0·8 ml of cholera filtrate—either kept in the liquid state or freeze-dried and reconstituted. These mixtures are incubated overnight at 37° C in a water-bath or incubator and then heated at 56° C to inactivate the enzymes of the filtrate, particularly the neuraminidase, which would otherwise destroy the virus receptors on the red cells. These inactivated serum dilutions may be stored for some time, months if frozen,

TABLE 24.1

Treatments used for removing from serum the 'non-specific' inhibitors of haemagglutination by certain viruses

α inhibitors	Influenza viruses β inhibitors	Parainfluenza viruses	Adenoviruses and enteroviruses	Arboviruses
V. cholerae filtrate [28] Periodate [29] Treatment with CO_2 [30]	Heat at 56° C—some species Trypsin [31] *V. cholerae* filtrate	*V. cholerae* filtrate [31]	Absorption with kaolin [32]	Treatment with acetone or absorption [33]

without loss of antibody activity. The virus suspension, however, is much less stable. Serial dilutions of serum are prepared as above and to each cup is added 0·25 ml of a dilution of virus calculated to contain four agglutinating doses (AD) of virus. The mixtures are allowed to stand at room temperature for 30 minutes and then 0·25 ml of red cell suspension is added and the mixtures are placed on the bench as before. Owing to the presence of serum the red cells settle more quickly and the pattern of agglutination may be seen readily after 45–60 minutes. A check titration of the virus suspension

TABLE 24.2

Protocol of representative haemagglutination-inhibition test with influenza virus

Virus titration

Virus dilution	1/10	1/20	1/40	1/80	1/160	1/320
Results* {	+ +	+ +	+ +	+ +	+	0
	+ +	+ +	+ +	+ +	+	0

Virus titre   1/160
   4 AD in 1/40 dilution ∴ use 1/4 dilution of stock 1/10 dilution in broth

Serum titration Dilutions of sera treated with *V. cholerae* filtrate

		1/10	1/20	1/40	1/80	1/160	Serum control	Titre
Normal rabbit serum		+ +	+ +	+ +	+ +	+ +	0	< 10
Patients' serum	A	+ +	+ +	+ +	+ +	+ +	+	?
	B	0	0	0	0	+ +	0	1/120
	C	0	+	+ +	+ +	+ +	0	1/20

Conclusions
1. The cholera filtrate is active and has destroyed non-specific inhibitors in normal rabbit serum.
2. Patient A's serum must be absorbed with red cells.
3. The tests with the sera of patients B and C are valid.

* Agglutination patterns are recorded thus: + + full agglutination; + partial agglutination; 0 no agglutination. Where no partial agglutination is seen end-points may be interpolated approximately by eye—e.g. patient B serum.

added to the cups is performed in order to confirm that the calculated four doses were actually used. Sometimes sera agglutinate red cells, and this is revealed by including a mixture of the initial dilution of each serum and red cells without virus in the test. If such serum agglutination occurs the serum dilution is absorbed with about 10 per cent of red cells, roughly as outlined earlier, and then retitrated. Typical haemagglutination patterns are shown in Fig. 24.1 and a representative protocol is shown in Table 24.2.

Haemagglutination tests of this type are satisfactory with influenza and parainfluenza viruses, but it is necessary to vary the red cells and temperature for some viruses. For instance, influenza C virus agglutinates to high titre only at 4° C. If by using inappropriate conditions or allowing the virus to

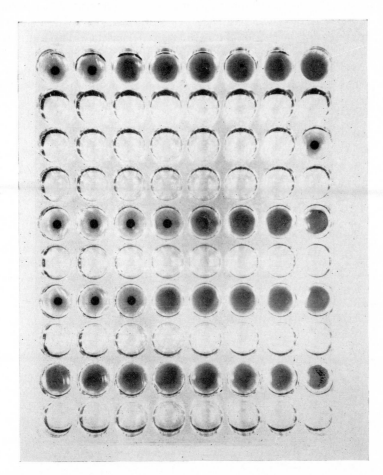

Fig. 24.1. A haemagglutination-inhibition test using adenoviruses. Haemagglutination is shown by the sheets of cells on the bottom of the cups of the plastic tray. Unagglutinated cells form a button. Dilution series start at the left. Three sera are inhibitory and one is not. (Courtesy of H.G.Pereira.)

become partly inactivated the titre of haemagglutinin used is reduced then the sensitivity of the test for antibodies will fall also. In the case of arboviruses it is necessary to use both an appropriate temperature and a buffer system adjusted to within 0·1 pH unit in order to get satisfactory results [33].

Alternative forms of the haemagglutination-inhibition test

In the original HI test described by Hirst the extent of haemagglutination was measured in a photoelectric colorimeter by recording the optical density in the middle of a tube containing the mixture of virus, serum and red cells. A slow rate of settling indicated the absence of haemagglutination and therefore the presence of antibody. The method is quite objective and quantitatively interpolated end-points can be easily obtained. However, it is more cumbersome than the pattern test and not much more accurate. The pattern test can in fact be made quite precise by making serial dilutions of $0.1 \log_{10}$ intervals instead of $0.3 \log_{10}$ [34, 35].

The methods of Fazekas and Drescher

Recently methods based on haemagglutination inhibition have been developed which though unsuitable for general use have proved powerful tools for giving more quantitative and precise information about antiviral antibodies.

TABLE 24.3

Representative results of measurements of haemagglutination-inhibiting antibodies against influenza A virus strain MEL in a rabbit immune serum (Fazekas & Webster) [37]

Concentration of virus	$2.62(\pm 0.11) \times 10^{10}$ particles/ml
Concentration of antibody	$2.24(\pm 0.48) \times 10^{14}$ molecules/ml
Equilibrium constant	$9.18(\pm 2.38) \times 10^{10}$
Number of antigenic sites	$2.15(\pm 0.49) \times 10^{3}$ per virus particle

The first of these was developed by Fazekas de St Groth and his colleagues as part of an investigation intended to measure the number of antibody molecules present and the equilibrium constant of their reaction with the virus [36, 37]. The method is basically to prepare a series of mixtures of known amounts of virus with antibody and allow these to react for a measured period of time before removing the virus by centrifuging or passing the mixture through a virus-retaining filter. The proportion of free antibody was then measured by a standard pattern type haemagglutination-inhibition test. In associated experiments they also measured the amount of antibody in serum by labelling the γ globulin with radioiodine and observing the amount specifically bound to virus. They also determined the number of particles represented by a haemagglutinating dose of each of the viruses used. It was then possible to calculate the number of antibody molecules present and their equilibrium constant with the virus used. Some representative results are shown in Table 24.3.

The second method is due to Drescher [38] who allowed virus and antibody to react together and measured the agglutination with a photometer. He showed that the reaction between homologous antibody and virus can be expressed in the form of the equation of the Freundlich isotherm. It is well known and was mentioned earlier that viruses do not produce really specific

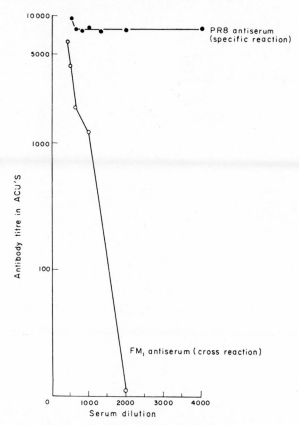

FIG. 24.2. The reaction between influenza virus and homologous and heterologous antibodies (PR8) as shown by the Drescher technique. The trite of specific antibody is independent of the dilution of serum used in the test. (By permission of J. Drescher and the *Journal of Immunology*.)

antibody responses, for example, related influenza viruses elicit antibody against each other when the sera are tested by the standard HI test. However, such cross-reacting sera show entirely different results in the Drescher test (Fig. 24.2). Homologous virus reacts with antibody in the form of the Freundlich isotherm, while the heterologous virus reacts less strongly so that the two types of antibody may be reliably distinguished [39]. The value of the test has only been established so far with influenza virus haemagglutinins, but it is likely that it will be useful in characterizing the antibodies against other haemagglutinating viruses.

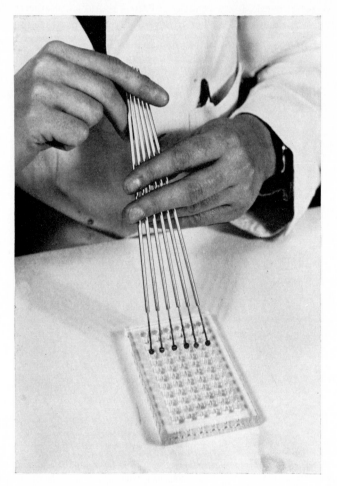

Fɪɢ. 24.3. The equipment for the Takátsy micromethod of performing haemagglutination-inhibition and similar serological tests.

Takátsy microtechniques

Takátsy [40] described simplified micromethods of performing haemagglutination-inhibition tests which have subsequently been widely adopted. He designed plastic plates in which small holes with conical bottoms were drilled. The smallest size of these are filled by adding saline with a calibrated dropper delivering volumes of 0·025 ml. To this serum is added by means of a flamed spiral metal loop which picks up 0·025 ml. The loop, either alone or as part of a group of six to eight, can be twirled in the cup to mix the saline and serum thoroughly and the mixture can then be transferred to the next set of cups in the same way to make serial twofold dilutions. Virus and red cells are added with the dropper. The test is sensitive and very reproducible, saves up to 90 per cent of the amount of reagents required in standard techniques and is quicker and less fatiguing to perform. The necessary equipment is now made commercially and the plastic plates may be obtained in a disposable form (Fig. 24.3).

Takátsy [42] also described a method of precipitating influenza viruses by dilution and using the precipitate for absorbing antibodies, but this technique is not of such wide application as the procedures mentioned above.

The neutralization test
It is a fundamental observation of virology that serum from an animal recently infected with a virus can neutralize the infectivity of that virus if the virus and serum are allowed to react together for a time. Neutralization was thus the first technique to be used for detecting antibody against viruses; it has been studied exhaustively over many years and it is still the basic method for the measurement of antiviral antibodies when a new virus is discovered and often remains the best when others are found later. The test can be done with virtually any virus even if it is of low titre and large amounts of tissue debris and other inert materials are present.

There are numerous techniques and variants of these so a few basic methods will be outlined here. These can readily be adapted to different viruses by using the appropriate host cells or animals and methods of assessment.

6. In ovo *neutralization test of influenza virus*
A pool of infected allantoic fluid is diluted tenfold in sterile neutral buffered saline in tubes kept in an ice-bath. It is convenient and accurate to use volumes of 4·5 ml in each tube and to transfer 0·5 ml after mixing thoroughly with a 1 ml pipette. A new pipette is used after the mixture from one tube has been added to the next. The contents of each tube are inoculated into eggs which have been incubated at 4° C for 10–11 days and candled and drilled for allantoic inoculation. Starting with the highest dilution, virus suspension is drawn up into a tuberculin syringe and 0·2 ml volumes are inoculated into each of groups of at least three eggs. The eggs are sealed with wax, incubated at 35° C for 2 days and then chilled at −20° C for 30 minutes. Each egg is then opened and 0·1 ml of allantoic fluid is removed and mixed with 0·5 ml of 0·5 per cent chick red cell suspension in a cup of a haemagglutination tray in order to detect the presence of virus haemagglutinin.

From this experiment the virus titre is calculated in egg-infectious doses per millilitre (Table 24.4). Then the serum to be tested is inactivated by heating at 56°C for 30 minutes and serially diluted in buffered saline using twofold steps and a sterile technique. A tube of virus is taken from the previously titrated pool which has been kept without thawing at $-70°$ C since the day it was prepared; this tube is thawed and diluted to give a suspension containing a calculated 100 EID_{50} in 0·1 ml. This dilution is then added to each serum dilution—the volume added is equal to the volume of the dilution so that the 100 EID_{50} is now contained in 0·2 ml of mixture. The mixtures are shaken

TABLE 24.4

Protocol of an end-point neutralization test

Results of virus titration 0·2 ml inoculated into eggs

Virus dilution	10^{-2}	10^{-3}	10^{-4}	10^{-5}	10^{-6}
Proportion of eggs infected	4/4	4/4	4/4	2/4	0/4

Therefore   1 $EID_{50} \equiv$ 0·2 ml of 10^{-5} dilution

∴ 100 EID_{50} in 0·2 ml of 10^{-3} dilution or 0·1 ml of 1/500

Serum titration Virus diluted 1/500 mixed with serial dilutions of serum

Initial dilution of serum	1/10	1/20	1/40	1/80	1/160
Proportion of eggs infected	0/3	0/3	0/3	3/3	3/3

Control virus titration

Further dilution of virus suspension used	10^{-1}	10^{-2}	10^{-3}
(0·1 ml inoculated to each egg)	4/4	1/4	0/4

Conclusions
1. The serum used neutralized virus.
2. The end-point of complete neutralization was 1/40. This may be used as the titre, or a 50 per cent end-point may be interpolated—approximately 1/120 more exactly by Reed Muench, Karber or other methods.
3. This neutralization titre was obtained with slightly less than the calculated 100 infectious doses.

vigorously to mix and are allowed to stand at room temperature for 20 minutes for serum and virus to react. At the end of this time, using a separate syringe for each mixture, 0·2 ml of each one is inoculated into a group of three eggs. These are incubated and tested as before and from the results the 50 per cent neutralization end-point is calculated by interpolation. A protocol is shown in Table 24.4.

A variant of this test is sometimes called the constant serum-varying virus test in which tenfold dilutions of virus are each mixed with the same dilution (say 1/10) of serum or of normal serum. This gives the results of two titrations in the presence or absence of serum and if the titres are significantly different then neutralization has occurred. If the titre with normal serum is 10^5 and that with test serum is 10^2 then the ratio between these, 10^3, is the neutralization index. This is a workable test when the virus titre is very variable; it can detect low antibody activity, but it is extravagant of serum, it really works well only when high titre virus is available and it does not distinguish reliably or quantitatively between the antibody activity of sera with high titres. The relation between the two tests can be seen in Fig. 24.4 which shows that the relationship between the logarithms of the dilution of virus

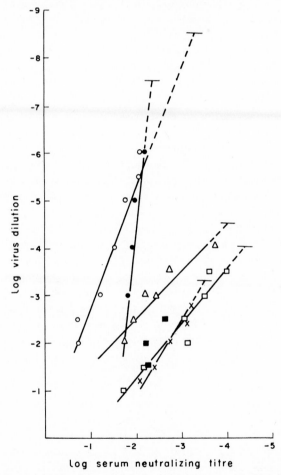

Fig. 24.4. Serum neutralization end-points obtained using a variety of doses of a neurotropic influenza virus and rabbit antiserum and assessing the result in different hosts [43]. The host systems which are more sensitive to virus are less sensitive to antibody. ● Allantoic cavity. ○ Chorioallantoic membrane. □ Mouse lung. △ Mouse brain. ■ Membrane *in vitro*. × Haemagglutination inhibition *in vitro*. − Titre of virus.

and of serum used at the end-point is apparently linear. The slope of the line is different in different hosts—the relation between dose of virus and dilution of serum is rarely really 1 to 1 as it is in the haemagglutination-inhibition test and this is why the neutralization index does not bear a simple quantitative relation to the amount of antibody in a serum. Also the hosts which are less sensitive for the detection of virus are usually more sensitive for the detection of antibody at any given virus dilution. The neutralization line may be very steep in some hosts, such as the allantoic cavity of the chick embryo and certain tissue cultures, and this is probably due to the fact that in these situations virus which escapes neutralization in the test tube and infects cells may yet be eliminated because its progeny are neutralized by antibody which is still present in the allantoic cavity or culture medium. The steep slope may be a valuable feature in the practical use of a neutralization test since in a test where such a relation holds the antibody titre obtained is practically unaffected by small errors in the dose of virus used.

A great many variations in these basic tests are possible; for example, the surviving virus may be detected by inoculation of a variety of host species by various routes or by inoculation of tissue cultures. Infection may be detected in various ways, such as the death of an animal, the presence of lung lesions or inclusions, and degeneration or haemadsorption in tissue cultures. It is important to remember that changing the host used may change markedly the results of the neutralization test as mentioned above.

Some viruses, vaccinia, for example, produce discrete lesions, such as pocks on the chorioallantoic membrane of embryonated eggs. With these viruses it is possible to increase the sensitivity of the neutralization test which, in the form described above, only detects neutralization when less than 1 per cent of the virus survives. When pocks are counted it may be possible to detect reliably a reduction of 50 per cent in the pock count and to use this as the index of significant neutralization; this may be especially useful when, as in the case of vaccinia virus, there is a proportion of more than 1 per cent of virus which even a very large dose of antiserum does not neutralize [44].

Kinetic neutralization tests
Virus is often inactivated by serum according to the equations of a simple bimolecular reaction with one component, antibody, in great excess. The rate of inactivation therefore depends on the concentration of this serum and an arbitrary constant (K) can be used to represent the effectiveness with which a particular serum is able to neutralize virus—it may be called its neutralizing activity.

7. Kinetic virus neutralization test of antibody against poliovirus
Heat-inactivated serum is used and diluted to a concentration which shows

partial inactivation of the virus. The virus is used at a concentration which will give countable, but large numbers of plaques in the assay system; poliovirus may be assayed in monolayers of primary monkey kidney or transformed

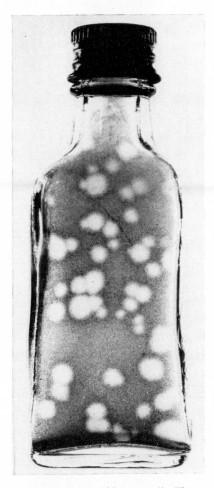

FIG. 24.5. Virus plaques in monolayers of human cells. These are each initiated by one virus particle and provide accurate assays of the number of such particles in a mixture. This assay is of poliovirus in HeLa cells. (Courtesy of N.J.Dimmock.) Such plaques form the basis of the kinetic virus neutralization test with poliovirus.

human cells such as HeLa cells, which are overlaid with agar by some modification of the method originally used by Dulbecco. Dilutions are made in phosphate buffered saline. A series of bottles are prepared with, say, 0·25 ml of serum dilution in each. To these at an accurately recorded time are added equal volumes of virus dilution and each mixture is immediately shaken vigorously. At an accurately measured time 0·2 ml of each mixture is added to 19·8 ml of saline and the whole shaken vigorously. This dilution stops the reaction, and in order to assay the amount of virus surviving at the moment

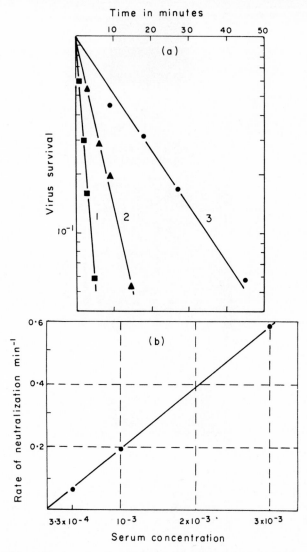

Fig. 24.6. Neutralization of poliovirus by homologous antiserum [45]. (a) shows the exponential inactivation curve of virus infectivity by antiserum while (b) shows that the rate of inactivation is proportional to the amount of antiserum used. (By permission of R. Dulbecco, *Virology*, and Academic Press.)

of dilution the diluted mixtures are then added to monolayers and overlaid in the standard manner prior to incubation at 36° C. After incubation neutral red is added and the number of virus plaques (Fig. 24.5) counted. The logarithm of the number of plaques may then be plotted against time as in Fig. 24.6. The best line drawn through these points may then be used to calculate the constant K for the serum used. A convenient method is shown in Table 24.5.

The calculation is not valid if virus inactivation does not follow first-order kinetics, and in fact the rate of inactivation usually decreases after an initial

TABLE 24.5

Calculation of results of kinetic neutralization test

We assume that the inactivation of the virus is described by the equation

$$\frac{Vt}{Vo} = e^{-ktc} \quad \text{or} \quad Log_e \frac{Vt}{Vo} = -ktc$$

where Vo = concentration of virus added to mixture

Vt = concentration detected after reaction

for t minutes with a concentration c of serum.

For simplicity suppose a 'single point' test is performed in which a mixture of 1/1000 dilution of serum is held for 120 minutes with virus and the plaque count shows 23 in unit volume of mixture and 137 in the virus control incubated with medium instead of serum then

$$\frac{Vt}{Vo} = \frac{23}{137} \quad C = \frac{1}{1000} \quad \text{and } t = 120 \text{ minutes}$$

Whence K = 15.

If many tests are performed with standard conditions of concentration and time it is convenient to plot a graph of $\frac{Vt}{Vo}$ against K which is a straight line if $\frac{Vt}{Vo}$ is plotted on a logarithmic scale.

period. It is important therefore when applying the test to a new virus to determine for how long the virus concentration declines exponentially. If this is known, however, it is often simple and satisfactory to determine the initial inactivation rate by assaying virus after a single fixed period of exposure to a few dilutions of serum. Such a method has been developed for use with rhinoviruses and was particularly valuable when the sensitivity of the virus assays was found to vary from one test to the other [46].

Tests of this type were first performed many years ago with certain animal viruses and with bacteriophage and have proved of great value. However, it is clear that the simple assumptions on which the interpretation is based are

CC*

not always valid. For instance, dilution of virus-serum mixtures may under certain circumstances dissociate antibody from virus [47, 48]. Certain sera may combine with vaccinia virus in such a way as to protect it from neutralization. (This may account for the unneutralizable fraction observed in some systems.) It is important to remember therefore that kinetic neutralization tests are still really empirical tests and to interpret them with care.

Further variants of the neutralization test

Antibodies and antiviral substances may be assayed by soaking small beads or filter paper disks in them and then adding the beads to agar plates in which monolayers have been infected with virus. Porterfield [50] has recently shown that this method may be of value in testing several sera against an arbovirus which produces plaques in chick embryo fibroblasts (Fig. 24.7). However, the technique is not easy and may be difficult to quantitate; for example, when two viruses grow up at different speeds, there may be much more time for antibody to diffuse out in tests with one virus than in tests with the other.

In order to differentiate very similar viruses, such as variants of poliovirus vaccine strains, use has been made of a test in which antiserum is incorporated in the agar overlay. The virus which is close antigenically to that against which the serum was made gives a low plaque count, whereas a virus which is antigenically different gives the same plaque count as with a normal overlay [51].

In the presence of low concentrations of antibody virus neutralization may take many hours and therefore it may be possible to detect very small amounts of antibody by prolonging the test or by increasing the temperature. This is only possible with viruses which are stable and are only slowly inactivated at 4° C or 37° C. One such modified test has been called immune-inactivation [52]: mixtures of virus and serum are held in the icebox overnight, then at 37° C for several hours next day and finally the reduction in infective virus is measured by plaque count. Using such a technique it has been shown that hypogammaglobulinaemic children actually make very small amounts of antiviral antibody in response to vaccination [53] and that the first antibody to be produced by a rabbit appears a few days after a small dose of poliovirus is injected [54].

Colour test

If a virus destroys cells their metabolism ceases and this may be detected because acid is no longer produced and so the medium is more alkaline than that of control cultures. The difference in pH may be revealed by the use of a suitable indicator [55]. Thus a virus neutralization test may be performed, for example, in disposable plastic plates [56], by a procedure very similar to that used for haemagglutination-inhibition test.

8. *Colour tests for antibody against poliovirus*

All dilutions are made in culture medium. Serial dilutions of serum are prepared in the cups of a plastic plate. Then to each cup is added more medium containing a calculated 100 infectious doses of virus. A control virus titration is put up as in the standard neutralization test described earlier. The mixtures

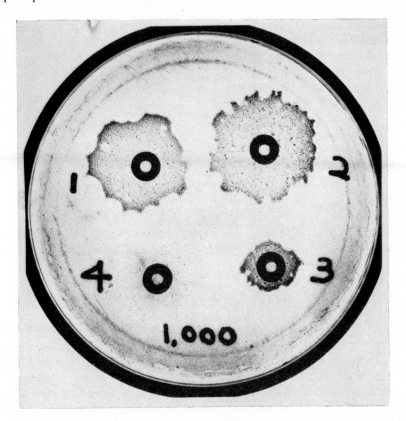

FIG. 24.7. Beads impregnated with antiserum have been used to produce zones of inhibition of cytopathic effect in this test of antibody activity against WEE virus growing in chick-embryo fibroblast cells. (J.S.Porterfield.)

are allowed to react for an hour and then a suspension of tissue culture cells is added to each cup, which is finally sealed by a layer of liquid paraffin or some other method. The cultures are incubated and the colour of the phenol red indicator in the medium is recorded at intervals. If the composition of medium, the amount of buffer and the concentration of cells are correctly judged the medium becomes definitely acid and the medium goes yellow in 4 or 5 days in uninfected cultures. (It may require a good deal of preliminary work to achieve this.) In cups infected with virus the cells are killed and produce no acid and so the medium is red. If the virus has been neutralized the medium becomes yellow. Thus virus infection and neutralization can be detected without the use of the microscope, although some workers use the instrument to check the reading in doubtful cups.

Other methods of detecting antigen–antibody complexes

This section deals with the application to viruses and their antigens of methods widely used in other fields of immunology. Little will be said in most instances about the principles or technical details. However, the virologist often finds that certain versions of these tests have particular advantages and these will be indicated where possible.

Complement fixation

This test is sensitive and applicable to a great many virus systems and is widely employed in diagnostic virology, since by its use antibodies directed against many diverse viruses may be detected using stable non-infectious antigens and a simple procedure.

The surfaces of virus particles contain antigenic proteins which can be detected in a CF test. However, care must be taken in preparing the antigens. When infectious poliovirus is heated the antigen is transformed from the D to the antigenically distinct C type which is found in the naturally occurring incomplete or non-infectious form of the virus [57]. If the virus is made non-infectious by careful treatment with formalin the D antigen activity is not changed [58].

Certain viruses also produce 'soluble' or non-particulate antigens. For example, the influenza A viruses all contain an internal ribonucleoprotein component which can be released by treating the virus particles with ether or can be extracted from infected tissue. In a similar way all influenza B viruses produce another antigen. These 'soluble' antigens may be readily detected by complement-fixation tests with a suitable immune serum and they are valuable reagents for diagnostic tests since whichever of the many influenza A or B viruses has infected a patient an increase in CF antibody against one or other of the two soluble antigens is likely to occur. There is also a common soluble antigen to all the human adenoviruses as well as distinct type-specific antigens which are unique to each serotype; both of these can be detected by complement fixation or in other ways. No common antigens for other groups of viruses, such as parainfluenza and picornaviruses have been demonstrated although myxoviruses in general have internal nucleo-protein complement-fixing antigens.

Many methods of complement fixation have been used in virology. A test using volumes of 0·25 ml, two 'full' units of complement and fixation at 37° C for 30 minutes is often used for diagnostic tests, although overnight fixation at 4° C may increase the sensitivity. Many virus antigens are very difficult and expensive to make and this has encouraged the use of micromethods. One method described by Fulton & Dumbell [59] employed a humidified metal box and engraved flat plastic sheets. The original purpose was to make 'three dimensional' tests with varying dilutions of antigen, serum and complement which were added in volumes of 0·025 ml with a dropping pipette. However, the equipment also proved suitable for testing a number of sera against a series of different viral antigens. More recently plastic haemagglutination trays kept in a plastic bag have been found to be more convenient than the plastic sheets and box [60]. Finally, the Takátsy method described earlier [40] is suitable for this type of CF test and has the advantage that when needed serial dilutions of small amounts of sera can be made in the plate whereas in the other micromethods serial dilutions must be made in large volumes and then transferred by dropper to the plate for the test.

To arrive at the end-point all the above methods depend on a rough grading of the amount of haemolysis by inspection of the tube or drop whereas it is possible to measure the degree of haemolysis by comparing the supernatant of the reaction mixture in a test tube with standard solutions of haemoglobin either by eye or by colorimeter. With tests of this type, such as that of Wadsworth, the titres can be expressed as the amount of complement fixed by serum and antigen; such titres are more precise and reproducible than those obtained with methods described previously, but are more cumbersome and require more antigen [61]. The technique of complement-fixation is further discussed in Chapter 20.

Agglutination and precipitation

Agglutination and precipitation methods have been widely used in virology. Agglutination of vaccinia viruses by immune serum was observed many years ago, but is a difficult test to perform particularly because it is difficult to prepare enough purified particle suspension and to avoid spontaneous agglutination. Agglutination of poliovirus particles has also been observed under the electron microscope [62], but this is also a technically difficult test, although it is possible in this way to agglutinate separately the C and D particles. It is easier to perform a small-scale flocculation test with poliovirus using virus purified and concentrated from tissue culture fluids [63]. Similar tests with influenza viruses were also successful, but ran into difficulties with non-specific inhibitors of precipitation [64]. The most valuable method by far has been the Ouchterlony agar-gel diffusion method or some modification of it.

The value of the method may be illustrated by a series of experiments on adenoviruses by Pereira and his colleagues. They were able to separate three distinct antigenic components of adenovirus type 5, to convert one into another, to demonstrate the purity of chemically separated fractions and so on, and to control all these procedures by precipitation tests in agar; representative patterns obtained by them are shown in Fig. 24.8 [65, 66, 67]. The much

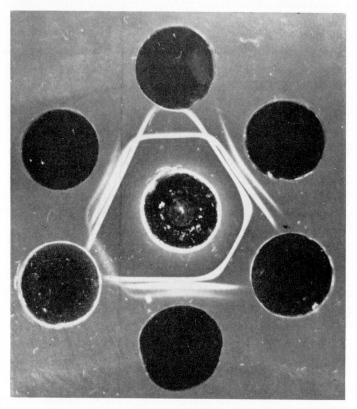

Fig. 24.8. Antigens of adenovirus type 5 demonstrated by gel precipitation. (H.G. Pereira.) There are three different viral antigens in infected cells, the cups in the outer rings contain alternately a single purified antigen and unfractionated material. It can be seen that the lines due to each purified antigen each fuse with one of the three produced by the crude material [94] (Courtesy of H.G.Pereira.)

larger number of antigens produced by cells infected with vaccinia virus can be detected with the same technique, and the time-sequence of their appearance and their selective inhibition by antiviral drugs can be shown in a way which would be impossible with other less discriminating methods such as complement fixation [68]. The method was also used to detect antibodies against adenoviruses in the sera of infected patients and cross-reactions between animal and human strains of adenoviruses [69, 70].

Fluorescence

Fluorescent antibody methods have been shown to be capable of identifying viral antigens within infected cells. In early studies the globulin from an immune serum was conjugated directly and used with the original techniques of Coons & Kaplan [23] (see Chapter 16). Later studies have used the two-stage method (indirect) [71] or the complement-staining three-stage method [72]. The latter two are important advances as there is a reduction of the number of conjugates required with each layer employed, and sensitivity may be increased. With the two-stage method (indirect) one needs a conjugate against each species, the serum of which is to be tested, while with the three-stage method only anti-guinea-pig conjugate is needed. However, the last-named method will not work with virus-antibody complexes which do not fix complement.

It has been possible to detect infection in tissue with a great variety of viruses, influenza, mumps, rabies, poliomyelitis, adenovirus and others, but in spite of the passage of time and the need for rapid diagnostic techniques the method has only found limited application. Influenza, ornithosis and a few other infections have been diagnosed by examining respiratory secretions [73], rabies by examining sections of brain, and recently coxsackievirus infections by examining sections of human appendix removed at operation. It was also observed recently that a specific diagnosis of enterovirus infections might be made by detecting antigen in leucocytes of the buffy coat of blood collected in the acute phase of the disease [74].

The fluorescent antibody method is too cumbersome for general use in measuring the antibody titre of serum, although antibody against *M. pneumoniae* was studied for some years in this way in the belief that it was anti-viral antibody. Frozen sections of infected chick-embryo lung were used and stained by adding dilutions of the human serum to be tested, followed by an anti-human globulin conjugate [75]. The highest dilution of serum giving clear staining was the antibody titre and it has subsequently been shown that antibody thus measured may be correlated quite well with that measured by complement fixation and with immunity to infection in the field [76].

Considerable use has been made of fluorescent antibody in studying the pathogenesis of experimental infections and the sites at which antigenic virus proteins accumulate within a cell. For example, the internal S antigen of the influenza viruses develop in the nucleus, while the surface V antigen develops in the cytoplasm near the nucleus, although the completed virus particles form at the cell surface [10]. In cells supporting the growth of the closely related parainfluenza viruses and Newcastle disease viruses the antigens appear only in the cytoplasm [77]. Polioviruses have been shown to develop in the cytoplasm although marked pathological changes take place in the nucleus; on the other hand adenoviruses and herpes virus antigens form in the nucleus which is also the site at which virus particles are seen to develop and the first pathological changes appear [78, 79]. Studies of this sort yield their maximum results when they are made part of a co-ordinated study in which the antigens are assayed quantitatively by some technique such as complement fixation or haemagglutination, infectious virus is titrated and conventional pathological examinations are also made.

The use of immunological methods in virology

Historically, one of the first uses of immunology in the study of viruses was the identification of viruses by their antigenic types. For this purpose two methods were used. One was the challenge of animals which had survived

TABLE 24.6

The relative use of certain methods in identifying the serotypes of some viruses of man

Virus group	Methods used		
	Neutraliz-ation	Haemagglu-tination inhibition	Complement fixation
Influenza	+	+ +	+
Parainfluenza	+	+ +	
Respiratory syncytial	+		+ +
Herpes simplex	+		+
Adenoviruses	+ +	+	(+)
Polioviruses	+ +		
Coxsackieviruses	+		+
Echoviruses	+	+	
Rhinoviruses	+ +		
Poxviruses	+		+ +
Arboviruses	+ +	+ +	+

+ + = frequently.   + = occasionally.

infection with the object of demonstrating immunity and the other was the neutralization test. The latter test is still widely used for this purpose although nowadays tissue cultures rather than animals are usually used as test objects. In addition, many viruses are now identified by haemagglutination-inhibition or by complement-fixation tests. Some of these are indicated in Table 24.6.

There are numerous serotypes of certain viruses, e.g. adenoviruses, cox-sackieviruses, rhinoviruses and arboviruses, and it may be a very laborious and wasteful procedure to test a single strain against many scores of sera. It is often valuable, therefore, to prepare pools of sera for neutralization tests. These may be simple combinations of several sera used so that the virus can be shown in one test to be unaffected by sera against perhaps ten viruses. If a pool does neutralize a virus then the virus can be set up in a separate test against each of the sera comprising the pool. A more efficient method is to use 'intersecting' serum pools [80], an example of which is given in Table 24.7. If properly designed it is possible to identify the virus for certain by the pattern of neutralization by the pools, e.g. a virus neutralized by pools A and C could only be serotype 9, although it is often desirable to confirm this by a further test with a single serum.

It is important to standardize the sera carefully. Obviously a very high titre virus may not be neutralized completely by a small dose of antiserum, therefore for critical work it is necessary to titrate the unknown virus first and to set it up against at least twenty units of antibody, i.e. twenty times the amount giving complete neutralization with the same dose of homologous

TABLE 24.7

An example of intersecting serum pools for the identification of virus serotypes (from Lim and Benyesh-Melnick)

Serum pool	Specific sera included (x) in indicated pool									
	1	2	3	4	5	6	7	8	9	10
A	x				x			x	x	
B		x			x	x				x
C			x			x	x		x	
D				x			x	x		x

virus; if it is neutralized it is, for critical work, necessary to titrate the unknown virus to find its end-point with the standard serum so that it may be compared with that given by the prototype. Quite often they are not the same and there are several reasons for this. In the first place the unknown virus may be antigenically rather different from the prototype. Some viruses seem to stimulate a rather wider range of antibodies than others, possibly because they contain more antigenic components. These 'broad' strains should really be chosen as prototypes because they may not be neutralized by sera against 'narrow' viruses although they induce antibodies which neutralize 'narrow' viruses quite well. A good example of this was the series of echovirus 6 'prime' strains which was found after the original type 6 virus had been designated [81].

Other viruses show frequent minor antigen variations so that even in the same epidemic several slightly different serotypes may be isolated in which the titre of both viruses is higher against the homologous virus than it is against the heterologous. It is a rather arbitrary matter, but viruses differing in titre by less than eight- or sixteen-fold are usually not thought to belong to different serotypes although the differences between them may be genuine and reproducible. It would be best if antigenic variants could be designated as distinct serotypes when their degree of variation shown is such that it has a definite effect on their behaviour in nature; for instance, inducing an antibody response which, at least on first infection, rendered the host immune to the virus and not to the variant. Generally speaking information of this sort is not available and so differences between strains are detected or not depending on the test used, and described as serotypes or not depending on the preferences of the investigator.

Some viruses are less well neutralized than are others although they carry exactly the same antigens. The most striking example of this sort of phenomenon, however, is the occurrence of Q [82], non-avid or '−' strains of influenza virus which are poorly inhibited by homologous antiserum in the

TABLE 24.8

Example of serological reactions of non-avid
or Q strains of influenza virus

Test performed with	Titre of antiserum against	
	Non-avid or Q virus	Avid or P virus
Q virus	30	20
P virus	240	320

haemagglutination-inhibition test. Sometimes these viruses can only be identified for certain by using an alternative test, such as strain-specific complement fixation or neutralization in which the virus will react normally (Table 24.8).

Another difficulty encountered in identifying viruses is the occurrence of mixtures. These may occur because a patient is infected with two viruses or because the virus he was excreting has been contaminated with another in the laboratory. Such mixtures may be recognized because each virus grows in a different sort of host; for example, Coxsackie virus A grows in suckling mice and adenovirus in tissue culture, so that they might both be isolated separately from one specimen of faeces. On the other hand there may be two viruses which can both grow in the same host. Inspection of Table 24.9 shows that a mixture of such viruses might appear to be a new serotype. To avoid this error it is first necessary to be aware of the possibility that it may occur, secondly to test viruses with pooled antisera, and then in cases of difficulty neutralize the viruses of both components.

Serological tests are very valuable in the diagnosis of virus infections. Complement-fixing antibody titres rise after infections and usually become positive 10–14 days after the onset of illness; they generally decline and become negative again after several months or a year or so have elapsed. Although the presence of high titre complement-fixing antibody is not a reliable sign that a patient has had a recent virus infection, titres of greater than 64 against influenza-soluble antigens and of 16 or more against poliovirus particle antigen have been used for this purpose. However, complement fixation can be used to detect antibody against the particle or V antigen which is similar to, if not identical with, the antibody which inhibits haemagglutination and neutralizes infectivity and persists for a long time after infection. It is therefore usually necessary and always desirable to test

TABLE 24.9

The results of neutralization tests with specific antisera and a mixed virus population

Test using virus	Result of test with antiserum		
	A	B	A+B
A	0	+	0
B	+	0	0
A+B	+	+	0

0 = no virus growth. + = virus growth

sera collected from the patient about the time of onset of disease and also 2 weeks later. The paired sera should be titrated in the same test and an increase of fourfold in titre is then regarded as indicating an antibody response to infection. Specific antibody responses are common when children are first infected with a virus, but later on the situation becomes more complex and there are often responses to viruses which may have a quite distant antigenic relationship to the virus with which the patient was infected. This has been particularly thoroughly studied in the case of influenza virus infections. Patients who have been infected with influenza A viruses produced antibody against this virus when infected or vaccinated later in life with influenza A1 or A2 virus. The antibody-producing mechanism had been conditioned by early experience, a phenomenon called by Davenport *et al* 'original antigenic sin' [84]. A similar phenomenon probably occurs with many infections other than those due to influenza, but it is more difficult to demonstrate since the patients are not regularly exposed to viruses in the same order and at the same time—however, it may be the reason that children infected with parainfluenza 1 virus tend to produce antibody against the parainfluenza 3 virus to which they are usually exposed very early in life. It is also well known that re-exposure to an antigen leads to the production of a broadly reacting antibody and this certainly occurs with viruses, possibly because minor antigenic components of the virus stimulate antibody after a time. For all these reasons, even if a fourfold increase in neutralizing or haemagglutination-inhibiting antibody titre has been demonstrated it is unwise to conclude that the patient has been infected with the virus used in the test; all that can safely be said is that he has been infected with a virus antigenically related to the one used in the test.

Sometimes antibody responses are observed to two viruses which are immunologically quite unrelated and then one can conclude that the patient has been infected simultaneously with two distinct infectious agents, but this is uncommon.

It has occasionally been suggested that it might be possible to use compound virus antigens in order to test one specimen of serum in one mixture with antigens from a variety of viruses. This is theoretically possible provided antigens of high titre are available, and the test has been used successfully with some arboviruses. However, it would only be of practical advantage if the majority of tests to be done with the serum were expected to yield negative results, or if it were not important to know the exact virus against which antibody was directed. This type of compound antigen cannot be used in the haemagglutination-inhibition test, since if, say, four haemagglutinating units are used two of which are influenza A and two are influenza B then agglutination will not be inhibited by either anti-A or anti-B serum [86]. It will only be inhibited by a mixture of both as was pointed out above when discussing the neutralization of mixtures of viruses. The complement-fixation test does not behave in this way and each component of a mixture of viruses will react with a specific antiserum in the presence of other antigens.

The avidity of antibody is not easy to measure in absolute terms, but it is clear that variations in the quality of antibody may affect the results of tests. For example, Sabin [87] has suggested that the 'colour' test measures the presence of a 'non-avid' antibody while the usual tube test measures 'avid' antibody and that these antibodies are produced in different amounts following vaccination. It has been shown that antibody produced shortly after poliovirus infection is more readily dissociated from virus by acid than that which is produced later [88]. Similarly, early antibody against influenza A2 may combine rather weakly with virus and therefore not inhibit agglutination when chicken cells with a strong affinity for virus are used; the same sort of antibody can only neutralize virus efficiently in the presence of fresh serum [89] and likewise a 'complement-requiring' antibody is found in the early stages of immunization of animals against herpes virus.

Conclusion

It is impossible to summarize adequately a subject as varied and extensive as the use of immunological methods in virology, but several points should have emerged from the foregoing pages. In the first place, it is clear that immunological techniques have always made a considerable contribution to virological practice and research, particularly in investigations on the infection of a whole organism, or when a sensitive and specific means of identifying a viral protein in the laboratory was required.

On the other hand, some virological techniques and experimental situations have provided results which contribute to the solution of the general biological problems of the immune response. Also some procedures which were evolved for use in virology may be adapted for use in related fields—a recent example is a colour-change method of titrating antibodies against mycoplasma which was developed from the colour test for poliovirus antibodies [90].

Finally, it seems that there is plenty of room for further development.* For instance, we need better micromethods so that antibodies in children's sera may be readily titrated against many specific antigens, perhaps using no more blood than can be picked up with a filter paper disk [91] from a prick in the skin. Some workers would like to develop fully mechanized and automated antibody assays for use in busy hospitals and in large-scale surveys. Others see a need for sensitive and specific *in vitro* methods for detecting the antigens of viruses which do not haemagglutinate. The complement-fixation test, for example, is insensitive and non-specific for the rhinoviruses, and neutralization is very tedious. Sensitized red cell methods have been used [92], but many have found them to be unsatisfactory. It may be possible to sensitize some particle other than red cells, or find some surface of biological or synthetic origin with which the viral protein will specifically combine as it does with susceptible cells during virus adsorption. Perhaps more use of radioactively labelled antibodies might give extra sensitivity to such methods.

More refined and effective methods might be more easily achieved if more was known about virus immunology at a molecular level; if the amino-acid sequences which define a virus antigen were known, and also the specific complementary chemical configurations on cells and antibodies with which this particular part of the viral surface can react. One would also like to know in precise terms what are the immunologically important changes which viruses induce when transforming normal into malignant cells. The localization of

* Several new methods of measuring anti-viral antibodies have appeared since this chapter was written (see refs. 95–97).

viral antigens under the electron microscope with ferretin-labelled antibody may have a part to play in this field [93] (see also Chapter 15). This is not the place to speculate on the solutions to such specific problems, but to point out that they and others like them represent the areas in which we may expect the methods of viral immunology to develop in the future.

References

[1] *Viral and Rickettsial Diseases of Man*, 4th ed. (1965) ed. HORSFALL F.L. JR. & TAMM I. Philadelphia: Lippincott

[2] *Diagnostic Procedures for Virus and Rickettsial Diseases*, 3rd ed. New York: American Public Health Association Committee

[3] SMITH W. & ANDREWS C.H. (1938) Serological races of influenza virus. *Brit. J. exp. Path.* **19,** 293

[4] JENSEN K.E., PEELER B.E. & DULWORTH W.G. (1962) Immunization against parainfluenza infections. Antigenicity of egg-adapted types 1 and 3. *J. Immunol.* **89,** 216

[5] COOK M.K., ANDREWS B.E., FOX H.H., TURNER H.C., JAMES W.P. & CHANOCK R.M. (1959) Antigenic relationships among the 'newer' myxoviruses (parainfluenza). *Am. J. Hyg.* **69,** 250

[6] WALKER D.L. & HORSFALL F.L. JR. (1950) Lack of identity in neutralization and haemagglutination-inhibiting antibody against influenza viruses. *J. exp. Med.* **91,** 65

[7] HALONEN P. (1961) Immunization with ECHO viruses grown in monkey kidney cell culture. Responses of mice, guinea pigs and rabbits. *Ann. Med. exper. Biol. Fenn.* **39,** 15

[8] PEREIRA H.G. (1956) Typing of adenoidal-pharyngeal-conjunctival (APC) virus by complement fixation. *J. Path. Bact.* **72,** 105

[9] ROSEN L. (1960) Serologic grouping of reoviruses by haemagglutination-inhibition. *Amer. J. Hyg.* **71,** 242

[10] BREITENFELD P.M. & SCHÄFER, W. (1957) The formation of fowl plague virus antigens in infected cells, as studied with fluorescent antibodies. *Virology* **4,** 328

[11] HENLE S., LIEF F.S. & FABIYI A. (1958) Strain specific complement-fixation test in antigenic analysis and serodiagnosis of influenza. *Lancet* **i,** 818

[12] CHANOCK R.M. & PEREIRA H.G. Personal communication

[13] DOGGETT J.E. & TAYLOR-ROBINSON D. (1965) Serological studies with respiratory syncytial virus. *Arch. ges. Virusforsch.* **15,** 601

[14] TAYLOR-ROBINSON D. & CHAPPLE P.J. Unpublished.

[15] BEALE A.J. Personal communication

[16] HIMMELWEIT F. (1960) Serological responses and clinical reactions to influenza virus vaccines. *Brit. med. J.* **2,** 1690

[17] SALK J.E., BAILEY M.L. & LAURENT A.M. (1952) The use of adjuvants in studies on influenza immunization. II. Increased antibody formation in human subjects inoculated with influenza virus vaccine in a water-in-oil emulsion. *Amer. J. Hyg.* **55,** 439

[18] MILLER L.F., PECKINPAUGH R.O., ARLANDER T.R., PIERCE W.E., EDWARDS E.A., DE BERRY P., PHILLIPS I.A. & ROSENBAUM M.J. (1965) Epidemiology and prevention of acute respiratory disease in naval recruits. II. Efficacy of adjuvant and aqueous adenovirus vaccines in prevention of naval recruit respiratory disease. *Amer. J. Pub. Hlth* **55,** 47

[19] SCIENTIFIC COMMITTEE ON COMMON COLD VACCINES (1965) Prevention of colds by vaccination against a rhinovirus. *Brit. med. J.* **1**, 1344

[20] TINT H. & STONE J. (1961) An adenovirus vaccine potency test. *J. Immunol.* **86**, 253

[21] MUFSON M.A. & CHAPPLE P.J. Personal communication

[22] TIMBURY M.C. (1963) Inhibition of viral replication by anticellular serum. *Virology* **20**, 629

[23] COONS A.H. & KAPLAN M.J. (1950) Localization of antigens in tissue cells. II. Improvements in a method for the detection of antigens by means of fluorescent antibody. *J. exp. Med.* **91**, 1

[24] NIVEN J.S.F., ARMSTRONG J.A., BALFOUR B.M., KLEMPERER H.G. & TYRRELL D.A.J. (1962) Cellular changes accompanying the growth of influenza virus in bovine cell cultures. *J. Path. Bact.* **84**, 1

[25] JENSEN K.E. & FRANCIS J. JR. (1953) The antigenic composition of influenza virus measured by antibody-absorption. *J. exp. Med.* **98**, 619

[26] HARBOE A. (1960) Heterologous antibody absorption of sera from ferrets cross-infected with influenza virus of the A_2-type and other A-type. *Acta path. microbiol. Scand.* **94**, 493

[27] ISAACS A. (1957) Particle counts and infectivity titrations for animal viruses. *Advances Virus Research* **4**, 111

[28] ISAACS A. & BOZZO A. (1951) The use of *V. cholerae* filtrates in the destruction of non-specific inhibitor in ferret sera. *Brit. J. exp. Path.* **32**, 325

[29] FRANCIS T. (1947) Dissociation of hemagglutinating and antibody-measuring capacity of influenza virus. *J. exp. Med.* **85**, 1

[30] *World Health Organization Technical Report Series* (1959) **170**, 40

[31] SAMPAIO A.A. DE C. & ISAACS A. (1953) The action of trypsin on normal serum inhibitors of influenza virus agglutination. *Brit. J. exp. Path.* **34**, 152

[32] ROSEN L. (1960) A haemagglutination-inhibition technique for typing adenoviruses. *Amer. J. Hyg.* **71**, 120

[33] CLARKE D.H. & CASALS J. (1958) Techniques for haemagglutination and haemagglutination-inhibition with arthropod-borne viruses. *Amer. J. trop. Med. Hyg.* **7**, 561

[34] HIRST G.K. (1942) The quantitative determination of influenza virus and antibodies by means of red cell agglutination. *J. exp. Med.* **75**, 49

[35] HORSFALL F.L. JR. & TAMM I. (1953) Fractional dilution procedure for precise titration of haemagglutinating viruses and haemagglutination-inhibiting antibodies *J. Immunol.* **70**, 253

[36] FAZEKAS DE ST GROTH S., WATSON G.S. & REID A.F. (1958) The neutralization of animal viruses. I. A model of virus antibody interaction. *J. Immunol.* **80**, 215

[37] FAZEKAS DE ST GROTH S. & WEBSTER R.G. (1963) The neutralization of animal viruses. IV. Parameters of the influenza virus antibody system. *J. Immunol.* **90**, 151

[38] DAVENPORT F.M., HENNESSY A.V., DRESCHER J., MULDER J. & FRANCIS T. JR. (1964) Further evidence on the relevance of serological recapitulation of human infection with influenza virus. *J. exp. Med.* **120**, 1087

[39] DRESCHER J., HENNESSY A.V. & DAVENPORT F.M. (1962) Photometric methods for the measurement of hemagglutinating viruses and antibody. *J. Immunol.* **89**, 794

[40] TAKÁTSY G. (1955) The use of spiral loops in serological and virological micromethods. *Acta microbiol. Acad. Sci. hung.* **4**, 365

[41] SEVER J.L. (1962) Application of a microtechnique to viral serological investigations. *J. Immunol.* **88**, 320

[42] TAKÁTSY G. & HAMAR M. (1956) The antibody content of immune sera absorbed with

influenza virus as determined with different serological tests. *Acta microbiol. Acad. Sci. hung.* **3**, 299

[43] TYRRELL D.A.J. & HORSFALL F.L.JR. (1953) Neutralization of viruses by homologous immune serum. 1. Quantitative studies on factors which affect the neutralization reaction with Newcastle disease, influenza A and bacterial virus, T3. *J. exp. Med.* **97**, 845

[44] BOULTER E.A. (1957) The titration of vaccinial neutralizing antibody on chorioallantoic membranes. *J. Hyg. (Camb.)* **55**, 502

[45] DULBECCO R., VOGT M. & STRICKLAND A.G.R. (1956) A study of the basic aspects of neutralization of two animal viruses, Western equine encephalitis virus and poliomyelitis virus. *Virology* **2**, 162

[46] TAYLOR-ROBINSON D. & TYRRELL D.A.J. (1962) Serological studies on some viruses isolated from common colds (rhinoviruses). *Brit. J. exp. Path.* **43**, 264

[47] CLARKE S.K.R. & TYRRELL D.A.J. (1958) The neutralization of influenza and other viruses by homologous immune serum. Studies in roller tube tissue cultures. *Arch. ges. Virusforsch.* **8**, 453

[48] LAFFERTY K.J. (1963) The interaction between virus and antibody. I. Kinetic studies. *Virology* **21**, 61

[49] LAFFERTY K.J. (1963) The interaction between virus and antibody. II. Mechanism of the reaction. *Virology* **21**, 76

[50] PORTERFIELD J.S. (1964) The plaque inhibition test. In *Immunological Methods*, ed. ACKROYD Oxford: Blackwell

[51] WECKER E. (1960) A simple test for serodifferentiation of poliovirus strains within the same type. *Virology* **10**, 376

[52] GARD S. (1957) Immuno-activation of poliovirus. *Arch. ges. Virusforsch.* **5**, 449

[53] BARON S., NASOU J.P., OWEN G.M. & BARNETT E.W. (1960) Antibody response of hypogammaglobulinemic patients given poliomyelitis vaccine. *Amer. J. Dis. Child.* **100**, 566

[54] SVEHAG S-E. & MANDEL B. (1964) The formation and properties of poliovirus-neutralizing antibody. *J. exp. Med.* **119**, 1

[55] SALK J.E., YOUNGER J.S. & WARD E.N. (1954) Use of color change in phenol red as the indicator in titrating poliomyelitis virus or its antibody in a tissue culture system. *Amer. J. Hyg.* **60**, 214

[56] MELNICK J.L. & OPTON E.M. (1956) Assay of poliomyelitis neutralizing antibody in disposable plastic panels. *Bull. Wld. Hlth. Org.* **14**, 129

[57] LEBOUVIER G.L., SCHWERDT C.E. & SCHAFFER F.L. (1957) Specific precipitates in agar with purified poliovirus. *Virology* **4**, 590

[58] BLACK F. & MELNICK J.L. (1954) The specificity of the complement fixation test in poliomyelitis. *Yale. J. Biol. Med.* **25**, 385

[59] FULTON F. & DUMBELL K.R. (1949) The serological comparison of strains of influenza virus. *J. gen. Microbiol.* **3**, 97

[60] PEREIRA H.G. (1956) Typing of adenoidal–pharyngeal–conjunctival (APC) viruses by complement-fixation. *J. Path. Bact.* **72**, 105

[61] WADSWORTH A. (1947) *Standard Methods of the Division of Laboratories and Research.* Baltimore: Williams & Wilkins

[62] HUMMELER K., ANDERSON T.F. & BROWN R.A. (1962) Identification of poliovirus particles of different antigenicity by specific agglutination as seen in the electron microscope. *Virology* **16**, 84

[63] SMITH W. (1961) The immunological response to poliomyelitis viruses. *Virology* **13**, 280

[64] BELYAVIN G. (1956) Normal serum inhibitors of influenza virus floculation. *Brit. J. exp. Path.* **37**, 75

[65] PEREIRA H.G. (1960) Antigenic studies of non-infectious adenovirus materials. *Nature, Lond.* **186**, 571

[66] PEREIRA H.G., ALLISON A.C. & FARTHING C.P. (1959) Study of adenovirus antigens by immuno-electrophoresis. *Nature, Lond.* **183**, 895

[67] ALLISON A.C., PEREIRA H.G. & FARTHING C.P. (1960) Investigation of adenovirus antigens by agar diffusion techniques. *Virology* **10**, 316

[68] WESTWOOD J.C.N. (1963) Virus pathogenicity. In *Mechanisms of Virus Infection*, ed. WILSON SMITH. London and New York: Academic Press

[69] YIN-COGRAVE M. (1962) Identification of adenoviruses by microprecipitin agar-gel diffusion. *Lancet* **1**, 1273

[70] DARBYSHIRE J.H. & PEREIRA H.G. (1964) An advenovirus precipitating antibody present in some sera of different animal species and its association with bovine respiratory disease. *Nature, Lond.* **201**, 895

[71] WELLER T.H. & COONS A.H. (1954) Fluorescent antibody studies with agents of Varicella and Herpes zoster propagated in vitro. *Proc. Soc. exp. Biol. (N.Y.)* **86**, 789

[72] GOLDWASSER R.A. & SHEPARD C.C. (1958) Staining of complement and modifications of fluorescent antibody procedures. *J. Immunol.* **80**, 122

[73] HERS J.F.P. (1963) Fluorescent antibody technique in respiratory viral disease. *Amer. Rev. resp. Dis.* **88**, part 2, 316

[74] SOMMERVILLE R.G. & MACFARLANE P.S. (1964) The rapid diagnosis of virus infections by immunofluorescent techniques applied to blood leucocytes. *Lancet* **1**, 911

[75] LIU C., EATON M.D. & HEYL J.T. (1959) Studies on primary atypical pneumonia. II. Observations concerning development and immunological characteristics of antibody in patients. *J. exp. Med.* **109**, 545

[76] CHANOCK R.M., MUFSON M.A., SOMERSON N.L. & COUCH R.B. (1963) Role of mycoplasma (PPLO) in human respiratory disease. *Amer. Rev. resp. Dis.* **88**, part 2, 218

[77] TRAVER M.I., NORTHROP R.L. & WALKER P.L. (1960) Site of intracellular antigen production by myxoviruses. *Proc. Soc. exp. Biol. (N.Y.)* **104**, 268

[78] PEREIRA H.G., ALLISON A.C. & BALFOUR B. (1959) Multiplication of adenovirus type 5 studied by infectivity titrations and by the fluorescent antibody technique. *Virology* **7**, 300

[79] LEBRUN J. (1956) Cellular localization of herpes simplex virus by means of fluorescent antibody. *Virology* **2**, 496

[80] LIM K.A. & BENYESH-MELNICK M. (1960) Typing of viruses by combinations of antiserum pools. Application to typing of enteroviruses (coxsackie and echo). *J. Immunol.* **84**, 309

[81] KARZON D.T., POLLOCK B.F. & BARRON A.L. (1959) Phase variation in Echo virus type 6. *Virology* **9**, 546

[82] VAN DER VEEN J. & MULDER J. (1950) *Studies on the Antigenic Composition of Human Influenza Virus A Strains*. Leyden: Stenfert Kroese

[83] MELNICK J.L., PAUL J.R. & WALTON M. (1955) Serological epidemiology of poliomyelitis. *Amer. J. pub. Hlth.* **45**, 429

[84] DAVENPORT F.M. & HENNESSY A.V. (1957) Predetermination by infection and by vaccination of antibody response to influenza virus vaccine. *J. exp. Med.* **106**, 835

[85] CHANOCK R.M., WONG D.C., HUEBNER R.J. & BELL J.A. (1960) Serologic response of individuals infected with para influenza viruses. *Amer. J. pub. Hlth.* **50**, 1850

[86] SALK J.E. (1951) A critique of serological methods for the study of influenza viruses. *Arch. ges. Virusforsch.* **4,** 476

[87] SABIN A.B. (1959) Present position of immunization against poliomyelitis with live virus vaccines. *Brit. med. J.* **1,** 663

[88] BRUNNER K.T. & WARD R. (1959) Differences in stability of antigen–antibody complexes formed with poliovirus and acute and convalescent phase human serum. *J. Immunol.* **83,** 405

[89] STYK B. (1962) Cofactor and specific antibodies against influenza viruses. III. The potentiating effect of cofactor on specific antibodies of early immune and of hyperimmune sera and the differences in the character of these antibodies. *Acta Virol.* **6,** 327

[90] TAYLOR-ROBINSON D. Personal communication

[91] BRODY J.A. (1963) Haemagglutination-inhibition and neutralization tests using whole blood dried on filterpaper discs. *Lancet* **2,** 616

[92] MCKENNA J.M., ZUSCHEK F. & FRANKEL J.W. (1957) An haemagglutination test for titration of antibodies to polioviruses. *Proc. Soc. exp. Biol. (N.Y.)* **97,** 160

[93] RIFKIND R.A., HSU K.C., MORGAN C., SEEGAL B.C., KNOX A.W. & ROSE H.M. (1960) Use of ferritin-conjugated antibody to localize antigen by electron microscopy. *Nature, Lond.* **187,** 1094

[94] KLEMPERER H.G. & PEREIRA H.G. (1959) Study of adenovirus antigens fractionated by chromatography on DEAE-cellulose. *Virology* **9,** 536

[95] ESPMARK J.A. (1965) Rapid serological typing of herpes simplex virus and titration of herpes simplex antibody by the use of mixed hemadsorption—a mixed antiglobulin reaction applied to virus infected tissue cultures. *Archiv. für Virusforschung* **17,** 89

[96] MATHOT C., ROTHEN A. & SCHER S. (1965) Immunological electro-adsorption method as applied in the case of mice leukaemia. Nature, *Lond.* **207,** 1263

[97] SABURI Y. & MATUMOTO M. (1965) Assay of measles virus hemolysin and its antibody. *Archiv. für Virusforschung* **17,** 29

CHAPTER 25

Immunological Methods in Mycology

J.PEPYS & JOAN L.LONGBOTTOM

Introduction

The description of fungi as a 'mutable and treacherous tribe' by Albrech von Haller 200 years ago reflects the difficulties which face the mycologist, the taxonomist and, in the present case, the immunologist. The many natural and other sources of variation are probably responsible for one of the outstanding difficulties in fungal immunology, namely that of obtaining reproducible results. An admirably informative analysis of natural variations of fungi has been made by Foster [1] and will be quoted here. 'Axioms' of microbial metabolism reflect the gradations within and between species. For example, individual progeny from any culture of a single spore origin may vary within wide limits in regard to biochemical activity, even if morphologically indistinguishable, and the cells in any one culture are not homogeneous physiologically. Strains morphologically and physiologically indistinguishable on one medium may be quite different from each other on another medium. Different strains of the same species and even daughter colonies of any single spore parent culture may, and usually do, vary within great inherent morphological, cultural and physiological limits. The growth of a fungus is also accompanied by physiological changes. Spore formation is the source of genetic variations and cultures of uniform cellular composition can be observed only in growth in shake cultures, when the cell material consists of vegetative mycelium.

In addition to these sources of variability in the fungal antigens, antibody responses are also subject to considerable variation. The simplest antigens may, in experimental animals or in man, excite different individual patterns of antibody responses, although these usually have some features in common.

Uniformity of methods and better understanding of the chemistry of fungal antigens will help to overcome some of these problems. There are many extensive and detailed reports on large numbers of fungal genera, species and strains in which all of the available immunological techniques have been used. This chapter will deal with general aspects likely to be of use to the immunologist, illustrated by limited numbers of examples.

Cultural conditions for fungal antigens

A variety of cultural conditions, such as surface or shake cultures on liquid or solid media of different types and at temperatures appropriate to the particular fungi, have been used. Media containing peptone tend to give better growth of many fungi, but the presence of non-dialysable material in the peptone adds to the amount of non-specific material in antigenic extracts obtained from culture media. This can be overcome by using peptones which have passed through dialysis membranes. Synthetic media have the advantage of being dialysable.

Liquid culture media are traditional and often rich sources of both polysaccharide and protein antigens, emphasis being laid most commonly on polysaccharide-type antigens because of their amount and their immunological importance, although protein and glycoprotein antigens are also important [2, 3]. Solid media may be good sources of soluble antigen which can be obtained from the liquid expressed from the medium by freezing and thawing, as for example with cultures of *Micropolyspora faeni* (*Thermopolyspora polyspora*) [4].

Satisfactory yields of antigen have been obtained from both surface or submerged cultures of, for example, *Coccidioides immitis* [5], *Trichophyton mentagrophytes* [6], *Histoplasma capsulatum* [7], and *Aspergillus fumigatus* [2, 8, 9]. Comparison of shake and stationary cultures of *C. immitis* [5] showed that the peak of antigen production in the shake culture was during the third week and that more prolonged growth did not provide additional antigen. Shake cultures also gave reproducible results in antigenic content. The medium of the stationary cultures contained no antigen at 4 weeks, even with vigorous growth. The antigen from culture in a synthetic medium was anticomplementary.

The development of a single antigen was used to compare cultures of *C. immitis* on a number of different media. It appeared after 10 days, first in Sabouraud's and Roessler's media, and in greater amounts in cultures at 37° C than at room temperature. No consistent relationship was found between the formation of antigen and the rate of growth or the accompanying rise in pH. Dialysable and non-dialysable anticomplementary factors in the cultures on synthetic media were attributed in part to the presence of ammonium ions and primary amines in Roessler's medium for example, or to citrate ions in asparagine medium which may combine with magnesium or calcium, both of which are needed for complement fixation. The antigen was present in the mycelium of cultures of all ages and its liberation was attributed to autolysis without cellular destruction [10, 11, 12]. Autolysis of 3-day-old mycelium of *C. immitis* in the presence of toluene yielded cell-free soluble antigen, about 60–70 per cent of the cell weight being liberated [13].

Antigens from *Aspergillus fumigatus* capable of giving precipitation reactions with strongly reacting human sera were present in the culture medium on the second day of surface culture at 37° C, on Sabouraud's medium. Antigen appeared early in the medium and the highest yield of antigens was present between 2 weeks and up to 6 weeks [2, 8, 14]. The medium from older cultures contained somatic polysaccharides which behaved like C-substance by combining with C-reactive protein [2, 14].

In shake cultures of *Histoplasma capsulatum* the maximum weight of organisms was present at 5 days and did not increase thereafter. Polysaccharide antigen appeared in the medium on the seventh day and was maximal at the twentieth day, suggesting that soluble antigens were being liberated by autolysis [7]. Variations of the antigens of *H. capsulatum* occur depending upon changes in nutritional factors and conditions of culture, and are shown by differences in the reactions of crude antigens prepared from yeast and filamentous growth phases [15].

Preparation of fungal antigens in general
A variety of fungal products, ranging from whole or disintegrated cellular material to crude or purified antigens obtained from autolytic or metabolic products in cellular material and culture media, have been used for immunological investigations. The cells or mycelium have been variously treated, being heated, dried and/or defatted prior to extraction. Among the physical methods used for disruption of cellular material are simple grinding in a pestle and mortar, homogenization in suitable blenders, repeated freezing and thawing, Mickle cell disintegration and ultrasonic vibration.

The physical properties of fungal antigens are important for serological tests. Wider use has been recommended of agglutination tests of fungal cells or particles [16]. Such tests require homogeneous suspensions which can be prepared from the conidia of certain fungi, from yeasts and from the yeast phase of dimorphic fungi. Surface-active agents may be needed to give good suspensions of conidia from hyphomycetes and ultrasonic treatment has been used for *Nocardia* preparations [17]. Complement-fixation tests with such preparations have been widely used, being most effective with somatic antigens which are more protein-like in character, as against the polysaccharide capsular antigens which react well with precipitating antibody.

The ready solubility of many of the fungal antigens has made simple extraction with isotonic saline or dilute buffered solutions, such as Coca's fluid, satisfactory for many purposes. On the other hand the use of untreated culture filtrates has also been quite general, e.g. histoplasmin, coccidioidin and blastomycin.

Polysaccharide antigens
The immunological interest and importance of polysaccharide antigens of

fungi, as of bacteria, has stimulated attempts to obtain purified, protein-free polysaccharides. A great variety of polysaccharides are produced by fungi. Some of these serve as reserve foods whereas many are fabricated into the structural framework or the capsular sheath. Other polysaccharides appear to have no definite function in the organism, but seemingly are simply by-products of metabolism.

There are often close relationships between the fungal polysaccharides and the pneumococcal polysaccharides studied by Heidelberger in his fundamental work on the mechanism and quantitative aspects of the antigen–antibody precipitation reaction. These were based on the fact that all the nitrogen in antigen–antibody precipitates produced by nitrogen-free polysaccharide could be attributed to specific antibody. Recent investigations of fungal polysaccharides along the same lines has shown that they provide a number of valuable reagents for the production of specific antigen–antibody reactions which are useful for the morphological study of polysaccharide antigens in the structural formation of fungi.

As with pneumococcal antigens, the fungal polysaccharide antigens are in general responsible for type specificity, whereas the protein antigens are responsible for broad species specificity. Purified fungal polysaccharides as a rule tend to be haptenic, reacting well with antisera but themselves failing to stimulate, or stimulating only weakly, the appearance of antibodies in experimental animals [18, 19, 20], although injection in Freund's adjuvant of the β-naphthol extract of *Candida* has given good antibody responses [21].

Most, if not all, of the various techniques for the specific extraction and purification of polysaccharides have been applied to fungi. These techniques have been brought together in a most practical manner in *Methods in Carbohydrate Chemistry, Volume 5: General Polysaccharides* [22]. The crude polysaccharide extracts are often 'deproteinized' by Sevag's method with chloroform and butyl (or amyl) alcohol followed by precipitation from the aqueous phase with ethanol or acetone. The deproteinizing action of trifluorotrichloroethane, used to obtained protein-free polysaccharides from pneumococci and streptococci, may be of interest with regard to fungi in which antigens of similar chemical structure are to be found. Other methods of deproteinization have included precipitation of the protein with perchloric or trichloroacetic acids, and also prolonged enzymatic digestion, e.g. by trypsin and pepsin, of the cellular material prior to extraction in alkali.

Separation of the polysaccharide and protein antigens in culture media of *A. fumigatus* [2, 14] and of *Candida* [25] was satisfactorily achieved by ammonium sulphate precipitation and of *Micropolyspora faeni* (*Thermopolyspora polyspora*) by trichloroacetic acid precipitation [3, 4].

An important example, for fungal immunology, of methods of extraction of specific polysaccharides, is fractionation with copper complexes [23].

Fehling's solution has been used to precipitate polymers containing D-mannose or D-xylose, the insoluble polysaccharide–copper complex being decomposed with an alcoholic solution of acid or by a chelating agent. This method was used to separate mannan from glycogen in extracts of yeast cells, which were disrupted by heating in an autoclave at pH 7 to avoid the degradation caused by alkaline extraction. The mannans extracted in this way from *Candida* and other species were not denatured and the whole yeast cells from which they were prepared remained intact after the extraction of the capsular material [24]. Traces of glucose present in the isolated mannans were considered to be due to an impurity from cell wall glucan.

Quaternary ammonium salts are also useful as specific precipitating agents since they are able to form insoluble salts with acidic polysaccharides and can therefore be easily separated from neutral polysaccharides. The latter do not react except as borate complexes. Purified glycopeptide has been prepared from ethylene glycol extracts of acetone-dried, powdered mycelium from *Trichophyton mentagrophytes* by precipitation with Cetavlon (cetyltrimethyl ammonium bromide) from borate buffered solutions by gradually increasing the pH [26, 27].

Somatic glycopeptide material from *Aspergillus fumigatus* has been extracted using the phenol/water method of Westphal for preparation of bacterial lipopolysaccharides [2, 8, 14] (see Chapter 9). This glycopeptide proved to be similar to glycopeptide extracted from the same batch of mycelium by heating in weakly acidic saline with subsequent alcohol precipitation, as for the preparation of C-substance polysaccharide of the pneumococcus [28]. Amongst other common methods used are alkaline, β-naphthol, sulphosalicylic acid and formamide extractions of mycelial material.

For further purification of fungal antigens more recent methods such as Sephadex gel filtration, resin and DEAE-cellulose ion-exchange column fractionation are now being extensively applied [2, 8, 14, 26, 27, 29 30].

Most of the polysaccharides have been shown to be branched chain molecules, usually containing three or more different monosaccharide types. The most common monosaccharide constituents of the polysaccharides isolated from fungi have been mannose, galactose and glucose [20, 27], and in many instances the presence of at least a small amount of bound nitrogen, often not detected by tests for protein, has been recorded. Several yeast mannans have been studied in detail, especially one from *Saccharomyces rouxii* which contained as much as 15 per cent protein. Recently the galactomannanpeptide isolated from *T. mentagrophytes* [27] was shown to contain D-galactose (9 per cent,) D-mannose (73 per cent) and protein (9 per cent) and a molecular weight of 40,000 was suggested, indicating a basic structure of about 200 mannose units. The predominant linkages in the chain were 1--2 and 1--4 with equal numbers of mannopyranose and galactofuranose terminal units, the N-terminal aminoacid assay indicating the presence of at least three major peptide chains ending in threonine, glycine and alanine. This was contrasted with the galactomannan from *T. granulosum* which was found to consist of a highly branched mannan with chiefly 1--2 and 1--6 linkages [30]. This molecule contained no nitrogen, however, presumably because of prolonged trypsin digestion and extraction with alkali.

Fractionation of the glycopeptide isolated from *A. fumigatus* showed several fractions containing increasing amounts of bound nitrogen linked to a glucogalactomannan (ratio 1 : 5 : 20) polysaccharide moiety [2, 14]. The electrophoretic mobility of these fractions increased with their increase in N content, which consisted of a high proportion of the hydroxy-amino acids, serine and threonine, together with alanine. Although ficin was able to remove the peptide moiety of the *T. mentagrophytes* glycopeptide [26], it was found to have no effect on the glycopeptide of *A. fumigatus* [14].

Different methods of extraction may yield polysaccharides with different specificity. Thus, sulphosalicylic acid extraction of *Nocardia* gave species or type-specific reactions, acetic acid extracts gave genus-specific reactions and formamide extraction gave group-specific reactions [31]. The polysaccharide extracted by sulphosalicylic acid was the most informative and contained, depending on the *Nocardia* species, glucosamine, galactose, glucose, arabinose and rhamnose [32].

Antisera

The methods employed in other fields of immunology have been adopted for the production of fungal antisera. These consist of the injection by various routes, with or without Freund's complete or incomplete adjuvant, of live or killed, intact or disintegrated fungi or of their soluble antigens. Antisera are also produced by active infection with appropriate fungi. Antibodies usually make their appearance, as expected, within 2–4 weeks. As with other complex antigenic mixtures short courses of immunization tend to give more specific antisera with limited cross-reactivity, whereas long intensive courses result in antisera with wide ranges of antibodies and often considerable cross-reactivity. Intensive immunization has been employed for many fungi, and where an antiserum is intended for 'finger-printing' the fungi, it is regarded as suitable when continued immunization ceases to evoke additional antibodies, usually of the precipitating type [8, 25].

The most effective method of producing antisera is the injection subcutaneously into multiple sites of fungal antigen in Freund's adjuvant, complete or incomplete. In some cases this injection is given weekly until maximum antibody production is reached, or it may be followed by injections intravenously or subcutaneously of aqueous or saline solutions or suspensions of fungal antigen. The administration of aqueous suspensions or solutions of antigen in this way is also effective in boosting the antibody titre in animals sensitized even months before. Amounts of antigen of the order of 20–100 mg are usually appropriate both for the initial and for subsequent injections. The addition of Zymosan to Freund's adjuvant is said to give more rapid and better antibody responses. Satisfactory antisera have been produced in this way against fungal genera, such as *Trichosporon* [69], *Geotrichum* [33], *Aspergillus* [8], *Candida* [25] and *Penicillium notatum* [34]. Antisera have been prepared by the same methods by the authors against *Aspergillus* species, *Mucor* sp., *Cladosporium herbarum*, *Penicillium notatum* and *Micropolyspora faeni* (*Thermopolyspora polyspora*).

The 'finger-printing' of fungi so as to determine their antigenic pattern has progressed rapidly with the use of antisera resulting from intensive immunization, and with the use of monospecific sera and sera absorbed with heterologous fungi. Precipitin, slide or tube agglutination, and complement-fixation tests have all been used. It should be noted that human sera from patients with pulmonary aspergilloma or farmer's lung may give as many arcs of precipitation against the appropriate extracts as the antisera from intensively immunized rabbits. Such sera are quite commonly found in affected subjects, and they are useful for studying antigenic relationships.

Immunofluorescence tests

The immunofluorescence test has a potentially wide application in fungal immunology [20, 35, 38]. Most of the usual methods have been employed, such as direct testing of fungal material with labelled fungal antisera, indirect testing with labelled antiglobulin sera to show the combination of antibody with fungal antigen, and fluorescence inhibition tests (see Chapter 16). An extension of these studies to the use of labelled antisera prepared against the individual immunoglobulins (IgA, IgM and IgG) is indicated in order to identify which of the immunoglobulins is reacting with particular fungal antigens.

Labelled antisera have been prepared from globulin fractions obtained by ammonium sulphate precipitation or by column fractionation of rabbit antisera. Simple and rapid filtration of the conjugates through Sephadex is being widely used for the removal of excess fluorescein and has been applied, for example, to rabbit antisera against *C. albicans* [36].

Autofluorescence of the fungi *in vivo* and *in vitro* can be a problem, as with the arthrospores of *C. immitis* and the tuberculate spores of *H. capsulatum* [37]. The autofluorescence can be diminished by using a 5113 Corning glass primary filter 3 mm thick, and a Wratten 2A secondary filter 2 mm thick [38]. Air drying or ethanol fixation on the slides of dermatophytes gave less autofluorescence than heat fixation [39, 40].

The problem of autofluorescence of the outer of the double walls of

B. dermatitidis has been resolved by adding white light to the ultra-violet field. This made the inner wall brightly refractile and easily distinguishable from fluorescein-stained and unstained *H. capsulatum* cells which do not show this [35].

Immunofluorescence tests are useful for many purposes. For example, anticomplementary sera from patients with histoplasmosis gave positive reactions by means of fluorescence inhibition tests in 97 per cent of patients whose subsequent sera gave positive complement-fixing reactions [41].

They are useful for the study of organisms which, because they are rough and filamentous are therefore not suitable for agglutination tests, and for organisms which grow poorly, yielding little antigen. Thus, they have been used for grouping actinomycetes [42]. Tests have also been made on isolates from patients and animals with actinomycosis and from healthy subjects. Dried smears were stained with labelled globulins obtained from rabbit antisera [43]. Young cultures, too immature for morphological identification, can be rapidly identified by immunofluorescence tests as can small numbers of viable or non-viable cells, or cells mixed with other types of cell as in contaminated cultures. The behaviour of antigens during fungal growth has been studied in *C. albicans* where, by means of fluorescein-labelled antibody, it was found that the cell wall material of the parent cell was incorporated in the walls of daughter cells and hyphae. Diminution of intensity of stain showed that the parent cell wall material was diluted by continued growth [44]. Such tests are of interest because they indicate the morphological loci of antigens.

Caution is necessary in the interpretation of immunofluorescence results since labelled normal rabbit sera were found with a number of fungal species to give fluorescence reactions not attributable to free fluorescein. Absorption with *B. dermatitidis* and *C. immitis* eliminated the reaction. Complement-fixation and agar-gel tests were negative, but the immunofluorescence tests are more sensitive. It was considered possible that the 'normal' rabbits had antibodies against related antigens, and shows the need for careful controls [38]. A similar problem is present in man, in whom antibodies against the dermatophytes, *Trichophyton mentagrophytes* and *T. rubrum*, were shown by immunofluorescence tests in uninfected, as well as infected, subjects. Cross-antigenicity was shown by absorption of the sera with related and unrelated organisms including *A. niger*, *Mycobacterium butyricum* and *C. albicans*, all of which reduced or inhibited the reactions in seven out of ten cases [45].

Cross-reactions are important in the differentiation of *H. capsulatum*, *B. dermatitidis* and *C. immitis*. Absorption of labelled immunoglobulins against *H. capsulatum* with *C. immitis* and *B. dermatitidis* gave a specific conjugate which stained the yeast phase cells but not the mycelium of *H.*

capsulatum. In the process of absorption more than 80 per cent of antibody protein, probably non-specific, was lost [46]. Similarly, *C. immitis* antiserum cross-reacted with *H. capsulatum*, *B. dermatitidis* and other heterologous fungi. Absorption with yeast cells of *H. capsulatum* eliminated the non-specific activity and the absorbed serum gave strong reactions with the tissue forms of *C. immitis* [49].

It has also been found, that an absorbed conjugate of antiserum to the yeast-phase of *H. capsulatum* gave specific reactions for *H. capsulatum* and seldom reacted with the yeast phase of *H. duboisii* [47]. Comparisons of the antigens of *H. capsulatum*, and *Chrysosporium* and *Sepedonium* species showed cross-reactions with non-absorbed, and specific reactions with absorbed, antisera. There was a varying pattern of shared antigens. *H. capsulatum* and *H. duboisii* were clearly distinguished. Relationships of interest were shown with other fungi, presenting an example of the taxonomic problems arising from antigen studies [48].

B. dermatitidis rabbit antiglobulins stained yeast and mycelial phases of ten strains of *B. dermatitidis*. Cross-reactions occurred with yeast and mycelial phases of *H. capsulatum* and other heterologous fungi. Absorption with yeast cells of *H. capsulatum* on two occasions and once with *Geotrichum candidum* gave a specific conjugate for the yeast phase cells of *B. dermatitidis* and no reactions occurred with the mycelial phase [50].

Dried smears of yeast-like organisms were tested with labelled rabbit antisera to *C. albicans*. The globulin fractions of the antiserum were separated by ammonium sulphate precipitation, and were then absorbed with *C. parakrusei* (*C. parapsilosis*) cells to remove antibodies against *C. stellatoidea*, since the latter absorbed out too much of the reactivity against *C. albicans*. All twenty-eight strains of *C. albicans* tested and eight strains of *C. tropicalis* gave positive reactions, whereas twenty-one other *Candida* species gave negative reactions, and forty-six other yeast-like organisms belonging to fifteen other genera gave negative or weak reactions and were readily distinguishable [51].

Cells of *Cryptococcus neoformans* and *C. neoformans* var. *innocuous* were tested against conjugated antisera to three strains of *C. neoformans*. Ninety-five out of ninety-six strains gave positive results with all three sera regardless of the amount of capsule present. Variations in capsular size were shown by differences in the width of the fluorescent staining. No cross-reactions were given between *C. neoformans* and twenty-three species of heterologous yeasts or between *C. neoformans* and antisera to other fungi [52]. The test was advantageous in that the fluorescence was not dependent upon the amount of capsular material, which may vary greatly.

In tests with labelled antiglobulin sera for the presence, on heat-killed *C. neoformans* cells, of antibody globulin in sera from culturally proven cases, antibodies against cryptococci were found in sera containing high titres of antibodies to *Candida albicans*. Absorption with *C. albicans* did not remove the cryptococcal antibodies, suggesting that certain strains of *C. neoformans* may stimulate appearance of both *C. neoformans* and *C. albicans* antibodies [53].

Immunofluorescence tests are of assistance in the study of cultures of pathogenic dematiaceous fungi which are difficult to distinguish because of their polymorphism and confusing similarity [17, 74]. Labelled antisera to *Cladosporium carrionii* and *C. bantianum* (*C. trichoides*) cross-reacted with a number of dematiaceous species but absorption gave specific sera. The findings showed that the antigen diffused centrifugally from the hyphae. The age of the culture influenced the affinity of the antibody for the hyphae and spores, young portions of mycelium staining more intensely than the older, probably because of diffusion of soluble polysaccharide and other antigens into the culture medium. This was probably responsible for the diffuse outward halo seen around the mycelia. The use of cultures of more than 1–2 weeks in age could therefore lead to false negative results [54].

In the fluorescence inhibition test the reaction of specific labelled fungal antisera is blocked by the reaction of specific antibodies in the test serum with the fungal antigens. This fluorescence inhibition test was compared with other tests with rabbit antiserum to *H. capsulatum*. The antiserum was absorbed with cells of *C. immitis* and *B. dermatitidis*. The conjugated antiserum was added together with the patient's serum to heat-fixed smears of formalin-killed, 7-day-old yeast-phase cultures of *H. capsulatum*. These were incubated at 37° C for 30 minutes. Positive fluorescence inhibition reactions were given with twenty-six out of thirty sera containing antibodies against the yeast phase, and with two out of eleven sera containing antibodies against histoplasmin only, whereas nine out of eleven of the latter sera, and sixteen out of thirty of the former sera gave positive reactions in agar-gel tests. The fluorescence inhibition test was simple and effective for the rapid detection of yeast-phase antibody and for the differentiation of histoplasmosis from other serologically related mycotic infections. The complement-fixation test was best for showing antibodies against both the histoplasmin and yeast-phase antigens. Of the sera giving complement-fixation titres of 1 in 8 or more, 87 per cent gave positive fluorescence tests and 53 per cent positive agar-gel tests [55].

Methods for immunochemical classification of fungi

Among the immunological methods used for the differentiation and classification of fungi are the agglutination tests on fungal cells, precipitation tests in agar-gel or quantitative precipitin tests, and complement-fixation tests. Similar results have been obtained with the various methods, yet the differences are important enough for more than one method to be required for definitive conclusions. In some cases attempts have been made to codify the findings into antigenic formulae. This needs to be supplemented, and probably will be in the near future, by the chemical characterization of the factors in the antigenic formulae. Selected examples only will be given of this important aspect of fungal immunology.

The agglutination test which characterizes the surface antigens *in situ* has been used by the slide agglutination method for the detailed study of four species of *Torulopsis*, with the use of monospecific and absorbed sera prepared against the genera *Torulopsis*, *Candida*, *Saccharomyces* and *Hansenula*. A total of thirty-four antibodies against thermostable and eleven against thermolabile antigens were tested. This battery of serological reagents was found to be useful for rapid identification. For example, *T. glabrata* could be identified by the possession of antigens corresponding to thermostable antigen 34, the corresponding antiserum being prepared from heated antiserum to *T. glabrata* which was absorbed with heated cells of *C. albicans* and *C. robusta*, and by the possession of thermolabile antigen 'k' which was an independent antigen not included in the series 'a' to 'j' already identified [56]. A similar analysis of the genus *Hansenula* was made with monospecific and absorbed sera, prepared against the genera *Candida*, *Torulopsis*, *Hansenula* and *Debaryomyces* [57]. These studies are of value for systematic classification based on the antigens of the yeasts.

Immunoelectrophoresis tests in agar gel are a very effective method for the discrimination of fungal antigens in terms of precipitating antibodies [8, 25]. In these tests crude antigens were prepared by saline extraction of freeze-dried homogenized cultures. Culture filtrates were used as the source of metabolic products, and contained in certain cases, for example *A. fumigatus*, all the antigens to be found in the cell extract, except one [8]. Comparison of culture filtrate with cell-sap antigens against human sera from patients with pulmonary aspergilloma shows, however, a much richer antigenic content in the cell sap extract [2, 14].

The rabbit antisera for immunoelectrophoresis tests were obtained by intensive immunization with crude antigen in Freund's incomplete adjuvant. This was carried on to the point where no further precipitins were produced [8]. Precipitation arcs obtained in immunoelectrophoresis tests were numbered to provide an antigenic mosaic for examination of the various fungal species by direct and absorption tests. A study was made of thirteen *Aspergillus* species, three *Penicillium* species, *Mucor mucedo*, *Cladosporium herbarum*, *Cladosporium trichoides*, *Epidermophyton floccosum*, *Trichophyton* (*Ctenomyces*) *mentagrophytes*, *T. soudanense*, *Candida albicans*, *C. pseudotropicalis* and *Geotrichum candidum*. The *A. fumigatus* extract gave sixteen precipitation arcs with the homologous rabbit antiserum, with which *A. fischeri* gave eight arcs, and the other fungi from one to three arcs, except for the *Cladosporium* species, *T. mentagrophytes*, *Candida* and *Geotrichum* which were negative. In tests against human sera from patients with aspergillosis, precipitins were also found against an antigen of *T. mentagrophytes*. In other studies [2, 14, 58, 59] important related antigens were found between *A. fumigatus* and *C. herbarum* in tests on the sera of patients with pulmonary aspergillosis, and varying patterns of related antigens between *Mucor*, *C. herbarum* and *A. fumigatus* in tests on the sera of patients with farmer's lung. The value of antisera from fully immunized rabbits is evident, but the even more extensive variety of antibodies against fungal antigens from *A. fumigatus*, for example, in human subjects makes it difficult to extrapolate from animals to man, who, it would seem, compares more than favourably with the rabbit as a producer of precipitating antibody.

Similar studies with hyperimmunized rabbit antisera have been made with the genus *Penicillium* [34], including nine *Asymmetrica* (*P. notatum*, *P. chrysogenum*, *P. digitatum*, *P. commune*, *P. terrestre*, *P. cyclopium*, *P. expansum*, *P. italicum* and *P. nigricans*), two *Monoverticillata* (*P. restrictum*, *P. frequentans*), two *Biverticillata-symmetrica*(*P. funiculosum*, *P. novaezeelandiae*). *P. notatum* had only two to three common antigens with the *Monoverticillata* and *Biverticillata-symmetrica*. The relationship of *P. notatum* with the other *Asymmetrica* was closer with five to eight antigens in common, except for *P. nigricans* which had four. As expected, because it belongs to the same series, *P. chrysogenum* had fourteen antigens in common, but a problem in systematics is suggested by the presence of only two common antigens in *P. digitatum* which is considered to be close to *P. notatum*.

The antigens of *Candida albicans*, *C. tropicalis*, *C. zeylanoides*, *C. krusei*, *C. pseudotropicalis*, *C. macedoniensis*, *C. stellatoidea* and other species were examined [25, 63] against hyperimmunized rabbit sera, providing a total of forty-eight specific factors for comparison [63]. *C. albicans* and *C. stellatoidea* were found to be closely related, *C. tropicalis* was related antigenically to *C. zeylanoides*, and all were different from the other species tested.

Whilst these tests gave similar taxonomic results to the slide agglutination tests, double the number of antigens were demonstrated by immunoelectrophoresis, and differences were shown between *C. pseudotropicalis* and *C. macedoniensis* which, it was claimed, were not revealed by the agglutination tests. Different agglutination patterns have, however, been obtained with these two species of *Candida* [65]. Chromatographic fractionation of *C. albicans* antigens on Amberlite XE64 provided an antigen, regarded as specific, giving a single precipitation arc against absorbed *C. albicans* antisera [60].

Immunochemical investigations are also being made, and it is to be expected that chemical characterization of specific factors will lead to rapid expansion of our knowledge. The outer cell-wall antigens of *Candida* have been shown to be soluble thermostable polysaccharides containing glucose and mannose [61]. These antigens were studied in mechanically disrupted cells by means of monospecific sera. Thermolabile cytoplasmic antigens are also present and yet other antigens are present both in the cell wall and the cytoplasm [64].

The identification of mannans as major surface antigens of *Candida* is important in their study. This has been shown with purified mannans by the quantitative precipitin test. The findings are valuable for the immuno-chemical analysis of highly branched polysaccharides and for resolving the antigenic structure of yeast mannans, although a number of complex questions have arisen from these studies [21, 24].

Antisera were prepared in rabbits and sheep by the injection, in Freund's adjuvant, of cell walls, and of a polysaccharide antigen obtained by β-naph-thol extract [19] of the cell wall. The mannans were extracted by fractionation with copper complexes by the method used to separate mannans from gly-cogen in yeast-cell preparations [23]. Of the various yeast genera from which mannans were extracted, 0·5–0·7 per cent N was found in the *Candida* man-nans only. Their immunological reactivity showed that they were not dena-tured, although the possibility of polymerization was not excluded.

Mannans from *Candida*, *Cryptococcus*, *Hansenula*, *Saccharomyces* and *Torulopsis* were tested against antisera to *Candida albicans* groups A and B. Mannans from *C. tropicalis* and *C. albicans* group A were very similar, whereas mannans from *C. albicans* group B and phosphomannan from the strain of *Hansenula capsulata* precipitated only 40 per cent of the amount of antibody protein which was precipitated by the homologous mannan, and mannans from the other genera precipitated even less. Tests with an antiserum to *C. albicans* group B showed that the same amount of antibody protein was precipitated by mannans of *C. albicans* group A, *C. albicans* group B, and *C. tropicalis*. Thus, *C. albicans* group A contained all the determinants of group B, together with additional determinants [21], although there is other evidence that group B has other antigens not present in group A [65]. Some or all of the antigenic differences were attributable to the mannans [21].

Many problems were revealed in this investigation. Whilst other man-nans obtained from *S. cerevisiae* and *S. rouxii*, both highly branched mole-cules, contained α-1-2 and α-1-6 linked mannose units, similar to those of *C. albicans* group A, they have the lowest levels of cross-reactions. In the case of the phosphomannan of *H. capsulata*, which contained a β-1-2 linked mannose backbone with single α-1-2 linked mannose residues occurring every fifth disaccharide unit, no significant cross-reactions were given and it was concluded that the antibody was reacting with the α-1-2 linked side units. Other phosphomannans, e.g. *H. holstii*, also contain both α-1-3 and α-1-2 linked mannose units but did not cross-react.

A mannose containing heteropolysaccharide of *Cryptococcus laurentii* var. *flavescens* was of interest. This acidic polysaccharide consists of a mannose backbone with xylose and glucuronic acid units as terminal sugars. Cross-reaction with anti-*Candida* serum suggests either that mannose is a terminal sugar in this polysaccharide or that the antibody combines with internally situated mannose residues, a possibility for which some evidence has been obtained [66].

Another problem requiring explanation is that double-diffusion tests with homologous and heterologous *C. albicans* anti-sera against crude cell-wall extracts (β-naphthol type) and mannans failed to give constant or predictable numbers of lines. The problem of whether this is due to different chemical groupings acting as antigenic determinants, or whether the antibody responses to these antigens differed because of heterogeneity of the animals providing the antisera remains to be answered.

Consideration also has to be given to whether the mannans contain units of several different molecular weights. There is evidence in favour of such a possibility from the multiple precipitation lines produced by dextrans of different molecular weights [67].

Quantitative precipitin and agar-gel tests were made on sheep antisera to *C. albicans* group B, *C. stellatoidea* and *C. tropicalis* with polysaccharides from eleven different species of fungi [24]. Whereas in tests against the antiserum to *C. albicans* group B, the mannans of *C. albicans* group A, *C. stellatoidea*, *C. tropicalis*, *H. capsulata* and *T. pinus* precipitated 80–120 per cent as much antibody protein as the homologous mannan, the mannans of *C. albicans* group B and *C. stellatoidea* precipitated 80–100 per cent, the other mannans precipitated from 44 down to 18 per cent. The other mannans tested also showed differences with the different antisera.

The problems here were that the *Candida* mannans gave reactions of identity with antisera to *C. albicans* group B and to *C. stellatoidea*, yet in tests against the antiserum to *C. tropicalis* definite differences were shown. In tests against *C. tropicalis* antiserum, *C. stellatoidea* mannan gave no precipitation in the tube precipitin test, yet it gave a precipitation reaction in the agar-gel test, and conversely the mannans from *S. cerevisiae*, *S. pini* and *T. pinus* precipitated 50 per cent or more of the antibody protein in the tube precipitation test but gave no reactions in the agar-gel test.

The results of these two investigations suggest that the possession of common monosaccharides and glycosidic linkages are not enough to predict antigenic crossreactivity, particularly with highly branched polysaccharides. An explanation is needed for the failure of certain mannans with the mannosidic linkages in unbranched and branched linkages to cross-react.

The complement-fixation test has been used for the serological classification of *Nocardiae* [32] using polysaccharide fractions extracted from mechanically disrupted cells with sulphosalicylic acid, formamide and 70 per cent acetic acid [31]. The descriptive terms for the *Nocardia* species used by the authors are not generally agreed, and here, too, antigenic analyses will need to be correlated with the more usual taxonomic criteria. A more widely accepted classification has been prepared [62]. Antisera were produced by intravenous injection of rabbits and intraperitoneal injection of guinea-pigs with saline suspensions of cell walls, and absorption tests were performed by adding wet cell-wall sediment to them. The polysaccharides of most of the *Nocardia* tested contained glucosamine, galactose, glucose and arabinose. Other *Nocardia* species also contained rhamnose, and one, referred to by the authors as *N. turbata*, contained rhamnose but not arabinose.

The tests showed four serological groups (A–D) and twenty-one serological types. Seven antisera were prepared for characterization of the antigens present in the polysaccharide extracted by sulphosalicylic acid. The antisera and their corresponding antigenic factors were as follows, the group factors being starred, *N. asteroides* No. 60 (1)*, *N. asteroides* No. 72 (2), *N. asteroides* No. 58 (3), *N. turbata* No. 152 (4)*, *N. sebivorans* No. 8595 (5)*, *N. farcinica* No. 4524 (6)*, *N. blackwellii* No. 81 (7). Types were identified by means of the antigenic factors corresponding to 2, 3 and 7.

The tentative scheme for the group classification of *Nocardia* based on factors 1, 4, 5 and 6 was as follows:

Tentative scheme of the group classification of *Nocardiae*

| Group designation | Antigenic factor | | | |
	1	4	5	6
A	+	(+)*	(+)	−
B	−	+	−	−
C	−	+	+	(+)
D	−	(+)	−	+

* The factor may or may not be demonstrable.

Sero-group A consisted of morphologically typical strains of *N. asteroides* and *N. corallina*. Sero-group B contained *N. brasiliensis*, *N. polychromogenes*, *N. caprae*, *N. leishmanii*, *N. erythropolis* and *N. rubra* (?). Sero-group C contained *N. farcinica*, *N. turbata*, *N. madurae*, *N. lutea*, *N. rubra*, *N. caviae*, *N. sebivorans*, *N. blackwellii* and atypical strains of *N. asteroides*. Sero-group D contained *N. eppingeri*, *N. pelletieri*, *N. rangoonensis*, *N. pretoriana*.

The findings confirmed the results obtained in tests with cell wall preparations [31], but the polysaccharides extracted with sulphosalicylic acid from defatted cells gave clearer results. Contributing to this was the extraction from

DD*

the cell wall by sulphosalicylic acid of sugars containing rhamnose. This is present in very small amounts and is probably involved in the serological specificity of some strains, and it was not found on hydrolysis of the cell walls. The serological classification corresponded in general with morphological classifications, and whilst no attempt was made to use it for definitive classification, the methods employed are a good example of how to conduct this sort of study.

Immunologically active polysaccharides extracted from cell extracts of *N. asteroides* and *N. brasiliensis*, showed that two from *N. asteroides* had the same molar ratios of arabinose and galactose, giving cross-reactions against each other in double-diffusion tests with the homologous and heterologous rabbit sera, and each absorbed out the antibodies against the other. Two polysaccharides from *N. brasiliensis*, however, were species-specific, containing arabinose, galactose and mannose in different molar ratios, and reacted only with homologous antisera [68].

In studies on the genus *Trichosporon* [69] evidence was obtained in support of the hypothesis that the hereditary antigenic pattern might be more stable than the form of the fungus, and that immunological characteristics are likely to be of importance in systematic classifications. These studies illustrate many of the immunological problems of fungi. For example, satisfactory antisera were obtained without difficulty with certain strains after repeated intravenous injection of formolized, heat-killed suspensions of 3-day-old cultures. Other strains such as *T. margaritiferum* evoked no antibody and *T. cutaneum* and *T. serviceum* which were poorly antigenic also tended to give spontaneous agglutination which made the interpretation of agglutination tests difficult. However, an initial injection of the antigen in Freund's adjuvant followed by intravenous injection of living cells resulted in antisera which were strongly precipitating.

Tests showed that the agglutination tests alone were not sufficient for antigenic analysis, since whilst the antigens of *T. pullulans* reacted strongly with the antiserum to *T. infestans*, there was no reaction of the *T. infestans* antigen to the *T. pullulans* antiserum. Agar-gel diffusion tests gave the best results with this genus, haemagglutination tests with sensitized red blood cells being regarded as too sensitive.

Three different antigenic formulae for these serological groups were tentatively assumed. *T. pullulans* which hydrolyses urea strongly was found to be serologically related to a sero-group containing *T. cutaneum*, *T. infestans* and *T. margaritiferum*, all of which hydrolysed urea, and it appeared also to be related to another group, thus holding an intermediary position. Cross-reactions were found between the urea-hydrolysing group and various species of *Cryptococcus*, *Candida curvata* and *C. humicola*. All these latter organisms had similar biochemical properties, such as lack of carbohydrate fermentation, hydrolysis of urea and synthesis of starch. The serological and biochemical relationships were thought to indicate true phylogenetic relationships among morphologically different yeasts, which at present are classified under several form genera.

A few of the growing number of attempts at immunochemical correlation will be given.

Three antigenic types, A, B and C, have been described in *Cryptococcus neoformans* [70, 71, 72]. All the antigens contained xylose, galactose, mannose and a uronic acid and were quantitatively similar on chromatographic analysis. They were obtained by fractionation with alcohol and were distinguished from each other by agglutination, capsular reaction and agglutinin absorption tests.

Polysaccharide antigens from eight strains of fungi in the genera *Geotrichum*, *Endomyces*, *Trichosporon* and *Endomycopsis*, prepared in various ways, contained galactose, glucose and mannose, three contained xylose as well, and one contained glucose and mannose only. The polysaccharides consisting of galactose, glucose and mannose cross-reacted with those containing xylose as well. The polysaccharides containing only glucose and mannose showed no cross-reaction with the others. No conclusions were come to regarding specific reacting groups [33].

The preparation of antigenic formulae is illustrated by several examples.

Four out of five antigens which have been described [73] in *H. capsulatum* and *B. dermatitidis* provide the following antigenic formulae for these fungi, the mycelial phase having a far less complicated antigenic structure.

	Growth phase	Antigens				Specific antigens
H. capsulatum	Yeast	A	B C		E*	B
	Mycelial	A	C			None
B. dermatitidis	Yeast	A	C*D	E		D
	Mycelial	A				None

* not detected in homologous antiserum

The following relationships are shown by the antigenic analysis of the dimorphous black pigment producing yeast-like fungi, the dematiaceous fungi which present difficult and controversial problems to the mycologist and taxonomist because of their morphology and cultural properties [17, 74].

Antigenic scheme of black yeast-like fungi

Pullularia pullulans .	.	.	.	A B C		
Pullularia bergeri	.	.	.	B	D	
Pullularia werneckei	.	.	.	C	E	
Sporotrichum gougerotii	.	.	.		F	
Phialophora jeanselmei	.	.	.		F	
Sporotrichum schenckii	.	.	.			G

For example, the nomenclature given by these authors is not regarded as standard.

Detailed and thorough application of immunoelectrophoresis to the study of fungi has led to the following conclusions. Each fungal species has its own immunoelectrophoretic picture which is reproducible under identical conditions [9]. This depends upon the use of hyperimmune rabbit sera, yet as has been shown, human sera may reveal antigens in excess of those found in the animal sera [2, 14]. The heterogeneity of some genera and homogeneity of others based on morphological criteria are shown by immunoelectrophoretic analysis, which as a method holds much promise for the future.

Capsular reactions

Capsular reactions similar to, but not identical with, those of bacteria are described in response to specific antibodies and the capsule of *C. neoformans*. The accentuation of the capsular outline which takes place is attributed to a line of precipitate formed at the interface of the capsular gel and the surrounding fluid and not to actual swelling of the capsule [75, 76]. A similar non-specific accentuation of bacterial capsules due to non-specific proteins is described and consists of a reversible salt-like combination of the proteins with the capsule under appropriate pH conditions [77].

Accentuation of the capsular outline of *C. neoformans* by a basic polysaccharide from *Aspergillus parasiticus* has also been observed. The positively charged polygalactosamine caused precipitation of acidic, negatively charged polysaccharides, including gum acacia, pneumococcus polysaccharide and cryptococcus polysaccharide [78, 79, 80]. This suggests that the possibility of complications arising from this phenomenon should be considered where sera are absorbed with polysaccharides of this type and are then tested against fungal elements.

Modifications of the capsule are of interest where there are difficulties in producing good antisera with certain capsulated strains. This has been attributed to capsular factors, since weakly encapsulated forms of *C. neoformans* (*T. histolytica*) and of *Sporotrichum schenckii* more readily stimulated antibodies capable of reacting with highly encapsulated strains [75]. On the other hand, it has also been found that certain strains may give a very good antibody response which is unrelated to the capsular thickness [20]. Decapsulation of the cells of *C. neoformans* by an enzyme from the organism *Alcaligenes* made the cells more potently immunogenic, high titre antisera being produced with them in mice. The enzyme also appeared to have some protective effect against infection of mice with this fungus [81, 82]. Uncovering of antigens was probably also responsible for the improved immunogenicity and higher agglutination titres of cells of *C. neoformans* after their treatment by mild acid hydrolysis with N/20 HCl [83].

Fungal antigens in tissues and body fluids

Both soluble and insoluble fungal antigens have been demonstrated in tissue and body fluids of animals and man by a variety of techniques. Large amounts of thermostable antigens were extracted from tissues of mice infected with *C. neoformans* and *S. schenckii*. They were found in the washings of the peritoneal cavity and in extracts of spleen, testis and lung. Soluble antigen was also found in the blood of mice infected with *C. neoformans*. Specific precipitation reactions were given by these antigens with rabbit antisera [84]. Soluble antigens of *C. neoformans* have been found in the cerebrospinal fluid, blood and urine of a patient with cryptococcosis. The reactive substance was relatively thermostable and gave precipitin and complement-fixing reactions with rabbit antiserum [85]. Antigens of *C. neoformans* have been detected in the serum and cerebrospinal fluid of seven out of nine patients with cryptococcosis of the central nervous system using a slide test with antibody-coated latex particles [86]. Immunofluorescence tests are as effective as histological stains in demonstrating the presence of polysaccharides of *C. neoformans* in the kidneys, though the technique has some limitations [98]. The presence of cryptococcal antigen in infected mice or of purified capsular polysaccharide injected into mice has been shown by intracutaneous injection of a homologous antiserum, that is, by reverse cutaneous anaphylaxis [87].

Antisera against mycelial components of *S. schenckii* have been used to give specific staining of cells in culture, in frozen sections, in 'dabs' from infected animals, and also to stain disintegrated detritus or phagocytosed elements [88]. Fluorescein-labelled immunoglobulins from antisera to *S. schenckii* stained both yeast and mycelial phases and revealed the organisms in exudates from lesions in mice and man [89]. *S. schenckii* has been identified in lesion exudates in twenty-four out of twenty-seven instances in which positive cultures were obtained. This test can be regarded, therefore, as a rapid and useful screening procedure [90].

Immunofluorescence tests on the sputum are a useful adjunct to cultural and clinical methods of diagnosis of *H. capsulatum* infections. Cross-reactions with *B. dermatitidis* may create difficulties and autofluorescence of *C. albicans* needs to be eliminated [91]. The test has been found to be an effective and rapid screening test, giving positive reactions in 85 per cent of sputa which were positive on culture and in seven proven cases which were negative on culture [92]. The tissue forms of *H. capsulatum* were differentiated from other pathogens by fluorescein-labelled globulins from a rabbit antiserum. Autofluorescence of spherules and endospores of *Coccidioides immitis* may cause difficulty [93]. *C. immitis* has been shown in the tissues by means of fluorescein-labelled antisera which had been absorbed with yeast cells of *H. capsulatum* to eliminate cross-reactions [94].

C. albicans has been demonstrated in the tissues of man and animals [95] and the course of infection in mice has been followed, showing that the fungus is present transitionally in the lungs and spleen and becomes localized in the kidneys and heart [96]. *C. albicans* has been demonstrated in oral smears by immunofluorescence tests, the claim being made that the reactions were serologically specific and the method superior to microscopy [97].

A specific conjugated antiserum against *Dermatophilus congolensis* has been used to identify this organism in suspensions of exudates from lesions of natural infection in cattle [99].

Cross-reactions between fungi, bacteria and other substances

The cross-reactions between fungal genera which have been mentioned represent only a part of the complex interrelationships [16]. The wide distribution of the polysaccharide antigens and their complex nature leads, as might be expected, to extensive cross-reactions with bacteria, which will be better understood when the detailed chemistry is unfolded. For example, type-specific polysaccharides of *C. neoformans* A contain xylose, galactose, mannose and glucuronic acid. They cross-react with antisera to types II and XIV pneumococcus, and a mixture of at least two polysaccharides is considered to be present because, on fractional precipitation with type XIV pneumococcus antiserum, the proportion of galactose in the mixture was increased. The cross-reaction with type II pneumococcus polysaccharide indicated that at least some glucuronic acid was present as an end-group. Concentration of galactose by the use of type XIV antiserum might be due to galactose end-groups in a xylo-glucurono-galactan [100]. Serological cross-reactions, albeit of a low order, of *C. neoformans* polysaccharide with polysaccharides of *Candida albicans*, *Saccharomyces cerevisiae*, *Trichophyton* and tragacanth gum are described [101, 102]. Serological relationships between *Sporotrichum schenckii* and pneumococci have been found. The specific capsular polysaccharide of *S. schenckii* and its type-specific antiserum gave cross-reactions with purified pneumococcal soluble antigens and pneumococcal antisera from types 10, 22, 23, 31, 32. *Leuconostoc mesenteroides* was found to be serologically related to *S. schenckii* and to a number of strains of streptococcus [103].

Common antigens between lipopolysaccharide antigens of *Candida* species and related yeasts and *Salmonella–Arizona* organisms have been found, attributable to minor antigens which are not included in the antigenic tables for the serological diagnosis of *Salmonella–Arizona* [104].

A remarkable cross-reaction has been found between certain polysaccharides of *A. fumigatus*, the purified galactomannanpeptide of *T. mentagrophytes* [26], and polysaccharides in extracts of *Epidermophyton floccosum*, which are all capable of acting as antigens and combining with related specific precipitins found in the sera of certain patients with aspergillosis [2, 14]. Furthermore, these polysaccharides combine with C-reactive protein, in the same way as pneumococcal C polysaccharide, to give a precipitation reaction which, in the case of *A. fumigatus* extracts, may be mistaken for a specific immunological reaction [2, 8, 14].

All these C-substance-like polysaccharides from the fungal and bacterial sources are allergenic for patients with the hypersensitive form of aspergillosis, giving immediate wealing reactions on skin testing. Similar C-substance-like polysaccharides are present in a number of nematode parasites [105]. They, too, are allergenic, on skin testing, for the patients with aspergillosis. There is evidence that the C-substance action and allergenic activities are related to the peptide content of the polysaccharide [2, 14].

Pulmonary aspergillosis in man

The variety and importance of immunological, clinical and pathological phenomena encountered in aspergillosis in man suggests that it may serve as a basic model for the study of hypersensitivity and infection due to other fungi, pathogenic and nonpathogenic [2, 14]. Antibody responses comparable with those in hyperimmunized animals are present in the sera of patients with pulmonary aspergilloma due to *A. fumigatus*. Specific reactions to other species may be obtained in occasional patients in whom the aspergilloma is due to other species, such as *A. nidulans*, *A. niger* and *A. flavus* [106].

Polysaccharide antigens are of major importance in particular for precipitation reactions with animal antisera to fungi in general. In aspergillosis in man, however, protein antigens are of greater importance. Two types of precipitation reaction in agar gel are observed; a broad diffuse band or arc produced by polysaccharide antigens and regarded as the 'H', or horse, type, and clearly defined arcs produced by protein and glycoprotein antigens and regarded as the 'R', or rabbit, type. Both types of reaction are due to IgG antibody, the 'R' reactions being multiple and more important for diagnosis.

Separation of the polysaccharide and protein antigens was best obtained by ammonium sulphate precipitation (55–75 per cent). Agar-gel electrophoresis of the antigens with staining of polysaccharide by PAS and of protein by amido-black showed clear separation of the polysaccharide and protein. The precipitate produced by the ammonium sulphate contained 66 per cent of protein and made up 17 per cent by weight of the culture filtrate. Other attempts at fractionation by alcohol, trichloracetic acid, or Cetavlon-borate precipitation, or by Sephadex filtration or DEAE-cellulose column chromatography were not as effective, although the latter methods were of value for fractionating the separated antigens.

The polysaccharide antigens were more stable than the protein antigens. They were isolated both from the culture filtrate (CF) and from the mycelium

(S) by phenol extraction [22] (Westphal method) or acidified saline [28]. Both CF and S polysaccharides were found to be gluco-galacto-mannan-peptides. The monosaccharides of the gluco-galacto-mannan were present in the ratio of 1 : 5 : 20. The peptide moiety contained particularly the hydroxy-amino acids, serine and threonine, together with alanine. The polysaccharide and peptide moieties play different and important roles. Degradation of the polysaccharide by periodic acid destroyed its capacity to react with the 'H' type precipitin, but did not destroy the capacity of the S polysaccharides to behave like pneumococcal C-substance and to combine with C-reactive protein. Absorption of a suitable serum containing both 'H' type precipitins and C-reactive protein, with the CF polysaccharide which does not combine with C-reactive protein, results in the inhibition of the 'H' type reaction to the S polysaccharide, but no inhibition of the C-substance/C-reactive protein reaction. Absorption of the serum with another C-substance-containing extract, that of *E. floccosum*, inhibits the C-reactive protein reaction but does not inhibit the specific precipitation reactions. The complex relationship of these polysaccharides to those of the dermatophytes has been discussed in the previous section.

It must be pointed out, however, that the capacity to combine with C-reactive protein of the *Aspergillus* S polysaccharide is dependent on its peptide moiety, and that this also applies to its capacity to act as allergen. That is, degradation of the polysaccharide moiety destroys its precipitating, but not its allergenic activity, thus throwing some doubt on the role of carbohydrates as the allergens responsible for the immediate reaction. The carbohydrates for which this is claimed all have peptide moieties of varying sizes, and should be re-examined to see how far these are essential for the immediate reaction.

Farmer's lung

Farmers exposed to the abundant microflora of mouldy hay reflect this in the variety of fungal antibodies in their sera. This is especially evident in farmers suffering from farmer's lung [3, 4, 58, 59, 107]. Their sera contain precipitins against thermophilic actinomycetes, notably against *Micropolyspora faeni* (*Thermopolyspora polyspora*) and *Thermoactinomyces* (*Micromonospora*) *vulgaris* and against the commoner fungal genera of mouldy hay such as *Aspergillus*, *Mucor* and *Cladosporium*. The fungal antibody appears to be related to antigens present in *Mucor*, and cross-reacts with related antigens in the other fungi. Absorption of the sera with *Mucor* is effective in inhibiting the reactions of the other fungi. Precipitins against antigens of *T. polyspora* and of fungi are also present in cattle suffering from fog-fever due to mouldy hay [108].

The presence in extracts of mouldy hay of antigens from *M. faeni* is best shown by immunoelectrophoresis in which precipitation arcs form in three main regions labelled A, B and C, although there may be a number of arcs in other regions as well. Fractionation of the antigens was best achieved in this case by trichloroacetic acid precipitation. This provided a precipitate containing antigens A and B, which are predominantly protein, and antigen C, which is predominantly polysaccharide. As in the reactions to *A. fumigatus* in pulmonary aspergillosis, the polysaccharide antigen gives a diffuse 'H' type reaction. Extracts prepared by trichloroacetic acid extraction of mouldy hay itself yields the C antigen [109]. The protein antigens are the more important, since less than half the positive sera gave reactions to the C antigen. Both fractions provoke farmer's lung type reactions in inhalation tests in affected subjects, the protein fraction being the more potent.

Fungal antigens, chiefly of the *Mucor* type, are present in a number of vegetable dusts as shown by tests against the sera of subjects working with these dusts and against the sera of patients suffering from aspergillosis and farmer's lung. Other antigens related to the particular vegetable dust itself are also present [3, 58].

Application of serological tests to diagnosis

The many variables to be taken into account are reflected in the problems of serological diagnosis for coccidioidomycosis, histoplasmosis and blastomycosis, and in many ways for fungal diseases in general [15]. The variations in individual antibody response make it likely that crude extracts containing the widest possible range of antigens will continue to be of practical value, although purified and standardized antigens are, of course, desirable objectives.

The antigenic content of crude extracts may not only be unknown, but the antigens may vary in concentration with each preparation. For example, the number of reactive components in agar-gel diffusion tests of four lots of histoplasmin varied from one to six [15]. Similarly, variations in individual antibody response to different antigens are also important. The number of precipitation arcs produced by one extract of histoplasmin varied from patient to patient.

A good example of these problems is seen in pulmonary aspergillosis where a battery of extracts is needed to obtain the greatest number of positive reactions, notably with weakly reacting sera of the type found in hypersensitive patients with asthma and pulmonary eosinophilia due to *A. fumigatus*. Indeed, in these subjects, positive reactions may on occasions be given with only one of many test extracts. By contrast, in the group with aspergilloma, that is the saprophytic group, the serological reactions are so strong that most extracts will give positive reactions.

Variations of antibody response may be due to slow growth of fungi as compared to rapid generation of bacteria, so that the differences in the antigens to which the host is exposed may be considerable [15]. Detailed understanding of the antigenic formulae should help to minimize the problems of cross-reactivity and this would be made more satisfactory by precise immunochemical characterization of fungal antigens.

Assessment of the value of serological tests for the diagnosis of fungal diseases as distinct from the skin tests shows that they fall into three groups, those in which useful and reliable tests exist, those in which the tests fail for one reason or another, and those for which there are no immunological tests [110, 16]. In the first group are coccidioidomycosis, histoplasmosis, and blastomycosis, for which serological tests are useful. In most instances changes in the intensity of the serological findings are of diagnostic and even of prognostic value.

Precipitin tests are of diagnostic value in aspergillus mycetoma due, in most cases, to *A. fumigatus* [2, 8, 14, 111] and due on rare occasions to other *Aspergilli* such as *A. nidulans*, *A. flavus* and *A. niger* [106]. Multiple precipitin arcs are the rule, though proven cases may be found to give only two to three arcs. In patients with the hypersensitive form of pulmonary aspergillosis, weak precipitation reactions of one to two arcs which, however, appear to be of immunopathological importance are obtained in many cases. In skin tests, and particularly intracutaneous tests with the protein antigens of *A. fumigatus*, dual reactions consisting of immediate wealing reactions followed by a second reaction appearing several hours later are obtained in patients with both reagins and precipitins. The presence of precipitins in patients without evidence of an aspergilloma or who are not suffering from asthma and pulmonary eosinophilia is probably evidence of infection at some time or another, and is usually associated with lung damage which favours such infections. Care must be taken in testing to avoid confusion of C-substance/C-protein reactions with a positive aspergillus reaction. This can be achieved either by using extracts free of C-substance-like polysaccharides or by the use of citrates or versene which reverse or inhibit C-protein reactions, because they chelate calcium on which this reaction is dependent.

In precipitin tests in patients suffering from maduromycetoma and actinomycetoma with antigens from *Streptomyces somaliensis*, *S. madurae*, *S. pelletieri* and *S. canescens* and from *Madurella mycetomi*, specific reactions were given by the homologous antigen. Thus, all but one of fourteen sera from the patients with actinomycetoma reacted with the *Streptomyces* but not the *Madurella* antigens, and, conversely, nine sera from the patients with maduromycetoma reacted only with the *Madurella* antigens [112].

Precipitation reactions to the antigens of *Micropolypora faeni* (*Thermopolyspora*) *polyspora* are of value in the diagnosis of farmer's lung in man and 'fog-fever' in cattle due to mouldy hay [3, 4, 108]. Because these antigens are present in samples of mouldy hay responsible for farmer's lung they have been called 'farmer's lung hay' or FLH antigens. A total of 87 per cent of affected subjects have precipitins against the FLH antigens. From 17–18 per cent of exposed but unaffected farmers also have these precipitins against FLH antigens, so that a positive reaction is not in itself diagnostic of the disease. FLH precipitins are, however, not present in the sera of non-exposed persons. Similar findings have been obtained in 'fog-fever' in cattle. In affected animals exposed to mouldy hay, 71 per cent had FLH precipitins, whereas exposed but unaffected animals or animals suffering from other diseases 21–26 per cent had FLH precipitins. Non-exposed animals seldom had FLH precipitins.

In the group of fungal diseases in which immunological reactions are not definitely established is infection with *Candida* species. Infected persons may have a higher titre of agglutinins [113, 114]. Precipitation reactions which may be of more value in diagnosis were positive in five patients with visceral mycosis tested with polysaccharide antigens extracted with β-naphthol [19]. Precipitins against a formamide extract of *C. albicans* were found in a patient with systemic infection, but not in normal subjects or subjects with superficial infection [115]. Similar results were obtained in six patients with chronic systemic infection with *Candida*, as well as in two cases where the diagnosis could not be established. No reactions were obtained in terminal infections, or in superficial infections [116].

There remains the third group of fungal infections in which serological tests are being developed and have not yet been fully established. Many examples of attempts to devise specific tests for these other fungal diseases have been discussed here and have been reviewed in detail elsewhere [16, 117].

References

[1] FOSTER J.W. (1949) *Chemical Activities of Fungi.* New York: Academic Press

[2] LONGBOTTOM, JOAN L. & PEPYS J. (1964) Pulmonary aspergillosis: Diagnostic and immunological significance of antigens and C-substance in *Aspergillus fumigatus. J. Path. Bact.* **88**, 141

[3] PEPYS J. & JENKINS P.A. (1965) Precipitin (F.L.H.) test in farmer's lung. *Thorax* **20**, 21

[4] JENKINS P.A. (1964) Immunological studies in farmer's lung. Ph.D. thesis. University of London

[5] AJELLO L., WALLS K., MOORE J.C. & FALCONE R. (1959) Rapid production of complement fixation antigens for systemic mycotic diseases. I. Coccidioidin: Influence of media and mechanical agitation on its development. *J. Bact.* **77**, 753

[6] CODNER R.C., CRUICKSHANK C.N.D., TROTTER M.D. & WOOD S.R. (1961) The production of trichophytin antigen in submerged culture of *Trichophyton mentagrophytes. Sabouraudia* **1**, 116

[7] MARKOWITZ H. (1964) Polysaccharide antigens from *Histoplasma capsulatum*. *Proc. Soc. exp. Biol. Med.* (*N. Y.*) **115**, 697

[8] BIGUET J., VAN KY P.T. & ANDRIEU S. (1964) Analyse immunoélectrophorétique d'extraits cellulaires et de milieux de culture d'*Aspergillus fumigatus* par des immunsérums expérimentaux et des sérums de malades atteints d'aspergillome bronchopulmonaire. *Annls. Inst. Pasteur* (*Paris*) **107**, 72

[9] BIGUET J., VAN KY P.T., ANDRIEU S. & FRUIT J. (1965) Analyse immunoélectrophorétique des antigènes fongiques et systématique des champignons. Répercussions pratiques sur le diagnostic des mycoses. *Mycopath. Mycol. appl.* (*Den Haag*) **26**, 241

[10] ROWE J.R., NEWCOMER V.D. & WRIGHT E.T. (1963) Studies of the soluble antigens of *Coccidioides immitis* by immunodiffusion. *J. invest. Derm.* **41**, 225

[11] ROWE J.R., NEWCOMER V.D. & LANDAU J.W. (1963) Effects of cultural conditions on the development of antigens by *Coccidioides immitis*. *J. invest. Derm.* **41**, 343

[12] ROWE J.R., LANDAU J.W. & NEWCOMER V.D. (1965) Effects of cultural conditions on the development of antigens by *Coccidioides immitis*. II. Complement fixation and immunodiffusion studies with human serum. *J. invest. Derm.* **44**, 237

[13] PAPPAGIANIS D., SMITH C.E., KOBAYASHI G.S. & SAITO M.T. (1961) Studies of antigen from young mycelia of *Coccidioides immitis*. *J. infect. Dis.* **108**, 35

[14] LONGBOTTOM, JOAN L. (1964) Immunological investigation of *Aspergillus fumigatus* in relation to disease in man. Ph.D. thesis. University of London

[15] CAMPBELL C.C. (1960) The accuracy of serologic methods in diagnosis. *Ann. N.Y. Acad. Sci.* **89**, 163

[16] SEELIGER H.P.R. (1962) Serology of fungi and deep fungous infections. In *Fungi and Fungous Diseases*, pp. 158–186, ed. DALLDORF G. Springfield, Ill.: C.C.Thomas

[17] SEELIGER H.P.R. (1960) Advances in the serology of fungi. *Trans. Br. mycol. Soc.* **43**, 543

[18] THIJØTTA T., RASCH S. & URDAL K. (1951) Preparation of fungus antigens for immunization and for serological reaction. A preliminary report. *Acta path. microbiol. scand.* **28**, 132

[19] ELINOV N.P. & ZAIKINA N.A. (1959) The precipitation test in the serological diagnosis of moniliasis. *Zh. Mikrobiol.* (*Mosk.*) **30**, 40

[20] SEELIGER H.P.R. (1964) Immuno-chemistry of fungi. *Mykosen* **7**, 71

[21] SUMMERS D.F., GROLLMAN A.P. & HASENCLEVER H.F. (1964) Polysaccharide antigens of *Candida* cell wall. *J. Immun.* **92**, 491

[22] WHISTLER R.L. (ed.) (1965) *Methods in Carbohydrate Chemistry. V. General Polysaccharides*. New York and London: Academic Press

[23] PEAT S., WHELAN W.J. & EDWARDS T.E. (1961) Polysaccharides of Baker's yeast. Part IV. Mannan. *J. chem. Soc.* 29

[24] HASENCLEVER H.F. & MITCHELL W.O. (1964) Immunochemical studies on polysaccharides of yeasts. *J. Immun.* **93**, 763

[25] BIGUET J., HAVEZ R., VAN KY P.T. & DEGAEY R. (1961) Étude électrophorétique, chromatographique et immunologique des antigènes de *Candida albicans*. Caracterisation de deux antigènes spécifiques. *Annls. Inst. Pasteur* **100**, 13

[26] BARKER S.A., CRUICKSHANK C.N.D., MORRIS J.H. & WOOD S.R. (1962) The isolation of trichophytin glycopeptide and its structure in relation to the immediate and delayed reactions. *Immunology* **5**, 627

[27] BARKER S.A., CRUICKSHANK C.N.D. & MORRIS J.H. (1963) Structure of a galactomannan-peptide allergen from *Trichophyton mentagrophytes*. *Biochim. biophys. Acta* **74**, 239

[28] Tillett W.S., Goebel W.F. & Avery O.T. (1930) Chemical and immunological properties of a species-specific carbohydrate of pneumococci. *J. exp. Med.* **52,** 895

[29] Bishop C.T., Blank F. & Gardner P.D. (1960) The cell wall polysaccharides of *Candida albicans:* Glucan, mannan and chitin. *Can. J. Chem.* **38,** 869

[30] Bishop C.T., Blank F. & Hranisavljevic-Jakovljevic M. (1962) The water-soluble polysaccharides of dermatophytes. I. A galactomannan from *Trichophyton granulosum. Can. J. Chem.* **40,** 1816

[31] Kwapinski J.B. (1963) Antigenic structure of actinomycetales. VI. Serological relationships between antigenic fractions of *Actinomyces* and *Nocardia. J. Bact.* **86** 179

[32] Kwapinski J.B. & Seeliger H.P.R. (1965) Investigations on the antigenic structure of actinomycetales. IX. Serological classification of the *Nocardiae* with the polysaccharide fractions of their cell walls. *Mycopath. Mycol. appl.* (*Den Haag*) **25,** 173

[33] Torheim B.J. (1963) Immunochemical investigations in *Geotrichum* and certain related fungi. III. Gel precipitation studies of reaction between rabbit immune sera and polysaccharide extracted from fungi. *Sabouraudia* **2,** 292

[34] Biguet J., Van Ky P.T. & Delcroix C. (1964) Étude préliminaire de la structure antigènique des *Penicillium* appreciè par l'analyse immunoélectrophorétique. *Extrait du Bull. Soc. Franc. Mycol. Medicale* **8.**

[35] Gordon M.A. (1962) Differentiation and classification of yeasts by the Coons fluorescent antibody technic. In *Fungi and Fungous Diseases*, pp. 207–209 ed. Dalldorf G. Springfield, Ill.: C.C.Thomas

[36] Gordon M.A., Edwards M.R. & Tomkins V.N. (1962) Refinement of fluorescent antibody by gel filtration. *Proc. Soc. exp. Biol. Med.* (*N. Y.*) **109,** 96

[37] Gordon M.A. (1959) Fluorescent staining of *Histoplasma capsulatum. J. Bact.* **77,** 678

[38] Kaplan W. & Kaufman L. (1961) The application of fluorescent antibody techniques to medical mycology. A review. *Sabouraudia* **1,** 137

[39] Miura T. & Kasai T. (1964) Differences in the result of the fluorescent antibody staining of dermatophytes due to the difference of fixing procedure. *Tuhoku. J. Exp. Med.* **84,** 72

[40] Miura T. & Kasai T. (1964) Autofluorescence of pathogenic fungi. *Tuhoku J. Exp. Med.* **82,** 158

[41] Kaufman L. Brandt B. & McLaughlin D. (1964) Evaluation of the fluorescent antibody and agar-gel precipitin test for detecting *Histoplasma* antibodies in anticomplementary sera. *Am. J. Hyg.* **79,** 181

[42] Coons A.H. & Kaplan M.H. (1950) Localization of antigen in tissue cells. II. Improvements in a method for the detection of antigen by means of fluorescent antibody. *J. exp. Med.* **91,** 1

[43] Slack J.M., Winger A. & Moore D.W.J. (1961) Serological grouping of *Actinomyces* by means of fluorescent antibodies. *J. Bact.* **82,** 54

[44] Goos R.D. & Summers D.F. (1964) Use of fluorescent antibody techniques in observations on the morphogenesis of fungi. *Mycologia* **56,** 701

[45] Walzer R.A. & Einbinder J. (1962) Immunofluorescent studies in dermatophyte infection. *J. Invest. Derm.* **39,** 165

[46] Kaufman L. & Kaplan W. (1961) Preparation of a fluorescent antibody specific for the yeast phase of *Histoplasma capsulatum. J. Bact.* **82,** 729

[47] Pine, L., Kaufman L. & Boone C.J. (1964) Comparative fluorescent antibody staining of *Histoplasma capsulatum* and *Histoplasma duboisii* with a specific anti-yeast phase of *H. capsulatum* conjugate. *Mycopath. Mycol. appl.* (*Den Haag*) **24,** 315

[48] KAUFMAN L. & BRANDT B. (1964) Fluorescent antibody studies of the mycelial forms of *Histoplasma capsulatum* and morphologically similar fungi. *J. Bact.* **87**, 120

[49] KAPLAN W. & GIFFORD M.K. (1964) Production of fluorescent antibody reagents specific for the tissue form of *Coccidioides immitis*. *Am. Rev. resp. Dis.* **89**, 651

[50] KAPLAN W. & KAUFMAN L. (1963) Specific fluorescent antiglobulins for the detection and identification of *Blastomyces dermatitidis* yeast-phase cells. *Mycopath. Mycol. appl.* (*Den Haag*) **19**, 173

[51] GORDON M.A. (1958) Differentiation of yeasts by means of fluorescent antibody. *Proc. Soc. exp. Biol. Med.* (*N.Y.*) **97**, 694

[52] KASE A. & MARSHALL J.D. (1960) A study of *Cryptococcus neoformans* by means of the fluorescent antibody technique. *Am. J. clin. Path.* **34**, 52

[53] VOGEL R.A., SELLERS T.F. & WOODWARD P. (1961) Fluorescent antibody techniques applied to the study of human cryptococcosis. *J. Am. med. Ass.* **178**, 921

[54] AL-DOORY Y. & GORDON M.A. (1963) Application of fluorescent antibody procedures to the study of pathogenic dematiaceous fungi. I. Differentiation of *Cladosporium carrionii* and *Cladosporium bantianum*. *J. Bact.* **86**, 332

[55] KAUFMAN L., SCHUBERT J.H. & KAPLAN W. (1962) Fluorescent antibody inhibition test for histoplasmosis. *J. lab. clin. Med.* **59**, 1033

[56] TSUCHIYA T., KUKAZAWA Y. & KAWAKITA S. (1961) Serological classification of the genus *Torulopsis*. *Sabouraudia* **1**, 145

[57] TSUCHIYA T., KAWAKITA S. & YAMASE Y. (1964) Serological classification of the genus *Hansenula III*. *Sabouraudia* **3**, 155

[58] PEPYS J., RIDDELL R.W., CITRON K.M. & CLAYTON Y.M. (1962) Precipitins against extracts of hay and moulds in the serum of patients with farmer's lung, aspergillosis, asthma and sarcoidosis. *Thorax* **17**, 366

[59] PEPYS J., LONGBOTTOM J.L. & JENKINS P.A. (1964) Vegetable dust pneumoconioses. Immunologic responses to vegetable dusts and their flora. *Am. Rev. resp. Dis.* **89**, 842

[60] VAN KY P.T., BIGUET J. & ANDRIEU S. (1961) Isolement chromatographique d'une fraction antigènique spécifique de *Candida albicans*. *C. r. hebd. Séanc. Acad. Sci.* (*Paris*) **253**, 2288

[61] JONSEN J., RASCH S. & STRAND Å. (1955) Specific polysaccharides in genus *Candida*. I. Preparation and properties of water-soluble fractions. *Acta path. microbiol. scand.* **37**, 449

[62] GORDON R.E. & MIHM J.M. (1962) The type species of the genus *Nocardia*. *J. gen. Microbiol.* **27**, 1

[63] BIGUET J., VAN KY P.T. & ANDRIEU S. (1961) Étude électrophorétique et immunochimique comparée des antigènes de quelques levures du genre *Candida* (*C. albicans, C. stellatoidea, C. tropicalis, C. zeylanoides, C. krusei, C. pseudotropicalis, C. macedoniensis*). *Mycopath. Mycol. appl.* (*Den Haag*) **17**, 239

[64] KEMP G. & SOLOTOROVSKY M. (1964) Localization of antigens in mechanically disrupted cells of certain species of the genera *Candida* and *Torulopsis*. *J. Immun.* **93**, 305

[65] MURRAY I.G. & BUCKLEY H.R. (in press) Serological studies of *Candida* species. Symposium on Candidiasis arranged by E.R. Squibb, 1965

[66] UCHIDA T., ROBBINS P.W. & LURIA S.E. (1963) Analysis of the serologic determinant groups of the salmonella E-group O-antigens. *Biochem.* (*Wash.*) **3**, 663

[67] FINGER I., KABAT E.A., BEZER A.E. & KIDD A. (1960) Agar diffusion studies in the dextran–antidextran system. *J. Immun.* **84**, 227

[68] ZAMORA A., BOJALIL L.F. & BASTARRADEA F. (1963) Immunologically active polysaccharides from *Nocardia asteroides* and *N. brasiliensis*. *J. Bact.* **85**, 549

[69] SEELIGER H.P.R. & SCHRÖTER R. (1963) A serological study on the antigenic relationships of the form *Trichosporon. Sabouraudia* **2**, 248

[70] EVANS E.E. (1950) The antigenic composition of *Cryptococcus neoformans*. I. A serologic classification by means of the capsular and agglutinization reactions. *J. Immun.* **64**, 423

[71] EVANS E.E. & KESSEL J.F. (1951) The antigenic composition of *Cryptococcus neoformans*. II. Serologic studies with the capsular polysaccharide. *J. Immun.* **67**, 109

[72] EVANS E.E. & MEHL J.W. (1951) A qualitative analysis of capsular polysaccharides from *Cryptococcus neoformans* by filter paper chromatography. *Science* **114**, 10

[73] KAUFMAN L. & KAPLAN W. (1963) Serological characterization of pathogenic fungi by means of fluorescent antibodies I. Antigenic relationships between yeast and mycelial forms of *Histoplasma capsulatum* and *Blastomyces dermatitidis. J. Bact.* **85**, 986

[74] SEELIGER H.P.R., LACAZ C.DA SILVA & ULSON C.M. (1958) Identification of fungi by serologic tests. Further serologic studies with dematiaceous fungi. *Proc. 6th Int. Congr. trop. Med. Malar.* **4**, 636

[75] NEILL J.M., CASTILLO C.G., SMITH R.H. & KAPROS C.E. (1949) Capsular reactions and soluble antigens of *Torula histolytica* and *Sporotrichum schenckii. J. exp. Med.* **89**, 93

[76] EVANS E.E., SEELIGER H.P.R., KORNFELD L. & GARCIA C. (1956) Failure to demonstrate capsular swelling in *Cryptococcus neoformans. Proc. Soc. exp. Biol. Med.* (*N.Y.*) **93**, 257

[77] TOMCZIK J. & GUEX-HOLZER S. (1954) Demonstration of the bacterial capsule by means of a pH-dependent salt-like combination with proteins. *J. gen. Microbiol.* **10**, 97

[78] EVANS E.E. (1959) Reaction of an aspergillus polysaccharide with *Cryptococcus* capsules and various acidic polysaccharides. *Proc. Soc. exp. Biol. Med.* (*N.Y.*) **101**, 760

[79] EVANS E.E. (1960) Capsular reactions of *Cryptococcus neoformans. Ann. N.Y. Acad. Sci.* **89**, 184

[80] EVANS E.E. (1962) Reactivity of the cryptococcal capsule. In *Fungi and Fungous Diseases*, pp. 187–206, ed. DALLDORF G. Springfield, Ill.: C.C.Thomas

[81] GADEBUSCH H.H. & JOHNSON J.D. (1960) Specific degradation of *Cryptococcus neoformans* 3723 capsular polysaccharide by a microbial enzyme. II. Biological activity of the enzyme. *J. infect. Dis.* **107**, 402

[82] GADEBUSCH H.H. & JOHNSON J.D. (1961) Specific degradation of *Cryptococcus neoformans* 3723 capsular polysaccharide by a microbial enzyme. I. Isolation, partial purification and properties of the enzyme. *Canad. J. Microbiol.* **7**, 53

[83] BENHAM R.W. (1935) *Cryptococci*—their identification by morphology and by serology. *J. infect. Dis.* **57**, 255

[84] NEILL J.M. & KAPROS C.E. (1950) Serological tests on soluble antigens from mice infected with *Cryptococcus neoformans* and *Sporotrichum schenckii. Proc. Soc. exp. Biol. Med.* (*N.Y.*) **114**, 557

[85] NEILL J.M., SUGG J.Y. & McCAULEY D.W. (1951) Serologically reactive material in spinal fluid, blood and urine from a human case of cryptococcosis (torulosis). *Proc. Soc. exp. Biol. Med.* (*N.Y.*) **77**, 775

[86] BLOOMFIELD N., GORDON M.A. & ELMENDORF D.F. (1963) Detection of *Cryptococcus neoformans* antigen in body fluids by latex particle agglutination. *Proc. Soc. exp. Biol. Med.* (*N.Y.*) **114**, 64

[87] ABRAHAMS I., GILLERAN T.G. & WEISS C.B. (1962) Quantitative studies on reverse cutaneous anaphylaxis in mice with progressive cryptococcosis. *J. Immun.* **89,** 684

[88] KUNZ C. (1959) Fluorescenz-serologische Untersuchungen an einen pathogen en pilzstamm (*Sporotrichum schenckii*). *Arch. klin. exp. Derm.* **209,** 200

[89] KAPLAN W. & IVENS M.S. (1960) Fluorescent antibody staining of *Sporotrichum schenckii* in cultures and clinical materials. *J. invest. Derm.* **35,** 151

[90] KAPLAN W. & GÖNZALEZ-OCHOA A. (1963) Application of the fluorescent antibody technique to the rapid diagnosis of sporotrichosis. *J. lab. clin. Med.* **62,** 835

[91] CARSKI T.R., COZAD G.C. & LARSH H.W. (1962) Detection of *H. capsulatum* in sputum by means of fluorescent antibody staining. *Am. J. clin. Path.* **37,** 465

[92] LYNCH H.J.J. & PLEXICO K.L. (1962) A rapid method for screening sputums for *Histoplasma capsulatum* employing the fluorescent antibody technic. *New Engl. J. Med.* **266,** 811

[93] GORDON M.A. (1959) Fluorescent staining of *Histoplasma capsulatum. J. Bact.* **77,** 678

[94] KAPLAN W. & GIFFORD M.K. (1964) Production of fluorescent antibody reagents specific for the tissue form of *Coccidioides immitis. Am. Rev. resp. Dis.* **89,** 651

[95] KUNZ C. (1958) Untersuchungen mit fluorescein—markierten antikorpen an Hefen. *Schweiz Z. Path. Bakt.* **21,** 892

[96] KEMP G. & SOLOTOROVSKY M. (1962) Fluorescent antibody studies of pathogenesis in experimental *Candida albicans* infection in mice. *J. Immun.* **88,** 777

[97] SCHAMSCHULA R.G. (1964) The application of the fluorescent antibody technique to the detection of *C. albicans* in oral pathological material. *Aust. J. exp. Biol. med. Sci.* **42,** 173

[98] MARSHALL J.D., IVERSON L., EVELAND W.C. & KASE A. (1961) Applications and limitations of the fluorescent antibody stain in the specific diagnosis of cryptococcosis. *Lab. Invest.* **10,** 719

[99] PIER A.C., RICHARD J.L. & FARRELL E.F. (1964) Fluorescent antibody and cultural techniques in cutaneous streptothricosis. *Am. J. vet. Res.* **25,** 1014

[100] REBERS P.A., BARKER S.A., HEIDELBERGER M., DISCHE Z. & EVANS E.E. (1958) Precipitation of the specific polysaccharide of *Cryptococcus neoformans* A by types II and XIV of anti-pneumonococcal sera. *J. Am. chem. Soc.* **80,** 1135

[101] EVANS E.E., SORENSEN L.H. & WALLS K.W. (1953) The antigenic composition of *Cryptococcus neoformans.* V. A survey of cross-reactions among strains of *Cryptococcus* and other antigens. *J. Bact.* **66,** 287

[102] SEELIGER H.P.R. (1958) *Mykologische Serodiagnostik*. Leipzig: J.A.Barth

[103] NEILL J.M., CASTILLO C.G. & PINKES A.H. (1955) Serological relationship between fungi and bacteria. I. Cross-reactions of *Sporotrichum schenckii* with pneumococci. *J. Immun.* **74,** 120

[104] AKSOYCAN N., LE MINOR L. & LE MINOR S. (1960) Antigènes commun entre le *Candida* et les *Salmonella–Arizona. Annals. Inst. Pasteur (Paris)* **99,** 723

[105] CAPRON A., BIGUET J., VAN KY P.T. & ROSE G. (1964) Possibilites nouvelles dans le diagnostic immunologique de la distomatose humaine a *Fasciola hepatica. Presse Med.* **72,** 3103

[106] LONGBOTTOM J.L., PEPYS J. & TEMPLE-CLIVE F. (1964) Diagnostic precipitin test in *Aspergillus* pulmonary mycetoma. *Lancet* i, 588

[107] PEPYS J., RIDDELL R.W., CITRON K.M. & CLAYTON Y.M. (1961) Precipitins against extracts of hay and fungi in the serum of patients with farmer's lung. *Acta allerg.* (*Kbh.*) **16,** 76

[108] JENKINS P.A. & PEPYS J. (1965) Fog-fever. Precipitin (F.L.H.) reactions to mouldy hay. *Vet. Rec.* **77,** 464

[109] KOBAYASHI M., STAHMANN M.A., RANKIN J. & DICKIE H.A. (1963) Antigens in mouldy hay as the cause of farmer's lung. *Proc. Soc. exp. Biol. Med.* (*N.Y.*) **113,** 472

[110] MURRAY I.G. (1964) Some immunological aspects of mycoses. *Proc. R. Soc. Med.* **57,** 412

[111] VOISIN C., BIGUET J., VAN KY P.T., SCHOULLER A., SERGEANT Y.H. & GERNEZ-RIEUZ C. (1964) Aspergilloses latentes et tuberculose pulmonaire chronique. *Revue Tuberc.* (*Paris*) **28,** 1311

[112] MAHGOUB EL SHEIKH (1964) The value of gel diffusions in the diagnosis of mycetoma. *Trans. R. Soc. trop. Med. Hyg.* **58,** 560

[113] WINNER H.I. (1955) The study of *Candida albicans* agglutinins in human sera. *J. Hyg., Camb.* **53,** 509

[114] COMAISH J.S., GIBSON B. & GREEN C.A. (1963) Candidiasis—Serology and diagnosis. *J. invest. Derm.* **40,** 139

[115] STALLYBRASS F.C. (1964) *Candida* precipitins. *J. Path. Bact.* **87,** 89

[116] TASCHDJIAN C.L., KOZINN P.J. & LEONA C. (1964) Immune studies in candidiasis. III. Precipitating antibodies in systemic candidiasis. *Sabouraudia* **3,** 312

[117] SALVIN S.B. (1963) Immunologic aspects of the mycoses. *Prog. Allergy* **7,** 213

CHAPTER 26

Immunological Methods Applied to the Study of Tissue Antigens and Antibodies

D.M.WEIR

Introduction

The majority of the immunological techniques described in Section 3 of this handbook have been used for the demonstration of tissue antigens and antibodies to such antigens. There are, however, difficulties peculiar to working with tissues and it is the object of this chapter to attempt to delineate some of these difficulties and how they may be overcome—as far as this has been achieved. As many of the basic immunological techniques have already been described, this chapter will give precise procedural detail only where modifications have been made which are necessary because of the inherent problems associated with working with tissues. Methods not covered in other parts of the handbook will be described in detail where they have particular relevance or are considered to have potential value in tissue studies.

Except for studies of histocompatibility antigen systems which employ iso antisera (see Batchelor, Chapter 30), the localization or demonstration of particular tissue antigens using immunological methods depends on the successful production of a specific antiserum in an animal of a species different from that of the source of the tissue. Herein lies one of the greatest obstacles in such a venture. Tissue antigens are very difficult to prepare in a pure state. The reason for this appears to be that the methods for fractionation of tissue components have not reached the stage of sophistication and general application which, for example, serum fractionation procedures have attained. This is due not only to the wide variety of complex materials in cells and tissues, but also the fact that they exist in different physical states. Cell sap, for example, could be treated in much the same way as serum in fractionation procedures, but mitochondria would need an entirely different approach. Further complications arise due to the interaction of one cell component with another resulting in the inactivation of certain antigens; for example, the disruption of a cell will result in the release of lysosomal enzymes, which include enzymes capable of acting on ribonucleic acids, deoxyribonucleic acids, proteins, phosphate esters, polysaccharides and glycosides. Any attempt to extract active antigen from a lysosome-rich cell fraction is

844

likely to be extremely difficult and Table 26.1 shows the rapid loss of antigenic activity by such a fraction (Fr. 3) on heating at 37° C [1]. The antiserum prepared against a particular tissue extract is thus likely to contain antibodies against a variety of cell and even serum components and the degree of success in preventing enzymic and other degradative changes in the cell constituents will be reflected in the specificity of the antibody. So that the absence of certain cellular antigens in the injected material would mean that the resulting antiserum would not show the presence of the particular antigen in the tissue. Thus, a negative result in procedures of this type must be treated with caution.

TABLE 26.1

Effect of heating on whole rat liver homogenate (WLH) and three liver fractions: Fraction 1—'nuclear', Fraction 3—'mitochondrial', and Fraction 6—'microsomal'. Note marked loss of activity of Fraction 3 which is the lysozome-rich fraction. Tested by complement fixation with CCl_4 (0·03 ml/100g body weight) induced rat antibody.

Reproduced by permission of the Editor of *Clin. exp. Immunol.*

Percentage activity remaining after heating (37° C)

Fraction	Time (minutes)				
	0	30	60	120	180
WLH	100	100	100	50	50
1	100	100	100	50	50
3	100	50	25	12	0
6	100	100	100	50	50

All fractions, WLH, 1, 3 and 6 retain 100 per cent activity after 6 hours at 0° C.

Competition between antigens in a mixture such as a tissue homogenate must also affect the balance of the antibodies to each antigen in the whole antiserum. In addition, the obvious parts played by the quantity, foreignness and physical state of the individual components present must affect the antiserum produced. It is now becoming clear that particulate antigens are more readily taken up by the phagocytic cells of the lymphoid follicles than soluble antigens [2]. However, this does not necessarily mean that more active localization of antigen in follicles leads to enhanced antibody formation as in passively immunized animal, in which follicular localization was increased, antibody formation was depressed [3]. However, Frei *et al* [4] consider that phagocytosis of antigen is essential for the induction of a primary response and have shown the dependence of this on particulate antigen. At least some entirely soluble antigens fail to stimulate antibody production [5, 4]. Soluble bovine γ globulin antigen appears to contain a sufficient number of aggregated molecules to allow antibody production, but if these are removed no antibodies are made [5]. Certain particulate antigens or routes of immunization may preferentially stimulate a particular class of immunoglobulin to be produced and techniques which are designed to detect the interaction of an antigen with IgG antibody may be unsuitable when applied to IgM or IgA antibody and may only give restricted information as to the quality of the antiserum, or the number of antigens in a particular tissue. In the detection of autoreactive immunoglobulins against particulate mitochondrial antigens found in rats after toxic liver damage [6, 7, 8, 1], the class of immunoglobulin formed appears to be exclusively IgM, despite repeated stimulation by the release of cell breakdown products at intervals. Torrigiani & Roitt [9] have reported that thyroglobulin fixed on to acrylic particles resulted in a prolonged IgM response, whereas if given in soluble form IgG antibody and IgM antibody were both initially formed, the IgM, however, rapidly disappearing after about 16 days. See Chapter 13 for discussion of some pitfalls in investigation of sequential synthesis of antibodies.

A well-known difficulty which is come up against in working with tissues and antisera is the problem of so called 'non-specific' uptake of serum components by tissue cells. This has caused particular difficulty in the fluorescent antibody technique, and methods for dealing with it are described in Chapter 16. 'Non-specific' reactions have been ascribed to the presence in serum of charged proteins which react with oppositely charged proteins in tissue [10]. There is evidence accumulating which appears to cast doubts on the 'non-specific' character of this phenomenon and it is likely that some at least of the 'non-specific' uptake factors from serum by tissues is in fact due to specific antibody present in normal serum. The stimulus for such antibody production is in doubt, but it has been suggested [11] that this type of antibody may be the result of an immunological response to tissue breakdown products. Adult rats do not appear to be tolerant to their particulate subcellular components and cannot be made tolerant by injections of liver antigen soon after birth [120]. This absence of tolerance with respect to IgM antibody may be due to the particulate nature of the antigens [1]. Evidence is also available to support the possibility that certain antibacterial antibodies can cross-react with tissue components [12]. Using fluorescein-conjugated anti-complement serum it is possible to show the uptake by tissue cells of complement-fixing normal serum factors which sediment with the IgM globulins in sucrose density gradients [11]. Karush [13] has noted that the continuous production of normal IgM globulin results in a concentration of about 10^{-4} M. This raises the possibility that a wide range of antibody conformations are formed corresponding to a range of immunological specificities and Karush suggests that some particular conformations may be present in concentrations of about 10^{-10}–10^{-12} M. Such an explanation would account for the finding of 'natural' antibodies against tissue antigen.

Preparation and choice of tissue antigens for *in vitro* studies

For the localization of tissue antigens techniques are available which include fluorescent or isotope-labelling methods applied to microtome sections of the tissue. To allow preservation of the antigen, sections are most often cut in the frozen state in a cryostat (see Holborow & Johnson, Chapter 16). A free-substitution method as an alternative is also described there. Impressions of tissues may be made by laying the cut surface of a tissue on a clean microscope slide and fixing the cells by air drying or a chemical fixative such as alcohol, acetone or formalin, the concentration and time of exposure being determined for the particular antigen to be demonstrated. For example, individual samples of the material can be exposed to the fixatives made up in a range of concentrations, e.g. 70–100 per cent at 37° C in the cold and at room temperature. The time of exposure may be gradually increased from 10 seconds to 15 minutes.

Whole tissue homogenates can be used for screening purposes and are prepared as discussed in Chapter 11. For certain purposes such as, for example, the detection of thyroid complement-fixing microsomal antibodies [16], human thyroid gland from patients with thyrotoxicosis is to be preferred [17]. Tissue of young animals is frequently used in tests to demonstrate anti-tissue antibody; for example, in the demonstration of antinuclear antibody in human serum infant thyroid was found to be more suitable than adult tissues [18], which contained interstitial autofluorescent collagen and autofluorescent granules in the epithelial cytoplasm. In complement-fixation tests with tissue homogenates, for example liver, the organs from older animals were often found to be more anticomplementary than tissues from younger animals. This may be due to the naturally occurring complement-fixing anti-tissue antibodies described above. Certain species-specific antigens are extremely stable and can be extracted from tissue by boiling or by ether (see later).

Preparation of antisera to tissue antigens

Immunizing antigens:

Much of the experimental evidence on tissue-specific antigens has come from the work of Pressman and his colleagues [19–24]. These workers, for immunizing purposes, use organ homogenates which have been finally disintegrated by sonic vibration. As a first step a perfused organ, taken from a freshly killed animal, e.g. a rat or slaughterhouse material thoroughly washed free of blood clots using borate buffered saline pH 8·0 and stored at −20° C until required for use (in practice for not more than 6 months). The frozen material is thawed suspended in a small volume of the borate buffered saline (approximately an equal volume) and homogenized in a tissue homogenizer with metal cutting blades (Waring blender or M.S.E. tissue homogenizer) until no large pieces of tissue remain and a coarse suspension is produced. Alternatively a teflon and glass homogenizer may be used, the teflon pestle attached to a fractional horsepower variable speed motor. If no mechanical instrument is available, a hand-operated glass homogenizer will produce a satisfactory homogenate.

The homogenate is then centrifuged at 300 g for 15 minutes and the sediment washed repeatedly until the washings are almost clear. The washing procedures will wash out soluble tissue antigens at the same time as contaminating serum proteins and it is conceivable that certain tissue-specific antigens may be lost. The failure of Yagi *et al* [23] to remove all anti-kidney activity by absorption of their antiserum with kidney sediment may be accounted for in this way. Small subcellular components, e.g. microsomes, will also be lost in the supernatant at the low g values given here. These can be retained in the sediment by increasing the g values to 10,000 g for 1 hour [1]. The sediment which has been prepared is now dispersed by sonic vibrations between 9 and 20 kc/sec and the resulting homogeneous preparation stored frozen. Reaggregation occurs on freezing and thawing the homogenate but the aggregates are easily dispersed by further sonication.

To obtain a preparation of rat liver suitable for immunizing to obtain tissue specific antibodies Pressman and colleagues further extracted the sediment three times with the borate buffered saline at 55° C, each extraction lasting 20 minutes. The resulting sediment was finally sonicated and either lyophilized or stored at 4° C with 1 : 20,000 merthiolate as a preservative.

Milgrom and his co-workers [25–30] have described organ-specific thermostable antigens in certain tissues, e.g. adrenal, brain and testicle, and these are extracted by a boiling and ethanol extraction method and can be used for immunizing purposes. The first step is to prepare a 20 per cent organ homogenate as described above. This homogenate is then rehomogenized in saline close to 100° C. The supernatant collected after centrifugation (approximately 2000 g for 15 minutes) is autoclaved at 121° C for 45 minutes and the autoclaved preparation centrifuged at approximately 100,000 g for 30 minutes. The supernatant is mixed with three volumes of ethanol (72 per cent used for adrenal-specific antigen and 95 per cent for brain-specific antigen) and left overnight at room temperature. The precipitate which forms is sedimented at 200 g for 30 minutes and dried at room temperature *in vacuo*. Finally the material is ground to a powder and stored in a closed container at room temperature for periods up to 1 year. The material is readily soluble in saline.

Highly purified and crystalline preparations of enzymes and hormones can be extracted from tissues and used for immunizing purposes. The resulting antisera have had wide application in the fluorescent antibody technique for the cellular localization of these substances. It is outside the scope of this chapter to deal with the extraction procedures for substances of this type; the reader is referred to Nairn [10] where an extensive bibliography is given (see also Chapter 11).

Production of antisera
The most commonly used animal for the production of antisera to tissue antigens is the rabbit, which is given two or three injections of from 5 to 50 mg of antigen emulsified with Freund's complete adjuvant at intervals of 3–4 weeks' bleeding 7–10 days after the final injection. An important observation has been made by Good [31] who noted that following the intravenous injection of BSA antigen into a rabbit approximately 100 times as much antibody was obtained when a second injection was given 30 days after than if the injection was given 10 days after. It was found that giving a second injection at 10 days actually resulted in less antibody being produced than if only one injection was given. In their study of antigens in immunity, Nossal, Austin & Ada [32] have clearly demonstrated with Salmonella flagellar antigens given without adjuvant that a secondary response is only evoked when the second dose of antigen equals, or preferably exceeds, the first dose. If small doses of antigen are given as the secondary stimulus, the excess antibody was solely IgM, and IgG if given in larger doses. It is suggested that a secondary response can only occur when levels of antigen in phagocytic cells are raised. The possibility, particularly with tissue antigens, that the animal is already primed (see above) may influence the antibody response on first injection of the antigen, this response being in fact a secondary rather than a primary response. There appear to be genetic factors, varying between different strains within a species, which control the capacity of experimental animals to respond to antigens and these may have some importance in relation to tissue antigens. The strain differences have been brought to light in experiments on the responses to hapten conjugates with poly-L-lysine in guinea-pigs [33] and with synthetic polypeptides in mice and rabbits [34]. In the rabbit experiments Himalayan rabbits responded consistently well to the synthetic polypeptide, whereas Sandylops were consistently bad. Dutch rabbits came somewhere in between. For the production of precipitating antibody the rat is unfortunately a much less suitable animal than the rabbit both from the point of view of quantity and quality (see Minden & Farr, Chapter 13) of the antibody produced and this is our own experience also

[35]. Fowls do not seem to have been widely used for antibody production although being further back in the evolutionary scale it would be expected that they would readily be able to recognize mammalian tissue antigens as foreign.

The specificity required of the antiserum is an important consideration. If it is necessary to raise antibody to every antigen present in the tissue homogenate, a long course of immunization will be required so that antigens present only in small quantities will be able to induce a full antibody response. For example, in rabbits injected with chromatographically purified ovalbumin two or three injections of antigen with adjuvant resulted in an antiserum which showed only a single line on immunoelectrophoresis with the ovalbumen. However, on further stimulation the rabbit produced an antiserum which reacted also with a minor contaminant in the ovalbumen preparation. An important observation has been made by Nairn [10] with reference to the suitability of antisera for fluorescent antibody staining. Some of the strongest specific fluorescent staining has been obtained with non-precipitating serum (for further discussion see Holborow & Johnson, Chapter 16). It is possible that this effect may be due to the sera containing IgM antibody which would have more fluorescein groups per molecule than IgG antibody. Repeated courses of immunization in the same animal are well known to increase the ability of an antiserum to cross-react with related antigens although individual antibody molecules have a greater affinity for antigen.

Freund's complete adjuvant, preferably containing heat-killed human-type tubercle bacilli, should be used with the immunizing antigen. The high content of peptido-glycolipid in the wax D fraction of human-type bacilli appears to enhance the immunogenicity of the antigen–adjuvant mixtures [37]. White considers that this may be due to the high content of unnatural D amino acids of the peptide conferring resistance to attack by mammalian enzymes, thus increasing the stimulus to the macrophages to phagocytose and process the antigen.

The adjuvant should contain a non-toxic light oil, e.g. Drakeol VFR (Pennsylvania Refining Co. Ltd) or *light* liquid paraffin. Nine parts of the oil is mixed with one part of an emulsifying agent, e.g. Arlacel, and 2 mg/ml of dried heat-killed tubercle bacilli, e.g. H37Ra. To prepare an adjuvant–antigen emulsion equal volumes of antigen in physiological saline or equivalent should be mixed with the adjuvant mixture in the following way: A small portion, e.g. one-fifth, of the volume of the antigen is drawn up into a syringe of sufficient size to take the complete volume of antigen and adjuvant. The adjuvant is forced through a small-bore needle with the point below the surface of the adjuvant. The mixture is drawn up into the syringe and forced out about six times, forming a milky emulsion, and the procedure repeated with volumes of the remaining antigen until a viscous milky emulsion is formed. The object of this method is to form a water-in-oil emulsion and the resulting emulsion may be tested by placing a drop or two of the emulsion on the surface of a beaker of water. If the drops remain on the surface and do not disperse when the beaker is slightly agitated, the emulsion is of a water-in-oil type. Dispersal of the droplets, forming a cloudy suspension in the water, indicates that the emulsion is of an oil-and-water type (see also Appendix 2, for further details of this and other methods for preparing emulsions).

Site and frequency of injection

Injections of antigen–adjuvant emulsion are usually given subcutaneously, sometimes into the footpads and occasionally intramuscularly or intra-venously. To take some examples—for production of antisera to thermo-stable ethanol insoluble antigens of brain and adrenal, Milgrom and his co-workers [25, 27] used albino rabbits of 3–4 kg, giving adjuvant emulsion containing up to 10 mg/ml of their brain antigen (see above) or 3 mg/ml of adrenal antigen. The first three injections were enriched with mycobacteria (*M. butyricum* or *M. smegmatis* was used in this case—see note above about value of human type), adding 8, 6 and 4 mg of the dried killed organisms to each millilitre of adjuvant for the first three inoculations given at weekly intervals, each inoculation in 0·7–1 ml volume intradermally into several sites in the footpads and the shaved back. A further three inoculations were given with adjuvant without mycobacteria at intervals of 1–3 weeks and the animals bled 7–10 days after the last inoculation.

For the production of tissue-specific anti-kidney antibodies Pressman and his colleagues [24] gave rabbits two subcutaneous injections of 10 mg of lyophylized kidney sediment in borate buffered saline with an equal volume of Difco complete adjuvant (i.e. containing *M. butyricum*) at intervals of 3 weeks. The animals were bled 10 days after the last injection. Goats were injected with rabbit kidney—50 mg of lyophylized sediment with an equal volume of complete adjuvant subcutaneously, followed 40 days later by a similar injection with complete adjuvant. Guinea-pigs were given 2 mg of lyophylized sediment subcutaneously and a further injection 40 days later. It is interesting to note that in some of their earlier work Pressman and his colleagues [21] gave much more intensive courses of immunization; for example, three injections of liver antigen at 14 day intervals with adjuvant, followed 6 weeks later by a course of ten injections without adjuvant over 6 weeks. Recent studies on the mode of action of adjuvants have given a rational basis for the use of much shorter courses of immunization. Depot-forming adjuvants appear to stimulate a secondary immune response reach-ing a similar level to that produced by frequent very small injections of antigen without adjuvant—for example, the administration of 2 mg of ovalbumen

EE

with incomplete adjuvant gave antibody levels measured by tanned-cell haemagglutination in mice identical to those achieved by injection of a total of 171 μg daily in divided doses over 50 days [36]. This confirms that the slow release of very small quantities of antigen is the main stimulus to the antibody response. The secondary response reaching a plateau of antibody production which can only be exceeded very temporarily by further doses of antigen, the level rapidly returning to the plateau level of the secondary response. This and other studies also carried out in the author's laboratory with influenza B, *Shigella sonnei* and BSA in rats suggest that provided the antigen persists within the depot for some months (and in the case of oval-bumen it could be detected after 544 days) there is little point in giving frequent doses of antigen with adjuvant and that after the initial dose with adjuvant all that is required is a booster dose after 3–4 weeks followed by bleeding 7–10 days after.

Non-organ and non-species specific antigens
An experimental model is available in which it is possible to induce the forma-tion of anti-tissue antibodies of the type found in various human disease states. These antibodies are non-organ and species non-specific and have been detected using primarily the complement-fixation test. Antibodies of this type were first described in human sera by Gajdusek [38] and were termed autoimmune complement-fixing antibodies (AICF). AICF antibodies have been found in sera from cases of systemic lupus erythematosus and various liver disease sera occurring in most sera from patients with primary biliary cirrhosis [39]. Antibodies of this type are readily induced in rats by the injection of carbon tetrachloride (0·03 ml/100 g body weight subcutaneously) [6, 7]. Sera taken on the third and fourth day after CCl_4 injection contain high titres of com-plement-fixing IgM antibody [7] directed primarily against the mitochon-drial fraction of the cell [1].

Production of antisera to DNA
Until recently there has been a lack of decisive data dealing with the anti-genicity of nucleic acids and there have been many conflicting reports [40, 41, 42, 43, 44]. Plescia *et al* [45] have resolved the difficulties of inducing anti-DNA antibodies by immunizing rabbits with complexes of DNA and methylated bovine serum albumin (MBSA). The complex was found to elicit consistently the formation of antibodies that react in complement-fixation tests with pure thermally denatured DNA from many species, rather like the antinuclear serum factor of systemic lupus erythematosus [46, 41, 47, 48]. The antigen calf thymus DNA (Worthington) is dissolved in 0·15 M NaCl to a concentration of 500 μg/ml. The solution is boiled at 100° C for 10 minutes, chilled rapidly in an ice-bath and after which a 1 per cent

solution of methylated BSA in water is added with mixing to give a ratio of MBSA to DNA of 1. For immunization one volume of the complex is emulsified with an equal volume of complex adjuvant and injected into rabbits at a concentration of 0·25 mg DNA/ml. The animals are given three injections at weekly intervals, each dose divided into 1·0 ml given intramuscularly and 0·4 ml into the footpads, giving a total of 1·05 mg/DNA. The animals are then bled 7–10 days after the last injection.

Preparation of antisera to low molecular weight tissue antigens

A special problem exists here in that low molecular weight materials do not readily induce an antibody response. The reasons for this are by no means clear and cannot entirely be accounted for by the related paucity of antigenic determinant groups in small molecules compared with large ones or by the more rapid clearance of small molecules from the body. Strain variation in response within a species, as mentioned above, have been noted in work with small molecular weight materials, and important also is the rigidity of the molecule evidenced by the enhanced antigenicity of the gelatin molecule when conjugated to extra tyrosine [49, 50]. To ensure a good supply of antisera it may be worth breeding from those animals in a group which give the best response. With low molecular weight hormone antigens it is desirable to select a species for immunization where it is known that the hormone in question is of different chemical composition to that occurring in the tissues of the animal itself.

The low molecular weight tissue antigens, glucagon (mol. wt. 3800) and insulin (mol. wt. 6000) have been shown to induce antibody responses provided they are given with adjuvants [51, 52]. Classical immunological techniques are a limiting factor in the estimation and detection of antigen–antibody reactions with low molecular weight antigen. Electrophoresis of immune serum mixed with isotope-labelled antigen is valuable in that evidence of immunity can be obtained by the association of radioactivity with the immunoglobulin of serum from immunized animals and not with the immunoglobulin from non-immune animals (see Chapter 18). This method has shown that a synthetic octapeptide of oxytocin (mol. wt. 1000) appears to induce an immune response in rabbits when injected with complete Freund's adjuvant as follows: An emulsion containing 100–400 μg of the peptide per millilitre given 1·0 ml subcut., 0·1 ml intradermally, or 0·1 ml into the footpads. The injections were given thrice weekly for 2 weeks, then three additional weekly doses were given. Blood was collected 2–4 weeks after the last immunization [53]. However, work carried out in association with the author by Dr P. Ganguli failed using similar methods to show an immune response in rabbits, guinea-pigs, fowls and dogs to porcine gastrin (mol. wt. 2114).

Of considerable interest is the report of Berglund [54] who has induced an antibody response as demonstrated by immunodiffusion to human fibrinopeptide B with a molecular weight of about 1400. After failing to induce a response by conventional methods, the fibrinopeptide was combined with acrylic plastic particles. For immunization a 0·125 per cent solution of the fibrinopeptide in 0·05 M citrate buffer pH 4·1 was coated on poly-methylmethacrylate* particles of 0·6 μ diameter in an 11 per cent solution by incubating the solution in the proportion of 5 : 2 at 37° C for 1 hour.

After five immunizations at 10 day intervals either intravenously or sub-cutaneously, the subcutaneous injections were combined with equal volumes of Freund's complete adjuvant. 0·7 ml of the fibrinopeptide polymethyl-methacrylate emulsion was used and 10/10 of the rabbits injected responded, in most instances after only three injections [55].

Techniques used to measure interaction of tissue antibodies with antigens
In selecting a test for assessing the antibody response qualitatively or quanti-tatively or demonstrating an antigen in a particular tissue it is necessary to take into account the immunoglobulin class which is predominant in the antiserum in use. As has already been noted, the nature of the antigen plays a part in determining which particular class of immunoglobulin is stimulated [9]. The different classes of immunoglobulin are more or less effective in the different types of serological reaction, for example IgM globulins are more effective in bringing about haemagglutination than IgG globulins (see Herbert, Chapter 21) and it has recently been shown [56] that only one or two molecules of IgM antibody are required to lyse a red cell in the presence of excess complement compared with about 700 molecules of IgG. A potent virus-neutralizing IgG antibody may be much less able to fix complement than poorly neutralizing IgG globulin produced early after infection, illustrating that even within a particular class of immunoglobulin differences in reactivity may exist [57]. During the primary response to BSA in rabbits we have noted marked increases over 3 or 4 days in the haemag-glutination titres in the IgM fraction of serum with minimal change in its ability to bind antigen as measured by the Farr technique (Chapter 13) [58]. See Chapter 13 for further discussion on this point.

The most satisfactory solution for estimating an antibody–antigen inter-action is to measure the primary union between antibody and antigen and not to depend on secondary phenomena such as fixation of comple-ment, agglutination and precipitation. Unfortunately, with tissue antigens this is not always possible as many of the methods for measuring primary union, for example, the Farr technique or radioimmunoassay methods

* Obtainable from A.B. Bofors, Läkemedelsforskningen, Taljegårdsgatan 3, Mölndal, Sweden.

(see Chapters 13 and 18), depend on using a purified antigen labelled with an isotope marker, or equilibrium dialysis designed for use with haptens (see Chapter 14). Perhaps the best solution to this problem is that offered by Pressman and his colleagues in their work on tissue-specific antigens. These workers make use of a paired-label technique with a mixture of antiserum globulin labelled with ^{125}I and normal serum or antiserum directed against an unrelated antigen labelled with ^{131}I. The difference between the ^{131}I counts due to the non-specific uptake of normal serum components and the ^{125}I counts from the attached immune serum give a measure of the specific uptake of antibody. The technique can be applied both *in vitro* and *in vivo*.

Initial purification of the antiserum is achieved by precipitation of the globulins by ammonium sulphate at 1/3 saturation carried out in buffer at pH 7·0. The antibody preparation is then further purified by absorption on to tissue preparations followed by elution at 60° C. One hundred milligrammes of tissue sediment is used for every 10 mg of iodine-labelled globulin and the mixture is shaken continuously for 1 hour at 37° C for absorption of globulin to take place. The sediments are washed with borate buffered saline to remove unabsorbed globulin and then suspended in a volume of preheated (59° C) borate buffered saline equal to the volume of the globulin which had been added at the start of the absorption. The mixture is shaken continuously for 15 minutes at 50° C ±1° C to elute a portion of the absorbed globulin and after centrifugation the supernatant is taken for subsequent use. About 1 per cent of the added globulin is recovered after the elution procedure.

Using the paired-label technique with a mixture of antibody globulin labelled with one of the iodine isotopes and an unrelated antibody globulin from the same species labelled with the other an estimate can be obtained of the specific uptake by a particular tissue sediment, a direct comparison being made between the uptake of the specific and control globulins in each experiment.

The purified antibody globulin which has been eluted from the tissue sediment can be tested for uptake by particular organs by injecting it into an animal and estimating the uptake by the various organs. This is achieved in, for example, the rat by injecting 2 ml of the eluted globulins into the tail vein of three rats. A fourth 2 ml portion diluted to 100 ml with 2 per cent rabbit serum in buffer is used to determine the radioactivity of the injected dose. Sixteen to 20 hours after the injection the perfused organs are cut up into pieces of about 1 g and used for the determination of radioactivity. The control 2 ml diluted portion mentioned above is also counted before and after the tissues are assayed. It is therefore possible to estimate the percentage of the injected activity taken up by the various organs. This procedure has the disadvantage that certain tissue antigens are not exposed *in vivo* as they might be in an *in vitro* preparation. A possible way of getting round this difficulty might be to use chemical toxic agents to expose intracellular antigens.

In an antiserum purified by elution the amount of material eluted, as has been noted above, is very small, thus the amount of radioactivity injected is also very small and that recovered even less. To take an example from the work of Pressman and colleagues [20] using tumour-localizing antibodies against Murphy rat lymphosarcoma. In the initial purification step using tumour sediment to absorb the specific antibody and eluting it at 60° C about 1 per cent of the total globulin initially added was recovered and this amounted to approximately half that absorbed by the tissue. The eluted globulin was contained in a volume of 10 ml and 2 ml of this was injected in the *in vivo* assay. Thus the amount of radioactivity in each rat represented 0·2 per cent of the initial whole-labelled protein or about 20 γ of the initial 10 mg. Therefore, a net localization of 5 per cent of this material in a particular tissue or organ represents about 1 γ of antibody globulin and an uptake of 0·1 per cent represents 0·02 γ. With iodination at the level of 1 atom of iodine per molecule of globulin the activity in samples taken in this way is thus very small and the number of counts correspondingly few also. The error, calculated as the square root of the number of counts divided by the number of counts times 100, increases as the number of counts decreases. In the paired-label technique counts of 5000 per minute were achieved for 1 minute periods, giving an error of approximately 1·4 per cent.

The ^{131}I and ^{125}I isotopes are counted simultaneously in a single sample using a dual-channel scintillation counter with a sodium iodide well-type scintillation head. This is possible as 80 per cent of the γ rays from ^{131}I have an energy of 0·36 Mev and 100 per cent of ^{125}I an energy of 0·035 Mev. The ^{125}I count is corrected for the overlap of ^{131}I in the low-energy channel (i.e. 20 per cent). A single-channel system can also be used, each sample is passed twice through the system. The use of automatic sample changer counting systems has greatly simplified the handling of the large number of separate counts required in experiments of this type.

Other labels

Another method which indicates in a non-quantitative manner the primary union of antibody with cellular antigens is the use of ferritin-labelled anti-tissue antibody layered on tissue sections or mixed with cell suspensions and examined by electron microscopy. These methods are described in Chapter 15 and have been recently applied to the study of antibody uptake by subcellular organelles [59]. Ammonium sulphate-precipitated globulins were prepared from rabbit antiserum against mixed mitochondrial and lysosomal preparations from rat liver. After ferritin labelling (see Chapter 15) 1 ml of the labelled globulin at a concentration of 10 mg/ml of protein was mixed with 1 ml of fresh well-washed mitochondrial fraction, 1 ml of tris-HCl sucrose buffer and 1 ml of fresh guinea-pig serum as a source of complement. Control tubes were also set up containing 1 ml volumes of the unconjugated mixtures of globulin and ferritin together with the mitochondrial fraction. After incubation at 37° C for 40 minutes, 20 ml of ice-cold sucrose (0·25 M) was added to each tube and the suspension centrifuged at 6000 *g* for 15 minutes. The washing process was repeated and the pellets made up in four volumes of 0·88 M sources at 0° C. Fixation was carried out for 1 hour in ice by adding 4 ml volumes of Palade's osmium tetroxide fixative (2 per cent OsO_4 in barbiturate buffer). The fixed material was recovered by centrifugation at 6000 *g* for 10 minutes and the resulting pellets processed for electron microscopy.

Fluorescent antibody methods
This technique has contributed, probably more than any other method, valuable information on the basis of differentiation and specificity of tissue antigens and the detection of anti-tissue antibodies in disease. These applications have been fully reviewed recently by Nairn [10] and Chapter 16 of this handbook is devoted to a consideration of the techniques involved.

Detection methods depending on secondary phenomena following primary union of antigen and antibody
Complement fixation
Of all the methods in this category complement fixation has probably been used most extensively. Unfortunately the method is open more to criticism than other available methods due essentially to the large number of variables in the complement-fixation system. Thus, careful control and evaluation is particularly important in this technique (see Levine, Chapter 20).

Since the description by Gajdusek in 1957 [38] of complement-fixing antibodies against liver homogenate in certain human-disease states the method has been extensively used for the detection of antibody against various tissue components in human and experimental animal sera [60, 61, 62, 6, 7, 63, 64, 65]. The method has been used in studies of the thermostable organ-specific antigens mentioned above in the studies of Milgrom and co-workers [28] and in studies on the antigenic properties of microsomes [66].

It is well known that there are a number of situations not associated with antigen–antibody union in which complement is inactivated, including heat denaturation and aggregation of γ globulin [67, 68] and sera which have stood at room temperature for a few days are known to become anticomplementary [69]. A useful control for tests for anti-tissue antibodies is the inclusion of a series of antibody dilutions without antigen parallel to the test series, this control row containing twice as much antibody as the test itself. Any anticomplementary effects of the serum will show up quite clearly and can be taken into consideration when reading the result of the test itself. A further point which must be established is that serum, from experimental animals or humans with anti-tissue antibody of the type described by Gajdusek [38], does not fix complement due to the release into the circulation of anti-complementary tissue breakdown products. This can be achieved by the inclusion of an antibody control of the type just described and by ascertaining whether such an effect is present when the antibody response has been inhibited by prior irradiation or splenectomy of the animal [7]. It is also reassuring to be able to absorb the activity from serum by means of the antigen, to isolate the activity in a particular immunoglobulin fraction and, of course, to demonstrate the activity by other tests such as passive haemagglutination [70, 71]. Beall [72] has suggested that the complement fixation observed between serum and human liver extracts may be due to aggregation of a 'γ globulin like' liver component with serum γ globulin. This proposition has been refuted in the case of many anti-tissue antibodies by the isolation of the antigenic activity in purified subcellular fractions washed free of any soluble 'γ globulin like' protein [1, 65].

The micro complement-fixation test (see Levine, Chapter 20) is very suitable for use in situations in which only small quantities of serum are available, as is the case in work with small animals. A test using a four-drop system, each drop about 0·05 ml in volume, is particularly suitable for large numbers of tests and has been extensively used in the detection of antibodies to tissue components [60, 7, 1], and is recommended by the author. A dilution series of inactivated antiserum is made up using a volume calculated to give just sufficient to provide one drop of antibody for each tube of the test dilution series and two drops in the antibody control series. The tests are carried out in very carefully washed MRC pattern plates of the type used in virus work. Starting from the highest dilution of antibody, drops are transferred to the wells in the plate using a carefully prepared straight-ended Pasteur pipette giving about 20–22 drops/ml. The complement and then the antigen are added in the same way each at a dilution estimated from a prior complement titration with antigen, the complement may conveniently be used at 1·25 MHD. No antigen is, of course, added to the antibody control series of dilutions and as there are already two drops of antibody no extra buffer need be added to make up the volumes.

After incubation at 37° C for 30 minutes, (or at 4° C and 24 hours incubation if increased sensitivity is required), 3 per cent sensitized sheep cells are added and the tests are read after 40 minutes' incubation after having been carefully shaken at 20 minutes. The end-point can be taken as the last tube showing clearly visible red cells.

A modification of this test in which antigen is diluted and serum kept constant can be used to compare different fractions of a particular tissue or different tissues for their content of antigen. For example, with the anti-liver antibody induced by toxic liver damage, the mitochondrial fraction was shown to contain most of the antigenic activity [1] (Fig. 26.1). The results can be converted to give the minimum quantity of antigen in terms of dry weight which will give a positive test (Fig. 26.2).

Conglutinating complement-absorption test

The conglutinating complement-absorption test (CCTA) described by Streng in 1910 has recently been redeveloped by Coombs, Coombs & Ingram [73].

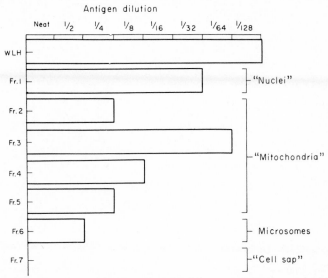

FIG. 26.1 Antigen dilution test using whole rat liver homogenate (WLH) and liver fractions with a constant dilution of a pool of rat serum taken from animals given CCl_4 subcutaneously, 0·03 ml/100 g body weight. Blocks represent positive complement-fixation test at respective antigen dilution.

Reproduced by permision of the Editor of *Clin. exp. Immunol.*

The basis of the test is as follows: When sheep red cells coated with anti-sheep cell antibody are mixed with fresh horse serum the horse complement is bound to the antibody-coated cells but will not lyse them, as horse complement is non-lytic. If such cells are exposed to bovine serum they will be agglutinated due to the presence of a β globulin component [74] which behaves like an anti-complement antibody, this component is known as conglutinin. Should, however, the horse complement have been used up by another antibody antigen system it will not be available to react with the sensitized sheep cells which will then not be agglutinated by the bovine

EE*

conglutinin. Coombs *et al* consider that the test is of greater sensitivity than the haemolytic complement-fixation system as horse complement which is used in the test was in their experience always superior in detecting antibodies in the sera of a wide variety of animal species. Evidence for this is provided by a comparison carried out by Dr Lachman between the haemolytic complement-fixation test and the conglutinating complement-absorption tests in their ability to detect antibodies against DNA in the serum of patients with systemic lupus erythematosus, which show the clear superiority of the conglutinating test [73]. The test has also been successfully used by Miesher *et al* to demonstrate antibodies against nuclear components in immunized

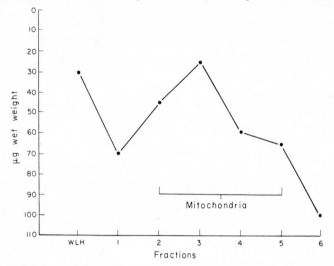

FIG. 26.2. Minimum weight of liver fraction shown in Fig. 26.1 which gave positive complement-fixation test results with the rat serum pool.
Reproduced by permission of the Editor of *Clin. exp. Immunol.*

guinea-pigs and rabbits. Table 26.2 shows the results of a comparison of the two tests carried out in the author's laboratory. Rat anti-liver antibody was tested against rat liver homogenate by both methods. Lachman's results and those on Table 26.2 although both demonstrating the increased sensitivity of the CCTT over the haemolytic complement-fixation test bring out one of the main disadvantages of the CCAT—the increased anticomplementary activity of the serum which appears in the test. The test therefore suffers from the disadvantage of any method which gives increased sensitivity in that the factors which interfere with specificity such as anticomplementary activity are also exaggerated. Coombs and his colleagues point out that earlier objections to the test based on difficulty in reading the results are overcome by a centrifugation and resuspension technique which they describe.

Method:

The method described by Coombs *et al* utilizes five unit volumes of 0·4 or 0·1 ml. In each tube of the test there is one unit volume of each of antigen, antiserum, complement, 0·5 per cent washed sheep red cell suspension and finally heat-inactivated bovine serum. This gives a total volume of either 2 ml or 0·5 ml. Isotonic saline is used for the dilutions and a unit volume of this replaces any reagent not required, as in the initial titration of complement, etc., or in the control tubes. Heat-inactivated serum (56° C 30 minutes) is used throughout. Prior to the actual test it is necessary to determine (1)

TABLE 26.2

Showing reciprocal of titres of four rat sera tested against rat liver antigen on third day after injection of 0·03 ml CCl_4/100 g body weight. Comparison of haemolytic complement-fixation test (37° C for 40 minutes for fixation) and conglutinin complement-absorption test (45 minutes at 37° C). Control rows are tests of anticomplementary activity of test serum.

Rat No.	1	2	3	4	
Control	0	0	0	0	Haemolytic complement-fixation test
Test	4	16	0	0	
Control	4	8	2	2	Conglutinin complement-absorption test
Test	16	64	8	4	

the titre of the anti-sheep cell antibody in the bovine serum, (2) the titre of the bovine conglutinin, (3) the titre of the horse complement, (4) the optimal antigen dilution for use in the test.

(1) The titre of anti-sheep cell antibody is first estimated by making a doubling dilution series of heat-inactivated bovine serum in unit volumes of saline. To each tube is added (a) a unit volume of three times washed 0·5 per cent sheep cell suspension, (b) a unit volume of heat-inactivated and diluted bovine serum (1/10 or 1/20) which has been absorbed with sheep cells (to remove the natural agglutinin) that acts as the source of conglutinin; (c) a unit volume of 1/5 horse serum (i.e. excess complement). Finally, to make up for the reagents not required for this test, two volumes of saline are added. The test is incubated at 37° C for 30 minutes and then centrifuged for 1 minute at 750 *g*. The tests are read by sharply flicking the tubes with the forefinger several times and estimating the degree of conglutination. Coombs describes five different appearances graded as follows: 4—a single large

clump of cells, the background remaining clear; 3—smaller clumps of cells, clear background, no clouding by free cells; 2—a few small clumps of cells, the background clouded by unconglutinated red cells; 1—very few small clumps with most of the cells free and unconglutinated; 0—homogeneous suspension of free red cells.

(2) The conglutinin titre of the bovine serum is estimated as above except that unsensitized sheep cells are replaced by sensitized sheep red cells (prepared by mixing 1 ml of 5% washed sheep cells and 1 ml of heat-inactivated bovine serum, incubated at 37° C for 15 minutes, washed once and made up with 10 ml of saline to give a 0·5 suspension). Coombs *et al* [73] recommend that a bovine serum is selected that when diluted 1/20 contains at least four to eight minimal sensitizing doses of antibody and four to eight minimal doses of conglutinin. It seems possible that bovine serum and horse serum varies in different areas, as bovine serum obtained from the local abattoir required to be used at 1/10 to achieve the requirements of the test and horse serum taken fresh and stored at −20° C never gave a complement titre of more than 1/8 in the three different samples tested.

(3) Titration of horse complement is achieved by the method recommended by Coombs *et al* (73) in which first a range titration (doubling dilution series) and then an exact titration (consecutive dilution series, e.g. 1/10, 1/20, 1/30, etc.) is carried out. The unit volumes are the same as for the previous tests and the indicator system is prepared by mixing equal volumes of the heat-inactivated bovine serum at a dilution dependent on the previous tests with a 0·5 per cent suspension of washed sheep cells incubated at 37° C for 15 minutes and added to the test. (Note—The sheep cells are not washed again after the addition of the bovine serum.) The complete test is incubated at 37° C for 30 minutes and read as described above.

(4) The optimal antigen dilution is determined by testing a doubling dilution series of known positive and negative sera against varying dilutions of antigen—like the chequerboard procedure used in haemolytic complement-fixation tests. The optimal dilution of antigen is the maximum concentration of antigen fixing the standard dose of complement with the smallest amount of antibody.

The test:

The final test is carried out in two stages in five unit volumes as described above. First the antiserum is titrated in a doubling dilution series with 2 MCD of horse complement. The mixture is kept at room temperature for 30 minutes to allow fixation of complement and then the indicator system of heat-inactivated bovine serum and 0·5 per cent sheep cells (previously inactivated at room temperature for 15 minutes). After 30 minutes at 37° C the test is read as described above.

Agglutination reactions

A variety of forms of agglutination reaction are applicable to the detection of antigens on the surface of tissue cells or for the demonstration of antibodies to such antigens. Many types of tissue cell are not suitable for the ordinary agglutination test because of a tendency for cells to aggregate spontaneously or because the cell in question is only one of a number of different types of cell in a mixture. The antiglobulin consumption test, the antiglobulin reaction, mixed agglutination and mixed antiglobulin reactions avoid these difficulties.

The mixed agglutination and antiglobulin reactions have been ingeniously elaborated by Coombs. Mixed agglutination has been specifically applied to the examination of tissue cells for blood group iso-antigens [75, 76]. For example, for the detection of blood group A antigen on their surface, cells are incubated with anti-A serum and then washed. Any antibody which remains adherent to the cells is detected by adding group A red cells and gently centrifuging the mixture. This allows free combining sites on the antibody adherent to the tissue cell to link with the A antigen on the red cell. The adherent red cells can be seen by placing a drop of the mixed cell preparation on a glass microscope slide sealing on a coverslip with paraffin wax and examining the preparation under the phase contrast microscope. The mixed antiglobulin reaction is a method for detecting antibody present on tissue cells. Such cells are mixed with another indicator cell or particle coated with antibody from the same species and an antiglobulin to the particular species globulin is added. In the presence of cells coated with antibody mixed agglutination will occur [77]. This test, like all types of antiglobulin test, suffers from the difficulty of the so-called 'non-specific uptake of globulins' (see previous discussion), which can interfere with the specificity of the test.

Mixed haemadsorption

This technique was originally described by Fagraeus & Espmark in 1961 [73] and is a modification of the mixed antiglobulin reaction. The method is an application of the mixed antiglobulin procedure to a situation where the antigen is sessile on a glass or other surface. The phenomenon is not strictly an agglutination test but rather an adsorption of red cells to the antigen adherent to the glass surface, the red cells being linked by an antiglobulin to the tissue cells, which are coated with an antibody to a surface antigen. The reaction can be read macroscopically and the iron staining of the red cells can be used to improve the photographic reproduction of the reaction. The test has been used as a test of species identity of cultured cells by Espmark & Fagraeus [79, 80], and organ-specific reactions were demonstrated with human serum from cases of thyrotoxicosis when tested on monolayer cultures of human thyroid cells [81]. It has been used for the study of antigens in tissue sections of brain and adrenal tissue [82] and antinuclear factor has also been traced in this way [83]. The test when applied to monolayer cultures only detects uptake of antibody by surface antigens; however, cellular extracts fixed on a glass surface would also be expected to be a suitable substrate. Fagraeus and her colleagues have shown that the test is one hundred to one thousand times more sensitive than the indirect fluorescent antibody technique or the cytotoxic test and in some experiments the titres obtained were equal to those obtained in a tanned-cell haemagglutination test.

The red cells—sheep erythrocytes or human group O Rh-positive cells after washing and making up to a 2 per cent suspension—are initially coated, 'first coating', with an equal volume of an appropriate amboceptor—e.g. rabbit anti-sheep cell serum or non-agglutinating human anti-Rh serum. After $1–1\frac{1}{2}$ hours' incubation at 37° C excess amboceptor is washed away and an equal volume of an appropriate dilution of antiglobulin serum is added to the 2 per cent suspension and left at room temperature for 2 hours. The cells are then finally washed and made up to a 2 per cent suspension. The preliminary procedures to make up the reagents required for the test involve trying out varying dilutions of the red cell coating antibody (amboceptor) used for the 'first coating' of the red cells with varying dilutions of the antiglobulin serum used for 'second coating'. These cells are used with a known positive serum and tissue-culture cells containing on their surface the specific antigen to be detected. When the test shows large clumps of indicator cells adsorbed on to the tissue-culture cells the combination of dilutions in this test is the correct one. Fagraeus *et al* found that concentration of the second coating antiglobulin above the level showing large clumps of indicator cells adsorbed on to the tissue-culture cells did not further affect the quality of the indicator cells.

The test itself is performed with washed tube cultures incubated with 0·3 ml of test serum for 1 hour at room temperature and after draining and washing once with a large volume of serum free medium the cultures are covered with 0·5 ml of a 0·2 − 0·4 per cent suspension of indicator cells and reading performed after $\frac{1}{2}$ – 1 hour. The test may be read macroscopically and for quantitation serial serum dilutions are made. Grading of results ranges from $+ + + +$ when the test cells are completely covered with indicator cells to $+$ when only scattered indicator cells are present.

A modification of the test for use with soluble antigens such as thyroglobulin has been described. Here a glass slide is layered with thyroglobulin at a concentration of 1 $\mu g/cm^2$ and fixed to the slide with acetone. A perspex template with holes serving as serum reservoirs is fixed over the slide with tape and the space between the template and slide filled with 0·75 per cent agar. Test serum is added to the holes in the template and after 40 hours the template and agar are removed and the suspension of indicator cells added.

After 10 minutes cells are poured off and the adsorption of indicator cells estimated.

The antiglobulin-consumption test

This technique described by Steffen [84] and Moulinier [85] depends on the uptake of antiglobulin antibodies by antibody globulin which is present on the surface of a cell. Cells coated with antibody are mixed with the antiglobulin and the depletion in the level of the antiglobulin antibody measured by titration against globulin-coated red cells.

After exposing the antiglobulin serum to the cell preparation which is coated with antibody the remaining antibody can be titrated by the method of Moulinier [85]. This technique has been used for the detection of antibodies on white cells and platelets by van Loghem *et al* [86], Dausset & Brecy [87] and Dausset, Colombani & Colombani [88]. It seems likely that this method would be applicable to the detection of antibody to tissue cells in general. The use of the technique to estimate the uptake of anti-tissue antibody is limited by the base-line consumption and if, for example, it is intended to detect an auto-reactive anti-tissue antibody the antiglobulin serum directed against the serum from which the tissue is derived will inevitably react with traces of serum in the tissue. The application of the technique to the detection of anti-mitochondrial antibodies in rat serum [1], even under strictly controlled conditions, was severely limited by the base-line consumption of the tissue itself even in the absence of added serum. Extended washing procedures carried out in the cold to remove traces of serum components from the tissue resulted in marked loss of antigenic activity of the washed material. The use of heterologous tissue would be likely to overcome, at least in part, the high level of base-line consumption found in such a situation. However, the question of 'non-specific' uptake of serum proteins, already discussed, remains a problem.

In theory, for the best results the antiglobulin serum should be specifically directed against the particular globulin class to be detected. Thus an anti-IgM globulin would be expected to be more sensitive an indicator in a system where the particular antibody reacting with the cell suspension was IgM in type. However, in practice an antiserum prepared against the partially purified 'globulins' would be likely to contain some anti-IgM antibody although most would be anti-IgG antibody.

Method:

The most important practical consideration for the setting up of a sensitive antiglobulin-consumption test is to use the antiglobulin serum at a concentration which is not far from the minimum required to agglutinate the sensitized cells. Thus, a small shift in the antibody content will be readily detectable.

Prior to the actual test it is necessary to titrate the anti-red cell (anti-sheep cell or human anti-Rh serum)—a small proportion of anti-D sera are not suitable [89]—using a 0·5 to 1 per cent suspension of washed erythrocytes. After the minimal agglutinating titre has been found the red cells can be made up with a subagglutinating dose (e.g. twice the minimal agglutinating titre). The antiglobulin serum is then titrated using the globulin-coated red cells. The test can be carried out in MRC pattern perspex plates in volumes of, for example, 0·2 ml and should be left at 37° C for at least 4 hours before reading the agglutination patterns. Overnight incubation at 4° C is a convenient alternative. The patterns are read and recorded.

The consumption test:

Careful consideration of the controls is required which must take into account the possible absorption of antiglobulin by the particular tissue cells being used in the test. It appears that the temperature at which the cells are washed may affect the base-line consumption of the antiglobulin [90]. The base-line consumption is minimized by washing at room temperature rather than at 4° C. Dausset and Colombani suggest that this effect may be due to cold incomplete antibody. The base-line consumption is also increased if the test serum is inactivated prior to use, presumably due to aggregated γ globulin which remains with the tissue suspension on centrifugation and later takes up antiglobulin. It also may be wise to wash the test cells with normal serum from the species used to prepare the antiglobulin serum, thus saturating the cells with normal serum so that they will only take up a specific antibody from the antiglobulin serum [91].

Having taken these factors into consideration, controls for the actual base-line consumption should be set up. Thus, the antiglobulin serum, diluted to the concentration to be used, should be exposed at room temperature or 37° C to the test cells which have been carefully washed. After recovery of the antiglobulin it is titrated against the coated red cells. Controls of the diluted antiglobulin should also be set up and these will show if any deterioration of the antiserum has occurred due to having been kept in a dilute state.

The washed test cells are mixed with test serum and incubated at 37° C for 1 hour and then excess serum carefully washed away, washing the cells at least six times. The washed deposit must now be made up to a concentration which will have sufficient adsorbed antibody to remove a detectable quantity of antiglobulin from the diluted antiglobulin serum. The less antibody there is in the test serum the more concentrated the cell suspension will need to be in order to take up sufficient antiglobulin. In testing for anti-leucocyte antibodies about 150 million cells have been found to be satisfactory [89]. The concentrated deposit of tissue cells is then exposed to the diluted antiglobulin serum and incubated again at 37° C for 1 hour. It is convenient to use a number of different antiglobulin dilutions ranging from one doubling dilution higher than the minimum agglutinating titre to three or four times this amount. This enables decreases in titre of only one tube to be taken as significant when they are found to be consistent in a number of different dilutions of antiglobulin. The more antiglobulin which is removed (reflecting the quantity of globulin derived from the test serum which has become attached to the tissue cells) the greater will be the shift in its titre, big reductions showing a shift in the end-point titre even in the higher concentrations of antiglobulin.

The results should be expressed as the number of units of antibody (one unit is present in the highest dilution of unabsorbed antiglobulin serum agglutinating the red cells) adsorbed by the test system as compared with the normal control.

Haemagglutination and coated inert particle agglutination reactions
The development and principles of these techniques are discussed in Chapter 21. These techniques have been widely used with tissue antigens, particularly with soluble antigens like thyroglobulin and nucleoprotein in tests for demonstrating antithyroid antibodies or antinuclear antibodies. Boyden's tanned red cell test is probably the most popular of all tests of this type and uses either sheep erythrocytes or human group O Rh-negative erythrocytes. Unmodified cells because of their ability to adsorb polysaccharide antigens have been used for the detection of antibodies to phenol–water extracts of human colon in the serum of patients with ulcerative colitis [92]. It is likely that this procedure could be used for most polysaccharide antigens from tissue although there appear to be some polysaccharides which are not taken up by red cells; for example, that of *Klebsiella aerogenes* [93]. The cells are washed three times (twice in physiological saline) and once in the phosphate buffered saline pH 7·2 (see Herbert, Chapter 21) and made up to about a 5 per cent suspension. An equal volume of the polysaccharide extract, at about 10 μg/ml, is added and the mixture incubated for 1–2 hours at 37° C. The cells are then washed free of excess polysaccharide—two washes in buffer and made up to a 1 per cent suspension. The test is set up and the patterns read like the tanned red cell test (see Herbert, Chapter 21). The cells may be used up to 2 days if refrigerated and the same procedure can be carried out with formalinized cells with slight reduction in sensitivity of the test.

Other red cell haemagglutination tests
Conjugation of various protein antigens to red cells following the modification of their surface by tannic acid was first described by Boyden in 1951 and the technique is fully described in Chapter 21. Protein antigens have also

been linked to the red cell surface by coupling with bis-diazotized benzidine (BDB) [94].

These methods have been quite extensively used with tissue antigens, particularly with thyroglobulin [95, 96, 97]. Milgrom & Witebsky [25] have also used the test as an inhibition test in their extensive studies on organ-specific antigens. Nuclear antigens have also been coated on to tanned cells and the test successfully used for detecting antibodies in serum of patients with systemic lupus erythematosus [98], although Seligmann [99] considers DNA not a suitable antigen for coating on to tanned cells. Liver antigens have also been coated on to such cells for the detection of anti-liver antibodies in rats [70, 71, 100, 101] and skin antigens have also been used for the demonstration of anti-skin antibodies in normal rabbit serum [102]. In the author's experience chemical linking of tissue antigens using BDB has proved considerably more reliable, the results being more reproducible and the coated cell preparation more stable than is the case with tannic acid treated cells. For a full description of the methods see Herbert, Chapter 21.

Inert particles

Polystyrene latex and bentonite have proved the most useful of the inert particles and have been coated successfully with a variety of tissue antigens including thyroglobulin [103, 95] and DNA [104, 105] and human γ globulin for the detection of rheumatoid factor [106].

Polystyrene latex particles are available commercially, average size 0·81 microns (Difco latex—Hyland—Baird and Tatlock, London). The particles are used at a 1/10 dilution from the suspension provided by the manufacturers made up in borate or glycine buffer pH 8·2. The suspension is mixed with an equal volume of the tissue-antigen preparation, e.g. the supernatant from thyroid homogenate or liver homogenate diluted about 1/30 w/v. Heavily particulate material is not suitable as this would interfere with the reading of the test, and thyroid microsomes which have been recently shown to be the cytoplasmic auto-antigen of the thyroid [65] make a very suitable antigen. The gland taken from a thyrotoxic patient, is cut into blocks and sliced with a razor prior to homogenization in a teflon and glass homogenizer. The resulting suspension is filtered through muslin and then differential centrifugation carried out (see Davies, Chapter 11) and the microsomes used as the antigen for coating the latex particles.

The mixture of latex particles and antigen are then added to serum dilutions each in a volume of 1 ml and after shaking, the tubes are incubated for 2 hours at 56° C. The tests are finally centrifuged for 3 minutes at 1000 *g* and read. An opaque suspension with no deposit negative test; opaque suspension with minimal deposit ± doubtful test; partially cleared suspension with granular deposit + ; clear or almost clear supernatant with granular deposit + +. An alternative method is to mix the serum and antigen in a capillary tube and after keeping the tests on the bench for 24 hours they are examined for agglutination [95].

Immune adherence

This is an immunological reaction in which a particulate antigen sensitized with antibody and complement becomes attached to human or monkey erythrocytes [107]. The technique has been applied particularly to bacteria, starch grains, vaccinia virus and rickettsiae. With cauliflower mosaic virus the test has been shown to have a sensitivity ten to one hundred times that of the immunodiffusion test in agar or the microprecipitin test previously used to detect antigenic activity [108]. The test does not appear to have been used successfully for particulate tissue antigens although in principle the technique should be applicable. An attempt in the author's laboratory to use the technique for the demonstration of antibody against rat liver antigens—whole cells or isolated subcellular components—was unsuccessful although the IgM antibody against the mitochondrial fraction could be clearly demonstrated by other methods [1]. A similar failure to detect antibodies against thyroid microsomes is reported by Roitt *et al* [65]. See also Chapter 28 pp. 949–952.

Precipitation tests

Precipitin tests, particularly immunodiffusion tests, have been used extensively for work with tissue antigens and antibodies. Antithyroid antibodies have been investigated by this method [109, 95, 110], antibodies to DNA in serum of patients with systemic lupus erythematosus [48, 111, 112] and antibodies to colonic extracts in children with ulcerative colitis [92]. Milgrom & Witebsky [25] have used the method in their intensive studies on organ-specific antigens, constituents of human gastric mucosa have recently been characterized by immunoelectrophoresis [113] and rat liver subcellular antigens by D'Amelio *et al* [114]. Tissue antigens have also been demonstrated in the serum following tissue breakdown [115, 116, 1].

The standard immunodiffusion techniques including immunoelectrophoresis are applicable to these problems and are described in detail in Chapter 19. The probable contamination of anti-tissue sera by antibodies to serum components will clearly require special attention and such antisera may have to be absorbed with serum. Another and probably better way round this problem is to use the modification proposed by Osserman [117] (Fig. 26.3). After electrophoresis of the antigen in agar between two longitudinal troughs, one trough is filled with antiserum raised against the antigen mixture and the other with the antigen which is contaminating the antigen mixture that has been electrophoresed. For example, if the antigen mixture is a tissue extract this would be likely to be contaminated with serum proteins and therefore the antigen put into the trough would be serum or perhaps a particular serum component. If a precipitin band was formed due to a reaction between antibody and a serum component in the electrophoresed antigen it would join and form at each end of the arc a line of identity with the longitudinal precipitin band formed between the antiserum and the serum in the trough. This method has been used successfully in studies on the antigenic constituents of lens extracts of various species [118]. Other variations include that described by Clausen & Heremans [119] in which two antigens are electrophoresed and an antiserum trough cut between them, leaving a small portion

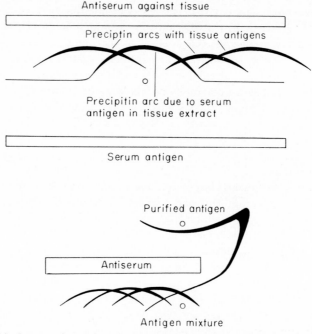

Fig. 26.3. Immunoelectrophoretic methods for testing tissue antigens for contamination by serum constituents or other contaminants (see text).

uncut. Lines of identity will then be formed between precipitin arcs which can link up through the uncut portion. Alternatively the trough may be cut short so that arcs can join round the shortened end. This latter method is, of course, only applicable to fast or slow migrating components.

Another problem peculiar to tissue antigens is the preparation of diffusible extracts of tissues. The standard tissue homogenizer has too much clearance between the teflon plunger and the glass barrel to break up subcellular components into a fine homogeneous material from which the antigenic components can be extracted suitable for diffusion in gel. In the studies on lens antigens mentioned above a very close fitting teflon and glass homogenizer is used and homogenization is aided by placing a small piece of fine glass tubing, e.g. from a finely drawn out Pasteur pipette, into the barrel with the antigen suspension. The glass which is ground up with the tissue helps to break up the cellular components.

The quantitative precipitin test has been used in studying reactions between DNA and serum of patients with systemic lupus erythematosus. The precipitin curves obtained were very similar to those obtained with classical antigen–antibody reactions except that the curve fell very slowly in the zone of antigen excess. The test gave optimal results when carried out at pH 8·0 [48, 44, 111]. Similar results were obtained in tests carried out with calf thymus nucleoprotein [112].

References

[1] PINCKARD R.N. & WEIR D.M. (1966) Antibodies against the mitochondrial fraction of liver after toxic liver damage in rats. *Clin. exp. Immunol.* 1 : 33.

[2] NOSSAL G.J.V., ADA C.L., AUSTIN C.M. & PYE J. (1965) Antigens in immunity. VIII. Localization of ^{125}I labelled antigens in the secondary response.

[3] UHR J.W. & BAUMANN J.B. (1961) Antibody formation. I. The suppression of antibody formation by passively administered antibody. *J. exp. Med.* **113**, 935

[4] FREI P.C., BENACERRAF B. & THORBECKE C.J. (1965) Phagocytosis of the antigen, a crucial step in the induction of the primary response. *Proc. nat. acad. Sci. (Wash.)* **53**, 20

[5] DRESSER D.W. (1962) Specific inhibition of antibody production. II. Paralysis induced in adult mice by small quantities of protein antigen. *Immunology* **5**, 378

[6] WEIR D.M. (1961) A complement fixation reaction with serum and tissue extracts after the injection of carbon tetrachloride into rats. *Lancet* **1**, 1147

[7] WEIR D.M. (1963) Liver auto-antibodies in the rat. *Immunology* **6**, 581

[8] WEIR D.M. (1964) Serum protein changes after administration of carbon tetrachloride in the rat. *Nature, Lond.* **202**, 307

[9] TORRIGIANI G. & ROITT I.M. (1965) The enhancement of 19S antibody production by particulate antigen. *J. exp. Med.* **122**, 181

[10] NAIRN R.C. (1964) *Fluorescent Protein Tracing*, pp. 125, 126. Edinburgh: Livingstone

[11] WEIR D.M. (1966) The immune response after tissue injury. *Path. europ.* **2**, 108

[12] KAPLAN M.H. & SUCHY M.C. (1964) Immunologic relation of streptococcal and tissue antigens. II. Cross reaction of antisera to mammalian heart tissue with cell wall constituents of certain strains of group A streptococci. *J. exp. Med.* **119**, 643

[13] KARUSH F. (1965) *Molecular and Cellular Basis of Antibody Formation*, p. 639, ed. STERZL J. Prague: Czechoslovak Acad. Sci.

[14] HIMSWORTH H.P. & GLYNN L.E. (1945) The gross chemical changes in the liver in dietetic necrosis. *Biochem. J.* **39**, 267

[15] NAIRN R.C., CHADWICK C.S. & McENTEGART M.G. (1958) Fluorescent protein traces in the study of experimental liver damage. *J. Path. Bact.* **76**, 143

[16] TROTTER W.R., BELYAVIN G. & WADDAMS A. (1957) Precipitating and complement-fixing antibodies in Hashimoto's disease, *Proc. roy. soc. Med.* **50**, 961

[17] IRVINE W.J., DAVIES S.H., DELAMORE I.W. & WYNN WILLIAMS A. (1962) Immunological relationship between pernicious anaemia and thyroid disease. *Brit. med. J.* 2, 454

[18] WEIR D.M., HOLBOROW E.J. & JOHNSON G.D. (1961) A clinical study of serum antinuclear factor. *Brit. med. J.* 1, 933

[19] KORNGOLD L. & PRESSMAN D. (1953) The in-vitro purification of tissue localizing antibodies. *J. Immunol.* 71, 1

[20] DAY E.D., PLANINSEK J., KORNGOLD L. & PRESSMAN D. (1956) Tumour localizing antibodies purified from antisera against Murphy rat lymphosarcoma. *J. Nat. Cancer Inst.* 17 517

[21] SULITZEANU D., YAGI Y. & PRESSMAN D. (1963) Separation of an antigenic fraction from rat liver responsible for the formation of liver localizing antibodies. *J. Immunol.* 90, 424

[22] SULITZEANU D., YAGI Y. & PRESSMAN D. (1964) Liver localizing antibodies—The limited contribution of Ag–Ab complexes. *J. Immunol.* 92, 724

[23] YAGI Y., KORNGOLD L. & PRESSMAN D. (1956) Purification of kidney components capable of neutralizing kidney localizing anti-rat kidney antibodies. *J. Immunol.* 77, 287

[24] GERY I., YAGI Y. & PRESSMAN D. (1965) Reactions of localizing anti-kidney antibodies with tissue of various species. *J. Immunol.* 94, 950

[25] MILGROM F. & WITEBSKY E. (1962) Immunological studies on adrenal glands. I. Immunization with adrenals of foreign species. *Immunology* 5, 46

[26] MILGROM F., TUGGAC M. & WITEBSKY E. (1963) Immunological studies on adrenal glands. III. Interspecies relations of thermostable adrenal-specific antigens. *Immunology* 6, 105

[27] MILGROM F., TUGGAC M., CAMPBELL W.A. & WITEBSKY E. (1964) Thermostable ethanol insoluble antigens of brain. *J. Immunol.* 92, 82

[28] MILGROM F., TUGGAC Z.M. & WITEBSKY E. (1964) Studies of species specificity. *J. Immunol.* 93, 902

[29] SHULMAN S., CENTENO E., MILGROM F. & WITEBSKY E. (1965) Immunological studies on adrenal glands. V. Chemical studies on the rabbit adrenal-specific autoantigen. *Immunology* 8, 531

[30] MILGROM F. (1965) Organ specific antigens of liver, testicle and pituitary. *J. Immunol.* 94, 157

[31] GOOD R.A. (1965) *Molecular and Cellular Basis of Antibody Formation*, p. 615, ed. STERZL J. Prague: Czechoslovak Acad. Sci.

[32] NOSSAL G.J.V., AUSTIN C.M. & ADA G.L. (1965) Antigens in immunity. VII. Analysis of immunological memory. *Immunology* 9, 333

[33] BENACERRAF B. (1965) *Molecular and Cellular Basis of Antibody Formation*, p. 57, ed. STERZL J. Prague: Czechoslovak Acad. Sci.

[34] HUMPHREY J.H. (1965) *Molecular and Cellular Basis of Antibody Formation*, pp. 85, 86, ed. STERZL J. Prague: Czechoslovak Acad. Sci.

[35] PINCKARD R.N. & WEIR D.M. Unpublished

[36] HERBERT W.J. (1966) The antigenicity of soluble protein in the presence of high levels of antibody; a possible mode of action of the antigen adjuvants. *Nature, Lond.* 210, 747

[37] WHITE R.G. (1965) The role of peptido-glycolipids of M. tuberculosis and related organisms in immunological adjuvance. *Molecular and Cellular Basis of Antibody Formation*, p. 71, ed. STERZL J. Prague: Czechoslovak Acad. Sci.

[38] GAJDUSEK D.C. (1957) An auto-immune reaction against human tissue antigen in certain chronic diseases. *Nature, Lond.* 179, 666

[39] WALKER J.G., DONIACH D., ROITT I.M. & SHERLOCK S. (1965) Serological tests in the diagnosis of primary biliary cirrhosis. *Lancet* **1,** 828

[40] MIESCHER P., COOPER N.S. & BENACERRAF B. (1960) Experimental production of antinuclear antibodies. *J. Immunol.* **85,** 27

[41] WEIR D.M. & HOLBOROW E.J. (1962) Serum antinuclear factor. Laboratory studies. *Ann. rheum. dis.* **21,** 40

[42] PHILLIPS J.H., BRAUN W. & PLESCIA O.J. (1958) Immunochemical study of a bacterial DNA. *J. Am. chem. Soc.* **80,** 2710

[43] ZALTA J.P. & KHOUVINE Y. (1956) Immunochime de ribonucléoprotéides de tissus normaux et cancéreux. *Compte. rend. soc. biol.* **150,** 339

[44] SELIGMANN M. (1960) *Ciba Foundation Symposia on Cellular Aspects of Immunity,* p. 411, ed. WOLSTENHOLME G.E.W. & O'CONNOR M. London: Churchill

[45] PLESCIA O.J., BRAUN W. & PALCZUK N.C. (1964) Nucleic acids as antigens. *Molecular and Cellular Basis of Antibody Formation,* p. 61, ed. STERZL J. Prague: Czechoslovak Acad. Sci.

[46] HOLBOROW E.J., WEIR D.M. & JOHNSON G.D. (1957) A serum factor in lupus erythematosus with an affinity for cell nuclei. *Brit. med. J.* **2,** 732

[47] BARBU E., SELIGMANN M. & JOLY M. (1960) Réactions entre des acides désoxyribonucléiques diversement dénatures ou degradés et les anticorps anti-acide désoxyribonucléique du serum de malades atteints de lupus erythémateux disséminé. *Ann. Inst. Pasteur.* **99,** 695

[48] HOLMAN H.R. & DEICHER H.R.G. (1959) The reaction of the lupus erythematosus (LE) cell factors with desoxyribonucleoprotein of the cell nucleus. *J. clin. Invest.* **38,** 2059

[49] SELA M. & ARNON R. (1960) Studies on the chemical basis of the antigenicity of proteins. 1. Antigenicity of polypeptidyl gelatins. *Biochem. J.* **75,** 91

[50] SELA M. & FUCHS S. (1965) On the role of charge and optical configuration in antigenicity. *Molecular and Cellular Basis of Antibody Formation,* p. 43, ed. STERZL J. Prague: Czechoslovak Acad. Sci.

[51] UNGER R.H., EISENTRAUT A.M., McCALL M.S. & MADISON L.L. (1961) Glucagon antibodies and an immunoassay for glucagon. *J. clin. Invest.* **40,** 1280

[52] YAGI U., MAIER P. & PRESSMAN D. (1965) Antibodies against the component polypeptide chains of bovine insulin. *Science* **147,** 617

[53] GILLILAND P.F. & PROUT T.E. (1965) Immunologic studies on octapeptides. II. Production and detection of antibodies to oxytocin. *Metabolism* **14,** 918

[54] BERGLUND G. (1965) Preparation of antiserum to an antigen of low molecular weight. *Nature, Lond.* **206,** 523

[55] BERGLUND G. (1965) Personal communication

[56] HUMPHREY J.H. & DOURMASHKIN R.R. (1965) *Complement. Ciba Foundation Symposium,* ed. WOLSTENHOLME G.E.W. & KNIGHT J. London: Churchill

[57] YOSHIMO K. & TANIGUCHI S. (1964) The appearance of complement-requiring neutralizing antibodies by immunization and infection with herpes simplex virus. *Virology* **22,** 193

[58] COHEN M.D., PINCKARD R.N. & WEIR D.M. (1966) Unpublished results

[59] DUMONDE D.C., ROODYN D.B. & PROSE P.H. (1965) The effects of antibodies on cells. III. Studies on the interaction of rat liver mitochondria and lysosomes with antibody and complement. *Immunology* **9,** 177

[60] ASHERSON G.A. (1959) Antibodies against nuclear and cytoplasmic cell constituents in systemic lupus erythematosus and other diseases. *Brit. J. exp. Path.* **40,** 209

[61] ASHERSON G.A. & DUMONDE D.C. (1962) Characterization of autoantibodies produced in the rabbit by the injection of rat liver. *Brit. J. exp. Path.* **43,** 12

[62] DEICHER H.R., HOLMAN H.R. & KUNKEL H.G. (1960) Anticytoplasmic factors in the sera of patients with systemic lupus erythematosus and certain other diseases. *Arthr. and Rheum.* **3,** 1

[63] SELIGMANN M. (1959) *Immunopathology 1st International Symposium,* p. 402, ed. GRABAR P. & MIESCHER P. Basel: Schwabe

[64] HIJMANS W. & SCHUIT H.R.E. (1959) Studies on the LE cell phenomenon. III. Complement fixation with nuclear substances and the LE cell factor. *Vox Sang. (Basel)* **4,** 376

[65] ROITT I.M., LING N.R., DONIACH D. & COUCHMAN K.G. (1964) The cytoplasmic auto-antigen of the human thyroid. I. Immunological and biochemical characteristics. *Immunology* **7,** 375

[66] WHITBECK E.G. & ROSENBERG L.T. (1964) Antigenic properties of microsomes from guinea-pig spleen, liver and lymph nodes. *Immunology* **7,** 363

[67] ISHIZAKA T. & ISHIZAKA K. (1959) Biological activities of aggregated gamma globulin. I. Skin reactive and complement fixing properties of heat denatured gamma globulin. *Proc. Soc. Exp. Brit. (N.Y.)* **101,** 845

[68] CHRISTIAN C.L. (1959) Studies on aggregated gamma globulin. I. Sedimentation, electrophoretic and anticomplementary properties. *J. Immunol.* **84,** 112

[69] ZINSSER H. & JOHNSON W.C. (1911) On heat sensitive anti-complementary bodies in human blood serum. *J. exp. Med.* **13,** 31

[70] WEIR D.M., PINCKARD R.N., ELSON C.J. & SUCKLING E.D.J. (1966) Naturally occurring anti-tissue antibodies in rat sera. *Clin. exp. Immunol.* **1,** 431

[71] RICHTER M., SARGENT A.U., MYERS J. & ROSE B. (1966) Production of autoantibodies in rats immunized with homologous or heterologous liver. *Immunology* **10,** 211

[72] BEALL G.N. (1963) The nature of the complement fixing antigen in normal human liver extracts. *J. Lab. Clin. Med.* **61,** 67

[73] COOMBS R.R.A., COOMBS A.M. & INGRAM D.G. (1961) *The Serology of Conglutination.* Oxford: Blackwell

[74] LACHMANN P.J. (1962) A comparison of some properties of bovine conglutinin with those of rabbit immuno-conglutinin. *Immunology* **5,** 687

[75] COOMBS R.R.A. & BEDFORD D. (1955) The A and B antigens on human platelets demonstrated by means of mixed erythrocyte-platelet agglutination. *Vox Sang. (Basel)* **5,** 111

[76] HOLBOROW E.J., BROWN P.C., GLYNN L.E., HAWES M.D., GRESHAM G.A., O'BRIEN T.F. & COOMBS R.R.A. (1960) The distribution of the human blood group A antigen in human tissues. *Brit. J. exp. Path.* **41,** 430

[77] COOMBS R.R.A., MARKS J. & BEDFORD D. (1956) Specific mixed agglutination : mixed erythrocyte-platelet antiglobulin reaction for the detection of platelet antibodies. *Brit. J. Haemat.* **2,** 84

[78] FAGRAEUS A. & ESPMARK A. (1961) Use of a 'mixed haemadsorption' method in virus-infected tissue cultures. *Nature, Lond.* **190,** 370

[79] ESPMARK J.A. & FAGRAEUS A. (1962) Detection of antigens in tissue culture with the aid of mixed haemadsorption. *Acta Path. Microbiol Scand.* Suppl. **154,** 258

[80] FAGRAEUS A., ESPMARK J.A. & JONSSON J. (1965) Mixed haemadsorption: A mixed antiglobulin reaction applied to antigens on a glass surface. *Immunology* **9,** 161

[81] JONSSON J., FAGRAEUS A. & ESPMARK J.A. (1964) Auto-antibodies to thyroid antigens studied by the mixed haemadsorption technique. *Proc. 10th Congr. Int. Soc. Blood Transf., Stockholm* 1964, Basel: Karger, 1965

[82] TÖNDER O., MILGROM F. & WITEBSKY E. (1964) Mixed agglutination with tissue sections. *J. exp. Med.* **119,** 265

[83] JONSSON J. & FAGRAEUS A. (1962) Studies on antinuclear factors with the mixed haemadsorption technique. *Acta Path. Microbiol. Scand.* **54,** 344

[84] STEFFEN C. (1955) Untersuchungen über die Verwendung des Antihumanglobulin-ablenkungs methode um nachweis von throbozyten antiköpern. *Wien. Z. inn Med.* **36,** 246

[85] MOULINIER J. (1955) Le test de consommation d'antiglobuline appliqué a la recherche des anticorps antithrombocytes. *Sang.* **26,** 811

[86] VAN LOGHEM J.J., VAN DER HART M., HIJMANS W. & SCHUITT H.R.E. (1958) The incidence and significance of complete and incomplete white cell antibodies with special reference to the use of the Coombs consumption test (CCT). *Vox Sang. (Basel)* **3,** 203

[87] DAUSSET J. & BRECY H. (1958) Test direct de consommation de l'antiglobuline sur les leucocytes et les plaquettes de certain malades atteints de pancytopénies idiopathiques. *Vox Sang. (Basel)* **3,** 197

[88] DAUSSET J., COLOMBANI J. & COLOMBANI M. (1961) Study of leucopenias and thrombocytopenias by the direct antiglobulin consumption test on leucocytes and/or platelets. *Blood* **18,** 672

[89] DAUSSET J. & COLOMBANI J. (1964) Detection of anti-leucocyte and anti-platelet antibodies by the antiglobulin consumption test. *Immunological Methods,* p. 375, ed. ACKROYD J.F. Oxford: Blackwell

[90] ENGELFRIET C.P. & VAN LOGHEM J.J. (1961) Studies on leucocyte iso- and auto-antibodies. *Brit. J. Haemat.* **7,** 223

[91] WALFORD R.L. (1960) *Leucocyte Antigens and Antibodies.* New York: Grune & Stratton

[92] BROBERGER O. & PERLMANN P. (1959) Autoantibodies in human ulcerative colitis. *J. exp. Med.* **110,** 657

[93] DAVIES D.A.L. CRUMPTON M.J., MACPHERSON I.A. & HUTCHISON A.M. (1958) The adsorption of bacterial polysaccharides by erythrocytes. *Immunology* **1,** 157

[94] PRESSMAN D., CAMPBELL D.H. & PAULING L. (1942) The agglutination of intact azo-erythrocytes by antisera homologous to the attached groups. *J. Immunol.* **44,** 101

[95] PHILP J.R., WEIR D.M., STUART A.E. & IRVINE W.J. (1962) A latex particle precipitation test in the diagnosis of thyroid disease. *J. clin. Path* **15,** 148

[96] ROITT I.M. & DONIACH D. (1958) Human auto-immune thyroiditis: Serological studies. *Lancet* **2,** 1027

[97] FULTHORPE A.J., ROITT I.M., DONIACH D. & COUCHMAN K. (1961) A stable sheep cell preparation for detecting thyroglobulin autoantibodies and its clinical applications. *J. clin. Path.* **14,** 654

[98] GOODMAN H.C., FAHEY J.L. & MALMGREM R.A. (1960) Serum factors in lupus erythematosus and other diseases reacting with cell nuclei and nucleoprotein extracts: Electrophoretic, ultracentrifugal and chromatographic studies. *J. clin. Invest.* **39,** 1595

[99] SELIGMANN M. (1964) Antinuclear antibodies in disseminated lupus erythematosus. *Immunological Methods,* ed. ACKROYD J.F. Oxford: Blackwell

[100] ARNASON B.G., SALOMON J. & GRABAR P. (1964) Anticorps antifoie et immuno-globulines sériques chez les souris classiques et axénignes, étude comparative après nécrose hépatique aigue provoquée par le tetrachlorure de carbone (CCl₄). *C.R. Ac. Sci. (Paris)* **259,** 4882

[101] SUCKLING D.E.J. & WEIR D.M. Unpublished

[102] BOYDEN S. (1965) Autoimmunity and inflammation. *Nature, Lond.* **201**, 200

[103] AGER J.A.M., HUTT M.S.R. & SMITH G. (1959) Detection of thyroid antibodies using bentonite particles. *Nature, Lond.* **184**, 478

[104] CHRISTIAN C.L., MENDEZ-BRYAN R.M. & LARSON D.L. (1958) Latex agglutination test for disseminated lupus erythematosus. *Proc. Soc. exp. Biol. (N.Y.)* **98**, 820

[105] BOZICEVICH J., NASOU J.P. & KAYHOE D.E. (1960) Desoxyribonucleic acid (DNA)— bentonite flocculation test for lupus erythematosus. *Proc. Soc. exp. Biol. (N.Y.)* **103**, 636

[106] SINGER J.M. & PLOTZ C.M. (1956) The latex fixation test. I. Application to the sero- logic diagnosis of rheumatoid arthritis. *Amer. J. Med.* **21**, 888

[107] NELSON R.A. (1953) The immune-adherence phenomenon. An immunologically specific reaction between micro-organisms and erythrocytes leading to enhanced phagocytosis. *Science* **118**, 733

[108] NELSON D.A. (1963) Immune adherence. *Advances in Immunology*, p. 131, ed. DIXON F.J. & HUMPHREY J.H. New York and London: Academic Press

[109] DONIACH D. & ROITT I.M. (1957) Auto-immunity in Hashimoto's disease and its implications. *J. clin. Endocrin.* **17**, 1293

[110] GOUDIE R.B., ANDERSON J.R. & GRAY K.G. (1959) Non-precipitating antithyro- globulin studied by the Ouchterlony technique. *Immunology* **2**, 309

[111] BARBU E., SELIGMANN M., JOLY M. (1960) Réactions entre des acides désoxyribo- nucléiques diversement dénaturés ou dégradés et les anticorps anti-acide désoxy- ribonucléique du sérum de malade atteints de lupus erythemateux disséminé. *Ann. Inst. Pasteur.* **99**, 695

[112] WEIR D.M. (1962) The anti-nuclear factor as an auto-antibody. M.D. thesis, Uni- versity of Edinburgh

[113] RAPP H.J. (1964) Constituents and antigen of normal human gastric mucosa as characterized by electrophoresis and immuno-electrophoresis in agar gel. *J. Immunol.* **92**, 579

[114] D'AMELIO V. & PERLMANN P. (1960) Distribution of soluble antigens in cellular structures of rat liver. *Exp. Cell Res.* **19**, 383

[115] ESPINOZA E. & INSUNZA I. (1962) Hepatic antigens in the blood of rats with toxic liver damage. *Proc. Soc. exp. Biol. (N.Y.)* **111**, 174

[116] GORDON A.H. (1961) Detection of liver proteins in circulating blood. *Nature, Lond.* **189**, 727

[117] OSSERMAN E.F. (1960) A modified technique of immunoelectrophoresis facilitating the identification of specific precipitin arcs. *J. Immunol.* **84**, 93

[118] CLAYTON R.M. (1966) Personal communication

[119] CLAUSEN J. & HEREMANS J. (1960) An immunologic and chemical study of the simi- larity between mouse and human serum protein. *J. Immunol* **84**, 128

[120] WEIR, D.M. & PINCKARD R.N. (1967) Failure to induce tolerance to liver antigen in rats. *Immunology* (in press)

CHAPTER 27

The Demonstration of Antibodies to Protozoa

W. H. R. LUMSDEN

Introduction

Protozoa, typically, exhibit more variety of morphological characteristics for the differentiation of species than do either the bacteria or the viruses, but nevertheless instances abound of morphologically identical parasites causing widely different clinical effects. Also the degree and character of multiplication of protozoal parasites in the vertebrate host vary widely and infections of individual or of epidemiological importance may be difficult or impossible to recognize by the usual protozoological methods of microscopy and inoculation into cultures or animals. In this situation the possibility that immunological approaches could provide convenient tools for the identification of pathogenic forms, and for the diagnosis of infection or past infection, has been an attractive one. Further, the possibility of artificial immunization against protozoal infection has invited interest.

The pursuit of these aims has produced a large body of immunological information relative to the Protozoa but in comparatively few instances have the desired objectives been attained, as regards either diagnosis or immunization. The main factors which have contributed to this result have been the complexities of the life histories of many of the parasites in their vertebrate hosts and arthropod vectors, the difficulty of the culture of the organisms in the forms infecting the vertebrate host, and the variations in antigenicity associated with these various transformations, and even with the course of infection with the same form.

The degree of application of the various possible immunological tests has varied widely among the Orders, tests being mainly developed pragmatically. It is usual to consider the immunology of individual parasites or parasite groups; in this review the opportunity is taken, as likely to afford useful comparisons, of classifying the subject instead according to the immunological tools used to detect and measure antigen–antibody reactions. The arrangement of these follows in substance the classification of specifically induced altered reactivity given by Humphrey & White [87].

The genera of organisms referred to, arranged according to the classification of Rothschild [142], are set out below. Most of the immunological information available refers to parasitic Protozoa, but mention is also made of some classical work on free-living forms.

Phylum Protozoa
  Class Mastigophora
    Sub-class Zoomastigina
      Order Protomonadina
        Leishmania
        Trypanosoma
        Bodo
      Order Metamonadina
        Trichomonas
  Class Rhizopoda
    Order Amoebina
      Hartmanella
      Entamoeba
  Class Sporozoa
    Sub-class Coccidiomorpha
      Order Eucoccidia
        Sub-order Eimeriidea
          Eimeria
        Sub-order Haemosporidia
          Plasmodium
        Sporozoa of uncertain systematic position
          Toxoplasma
          Sarcocystis
          Babesia
          Theileria
  Class Ciliata
    Sub-class Holotricha
      Order Trichostomatida
        Balantidium
      Order Hymenostomatida
        Sub-order Tetrahymenina
          Glaucoma
          Colpidium
        Sub-order Peniculina
          Paramecium

Definitions and abbreviations
Immunological terminology follows that of Humphrey & White [87]. The following definitions are made:

Isolate. A section of a wild population separated off by transference into artificial conditions of maintenance, usually by inoculation either into cultures or into laboratory animals [102].

Strain. A population, derived from an isolate, maintained in captivity by inducing it to reproduce continuously, by serial passage in cultures or in laboratory animals [105, 102].

Stabilate. A population of an organism whose reproduction has been arrested by viable preservation on a unique occasion. In stabilate material, selection of a continuously reproducing population, as occurs in a strain, is avoided, and selection is restricted to that exerted by the processes of preservation and retrieval from preservation [105, 102].

Other workers, e.g. Garnham [69], have used the term 'strain' to designate particular antigenic or behavioural types. A statement, according to that usage, that a given parasite existed as single or several strains, would be replaced, according to present definitions, by one that the strains of a parasite were similar, or diverse, in respect of some specific behavioural characteristic.

Premunition and sterile immunity. These terms distinguish, respectively:

(a) A situation of compromise between parasite and host, in which the parasite lives within the host in a latent state, the host being in a state of immunity or increased resistance to further infection by virtue of this latent infection.

(b) A state of immunity to further infection persisting after the complete disappearance of the infecting agent.

It is emphasized [173] that premunition, although descriptively a valid entity, does not stand apart as a fundamentally separate immunological phenomenon. In any case, the certain establishment of a state of specific acquired resistance as due to one or the other will often be impossible.

Some terms, constantly recurring, may for convenience be abbreviated:

Washing—indicates dilution of the concentration of some substances in the ambient fluid in which organisms are suspended, by centrifugation, rejection of the supernate and resuspension in a suitable medium. Although the number of washing procedures carried out is usually stated, the degree of removal of substances achieved is usually uncertain as this will depend on the dilution factor at each washing operation, which is determined by the volumes of diluent retained with the deposit and used for resuspension.

Inactivation—indicates heating at 56° C for 30 minutes. *PBS*—phosphate buffered saline. *ICe*—intracerebral. *ICu*—intracutaneous. *IM*—intramuscular. *IP*—intraperitoneal. *IV*—intravenous. *SC*—subcutaneous.

Protozoal antigens
Although there are many references to protozoal 'toxins' in the literature there

appear to be no established examples comparable with, for instance, the exotoxins of *Clostridium welchii*. McGregor [114] refers to immunity to malaria being acquired in two stages. In the first the host becomes able to deal with the pyrogenic products of erythrocytic schizogony and so to support an intense parasitaemia with few clinical effects. In the second stage the immunity becomes directed towards the elimination of the parasite. Perhaps the first stage is an immunological process analogous to the production of antibody to bacterial toxins.

Taliaferro [158] distinguished between: any or all of the antigens of a parasite which may be useful for diagnostic purposes; a restricted number of antigens of importance in relation to the induction of immunity in the host. The second group will be included in the first and, as mutually exclusive groups, internal antigens, only liberated on the disruption of the organisms, and external antigens, normally manifest on the surface of the organism, have been proposed [101]. The internal antigens will, clearly, be expected to include a large variety of materials—enzymes, and cytoplasmic and nuclear constituents. The external antigens will normally be presented to the host's immunological mechanism and there is evidence that certain protozoa may also release antigenic material into the ambient fluids in which they subsist. Thillet & Chandler (161) demonstrated this for *Trypanosoma lewisi* and called it metabolic antigen. Weitz [168, 169] demonstrated a similar, released, antigen in *Trypanosoma rhodesiense* infections in rats, which he called 'exoantigen'. Probably the released antigens are the same as one or other of the normally exhibited external antigens.

Characteristic of some protozoa, e.g. many of the *Trypanosoma* (*Trypanozoon*) spp., is a propensity for antigenic variation; the population of each successive relapse differs antigenically from those of most or all previous relapses in the same host. This variation appears to be related to alteration in the external and released antigens. How extensive is the range of variation within any given population is still uncertain but certainly it may be extensive. Also, culture forms differ antigenically from blood forms in the trypanosomes and antigenicity may vary from stage to stage in parasites which undergo complex cycles of development, such as *Plasmodium* [114].

Living organisms may be used as antigen. Where organisms are subject to antigenic variation, preservation of living material as stabilates or its rapid passage in laboratory animals will be required. When suspensions of organisms in their original ambient fluid are used, as for agglutination tests with *Trypanosoma*, both external or released antigens may be involved. Materials containing released antigen may be separated by removal of organismal bodies and tissue components by clotting, centrifugation or filtration. Separation of organismal bodies alone may be difficult and may involve disruption of host cells, the use of specific sera or phytohaemagglutinins for removal of tissue elements, and differential centrifugation and washing. The process of washing is not free from danger of affecting the antigen; Lumsden *et al* [182] have shown that rapid and catastrophic falls in the infectivity of trypanosome suspensions may follow exposure to certain hydrogen-ion concentrations. Once separated, organisms may be used alive or in suspensions killed with formalin or in other ways. Or antigens may be prepared from them by disruption in the Hughes press [85], in the Mickel disintegrator [78], by ultrasonication or by lyophilization and trituration [148], with or without further extraction or purification.

Preparation of antisera

Few special processes have been developed for the preparation of antisera against protozoal antigens. As regards the antisera developed to infections of living trypanosomes Cunningham & Vickerman [45] infected rabbits and bled them after about 14 days; this period is on the long side for antisera specifically related only to the infecting organism. A more satisfactory procedure is likely to be infection of the animal with a large dose and drug treatment at a time appropriate to suppress second and later parasitaemic waves possibly of different antigenic type [183]. As regards the preparation of sera to killed antigen the usual approaches have been employed, simple injection or the concomitant use of potash alum [169], or Freund's adjuvant [148].

Immunological tests of application in protozoology related to reduced host reactivity

Modification of the course of the infection *in vivo*

Knowledge of the susceptibility of the hosts under experiment is fundamental. The susceptibility of a given host species to particular parasites will usually be known but the establishment of the status of individual animals may be less straightforward. Some parasites may infect, but multiply at such low levels that their presence is difficult to detect and these infections, naturally acquired, may induce an active specific immunity which will affect the interpretation of subsequent challenge experiments. Such situations are likely to arise in experimentation with parasites whose only hosts are large animals difficult to isolate from natural transmission, such as *Theileria* spp. in cattle in Africa.

When specific modification of the course of the infection with a protozoal parasite has been demonstrated it may be uncertain to what extent humoral or cellular mechanisms are involved. That humoral mechanisms are operative when alteration in reactivity follows passive immunization procedures is a justifiable assumption. The corresponding assumption regarding active immunization procedures is more open to doubt, but there exist situations in which although humoral antibodies could not be demonstrated by passive procedures their existence can be deduced from other data. An example is the dissemination of immunity through the body from infections restricted to particular sites, such as occurs in *Eimeria* infection in fowls between experimentally infected and non-infected portions of the gut [26]. Also, there are many situations in which other evidence suggests the importance of humoral antibodies in actively induced resistance. Examples of active immunization will, therefore, be considered.

Immunity to challenge will not be expected to be absolute but will depend on the quality and quantity of the insult administered. Protozoa differ in their propensity to retain infectivity in culture and on serial passage. For instance, Adler [3] records that strains of *Leishmania tropica* retained infectivity for man, but not for *Cricetulus*, after maintenance in culture for 20 years. *Trypanosoma* spp. of the group Salivaria are typically non-infective in culture, reproducing the developmental stages occurring in *Glossina* but failing to reach metacyclic infective development. The antigenic changes taking place in trypanosomes maintained in laboratory animals are well known. Quantitation and quality-control of the challenge may be accomplished for favourable materials, such as some *Trypanosoma* spp., by setting up stabilate material, establishing its antigenic type and titrating its infectivity in small animals before experimental use [104]. But with many organisms, because of long prepatent periods, subclinical or latent infections, and other factors, challenge dose may be difficult to measure. In some protozoa another complication arises, that the organism performs more than one type of development in the host, each type differing in its propensity to stimulate antibody response. An example is *Plasmodium* in which antibody reaction to the sporozoite and pre-erythrocytic cycles are negligible and only the parasites of the erythrocytic cycle are significantly antigenic [33]. Also in these parasites, the factors of parasite multiplication in the pre-erythrocytic stage are typically large, so that a given sporozoite dose may be greatly multiplied before the parasites are exposed to any antibody reaction on the part of the host. The importance of these considerations with regard to the interpretation of challenge experiments has been very properly emphasized by McGregor [114].

Leishmania

The variability of infectivity to mammal hosts of *Leishmania* spp. maintained in culture is notorious [3]; *L. tropica* may lose infectivity for *Cricetulus*, a host to which it is invariably lethal on first isolation, after less than 2 years. However, it maintains its infectivity for man apparently unchanged for periods of 20 years and so challenge experiments carried out in man are less difficult to interpret than when made in other hosts. In this example, the introduction of parasites, either from natural lesions or from cultures, into the dermis of a non-immune subject stimulates a local histiocyte proliferation in which leishmania forms multiply. Later, lymphocyte and plasma cells infiltrate, the histiocytes diminish in numbers, and with them the parasites, which latter eventually disappear. This spontaneous cure is followed by lasting resistance to challenge by the infecting strain. The role of antibodies in this immunity is uncertain. Humoral antibodies have not been demonstrated by classical methods in cutaneous leishmaniasis but immunity, once established, is generalized throughout the dermis [10].

As regards visceral leishmaniasis, persons cured by chemotherapy do not undergo further attacks although some 70 per cent subsequently develop dermal leishmaniasis. Intradermal and subcutaneous inoculation of East African dermatropic *Leishmania donovani* may induce an immunity not only to the same dermatropic material but also to *L. donovani* from other parts of the world, but not to *L. tropica* [120, 121]. This freedom from, or modification of, infection is due to the immune response of the host [3]. Humoral antibodies to *Leishmania* can be demonstrated in the serum by complement-fixation tests. There is also a large increase in serum γ globulin [3].

Trypanosoma
The normal course of the infection of *T. lewisi* in the non-immune rat host consists of an initial period of about 6 days, during which multiplication is intense and the organisms are highly variable in size, followed by a crisis which reduces the population to a few individuals of uniform large size, the so-called 'adult' trypanosomes; this latter population persists for a few weeks before a second crisis ends the infection. To account for these events Taliaferro, and his colleagues, in an extensive series of papers [158], suggested that the antibodies formed by the host consist of (a) a lytic antibody responsible for the first crisis, (b) an antibody producing metabolic effects, in particular inhibiting reproduction without being immediately lethal, so controlling the population to low levels but not extinguishing it, and (c) a second lytic antibody causing the termination of the infection [46]. The evidence for the reproduction-controlling antibody, called 'ablastin', comprises changes in the mean and in the variability of the length of organisms in the blood during the course of the infection, the demonstration that reproduction of inoculated organisms can be inhibited by the concurrent inoculation of a serum from an animal with an established infection, but apparently without the inoculated organisms being destroyed, and that the inhibiting action of such a serum cannot be absorbed by incubation with trypanosomes even though trypanocidal activity *in vitro* is abolished. Thillet & Chandler [161], however, recorded that the passive protection afforded by such sera could be absorbed

by the metabolic products accumulating in the ambient fluid of a trypano-some suspension incubated *in vitro*. They regarded ablastin as an antibody against metabolic products. The ablastin concept has been criticized by Ormerod [130] who points out that a change in antigenicity between the 'developmental' and 'adult' stages could account for the observed effects. In particular he suggests that the apparent non-absorbability of ablastin-containing serum could be accounted for by the trypanosomes used for absorption having been harvested at peak parasitaemia, when they might already have been saturated with antibody, and that the continued infectivity of suspensions exposed to ablastin-containing serum might be due to the presence of adult forms of different antigenic type not susceptible to the antibodies to developing forms contained therein.

D'Alesandro [46] investigated the effect of inoculation of individual frac-tions of the sera of *T. lewisi*-immune rats, separated by ultracentrifugation or by starch electrophoresis, in the course of the infection in non-immune hosts. Experimental rats were inoculated intra-peritoneally with trypano-somes and 1 day later, when parasitaemias were still low, received the serum fractions by the same route. Ultracentrifuge fractions were titrated on a serum protein/body weight basis; after preliminary similar titration to locate the main area of activity, electrophoretic fractions were inoculated as whole individual eluates to single infected animals. Estimates of trypanocidal acti-vity were made by comparing the trypanosome concentrations in the peri-pheral blood immediately before the administration of the serum fraction with those obtaining 24 hours later. For studies of ablastic activity, sera were absorbed prior to electrophoresis with 10^9 organisms per ml of serum. Reproductive activity of the trypanosome population in rats passively treated with the electrophoretic fractions was assessed by comparing the proportion of dividing forms, and organisms less than 20 μ long among total population, during the 4 days following the administration of the fraction, with the same proportion observed in control rats.

As regards the recognition of actively induced immunity, Corradetti [184] showed that, following a primary attack of *T. lewisi*, rats were refractory to reinfection. Even splenectomized such animals showed no parasitaemia, or only a transient one, following further challenge. Thillet & Chandler [161] compared the immunogenicity of homogenates of *T. lewisi* organisms with that of the metabolic products released by organisms to the ambient. The trypanosomes, in the blood of infected rats during the phase of intense multi-plication, were washed, suspended in 50 per cent rat serum in saline at a concentration of 2×10^8 parasites per ml, and incubated at 27·5° C for 24 hours. The organisms and supernate were separated by centrifugation, the former being washed and disrupted by freezing and thawing until non-infec-tive, the latter filtered through sintered glass filters. The two products were used to immunize rats, injections were made into one group of rats of 4×10^9 disrupted organisms, into another of the metabolic products of the same organisms. These groups, and appropriate controls, were challenged. Intense parasitaemias occurred in the control animals, modified parasitaemias in those animals receiving disrupted organisms, but the rats receiving metabolic products never became parasitaemic at all.

Results with the salivarian trypanosomes were similar. Animals may be passively protected by immune sera. For instance, Seed [148] inoculated mice IP with such a number of washed trypanosomes as would produce low parasitaemias 24 hours later. At that time he inoculated the infected mice with normal rabbit serum and antisera prepared in rabbits to homologous and other antigenic variants. Protection was judged by average survival time and homologous protection was shown. Lourie & O'Connor [100] and Fulton & Lourie [65] infected mice with *T. brucei* Subgroup organisms and *T. congolense*, cured them with drugs, and challenged them by IP inoculation of living organisms. Resistance was judged by the subsequent incidence of parasitaemia, whether or not it occurred, or by the duration of the prepatent period. Mice might be completely immune to such challenge for more than 200 days after the cure of the infection. In experimentation of this sort it is to be remembered that some drugs have remarkably long prophylactic effects [165, 106]. Weitz [169] demonstrated that the serum of rats at the height of the infection with *T. brucei* Subgroup organisms contains a released soluble antigen—exoantigen—and if inoculated into non-immune hosts would immunize them against homologous challenge.

Eimeria

Unsuccessful efforts to immunize susceptible animals by passive methods or by active methods using non-infective antigens have been summarized [84, 12]. Horton-Smith and colleagues [84] demonstrated specific homologous resistance to a challenge of 2×10^7 oocysts following two immunizing infections initiated with 5×10^5 and 5×10^6 oocysts, successively, of *Eimeria acervulina*. Similarly, fowls immunized with 5×10^2 and 5×10^3 oocysts, successively, withstood challenges of 1×10^7 oocysts of *E. tenella*, *necatrix* and *maxima*. There were no clinical signs of infection and reproductive indices (the number of oocysts produced divided by the number of oocysts fed) diminished with succesive infections, from thousands in the first, to zero in the third infection. Similar results were obtained with *E. meleagrimitis* [12] and, after a single infection, with *E. stiedae* in the rabbit [84].

Experiments with *E. tenella* in fowls with ligated caeca demonstrated that the distribution of infection is solely by the lumen of the gut, and that sporozoites do not migrate between the caeca by the circulation or by any other route. Nevertheless, resistance, sometimes complete, could be induced in a ligated and, therefore, uninfected caecum, by an infection elsewhere in the gut, or in the main gut by infection of a ligated caecum, indicating that humoral antibody is involved in resistance [26, 82, 84]. On the other hand, administration of whole sera, or the γ globulin fraction of the serum from resistant animals, did not protect susceptible subjects from challenge, either with *E. stiedae* or *E. tenella*. Nor did the injection of antigen prepared from these species protect against subsequent challenge although precipitating, and in *E. stiedae*, complement-fixing antibodies, as demonstrable after natural infections, were produced.

Plasmodium

Garnham & Bray [70] describe the mechanism of immunity against *P. cynomolgi* in *Macaca mulatta*. The host reaction is ineffective against pre-erythrocytic schizonts in the liver and also against the first-generation erythrocytic schizonts; second and subsequent generations of the latter, however, are suppressed. The importance of quantitative aspects of challenge in plasmodial infections, particularly the factor of multiplication in the pre-erythrocytic stage, has been emphasized by Coggeshall [31] and McGregor [114]. McGregor suggests that the general belief that immunity in human malaria is specific for parasite strains [34] may be untrue, as the investigations on which it is based were made in ignorance of the reproductive capacity of pre-erythrocytic forms, and the challenge used may have overwhelmed the measure of immunity possessed by the hosts.

The passive transfer of immunity in simian malaria by means of serum is reviewed by Coggeshall [31]. Essentially, immune serum from chronically infected monkeys protected, but against only minimal numbers of homo-logous parasites. The transfer of immunity required large quantities of serum, about 26 ml per kg body weight [33]. Garnham & Cohen [unpublished, quoted by 34], working with *Plasmodium cynomolgi*, showed that protective activity was associated with the γ globulin, not with other serum protein fractions; the IV inoculation of 150 mg/kg body weight suppressed infections if given at the beginning of visible parasitaemia but was inactive against established infections. The IgG fraction of the serum of adult humans, living in a hyperendemic area in West Africa was found to be protective to children suffering from severe parasitaemia resident in the same areas [35, 34]. The IgG fraction was prepared from the serum of healthy adult Africans by chromatography on a diethylaminoethyl (DEAE) cellulose column. The γ globulin fraction, judged pure by paper and starch-gel electrophoresis, was injected IM (total dose 1·2–2·5 g per child) to children weighing 5·4–12·6 kg with *P. falciparum* parasitaemias of $10–230 \times 10^6$ parasites per ml. The course of the parasitaemia was little affected for 2 days following the injection but by 4 days afterwards parasitaemias were drastically reduced and by 9 days practically abolished. There was, also, alleviation of the clinical illness. In control children treated similarly, but with the other serum protein fraction of low IgG content, or with γ globulin from United Kingdom donors, still showed high parasitaemias on day 9 after treatment.

There is some other evidence of the presence of passively acquired immunity to malaria. The relative resistance to natural challenge of infants born in hyper-endemic areas is ascribed to the acquisition of antibody from their mothers [34]. Parallel examples occur in laboratory animals, e.g. in rats born to mothers immune to *Plasmodium berghei* [160]. Manwell & Goldstein [122] found that birds receiving inoculations of serum from birds immune to *P. circumflexum* withstood infective inoculation and parasites could not be recovered from them by inoculation of blood into susceptible hosts. Birds receiving immune serum after inoculation were less protected, but a higher degree of homologous, as compared to heterologous, immunity was distinguished. Hegner & Eskridge [81] obtained similar results with *P. cathemerium.*

As regards active immunization there are many examples in laboratory animals. Manwell & Goldstein [122] found that chronic infection of birds with *P. circumflexum* protected against subsequent infection. Cowper & Woodward [39] and Corradetti [184] showed that in rats surviving a primary attack of *P. berghei* further inoculations of parasites induced only a slight parasitaemia or none at all. Cox [40] treated the initial infection of *P. vinckei* in mice with chloroquine and, provided the initial parasitaemia had been sufficiently long, could only induce fleeting parasitaemias by subsequent challenge. Coggeshall [31] found that *Macaca* monkeys recovered, following treatment, from an acute infection of *P. knowlesi*, could withstand the IV inoculation of large numbers of homologous organisms; they were removed within a few hours from the blood stream. The immunity was homologous only; a few parasites of the morphologically similar *P. inui* gave rise to an infection typical of that expected in a normal monkey.

In human malaria, observation of the effects of natural challenge shows that children in hyper-endemic areas undergo severe clinical attacks soon after the third month of life when the maternal antibodies are dissipated. Later there is again a reduction in frequency and severity of clinical attack which is ascribed to the acquisition of antibodies following infection. McGregor *et al* [116, 115] and Gilles & McGregor [73] showed that the percentage of γ globulin in total protein as determined by electrophoresis paralleled this acquisition and that there was significant difference between subjects protected from malarial attack by drugs and those given only a placebo. A further demonstration of the acquisition of immunity is the discrepancy, in the estimates of inoculation rate in nature, between the high estimates derived from entomological data and the low estimates derived from a mathematical analysis of the infant parasite rate [110, 25]. Zuckerman *et al* [180] demonstrated resistance induced by the inoculation of non-living plasmodial material. They treated highly infected mouse blood with saponin to remove the erythrocytes, washed the parasites and disrupted them by means of the Hughes press. The product was stored at 4° C and inoculated subcutaneously into rats within 3 days on up to five occasions. Rats so treated, when challenged, exhibited lower parasitaemias, lower mortality rates and shorter patent periods, and longer prepatent periods, than did control rats.

Toxoplasma
Antiserum has little effect in preventing or curing *Toxoplasma* infection in experimental animals; parasitaemia and antibody may co-exist and hosts may die despite their possessing high-titre antibody [16]. Indeed, in rabbits immunized with killed organisms, and showing high dye-test and complement-fixation titres, infections following challenge might even be enhanced. However, following natural infection, rabbits were immune to further challenge [86].

Babesia
Hall [80] showed the progeny of cows exposed to *B. argentina* and *B. bigemina* to be less susceptible to infection with *B. argentina*, either by blood inoculation or by tick-bite, than the calves of cows with no history of infection. This is correlated with complement-fixing antibody content of the colostrum and of the serum of the calf after suckling [138].

As regards active immunity Riek [138] records that recovery from clinical infection with *Babesia* sp. in cattle leads on to a state in which further infection with the homologous parasite does not cause clinical signs although parasitaemia may occur. Schindler [147] found dogs, whole or splenectomized, resistant to further infection with *B. canis* after undergoing an induced infection; this resistance was not correlated with the presence of complement-fixing antibodies.

Theileria
Modification of the course of *Theileria* infection *in vivo* provides the main evidence for the existence of antibodies against these parasites. With some species, *T. mutans*, *T. annulata* and *T. parva*, there is a clearly defined immunity to further homologous challenge after infection but not to heterologous challenge [126, 14]. With other named species the situation may be less clearly defined and definitive results are often lacking because of difficulties in providing standard animals for experiment, in assessing the severity of the attack following challenge and of variations in the cycle of development

of the parasite in the vertebrate host. All parasite species are not uniform in their propensity to produce both exoerythrocytic and erythrocytic forms and antigenicity may vary between these forms [14]. As regards the definition of the challenge dose this presents particular difficulties. Serial blood passage of *Theileria* may result in the loss of erythrocytic forms, sometimes transmission either by blood or by tissue inoculation is difficult and it is necessary to transmit by tick-bite [14]. Thus the provision of a reproducible standard challenge for experimental purposes is not yet possible. To aid the assessment of the intensity of reaction of animals under challenge Sergent *et al* [150] have proposed a 'crisigramme', a graphic method by which observations on parasitaemia and pyrexia are summed; but decisions as to immunological identity may still be questioned because of the wide differences in the virulence of strains [149, 150, 5, 6].

As regards passive immunization against *Theileria* by the injection of serum, the results are contradictory and confused and it is concluded [14] that the evidence for the existence of protective antibody in the serum of animals which have undergone *Theileria* infection is not yet conclusively proven. That recurrence of parasitaemia usually follows splenectomy in immune animals [126] is, however, indicative of its occurrence.

In vitro demonstration of humoral antibody

Directly observable effects of antibody on the organismal body
Morphological modification
Leishmania
Specific antisera to *Leishmania* spp., prepared in rabbits, show no appreciable parasiticidal properties, but they change the morphology of the organisms, affecting flagellar growth and activity, cell division and cell agglomeration. The organisms grow in clumps of leishmania forms alone, or of leptomonads with incompletely developed flagella, or of agglomerated leptomonads with normal flagella, depending on the concentration of serum used; large multinucleated aflagellar syncytia may be formed [3].

Trypanosoma
Adler [2] observed the effects of specific antiserum on the behaviour of *T. cruzi* in culture. Two approaches were used, adding specific antiserum to fully grown cultures, and growing the organisms in the presence of specific antiserum. Culture media were chosen in which the organisms typically produced a uniform growth, not forming rosettes, clumps or leishmania forms. Semi-solid Locke-serum-agar was one suitable medium. Specific

antisera were prepared in rabbits by IV inoculation. To observe the effect on fully grown cultures, the antiserum was distributed in the desired concentrations to culture medium in tubes and then organisms were added in quantities exceeding the maximal growth on normal medium. To avoid agglutination of organisms in growing cultures, the inoculated organisms were distributed in 2 ml of the medium by shaking and rolling, the antiserum then added and distributed in the medium by the same treatment. Specific antisera added to normal cultures caused agglutination, chain-formation and immobilization of most, but not all, of the organisms; antiserum titres were expressed as the highest dilution causing such effects. In fully developed normal cultures antiserum caused immobilization, clumping and network formation, and discard of flagella; multicellular masses without trace of cell walls were formed rapidly. In cultures grown in the presence of antisera, at concentrations which still, however, permitted growth, irregular syncytial masses of organisms were formed, with flagella projecting at various points or submerged in the interior of the mass. After this period of chaotic growth, reorganization again took place and leishmanial, crithidial or trypanosome forms were developed, leishmania and trypanosome forms at higher, crithidia at lower, antiserum concentrations.

Toxoplasma

Strannegård [156] used morphological alteration of *T. gondii* in cell culture to study the effect of specific antibodies. Activator (properdin) was important in the reaction. Activator alone produced morphological alteration, which, however, differed from that caused by the complete system.

Immobilization

Entamoeba

Zaman [176] comments that as some *Entamoeba* spp. cannot be grown axenically, and as it is not possible to wash the organisms free of bacteria, that an immobilization test, involving only direct observation of the effect of antibody on the organisms, avoids complications caused by the presence of bacterial antigens. Antisera were prepared by injecting rabbits IV with organisms washed four times in normal saline. Each animal received $3–4 \times 10^6$ organisms. Sera were inactivated. Organism suspensions containing about 5×10^4 organisms per ml were added to the serum dilutions. It was found important to use young cultures with active trophozoites as cysts and precysts could be mistaken for immobilized organisms. The state of 100 organisms was observed in a haemacytometer cell and the highest concentration producing complete immobilization was regarded as the titre of the serum. Tests were made at room temperature, except with *Entamoeba coli* and *histolytica*, which were made at 37° C. Cross-reactions were studied by observing the degree of immobilization of heterologous organisms at a dilution corresponding to the homologous immobilization titre [176].

The reaction took place in three phases—an initial phase in which organisms became rounded, an intermediate one in which they were immobilized and a terminal phase when they were again released. If the sera were not inactivated, lysis occurred. *Entamoeba* sp. of restricted activity, such as *E. coli*, were found unsuitable for this approach. Immobilization titres were comparatively low, 1/30 being the highest obtained, as compared with titres of 1/1000 or more with *Paramecium* spp. [176]. Adam [1] used the technique to illuminate the taxonomy of the hartmanellid amoebae.

Eimeria

Augustin & Ridges [12] studied the motility of the merozoites of *E. meleagrimitis* in the sera of the immune and non-immune turkeys and in other fluids. Three- to four-week-old birds were given each 75×10^4 sporulated oocysts and were killed about 98 hours later after being starved for at least 6 hours. The duodenum was removed, cut to expose its mucous lining, and immersed in physiological saline or Ringer's solution at 37° C. The pieces of duodenum were agitated to detach the merozoites, and then removed. The suspension was centrifuged to concentrate the merozoites and was used immediately afterwards for experiment. The suspension was added to saline, Ringer's solution with or without 0·5 per cent gelatine, unheated fresh normal turkey serum (containing complement), inactivated or stored normal turkey serum (complement-free), and immune turkey serum, both fresh and inactivated. The mixtures were incubated at 37° C and samples were removed at intervals for examination by phase-contrast microscopy on a warm stage. In saline or in Ringer's solution or in inactivated normal serum, merozoites remained active for 2–3 hours. In inactivated immune serum, the merozoites became sluggish after 20 minutes' exposure and a precipitate began to form at their pointed ends. The precipitate thereafter increased, the merozoites shortened, and their cytoplasm appeared to be extruded through pores at their pointed ends. By $2\frac{1}{2}$ hours the merozoites had practically disappeared. In non-inactivated sera, whether immune or not, merozoites disappeared in less than an hour.

Balantidium

Zaman [177] used *Balantidium* strains isolated in laboratory culture from pigs and from man, and antisera prepared in rabbits by the inoculation of about 8×10^4 cells. Test and control sera were inactivated, otherwise the organisms were lysed. 0·25 ml of *B. coli* suspension of a concentration of 5×10^4 organisms per ml was added to serial dilutions of the serum in saline. Tubes were incubated at about 20° C. The highest serum dilution producing immobilization in 30 minutes was regarded as the serum titre. The highest titres obtained were 1/64, as compared with 1/1000 or more with *Paramecium* [15].

Glaucoma-Colpidium

Robertson [140] found these organisms delicate and difficult to separate undamaged from culture medium for serological use by centrifugation and resuspension; she therefore used as living antigen suspensions 3- to 4-day-old cultures in peptone water diluted with 0·2 per cent peptone in 0·5 per cent NaCl so as to give concentrations of $5–10 \times 10^3$ per ml. Antisera were prepared by the IV inoculation of $13–33 \times 10^6$ washed living organisms into a rabbit. Mixtures of antigen suspension and of serum dilutions in 0·5 per cent NaCl were made both in tubes and in petri dishes. The organisms required to be shielded from light. Normal, complement-containing, sera of rabbits, guinea-pigs and rats killed, agglutinated or lysed organisms up to dilutions of 1/160; inactivated, they were without direct effect. Moderately potent antisera immobilized organisms in 5–10 minutes. There was also an emission of a transparent exudate, containing refractive particles, which held the slightly motile organisms together. With more potent antisera the pellicle of the organisms was thickened either in a fragmentary way or as a uniform sheath to the organism. 'Agglutination' with exudate was well developed but the organisms were rarely completely immobile. Although some individuals were killed, progressive recovery took place after about 6 hours and ultimately the organisms escaped from the sheaths, which were left as delicate perfect shells adherent to each other. With highly potent antisera thick sheaths were rapidly produced; recovery was later and frequent only at the higher dilutions, beyond 1/640. Additions of complement to the reaction enhanced the effect and caused lysis at high dilutions.

Paramecium

Antisera were prepared in rabbits by the IP inoculation of about $10^{4·9}$ washed living organisms [18] or by the IV inoculation of suspensions of fragments of 'a few thousand' individuals, washed and then broken up by being passed through a fine injection needle [15]. Several (up to 7) injections were made at 3- to 4-day [15] or weekly [18] intervals. Antisera so prepared were inactivated before use and stored at 0° C with or without the addition of phenol. Serum dilutions were made in a salt solution imitative of the constitution of spring water [18] or in Ringer's solution [15]. The organisms to be used for testing were stranded on filter paper and washed with the same diluent as used for the serum, then suspended in diluent and washed two or three times, the final suspension being adjusted to contain about 500 organisms per ml. 0·02 ml quantities of this suspension, containing 5-20 organisms, were added to 0·2 ml quantities of the serum dilutions and the mixtures were incubated at 28° C for 2 hours. A serum-free control was included. The titre of a serum was taken as the highest dilution at which immobilization occurred [18, 15].

The sequence of events following the introduction of *Paramecium* into a solution containing homologous antiserum is characteristic. Organisms first show an 'avoiding' reaction, making irregular reversals in their direction of movement and rapid motions from side to side. Forward movement slows and finally ceases. Ciliary movement continues for some time after the organism comes to a standstill; it persists longest in the gullet. Cytoplasmic circulation endures longer than ciliary movement, but finally death supervenes. Agglutination does not take place. Antisera are typically specific for particular antigenic types and can often be used without absorption [15].

Agglutination

Leishmania

Noguchi [128] and Adler & Theodor [7] used agglutination reactions to study the relationships between the *Leishmania* spp. affecting man and *Herpetomonas* spp. isolated from insects and plants. Suspensions of culture organisms in saline (1 ml) were tested against 0·05 ml quantities of antisera prepared by the IV inoculation of culture material to rabbits. Gross examination and dark-ground microscopy were carried out on the suspension for up to 24 hours. Agglutination was recognizable macroscopically by clearing of the turbid suspension and formation of a sediment, microscopically by the swelling and distortion of the cell body and twisting and adherence of the flagella, leading on to lysis.

Trypanosoma

Soltys [154] demonstrated agglutinating antibody to *T. brucei* Subgroup organisms and to *T. congolense* in the sera of rabbits which had been infected and which had received formalinized trypanosome suspensions. As antigen he used suspensions of living trypanosomes harvested from infected mice at peak parasitaemia, separated and suspended in Alsever's solution with horse serum. Cunningham & Vickerman [45] refined the method by using stabilate material as antigen. The blood of infected mice, on the second or third day of infection, having about 4×10^8 organisms per ml, was preserved in capillary tubes [43]. Antisera were prepared in rabbits. The test was performed on glass plates, 1 μl of the thawed stabilate material being added to 0·1 ml quantities of the serum dilution; the plates were incubated at 25° C in a humid atmosphere for 1 hour. Cunningham & Grainge [41] carried out tests in small drops of antiserum dilution laid out on siliconed glass slides; seventy-five tests could be made on one slide, antigen being added to the drops by means of a glass capillary drawn out finely. Agglutinating antibodies to trypanosomes have been detected in the meals of blood-sucking insects by this method; the host species from which blood meals are derived may be determined serologically [170] so that a possibility is opened of studying the antibody status of wild animals without their capture.

Weitz [168, 169] showed that the antibody response of hosts to trypanosome infection was not only to the bodies of the organisms. Normal rats were inoculated with trypanosome-free serum prepared from infected rats. Antisera so prepared agglutinated homologous living trypanosomes *in vitro*. The reaction was inhibited by the serum of infected, but not of uninfected rats [171]. Weitz interpreted these effects, together with evidence of precipitating antibody, as indicating that trypanosome populations released antigenic material—'exoantigen'—into the ambient.

Bodo

The action of antibody to *B. caudatus* was studied by Robertson [139]. The organism required a bacillus as food supply but, this supplied, could be cultivated in simple salt solutions or in distilled water. Antisera were prepared most satisfactorily by IV inoculation of washed organisms suspended in 0·1 per cent formol saline into rabbits; inoculation was commenced with 10^7 organisms, rising to 2×10^8 organisms per dose later. Living organisms from cultures were washed and suspended at a concentration of 5–7×10^5 per ml. Antisera were serially diluted and 2 ml quantities of the dilutions and of the antigen suspension were mixed in tubes and then poured into petri dishes. Incubation was at about 20° C, shielded from light, and observation by microscope, was extended to 24 hours. Agglutination of the accompanying bacteria took place in the higher serum concentrations but did not confuse observation of the *Bodo*. Reactions were complex. In the first place *Bodo* may aggregate spontaneously under the influence of various factors such as CO_2 accumulation, and also attach naturally by the longer flagellum to certain particles. In inactivated homologous antisera agglutination took place to titres as high as 1/6400, but the reactions were complicated by immobilization; when immobilization took place the organisms stuck to the glass and so agglutination was reduced. Death of organisms was considered a more consistent index of antibody activity; inactivated normal sera were not lethal even at 1/5 dilution though they might agglutinate organisms to titres not far short of those obtained with homologous antisera.

Trichomonas

Pierce [135] described extensive experience with the test devised by Kerr & Robertson [94] with *T. foetus*. The antigen suspension was prepared from cultures towards the end of the phase of rapid cell division. The organisms were washed in glucose saline and a suspension of concentration 10^5 organisms per ml made up. 1·5 ml quantities of this antigen were mixed with equal volumes of the test serum dilutions and the mixtures poured into petri dishes which were then incubated. The test was read under the low-power microscope. Normal serum, positive serum and saline controls were included, as *T. foetus* suspensions were found to vary in sensitivity. Sera for test were centrifuged and inactivated; no preservatives were admissible. Because normal cattle sera, even inactivated, contained agglutinins for *T. foetus* a system of scoring of reactions was necessary to distinguish positive results. Reactions varied from 'pre-agglutination', characterized by immobilization without clumping, and 'echelon', leaf-like, clumping at high, to occasional small aggregations at low, antibody concentrations. An index of agglutinating activity was calculated for each serum on these bases. *T. foetus* strains varied widely in their agglutinability, particularly recently isolated strains; but even strains regularly used for test might temporarily increase in sensitivity.

Pierce [135] developed the test to demonstrate agglutinins in vaginal mucus or uterine secretion [95]. 2 ml quantities of serial dilutions of the test material were mixed with 2 ml quantities of an agar solution fluid at 60° C. The mixtures were poured into petri dishes and allowed to solidify. 1·5 ml quantities of a *T. foetus* suspension, prepared as described above, were then pipetted on to the agar surface. The plates were incubated and examined under the low-power microscope. The intensity of the reaction was scored; agar, agar-saline, uninfected and infected mucus and normal serum controls were included.

Eimeria

McDermott & Stauber [109] prepared suspensions of second-generation merozoites of *Eimeria tenella* from the caeca of chickens killed 5 days after being infected. The caeca were washed out with saline, and the caecal mucosa scraped off. This material was homogenized and digested with trypsin. From this suspension, by washing and suspension in formol saline, a concentrated suspension of merozoites with minimum extraneous material was prepared; it was stored refrigerated. The merozoites were agglutinated by the sera of chickens and rabbits inoculated with the suspensions and also by the sera of experimentally infected chickens. Agglutination titres were highest, reaching 1/320, between days 10 and 15 after infection and persisted for at least 30 days after infection. Absorption of antisera with suspensions of uninfected mucosa did not reduce their agglutinating capacity.

Plasmodium

Eaton [55] described a test for antibody agglutinating *Plasmodium knowlesi*. The antigen was prepared from the citrated blood of *Macaca mulatta*, moribund with acute infections, in which 20 per cent or more of the erythrocytes were parasitized. The erythrocytes were deposited by centrifugation, separated from plasma, resuspended in saline, and redeposited by slow centrifugation or allowed to settle by gravity. The brown layer of parasitized cells and leucocytes above the more rapidly settling unparasitized cells was used as antigen. The cells were resuspended in saline at an opacity equivalent to that of a 0·5 per cent suspension of erythrocytes. At least 50 per cent of the erythrocytes of the suspension should be parasitized and the suspension should be free of clumps, not contain an excess of leucocytes and be brown rather than red in colour; a red colour indicated that too many normal cells and young parasites were present. Sera to be tested for antibody were inactivated. 0·3 ml quantities of antigen suspension were mixed with serum dilutions and allowed to stand for 2 hours. Agglutinated cells settled as granules, unagglutinated cells settled compactly without granule formation. Microscopical examination of the deposits was used to confirm the result. Or the test was performed as a hanging drop; in this case agglutination was evident, with strongly positive sera, in 15–30 minutes. The macroscopic technique required suspensions in which over 50 per cent of the cells were parasitized. The microscopic test recognized agglutination at higher serum dilutions and was effective with suspensions containing only 5–10 per cent of infected cells; in addition it distinguished specific agglutination of parasitized cells from non-specific agglutination of erythrocytes and spontaneous clumping of cells. Sera from twelve infected *Macaca* showed agglutinin titres of 1/4 to 1/1024. Sera from uninfected *Macaca* showed no agglutinating activity against *P. knowlesi* antigen; nor did sera from monkeys infected with *Plasmodium inui*.

The antigen was difficult to prepare as standard suspensions of predictable sensitivity; equivocal results occurred with weakly reacting sera. It deteriorated rapidly at 0° C. Suspensions of free parasites were agglutinated in a similar way but were not more sensitive than antigen prepared from unhaemolysed parasitized cells.

Toxoplasma

Suspensions of parasites free from other cells for agglutination and other tests have been prepared by Fulton & Turk [68], Fulton & Spooner [66] and Fulton [64]. *Sigmodon* (cotton rat) of 100–200 g weight were inoculated with about 2×10^6 *Toxoplasma gondii* and killed on day 3. The peritoneal exudate, of volume about 4 ml per rat, was collected by pipette, passed through 'gauze', and centrifuged for 15 minutes at 2500 *g*. The deposit, after rejection of the supernate, was resuspended in buffered saline by shaking gently with glass beads, and allowed to stand for a few minutes. Many leucocytes agglutinated and could be removed by pipette. The suspension was then passed through a sintered glass filter of pore size 15–40 *μ* by gentle suction and the filter washed with a volume of saline equal to that of the suspension. The suspension, now free of leucocytes, was centrifuged at 1800 *g* for 5 minutes and the parasites resuspended in saline. Any erythrocytes present were agglutinated by anti-erythrocyte rabbit serum or haemolysed by guinea-pig serum, refiltering being carried out if necessary. The parasites, now free from other cells, were washed several times and suspended in 0·5 per cent formalin in buffered saline (pH 7·4) to a specified optical density. The suspensions were kept at 2° C and shaken gently with glass beads before use. They were diluted 1/4 in formal saline for use and 0·4 ml quantities were added to similar quantities of twofold dilutions ranging from 1/10 to 1/10,240 of the serum under test, in glass tubes scrupulously cleaned. Controls, without serum and with a serum of known activity, were included. After shaking, the mixtures were incubated. The test was then read from below by means of a mirror. The range of titres for sera from people known to be infected was above those for sera from healthy populations. Good correlation between the results of the test and those of the dye-test was found with a series of sera of high titre. Raised agglutination titres to *T. gondii* did not occur in the sera of men or of *Cricetulus* infected with *Leishmania donovani* or in the sera of animals infected with *Trypanosoma lewisi, T. cruzi, T. vivax, T. gambiense, Plasmodium berghei* or *Spirochaeta recurrentis*. In absorption experiments, only the homologous organisms reduced titres to *Toxoplasma* antigen [62, 64]. A microtechnique has been developed [64].

Lysis
Trypanosoma
Lourie & O'Connor [100] reviewed the subject of lysis of trypanosomes by immune serum and themselves studied the matter in relation to *T. brucei* Group organisms. Antisera were prepared by the inoculation of mice, curing the infection with drug 2 days later, and harvesting the serum of the mice after another 5 days. Serum dilutions were made in 50 per cent unheated guinea-pig serum in Ringer–glucose solution. 0·45 ml quantities of the dilutions were distributed to tubes and sown with 0·025 ml quantities of suspensions in Ringer-glucose solution of washed trypanosomes at concentrations of about 2×10^7 per ml. Tubes were incubated at 37° C and samples of the suspensions withdrawn and introduced into a haemacytometer cell for counts to be made of living trypanosomes at intervals up to 24 hours. By modifications of this technique Lourie & O'Connor [100] showed: that lysis took place in the absence of complement but that rapid lysis depended on its presence; that mouse serum is anticomplementary; that guinea-pig serum dilutions of up to 1/32 are sufficient for rapid lysis; that trypanolytic titres of 1/1024 or more may occur in mouse sera collected between days 4 and 11 after infection and that thereafter, although a decline takes place, trypanolytic

activity may be detected for at least 8 months; that trypanolysis is type specific.

Le Page [personal communication] has developed a micro-method based on the immune lysis technique of Lourie & O'Connor [100]. Antiserum dilutions, in 0·025 ml aliquots, are prepared on siliconed ceramic ring slides using the micro-titre (Adams Co., U.S.A. Agents: V.A. Howe, 46 Pembridge Road, London, W.11) apparatus. 0·025 ml amounts of the trypanosome suspensions containing $1–5 \times 10^5$ organisms per ml and premixed with four lytic doses of guinea-pig complement are then added to the antiserum dilution series and, following mixing, the plates are incubated in a moist atmosphere at 37° C for 90 minutes. Coverslips are then placed on each drop and the proportion of lysed organisms in each estimated by direct observation under the phase-contrast microscope. Appropriate controls are set up to establish the complement dependence of the reaction. The diluent used for the dilution series is tris (0·01 M) buffered T.C. 199 pH 7·6 plus crystalline bovine serum albumin 0·5 per cent with penicillin 100 units per ml and dihydrostreptomycin 100 μg per ml. The diluent is membrane filtered before use, and all sera are centrifuged to remove any contaminating debris. The technique may be particularly useful for *Trypanosoma* spp. which are difficult to obtain in concentrated suspensions or which tend to auto-agglutinate, such as *T. congolense*.

Eimeria

Horton-Smith & Long [83] separated second-generation merozoites of *E. tenella* from caecal tissue of fowls by washing and centrifugation and used these and sporozoites to demonstrate lysins in the sera of immune fowls. Antigen–serum mixtures were incubated at 37° C and examined microscopically. Sera from non-immune fowls were never lytic. Nor were heated sera from immune birds, though merozoites became distorted. In unheated sera or after the addition of fresh normal fowl serum (as a complement source) to treated immune sera, lysis occurred. Sporozoites were lysed under the same conditions. However, sporocysts, obtained by the mechanical rupture of sporulated oocysts, were unaffected by immune serum with or without complement.

Indirect demonstration of humoral antibody

Neutralization of infectivity

Trypanosoma

Soltys [153] separated the organisms in infected mouse blood, taken at peak parasitaemia, and suspended them in Alsever's solution for use in neutralization tests with *T. brucei* Subgroup organisms and *T. congolense*. The antigens were tested against antisera prepared in rabbits by infection with living organisms, with or without drug treatment, and by the injection of forma-linized suspensions. The antigen suspension was added to serum dilutions and the mixtures incubated; thereafter groups of mice were inoculated with each mixture. Soltys was able to show neutralization of infectivity up to serum dilutions of 1/320 with homologous antigen–serum mixtures but not with any heterologous mixture. Since Soltys's work two developments have refined the method. The development of simple standard methods for the preservation of viable trypanosomes at low temperatures [136, 43] has allowed the long-term storage of standard material not subject to the continuous selection, and the consequent changes in characteristics, which occur during serial passage, now called 'stabilate' material [105] to distinguish it from 'strains' maintained by serial passage. Secondly, more precise ways of estimating the infectivity of trypanosomes have been developed [104] by serial dilution of suspensions and inoculation of standard quantities of each of the various dilutions into groups of mice. On the basis of the infections occurring in these groups of mice the infectivity of the suspension is estimated; it is expressed in 63 per cent infective doses for mice (ID_{63}). With tenfold dilutions and six mice at each dilution differences in infectivity of about tenfold may be recognized. The method was used to compare infectivity and numbers in trypanosome suspensions and the two parameters were found not to be constantly related; e.g. the relation varied widely from day to day during the course of the infection [185]. In combination, viable preservation and infectivity titration offer possibilities for the standardization of experiments in that previously titrated infective material is made available. Cunningham *et al* [44] have used these approaches to demonstrate the successive development of antigenic variants in a trypanosome infection in a cow, and the successive development of antibodies to these variants. Neutralization tests, also, may be applied at parasite concentrations below those possible with visual methods. Trypanosomes can be easily observed in the blood of animals only when the concentrations are about 10^6 per ml or more; infection of susceptible hosts may be obtained with only a few organisms.

Trichomonas

Teras *et al* [159] demonstrated neutralizing antibodies in the sera of human beings infected with *T. vaginalis* by intraperitoneal inoculation of mice with cultures. Lumsden *et al* [107] have developed a method for the titration of the infectivity to cultures of fresh and stabilate material of *T. vaginalis* which should have application in neutralization procedure.

Eimeria

Horton-Smith *et al* [84] record experiments in which the sporozoites of *E.*

tenella were incubated at 37° C for 1 hour in 1/3 dilutions of the sera of birds resistant to *E. tenella* and similarly in the sera of non-immune birds, and then administered to susceptible hosts. The subsequent infections were judged on mortality, on the caecal lesions induced and on oocyst production. There were no lesions in the birds receiving the suspensions incubated with immune sera; oocyst production in these birds was less than in birds receiving the non-immune serum suspension.

Similar experiments with second-generation merozoites introduced into the recta of susceptible birds gave similar results. Merozoites incubated in serum from immune birds did not develop to produce oocysts, while those incubated in serum from non-infected birds did so. There was evidence of immobilization or lysis of merozoites in immune, but not in non-immune, serum.

Augustin & Ridges [12] inoculated merozoite suspensions, prepared as described for immobilization tests (*v.s.*), mixed with saline, or with Ringer's solution containing 0·5 per cent gelatine, and immune and non-immune sera, into the duodenum exposed by laparotomy. They judged the effect of these materials by comparison of the numbers of merozoites inoculated (estimated by haemacytometer counts of formalinized samples of the suspension) and the number of oocysts produced up to 120 hours after inoculation. The peak oocyst production was between 48 and 72 hours after inoculation and there were hardly any after 96 hours. With inactivated normal serum, values of 10–12 merozoites per oocyst were obtained, with inactivated immune serum, values of 50–120. However, fresh untreated normal serum, and saline also, were effective in reducing oocyst production.

Plasmodium

Coggeshall [30, 31] described a neutralization test with *Plasmodium knowlesi* in *Macaca* monkeys. He emphasized the need to control the number of parasites in the experiment, otherwise the protective effect of a serum was obscured. The protection demonstrated was specific for *Plasmodium* spp. Samples of *P. knowlesi*, each containing 10^4 parasites, were incubated severally with 2·0, 0·2, 0·02 and 0·002 ml quantities of immune serum and with 2·0 and 0·002 ml quantities of normal serum and the suspension then inoculated individually into *Macaca* monkeys. Those monkeys receiving the suspensions containing 2·0 and 0·2 ml of immune serum were protected and survived; all the others died. Absorption of the immune serum with an excess of viable *P. knowlesi* parasites or heating to 56° C removed its neutralizing activity [30].

Toxoplasma

Sabin & Ruchman [145] and Sabin [143] assessed the neutralization of *T. gondii* by immune serum by observation of the skin reaction in rabbits following ICu inoculation. Suspensions, prepared from mouse brains 4 days after ICe inoculation, were shown by microscopy to contain large numbers of *T. gondii* and no bacteria. A 10 per cent brain suspension was prepared by grinding and allowed to sediment. The opalescent supernate was regarded as the 1/10 antigen dilution. 0·15 ml quantities of it, and of 1/50, 1/500 and 1/5000 dilutions made from it, were put up severally with 0·15 ml quantities of serum to be tested and 0·15 ml quantities of Tyrode solution as control, giving final concentrations of *T. gondii* antigen of half the above quoted values. After shaking and standing at about 20° C for 30 minutes the mixtures were injected ICu into the back of clipped rabbits; 0·2 ml of each of the mixtures was inoculated. A control series and four sera could be accommodated on one rabbit. Some rabbits were found naturally immune; insignificant lesions developed with the control mixtures and the animals survived. Skin lesions began to appear about day 4 after inoculation, after the erythema and oedema generally produced by the inoculation of human sera into rabbits, and were raised and indurated, with central necrosis in the case of the higher concentrations of organisms. They were fully developed by day 7 or 8. Sera lost neutralizing activity in 30 minutes at 56° C, in a few weeks at 4° C but not when lyophilized or stored at −79° C. The addition of complement did not restore activity to sera which had lost it. Neutralizing activity following infection was found in the sera of men and *Macaca* but not in those of mice, rabbits, dogs or cats.

Strannegård [156] showed that specific antibodies would impair the ability of *T. gondii* to penetrate cells in tissue culture; without the presence of properdin, however, only a minor antibody effect was demonstrable.

Macdonald [186] developed a test in which a suspension of *T. gondii* was exposed to dilutions of heat-inactivated sera and the number of pocks caused on the chorioallantoic membrane of embryonated hens' eggs was compared with controls. Jacobs *et al* [91] filtered *T. gondii* from mouse peritoneal exudate through a large pore filter to remove infected leucocytes, incubated the suspensions with immune sera, and then titrated the infectivity of the mixtures to mice.

Inhibition of metabolism

Trypanosoma

Desowitz [49, 50] demonstrated inhibition of the respiratory rate of *T. vivax* suspensions when exposed to homologous serum. 2 ml quantities of serum or serum dilution were placed in 20 ml Warburg respirometer flasks together with sufficient organisms, in whole citrated blood, to give concentrations of $3-6 \times 10^7$ organisms per ml. Glucose was added to raise the blood-sugar level to 350 mg per 100 ml. The oxygen consumption of the mixture was observed over a period of 1 hour at 36·5° C. Reduction of oxygen consumption was accompanied by lysis of the organisms. Inhibition of respiration was marked in undiluted serum and at a dilution of 1/10, little at a dilution of 1/50. In studies using undiluted serum [50] an index was calculated, as $100 - t/c$ (100), where t and c were the O_2 consumptions per hour in the test and control sera, respectively.

In later studies Desowitz [51] used, instead of whole infected blood, try-panosomes, separated from blood cells, washed and resuspended in the proportion of 1 volume of packed organisms to 20 volumes of saline. 0·2 ml of this suspension, with 0·25 ml of a 4 per cent glucose solution, was incubated with 2·0 ml of the serum component in the Warburg respirometer. Titres of respiratory inhibition of, usually, 1/50 to 1/70, were obtained with homologous materials.

Thurston [162], using *T. brucei* from the blood of infected rats, compared the sensitivity of the method with that of the neutralization tests of Soltys [154]. She found that O_2 consumption was reduced only by concentrations of serum which caused immobilization and lysis; little effect was caused by lower concentrations which did, however, reduce infectivity.

Toxoplasma

Fulton & Spooner [66], using pure suspensions of *T. gondii* (for preparation see agglutination, above), showed that the inhibition of respiration caused by the normal sera of some animals (but not by those of mice or man) could be largely abolished by inactivation. Anti-*Toxoplasma* sera, which gave high titres in the dye-test, also inhibited respiration in *Toxoplasma*, but there was no obvious correlation of the results of the two tests. It appears that the labile 'activator', possibly properdin, factor may be of importance in this reaction [62].

Modification of staining reaction

Toxoplasma

The dye-test of Sabin & Feldman [144] depends on the alteration of the stain-ing reaction of the organism after exposure to specific antibody. The antigen used is living *T. gondii* from the peritoneal exudate of infected mice. Besides specific antiserum, 'activator', derived from certain human sera, is necessary. Activator is stable at $-20°$ C but is destroyed by exposure to $56°$ C for 30 minutes or by 2 per cent NaCl; it appears to involve the properdin system; indeed, some authors imply that properdin alone may give a reaction with-out antibody [62]. Beverley & Beattie [20] proposed a standard test. The *Toxoplasma* antigen was maintained by IP passage in mice; the peritoneal exudate of mice 8–10 weeks old on day 3 after inoculation was used for the test: earlier, the *Toxoplasma* content was too low; later, antibody production of the mouse interfered. The exudate, reinforced by peritoneal injection of saline, if necessary, was heparinized (about 1 unit per mouse) and films were stained and examined to check that sufficient extracellular organisms were present. Intracellular *Toxoplasma* were excluded from consideration. Suspensions of widely different organismal concentrations might be used; the concentration was determined later and the results adjusted to a standard. It was important not to delay by adjusting the suspension to any standard concentration as the susceptibility of organisms to antibody rose rapidly at room temperature. The dye solution [144] consisted of 3 ml of a saturated alcoholic solution of methylene blue added to 10 ml of sodium carbonate–sodium borate buffer of pH 11; it was made fresh daily. Suitable donors were identified as sources of 'activator'-containing sera, by mixing fresh sera with the antigen, incubating and staining; only donors whose sera resulted in few or none of the *Toxoplasma* being unstained were admitted. Sera stored at $-20°$ C retained their potency for 3 or more months. Test sera were used without inactivation and dilutions were made in saline. Tubes were set up containing serum dilutions, activator and antigen with a saline control and incubated at $37°$ C for 1 hour, methylene blue was added, and the test kept at $4°$ C until read, best on the same day. The end-point was taken as the highest dilution of serum which prevented staining of 50 per cent of the *Toxoplasma* not affected by mouse antibody. One correction was applied graphically to adjust for the effect of mouse antibody and a second, based on the count of stained extracellular *Toxoplasma* in the control, to adjust to the standard—an antigen suspension containing 3×10^7 organisms per ml. The specificity of the test has been frequently called in question [62]; Awad & Lainson [13] encountered positive results with *Sarcocystis* as well as with *Toxoplasma* antisera.

Labelled antibody techniques

Techniques for labelling antibody molecules by conjugating them to fluorescein are reviewed in general by Coons [37] and described by Holborow & Johnson in Chapter 16. Problems involved in obtaining objective measurements of fluorescein-stained organisms are discussed by Goldman [77]. For electron microscope studies antibody has been labelled with ferritin [125] (see Andres, Hsu & Seegal, Chapter 15).

Leishmania
Shaw & Voller [151] used as slide antigens thin smears made from 10-day-old cultures of *L. infantum* and liver smears of hamsters infected with *L. donovani*. Slides were air dried, immersed in $0·3$ N HCl for 5 minutes, and washed twice in $0·15$ M PBS. The slide antigens were overlayed with dilutions of test sera for 45 minutes, washed for 15 minutes in PBS, overlayed with fluorescein-labelled anti-human globulin, washed again, and mounted in 10 per cent

glycerol in buffered saline. The same process was used for *L. brasiliensis* in tissue sections. The intensity of fluorescence of the parasites was estimated and the end-point was recorded as the serum dilution at which organisms were just detectable. Non-specific staining occurred only with undiluted sera. Serum from a known infected individual gave an end-point titre of 1/500. The test was only group specific, as *Trypanosoma cruzi* antigen also fluoresced after treatment with *L. infantum* serum.

Bray & Lainson [23] found that no differentiation of *Leishmania* spp. was possible by serial dilution of sera in the fluorescent antibody test; all sera stained all antigen preparations and absorption of sera extinguished the reaction irrespective of the antigen used. As regards use of the test for diagnosis of *Leishmania* infections in the field, Bray & Lainson [22] conclude that it might be useful for the diagnosis of visceral leishmaniasis, but only where trypanosomiasis was absent, and not for the diagnosis of cutaneous leishmaniasis.

Trypanosoma

Williams *et al* [174] and Sadun *et al* [146] used the indirect fluorescence technique to demonstrate antibody to *T. cruzi*, *T. gambiense* and *T. rhodesiense*. They studied both blood and culture forms and concluded that the blood forms gave in general more consistent results and brighter fluorescence. Thin blood films were made on slides from the tail blood of infected rats and an area 2 cm in diameter was defined by paint, to confine and economize reagents. First, 5 per cent formalin–rhodamine bovine albumin was added to the defined area and after 10 minutes' fixation the antigen film was washed three times with 0·1 M PBS (pH 7·0–7·2). 0·1 ml of the test serum dilution was then allowed 10 minutes' contact. After again washing with PBS the test area was exposed for 5 minutes to fluorescein-labelled anti-rabbit globulin serum, diluted so as to give brilliant fluorescence with specific antisera and practically none with normal serum, usually 1/40 or 1/60. After washing again in PBS the specimen was mounted in buffered glycerol for examination. Antisera were derived from rabbits bled at various intervals after being infected by a single IP inoculation; also sera from patients, proved to be trypanosomiasis cases by recognition of the organism, were examined using an anti-human globulin conjugate. There were extensive cross-reactions between the different antigens; cross-reactivity existed also with *T. lewisi* and it was suggested that this species might be used for laboratory diagnostic procedures, having the advantage that it is not infective to man. The technique was applicable to minute amounts of dried blood on absorbent paper using the extraction method described by Anderson *et al* [9]. Voller [166] successfully used slide antigen of *T. cruzi* fixed with acetone.

Weitz [172] conjugated antisera to the exoantigens of *T. brucei* and *T.*

vivax, respectively, with fluorescein and rhodamine and demonstrated the specificity of these antigens with organisms mixed in blood films; the organisms fluoresced, respectively, green or blue. This specificity extended to antigenic variants of the same parent strain; results paralleled agglutination tests. Conjugated antisera to the antigens of washed disintegrated organisms, on the other hand, did not distinguish the species.

Trichomonas

McEntegart *et al* [113] found that *Trichomonas vaginalis* could be differentiated from *T. foetus* (Belfast serotype) by immunofluorescence. Organisms from young cultures were deposited on slides, fixed with acetone, and dried. Antisera were prepared as described for passive haemagglutination tests for this organism. The globulin fraction was separated and conjugated to fluorescein isocyanate; the conjugate was purified by repeated ethanol fractionation and absorbed twice with liver powder. The acetone-fixed films were flooded with conjugated anti-serotype globulin, washed, and mounted in buffered glycerol for examination. Exposure to unconjugated immune globulin inhibited the attachment of subsequently applied homologous conjugate.

Kučera & Kramàř [98] demonstrated antibody in the sera of trichomoniasis patients by the indirect fluorescent method. *T. vaginalis*, from cultures washed in saline and resuspended in neutral 1 per cent formalin in saline, was used as antigen. Serum antigen mixtures were incubated at 20° C for 30 minutes and the antigen–antibody complex washed in saline and water and then dried on the slide for exposure similarly to fluorescein-conjugated anti-human γ globulin. Complementary staining was carried out with rhodamine-tagged bovine albumin. Preparations were examined in buffered glycerol.

Entamoeba

Goldman [74] found that living *E. histolytica* would not stain with fluorescein-isocyanate conjugated specific antiserum; of various killing agents tried, methyl alcohol led to the brightest fluorescence. Culture amoebae were used, washed, fixed with absolute methyl alcohol and washed and suspended in saline. Antisera were prepared in rabbits by the SC inoculation of 10^7 living culture organisms, washed so as to reduce bacterial content. Conjugates were prepared by precipitating globulins from normal and specific sera with half-saturated $(NH_4)_2SO_4$ (see Chapter 16). The globulins were reacted with fluorescein at 1–2° C overnight and purified by dialysis against normal saline until the dialysate showed little fluorescence; precipitation of the saline solution with half-saturated $(NH_4)_2SO_4$ was carried on until all the fluorescence was associated with the precipitate and none with the supernate; then dialysis against saline was carried out to remove $(NH_4)_2SO_4$.

Two to three absorptions of the material with liver powder were required to abolish non-specific staining. For use, the organisms were deposited from suspension by centrifugation, and saline dilutions of the conjugated sera were added to them after removal of the supernate. The reaction was allowed to proceed at about 20° C for a few hours or at 0° C overnight. Thereafter the organisms were deposited by centrifugation and washed for examination. Controls were included: normal serum conjugate; absorption of specific antiserum with *E. histolytica* and bacterial suspensions; precipitation of specific antibody with soluble *E. histolytica* antigen; blocking of fluorescence with unconjugated specific antiserum. *E. coli* were stained with *E. histolytica* conjugate but absorption with *E. coli* practically abolished staining with that organism while leaving that from *E. histolytica* essentially unchanged. The test necessitated subjective estimates by the examiner of the degree of fluorescence but absorption facilitated decisions.

Plasmodium

Tobie & Coatney [164] attempted to develop fluorescent antibody staining of *Plasmodium* spp. of man so that only the parasites would be visible and so the films could be scanned automatically. Antigen was prepared as thin blood films fixed in 0·1 per cent HCl and washed thereafter in PBS (pH 7·0). Antibody was provided by the globulin fraction of the serum of a long-term *P. vivax* patient, precipitated by half-saturation with $(NH_4)_2SO_4$. The precipitated material was separated by centrifugation, redissolved in PBS, dialysed till free of $(NH_4)_2SO_4$, and diluted in carbonate–bicarbonate buffered saline (pH 9·0) to 10 mg protein per ml. It was then conjugated at 40° C for 18 hours and dialysed at 4° C against PBS until the dialysate showed no fluorescence. The labelled antibody solution was stored at 4° C and absorbed twice with rabbit liver powder before use. It was allowed to react at about 20° C for 30 minutes; the films were washed in PBS and mounted in buffered glycerol for examination. Controls were of labelled normal rabbit globulin, anti-*Leptospira* globulin, and human anti-amoeba globulin. The reaction was inhibited by unlabelled specific globulin. The cytoplasm of the parasites, not the nuclei, fluoresced, best with blue-violet light. Leucocytes showed faint staining: anti-*Leptospira* and anti-amoeba sera gave no reaction. Antibody to *P. cynomolgi bastianelli* yielded fluorescence similar to that elicited by antibody to *P. vivax*. Fluorescent stippling on erythrocyte ghosts was considered likely to represent plasmodial antigen.

Voller & Bray [167] used the indirect fluorescent method to measure humoral antibody to the parasites *P. falciparum*, *P. malariae* and *P. ovale*. Air-dried thin blood films from infected children were used for antigen; fixation in dry acetone for 5 minutes and rapid drying at an atmospheric humidity of under 50 per cent, or in 0·1 per cent HCl in water or saline and transfer to PBS (pH 7·2), gave preparations which could be stained, but false positives occurred with acetone-fixed material. Test sera were from naturally infected humans and included umbilical cord blood. A commercial antiserum to human globulin conjugated to fluorescein isothiocyanate was absorbed once with liver powder before use. The antigen film was washed with PBS, exposed to test serum dilution at 23° C for 20 minutes, washed again in PBS and then exposed to 1/20 dilution of antiglobulin serum at about 20° C for 30 minutes. The film was washed for 15 minutes in PBS, and mounted in that fluid for fluorescent examination. End-points were defined, for acetone-fixed material, visible but indistinct fluorescence of parasite cytoplasm, for HCl-fixed material, the highest dilution giving brilliant fluorescence of parasite cytoplasm. Although acetone-fixed films gave positive results up to 1/120 dilution with non-immune sera, positive results up to 1/6400 occurred with immune sera. Although HCl-fixed films gave fewer false positives they suffered from the disadvantage that they would keep for only a few days as compared to weeks for acetone-fixed material. The technique failed to stain oocyst or sporozoite material from mosquitoes. Antibody was demonstrated in the sera of naturally infected individuals and in the cord blood of African infants; but the test was regarded as not entirely consistent and emphasis was placed on standardization of materials.

Toxoplasma

Goldman [75, 76] developed a test for antibodies to *T. gondii*, based on the inhibition of staining of the organism with fluorescein-labelled antibody. *T. gondii* was procured in the peritoneal exudate of mice infected 3–4 days earlier. 0·5–1·0 ml of exudate was added to 10 ml of 1 per cent formalin in 0·65 per cent saline. After standing at about 20° C for 30 minutes, the suspension was centrifuged slowly to throw down heavier particles and then the supernate removed and centrifuged to deposit the *T. gondii*. The deposited organisms were resuspended in 3 ml saline. Small drops of this suspension were allowed to dry on glass slides as areas 4–5 mm in diameter. Prepared slides were stored at −20° C. Labelled antibody was prepared from both infected human and rabbit sera. The serum was fractionated with half-saturated $(NH_4)_2SO_4$ to obtain the globulin portion. The globulin was labelled with fluorescein and the conjugate was dialysed and repeatedly precipitated with half-saturated $(NH_4)_2SO_4$ to remove uncombined fluorescein. The final product was dialysed against alkaline buffered saline and stored at −20° C. Sera were stored at −20° C and tested undiluted.

Antigen smears were removed from storage and allowed to dry thoroughly. Test serum, 0·02 ml in volume, was mixed in a tube with 0·02 ml of labelled antibody, the latter diluted 1/3 or 1/4; the entire mixture was transferred to the smear. The dilution of choice of the labelled antibody was established by experiment. Smears were incubated at 37° C in a humid atmosphere for 1 hour and then washed. They were then dried and mounted in buffered glycerol for examination. The degree of fluorescence was assessed visually, with the aid of filters, and scored in five categories varying from 'no definite fluorescence' to 'brilliant yellow-green'. The results of the test were compared with those obtained by the dye-test and by complement fixation. In the first comparison there was close correlation between the results, but not in the second. The author discusses the difficulties still involved in the application of this approach.

Carver & Goldman [27], investigating the possibility of staining *T. gondii* in tissues, found that formalin and other commonly used histological fixatives abolished staining capacity. One to seven days' fixation in an absolute ethanol–glacial acetic acid mixture (19 : 1), however, gave satisfactory results. Tissues were embedded in paraffin for sectioning. Sections were freed of paraffin and partially hydrated by passing them through xylol and ethanol dilutions and were dried in air from 70 per cent ethanol. Conjugate was added and staining allowed to take place at 37° C for 1 hour.

Babesia

Schindler [147] records the demonstration of antibodies to *B. canis* by immunofluorescence. Methods of measurement of humoral antibody to *Plasmodium* [167] have been applied to *B. divergens* infections in splenectomized *Macaca* monkeys [71].

Paramecium

Using antiserum conjugated with fluorescein isocyanate and essentially the same methods as used for immobilization studies (q.v.), Beale & Kacser [187] visualized the relation of antibody to *P. aurelia* both in living immobilized organisms and in material fixed with osmic acid, before or after fluorescent staining. Organisms were treated in suspension and after washing were examined in dilute (1/10) Ringer's solution. The technique was extended for sectioning of organisms by Beale & Mott [188]; the organisms were fixed with osmic acid, embedded in gelatine and sectioned at −8° C. Sections were treated with antibody conjugated with fluorescein or with rhodamine, or both.

Mott [125] labelled immobilizing antibody to *P. aurelia* with ferritin and exposed fixed organisms to its effect. Sections of the organisms examined by electron microscopy revealed ferritin granules on the pellicle and cilia in homologous organisms only. By counter-staining with potassium permanganate and uranyl acetate the globulin of the antibody was revealed as a fuzz on the pellicle and cilia.

Passive agglutination

Trichomonas

McEntegart [111] proposed a haemagglutination technique (for a full discussion of the methods see Herbert, Chapter 21) for the recognition of humoral antibodies to *Trichomonas vaginalis*. Antisera were prepared in rabbits by the IV inoculation of suspensions of washed organisms, a total of 5 ml, containing about 5×10^7 organisms being injected. For the sensitization of erythrocytes, antigen was extracted by the formamide method developed by Fuller [60] for the extraction of streptococcal group-specific polysaccharides. A 2 per cent suspension of sheep erythrocytes was added half to an equal volume of normal saline to provide a control suspension and half to an equal volume of a suitable dilution of the antigen in saline (usually 1/10). After mixing components, each suspension was incubated at 37° C for 1 hour. Sera for test were diluted 1/5 in saline, inactivated and absorbed at 37° C for 20 minutes, twice, with 0·1 ml of packed sheep erythrocytes per 2 ml of diluted serum. Serial dilutions of the absorbed serum were distributed in 0·2 ml volumes in tubes, 0·2 ml of sensitized erythrocytes added, the contents mixed and the tubes incubated at 37° C for 30 minutes. Controls were included to exclude heterophile and non-specific agglutination. Agglutination titres of 1/25 to 1/100 were obtained with rabbit antisera to *T. vaginalis*, lower titres with bovine antisera to *T. foetus*. A higher incidence of positive reactions, with titres up to 1/250, was obtained with sera from females shown infected with *T. vaginalis* than with 'normal' male and female sera, in which also titres never exceeded 1/20. Lanceley [99], however, found no correlation between the results of tests for humoral antibodies to *T. vaginalis* by agglutination of sensitized red cells and protozoological findings in a series of 174 male patients. There was, however, a closer correspondence in the case of female patients. McEntegart [112] showed that *T. vaginalis* and two serotypes of *T. foetus* could be distinguished by essentially the same test.

Entamoeba

Kessel *et al* [96] discuss the inconsistency of results of serological tests for *E. histolytica* when organisms grown in association with bacteria are used as antigen. They prepared antigen from *E. histolytica* grown in assocation with a non-intestinal organism—*Trypanosoma cruzi*. Culture growths were harvested, washed and centrifuged. After rejection of the supernate and upper sediment a grey mucoid sediment remained, containing large numbers of *E. histolytica*. This sediment was laked in distilled water, restored to isotonicity and centrifuged. The antigen diluted 1/20 was attached at pH 6·4 and 37° C to human O cells tanned at 20° C with concentrations of tannic acid of 1/80,000 to 1/120,000. The test showed good correlation with the

clinical and parasitological history of patients investigated and with complement-fixation results.

Plasmodium

Boyd *et al* [21] met with only limited success in their trials of techniques using
collodion particles. Stein & Desowitz [155] investigated haemagglutination
in relation to *P. berghei*, *P. cynomolgi*, *P. coatneyi* and *P. vivax* using the
infected blood of the appropriate host as antigen. The cells in heparinized
infected blood were deposited by centrifugation, washed twice, and then
haemolysed in five times their volume of distilled water. The supernate after
centrifugation being discarded, the deposit was again treated in the same way
and the deposit was washed twice in PBS (pH 7·2). The final deposit was
resuspended in 1 ml of PBS and ground in an all-glass homogenizer. The
product was centrifuged and the supernate stored at −20 or −70° C for
use as antigen. Sheep erythrocytes were used for sensitization. Sheep blood
was collected in an equal volume of Alsever's solution; after storage at about
4° C for several days, erythrocytes were washed in saline and resuspended in
9 volumes of PBS. 200 ml of suspension were treated with 50 ml of 20 per cent
formalin, the latter being contained in a cellophane bag for the first 2 hours,
then released and mixed by magnetic stirrer for 18 hours (see Chapter 21).
The cells were then washed in PBS. The cells were tanned by mixing equal
volumes of 1/20,000 tannic acid in PBS with 2·5 per cent cell suspension in the
same medium, incubating at 37° C for 15 minutes, washing and resuspending
to a 2·5 per cent concentration. Cells were sensitized by mixing equal volumes
of this concentration with antigen dilutions (1/10 to 1/100) and 4 volumes of
PBS. After 15 minutes at about 20° C they were washed and resuspended in
0·125 per cent crystalline bovine albumin in PBS. One drop of the various
suspensions was added to 0·5 ml of crystalline bovine albumin solution in
PBS and the highest antigen concentration yielding a negative pattern after 24
hours was chosen for the test; usually this was 1/50. Test sera were inactivated
and absorbed overnight at 4° C with equal volumes of sheep erythrocytes.
Twofold dilutions of the sera were made in crystalline bovine albumin in
PBS; to 0·5 ml of the serum dilution was added 1 drop of sensitized cell
suspension. Tubes were shaken and read at 4 hours and 24 hours. Sera from
P. vivax patients reacted to higher titres than did control sera from persons
apparently uninfected; the highest titres were obtained with homologous
antigen but even with *P. berghei* the average titre of infected patients was five
times higher than that of the controls. The method has been applied for
survey in the field [52].

Toxoplasma

Jacobs & Lunde [90] used the peritoneal exudate of infected mice as the source of antigen, resuspending the cells deposited by centrifugation in a volume of distilled water ten times the weight of the deposit after rejection of the supernate. After 18 hours at 5° C, and centrifugation, the supernate was readjusted to isotonicity by the addition of its volume of 1·7 per cent saline. The antigen was used to sensitize tanned sheep cells. Sera were inactivated and absorbed overnight with equal volumes of packed sheep erythrocytes. Test sera were diluted in 1/50 normal rabbit serum saline. 0·05 ml of sensitized sheep cells was added to 0·5 ml of each serum dilution; the mixture was shaken and read after 2 hours at 37° C and again, after redisturbance, after standing overnight at about 20° C. Results paralleled dye test results fairly closely; in a developing infection the test did not reveal antibodies as early as did the dye test but earlier than did complement-fixation tests.

Lunde & Jacobs [108] found that antigen so prepared lost potency rapidly when stored in solution. However, when frozen (−15° C), lyophilized or precipitated with acetone and dried from ether, it was stable for at least 5 months.

Siim & Lind [152] obtained promising results with sensitized polymethyl methacrylic plast particles. The deposit from the peritoneal exudate of mice infected 5 days previously with *T. gondii* was washed, added to 10 parts of distilled water, and extracted by alternation between −70° C and 20° C and by grinding. The fluid was centrifuged at 14,000 rev/min for 1 hour in an angle centrifuge and the supernate used as antigen to coat the particles. The particles, of diameter 0·5 μ, were added in suspension to a 1/100 dilution in saline of the antigen, to a final concentration of 0·3 per cent. The suspension was shaken for 1 hour at 20° C and then stood at 4° C for 2 days. It was then centrifuged, the sediment resuspended in the original volume of saline, 0·01 per cent merthiolate added and stored at 4° C. Test sera were inactivated and diluted serially in saline with 2 per cent inactivated negative human serum (pH 7·0–7·2). Drops of serum dilutions were placed on slides and antigen suspension added in a ratio 1/20. The slides were shaken and stored at 4° C overnight. The reaction was read with a lens (×6). With the sera of infected mice, the test paralleled the results of dye tests and haemagglutination tests with tanned red cells, but was generally less sensitive.

Opsonization

Plasmodium

Zuckerman [179] discusses attempts to demonstrate opsonins against the avian malaria parasites *Plasmodium gallinaceum* and *P. lophurae*. She [178] resuspended washed erythrocytes from an infected animal in normal fowl serum and in hyperimmune homologous serum. She then exposed chicken macrophages in *in vitro* cultures to these two suspensions for 4 hours, thereafter fixing and staining the cultures. She found that the macrophages exposed to the suspensions in normal serum were only sluggishly phagocytic. Those exposed to the hyperimmune serum suspensions, on the other hand, were encased in a 'nap' of erythrocytes, and had ingested many of them. Red cells adhered also to the glass. It was notable, however, that the ingested or adherent red cells included normal as well as parasitized cells. When the macrophages were allowed to digest their contents before being fixed and examined, and the amount of included parasite pigment was used as the indicator of the total amount of parasite substance ingested, the indices with hyperimmune sera were never more than nine times those with normal, often less, and post-infection sera could not be distinguished from normal sera. Zuckerman [179] discusses this apparent demonstration of opsonization further in relation to the demonstrated involvement of unparasitized cells and to the fact that more erythrocytes are destroyed in malaria infections generally than can be accounted for by their rupture by parasites. Whether this effect is to be related to the alteration of the erythrocytes by the parasite and the production of antibody against erythrocytes, to the adsorption by erythrocytes of parasite antigens or to the existence of an antigen common to the parasite and the erythrocyte is yet unresolved.

Immune adherence

Trypanosoma

Various terms—the Rieckenberg, thrombocytobarin and *Beladung* reactions —have been applied to this phenomenon [48]. The reaction depends on the presence of organisms, specific antibody, complement and suitable particles. Brown & Broom [24] have studied the factors determining the reaction and have proposed standard procedures. *T. brucei* Subgroup organisms from the blood of infected rats were washed and resuspended, concentrations being adjusted according to haemocytometer counts. Human erythrocytes were washed and resuspended, concentrations being adjusted in the same way. Satisfactory results were obtained with erythrocyte suspensions of 3×10^8 and $1 \cdot 25 \times 10^9$ per ml, tested with trypanosome suspensions of concentrations between 3×10^6 and 1×10^8 per ml, after incubation at $37°$ C for 5 minutes in the presence of antiserum and complement. At lower erythrocyte concentrations, trypanosomes were lysed and at higher trypanosome concentrations adhesion did not occur. Complete complement was shown to be necessary for the reaction. Adhesion occurred only with human and monkey erythrocytes, not with those of other 'ordinary laboratory animals'. Two humans differed widely in the susceptibility of their erythrocytes to adhesion; the characteristic reaction of each was maintained substantially unchanged over periods of some months. Some Enterobacteriaceae in suspension showed adhesion, others did not. Possible reasons for these differences were investigated, but fruitlessly, and empirical trial of erythrocyte suspensions was required. Comparatively large quantities of complement were required for the reaction; in one case a 1/10 dilution was required for adhesion while haemolysis took place at 1/40. Adhesion was of two types: flagellar, in which the organism is attached to the cell by the flagellar tip, and 'caddis' in which the trypanosomes are enveloped in erythrocytes; the latter form tends to occur at higher antiserum concentrations and after longer incubation. Adhesion was detected by microscopy. Nelson [127] working with *Treponema* and other organisms detected adherence by centrifuging the suspensions to deposit the cells and estimating the content of organisms of the supernates.

Precipitation and immunoelectrophoresis

Trypanosoma

Gray [78] demonstrated precipitating antibody to trypanosomes by testing antigens prepared from laboratory infections in rats against the sera of naturally infected bovines. *T. vivax* and *T. brucei* Subgroup organisms were harvested from the citrated blood of infected rats with massive infections. The trypanosomes were separated by centrifugation from blood elements and washed repeatedly in saline. The washed organisms were disrupted in twice their volume of saline in the Mickel disintegrator. The product was centrifuged and the opalescent supernate used as antigen. The antigen was tested against the bovine sera by double diffusion in agar.

Weitz [168, 169] used double diffusion in agar gel (see Ouchterlony, Chapter 19), and starch-gel electrophoresis to demonstrate the antibodies to the various antigens of *T. brucei* Subgroup organisms. He inoculated the serum of infected rats, freed from trypanosomes by filtration or centrifugation, into rats. The sera of these rats when tested by double diffusion gave a single line of precipitation against the infected rat serum, none against the serum of uninfected rats. Weitz attributed this result to an antigen released from the trypanosomes into the ambient—exoantigen. He used precipitin ring tests with constant antiserum against dilutions of infected rat serum to measure amounts of exoantigen, obtaining titres as high as 1/1280. Immunoelectrophoresis of normal and infected rat serum was made in starch gel. The strips were sliced horizontally into two portions; one portion was stained with naphthalene black, and the other by embedding in agar on plate glass and cutting channels in the agar for antiserum, was used for immunodiffusion. Infected and normal rat sera were electrophoretically identical but on immunodiffusion the exoantigen could be distinguished as a precipitation arc near the serum γ globulin component. With antisera to trypanosome homogenates Weitz showed that the lines of precipitation attributed to exoantigen were separate from those attributed to homogenate components. These methods have been further applied to highly sophisticated studies of the trypanosomal antigens [e.g. 148, 175, 124].

Trichomonas

The material obtained from *T. foetus* by extraction with anhydrous diethylene glycol (see Anaphylaxis, below) precipitated specifically with *T. foetus* immune rabbit serum to titres as high as 1/64,000, only to 1/1000 or less with heterologous immune or normal sera [58].

Entamoeba

Goldman [74] washed and lyophilized culture *E. histolytica* and extracted the product in saline. Precipitation was obtained in ring tests with specific antisera prepared by the inoculation of rabbits with living organisms (see labelled antibody techniques) but not with a control preinoculation serum.

Maddison [117] used an antigen prepared from ultrasonically disrupted culture *E. histolytica* against the sera of clinical cases of amoebiasis and antisera raised in rabbits in double diffusion systems in agar gel. Specific antibodies to *E. histolytica* were demonstrated but there were also lines attributable to other antigens, perhaps *Clostridium welchii* and indicative of gut tissue destruction. The specific reaction was less sensitive than the passive agglutination method of Kessel *et al* [96]. Atchley *et al* [11] have devised a micro-technique.

Eimeria

Rose [141], working with *Eimeria stiedae*, used two kinds of antigen, bile-duct exudate and oocyst. The clear supernate of the exudate from the bile ducts of infected rabbits at various stages of the infection was stored in small quantities at $-20°$ C. Packed oocysts, from heavily infected rabbit livers between the twenty-second and twenty-sixth days of the infection were washed in water and in 0·9 per cent saline, inspected microscopically for purity, suspended at a concentration of 10 per cent v/v in saline and frozen and thawed rapidly; the suspension was then ground in a glass tissue-grinder, adjusted to pH 7·6 and centrifuged; the milky supernate was used, being stored in small quantities at $-20°$ C. Antisera were derived from rabbits which had undergone oral infections, with or without clinical signs, and from rabbits inoculated with bile-duct antigen, with or without alum precipitation. Tests were carried out by double diffusion in agar gel. Quantitative precipitation tests, also, were performed, following Kabat & Meyer [92]. The strongest reactions were given by sera prepared by the subcutaneous inoculation of alum-precipitated bile-duct antigen, tested against homologous antigen and against oocyst antigen. With orally infected rabbits the strongest reactions were given by sera from animals recovering from heavy infections, usually 40 to 60 days after initial infection.

Similar approaches have been used to demonstrate antibody in *Eimeria tenella, necatrix, acervulina* and *maxima* infections in fowls [83, 84]. Antigens were prepared from asexual stages, from gametocytes and from oocysts, mostly from the first. Antisera were prepared from fowls which had received three graded doses of oocysts. Agar was made up in 8 per cent NaCl. The time of the infection at which responses could be detected by precipitation varied among the *Eimeria* spp., being latest, after 21 days, with *E. necatrix*.

Augustin & Ridges [12] studied the antibodies developed against *E. meleagrimitis* using as sources of antigen oocysts and gut material taken appropriately in the course of the infection to be representative of particular stages—sporozoites or merozoites—as well as pancreas, liver and other tissues from infected and non-infected birds. Tissues were cut into pieces, and extracted with physiological saline with 0·1 per cent sodium azide. The extracts were filtered and the filtrates concentrated three- to thirty-five-fold by pressure dialysis and then immediately used for experiment. With the sera of immune turkeys, no precipitation was detected in double-diffusion tests against oocysts, whether trypsin-digested or not. The sera, however, contained precipitating antibody to tissue antigens particularly abundant in infected, probably enzymatically degraded, tissues. Antibodies to parasite antigen could be detected with sporozoite preparations. Electrophoresis of antigen preparations and testing against antisera prepared in rabbits against infected guts, unabsorbed or absorbed with normal host tissues, demonstrated precipitation lines attributable to sporozoites or their metabolic products.

Plasmodium

Boyd *et al* [21] summarized various attempts to develop precipitation techniques for *Plasmodium* but considered them unpromising. Zuckerman *et al* [180] have, however, demonstrated antibody to *P. berghei* in the sera of infected rats by double diffusion in agar; they used as antigen parasites separated from host erythrocytes by treatment with saponin, disrupted in the Hughes press.

Toxoplasma

O'Connor [129] prepared antigen from the peritoneal exudate of mice infected 3 days previously with about 10^6 *T. gondii*. The exudates from several mice were pooled, diluted twofold with 0·85 per cent NaCl and centrifuged. The supernate was removed and stored frozen for use as antigen. Gamma globulin fractions were derived from human and rabbit antisera to *T. gondii* of known high dye-test titres (1/50,000 or higher), by electroconvection [137]; homogeneous protein solutions containing 0·62 mg N per ml, with dye-test titres of 1/1024, were tested against the antigen by double diffusion in agar gel. Precipitation lines were obtained up to dilutions of 1/4 to 1/32 after 24–48 hours' incubation. Undiluted aqueous humour obtained by paracentesis bulbi from cases of uveitis was tested against the *T. gondii* antigen, against mouse tissue protein and against other antigens possibly aetiologically related to the disease. Precipitation lines were obtained against *T. gondii* antigen, though sometimes only after 3–4 weeks' diffusion.

Babesia

Schindler [147] demonstrated antibodies against *B. canis* by double diffusion in agar gel, using as antigen extracts from isolated organisms.

Theileria

Barnett [14] quotes unpublished work by K.P.Bailey to the effect that agar-gel precipitation techniques, using gland extracts and the serum from reacting and recovered cattle, were insufficiently sensitive for practical application.

Paramecium

Bernheimer & Harrison [18] forced *Paramecium* (2000 organisms per ml) in water through fine needles to produce suspensions of fine fragments and investigated the precipitation of these suspensions by homologous antisera. Although precipitation was obtained results were inconsistent.

Complement fixation

Leishmania

Noguchi [128] demonstrated fixation of complement by culture forms of *Leishmania* spp. and of *Herpetomonas* spp. with homologous antisera prepared in rabbits. Complement-fixing antibodies have not been demonstrated in *L. tropica* infections but have been reported in mucocutaneous leishmaniasis with *L. brasiliensis* antigen. They have been found also in *L. donovani* infections though there is no consistent relation between complement-fixing titre and the γ globulin content of the serum [3, 4].

Trypanosoma

Fife & Kent [59] having encountered unexplained reactions in previous studies of complement fixation by *T. cruzi*, extracted the antigen with ether to remove lipids, fractionated it and compared the activity of the fractions. *T. cruzi* was grown in culture in cellulose sacs suspended in medium, harvested at 30–35 days. The organisms were washed and lyophilized. The desiccated organisms were extracted with ether, then with veronal-acetate buffered saline. The latter extract was then fractionated with chloroform gel into carbohydrate and protein antigens. Specific reactivity was reduced in both the fractions as compared with the unfractionated antigen, but non-specific reactivity was practically abolished. Cross-reactions with helminthic sera were eliminated and the frequency of cross-reactions with sera from *Leishmania brasiliensis* and *L. tropica* patients were much reduced. For the demonstration of specific antibodies to *T. cruzi* the protein antigen is preferable being less reactive with *Leishmania* antisera and having a higher optimal dilution.

Trichomonas
Teras *et al* [159] record the demonstration of complement-fixing antibodies in the sera of infected human beings.

Hartmanella
Cerva [28] demonstrated complement fixation by *Hartmanella* spp. with antisera prepared in rabbits.

Entamoeba
The antigen prepared by Kessel *et al* [96] from *E. histolytica* grown in association with *Trypanosoma cruzi* instead of with gut organisms, for use in passive agglutination, was also used for complement fixation. Results correlated well with clinical and parasitological history and with the haemagglutination test results.

Eimeria
Complement-fixation procedures for *Eimeria stiedae* were developed by Rose [141] using the same antigen and antiserum materials as for precipitation techniques (q.v.), and a 50 per cent end-point technique. The pattern of response followed that shown by the precipitation studies, the highest values being given by antisera to alum-precipitated bile-duct antigen, and the next highest by the serum of an animal recovered from a severe clinical infection.

Plasmodium
Attempts to demonstrate complement fixation by plasmodial antigen–antibody reactions have been reviewed by Coggeshall & Eaton [32] who themselves developed a complement-fixation reaction with *Plasmodium knowlesi*. Antigens were prepared from the spleen or blood of *Macaca* monkeys dying from *P. knowlesi* infection. Spleens were chopped, frozen, and dried in a vacuum desiccator; the dried material was ground at $-70°$ C, extracted with saline and the mixture centrifuged; the supernatant was used as antigen. Blood in which the erythrocytes were 20–50 per cent parasitized was collected in 2 per cent sodium citrate solution and then treated in several ways. In one, packed washed erythrocytes and parasites were suspended in an equal volume of saline; this suspension was frozen, dried, ground and extracted with saline in the same way as for the spleen material. In another, the washed blood cells were resuspended, mixed with 3 volumes of distilled water, toluene added as a preservative, and the material then allowed to autolyse for 48

hours; the suspension was then centrifuged and the supernate, readjusted to isotonicity, used for antigen. Antigen was prepared also from mixtures of distilled water and parasitized blood which had been allowed to autolyse in the refrigerator for several weeks. Antigens prepared by these various methods did not differ much among themselves but those prepared from blood were slightly the more sensitive. Antigens were used at four times the dilution showing slight, and eight times the dilution showing marked, anticomplementary activity; in most cases this was a dilution of 1/10 or 1/16 of the original antigen solution. Sera for testing were inactivated and stored at 0° C. The haemolytic system was a 5 per cent sheep erythrocyte suspension and an antiserum prepared in rabbits. Tests were read as soon after the addition of the haemolytic system as the controls had cleared, usually 15–30 minutes. Serum titres were expressed as the highest serum dilution which fixed complement, demonstrable by the presence of unhaemolysed erythrocytes. Some complication was imposed by the frequent anticomplementary character of the monkey sera. It was necessary to increase the amount of complement used to $2\frac{1}{2}$ units, and weak reactions might fade quickly. Also, the serum controls might not clear completely. In this case the tests were read at 30 minutes if the normal serum and antigen controls showed complete haemolysis and an adjustment was made if the serum was significantly anticomplementary at a dilution of 1/2. If a serum was anticomplementary at the 1/4 dilution, the result was excluded. There were wide variations in the titres shown by different monkeys during the course of *P. knowlesi* infection. Generally titres between 1/4 and 1/16 occurred, but some monkeys only attained titres of 1/2 or 1/4. Titres of 1/32 or 1/64 sometimes occurred, especially following super-infection with massive doses of parasites.

Eaton & Coggeshall [56] explored the application of complement-fixation tests, using *P. knowlesi* antigen, to the diagnosis of *Plasmodium* in man. They found antigen prepared from dried parasitized erythrocytes by extraction with saline, freezing and thawing the most sensitive and specific; some spleen-derived materials fixed complement non-specifically and could not be used for *Plasmodium* diagnosis, especially with luetic sera. Some human sera gave weak complement fixation with antigens prepared from normal monkey erythrocytes and a control antigen made from normal monkey erythrocytes and the same effective dilution as the malaria antigen is recommended. *P. knowlesi* antigens fixed complement with sera of human patients infected with *P. vivax* and *P. falciparum*.

Stratman-Thomas & Dulaney [157] examined the diagnostic application of the complement-fixation test in human malaria. Although they regarded their antigen as more sensitive than those prepared by other workers, they failed to show complement-fixing antibody in the sera of many patients found infected by parasitological methods. Demonstrable complement-fixation was correlated with presence or recent presence of parasites in the blood, titres falling as parasites disappeared. On the other hand, no strong fixation was found with sera of any uninfected subjects. Also, in extensive practical application [21], although fixation was found to be practically always absent with sera from known uninfected persons, it was present in only 30–40 per cent of known infected persons. Kligler & Yoeli's [97] study of the time of appearance of complement-fixing antibody may explain some of these inconsistencies; complement-fixing antibody appeared only after two or more clinical attacks and disappeared again by 4 months after the last attack. Pautrizel & Nguyen-Vinh-Nien [133] demonstrated complement fixation by *P. berghei* antigen and the serum of infected rats. This antigen was prepared by the separation of infected erythrocytes by centrifugation in a solution of polyvinyl pyrrolidone, lysis of these erythrocytes by the addition of distilled water and tryptic digestion of the result to remove blood cell stromata. The residual organisms were washed in glucose-saline and lysed by freezing and thawing. Fixation was carried out at 6–8° C for 18 hours.

Kligler & Yoeli [97] found that the sera of human malaria patients which fixed complement with *P. knowlesi* antigen also did so with *P. gallinaceum* antigen.

Toxoplasma

Many different antigens derived from infected hosts have been tried in attempts to increase sensitivity and avoid anticomplementary action, brain and spleen extracts, chicken chorioallantoic membrane, peritoneal exudate, lung, *T. gondii* separated from other cells [62]. The last appears likely to be the most able to be standardized and has been applied in complement-fixation procedures [67]. The suspension of organisms was prepared as described above for the agglutination test with *T. gondii* except that the organisms after suspension in 10 per cent formol saline for 24 hours were transferred to saline with only a trace of formalin. Suspensions of this sort gave consistent results for up to 6 months. Sera were diluted 1/4 in veronal buffer and inactivated at 60° C for 30 minutes before being tested in three dimensional complement-fixation tests (concentrations of antigen, antibody and complement all being varied) by the plastic plate method of Fulton & Dumbell [61]. Sera which at a dilution of 1/4 fixed 2 or more units of complement in the presence of the optimal amount of antigen were regarded as positive. The antigen was not anticomplementary.

Close agreement was shown between the results of this test and those obtained from agglutination and dye tests with a series of experimental rat sera. Agreement was not so close in the case of a series of human sera of miscellaneous provenance perhaps because of differences in the time of appearance of complement-fixing and other antibodies or because of the antigens used differing. However, the standardized antigen should allow comparison of antigens.

Sarcocystis

Awad & Lainson [13] prepared a 10 per cent suspension in saline of sarco-cysts dissected from the oesophagi of sheep, by grinding with sterile carbo-rundum. The suspension was frozen and thawed four times, kept at 4° C for at least 15 hours and centrifuged. The clear supernate was separated, and stored at −70° C, after the addition of 1/10,000 sodium merthiolate, for use as antigen. A control antigen was made in the same way but from heart or diaphragm muscle found free from *Sarcocystis* on microscopical examina-tion. Antiserum was raised in guinea-pigs by the IP inoculation of antigen. The optimum antigen concentration was determined by titration and was usually 1/40. Sera were inactivated and tested at 1/5, 1/10 and 1/20. 3 MHD of complement were allowed and fixation was allowed to proceed for $1\frac{1}{2}$ hours, the last half-hour at 37° C. Three per cent sheep cells sensitized at 37° C for 30 minutes was used as indicator. A control was provided, with positive serum but with the same dilution of the non-infected antigen. Results agreed well with parasitological findings; *Sarcocystis* antigen did not react with *Toxoplasma* antisera.

Babesia

Schindler [147] reported complement-fixing antibody in dogs infected with *B. canis*; he used organism extracts as antigen.

Theileria

Barnett [14] quotes work in which fixation of complement was obtained using an antigen extracted from the lymph nodes of animals dying of theile-riosis and the sera of animals infected with *T. parva*, but records that attempts to repeat these results have failed because of the anticomplementary nature of the antigen. He quotes also unpublished work by K.P.Bailey and K.Cowan who found that the serum of rabbits, hyperimmunized against erythrocytic forms of *Theileria*, fixed complement when put up against material prepared from lymph nodes infected with *T. parva* but not with uninfected lymph-node material. But no fixation was obtained with infected lymph-node antigen and the sera of bovines recovered from the infection.

Paramecium

Bernheimer & Harrison [18] incubated 0·5 ml of *Paramecium* suspensions, containing 2000, 1000, 500, etc., organisms per ml with 0·5 ml quantities of homologous antiserum dilutions and 0·5 ml quantities of guinea-pig serum. Addition of sensitized sheep erythrocytes and further incubation at 38° C for half an hour indicated fixation of complement at all serum dilutions up to 1/200 and at antigen dilutions containing 250 or more organisms per ml.

Immunoconglutination

Although immunoconglutinins are to be regarded as immune bodies to complement adsorbed on the antigen–antibody complex rather than specific antibodies to the particular antigen concerned [36] (see Weir, Chapter 26) they have been shown to be particularly prolifically produced by auto-stimulation in trypanosome infections [88] and therefore cannot be passed without remark.

Trypanosoma

Rabbits were infected by the IV inoculation of 2×10^5 living washed *T. brucei* Subgroup derived from infected mice. The rabbits were bled at intervals up to day 18 after inoculation, their sera being stored at $-20°$ C. All sera from an experiment were tested at one time against a single preparation of reagents. Alexinated cells (cells sensitized with antibody which have also adsorbed complement) were prepared: equal volumes of a 4 per cent sheep cell suspension and of inactivated bovine serum diluted 1/2 were mixed and incubated at 37° C for 15 minutes; the cells were washed and resuspended; equal volumes of this sensitized cell suspension were mixed with undiluted horse serum (complement) and undiluted inactivated horse serum (to ensure ample C′4) and 17·5 ml of saline; the mixture was incubated; the cells were washed and suspended in saline to a 0·4 per cent concentration. For the test, sera were first absorbed with sheep cells; then 0·1 ml of the serum dilutions were mixed with 0·3 ml of saline and 0·1 ml of 0·4 per cent suspension of alexinated cells. The mixtures were incubated at 37° C for 30 minutes, centrifuged, and the sedimented cells resuspended to observe clumping [89]. Immunoconglutinin titres of 1/128 to 1/256 were obtained on day 24 of the infection.

Quantitation of immunoglobulins

A variety of non-specific tests have attracted attention for the diagnosis of protozoal infection—the formol-gel, gum-mastic and thymol turbidity tests for trypanosomiasis and the cephalin-flocculation test for malaria and many others. These tests appear to depend in part at least on the increase in immunoglobulins in the serum of the infected host but are affected by changes in other serum protein constituents and suffer from the drawback that similar changes may be caused by various different infecting agents. For instance, the cephalin flocculation occurring in *Plasmodium vivax* infection was considered by Guttman *et al* [79] to be determined by hypoalbuminaemia and a decreased capacity of the serum albumin fraction to inhibit the flocculating action of γ globulin as well as an increase in the γ globulin content of the serum. More sophisticated methods are now available and have been applied particularly in trypanosomiasis.

Trypanosoma

Desowitz [50, 51], by means of Antweiler moving boundary electrophoresis, showed increase in the γ globulin amounts in the serum of sheep, of various breeds of cattle, and of *Gazella* and *Sylvicapra* (duiker) following infection with *T. vivax* and *T. brucei* Subgroup organisms.

Mattern [123] drew attention to the large increase in IgM immunoglobulins occurring in *T. gambiense* infections in man. He estimated the serum concentration of IgM by setting up a series of pairs of wells in agar gel and charging one well of each pair with specific IgM antiserum, the other with a serum dilution. The dilution to which a discernible line of precipitation extended was a measure of the amount of IgM in the serum. Mattern found the serum IgM level in *T. gambiense* patients to be as much as sixteen times that of a pool of normal healthy persons.

Other methods for estimating particular immunoglobulins have been proposed. Darcy [47] calibrated the position of the line of precipitation between the two wells, one containing the test serum and the other specific antiserum, in double diffusion in agar gel. Benz [17] devised a special immunoelectrophoretic arrangement which obviated the need for immunoglobulin class-specific antiserum. Fahey & McKelvey [57] described the quantitative determination of serum immunoglobulins by a radial diffusion method; the serum to be determined was introduced into a well in a plate of agar containing antibody to a particular immunoglobulin class. The immunoglobulin concentration was estimated by comparison of the diameter of the precipitation zone developing with those of the zones produced by standard preparations.

Mancini *et al* [118] have examined the method of radial immunodiffusion for the quantitation of antigen and have proposed standardizations of technical procedure. They found that the final area reached by the precipitate was directly proportional to the amount of antigen employed and inversely proportional to the antibody concentration. The temperature at which the plates were incubated was unimportant. The method was sensitive and, also, highly reproducible, the standard deviation of antigen determinations being less than 2 per cent of the mean.

The application of radial immunodiffusion to serum samples for the diagnosis of trypanosomiasis in the field was examined [103]. No useful peculiarities were found in the IgG or IgA but the IgM was characteristically increased to levels clearly distinguishable from the normal range. Several other infections—tuberculosis, leprosy, syphilis, leishmaniasis—were not characteristically associated with high serum IgM values, though occasional patients did show increased values. Patients with idiopathic splenomegaly, a condition likely to be caused by *P. malariae* [72], frequently showed increased values.

Plasmodium
Radial immunodiffusion has been used to estimate the IgM contents of the sera of patients during the course of the infection with *P. vivax*. The results paralleled closely anti-plasmodial antibody estimates made by the method of immunofluorescence [163].

Related to increased host reactivity

Immediate-type hypersensitivity
Augustin & Ridges [12] suggest that local immune reactions may be hypersensitivity reactions, pointing out that coccidiosis is associated with a local infiltration of leucocytes as is the case in the immediate-type hypersensitivity reactions in man and animals. They cite the 'self-cure' phenomenon in nematode infections in sheep as likely to be mediated by reaginic antibodies, and consider that they may be important in parasitic infections and would merit study.

Leishmania
Adler & Zuckerman [8] record some skin reactions to leishmanin antigen (see delayed hypersensitivity, below) which appear likely to be immediate-type hypersensitivity reactions. Two humans were inoculated ICu with *L. tropica* and 9 months later, when the cutaneous lesions still contained parasites, they were inoculated ICu with 0·1 ml quantities of homologous leishmanin antigen and of a control material. Diffuse erythema was present at the site of antigen inoculation 1 hour after inoculation and faded after 2 hours. Erythematous reactions appeared again on the day following antigen inoculation and persisted for 7–9 days. Reactivation of the reaction occurred 20 days after inoculation. Organisms were absent from the reaction sites. In another patient an Arthus-type reaction was elicited. A patient, originally inoculated with flagellates from a naturally infected *Phlebotomus*, developed a lesion which underwent spontaneous cure after 2 years. At various times during the 19 years following cure the patient was reinoculated, and found immune, and tested with leishmanin antigen, and found positive. A later ICu inoculation of 6×10^6 organisms, however, was followed in 6 hours by a rigor and in 24 hours by extensive oedema around the site of inoculation, with central necrosis and haemorrhage, which lesion lasted for more than 2 months before healing. The lesion was bacteriologically sterile on several

occasions and *Leishmania* were found in it only in the first 24 hours. Manson-Bahr [119] records similar experiences with *L. donovani*.

Bray & Lainson [23] indicated that a Prausnitz-Küstner type reaction, the passive cutaneous anaphylaxis reaction [132], may be elicited in monkeys and guinea-pigs by the ICu inoculation of immune serum followed by the IV inoculation of antigen and Evans blue.

Trichomonas

Feinberg & Morgan [58] extracted a specific material which induced an immediate-type skin reaction in sensitized cattle, by extraction of *T. foetus* with anhydrous diethylene glycol. Organisms from pure culture were washed in saline and lyophilized. The material was extracted successively with alcohol, ether, acetone, chloroform and pentane and freed of solvent *in vacuo*. It was then ground with diethylene glycol and extracted at room temperature in the dark for several days. The extract was recovered by centrifugation and filtered, poured into four times its volume of cold acetone, stirred and allowed to flocculate at 1–2° C for 24 hours. The deposited material was collected by centrifugation, washed with 1 : 4 diethylene glycol-acetone mixture and with acetone, dissolved in water, dialysed and lyophilized. The most active material serologically was that precipitated from aqueous solution by 43–75 per cent acetone. The extracted material did not induce any demonstrable specific agglutinin or precipitin on inoculation into rabbits. ICu inoculation of 0·1 ml of solutions of the material containing as little as 0·125 mg/ml induced skin reactions in sensitized cows as compared with a normal control. The reaction became evident in 10 minutes, reached a peak at 30–60 minutes and disappeared by 6 hours; the reaction was an increase in skin fold thickness as compared with a control animal. It was not established that the reaction was entirely specific as heterologous and other control materials were not available. The material was identified as a polysaccharide–amino acid complex.

Kerr [93] has recorded similar immediate-type skin reactions, in infected cattle, to material precipitated with trichloracetic acid from a suspension of *T. foetus* laked by the addition of water. The reaction is described as a 'shallow plaque' more obvious to the eye than to measurement. Feinberg & Morgan [58] considered this reaction likely to be mediated by nucleoproteins.

Kerr & Robertson [95] describe active and passive sensitization of the uterus by intra-uterine instillation. The antigens used were lyophilized washed organisms or extracts from organisms disrupted by laking in distilled water or heat-killed. Successive instillations of antigen were made and a high proportion of animals reacted. The reaction was an increase in uterine size, tenseness and, in severe cases, a mucous secretion; maximum development was about 2 hours after stimulus and the reaction often disappeared by 4 hours. Similar reactions were elicited by the instillation of antigen into the uterus 9–14 days after the intra-uterine inoculation of 60 ml of high agglutinating titre antiserum.

The reaction appears to be related to local, not serum, antibody; it could not be elicited by the primary instillation of antigen into the uteri of animals with high serum antibody levels induced by IM inoculation.

Delayed-type hypersensitivity
Although these reactions are mediated by sensitized cells and not by antibodies, they may constitute stages in the development of the same process [87] and so, as they are of diagnostic significance in some protozoal conditions, they are here included.

Leishmania
Most of the antigens in common use for delayed-type hypersensitivity skin tests for infections other than protozoa are cell-free preparations [87]. The 'leishmanin' antigen used for the diagnosis of *Leishmania* infection is a phenolized suspension of culture organisms. Dostrovsky & Cohen [53] prepared their antigen as follows: *Leishmania tropica* was grown on semi-solid Locke-serum-agar medium; the organismal growth, in the top layers of the culture, was removed and washed in three changes of saline; the washed organisms were resuspended in 0·5 per cent phenol saline at a concentration of 10^6 organisms per ml. The concentration of organisms was adjusted on the basis of haemacytometer counts.

The test dose used was 0·1 ml inoculated ICu. An infiltrated erythematous area of diameter greater than 5 mm, 48 hours after inoculation, was regarded as a positive reaction. The positive reaction lasted 2–3 or more weeks. Histological examination showed the epidermis normal except for some intracellular oedema and scattered foci of cellular aggregations in the dermis, particularly in the deeper layers. These aggregations, mainly of round cells, histiocytes, fibroblasts and granulocytes, were located mainly round blood vessels, sweat ducts and glands, muscles and nerves.

The reaction may be positive as early as 2 days after the inoculation of parasites [54]. Manson-Bahr [120] considers the positive test to develop about 6 weeks after treatment. The reaction probably persists for life; it is not species specific [3]. Although the reaction is generally classed as a delayed-hypersensitivity one [87], Dostrovsky & Sagher [54] succeeded in transferring it passively by the injection of serum from patients with positive reactions. Bray & Lainson [23[discuss their own, and other workers', failure to transfer hypersensitivity to *Leishmania* by washed leucocytes and are reluctant to abandon the belief that a cell-bound factor is responsible;

they consider that cells other than peripheral blood leucocytes may be concerned.

Trichomonas

The material derived from *T. foetus* by extraction with diethylene glycol which gave anaphylactic skin reactions with sensitized cattle gave delayed-type reactions with homologously immunized rabbits [58].

Toxoplasma

Antigen was prepared from the centrifugate of the peritoneal exudate of infected mice or hamsters; it was frozen and thawed, extracted with saline, and preserved with phenol. An antigen prepared from mouse spleen was used as a control. The antigen was used at a dilution of 10^{-3} to 10^{-4}. The reaction appeared 24–48 hours after ICu inoculation and persisted for 4–10 days. It may not become positive till 1 year after infection [62].

Conclusion

The wide range of the subject, the multifariousness of the approaches which have been employed in its study and the necessarily limited experience of one person prevent any fully balanced assessment of the field. The work noted is believed, however, to be a fair sample of the information available and to provide representative examples of most of the methods so far employed. Although inevitably superficial, it may assist progress by indicating areas in which new attack would be profitable. Although many tests for antibody to protozoa have been described, it is frequently difficult to assess their significance because they have not passed into more general application so that extended data on performance are built up. Perhaps the very multiplicity of tests is indicative that methods are still in the main unsatisfactory. The field certainly presents many more difficulties than do those of the bacteria or viruses, for many reasons, e.g. variation of antigen associated with the often complex life histories of the protozoa, the difficulty of culture of many parasitic protozoa *in vitro* and the small quantities of antigen produced therein, the difficulty of separating parasitic protozoa from the tissues in which they live, or from other organisms inhabiting the same host environment, the protection from the host's antibody afforded to organisms which have adopted an intracellular habitat.

The field has also, perhaps, been regarded as basically different from that of the immunology of bacterial and virus infections, for example, in the concepts of premunition and of ablastic antibody. However, it seems unlikely that this is the case [W.H.O., 1965].

Some general points should be made:

(a) A main need in the field at present is for the standardization and purification of antigens. As regards living antigens it is now possible in most cases to relate experimentation to stabilate material. Dead antigens are too frequently crude tissue or organism extracts in which many adventitious antigenic materials exist, many certainly irrelevant to the main problems; separation of organisms, extraction and purification of antigens require to be improved.

(b) Modification of the course of the infection *in vivo* is an ultimate aim but as an experimental method it has limitations especially with large animals. In some infections, e.g. *Theileria*, however, it may be the only tool available.

(c) Morphological modification is clearly of interest in relation to antibody action but its inherent requirement for expert observation limits its general application.

(d) Immobilization, agglutination, lysis and death of organisms are probably successive or related events caused by the same mechanism and which is chosen is a matter of convenience of observation.

(e) Neutralization of infectivity is of particular importance as this relates to a primary ability of the host to protect itself from parasitic organisms. Tests based on neutralization can be applied at very low parasite concentrations, and have special applications, therefore, for parasites which cannot be produced at high concentrations.

(f) As regards labelled antibody techniques, staining with fluorescein-conjugated antibody often presents problems in the objective estimation of the degree of fluorescence.

(g) Opsonization and immune adherence methods have been little exploited and their applications are still uncertain.

(h) Antibody-induced modification of staining has been applied only to *Toxoplasma* and although widely used has not received universal acceptance.

(i) Most of the methods discussed above necessitate the use of living antigen, a process often not free from hazard, and offering problems of maintenance of antigen. Passive agglutination, precipitation and complement fixation offer advantages in these respects. The specificity and sensitivity of passive-agglutination and complement-fixation tests require more study in parallel. Precipitation and immunoelectrophoresis offer great potentiality for antigenic analysis but elimination of adventitious antigens from the systems may present problems.

(j) Immunoconglutination and quantitation of immunoglobulins may offer valuable evidence of the process of infection but have shortcomings as regards specific parasite diagnosis.

(k) Hypersensitivity reactions to protozoal antigens deserve more attention, not only from their application in diagnostic purposes but for the light they may shed on the pathogenesis of protozoal infections.

(l) Miniaturization of methods appears to have great advantages. In the first place, some of the protozoal infections here treated are diseases of primitive peoples. Methods which can be applied to finger-prick blood dried on filter paper have manifest advantages in this context. Microprecipitation and microagglutination tests have been designed and offer great advantages in economy of materials and of operation.

Acknowledgments

I am indebted to Mrs K.M.G.Adam who has put her comprehensive knowledge of the protozoal literature freely at my disposal. My wife, Pamela Kathleen Lumsden constituted an indispensable link by interpreting my handwriting into typescript.

References

[1] ADAM K.M.G. (1964) A comparative study of hartmanellid amoebae. *J. Protozool.* **11**, 423

[2] ADLER S. (1958) The action of specific serum on a strain of *Trypanosoma cruzi*. *Ann. trop. Med. Parasit.* **52**, 282

[3] ADLER S. (1963) Immune phenomena in leishmaniasis. In *Immunity to Protozoa*, ed. GARNHAM P.C.C., PIERCE A.E. & ROITT I. Oxford: Blackwell Scientific Publications

[4] ADLER S. (1964) *Leishmania. Advances in Parasitology*, **2**, 35–96. London: Academic Press

[5] ADLER S. & ELLENBOGEN V. (1935) Observations on theileriosis in Palestine. *Arch. Inst. Pasteur Alger.* **13**, 451

[6] ADLER S. & ELLENBOGEN V. (1936) Remarks on the relationship between the Palestinian and Algerian pathogenic *Theileria. Arch. Inst. Pasteur Alger.* **14**, 66

[7] ADLER S. & THEODOR O. (1926) The identity of *Leishmania tropica* Wright, 1903, and *Herpetomonas papatasii* Adler, 1925. *Ann. trop. Med. Parasit.* **20**, 355

[8] ADLER S. & ZUCKERMAN A. (1948) Observations on a strain of *Leishmania tropica* after prolonged cultivation: Notes on infectivity and immunity. *Ann. trop. Med. Parasit.* **42**, 178

[9] ANDERSON R.I., SADUN E.H. & WILLIAMS J.S. (1961) A technique for the use of minute amounts of dried blood in the fluorescent antibody test for schistosomiasis. *Expl Parasit.* **11**, 111

[10] ANSARI N. & MOFIDI C. (1950) Contribution a l'étude des 'formes humides' de leishmaniose cutanée. *Bull. Soc. Path. exot.* **43**, 601

[11] ATCHLEY F.O., AUERNHEIMER A.H. & WASLEY M.A. (1963) Precipitate patterns in agar gel with sera from human amoebiasis and *Entamoebae histolytica* antigen. *J. Parasit.* **49**, 313

[12] AUGUSTIN R. & RIDGES A.P. (1963) Immunity mechanisms in *Eimeria meleagrimitis*. *Immunity to Protozoa*, ed. GARNHAM P.C.C., PIERCE A.E. & ROITT I. Oxford: Blackwell Scientific Publications

[13] AWAD F.I. & LAINSON R. (1954) A note on the serology of sarcosporidiosis and toxoplasmosis. *J. clin. Path.* **7**, 152

[14] BARNETT S.F. (1963) The biological races of the bovine *Theileria* and their host-parasite relationship. In *Immunity to Protozoa*, ed. GARNHAM P.C.C., PIERCE A.E. & ROITT I. Oxford: Blackwell Scientific Publications

[15] BEALE G.H. (1954) *The Genetics of* Paramecium aurelia. Cambridge: University Press

[16] BEATTIE C.P. (1963) Immunity to *Toxoplasma*. In *Immunity to Protozoa*, ed. GARNHAM, P.C.C., PIERCE A.E. & ROITT I. Oxford: Blackwell Scientific Publications

[17] BENZ M. (1964) Technique de titrage de la Beta-2-macroglobuline dans le sérum sanguin. *Rev. franc. Et. clin. biol.* **9**, 657

[18] BERNHEIMER A.W. & HARRISON J.A. (1940) Antigen–antibody reactions in *Paramecium*: The *aurelia* Group. *J. Immunol.* **39**, 73

[19] BERNHEIMER A.W. & HARRISON J.A. (1941) Antigenic differentiation among strains of *Paramecium aurelia*. *J. Immunol.* **41**, 201

[20] BEVERLEY J.K.A. & BEATTIE C.P. (1952) Standardization of the dye test for toxoplasmosis. *J. clin. Path.* **5**, 350

[21] BOYD M.F., CHRISTOPHERS SIR R. & COGGESHALL L.T. (1949) Laboratory diagnosis of malaria infections. In *Malariology*, ed. BOYD M.F. London: W.B.Saunders Co.

[22] BRAY R.S. & LAINSON R. (1965) Failure to transfer hypersensitivity to *Leishmania* by injection of leucocytes. *Trans. R. Soc. trop. Med. Hyg.* **59**, 221

[23] BRAY R.S. & LAINSON R. (1965) The immunology and serology of leishmaniasis. I. The fluorescent antibody staining technique. *Trans. R. Soc. trop. Med. Hyg.* **59**, 535

[24] BROWN H.C. & BROOM J.C. (1938) Studies in trypanosomiasis. II. Observations on the red cell adhesion test. *Trans. R. Soc. trop. Med. Hyg.* **32**, 209

[25] BRUCE-CHWATT L.J. (1963) Congenital transmission of immunity to malaria. In *Immunity to Protozoa*, ed. GARNHAM P.C.C., PIERCE A.E. & ROITT I. Oxford: Blackwell Scientific Publications

[26] BURNS W.C. & CHALLEY J.R. (1959) Resistance of birds to challenge with *Eimeria tenella*. *Expl Parasit.* **8**, 515

[27] CARVER R.K. & GOLDMAN M. (1959) Staining *Toxoplasma gondii* with fluorescein-labelled antibody. III. The reaction in frozen and paraffin sections. *Amer. J. clin. Path.* **32**, 159

[28] ČERVA L. (1965) Immunological studies of hartmanellid amoebae. *Progress in Protozoology*, p. 255. Amsterdam: Excerpta Medica Foundation

[29] COGGESHALL L.T. (1940) The occurrence of malaria antibodies in human serum following induced infection with *Plasmodium knowlesi. J. exp. Med.* **72**, 21

[30] COGGESHALL L.T. (1940) The action of immune serum in *Plasmodium knowlesi* malaria parasites *in vitro*. *Proc. 3rd Internat. Congr. Microbiol.* pp. 469

[31] COGGESHALL L.T. (1943) Immunity in malaria. *Medicine* **22**, 87

[32] COGGESHALL L.T. & EATON M.D. (1938) The complement fixation reaction in monkey malaria. *J. exp. Med.* **67**, 871

[33] COGGESHALL L.T. & KUMM H.W. (1937) Demonstration of passive immunity in experimental monkey malaria. *J. exp. Med.* **66**, 177

[34] COHEN S. & McGREGOR I.A. (1963) Gamma-globulin and acquired immunity to malaria. In *Immunity to Protozoa*, ed. GARNHAM P.C.C., PIERCE A.E. & ROITT I. Oxford: Blackwell Scientific Publications

[35] COHEN S., McGREGOR I.A. & CARRINGTON S.P. (1961) Gamma-globulin and acquired immunity to human malaria. *Nature, Lond.* **192,** 733

[36] COOMBS A.M. & COOMBS R.R.A. (1953) The conglutination phenomenon. IX. The production of immunoconglutinin in rabbits. *J. Hyg. (Camb.)* **51,** 509

[37] COONS A.H. (1956) Histochemistry with labelled antibody. *Internat. Rev. Cytol.* **5,** 1

[38] CORRADETTI A. (1955) Studies on comparative pathology and immunology in *Plasmodium* infections of mammals and birds. *Trans. R. Soc. trop. Med. Hyg,* **49,** 311

[39] COWPER S.G. & WOODWARD S.F. (1958) Observations on *Plasmodium berghei* infection in white rats: Blood changes and acquired resistance. *Ann. trop. Med. Parasit.* **53,** 103

[40] COX F.E.G. (1965) Acquired immunity to *Plasmodium vinckei. Progress in Protozoology,* p. 167. Amsterdam: Excerpta Medica Foundation

[41] CUNNINGHAM M.P. & GRAINGE E.B. (1963) A microagglutination test. *East African Trypanosomiasis Research Organization, Report, 1961,* p. 20

[42] CUNNINGHAM M.P. & HARLEY J.M.B. (1963) Detection of antibodies against trypanosomes in blood meals of wild *Glossina. East African Trypanosomiasis Research Organization, Report, 1961,* pp. 22–23

[43] CUNNINGHAM M.P., LUMSDEN W.H.R. & WEBBER W.A.F. (1963) The preservation of viable trypanosomes in lymph tubes at low temperature. *Expl Parasit.* **14,** 280

[44] CUNNINGHAM M.P., VAN HOEVE K. & GRAINGE E.B. (1965) A new method for the investigation of the immune response of animals infected with trypanosomes. *East African Trypanosomiasis Research Organization, Report, 1963–64,* pp. 35

[45] CUNNINGHAM M.P. & VICKERMAN K. (1962) Antigenic analysis in the *Trypanosoma brucei* Group, using the agglutination reaction. *Trans. R. Soc. trop. Med. Hyg.* **56,** 48

[46] D'ALESANDRO P.A. (1959) Electrophoretic and ultracentrifugal studies of antibodies to *Trypanosoma lewisi. J. infect. Dis.* **105,** 76

[47] DARCY D.A. (1960) A quantitative application of the agar diffusion plate. The estimation of specific proteins in serum. *Immunology* **3,** 325

[48] DAVIS L.J. & BROWN H.C. (1927) The adhesion phenomenon, a specific serological reaction occurring in trypanosomiasis. *Trans. R. Soc. trop. Med. Hyg.* **21,** 113

[49] DESOWITZ R.S. (1956) Effect of antibody on the respiratory rate of *Trypanosoma vivax. Nature, Lond.* **177,** 132

[50] DESOWITZ R.S. (1959) Studies on immunity and host-parasite relationships. I. The immunological response of resistant and susceptible breeds of cattle to trypanosomal challenge. *Ann. trop. Med. Parasit.* **53,** 293

[51] DESOWITZ R.S. (1960) Studies on immunity and host-parasite relations. II. The immune response of antelope to trypanosomal challenge. *Ann. trop. Med. Parasit.* **54,** 281

[52] DESOWITZ R.S. (1965) Recent investigations on the use of the haemagglutination test in malaria. *Progress in Protozoology,* p. 169. Amsterdam: Excerpta Medica Foundation

[53] DOSTROVSKY A. & COHEN H.A. (1957) Inhibition of intracutaneous leishmanin reaction by hydrocortisone acetate. *J. investig. Dermat.* **29,** 15

[54] DOSTROVSKY A. & SAGHER F. (1946) The intracutaneous test in cutaneous leishmaniasis. *Ann. trop. Med. Parasit.* **40,** 265

[55] EATON M.D. (1938) The agglutination of *Plasmodium knowlesi* by immune serum. *J. exp. Med.* **67,** 857

[56] EATON M.D. & COGGESHALL L.T. (1939) Complement fixation in human malaria

with an antigen prepared from the monkey parasite *Plasmodium knowlesi. J. exp. Med.* **69,** 379

[57] FAHEY J.L. & McKELVEY E.M. (1965) Quantitative determination of serum immunoglobulins in antibody-agar plates. *J. Immunol.* **94,** 84

[58] FEINBERG J.G. & MORGAN W.T.J. (1953) The isolation of a specific substance and a glycogen-like polysaccharide from *Trichomonas foetus* (var. Manley). *Brit. J. exp. Path.* **34,** 104

[59] FIFE E.H. & KENT J.F. (1960) Protein and carbohydrate complement fixing antigens of *Trypanosoma cruzi. Amer. J. trop. Med. Hyg.* **9,** 512

[60] FULLER A.T. (1938) The formamide method for the extraction of polysaccharides from haemolytic streptococci. *Brit. J. exp. Path.* **19,** 130

[61] FULTON F. & DUMBELL K.R. (1949) The serological comparison of strains of influenza virus. *J. gen. Microbiol.* **3,** 97

[62] FULTON J.D. (1963) Serological tests in toxoplasmosis. In *Immunity to Protozoa,* ed. GARNHAM P.C.C., PIERCE A.E. & ROITT I. Oxford: Blackwell Scientific Publications

[63] FULTON J.D. (1965) Micro-agglutination test for *Toxoplasma* antibodies. *Immunology* **9,** 491

[64] FULTON J.D. (1965) Studies on agglutination of *Toxoplasma gondii. Trans. R. Soc. trop. Med. Hyg.* **59,** 694

[65] FULTON J.D. & LOURIE E.M. (1946) The immunity of mice cured of trypanosome infections. *Ann. trop. Med. Parasit.* **40,** 1

[66] FULTON J.D. & SPOONER D.F. (1960) Metabolic studies on *Toxoplasma gondii. Expl Parasit.* **9,** 293

[67] FULTON J.D. & SUTTON R.N.P. (1962) Pure suspension of *Toxoplasma gondii* for use in complement-fixation test. *Immunology* **5,** 621

[68] FULTON J.D. & TURK J.L. (1959) Direct agglutination test for *Toxoplasma gondii. Lancet* **2,** 1068

[69] GARNHAM P.C.C. (1963) An introduction to protozoal immunity. In *Immunity to Protozoa,* ed. GARNHAM P.C.C., PIERCE A.E. & ROITT I. Oxford: Blackwell Scientific Publications

[70] GARNHAM P.C.C. & BRAY R.S. (1956) The influence of immunity on the stages (including late exo-erythrocytic schizonts) of mammalian malaria parasites. *Rev. bras. Malariol.* **8,** 151

[71] GARNHAM P.C.C. & VOLLER A. (1965) Experimental studies on *Babesia divergens* in rhesus monkeys with special reference to its diagnosis by serological methods. *Acta Protozool.* **3,** 183

[72] GEBBIE D.A.M., HAMILTON P.J.S., HULL M.S.R., MARSDEN P.D., VOLLER A. & WILKS N.E. (1964) Malarial antibodies in idiopathic splenomegaly in Uganda. *Lancet* **2,** 392

[73] GILLES H.M. & McGREGOR I.A. (1959) Studies on the significance of high serum-gamma-globulin concentrations in Gambian Africans. I. Gamma-globulin concentrations of Gambian children in the first two years of life. *Ann. trop. Med. Parasit.* **53,** 492

[74] GOLDMAN M. (1953) Cytochemical differentiation of *Entamoeba histolytica* and *Entamoeba coli* by means of fluorescent antibody. *Amer. J. Hyg.* **58,** 319

[75] GOLDMAN M. (1957) Staining *Toxoplasma gondii* with fluorescein-labelled antibody. I. The reaction in smears of peritoneal exudate. *J. exp. Med.* **105,** 549

[76] GOLDMAN M. (1957) Staining *Toxoplasma gondii* with fluorescein-labelled antibody. II. A new serological test for antibodies to *Toxoplasma* based upon inhibition of specific staining. *J. exp. Med.* **105,** 557

[77] GOLDMAN M. (1960) Antigenic analysis of *Entamoeba histolytica* by means of fluorescent antibody. I. Instrumentation for microfluorimetry of stained amoebae. *Expl Parasit.* **9,** 25

[78] GRAY A.R. (1960) Precipitating antibody in trypanosomiasis in cattle and other animals. *Nature, Lond.* **186,** 1058

[79] GUTTMAN S.A., POTTER H.R., HANGER F.M., MOORE D.B., PIERSON P.S. & MOORE D.H. (1945) Significance of the cephalin-cholesterol flocculation test in malarial fever. *J. clin. Invest.* **24,** 296

[80] HALL W.T.K. (1960) The immunity of calves to *Babesia argentina* infection. *Aust. vet. J.* **36,** 361

[81] HEGNER R. & ESKRIDGE L. (1938) Passive immunity in avian malaria. *Amer. J. Hyg.* **28,** 367

[82] HORTON-SMITH C., BEATTIE J. & LONG P.L. (1961) Resistance to *Eimeria tenella* and its transference from one caecum to the other in individual fowls. *Immunology* **4,** 111

[83] HORTON-SMITH C. & LONG P.L. (1963) Coccidia and coccidiosis in the domestic fowl and turkey. *Advances in Parasitology* **1,** 67

[84] HORTON-SMITH C., LONG P.L., PIERCE A.E. & ROSE M.E. (1963) Immunity to Coccidia in domestic animals. In *Immunity to Protozoa*, ed. GARNHAM P.C.C., PIERCE A.E. & ROITT I. Oxford: Blackwell Scientific Publications

[85] HUGHES D.E. (1951) A press for disrupting bacteria and other micro-organisms. *Brit. J. exp. Path.* **32,** 97

[86] HULDT G. (1965) Immunity in experimental toxoplasmosis. *Progress in Protozoology*, p. 186. Amsterdam: Excerpta Medica Foundation.

[87] HUMPHREY J.H. & WHITE R.G. (1964) *Immunology for Students of Medicine.* Oxford: Blackwell Scientific Publications

[88] INGRAM D.G., BARBER H., McLEAN D.M., SOLTYS M.A. & COOMBS R.R.A. (1959) The conglutination phenomenon. XII. Immunoconglutinin in experimental infections of laboratory animals. *Immunology* **2,** 268

[89] INGRAM D.G. & SOLTYS M.A. (1960) Immunity in trypanosomiasis. IV. Immunoconglutinin in animals infected with *T. brucei. Parasitology* **50,** 231

[90] JACOBS L. & LUNDE M.N. (1957) A haemagglutination test for toxoplasmosis. *J. Parasit.* **43,** 308

[91] JACOBS L., REMINGTON J.S., KAUFMAN H., MELTON M.L. & LUNDE M.N. (1959) The relationship of *Toxoplasma* dye test and neutralization antibodies. *J. Parasit.* **45,** Suppl., 52.

[92] KABAT E.A. & MAYER M.M. (1961) *Experimental Immunochemistry.* Springfield: C.C.Thomas

[93] KERR W.R. (1944) The intradermal test in bovine trichomoniasis. *Vet. Rec.* **56,** 303

[94] KERR W.R. & ROBERTSON M. (1941) An investigation into the infection of cows by *Trichomonas foetus* by means of the agglutination reaction. *Vet. J.* **97,** 351

[95] KERR W.R. & ROBERTSON M. (1953) Active and passive sensitization of the uterus of the cow *in vivo* against *Trichomonas foetus* antigen and the evidence for the local production of antibody at that site. *J. Hyg. (Camb.)* **51,** 405

[96] KESSEL J.F., LEWIS W.P., MA S. & KIM H. (1961) Preliminary report on a haemagglutination test for entamoebae. *Proc. Soc. exp. Biol. Med.* **106,** 409

[97] KLIGLER I.J. & YOELI M. (1941) The diagnostic and epidemiological significance of the complement fixation test in human malaria. *Amer. J. trop. Med.* **21,** 531

[98] KUČERA K. & KRAMÁŘ J. (1965) Indirect immunofluorescent test for the sero-

diagnosis of *Trichomonas vaginalis* infections. *Progress in Protozoology*, p. 198. Amsterdam: Excerpta Medica Foundation

[99] LANCELEY F. (1954) Laboratory aspects of *Trichomonas vaginalis*. *Brit. J. ven. Dis.* **30**, 163

[100] LOURIE E.M. & O'CONNOR R.J. (1936) Trypanolysis *in vitro* by mouse immune serum. *Ann. trop. Med. Parasit.* **30**, 365

[101] LUMSDEN W.H.R. (1965) Biological aspects of trypanosomiasis research. *Advances in Parasitology* **3**, 1–57. London: Academic Press

[102] LUMSDEN W.H.R. (1965) Implications and potentiality of viable preservation of protozoa and other organisms. *Progress in Protozoology*, 58. Amsterdam: Excerpta Medica Foundation

[103] LUMSDEN W.H.R. (in press) The estimation of IgM immunoglobulin in serum in the diagnosis of human trypanosomiasis. *Bull. Wld Hlth Org.*

[104] LUMSDEN W.H.R., CUNNINGHAM M.P. WEBBER W.A.F., VAN HOEVE K. & WALKER P.J. (1963) A method for the measurement of the infectivity of trypanosome suspensions. *Expl Parasit.* **14**, 269

[105] LUMSDEN W.H.R. & HARDY G.J.C. (1965) Nomenclature of living parasite material. *Nature, Lond.* **205**, 1032

[106] LUMSDEN W.H.R., HERBERT W.J. & HARDY G.J.C. (1965) *In vivo* prophylactic activity of Berenil against trypanosomes in mice. *Vet. Rec.* **77**, 147

[107] LUMSDEN W.H.R., ROBERTSON D.H.H. & MCNEILLAGE G.J.C. (1966) Isolation, cultivation, low temperature preservation and infectivity titration of *Trichomonas vaginalis* Donné 1837. *Brit. J. vener. Dis.* **42**, 145

[108] LUNDE M.N. & JACOBS L. (1959) Characteristics of the *Toxoplasma* haemagglutination test antigen. *J. Immunol.* **82**, 146

[109] MCDERMOTT J.J. & STAUBER L.A. (1954) Preparation and agglutination of merozoites of the chicken coccidian. *J. Parasit.* **40**, Suppl. 23

[110] MACDONALD G. (1957) *Epidemiology and Control of Malaria*. London: Oxford University Press

[111] MCENTEGART M.G. (1952) The application of a haemagglutination technique to the study of *Trichomonas vaginalis* infections. *J. clin. Path.* **5**, 275

[112] MCENTEGART M.G. (1956) Serological comparison of a strain of *Trichomonas vaginalis* with the Belfast and Manley strains of *Trichomonas foetus*. *J. Path. Bact.* **71**, 111

[113] MCENTEGART M.G., CHADWICK C.S. & NAIRN R.C. (1958) Fluorescent antisera in the detection of serological varieties of *Trichomonas vaginalis*. *Brit. J. vener. Dis.* **34**, 1

[114] MCGREGOR I.A. (1965) Consideration of some aspects of human malaria. *Trans. R. Soc. trop. Med. Hyg.* **59**, 145

[115] MCGREGOR I.A. & GILLES H.M. (1960) Studies on the significance of high serum γglobulin concentrations in Gambian Africans. II. Gamma-globulin concentrations of Gambian children in the fourth, fifth and sixth years of life. *Ann. trop. Med. Parasit.* **54**, 275

[116] MCGREGOR I.A. GILLES H.M., WALTERS J.H., DAVIES A.H. & PEARSON F.A. (1956) Effects of heavy and repeated malarial infections on Gambian infants and children: Effects of erythrocyte parasitization. *Brit. med. J.* **2**, 686

[117] MADDISON S.E. (1965) Characterization of *Entamoeba histolytica* antigen–antibody reaction by gel-diffusion. *Expl Parasit.* **16**, 224

[118] MANCINI G., CAREONARA A.O. & HEREMANS J.F. (1965) Immunochemical quantitation of antigens by single radial immunodiffusion. *Immunochemistry* **2**, 235

934   *Antigen–Antibody Interactions*

[119] MANSON-BAHR P.E.C. (1959) East African kala-azar with special reference to the pathology, prophylaxis and treatment. *Trans. R. Soc. trop. Med. Hyg.* **53**, 123

[120] MANSON-BAHR P.E.C. (1961) Immunity in kala-azar. *Trans. R. Soc. trop. Med. Hyg.* **55**, 550

[121] MANSON-BAHR P.E.C. (1963) Active immunization in leishmaniasis. In *Immunity to Protozoa*, ed. GARNHAM P.C.C., PIERCE A.E. & ROITT I. Oxford: Blackwell Scientific Publications

[122] MANWELL R.D. & GOLDSTEIN F. (1938) Life history and immunity studies of the avian malaria parasite, *Plasmodium circumflexum*. *Proc. Soc. exp. Biol. Med.* **39**, 426

[123] MATTERN P. (164) Techniques et interêt épidémiologique du diagnostic de la trypanosomiase humaine africaine par la recherche de la β_2-macroglobuline dans le sang et dans le L.C.R. *Ann. Inst. Pasteur (Paris)* **107**, 415

[124] MILLER J.K. (1965) Variation of the soluble antigens of *Trypanosoma brucei*. *Immunology* **9**, 521

[125] MOTT M.R. (1965) Electron microscopy studies of the immobilization antigens of *Paramecium aurelia*. *J. gen. Microbiol.* **41**, 251

[126] NEITZ W.O. (1957) Theilerioses, Gonderioses and Cytauxanoses: A review. *Onderstepoort J. vet. Res.* **27**, 275

[127] NELSON R.A. (1953) The immune-adherence phenomenon. *Science* **118**, 733

[128] NOGUCHI H. (1926) Comparative studies of herpetomonads and leishmanias. II. Differentiation of the organisms by serological reactions and fermentation tests. *J. exp. Med.* **44**, 327

[129] O'CONNOR G.R. (1957) Anti-*Toxoplasma* precipitins in aqueous humour. *Arch. Opthalm.* **57**, 52

[130] ORMEROD W.E. (1963) The initial stages of infection with *Trypanosoma lewisi;* control of parasitaemia by the host. In *Immunity to Protozoa*, ed. GARNHAM P.C.C., PIERCE A.E. & ROITT I. Oxford: Blackwell Scientific Publications

[131] OUCHTERLONY Ö. (1964) Gel diffusion techniques. In *Immunological Methods*, ed. ACKROYD J.F. Oxford: Blackwell Scientific Publications

[132] OVARY Z. (1964) Passive cutaneous anaphylaxis. In *Immunological Methods*, ed. ACKROYD J.F. Oxford: Blackwell Scientific Publications

[133] PAUTRIZEL R. & NGUYEN-VINH-NIEN (1953) Mise en evidence d'anticorps chez le rat parasité par *Plasmodium berghei* à l'aide d'un antigène preparé avec le sang de rat impaludé. *Bull. Soc. Path. exot.* **46**, 671

[134] PIERCE A.E. (1947) The serum agglutination reaction of *Trichomonas foetus* Riedmuller, 1928. *Lab. J.* **8**, 238

[135] PIERCE A.E. (1947) The demonstration of an agglutinin to *Trichomonas foetus* in the vaginal discharge of infected heifers. *J. comp. Path.* **57**, 84

[136] POLGE C. & SOLTYS M.A. (1957) Preservation of trypanosomes in the frozen state. *Trans. R. Soc. trop. Med. Hyg.* **51**, 519

[137] RAYMOND S. (1952) New design of electrophoresis-convection apparatus. *Proc. Soc. exp. Biol. Med.* **81**, 278

[138] RIEK R.F. (1963) Immunity to babesiosis. In *Immunity to Protozoa*, ed. GARNHAM P.C.C., PIERCE A.E. & ROITT I. Oxford: Blackwell Scientific Publications

[139] ROBERTSON M. (1934) An *in vitro* study of the action of immune bodies called forth in the blood of rabbits by the injection of the flagellate protozoon *Bodo caudatus*. *J. Path. Bact.* **38**, 363

[140] ROBERTSON M. (1939) A study of the reactions *in vitro* of certain ciliates belonging to the *Glaucoma-Colpidium* Group to antibodies in the sera of rabbits immunized therewith. *J. Path. Bact.* **48**, 305

[141] ROSE M.E. (1959) Serological reactions in *Eimeria stiedae* infection in the rabbit. *Immunology* **2**, 112

[142] ROTHSCHILD, LORD (1965) *The Classification of Living Animals.* London: Longmans

[143] SABIN A. (1942) *Toxoplasma* neutralizing antibody in human beings and morbid conditions associated with it. *Proc. Soc. exp. Biol. Med.* **51**, 6

[144] SABIN A.B. & FELDMAN H.A. (1948) Dyes as microchemical indicators of a new immunity phenomenon affecting a protozoon parasite (*Toxoplasma*). *Science* **108**, 660

[145] SABIN A. & RUCHMAN I. (1942) Characteristics of the *Toxoplasma* neutralizing antibody. *Proc. Soc. exp. Biol. Med.* **51**, 1

[146] SADUN E.H., DUXBURY R.E., WILLIAMS J.S. & ANDERSON R.I. (1963) Fluorescent antibody test in the diagnosis of African and American trypanosomiasis in man. *J. Parasit.* **49**, 385

[147] SCHINDLER R. (1965) Serological and immunological investigations in babesiosis. *Progress in Protozoology*, pp. 34–35. Amsterdam: Excerpta Medica Foundation

[148] SEED J.R. (1963) The characterization of antigens isolated from *Trypanosoma rhodesiense*. *J. Protozool.* **10**, 380

[149] SERGENT E., DONATIEN A., PARROT L. & LESTOQUARD F. (1935) Theilerioses bovines de l'Afrique du Nord et du proche-orient. *Arch. Inst. Pasteur Alger.* **13**, 472

[150] SERGENT E., DONATIEN A., PARROT L. & LESTOQUARD F. (1945) *Etudes sur les piroplasmoses bovines.* Algiers: Institut Pasteur d'Algérie

[151] SHAW J.J. & VOLLER A. (1964) The detection of circulatory antibody to kala-azar by means of immunofluorescent techniques. *Trans. R. Soc. trop. Med. Hyg.* **58**, 349

[152] SIIM J.C. & LIND K. (1960) A *Toxoplasma* flocculation test. *Acta path. microbiol. scand.* **50**, 445

[153] SOLTYS M.A. (1957) Immunity in trypanosomiasis. I. Neutralization reaction. *Parasitology* **47**, 375

[154] SOLTYS M.A. (1957) Immunity in trypanosomiasis. II. Agglutination reaction with African trypanosomes. *Parasitology* **47**, 390

[155] STEIN B. & DESOWITZ R.S. (1964) The measurement of antibody in human malaria by a formolized tanned sheep cell haemagglutination test. *Bull. Wld Hlth Org.* **30**, 45

[156] STRANNEGÅRD Ö. (1965) Kinetics of the *in vitro* inactivation of *Toxoplasma gondii* by specific antibodies. *Progress in Protozoology*, p. 186. Amsterdam: Excerpta Medica Foundation

[157] STRATMAN-THOMAS W.K. & DULANEY A.D. (1940) Complement fixation in human malaria II. Diagnostic application. *J. Immunol.* **39**, 257

[158] TALIAFERRO W.H. (1963) Cellular and humoral factors in immunity to Protozoa. In *Immunity to Protozoa*, ed. GARNHAM P.C.C., PIERCE A.E. & ROITT I. Oxford: Blackwell Scientific Publications

[159] TERAS J., JAAKMEES H., NIGESON U., ROIGAS E. & TOMPEL H. (1965) Immunity due to infestation with *Trichomonas vaginalis*. *Progress in Protozoology*, pp. 49–50. Amsterdam: Excerpta Medica Foundation

[160] TERRY R.J. (1955) Transmission of antimalarial immunity (*Plasmodium berghei*) from mother rats to their babies during lactation. *Trans. R. Soc. trop. Med. Hyg.* **49**, 302

[161] THILLET C.J. & CHANDLER A.C. (1957) Immunization against *Trypanosoma lewisi* in rats by injections of metabolic products. *Science* **125**, 346

[162] THURSTON J.P. (1959) The effect of immune sera on the respiration of *Trypanosoma brucei in vitro*. *Parasitology* **49**, 463

[163] TOBIE J.E. (1965) Quantitative determination of the serum IgM macroglobulins in human malaria infections. *Progress in Protozoology*, pp. 164–165. Amsterdam: Excerpta Medica Foundation

[164] TOBIE J.E. & COATNEY G.R. (1961) Fluorescent antibody staining of human malaria parasites. *Expl Parasit.* **11**, 128

[165] VAN HOEVE K. & CUNNINGHAM M.P. (1964) Prophylactic activity of Berenil against trypanosomes in treated cattle. *Vet. Rec.* **76**, 260

[166] VOLLER A. (1963) Immunofluorescent observations on *Trypanosoma cruzi*. *Trans. R. Soc. trop. Med. Hyg.* **57**, 232

[167] VOLLER A. & BRAY R.S. (1962) Fluorescent antibody staining as a measure of malarial antibody. *Proc. Soc. exp. Biol. Med.* **110**, 907

[168] WEITZ B.G.F. (1960) A soluble protective antigen of *Trypanosoma brucei*. *Nature, Lond.* **185**, 788

[169] WEITZ B. (1960) The properties of some antigens of *Trypanosoma brucei*. *J. gen. Microbiol.* **23**, 589

[170] WEITZ B. (1963) The feeding habits of *Glossina*. *Bull. Wld Hlth Org.* **28**, 711

[171] WEITZ B. (1963) The antigenicity of some African trypanosomes. In *Immunity to Protozoa*, ed. GARNHAM P.C.C., PIERCE A.E. & ROITT I. Oxford: Blackwell Scientific Publications

[172] WEITZ B. (1963) Immunological relationships between African trypanosomes and their hosts. *Ann. N.Y. Acad. Sci.* **113**, 400

[173] W.H.O. (1965) *Expert Committee on Immunology and Parasitic Diseases*. World Health Organization, Technical Report Series, No. 315. Geneva

[174] WILLIAMS J.S., DUXBURY R.E., ANDERSON R.I. & SADUN E.H. (1963) Fluorescent antibody reactions in *Trypanosoma rhodesiense* and *T. gambiense* in experimental animals. *J. Parasit.* **49**, 380

[175] WILLIAMSON J. & BROWN K.N. (1964) The chemical composition of trypanosomes. III. Antigenic constituents of *brucei* trypanosomes. *Expl Parasit.* **15**, 44

[176] ZAMAN V. (1960) Studies with the immobilization reaction in the genus *Entamoeba*. *Ann. trop. Med. Parasit.* **54**, 381

[177] ZAMAN V. (1964) Studies on the immobilization reaction in the genus *Balantidium*. *Trans. R. Soc. trop. Med. Hyg.* **58**, 255

[178] ZUCKERMAN A. (1945) *In vitro* opsonic tests with *Plasmodium gallinaceum* and *Plasmodium lophurae*. *J. infect. Dis.* **77**, 29

[179] ZUCKERMAN A. (1963) Immunity in malaria with particular reference to red-cell destruction. In *Immunity to Protozoa*, ed. GARNHAM P.C.C., PIERCE A.E. & ROITT I. Oxford: Blackwell Scientific Publications

[180] ZUCKERMAN A., HAMBURGER Y. & SPIRA D. (1965) Active immunization of rats against rodent malaria with a non-living plasmodial product. *Progress in Protozoology*, pp. 50–51. Amsterdam: Excerpta Medica Foundation

[181] ZUCKERMAN A., RON N. & SPIRA D. (1965) The demonstration of antiplasmodial antibody in rats by means of gel diffusion. *Progress in Protozoology*, pp. 167–168. Amsterdam: Excerpta Medica Foundation

[182] LUMSDEN W.H.R., CUNNINGHAM M.P., WEBBER W.A.F., VAN HOEVE K., KNIGHT R.H. & SIMMONS V. (1965) Some effects of hydrogen ion concentration on trypanosome numbers and infectivity. *Expl Parasit.* **16**, 8

[183] CUNNINGHAM M.P. & GRAINGE E.B. (1963) Preparation of high titre specific agglutinating sera against antigenic variants of the *T. brucei* Subgroup. *East African Trypanosomiasis Research Organization, Report, 1961*, p. 19

[184] CORRADETTI A. (1963) Acquired sterile immunity in experimental protozoal infec-

tions. In *Immunity to Protozoa*, ed. GARNHAM, P.C.C., PIERCE A.E. & ROITT I. Oxford: Blackwell Scientific Publications

[185] CUNNINGHAM M.P., VAN HOEVE K. & LUMSDEN W.H.R. (1963) Variable infectivity of organisms of the *T. brucei* Subgroup during acute relapsing infections in rats, related to parasitaemia, morphology and antibody response. *East African Trypanosomiasis Research Organization, Report, 1961*, p. 21

[186] MACDONALD A. (1949) Serological diagnosis of human toxoplasmosis. *Lancet* **1,** 950

[187] BEALE G.H. & KACSER H. (1957) Studies on the antigens of *Paramecium aurelia* with the aid of fluorescent antibodies. *J. gen. Microbiol.* **17,** 68

[188] BEALE G.H. & MOTT M.R. (1962) Further studies on the antigens of *Paramecium aurelia* with the aid of fluorescent antibodies. *J. gen. Microbiol.* **28,** 617

CHAPTER 28

The Demonstration of Antibodies to Helminths*

E.J.L.SOULSBY

Introduction

The immunology of helminth infections, in general, has not reached the degree of sophistication of that in other fields: several factors have contributed to this, but a major one has been the difficulty of obtaining and preparing sufficient quantities of material for antigen analysis and other purposes. However, the increasing emphasis on helminth disease stimulated by the World Health Organization [1] and other agencies has highlighted the need for much improved immuno-diagnostic tests for the widespread helminth infections, especially in the tropical areas, and this has led to a marked improvement of immunological procedures and techniques associated with helminthology.

It would be impossible in this chapter to cover all which has been done in the field of helminthology and consequently only the major areas of interest have been considered. Nevertheless, the techniques mentioned should serve as a guide to the possibilities for various other host-helminth systems and with a little modification be readily applied to them. Because of the ever-present problem of the production of antigen a section has been devoted to this and then the various techniques which can be used are considered separately.

The application of immunological tests in helminthology

The major use of immunological tests has been in the diagnosis of natural infections or the experimental study of the host response to artificial infection. They have been little used for the specific identification of organisms since, generally, the morphology of helminths is such that they can be readily recognized microscopically. Nevertheless immunological procedures have been used to localize, and sometimes characterize, specific materials possibly of physiological importance to the parasite. Examples of such are the detection

* Some of the techniques described in this chapter have been developed with financial assistance from U.S.P.H.S. Grant AI 06262.

of excretions and secretions at the orifices or pores of development stages such as nematode larvae, the embryos of tapeworms and eggs of schistosomes while the significance in the immune response of physiologically functional materials such as exsheathing fluid of gastro-intestinal nematodes and the enzymes of the oesophageal glands of hookworms have received study. More recent applications have been the fluorescent antibody technique, immune adhesion and mixed agglutination for the demonstration of the antigenicity of the cuticle and other structures.

The greatest use of immuno-diagnostic tests has been in the human field and these have been subject to many problems such as the provision of satisfactory homologous antigens, the wide range of cross-reactions between helminths and the different levels of sensitization in a population. Since helminths do not multiply in the host a minimal infection may stimulate little antibody response with a consequent lack of correlation between the immuno-diagnostic test and the presence of infection. In areas where helminth infection rates are low, or in a defined experimental infection, few problems exist with cross-reactivity between helminths but in endemic areas of helminth infection, for example the tropics, cross-reactions may be troublesome.

Production of helminth antigens

One of the major problems in the immunology of helminth infections has been the provision of adequate amounts of antigen. Only in a few instances have helminths been successfully cultivated *in vitro* and even in these synchronous growth and development comparable to that in the normal host is lacking. The recent developments in this area with *Trichinella spiralis* [2], *Spirometra* [3] and various gastro-intestinal nematodes of domestic animals are most encouraging, especially since the intermediate developmental stages of helminths, which may be important in the immune response and in the pathogenic process, are not yet readily available and must be obtained from artificially infected animals, frequently with host protein, if not tissue, contamination. In the absence of adequate cultivation techniques antigen sources have been restricted to mature parasites obtained at post-mortem of animals or the infective stages of these parasites. With the latter the facility with which they may be obtained varies greatly. In those helminths with a direct life cycle the infective stages may be cultured from eggs on a variety of media (sterile faeces, peat moss, etc.) and then separated from the culture material for antigen preparation. Where an intermediate host is required in the life cycle the problem may be more difficult, necessitating maintenance of colonies of the vector organisms. Despite this, laboratory procedures are now available for the large-scale production of cercariae of the human schistosomes from the vector snails, adult schistosomes from infected mice, *Trichinella* larvae from rats, mice, and guinea-pigs, etc., and various developmental stages of ascarids from laboratory animals. (Information is available from the author indicating where supplies of various parasites and their antigens can be obtained.)

An advantage of using infective larvae as a source of antigen is that contamination by host protein is avoided, this being a constant problem with materials obtained at post-mortem of an animal. Much of this can be removed by adequate washing, but in some instances the sharing of antigens between host and helminth, as in hydatid infection [4], may lead to difficulties in the interpretation of diagnostic tests.

Despite the above difficulties there are a variety of immunological tests which can be performed using a minimum of antigen and which can be used when it is not possible to obtain large numbers of a helminth species. These are discussed in the section dealing with tests on living organisms.

Antigen preparations usually consist of an extract of the homogenized parasite (larvae or adults) but with larger species dissection may provide more defined tissues (e.g. oesophageal glands of dog hookworms [5]) while specific physiological substances (e.g. exsheathing fluid [6]) may be obtained under appropriate conditions.

For many serological procedures a simple phosphate buffered (pH 7·2) saline extract of homogenized fresh or lyophilized helminths is adequate. This is preserved at 4° C with the addition of merthiolate in a concentration of 1:10,000. In diagnostic tests there is much to be gained by more specific and less heterogeneous preparations and the two main techniques for this are those of Melcher [7] (acid soluble fraction) and Chaffee *et al* [8] (ether extraction). These will be discussed later.

Basic studies in helminth immunology have produced recent developments in the techniques of extraction and isolation of helminth antigens allowing high yields of materials which give much more consistent results than previously. Since many of the proteins of helminths (e.g. of *Schistosoma mansoni* [9]) appear to be extremely sensitive to freezing and thawing and to heat treatment great care should be taken in the extraction procedures. For protein antigens better extraction is achieved following defatting, which should be done in chilled anhydrous ether, preferably at $-70°$ C, using ultrasonication. Centrifugation and separation of soluble lipids is preferably done in a refrigerated centrifuge at $-20°$ C and the defatted residue stored at $-20°$ C. For extraction of the residue (at 3° C) distilled water buffered at pH 7·0–7·2 with 0·02 M EDTA buffer [9] has been found to be superior to phosphate and borate buffers and yields of up to 80 per cent extraction from defatted material have been obtained [9]. Equilibration is carried out by dialysis or by filtration through Sephadex. Subsequent column chromatography and other procedures have been detailed by various authors [9, 10, 11].

It is necessary to determine the protein content of various fractions and since polysaccharides are abundant in helminths, determinations of free and protein-bound carbohydrates are also of value.

The specific chemical identification of antigens prepared by the above techniques has occasioned almost no study, but investigations in this general direction are illustrated by a study of the antigenic structure of *Trichinella spiralis* larvae using immuno-electrophoresis as the principal analytic method. This showed eleven distinct antigens in buffered saline extracts [12], ten of which were proteins and the remaining one contained some polysaccharide associated with the protein molecule. In no instance was it found that acid or alkali extraction of material yielded antigens different from those found in the buffered saline extract. One major antigen of the parasite appeared to have an isoelectric point similar to that of normal human serum γ globulin and subsequent work using enzymatic degradation techniques revealed that it was rapidly and completely hydrolysed by lysozyme, the other protein antigens being unaffected [13]. It was therefore suggested that this major antigen was mucoprotein in nature, but at present no further information is available about it.

Extensive and detailed work on antigens used for skin tests in filarial and *Clonorchis sinensis* infections [10, 11] has produced materials of high specificity and reactivity. Thus an antigen from the dog heartworm, *Dirofilaria immitis*, prepared from a phosphate buffered extract of lyophilized worms and subsequently separated by Sephadex and DEAE-cellulose column chromatography produced an immediate skin reaction in filarial patients when injected in 0·05 $\mu\mu$g amounts. The final purified antigen was a protein with a small amount of carbohydrate [2·5 per cent] which gave a single broad band on electrophoresis. An acid hydrolysate analysed by paper electrophoresis revealed the amino acids lysine, arginine, glycine, alanine, glutamic and aspartic acids and valine, while degradation by proteolytic enzymes greatly reduced the antigenic activity of the preparation. Similar studies with a skin antigen from *Clonorchis sinensis* produced an active substance which in quantities of 0·3 $\mu\mu$g of protein gave an immediate skin reaction [11]. The antigen contained 55 $\mu\mu$g of protein and 62·5 $\mu\mu$g of carbohydrate per ml and various tests indicated that the protein moiety was the substance responsible for the skin reaction.

Over the years much emphasis has been placed on the importance of the antigens produced by living parasites. These have been referred to as 'metabolic products' (excretory and secretory materials is more satisfactory) and though it is likely they play an important part in the immune response such materials are difficult to collect in any substantial quantity. The ready provision of these by *in vitro* techniques is a goal which has yet to be realized and at present they are obtained by maintaining the parasites in buffered saline or some nutrient medium. Their subsequent storage, concentration

and isolation depend on existing techniques of lyophilization and fractionation.

Immunological tests of value in helminth infections

By no means all the presently available immunological tests have been applied
to helminth infections and in some cases, because of the lack of defined
antigens, it would be difficult to envisage that they could be used. Consequently
the techniques in present use are those which can be employed without any
clear knowledge of the character of the antigen other than that it contains
protein, lipid or polysaccharide or complexes of these.

Complement fixation

This technique has a long history of usefulness in helminth infections dating
from early work with hydatid disease and schistosomiasis; it is also used
extensively in studies of experimental helminth infections. At one time it was
the only test of any significance even though the 100 per cent end-point technique was used. The use of quantitative methods [14] has led to much more
satisfactory results, especially in the human field, but with experimental
animals such as horses, cattle and sheep the direct application of such techniques may not be entirely satisfactory due to the variation in their ability to
fix guinea-pig complement [15]. Alternative complement-fixing techniques
are necessary and in swine, horses and cattle the conglutinin complement-
fixation technique [16], using horse complement, is more applicable (see
Weir, Chapter 26).

Substantial advances have been made in the preparation of antigens which
lack anticomplement activity and show good specificity with the homologous
species. Though antigen purification will almost always produce lower yields
of antigen the increased specificity which results is of great advantage. The
most advantageous technique for antigen preparation must be determined
for each system but the antigens which are in more common use for complement-fixation tests are a saline extract, an acid-soluble fraction and an
acetone-extracted fraction.

The simple saline extraction of parasites may be done with fresh or lyophilized parasites and buffered saline, worms being ground in a hand tissue
grinder or by a teflon pestle connected to an electric motor. These procedures
are best performed in an ice-bath and the latter is essential where a motor-
driven tissue grinder is used. The weight of worms to extractant is a factor
which must be determined by experimentation, but usually a 10 per cent stock
antigen is prepared, various dilutions, as necessary, being made from this.
Where large-scale antigen production is in process it is advantageous to lyo-

philize worms in known aliquots and given quantities are then homogenized with saline. More satisfactory results may be obtained by overnight extraction at 4° C and in all cases the material is centrifuged in the cold for 30 minutes and the supernatant used as the antigen. It is advisable that a nitrogen determination be performed on all antigens before use. As a replacement for buffered saline Coca's solution (0·5 per cent NaCl; 0·05 per cent NaHCO$_3$; 0·4 per cent phenol) may be used. It is desirable that saline extracts are stored in the refrigerator at 4° C since freezing at −20° C causes precipitation and antigenicity may be lost by further lyophilization.

The use of an acid-soluble protein fraction (Melcher) [7] represents an attempt to produce a more specific antigen and it has been used successfully in trichinosis [17] and is of value for other helminths. The preparation is as follows:

Five hundred milligrammes of lyophilized parasites are extracted for 7 days with petroleum ether in a soxhlet apparatus. The material is dried and then ground in a tissue grinder with 25 ml of borate buffer at pH 8·3, being extracted overnight at 4° C with constant shaking. Following centrifugation for 15 minutes at 4° C the supernatant is precipitated with 0·2 N HCl in the cold at pH 4·8 and the supernatant recovered by centrifugation in the cold. This is the acid-soluble fraction which is used as antigen and it may be stored lyophilized for at least a year without losing its antigenicity.

The development of the Chaffee antigen [8] for the complement-fixation test in schistosomiasis has produced an antigen which is relatively free of nonspecific reactions. It was originally developed for *Schistosoma mansoni* when it was found necessary to treat materials from adult schistosomes with ether at low temperature to remove non-specific fixation factors with syphilitic serum. The technique, though originally described for schistosomes, is probably applicable to any parasite.

One hundred milligrammes of lyophilized parasites are placed in a tissue grinder and homogenized with 10 ml of chilled anhydrous ether. The ether must be free of water and preferably from a newly opened bottle. To avoid denaturation of the proteins the whole operation should be carried out at a low temperature, the ether and grinder being precooled to −20° C and the operation carried out in a calcium chloride or alcohol ice-bath at −18 to −15° C. Grinding may be done by hand or motor and is continued for 10 minutes until all the material is in suspension. The suspension of ground worms in ether is then transferred to a precooled centrifuge tube and centrifuged in a refrigerated centrifuge for 30 minutes at about 800 *g*. The supernatant is decanted and the sediment dried by suction from a water vacuum pump. The dry residue is transferred to a grinder and homogenized for 10 minutes with 15 ml of veronal buffer in an ice-bath at 0–3° C. The suspension is left in the refrigerator at 3–6° C for several hours or overnight and it is then centrifuged for 30 minutes in a refrigerated centrifuge at 3–6° C and the supernatant liquid, which represents the antigen, is carefully transferred to a previously chilled tube. The antigen is most satisfactorily preserved in the lyophilized state at −20° C but may also be stored frozen at −20° C.

Precipitation techniques

Due to the complexity of helminth antigens little work has been done on quantitative precipitin techniques but the advent of immuno-diffusion procedures has given a great impetus to the studies of helminth immunology. Early work using double-diffusion procedures [Oudin] was carried out on *Ascaris* [18] and *Toxocara* [19] and the more recent application of these techniques, along with immuno-electrophoresis, has led to a demonstration of the great complexity of the helminth organism. Thus in *Trichinella* larvae at least eleven antigens have been recorded [12], in *S. mansoni* at least fourteen [20] and in *Fasciola hepatica* at least seven [21]. The usefulness of immuno-diffusion and immuno-electrophoretic methods cannot be over-emphasized. Not only can the multiplicity of the antigenic mosaic be determined but the relations with other species may be determined, and using a combination of fractionation procedures, such as chromatography and immuno-diffusion, the plurality and specificity of antigens can be checked during isolation procedures (see Ouchterlony, Chapter 19).

Thus, as previously mentioned, the chemical nature of one *T. spiralis* antigen has been studied by enzyme degradation techniques, specific antigens have been isolated from *Ascaris* [22] and a detailed analysis of hydatid fluid showed the presence of host proteins in material prepared from pig hydatid cysts [29].

Immuno-diffusion tests have been valuable in determining the composition of physiologically functional antigens such as exsheathing fluid of strongyle larvae and an illustration of their use in experimental immunology of helminth infections occurs in the self-cure phenomenon to *Haemonchus contortus*. This mechanism is produced when previously infected and sensitized sheep are subject to reinfection with infective larvae, this resulting in a spontaneous and dramatic elimination of the existing burden of parasites. Experimental work has demonstrated this to be associated with the moulting of larvae from the third to fourth larval stage and a strong precipitin response occurs to exsheathing fluid at this time (Fig. 28.1). The production of exsheathing fluid by infective larvae is stimulated by a dialysable component in the digestive tract of sheep which then initiates the secretion or release of preformed exsheathing fluid from an area near the base of the oesophagus of the infective larva, the fluid being excreted at the excretory pore [23]. This material contains a leucine amino peptidase which is specific for the individual parasite and acts on its substrate on the interior wall of the sheath particularly in a narrow area encircling the sheath about 20 μ from the anterior end of the larva. This results in the splitting of the sheath and the anterior part is thrown off in the form of a cap. Immuno-diffusion tests have shown 'sheath free' exsheathing fluid to consist of at least three antigens while normal exsheathing fluid (i.e. with sheaths) showed several additional systems which presumably represented breakdown products of the sheath. Comparison of normal and inactivated (mercuric chloride 10^{-3} M) exsheathing fluid identified a precipitating system absent in the latter, the antigen of which possibly represented the

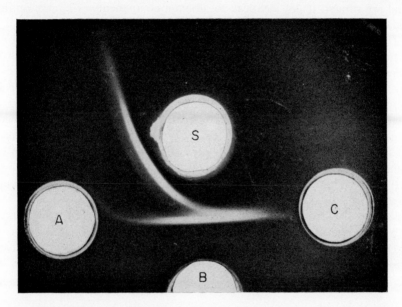

Fig. 28.1. Precipitin response of a sheep 5 days after self-cure to *Haemonchus contortus* had occurred. S = serum. A = exsheathing fluid. B = antigen prepared from homogenized infective larvae. C = 'metabolic' excretions of larvae (1 million incubated in saline for 24 hours).

active component of exsheathing fluid [24]. Apart from being excreted at the time of ecdysis exsheathing fluid is also present in homogenates of the infective larvae but not present in the excretions and secretions of unstimulated larvae [24, 25]. This work, which would have been impossible without the aid of the immuno-diffusion techniques, probably represents the first demonstration of a material which serves both a functional capacity in the physiology of the parasite and in the immune mechanism of the host. It is likely that further work along these lines will be most rewarding especially with substances specifically isolated from the life cycle of the parasite.

The extreme usefulness of immuno-diffusion and immuno-electrophoretic techniques is further illustrated by their use in comparing the antigen antibody systems produced by immunization with homogenates of worms with those induced by natural infection. Such procedures may reveal 'internal' antigens which are never presented to the host immunological mechanism and also determinants which are common to both host and parasite [26, 27], the latter allowing a more sophisticated interpretation of the phenomenon of parasitism. Using the technique of Allison & Humphrey [28] it has been shown that the diffusion coefficients of four of the antigenic components of hydatid fluid are similar, if not identical, to albumin components of human serum, while one was related to γ globulin [29].

The techniques of course have drawbacks, one of which is the interpretation of the vast multiplicity of systems demonstrable by them. Thus studies with *S. mansoni* revealed seven specific adult worm antigens, three cercarial and five egg antigens but there remained some twenty-five precipitating systems which could not be identified [29]. Another difficulty is that to obtain satisfactory precipitating sera it is often necessary to immunize animals with large amounts of antigen since the level of precipitating antibodies in natural infection may be extremely low and only a single precipitating system may be found at the peak of the immune response.

It has been found in work with sheep and cattle that an increase in the ionic strength of agar, to 12–14 per cent sodium chloride, greatly enhances the speed with which antigen antibody precipitates form and also their density [30]. The same situation pertains in the case of fowl sera.

The immuno-diffusion techniques used in helminthology do not differ from those applicable to other studies and their application is chiefly a matter of the choice of antigen and a satisfactory precipitating serum.

Agglutination

Because of the relatively large size of helminths there are only few instances where direct agglutination of organisms can be employed in serological tests, examples of this being the cercariae and miracidia of trematodes. Attempts have been made by some workers to produce agglutinable particles by grinding up parasites, but in general these procedures are of little value. Consequently the techniques developed in other areas for the attachment of antigens to various 'carrier' particles such as tanned red cells, bentonite, cholesterol, etc., have been exploited and expanded within recent years. Substantial work on this has been carried out with regard to immuno-diagnostic tests as well as experimental investigation of laboratory infections and these techniques are in regular use for epidemiological work with schistosomiasis, trichinosis, hydatid disease, etc.

The Boyden [31] technique (see Herbert, Chapter 21) has been widely used in the study of the immunology of gastro-intestinal nematode infections of sheep. Modifications from the original technique are that veronal buffer at pH 7·2 may be substituted for the two buffers at pH 6·4 and pH 7·2 and normal guinea-pig serum in a dilution of 1 in 250 can replace normal rabbit serum. This was used initially because of problems with antibodies to helminth infections in 'normal' rabbits and subsequently it has been a standard diluent in the author's laboratory, being prepared periodically from batches of guinea-pigs. It is as well to stress that it is wise to examine 'standard sera', e.g. complement, antiglobulin sera and type-specific sera, for their content of helminth antibodies, especially if they have been produced by a commercial organization. On a number of occasions the author has found that anomalous results with such reagents could be traced to such antibodies. If found they should be removed by absorption.

The use of formalized cells has allowed standardization of cell suspensions and tanned formalized cells exposed to antigen have retained their sensitivity when stored lyophilized in the freezer at $-20°$ C (see Herbert, Chapter 21) [32]. The choice of antigen depends on the system under examination. For gastro-intestinal nematodes a distilled-water extract of homogenized infective larvae subsequently heated to 105° C and then made isotonic has been found satisfactory [33] but other suitable antigens consist of extracts of sonicated larvae, the metabolic products of larvae cultured in a nutrient medium or exsheathing fluid. Nitrogen concentrations of 2–8 μg per 1 ml are satisfactory. In *Ascaris* infection an extract of homogenized whole worm has been used routinely by the author, while in human hydatid infection hydatid cyst fluid of pig origin is the antigen choice, though low-level non-specific reactions may be seen in a small number of patients ill with other diseases, particularly those of the liver [4]. Such reactions are traceable to cross-reaction between host proteins in the tissues and fluid of the hydatid parasite and auto-antibodies which are frequently present in sera of patients suffering from chronic liver infections. With schistosomes, a variety of antigens have been shown to be active in the haemagglutination test and it is likely that the system can be utilized in almost any helminth infection provided a satisfactory protein antigen is prepared.

A variety of flocculation tests have been developed for the detection of antibody. Work on this was initiated by the modification of the Kline technique, for the diagnosis of syphilis, to the diagnosis of trichinosis [34]. It was shown that an alkaline extract of lyophilized *Trichinella* larvae coated on cholesterol provided a satisfactory antigen and since then it has been successfully used in the detection of infections in both man and pigs. It will, for example, give a positive reaction as early as the eighth day after experimental infection and antibodies persist for at least 903 days. Following the adoption of this test for trichinosis, other particles such as collodion and carmine were assessed as antigen carriers but bentonite particles were found to be the most

HH

useful. The latter has advantages over the cholesterol technique, which suffers from instability, since it is simple, easy to perform and the reagents are stable. The technique for preparation of reagents is as follows [35]:

Stock bentonite particles are prepared by homogenizing 0·5 g of No. 200 standard bentonite in 100 ml of glass-distilled water in a blender for 1 minute. The suspension is transferred to a glass-stoppered cylinder or bottle, distilled water being added to 500 ml. It is well shaken and allowed to stand for 1 hour and the supernatant suspension centrifuged at 500 *g* for 15 minutes. The resulting supernatant is removed and centrifuged at 750 *g* for 15 minutes, the supernatant discarded and the sediment resuspended in 100 ml of distilled water by blending for 1 minute. This stock suspension may be stored at 4° C for up to 6 months. It may be lyophilized, being reconstituted to give the same preparation as above.

A stock antigen–bentonite suspension is prepared by thoroughly mixing the bentonite suspension with the helminth antigen (the concentration must be determined by trial and error, but usually an equal mixture is satisfactory with antigens with a nitrogen content of 5–10 μg per 1 ml). The mixture is left overnight at 4° C during which time the antigen is absorbed on to the bentonite particles. The particles may be stained with methylene blue or thionine blue (0·1 per cent solution), being exposed for at least 1 hour to the dye. This stock antigen–bentonite suspension can be stored at 4° C for several weeks.

For use in serological tests the above stock antigen suspension is thoroughly mixed and the desired quantity removed, e.g. 10 ml. This is washed twice with 10 ml of 0·85 per cent saline by centrifugation at 1000 *g* for 5 minutes. The sediment, now cleared of free antigen, is resuspended in 5 ml of saline. To stabilize the suspension in saline a small amount of Tween 80 (e.g. 0·1 ml of 1 in 200 solution in distilled water) is added and the stability tested by agitating the suspension on a slide as in the test described below. Small quantities of Tween 80 are added until no flocculation occurs with normal serum. If too much Tween is added it may interfere with the test and this should be assessed with a known positive serum. In this case the suspension is washed once in saline and stabilization repeated. Once adjusted, the antigen-coated particles are stable for several weeks at 4° C.

Sera for test are inactivated at 56° C for 30 minutes and serially diluted in saline: 0·1 ml of test serum is placed on a wax-ringed slide and a drop (0·025 ml) of antigen-coated bentonite particles is added to each serum sample and the slide agitated on a rotating shaker for 15 minutes at 100 rev/min. Flocculation is assessed by examination under a dissecting microscope and the reactions scored according to the degree of clumping.

The bentonite flocculation technique, using *T. spiralis* antigen, has been used for several years by the Communicable Diseases Center, Atlanta, Georgia, for the diagnosis of human trichinosis, where it is considered the test of choice. A Melcher-type antigen is used but this may be replaced by a metabolic antigen prepared from living *T. spiralis* larvae, giving even greater sensitivity [36].

A further flocculation technique principally employed for the diagnosis of *Schistosoma mansoni* infections has been developed as a modification of the VDRL for syphilis and consists of cholesterol–lecithin crystals coated with a cercarial antigen prepared in the Chaffee manner [37]. It is simple and sensitive and probably could be used with advantage in other helminth infections. The technique is as follows:

An antigen is prepared from lyophilized cercariae, essentially following the method described by Chaffee, but veronal buffer is substituted by triethanolamine buffer salt (TBS) solution. The antigen is lyophilized in 1 ml amounts. A stock solution of 1 per cent cholesterol and 0·1 per cent lecithin is prepared in absolute alcohol and stored at room temperature in the dark. Cholesterol may precipitate from the solution in time and if this occurs it should be discarded and a fresh batch made. The antigen is reconstituted in distilled water and to 0·6 ml of dissolved antigen is slowly added 0·3 ml of the cholesterol–lecithin mixture, the tube being rotated continuously and rotation continued for about 10 seconds after all the solution has been added. The container is then shaken vigorously for 1 minute, 1·1 ml of triethanolamine buffer salt solution is added and again the suspension is shaken for 1 minute. The tube is allowed to stand for 1–2 minutes and the mixture is then centrifuged at approximately 1000 *g* for 15 minutes. The supernatant is discarded and the tube inverted to drain the sediment, the sides of the tube being cleaned with a gauze-wrapped applicator stick. Two millilitres of TBS saline are added and the antigen mixed thoroughly in this. This is the antigen emulsion. For the performance of a test 0·05 ml of heated serum is placed on a well slide and to this one drop of antigen emulsion is added; it is then rotated at 180 rev/min on a slide rotator for 5 minutes and then read under the low power of a compound microscope when various degrees of flocculation can be seen and extent of the reaction scored.

Haemagglutination techniques with living parasites

A variety of these exist and some have proved most useful in the investigation of certain antigen structures of helminths. It is very likely that these techniques can be applied to a variety of problems in helminth immunology and their use is illustrated here with reference to the surface reactions on the cuticle but it is anticipated that other structures of parasites could well be examined in this manner.

Immune adherence

Though known for some considerable time the details of this reaction were first put on a sound footing by Nelson [38] who defined the reaction as the attachment of antigen–antibody–complement complexes to the surface of untreated primate erythrocytes or non-primate platelets. Some of the earliest work with this reaction was with trypanosomes when leucocytes were seen to adhere to the parasites *in vitro* and platelet adhesion, using various bloods, was observed with *Trypanosoma brucei* and *Trypanosoma equiperdum*. Immune adherence has been demonstrated with microfilariae and leucocytes in the presence of homologous immune serum. Its use as an investigational tool in helminthology was reintroduced by the present author who used it to demonstrate the antigenicity of the nematode cuticle and to determine that complement was fixed in the reaction [39]. Though alternative tests such as the fluorescent antibody technique are available for this type of work the immune adherence system allows extensive screening of parasites to be done fairly rapidly and obviates the necessity for specialized equipment or reagents.

The following detail is applicable to the technique for demonstration of the antigenicity of the nematode cuticle and in this red cells adhere to the parasite, producing a coating of cells on the surface.

Helminths, for example infective larvae from a faecal culture, ascarid larvae hatched from eggs and grown *in vitro* or free-living nematodes such as *Turbatrix aceti*, are washed three times by centrifugation in an excess of veronal buffer. A given quantity (e.g. 200 in 0·2 ml) are exposed to heat-inactivated serum [0·2–0·5 ml] in various dilutions at 37° C for 30 minutes. The tubes are then centrifuged at low speed [500 rev/min] the supernatant removed and larvae washed three times in an excess of veronal buffer. (Tubes with a capacity of 5 ml are usually used and larvae are washed with at least 4 ml of veronal buffer at each wash.) Larvae may now be exposed to guinea-pig complement at a dilution of 1 in 30 (or greater, depending on the complement titre) for 30 minutes at 37° C and subsequently washed as previously described. The parasite now theoretically possesses antibody globulin attached to the surface antigenic determinants on the cuticle and complement is fixed to the antigen–antibody complex. This may then be detected by placing the sensitized larvae in a suspension of primate cells. The author uses his own (AB Rh negative) cells but there does not appear to be any marked differences with other blood-group systems. The cells are collected in Alsever's solution and after three washes are made up to a 3 per cent suspension in veronal buffer.

A drop of larval suspension sensitized with the test serum is placed on a siliconed slide (or alcohol clean slide with two thin lines of paraffin wax painted across so that a cover glass will rest on them) and a drop of the suspension of human cells is mixed with them using the corner of a clean slide. A cover glass is placed over the preparation and it is observed under 100 × magnification using phase or dark-ground illumination. The vigorous movements of larvae assist in the reaction since they come into contact with many more erythrocytes than they would if they were immobile. If larvae have not previously been sensitized to complement, a drop of complement may be added at this stage of the test with essentially the same results. Within a minute or so of mixing the reagents red cells become adherent to the surface of the cuticle and remain fairly firmly fixed there despite the violent lashings of

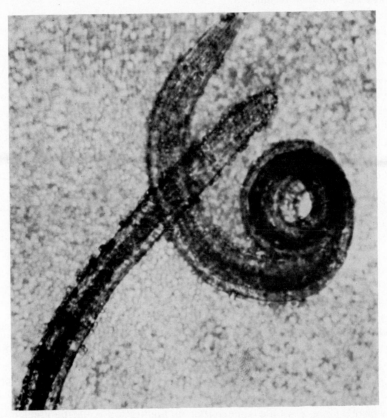

FIG. 28.2. Immune adherence with larvae of *Ascaris suum*. Larvae have been sensitized to homologous antibody, washed and then exposed to guinea-pig complement, washed and then exposed to human red blood cells.

the larvae. Several preparations can be made and there is no necessity to observe the preparation continuously since in a few minutes (3–4) unattached red cells lie in a carpet and out of focus on the surface of the slide, those adherent to the larvae being sharply in focus when the preparation is examined microscopically (Fig. 28.2). Using this technique it has been possible to demonstrate antibodies in high dilution in serum and also to show a quantitative difference in the antigenicity of various larval stages of *Ascaris suum*.

The specificity and sensitivity of the reaction and its lack of requirement for special apparatus should lend it to a variety of uses with various developmental stages and isolated tissues and using absorption techniques it may be possible to indicate the antigenic composition of various organs.

Mixed agglutination techniques

Direct mixed agglutination, for the specific identification of antigenic determinants on cells, etc., has been extensively developed by Coombs *et al* [40]. In this technique the test material (cells) is exposed to specific antibody and after washing a known particulate homologous antigen (e.g. A cells, sheep cells, etc.) is added. There is mixed clumping or mixed agglutination between the test particulate antigen and the test material. This technique has been developed in the author's laboratory for the identification of the Forssman antigen on the cuticle of nematodes, the technique being as follows. Sheep red cells are treated with papain (0·25 per cent papain; 3·6 per cent Na_2HPO_4. $12H_2O$; 0·2 per cent l cystein HCl) for 10 minutes at 37° C and afterwards are washed three times and resuspended in veronal buffer to give a concentration of 3 per cent.

Test organisms such as second-stage larvae of *Ascaris* grown in culture, or *Turbatrix aceti*, are exposed to a strong anti-Forssman antiserum preparing in rabbits against the heated stromata of sheep red blood cells. Incubation is for 30 minutes at 37° C and the larvae are then washed three times in an excess of veronal buffer.

The test is performed by placing a drop of larvae on a slide with a drop of sensitized cells and a positive reaction is indicated by an even coating of cells on the surface of larvae in a manner comparable to that in immune adherence.

Using this technique it has been possible to demonstrate that some stages of development of *Ascaris* and *Turbatrix* possess surface determinants which are likely to be Forssman in character. The reaction is, of course, a reflection of antibody fixed to the cuticle, but by inference such antibody is attached to the antigenic determinants. Though the technique has been used so far for one system only, it would appear that its application could be great in the field of helminthology, especially with surface determinants. The attachment of other determinants to red cells by, for example, diazotized benzidine, difluorodinitrobenzene or by photo-oxidation may provide indicator particles with the specificity of interest. Preliminary trials in this direction have indicated that an antigen prepared from the cuticle of *Ascaris* can be linked by photo-oxidation (using rose bengal) [41] to erythrocytes which then produce mixed agglutination with *Ascaris* larvae coated with antibody. (See also Chapter 21.)

Mixed antiglobulin agglutination

This is a further step in the reaction in which antiglobulin is used as an intermediary to link globulin on the cuticle of the parasite with another globulin from the same species, but of unrelated specificity, attached to a red cell which serves as an indicator particle. Using this technique, globulin, possibly of antibody nature, derived from serum, has been demonstrated on the cuticle of the free-living nematode *Turbatrix aceti* [42]. This shows specificity and can be absorbed from the serum by living or dead worms. A similar technique has been used in *Ascaris* infections with good success. The potential of this technique is great since by absorption tests and the use of specific antisera to defined antigens it would be possible to determine the existence of a variety of antigens on and in the parasite and perhaps even to localize them to specific areas of the body. The technique of the test is as follows:

Parasitic stages such as larvae of *Ascaris* or adults of *T. aceti* are exposed to serial dilutions of antibody at 37° C for 30 minutes and are then washed three times in an excess of veronal buffer.

Indicator cells consist of a 2 per cent suspension of three times washed sheep erythrocytes sensitized with a rabbit anti-sheep red blood cell serum of high titre which has been photo-oxidized using eosin Y [43] or rose bengal [41]. Photo-oxidation is carried out until direct agglutinating activity of the rabbit serum globulin is completely removed and only sensitizing ability remains. Such photo-oxidized globulin can be stored in the frozen condition for at least 1 year. Cells so treated are washed three times to remove the surplus globulin and prior to the test their agglutinability is tested on a slide with a drop of dilute goat (or sheep) anti-rabbit globulin. (Since the test is sensitive the anti-globulin serum should be absorbed with parasites before use.)

For the test one drop of sensitized larvae is placed on a siliconed slide (or one with two wax marks which will support a cover glass) plus one drop of sensitized cells and one drop of dilute (1 in 20) species antisera. The suspension is mixed and a cover glass placed over the preparation and it is observed under 100× power of a microscope by phase or dark-ground illumination. With a strong system the reaction is evident within a few seconds, cells clumping strongly to the larvae and also to each other in the surrounding medium due to the antiglobulin reacting with the globulin both on the parasite and cells (see Fig. 28.3). The larvae assist in the reaction since they move actively through the suspension, coming into contact with a large number of cells in the process. A negative reaction consists of agglutinated cells in the preparation but no attachment of these to the larvae.

In the system a nice balance between agglutination and the size of clumps of cells is essential, since where large clumps form, the vigorous action of larvae may dislodge them. This may be avoided if a further step is taken in the preparation. Larvae sensitized by antibody and washed free of serum are further exposed to an antiglobulin (1 in 20 to 1 in 40) serum for 30 minutes at

37° C and subsequently are washed three times. When larvae are exposed to sensitized cells agglutination is avoided in the preparation and in a positive reaction cells are attached only to the larvae and not to each other. Preparations can be left on the bench before being read and since the unattached cells lie out of focus in an even carpet on the floor of the slide the reaction is easy to read. Using this latter technique it has been possible to titrate serum for the mixed anti-globulin agglutination reaction to high levels and also to investigate the cross-reactivity between other parasites.

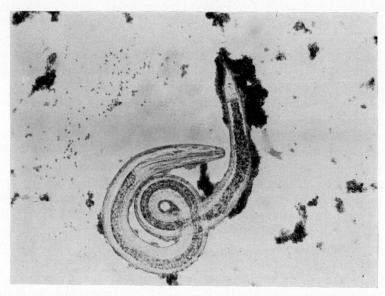

Fig. 28.3. Mixed anti-globulin agglutination with *Ascaris suum* larvae. Larvae have been sensitized to homologous antibody and then washed. Sheep red cells sensitized with a photo-oxidized rabbit anti-sheep red cell globulin and washed. When sensitized larvae and cells are mixed in the presence of goat anti-rabbit globulin, cells agglutinate with the cuticle of the parasite and with each other.

The test, of course, only detects fixed globulin and does not give any indication of the specificity of it. Nevertheless, with known antibodies and antigens it has proved to be a most useful technique and with a little thought many useful systems could be proposed for the test.

Fluorescent antibody techniques (see Holborow & Johnson, Chapter 16)
The application of these techniques is widely known and they have been used both as diagnostic tools and in experimental work on helminth immunology. Their use in diagnostic work has received extensive study and along with the developments of micro methods of obtaining serum samples (such as the

finger-prick technique and the filter-paper method of storing small samples [44]) the fluorescent-antibody technique used in conjunction with these procedures provides a method whereby large numbers of samples may be readily collected with the minimum of objection, especially from primitive people, and the samples may be easily mailed to a central laboratory and there examined.

Fluorescent-antibody techniques for the immuno-diagnosis of schistosomiasis in humans initially required the use of freshly killed cercariae as antigen. However, such cercariae if stored for periods of 24 hours or longer were unsuitable since they showed an increasing tendency, non-specifically, to take up the fluorescein-labelled anti-species serum used in the test. The use of lissamine rhodamine as a counter-stain eliminates the non-specific staining effect by the fluorescein-labelled serum. A standard suspension of cercariae for use in the test is now prepared as follows. *Schistosoma mansoni* cercariae, freshly emerged from laboratory-reared and infected *Australorbis glabratus*, are collected by standard methods [45] and are then exposed to a 1 in 25 dilution of lissamine rhodamine R.B. 200, conjugated to bovine albumin, for 5 minutes. Following this, cercariae are fixed by the addition of an equal volume of 20 per cent formalin. Samples of cercariae in formalin and the rhodamine-bovine albumin may be stored at 3–6° C after shell freezing in a dry ice-bath or stored lyophilized. Such cercariae provide a standard suspension which may be transported at normal temperatures over a long distance without losing its effectiveness.

The test procedure for the fluorescent-antibody technique in schistosomiasis is as follows [46]; all reactions being carried out in 13×100 mm test tubes. One millilitre of cercarial suspension containing 200–400 cercariae is washed twice in phosphate buffered saline and then 0·1 ml of test serum dilution is added to the sedimented cercariae and incubated for 30 minutes at room temperature, being gently agitated periodically. The sensitized cercariae are then washed with phosphate buffered saline and treated with 0·1 ml of fluorescein-labelled anti-human globulin for 15 minutes. Subsequently the cercariae are washed a further twice in saline and suspended in 0·1 ml of 90 per cent buffered glycerine and then a sample is placed on a slide and examined microscopically using ultra-violet light. Using this test cross-reactions occur with sera from patients with other schistosome infections such as *Schistosoma japonicum* and *Schistosoma haematobium*, indicating the group specificity of the reaction; however, sera from patients infected with other parasitic helminths show no reaction. One of the advantages of the fluorescent-antibody technique for the diagnosis of schistosomiasis is that the test is relatively easy to perform, antigen may be preserved for use and only small quantities of serum and antigen need be used.

A similar technique has been developed for the diagnosis of trichinosis in

HH*

man and animals [47]. The results indicate that the test shows considerable promise as a diagnostic procedure, especially since small quantities of reagents are necessary. The test antigen consists of formalized suspension of larvae obtained by digestion of infected muscle.

More general use of fluorescent-antibody techniques in experimental work using both the direct and indirect techniques has demonstrated the antigenicity of various tissues of parasites [48]. For example, the cuticle of *Ascaris* and *Trichinella* and the intestine of *Trichinella* have been shown to fix antibody and the precipitates demonstrable at orifices of larvae and around the eggs of schistosomes, when these are placed in immune serum, are seen to be of antibody origin. In the absence of defined isolated antigens, and hence specific antisera, whole worm preparations or sections of these have been used in such tests with a resulting multiplicity of reactions. With the production of more specific antigen fractions, both those which are recognized as specific tissues and organs and subcellular fragments such as mitochondria, lyosomes and nuclear elements, it should be possible to delineate more precisely the location of antigens within the organism.

A further application of the fluorescent-antibody technique has been used to demonstrate that helminths, placed in Millipore diffusion chambers and implanted in hosts, became stained with fluorescent antibody when this is injected intravenously [49]. Approaches such as these, particularly with more defined antisera and the different immunoglobulin fractions of serum, should reveal valuable information on the immunological responses to helminths, particularly the bowel forms.

Fluorescent-antibody techniques have been little used in the specific identification of helminths but they should prove to be of value in the demonstration of the migratory stages in the life cycle or the identification of material in tissues which cannot be readily identified morphologically.

Skin tests and anaphylactic reactions (see Chapters 22 and 35)
For many years skin tests have been used in the diagnosis of helminth infections and they are particularly used in trichinosis and schistosomiasis. In the latter, the response is of the immediate type, the optimal time for reading the reaction being 15 minutes, while in trichinosis, both early and delayed skin sensitivity has been reported, delayed skin reactions having been observed in rabbits and guinea-pigs and in early infection in man. There are varying reports of the efficacy of the skin test in trichinosis and it still needs critical evaluation, especially since a wide variety of antigens have been used. Skin sensitivity may persist for at least 10 years and some reports suggest that a positive reaction may be present even 20 years after infection. When used for survey purposes it is extremely difficult to correlate positive results with the presence of infection. Cross-reactions may occur with other helminths and a

marked sensitivity to *Ascaris* may lead to positive reactions with *Trichinella spiralis* antigen [50].

In schistosomiasis the principal antigens which have been used consist of a saline extract of adult worms or an antigen prepared by the Melcher or the Chaffee method. In humans the intradermal test is usually performed on the flexor surface of the forearm but it has also been shown that skin tests carried out on the back are more reactive. The volume of fluid injected varies from 0·01 to 0·05 ml, the latter being more satisfactory, and the antigen should be standardized to contain between 20 and 40 μg of nitrogen per ml of antigen.

Active cutaneous anaphylaxis techniques may be used in the assessment of antigenic fractions of helminths thereby providing a ready method of screening large numbers of fractions in immunized animals. In particular they should be of value in obtaining species-specific antigens which do not cross-react with heterologous helminth systems. One aspect of the use of skin tests in the examination of helminth antigens is that the antigens should be checked for non-specific reactions due to pharmacologically active substances present in the worm or created during the extraction process. For example, extracts of *Ascaris* contain histamine-releasing substances which degranulate mast cells and hence produce skin reactions of the immediate type in normal subjects [51]. Such extracts also contain material which produces a slow contraction of smooth muscle [52].

Other tests based on active anaphylaxis phenomena have been utilized by various authors in the investigation of helminth immunological mechanisms. For example, Schultz-Dale tests with isolated segments of ileum of guinea-pigs and antigen extracted from the eggs of *Toxocara* demonstrated a dose-dependency between the post-infection time and the number of infective eggs of *Toxocara* given to guinea-pigs [53]. Heavily infected animals were positive to Schultz-Dale reaction as early as 8 days while the lightest infected animals were not positive until the twentieth day of infection. The ability to detect an immune response as early as the eighth day is to be compared with the inability to detect circulating antibody before the twenty-eighth day by the use of living larvae placed in immune serum.

Similar techniques utilize the local allergic damage produced by the injection of specific antigen into the subcutaneous tissues of sensitized mice which results in the degranulation of mast cells and the release of pharmacologically active substances. The mouse infected with *T. spiralis* is a suitable subject for this since it contains relatively large numbers of mast cells in the subcutaneous connective tissue. When the skin of *T. spiralis* infected mice is injected with the homologous antigen (30 μg N/ml) tissue-spreads reveal disrupted mast cells. Subsequent work has demonstrated that infective mice react to both the metabolic and somatic antigens of *T. spiralis* and the severity of degranulation depends to some extent on the period of sensitization [54], since antigen-induced reactions produced 2 weeks after infection were relatively minor but later in the course of the infection cell injury was more pronounced. Sensitization can be passively transferred to normal mice by the injection of specific antiserum. The reaction has a relatively high degree of specificity in that mice, maximally sensitized to *T. spiralis*, do not show mast cell disruption when tested with somatic antigens extracted from heterologous worms, such as *Nippostrongylus* or *Strongyloides*.

Local anaphylaxis mechanisms may be replaced by general anaphylaxis, this being induced by the intravenous injection of antigen in a sensitized animal. This technique has been used many years ago in guinea-pigs in the study of antigens from *Ascaris* [55] and more recently it was shown that 1 month after infection of mice with 200 *Trichinella* larvae an intravenous challenge with somatic antigen (300 μg N/ml) rapidly induced characteristic signs of anaphylaxis [54]. These techniques have obvious uses and provide very critical and specific methods for the examination of fractionated antigens and those produced in *in vitro* culture.

Passive cutaneous anaphylaxis (PCA) did not receive extensive attention until the demonstration of reagin-like antibodies in animals immune to helminth parasites [56]. As with other skin-test techniques, this should provide a satisfactory method of examining in detail the various antigens and methods of immunization. This is perhaps illustrated in the recent work with *Nippostrongylus braziliensis* and *Schistosoma mansoni* in which skin-sensitizing antibodies of the reagin type show a close correlation with the acquisition of protective immunity. In the case of the rat parasite, *N. braziliensis'* serum from an infected animal is injected into the skin of a normal worm-free rat and 3 days later a mixture of antigen and Evans blue is injected intravenously. At present, antigens prepared from adult worms are the best source of material though infective larvae have been shown to contain a lesser amount of antigen [57]. Following injection of antigen, and within 20 to 30 minutes, a discrete blue area approximately 1·5 cm in diameter appears at the site of the injection of the serum. It has been found that the skin-sensitizing antibody is induced only by actual infections and attempts to induce it artificially by vaccinating rats with freshly homogenized adult worms (with or without Freund's complete adjuvant) have been unsuccessful. Similarly no immunity to reinfection is stimulated by this method of immunization though precipitating antibodies are induced by it. This technique provides a satisfactory and specific method for the investigation of antigenic fractions of parasites and the antibodies which are associated with immunity. Since there appears to be a close correlation between the skin-sensitizing antibodies and protective immunity it is probable that a satisfactory experimental model has been established to examine the importance of various antigens and their method of administration in the production of protective immunity. Modifications of the passive cutaneous anaphylaxis technique include the classical Prausnitz-Küstner reaction which has been studied in schistosomiasis and also in *Fasciola hepatica* infection in cattle.

Other *in vitro* techniques with whole living organisms
A wide variety of organisms, usually the larval stages, have been used in *in vitro* systems to investigate various effects of the immune response on parasites. In some instances these have formed the bases of diagnostic tests especially when it has been difficult or impossible to obtain enough soluble antigen for more quantitative techniques. Such tests have the advantage that they are simple to perform and read and may be carried out on a few organisms. Their disadvantage is the necessity for living stages and therefore they may be performed only in laboratories which maintain the parasites. The mixed-agglutination, immune-adhesion and the fluorescent-antibody techniques are, of course, applicable to living organisms but the techniques considered in this section are those with a more direct action on the parasite.

It is probable that any living stage which can be obtained and maintained for at least a limited period in a suitable medium would be satisfactory test antigen and the illustrations given below give some indication of the scope to which such techniques may be put.

Precipitin reactions with living parasites
The larval stages of *Trichinella spiralis*, *Ascaris* and human hookworms have been used for this and the following account illustrates the technique.

Parasitic stages obtained from the host (e.g. *T. spiralis* larvae by muscle digestion, or *Ascaris* larvae from the lungs of infected rabbits, guinea-pigs, etc.) are cleaned of tissue debris by sedimentation and decanting. Sterile saline is used in the latter stages and the final suspension of clean larvae may be made up in 1000 units of penicillin and 1 mg of streptomycin per ml. About 100 larvae are placed in a depression slide along with 0·2–0·5 ml of the test serum, diluted if necessary; the cavity is covered with a cover glass and sealed with wax or Vaseline and then incubated in a humid chamber at 36° C. The preparation is examined periodically (e.g. at 2, 5 and 24 hour intervals), attention being paid to the formation of refractile precipitates at the mouth, excretory pore and anus of the larvae. The technique employed should be sterile since the growth of bacteria, etc., interferes with the reaction and the reading of the result. Such a system has been used in the diagnosis of trichinosis [57], and is considered to be extremely sensitive, reactions becoming positive during the second to third week of illness. In addition to the species of parasites mentioned above, this technique has been used to measure antibody levels in guinea-pigs infected with *Toxocara*; it has also been used to determine the importance in the immune response of various developmental stages in sheep gastro-intestinal nematodes and undoubtedly it could be applied to a wide range of other species.

A similar technique has been used in investigation of immunological phenomena in cestode infections. Thus hatched hexacanth embryos from *Taenia* spp. eggs, when placed in homologous immune serum, develop a precipitate at one pole, which is the site of the orifice of a penetration gland [58], and workers in the Soviet Union have developed a serological test based on the formation of precipitates on the scolices of *Echinococcus* tapeworms when they are placed in homologous serum [59]. This latter observation can be correlated with that which demonstrated the existence of gland openings on the scolex of this tapeworm [60].

In vitro tests with schistosome developmental stages have been a profitable area of research and apart from their usefulness in investigating the mosaic of antibodies which are induced by infection, in some cases, they have been developed into diagnostic tests.

Cercarienhüllenreaktion (CHR)

This was originally described by Vogel & Minning [61] and has attracted attention as a diagnostic test in schistosomiasis. It is characterized by the formation of an encircling membrane or envelope, which is due to the swelling of the cercarial cuticle, when cercariae are placed in immune serum. The reaction is not species specific since infection with several other species of schistosomes induce the reaction but it is independent of other helminth infections. The reaction is capable of detecting infection as early as 40–47 days after experimental infection and it is positive with the sera of animals infected with parasites of one sex. It is not stage specific since all stages of the life cycle stimulate the reaction. There is some indication that the technique may be of value in assessing the cure of an infected person since the CHR becomes negative 5–7 months after successful therapy.

Apart from the intrinsic interest of the reaction of antibody with cercariae, the CHR has proved of great value in demonstrating the differences in antigenicity between cercariae before skin penetration and schistosomules immediately following skin penetration [62]. This latter application illustrates the exquisite nature of some of the reactions in helminth immunology and this, for example, is unlikely to have been detected by the more conventional techniques. It also illustrates the applicability of such a technique using small quantities of test material such as can only be obtained following the penetration of the skin by cercariae.

The technique for the CHR is as follows: Cercariae of *Schistosoma mansoni* are obtained from laboratory-reared *Australorbis glabratus* and concentrated so that a drop of suspension contains thirty to fifty cercariae. One drop is placed on a clean slide and mixed with one drop of serum and a cover glass placed on the preparation; this may be sealed with paraffin and the whole is placed in a Petri dish on moistened filter paper. The reaction is examined microscopically at 1, 2 and 4 hours, the formation of a dense envelope around the cercariae being noted and the reaction scored according to the degree of precipitation.

Cercarial agglutination test

This was first noted when the serum of monkeys infected with *S. mansoni* was found to agglutinate living cercariae of that species [63]. The appearance of agglutinins coincides with the appearance of eggs in the faeces of infected animals and occurs before the complement-fixation test is positive. There are usually more agglutinins in acute sera than in chronic. The test has yet to receive critical evaluation as a diagnostic test and it suffers from the disadvantage that non-specific agglutinins may be present in normal serum. These are frequently masked by a cercaricidal effect which can be eliminated by inactivation at 56° C.

Circumoval precipitin test

This was first reported by Oliver-Gonzáles [64] who observed precipitates around living schistosome eggs when they were placed in homologous serum from infected humans or monkeys. This is a reaction between specific antibodies and secretions which diffuse through the egg shell wall, being produced by the living miracidium inside the egg. The reaction is specific for the egg stage, being absorbable by eggs but not with adult or cercarial antigens. The reaction is also species specific, precipitates appearing around eggs in homologous serum only [65]. It seems likely that the antibodies are induced by the eggs which are deposited in the liver and venules of infected animals and may be due to a PAS-positive material from the glands of miracidia, this material diffusing through the egg shell. The reaction is stronger in chronic cases of schistosomiasis than in early stages and it may also be of value in assessing therapy since it has been noted to become weaker during therapy and negative 120–180 days after successful therapy [66].

The technique of the test is as follows: *Schistosoma mansoni* (or other species of schistosome) eggs are obtained from faeces and infected livers of animals and suspended in 1·75 per cent saline; this tonicity inhibits hatching. A given number of eggs [50] in a small volume of fluid is mixed with a drop of inactivated serum and the preparation sealed with wax or petroleum jelly. After incubation for 24 hours at 37° C in a humid chamber the preparation is examined under low magnification and the intensity of the precipitate on the eggs and the percentage of eggs affected are determined. The precipitates appear as long plumes or chain-like formations; in normal serum small blister-like reactions may be seen but these are readily distinguished from the reactions with immune serum.

Miracidal immobilization test

This phenomenon consists of a slowing or stoppage of the ciliary movement of miracidia when they are placed in immune serum [67]. Relatively high levels of the antibodies responsible are found in infected animals and humans and these appear much earlier than those responsible for the other serological tests. The reaction is positive with infection with all developmental stages of schistosomes and some degree of cross-reaction occurs between miracidia of heterologous schistosomes, but the reaction is strongest with the homologous species. Immobilizing antibodies may be found in many normal sera from various animals but usually these can be removed by heating. Such reactions are probably similar to the miracidal, complement dependent, component of normal serum which is reactive with the miradicia of *Fasciola hepatica* [68].

The technique of the miracidal immobilization test is as follows: miracidia are hatched in distilled water from a suspension of clean eggs obtained from the liver, digestive tract and faeces of infected animals. Suspensions (100 per 1 ml) are prepared in chlorine-free water and inactivated serum, serially diluted, is mixed with the suspension. The reaction is examined microscopically after 10 minutes.

While this reaction probably will never gain favour as a diagnostic test it would appear to offer a system of value for the study of cytotoxic effects of antibody on parasitic stages which are easily obtained. Furthermore, because of their free-living existence the miracidia can be maintained in simple solutions, thus lending themselves to detailed biochemical and manometric studies.

An extension of the above techniques is the study of immunological mechanisms on organisms developing in *in vitro* systems. Using such an approach it has been shown that the infective stages of the cattle nematode *Oesophagostomum radiatum*, grown in the presence of tissue extracts of immune animals, react with precipitate formation and a coating phenomenon (? immune adherence) only when they have developed in culture to the late third larval stage [69]. A delay in development of larvae in the presence of homologous immune serum was noted in this system and also with the *in vitro* growth of the rat nematode *Nippostrongylus braziliensis* in its homologous immune serum. However, comparable work with *Neoplectana glazeri*, an insect nematode, showed different results. This nematode can be cultured in defined media through successive generations, but serum from rabbits immunized artificially with the nematode failed to cause deleterious effects on growth or reproduction despite an abundance of precipitate on the parasites and in the medium [70]. The reaction was specific in that reaction did not occur when two related nematodes were grown in the presence of *N. glazeri* immune serum.

Unfortunately there are no parasitic nematodes of vertebrates which can be cultured with the facility of *N. glazeri* but even short-term culture or maintenance may be sufficient for many studies. Thus, a decrease in oxygen consumption of infective larvae of *N. braziliensis* was noted when they were placed in immune serum [71], similar results have been demonstrated with adult worms of this species and immune serum [72] and an alteration in their behaviour in a thermal gradient when exposed to immune serum has also been investigated [73].

It is unlikely that such procedures will ever be used as diagnostic tests but they do provide a most exquisite method of indicating the stages of development, the patterns of behaviour and the physiological processes which are affected by the immune mechanisms and hence they can be used for the detection of antibodies which are responsible for these effects.

References

[1] World Health Organization (1964) *Research in Immunology.* Wld Hlth Org. Techn. Rep. Ser. No. 286
World Health Organization (1965) *Immunology and Parasitic Diseases.* Wld Hlth Org. Techn. Rep. Ser. No. 315

[2] BERNTZEN A.K. (1965) Comparative growth and development of *Trichinella spiralis in vitro* and *in vivo*, with a redescription of the life cycle. *Exptl Parasitol.* **16**, 74

[3] BERNTZEN A.K. & MUELLER J.F. (1964) *In vitro* cultivation of *Spirometra mansonoides* (Cestoda) from the Procercoid to the early adult. *J. Parasitol.* **50**, 705

[4] KAGAN I.G., ALLAIN, DOROTHY S. & NORMAN, LOIS (1959) An evaluation of the hemagglutination and flocculation tests in the diagnosis of echinococcus disease. *Amer. J. Trop. Med.* **8**, 51

[5] THORSON R. E. (1956) Proteolytic activity in extracts of the esophagus of adults of *Ancylostoma caninum* and the effect of immune serum on this activity. *J. Parasitol.* **42**, 21

[6] SOULSBY E.J.L., SOMMERVILLE R.I. & STEWART D.F. (1959) Antigenic stimulus of exsheathing fluid in self-cure of sheep infected with *Haemonchus contortus. Nature, Lond.* **183**, 553

[7] MELCHER L.R. (1943) An antigenic analysis of *Trichinella spiralis. Jour. Infect. Dis.* **73**, 31

[8] CHAFFEE E.F., BAUMAN P.M. & SHAPILO J.J. (1954) Diagnosis of schistosomiasis by complement fixation. *Amer. J. Trop. Med.* **3**, 905

[9] KENT N.H. (1963) Comparative immunochemistry of larval and adult forms of *Schistosoma mansoni. Ann. N.Y. Acad. Sci.* **133**, 100

[10] SAWADA T., TAKEI K., KATAMINE D. & YOSHIMURA T. (1965) Immunological studies on filariasis. III. Isolation and purification of antigen for intradermal skin test. *Jap. J. Expt. Med.* **35**, 125

[11] SAWADA T., NAGATA Y., TAKEI K. & SATO S. (1964) Studies on the substance responsible for the skin test in clonorchiasis. *Jap. J. Expt. Med.* **34**, 315

[12] TANNER C.E. & GREGORY JUDITH (1961) Immunochemical studies of the antigens of *Trichinella spiralis*. I. Identification and enumeration of antigens. *Canad. J. Microbiol.* **7**, 473

[13] TANNER C.E. (1963) Immunochemical study of the antigens of *Trichinella spiralis* larvae. III. Enzymatic degradation of the major precipitating antigen. *Exptl. Parasitol.* **14**, 346

[14] WADSWORTH A.B. (ed.) (1947) *Standard Methods of the Division of Laboratories and Research of the New York State Department of Health*. Baltimore: Williams & Wilkins

[15] OSLER A.G. (1963) Skin reactions of the immediate and delayed types of hypersensitivity: Some aspects of their mechanisms. In *Immunodiagnosis of Helminthic Infections*, ed. JACKOWSKI L.A. Amer. J. Hyg. Monograph Series No. 22

[16] COOMBS R.R.A., COOMBS A.M. & INGRAM D.G. (1961) *The Serology of Conglutination and its Relation to Disease*. Oxford: Blackwell Scientific Publications

[17] FRISCH A.N., WHIMS C.B. & OPPENHEIM J.M. (1947) Immunologic reactions in trichinosis with purified antigen. *Amer. J. Clin. Path.* **17**, 29

[18] SOULSBY E.J.L. (1957) Antigenic analysis of *Ascaris* tissues by the double diffusion precipitin test. *Trans. Roy. Soc. Trop. Med. Hyg.* **51**, 9

[19] KAGAN I.G. (1957) Serum-agar double diffusion studies with *Ascaris* antigens. *J. Infect. Dis.* **101**, 11

[20] BIGUET J., CAPRON A. & TRAN VAN KY P. (1962) Les antigènes de *Schistosoma mansoni*. 1. Etude électrophorétique et immunoélectrophorétique. Characterization des antigènes specifiques. *Ann. Inst. Pasteur.* **103**, 763

[21] CAPRON A., BIGUET J., TRAN VAN KY P. & ROSE G. (1964) Possibilités nouvelles dans le distomatose humaine a 'Fasciola hepatica'. Mise en évidence d'anticorps sériques par immunoélectrophorèse. *La Presse Med.* **72**, 3103

[22] KENT N.H. (1963) Fractionation, isolation and definition of antigens from parasitic helminths. In *Immunodiagnosis of Helminthic Infections*, ed. JACKOWSKI L.A. Amer. J. Hyg. Monograph Series No. 22

[23] SOMMERVILLE R.I. (1957) The exsheathing mechanism of nematode infective larvae. *Exptl. Parasitol.* **6**, 18

[24] ROGERS W.P. & SOMMERVILLE R.I. (1960) The physiology of the second ecdysis of parasitic nematodes. *Parasitology* **50**, 329

[25] SOULSBY E.J.L. & STEWART D.F. (1960) Serological studies of the self-cure reaction in sheep infected with *Haemonchus contortus*. *Austral. J. Agric. Res.* **11**, 595

[26] DINEEN J.K. (1963) Immunological aspects of parasitism. *Nature, Lond.* **197**, 268

[27] DAMIAN R.T. (1964) Molecular mimicry: Antigen sharing by parasite and host and its consequences. *Amer. Naturalist.* **98**, 129

[28] ALLISON A.C. & HUMPHREY J.H. (1959) Estimation of the size of antigens by gel diffusion methods. *Nature, Lond.* **183**, 1590

[29] KAGAN I.G. & NORMAN, LOIS (1963) Analysis of helminth antigens (*Echinococcus granulosus* and *Schistosoma mansoni*) by agar gel methods. *Ann. N.Y. Acad. Sci.* **113**, 130

[30] SOULSBY E.J.L. (unpublished observations)

[31] BOYDEN S.V. (1951) Adsorption of proteins on erythrocytes treated with tannic acid and subsequent hemagglutination by anti-protein sera. *J. expt. Med.* **93**, 107

[32] ALLAIN, DOROTHY S. & KAGAN I.G. (1961) The use of formalized red cells in the serology of hydatid disease. *J. Parasitol.* **47**, 61

[33] SOULSBY E.J.L. (1960) The use of the hemagglutination technique for the detection of antibodies in gastro-intestinal nematode infections of sheep. *Brit. Vet. J.* **116**, 1

[34] SUESSENGUTH H. & KLINE B.S. (1944) A simple rapid flocculation slide test for trichinosis in man and in swine. *Amer. J. Clin. Path.* **14**, 471

[35] KAGAN I.G. (1960) Trichinosis: A review of biologic, serologic and immunologic aspects. *J. Infect. Dis.* **107**, 65

[36] SADUN E.H. & NORMAN, LOIS (1959) Metabolic and somatic antigens in the determination of the response of rabbits to graded infections of *Trichinella spiralis*. *J. Parasitol.* **43**, 236

[37] ANDERSON R.I. (1960) Serologic diagnosis of *Schistosoma mansoni* infections. I. Development of a cercarial antigen slide flocculation test. *Amer. J. Trop. Med.* **9**, 299

[38] NELSON R.A. (1953) The immune-adherence phenomenon. An immunologically specific reaction between micro-organisms and erythrocytes leading to enhanced phagocytosis. *Science* **118**, 733

[39] SOULSBY E.J.L. (1962) The antigenicity of the nematode cuticle. *Parasitology* **52**, 5P

[40] COOMBS R.R.A. (1963) In *Immunological Methods*, C.I.O.M.S. Symposium, ed. ACKROYD J.F. & TURK J.L. Oxford: Blackwell Scientific Publications

[41] STEELE A.S.V. & COOMBS R.R.A. (1964) The red cell linked antigen test for incomplete antibodies to soluble proteins. *Int'l. Arch. Allergy* **25**, 11

[42] COOMBS R.R.A., POUT D.D. & SOULSBY E.J.L. (1965) Globulin, possibly of antibody nature, combining with the cuticle of live *Turbatrix aceti*. *Exptl. Parasitol.* **16**, 311

[43] COOMBS R.R.A. & FISET M.L. (1954) Detection of complete and incomplete antibodies to egg albumin by means of a sheep red cell–egg albumin unit. *Brit. J. exp. Path.* **35**, 472

[44] SADUN E.H., ANDERSON R.I. & WILLIAMS J.S. (1961) Fluorescent antibody test for the laboratory diagnosis of schistosomiasis in humans by using dried blood smears on filter paper. *Exptl. Parasitol.* **11**, 117

[45] PELLEGRINO J. & NUNES R.M.B. (1956) Tecnica de obtencao de cercarias dessecadas de *Schistosoma mansoni* para o preparo de antigenos. *Rev. bras. Malar.* **8**, 397

[46] SADUN E.H. (1963) Seminar on immunity to parasitic helminths. VII. Fluorescent antibody technique for helminth infections. *Exptl. Parasitol.* **13**, 72

[47] SADUN E.H., ANDERSON R.I. & WILLIAMS J.S. (1962) A fluorescent antibody test for the serological diagnosis of trichinosis. *J. Parasitol.* **Suppl. 48**, 17

[48] JACKSON G.J. (1959) Fluorescent antibody studies of *Trichinella spiralis* infections. *J. Infect. Dis.* **105**, 97

[49] COLEMAN R.M. & FOTORNY N.M. (1962) *In vitro* isolation of *Hymenolepis nana* and antibody-binding sites. *Nature, Lond.* **195**, 920

[50] SOULSBY E.J.L. (1962) The specificity of skin reactions in pigs using *Trichinella spiralis* antigen. In *Trichinellosis, Proc. 1st Int. Conf. on Trichinellosis*, ed. KOZAR Z. Warsaw: Polish Scientific Publishers

[51] UVNAS B. (1960) Mechanism of action of a histamine-liberating principle in jelly fish (*Cyanea capillata*). *Ann. N.Y. Acad. Sci.* **90**, 751

[52] UVNAS B. (1963) Mechanism of histamine release in mast cells. *Ann. N.Y. Acad. Sci.* **103**, 278

[53] OLSON L.J. & SCHULZ C.W. (1963) Nematode induced hypersensitivity reactions in guinea pigs: Onset of eosinophilia and positive Schultz-Dale reactions following graded infections with *Toxocara canis*. *Ann. N.Y. Acad. Sci.* **113**, 440

[54] BRIGGS N.T. (1963) Hypersensitivity in murine trichinosis. Some responses of Trichinella-infected mice to antigen and 5-hydroxytryptophan. *Ann. N.Y. Acad. Sci.* **113**, 456

[55] SPRENT J.F.A. (1949) On the toxic and allergic manifestations produced by the tissues and fluids of *Ascaris*. 1. Effect of different tissues. *J. Infect. Dis.* **84**, 221

[56] OGILVIE B.M. (1964) Reagin-like antibodies in animals immune to helminth parasites. *Nature, Lond.* **204**, 91

[57] ROTH H. (1946) Employment of serological and skin tests at outbreaks of trichinosis in the Ålingoas and Boras districts (Sweden). *Acta Med. Scand.* **126**, 17

[58] SILVERMAN P.H. (1955) A technique for studying the *in vitro* effect of serum on activated Taenied hexacanth embryos. *Nature, Lond.* **176**, 598

[59] SHULTS R.S. & ISMAGILOVA R.G. (1963) Scolex-precipitation reaction in the diagnosis hydatidosis. *Med. Parazit. Para. Bol. Moscow.* **32**, 678

[60] SMYTH J.D. (1964) The biology of the hydatid organisms. In *Advances in Parasitology*, Vol. 2, p. 169, ed. DAWES B. London and New York: Academic Press

[61] VOGEL H. & MINNING W. (1949) Hüllenbildung bei Bilharzia-Cercarien im Serum Bilharzia-infizierter Tiere und Menschen. *Zbl. Bakt.* **153**, 91

[62] STIREWALT M.A. (1963) Cercaria vs Schistosomule (*Schistosoma mansoni*): Absence of the pericercarial envelope *in vivo* and the early physiological and histological metamorphosis of the parasite. *Exptl. Parasitol.* **13**, 395

[63] LIU C. & BANG F.P. (1950) Agglutination of cercariae of *Schistosoma mansoni* by immune sera. *Proc. Soc. exp. Biol. Med.* **74**, 68

[64] OLIVER-GONZÁLEZ J. (1954) Anti-egg precipitin in the serum of humans infected with *Schistosoma mansoni. J. Infect. Dis.* **95**, 86

[65] OLIVER-GONZÁLEZ J., BAUMAN P.M. & BENENSON A.S. (1955) Immunological aspects of infections with *Schistosoma mansoni. Amer. J. Trop. Med.* **4**, 443

[66] OLIVER-GONZÁLEZ J., RAMOS F.L. & COKER C.M. (1955) Serological reactions against egg antigens as an aid in the evaluation of therapy in schistosomiasis. *Amer. J. Trop. Med.* **4**, 908

[67] SENTERFIT L.B. (1953) Immobilization of *Schistosoma mansoni* miracidia by immune serum. *Proc. Soc. exp. Biol. Med.* **84**, 5

[68] SOULSBY E.J.L. (1957) An antagonistic action of sheep serum on the miracidia of *Fasciola hepatica. J. Helminth* **31**, 161

[69] DOUVRES F.W. (1962) The *in vitro* cultivation of *Oesophagostomum radiatum*, the nodular worm of cattle. II. The use of this technique to study immune responses of host tissue extracts against the developing nematodes. *J. Parasitol.* **48**, 175

[70] JACKSON J.G. (1962) On axenic cultures of certain protozoan and worm parasites of insects. *Trans. N.Y. Acad. Sci.* **24**

[71] MULLIGAN W., URQUHART G.M., JENNINGS F.W. & NEILSON J.T.M. (1965) Immunological studies on *Nippostrongylus braziliensis* infection in the rat: The 'self cure' phenomenon. *Exptl. Parasitol.* **16**, 341

[72] SCHWABE C.W. (1957) The *in vitro* action of immune rat serum on the nematode *Nippostrongylus muris. J. Infect. Dis.* **62**, 337

[73] McCUE J.F. & THORSON R.E. (1965) Host effects on the migration of *Nippostrongylus braziliensis* in a thermal gradient. *J. Parasitol.* **51**, 414

SECTION 4

Methods for the Study of Cellular and Transplantation Immunity

CHAPTER 29

The Biometrics of the Spleen Weight Assay

D.MICHIE

Introduction

Simonsen [1] has developed a method for the bio-assay of immunological activity in suspensions of lymphoid cells. The method is based on the finding that the degree of splenomegaly which develops in the early stages of the graft-versus-host reaction is correlated with the number of immunologically competent donor cells. The method lends itself to application in two main fields of investigation, namely:

1. The analysis of all kinds of lymphoid cell chimeras, with the object of establishing the relative proportions, and immunological status, of the donor and host cells present, and

2. The quantitative measurement of the immunological effects of natural and experimental variables brought to bear upon lymphoid cell suspensions, lymphoid tissues or whole animals. The assay of transplantation antigen falls under this heading.

This chapter relates spleen assay methods to simple biometrical considerations, and in addition offers practical rules and suggestions. These have for the most part been derived from applying standard assay theory as outlined by Finney [2] to experimental data on the splenomegaly phenomenon in the mouse including original material kindly made available to me by Dr Simonsen.

The same general principles, and for the most part the same detailed procedures, should be applicable to any other species in which the splenomegaly reaction is well marked and in which sufficiently uniform material, from the immuno-genetic point of view, is available.

Graft-versus-host disease as a test of immunological activity

A graft-versus-host reaction occurs when the grafted cells are competent to react against the host, but the host, for one reason or another, is not competent to act against the graft. Any sign of the ensuing disease, e.g. growth-retardation or death, can in principle be used for testing the immunological activity of a donor cell suspension. The advantages in the mouse species offered by the spleen test are:

1. The rapidity with which a result is obtained (the time required ranges from 7 to 12 days, according to strain-combination).
2. Sensitivity to low doses of donor cells. $0.5 + 10^6$ lymphoid cells are readily detectable in donor–host combinations which require ten or twenty times that number to cause growth retardation, and even more to cause appreciable mortality.
3. The availability of a quantitative scale of measurement on which biological variation is reasonably small relative to effects of experimental variables.

The drawback of the method for some purposes is that the test animals require to be killed at a definite interval after injection, since the splenomegaly usually subsides after the second week. For continuous monitoring of graft-versus-host activity without sacrifice of the subject, the weight-gain test of Russell [3] and the phagocytic test of Howard [4] are available. The latter has a sensitivity comparable to that of the spleen test [5].

Spleen tests

A simple spleen test will now be described, as a step towards the more complex topic of the spleen assay. A *test* seeks to discover whether one preparation possesses more activity or potency than some other preparation, whereas an *assay* is more ambitious and seeks to estimate the *relative potency* of the one to the other and at the same time to set limits of accuracy to the estimate.

As an illustration Table 29.1 is made up of material abstracted from a large unpublished series of observations by Simonsen. The comparison here is between the efficacy of spleen cells from normal AKR-strain adult donors and from AKR donors which had been pre-immunized against C3H antigens. In each case the donor cells were injected intraperitoneally into F_1 hybrids between the two strains. The use of F_1 hybrid recipients is the standard practice. Such animals are genetically disqualified from rejecting the donor cells, none of whose antigens are foreign to them, but are at the same time fully qualified to stimulate the donor cells by virtue of the antigens inherited from the other parent strain. The use of infants rather than older mice is dictated by considerations of sensitivity.

In order to interpret the data of Table 29.1 we need to find quantities expressing the mean responses to the two donor types used. In the uninjected control mice there appears to be a correlation, even within the individual litters, between the spleen weights and body weights. This relation is generally found, so that some correction for body weight is called for. In practice it is

TABLE 29.1

A test of the effect of pre-immunizing adult AKR mice with C3H antigens on the power of their spleen cells to produce splenomegaly in infant C3H × AKR hybrids

Test inoculum	Litter No.	Age at injection	Age at sacrifice	Injected			Uninjected		
				Spl. wt. (mg)	Body wt. (g)	Rel. spl. wt.	Spl. wt. (mg)	Body wt. (g)	Rel. spl. wt.
10 million spleen cells from untreated adult AKR mice	256	0 d.	11 d.	9	3·4	26	9	3·7	24
				11	3·5	31	11	3·8	29
				11	3·6	31	10	3·7	27
	255	0 d.	11 d.	16	5·0	32	18	5·3	34
				21	5·3	40	23	5·6	41
	266	10 d.	21 d.	60	10·9	55	57	11·5	50
				40	10·4	38			
5 million spleen cells from adult AKR mice pre-immunized with C3H × AKR tissue	217	7 d.	17 d.	35	4·7	74	13	4·9	27
				41	4·8	85	11	4·7	23
				35	4·9	71	11	4·4	25
	218	7 d.	17 d.	33	4·0	83	7	3·8	18
				35	3·8	92	10	4·3	23
				39	4·0	97	9	3·9	23

found adequate to divide spleen weight by body weight, thus deriving a relative spleen weight expressible, for example, as milligrammes spleen per 10 g body weight. These ratios have been calculated and entered in the table. A second feature of the data, equally apparent after correction for body weight, is that the mice with obvious spleen enlargement show greater variability among themselves than do their litter-mate controls. It is desirable to find a scale on which variability is less dependent on the mean, and the logarithmic scale suggests itself. In Table 29.2 the data of Table 29.1 are shown as the logarithms of the relative spleen weights, a change of scale which has removed some at least of the discrepancy. The comparison between treated and control mice can now be expressed as a *difference* as shown in the table. The antilogarithm of this quantity estimates the relative spleen weight of the treated mice as a ratio to that of the controls, the 'spleen index' of Simonsen.

Although the difference between normal and pre-immunized donors seems obvious enough from inspection, an estimate derived from such data can only be given a very low level of precision. Indeed, unless the five litters have been assigned to the two treatments by strict randomization, no limits of error can validly be assigned at all. Supposing that proper randomization had been applied, the correct procedure would be a weighted analysis of variance, leading to a *t*-test with three degrees of freedom. The result would still have to be interpreted with caution owing to obvious discrepancies between the different litters in respect of age and the interval between injection and sacrifice.

Principles of weighting

Whether or not such an analysis were thought worth the trouble, it is likely that the investigator would wish to combine the estimates obtained from different litters to give a single combined estimate for each treatment. Here again a method of weighting is required.

The appropriate weight to be attached to a difference between the mean of n_1 treated and that of n_2 untreated mice in a litter is given by

$$w = \frac{n_1 n_2}{s_1^2 n_2 + s_2^2 n_1} \tag{1}$$

where s_1 is the intra-litter standard deviation of treated mice and s_2 that of untreated controls. When s_1 can be assumed equal to s_2 this reduces to

$$\frac{1}{s^2} \times \frac{n_1 n_2}{n_1 + n_2}.$$

For most purposes the constant factor $1/s^2$ can then be dropped, since only the relative, not the absolute, magnitudes of the weights are of importance.

Table 29.2

The data of Table 29.1 after logarithmic conversion

Test inoculum	Litter No.	Age at injection	Age at sacrifice	Log relative spleen weights			Antilogarithm of the difference, estimating 'spleen index'
				Injected	Uninjected	Difference	
10 million spleen cells from untreated adult AKR mice	256	0 d.	11 d.	1·415	1·380		
				1·491	1·462		
				1·491	1·431		
			Means:	1·466	1·424	+0·042	1·10
	255	0 d.	11 d.	1·505	1·531		
				1·602	1·613		
			Means:	1·553	1·572	−0·019	0·96
	266	10 d.	21 d.	1·778	1·699		
				1·602			
			Means:	1·690	1·699	−0·009	0·98
5 million spleen cells from adult AKR mice pre-immunized with C3H × AKR tissue	217	7 d.	17 d.	1·869	1·431		
				1·929	1·362		
				1·851	1·398		
			Means:	1·883	1·397	+0·486	3·06
	218	7 d.	17 d.	1·919	1·255		
				1·964	1·362		
				1·987	1·362		
			Means:	1·957	1·326	+0·631	4·28

A combined estimate of the average effect of treatment is obtained as $\Sigma wd/\Sigma w$ where d stands for the individual differences between means.

The assumption that s_1 is equal to s_2 is appropriately made when testing a null hypothesis according to which the treatment is without effect. This approach has been illustrated in the analysis of spleen tests by Michie, Woodruff & Zeiss [6]. Otherwise it is not applicable, for the variability among litter-mates receiving a given dose greatly exceeds that found among untreated control mice. In Table 29.3 are shown estimates of s_1^2 and s_2^2 obtained from ten litters of C3H + DBA-2 mice each containing some members injected with adult C3H spleen cells. s_1^2 is here estimated as $2 \cdot 25 \times s_2^2$, a ratio which is significantly greater than unity (Table V of Fisher & Yates [7]).

TABLE 29.3

Estimates of variability derived from log relative spleen weights in litters of C3H × DBA-2 mice injected intraperitoneally with adult C3H spleen cells. Ages at injection ranged from 0 days to 8 days. The variance of response, s^2, is estimated from the within-litter within-dose level mean square

	Mean spleen indices	s^2 estimated as the mean square deviation	Degrees of freedom	Variance ratio
Injected mice	1·66–2·70	0·00417	10	
	2·75–3·16	0·00459	10	
	3·39–4·37	0·00319	9	
	Combined	0·00401	29	
Uninjected litter-mates		0·00178	22	2·25

The fact that the logarithmic transformation has not entirely removed the discrepancy in variance is of no importance for the assay analyses which will later be described, since these are based on comparisons between treated mice at different dose-levels and do not utilize untreated litter-mates except for checking purposes. It will, however, be of the greatest importance that the transformation should remove any tendency among batches of treated mice for the variance of response to be correlated with the mean. The subdivision of the treated mice of Table 29.3 into three response levels shows that this criterion has been adequately met.

Split-litter tests

A large gain in information accrues when comparisons are made within instead of between litters, so that effects both of known variables such as age or litter-size, and of uncontrolled variables affecting litters as units, are balanced out between the treatments which are being compared. An example of a split-litter test of immune as compared with normal AKR donors is given in Table 29.4, for comparison with the data of Table 29.2. Although only two litters have been used, the test is far more informative and the result more conclusive.

In an analysis of variance, or a *t*-test, applied to these data, the comparatively low level of variation observed *within* treatment groups can now be utilized as the basis for tests of significance. Admittedly this approach makes the assumption that there is no interaction between litter-effects and treatment-effects. That is to say, although the levels of response to the two treatments are expected to fluctuate from litter to litter, they are assumed to be

TABLE 29.4

A split-litter test of the effect of pre-immunizing adult AKR mice with C3H antigens on the power of their spleen cells to produce splenomegaly in infant C3H × AKR hybrids. Interval between injection and sacrifice: 10 days. Numbers denote log relative spleen weights

Litter No.	Age at injection	2×10^6 cells from immune AKR	2×10^6 cells from normal AKR	Nil	Difference between immune donor and normal donor
277	7 d.	1·489	1·167	1·212	
		1·573	1·230	1·255	
		1·477	1·230		
	Means:	1·513	1·209		+0·304
278	9 d.	1·674	1·480	1·449	
		1·667	1·462	1·433	
	Means:	1·671	1·471		+0·200

affected to the same degree, the *relative* effects of the two treatments remaining unaltered. In the present instance this assumption, which will acquire great importance in the later analysis of assay results, is probably not warranted. The difference between the two values in the right-hand column of the table is suspiciously large, and the full analysis of variance confirms that the discrepancy, although not attaining formal significance, is suggestive ($0.05 < P < 0.10$). The likely explanation is that the 'responses' to normal donor cells probably do not represent responses at all, the dose-level being sub-threshold, as suggested by comparison with the untreated controls. Hence the assumption of non-interaction, applicable only to differences between true responses, is not valid. The above thus provides a good illustration of the usefulness of including uninjected controls ('blank' injections with host-type cells are even better) in split-litter tests and also, as we shall see, in full-scale assays. They do not themselves enter the analysis, but are there as a check that the validity-requirements have been met.

It may be emphasized in passing that this failure of parent-strain cells to provoke the splenomegaly response is characteristic of strain combinations, such as C3H and AKR, where there is no antigenic difference in respect of the H-2 group [8]. It should, therefore, be borne in mind that unless pre-immunization procedures are used the splenomegaly reaction, unlike the homograft reaction to skin grafts, is only applicable to the analysis of H-2 differences.

The dose-response line

Even if the foregoing split-litter test constituted a true comparison of response-levels, it would still be impossible to translate the result into an estimate of the relative potency of the two kinds of inoculum, unless by chance the standard (non-immunized) and test (immunized) preparations had been administered at different dosages which happened to yield the same mean response. It would then be possible to say that one million cells of the test were equivalent in spleen-enlarging potency to x million cells of the standard, but only on the assumption that on a logarithmic plot of dosage, the dose-response lines obtained with the two preparations would be found to run parallel. This can be seen intuitively from inspection of the assay illustrated in Fig. 29.1. It is evident that the horizontal distance between the two dose-response lines will give the same estimate of relative potency irrespective of the level on the response scale at which the distance is measured.

Two other characteristics of a good assay system, although not essential, as is parallelism, are none the less highly desirable in simplifying the analysis. The first of these is that measurements should be expressed on a scale which eliminates gross dependence of the variability of response upon the mean. The use of the logarithm of the relative spleen weight has already been discussed from this point of view and found, at least in the material there examined, to be adequate (see Table 29.3). The other criterion of a satisfactory scale is that the dose-response line should not depart detectably from a straight line in that part of the response-range over which it is proposed to use the assay. Unless these characteristics of the dose-response line have been carefully verified for the particular material and experimental conditions to be employed in an assay, the use of the standard methods for analysing the result is not justified and should not be attempted.

In Table 29.5 results are shown which take a form ideally suited for such preliminary verification, except that in practice a much larger series would be needed to yield firm conclusions. The small sample shown is presented merely in order to illustrate the structure of the analysis, which has been set out very fully for use as an exemplar.

The form of the dose-response relation can be displayed by plotting the three means at the foot of the table against dose-levels as has been done in Fig. 29.2. An estimate of the slope can obviously be obtained from a comparison of the mean responses to the top and bottom dose-levels: as shown

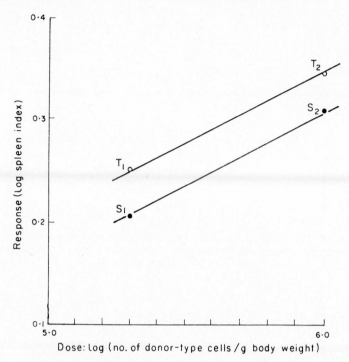

FIG. 29.1. Typical spleen assay results (means of four replicates). Horizontal distance between lines is approximately 0·3 on the log dosage scale, indicating in this case a twofold difference in potency between test and standard preparations.

Host type: $(CBA \times C57BL)F_1$
Donor type: S = Normal C57BL
        T = C57BL immunized by CBA tumour graft
$T_2 = 10^6$ cells of T per g body weight of host
$T_1 = 2 \times 10^5$ cells of T per g body weight + 8×10^5 cells of B
$S_2 = 10^6$ cells of S per g body weight
$S_1 = 2 \times 10^5$ cells of S per g body weight + 8×10^5 cells of B
B = host type $(CBA \times C57BL)F_1$

graphically in the figure these means indicate that an increase of two dose-levels has raised the response by 0·15, denoted by the symbol $\bar{U}$. The middle mean response has nothing to say about the slope, but is used to test the straightness of the line. The vertical distance of this point (or, more conveniently, twice the distance, $\bar{V}$) from a straight line connecting the upper and lower responses provides a measure of curvature. The main question to be answered is whether the value of $\bar{V}$ departs sufficiently from zero to contradict the assumption of linearity. If so, it suggests either that the logarithmic measure of response was a bad choice or that some systematic experimental

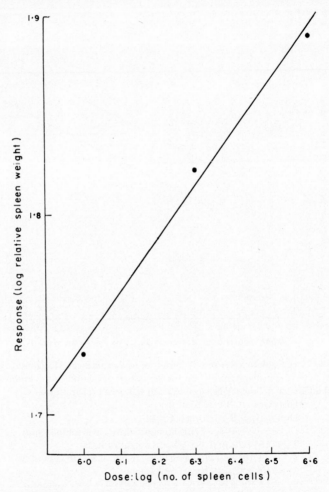

Fig. 29.2. Graphic presentation of the data of Table 29.5 showing the form of the dose-response line.

error is present, of which the most likely is failure to choose a dose-range which ensures that the responses fall within the linear part of the dose-response relation. A subsidiary question is whether the $\bar{U}$ and $\bar{V}$ values calculated from the individual litters show more litter-to-litter fluctuation than

TABLE 29.5

A dose-response test with duplicate doses. A response, y, is expressed as log relative spleen weight. $\bar{y}_B$ denotes the mean response in litter B, $\bar{y}_{A1}$ the mean response at dose-level 1 in litter A, etc. $\bar{y}$ is the general mean

Litter	Age at injection	(Uninjected controls)	Dose levels 1(= 1×10^6)	2(= 2×10^6)	3(= 4×10^6)	Coefficient of slope $\bar{y}_3-\bar{y}_1 = U$	Coefficient of curvature $\bar{y}_1+\bar{y}_3-2\bar{y}_2 = V$	Means for the different litters
A	1 d.	1·665	1·892	1·989	1·952			
		1·547	1·820	2·079	2·029			
		Means:	$1\cdot8560 = \bar{y}_{A1}$	$2\cdot0340 = \bar{y}_{A2}$	$1\cdot9905 = \bar{y}_{A3}$	$+0\cdot1345 = \bar{U}_A$	$-0\cdot2215 = \bar{V}_A$	$1\cdot9602 = \bar{y}_A$
B	5 d.	1·415	1·754	1·598	1·792			
		1·456	1·746	1·789	1·932			
		Means:	$1\cdot7500 = \bar{y}_{B1}$	$1\cdot6935 = \bar{y}_{B2}$	$1\cdot8620 = \bar{y}_{B3}$	$+0\cdot1120 = \bar{U}_B$	$+0\cdot2250 = \bar{V}_B$	$1\cdot7685 = \bar{y}_B$
C	3 d.	1·459	1·551	1·760	1·799			
		1·408	1·667	1·720	1·829			
		Means:	$1\cdot6090 = \bar{y}_{C1}$	$1\cdot7400 = \bar{y}_{C2}$	$1\cdot8140 = \bar{y}_{C3}$	$+0\cdot2050 = \bar{U}_C$	$-0\cdot0570 = \bar{V}_C$	$1\cdot7210 = \bar{y}_C$
Means for the different dose-levels:			$1\cdot7383 = \bar{y}_1$	$1\cdot8225 = \bar{y}_2$	$1\cdot8888 = \bar{y}_3$	$+0\cdot1505 = \bar{U}$	$-0\cdot0179 = \bar{V}$	$1\cdot8166 = \bar{y}$

II

can be attributable to sampling variation. A positive answer is a danger-signal that injection and dilution procedures may not have been properly standardized.

A test of the type illustrated in Table 29.5 thus represents a reconnaissance of the territory which later assays are to occupy. These assays, if the '6-point' design is adopted (see next section) will themselves afford further tests of linearity. But the 'fluctuation' test referred to above can only be performed

TABLE 29.6

Plan for the analysis of data of the type shown in Table 29.5. N is the total number of mice entering the analysis, i.e. 6k where k is the number of litters. n is the number in the category indicated by the attached subscript. A bar over a symbol, e.g. $\bar{y}_B$, denotes the mean for the category concerned

Source of variation	Sum of squares	Degrees of freedom
Total variation about the general mean	$\Sigma y^2 - N\bar{y}^2$	$N-1$
Differences between litter means	$n_A\bar{y}_A^2 + n_B\bar{y}_B^2 + n_C\bar{y}_C^2 - N\bar{y}^2$	$k-1$
Within litters (can be obtained by sub-traction of above two items)	$\Sigma y^2 - n_A\bar{y}_A^2 - n_B\bar{y}_B^2 - n_C\bar{y}_C^2$	$N-k$
Slope	$\bar{U}^2 k$	1 ⎫
Curvature	$\frac{1}{3}\bar{V}^2 k$	1 ⎪
Differences between litter slopes	$\bar{U}_A^2 + \bar{U}_B^2 + \bar{U}_C^2 - \bar{U}^2 k$	$k-1$ ⎬
Differences between litter curvatures	$\frac{1}{3}(\bar{V}_A^2 + \bar{V}_B^2 + \bar{V}_C^2) - \frac{1}{3}\bar{V}^2 k$	$k-1$ ⎪
Within dose-litter groups	$\Sigma y^2 - n_{A_1}\bar{y}_{A_1}^2 - n_{B_1}\bar{y}_{B_1}^2 - n_{C_1}\bar{y}_{C_1}^2 - n_{A_2}\bar{y}_{A_2}^2 \ldots$ etc.	$N-3k$ ⎭

when duplicate doses have been administered at each level. The required analysis will now be described, in the belief that the reader will think it worth performing at least one such test of his materials and methods before pro-ceeding to use them in large-scale assay work.

The appropriate statistical procedure is the Analysis of Variance, which seeks to assess the relative responsibility of the known variables for the total variation observed. Sums of squares are computed according to the plan shown in Table 29.6, and division of these by their corresponding 'degrees of freedom' yields estimates of variance in the form of mean squares. (See also p. 1113.)

Although Table 29.6 may seem to have a rather formidable appearance, it is in a form which can be easily and quickly applied to the data of Table 29.5, in which all items have been given labels corresponding to the symbols in the plan. The result is shown in Table 29.7, in which the mean squares reveal the relative contribution to the total variation of those variables which are of interest. The first step is to verify that the litter-to-litter fluctuation of the slope and curvature items is not significantly greater than the last item of the table which represents the 'irreducible' variance found among the litter-mates

TABLE 29.7

Application of the plan of Table 29.6 to the data of Table 29.5

Source of variation	Sum of squares	Degrees of freedom	Mean square
Total	0·342108	17	
Between litters	0·190256	2	
Within litters	0·151852	15	
Slope	0·067921	1	0·067921
Curvature	0·000320	1	0·000320
Slope differences	0·004709 ⎫	4	0·009676 ⎫ Variance ratio
Curvature differences	0·033992 ⎭		= 1·907
Within dose-litter groups	0·045657	9	0·005073 ⎭
	0·152599	15	

(checks, within the limits of rounding error)

exposed to the same dose. The observed ratio of 1·907 is not unduly great relative to sampling error, as verified from Fisher & Yates's Table V [7]. With a larger number of litters a ratio of this size would be a danger-signal, indicating the presence of some experimental error unevenly distributed between litters. In the present case the sums of squares and degrees of freedom of the last three items of the table can reasonably be pooled, yielding a combined estimate for 'error variance' of 0·006489 with thirteen degrees of freedom. This value is now used as a denominator in tests of significance of the slope and curvature items, according to the relations

$$t_{(13)} = \sqrt{\frac{0.067921}{0.006489}} \text{ and } \sqrt{\frac{0.000320}{0.006489}} \text{ respectively.}$$

(See Table III of Fisher and Yates for a table of t.)

Evidently the slope is highly significant, as it should be, whereas the curvature item is small relative to its sampling error. Since t expresses the ratio of a quantity to its standard error (s.e.) we have

$$\frac{\bar{U}}{\text{s.e.}} = \sqrt{\frac{\bar{U}^2 k}{0 \cdot 006489}}, \text{ and therefore s.e.} = \sqrt{\frac{0 \cdot 006489}{k}}$$

and hence $\bar{U} = +0 \cdot 1505 \pm 0 \cdot 0465$.

$\bar{U}$ represents the increase in mean response when the dose is raised two levels. On the logarithmic dose-scale, this is a rise of $0 \cdot 602$ units, so that the estimated true slope is $+0 \cdot 250 \pm 0 \cdot 077$.

A final check on validity which can be applied to data of this type, if a sufficient number of litters is available, is to test the independence of the variance of the response from the mean. This is done by summing separately the three components of the 'within dose-litter groups' item, thus obtaining three sums of squares, from which three estimates of variance, corresponding to different dose levels, can be calculated for comparison with each other.

The spleen weight assay

The importance of the slope of the dose-response line becomes apparent when we wish to compare the effects of a standard cell suspension with those of a second which is believed to behave as though it had been obtained by diluting or concentrating the standard to an unknown degree. The two preparations can then be titrated in parallel, to give an estimate of the *relative potency*, i.e. the unknown factor of dilution or concentration.

Inspection of Fig. 29.1 in which the results of a typical assay have been plotted shows that simple geometrical considerations lead to an estimate of the unknown factor, i.e. the relative potency of the test to the standard. Suppose that $\bar{y}_T$ and $\bar{y}_S$ represent the respective mean responses, and b the slope, i.e. the increment of response per unit increment of log dose: then the horizontal distance between the lines, or log potency ratio, can be estimated as

$$M = \bar{x}_S - \bar{x}_T + \frac{\bar{y}_T - \bar{y}_S}{b} \tag{2}$$

The reader can also easily verify that parallelism of the lines follows from the assumption that the test preparation can be regarded as a dilution or concentration of the standard in some inert medium. Standard methods for the design and analysis of such assays are described by Finney [2]. We shall briefly outline two commonly used designs, the 6-point assay and the 4-point assay as applied to spleen weight data.

The 6-point assay

The basic features are similar to those of the dose-response test analysed in the preceding section, except that, of the six treated mice in each litter, three receive serial dilutions of the test preparation and three receive serial dilutions of the standard. The three test dilutions bear a constant ratio to the three standard dilutions, and this ratio will be fixed by the experimenter's prior expectation concerning the relative potency. Suppose that we were comparing the potency of spleen cells from a normal and an immune donor for a given strain-combination we might guess the 'factor of immunization' [9] as x. A typical design would then be to administer, say, 1 million, 3 million and 9 million cells as the three standard doses and 1/x million, 3/x million, and 9/x million as the test doses. For ease of analysis it is essential to make the dose-levels of the two groups conform to the same geometric series. A specimen assay of this type is shown in Table 29.8.

Accepting these data as they stand, we would apply the standard form of analysis given in §5·1 and §5·4 of Finney.

Under some circumstances preliminary pruning or rearrangement of the raw data is called for, before proceeding with the standard analysis. The main indications for the omission of a litter from the series are the following:

1. The occurrence of one or more 'runts' in the litter as judged by body weight. These animals give anomalous spleen-weight responses. They should be recognized by Dixon's criterion for outliers, as applied by McLaren & Michie [10].

2. 'Undershoot' at lowest dose, i.e. failure of an animal to give a response, recognized by the occurrence of a negative log index at the lowest dose (i.e. spleen index less than unity).

3. 'Overshoot' at highest dose. The useful range of response is in the region lying between 0·00 and 0·45. Above values of about 0·45 the log index begins to lose its well-behaved relation to dose.

If these criteria lead to a substantial number of exclusions, then in the case of a 4-point assay the series should be discarded *in toto*, and a fresh attempt made after suitable adjustment of the dose-levels. In the case of a 6-point assay a rescue operation can often be performed by dropping the upper or the lower dose, according as overshoot or undershoot has occurred, from the treated and standard batches, thus reducing the assay to a valid 4-point assay which can be processed in the normal way.

It is worth aiming at setting up a 'production-line' system so that the whole chain of procedures, technical, clerical and statistical, run smoothly on a routine basis. The recommended design for this purpose is shown diagrammatically in Fig. 29.3, and the standard record format used by the author is set out in Table 29.8. Finally a complete 'cook-book' account of the preparation and injection of cell suspensions is given below.

TABLE 29.8

Standard record card, on which details of a litter are entered, first at injection, and second at sacrifice

Date 17/5   Assay No. 173

Host Litter

Genotype	No.	Born	Age
(A×B)F₁	7	14/5	3d.

Av. body wt. 4·2 g

Test

Genotype	Age	Sex
A (immun.)	12 w.	♂

Body wt. 25 g
Spl. wt. 122 mg
Total cells 249 × 10⁶

Standard

Genotype	Age	Sex
A	9 w.	♂

Body wt. 23 g
Spl. wt. 92 mg
Total cells 197 × 10⁶

Blank

Genotype	Age	Sex
(A×B)F₁	11 w.	♂

Body wt. 22 g
Spl. wt. 97 mg
Total cells 230 × 10⁶

$$1 \ (2\,\text{m. S} + 18\,\text{m. B})/\text{g} = S_1$$
$$2 \ (20\,\text{m. S})/\text{g} = S_2$$
$$3 \ (1\,\text{m. T} + 19\,\text{m. B})/\text{g} = T_1$$
$$4 \ (10\,\text{m. T} + 10\,\text{m. B})/\text{g} = T_2$$
$$5 \ (20\,\text{m. B})/\text{g} = B$$

Marks

No.	Marks
1	1
2	r
3	1+r
4	1+t
5	r+t

No.	Marks
6	—
7	—
8	
9	
10	

No.	Date	Days	Sex	B.W.	S.W.	R.S.W.	S.I.
1	22/5	8	♂	6·6	41		
2	,,	,,	♂♀	6·5	79		
3	,,	,,	♀	6·8	63		
4	,,	,,	♂♀	6·8	114		
5	,,	,,	♀	6·7	33		

No.	Date	Days	Sex	B.W.	S.W.	R.S.W.	S.I.
6	22/5	8	♂	6·4	28		
7	,,	,,	♀	6·7	37		
8							
9							
10							

Key: B.W. = body weight   S.W. = spleen weight   R.S.W. = relative spleen weight   S.I. = spleen index

Preparing spleen cell suspensions for spleen assay

1. Kill mouse.
2. Moisten fur round thorax with 70 per cent alcohol.
3. Nick the skin under the armpit.
4. Seize fore-paws in one hand and strip skin off with the other.
5. Open peritoneum and remove spleen into homogenizer.
6. Add approximately $\frac{1}{2}$ ml physiological saline per spleen.
7. Grind gently and pour suspension through stainless steel sieve into test-tube. The tube should immediately be marked 'T', 'S' or 'B' as the case may

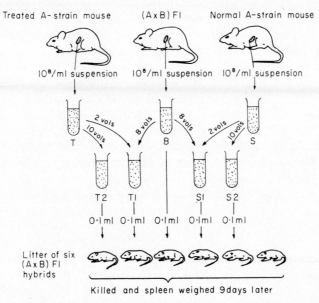

Fig. 29.3. Standard design for spleen assays, in terms of two hypothetical strains 'A' and 'B'. The effect of some treatment on the reactivity of A mice against B antigens is to be assayed.

be ('test donor', 'standard donor' or 'blank donor'). Test-tubes should be round-bottomed and not more than 4 in. long so that a 1 ml tuberculin syringe without needle can be used to suck suspension up and down. Whenever not in use the tube should stand in crushed ice to keep the suspension cool.

8. Wash through with another $\frac{1}{4}$ ml saline per spleen.
9. Suck up and down six times with tuberculin syringe.
10. Get 'Newton's rings' on haemocytometer slide.
11. Put a drop of suspension out on clean glass surface for cell count.
12. Draw suspension up to 0·5 mark in white-cell pipette.
13. Draw white-cell diluting fluid up to 11 mark.

14. Prise rubber tube off pipette. Hold pipette with thumb and forefinger, closing top and bottom, and shake for 1 minute.

15. Allow half of contents to run out; then blob cautiously on to edge of coverslip, until area of field exactly covered.

16. Count five of the central 4×4 fields. This gives concentration of suspension in millions/ml. Haemocytometer should not be allowed to stand before counting, because of evaporation.

17. Adjust suspension to final concentration of 100 million/ml. To do this, first measure volume of suspension by drawing it up into a syringe. Calculate total number of cells by multiplying this volume by the concentration estimated from the count. Then add a measured volume of saline from a syringe to make up the final concentration. For instance, take the following case:

   Original concentration estimated as 195 million/ml.

   Volume measured as 0·78 ml.

   Therefore total number of cells = 0·78 × 195 million = 152 million.

   Therefore final volume should be 1·52 ml, which means adding 0·74 ml.

18. Change the label from 'T' to 'T$_1$', 'S' to 'S$_1$', or 'B' to 'B$_1$' as the case may be.

19. When T_1, S_1 and B_1 are ready, make up T_2 and S_2 by appropriate mixture. We now have five tubes, in each of which a separate tuberculin syringe is standing. Use these to mix the suspensions thoroughly, draw up, fit needle, and adjust volume to 0·1 ml per g of average body weight of recipients. Lay each charged syringe with needle point in marked tube on operating table.

20. Discharge each syringe by intraperitoneal injection into individually marked members of the litter.

21. Recharge the syringes from their respective tubes ready for the next litter.

Dilution of cell suspensions: saturation and inactivation hazards

Analysis of unpublished observations have shown that the customary practice of adjusting doses by dilution in saline is not valid. It turns out that the proportion of injected cells which participate in the reaction is not constant, but falls as the total number of injected cells is raised, as though the host's capacity to absorb the donor cells were becoming 'saturated'. The practical consequence is that the test and standard doses administered in a given assay must all be adjusted to a constant cell number by mixing with appropriate amounts of a suspension of inactive (typically host-type F_1) cells, as shown in Fig. 29.3.

References

[1] SIMONSEN M. (1962a) Graft-versus-host reactions. Their natural history and applicability as tools of research. In *Progress in Allergy*, Vol 6, pp. 349–467. Basle: Karger

[2] FINNEY D.J. (1952) *Statistical Method in Biological Assay*, p. 22. London: Griffin

[3] RUSSELL P.S. (1960) The weight-gain assay for runt disease in mice. *Ann. N.Y. Acad. Sci.* **87,** 445

[4] HOWARD J.G. (1961) Changes in the activity of the reticulo-endothelial system (RES) following the injection of parental spleen cells into F_1 hybrid mice. *Brit. J. exp. Path.* **42,** 72

[5] HOWARD J.G. (1963) Immunological modification of graft-versus-host reactions. *Guy's Hospital Report*, **112,** 360

[6] MICHIE D., WOODRUFF M.F.A. & ZEISS I.M. (1961) An investigation of immunological tolerance based on chimaera analysis. *Immunology* **4,** 413

[7] FISHER R.A. & YATES F. (1963) *Statistical Tables*, sixth edition. Edinburgh: Oliver and Boyd

[8] SIMONSEN M. & JENSEN E. (1959) The graft-versus-host assay in transplantation chimaeras. In *Biological Problems of Grafting*, pp. 214–238. Oxford: Blackwell

[9] SIMONSEN M. (1962b) The factor of immunization: Clonal selection theory investigated by spleen assays of graft-versus-host reaction. *CIBA Foundation Symposium on Transplantation*, 1961, p. 185. London: Churchill

[10] McLAREN A. & MICHIE D. (1960) Congenital runts. *CIBA Foundation Symposium on Congenital Malformations*, pp. 178–194

II*

CHAPTER 30

Assays for Cytotoxic and Haemagglutinating Antibodies against Histocompatibility Antigens

J.R.BATCHELOR

Introduction

An understanding of histocompatibility (H) antigen systems has now become important to several fields of biological research and to clinical medical practice. However, information upon practical aspects of testing for these antigens and interpretation of results is scattered in a variety of journals. The purpose of this chapter is to discuss the principles upon which antigen detection tests are based, and to describe in detail how such tests may be carried out. A large number of different methods have been described, but the author will confine himself here to a discussion of haemagglutination and cytotoxic methods since these have been the most frequently used techniques.

Immunization procedures

For both haemagglutination and cytotoxic tests it is usual to employ iso-antisera, that is sera prepared by immunization with tissues from another member of the same species. Sera may be prepared by a number of different schedules. Most of our experience has been gained from studies upon antibodies which react with antigens of the H-2 system of the mouse. A schedule which is suitable for eliciting antibodies against this system obviously will not be universally applicable. It can, however, act as a guide for the production of antisera against other strong systems. If antisera reacting against antigens of weaker systems are required, more prolonged immunization schedules may be necessary. In the author's hands, the use of Freund's adjuvant has not led to any significant increase in titres of H-2 antibodies obtained, but adjuvants are used in some laboratories [1]. Possibly their value may be greater when raising antisera against weaker H system antigens, or in other species. Freund's complete adjuvant may also be used for inducing an antibody-rich ascites. The yield of antibody from small animals, e.g. mice, can be increased considerably by this means. A suitable method is

988

to complete the immunization schedule by injecting the mice intraperitoneally with an antigen/adjuvant emulsion every 4–5 days until sufficient ascites has accumulated. Over 10 ml of ascitic fluid may be harvested from a single adult mouse in contrast to the 1·0 ml of blood which may be obtained by cardiac puncture. Even if a mouse is subjected to serial bleedings, either from the tail, or from the retro-orbital venous plexus, the maximum yield of blood is in the region of 1·5–2·0 ml per animal.

So far attempts to concentrate antisera have been largely neglected. This is because the stronger H system antigens have claimed our attention almost entirely and high-titre sera against these may be produced easily. But as interest in weaker systems grows, it is likely that antibody-concentration techniques will become important. This applies particularly to sera against human H antigens, where opportunities for obtaining high-titre reagents are limited.

Normal, neoplastic, or foetal tissues may be used for immunization provided they contain the relevant antigens. The use of neoplastic tissue has the advantage that large amounts of a transplantable tumour can be obtained from a single animal, and when limited stocks of inbred animals are available, their economical use is an important consideration. Since tumour cells proliferate, the total antigenic mass which immunizes a recipient is much greater than the original inoculum given. On the other hand tumours, as they progress towards the autonomous state, tend to lose antigens, including H antigens. Highly malignant tumours which lack strain specificity are particularly suspect in this respect. In practice, if antigens of a strong system are being investigated, strain-specific tumours are usually satisfactory material for immunization. For weak systems, either normal tissues or newly arisen tumours are preferable since prolonged transplantation allows increased opportunities for antigenic loss to occur. A second disadvantage in the use of tumours for immunization is that some may continue to grow in the face of a recipient's immune response as a result of immunological enhancement [2, 3]. However, this problem does not arise very frequently. If antisera raised by immunization with tumours are being employed for genetic experiments, it is imperative that the tumour is carried in the native strain, and not hybrid animals. Obviously host cells will contaminate any tumour inoculum, and if these are of hybrid origin, unwanted antibodies will appear in the antiserum.

Normal tissues for immunization may be conveniently obtained from lymphoid tissues, e.g. spleen, thymus, and from liver and kidney. Like foetal tissues, they may be lightly homogenized with ease. Antigen preparations may be inoculated either as fresh tissue or in the lyophilized state. High doses of lyophilized tissue are frequently toxic if given in a single injection, but by giving a series of injections at 2 hourly intervals the same total dose may be administered without lethal effect. Some examples of different immunization schedules are given in Table 30.1.

Immunization may also be achieved by skin or organ grafting. If the object is merely to obtain an antibody response from an experimental animal, such procedures would be unnecessarily involved. However, in humans

TABLE 30.1

Some examples of immunization schedules to elicit antibodies against H antigens

Host	Antigenic material	No. of injections and intervals	Dose	Antibody	Reference
Mouse	Leukaemias and ascites tumours	3–4 injections given on days 0, 28, 42, 56	1st inj. 2–7×10^5 cells SC, the rest 10–100×10^6 cells IP	H-2	[4]
	Homogenates of solid tumours and normal tissues	3–10 injections at weekly intervals	10–100 mg wet weight IP	H-2	[5]
	Lyophilized normal or neoplastic tissue	4 injections at weekly intervals	10–20 mg dry weight IP	H–2	[6]
Rat	Lymphoid tissue	3 injections; intervals between injections not stated	Each injection 40×10^6 cells, 1st inj. SC, the remainder IP	Antigens 1 and 2	[7]
Dog	Myeloid and lymphoid tissue	Minimum of 3 injections at weekly intervals	1 ml in each of 10 sites intradermally, and 7·5–11 ml IP, cell concentration between 3–53×10^6/ml	Unknown H system	[8]

there are certain advantages in using skin grafts as a method of immunization. Firstly, if any violent immediate hypersensitivity reaction occurs during the immunization course, the reaction is limited to the neighbourhood of the graft and there is no danger of general systemic effects. Secondly, some estimate of the antigenic disparity that exists between the donor and recipient may be obtained from the survival time of the primary skin graft. Thirdly, full-thickness grafts contain very few red cells and thus the risk of immunizing against the known red cell antigens is reduced to a minimum. At present there is no evidence to indicate that human H antigens are represented on red cells,* so that immunity provoked by skin should not extend to red cells also. If other types of tissue are used for immunization, removal of red cells from them may be a difficult problem.

The number of skin grafts required to elicit an antibody response in man varies. Walford and his colleagues [9] have described the appearance of lymphocytotoxic antibodies in a pair of individuals who exchanged a series of skin grafts measuring 1·5 cm square. Antibodies were first detected after the second graft in both volunteers. In the author's experience with reciprocal skin grafts of approximately the same size exchanged between volunteers, cytotoxic antibodies were first detected after two grafts in two cases, after three grafts in one case, and after five grafts in another. A further two pairs in the process of being immunized have no antibodies after two grafts. Cytotoxic antibodies have also been found in the serum of a burned child, 2–3 weeks after she was grafted with five strips of paternal skin measuring 2·5 × 15 cm each.

Isoimmunization of human subjects may also be carried out with buffy coat leucocytes. Human white cells are known to carry some, possibly all, the H antigens of an individual since recipients can be immunized against skin grafts by leucocytes from the graft donor [10]. It is not known whether all leucocyte antigens recognized by isoimmune sera are H antigens, but certainly a proportion must be. Van Rood has commented on the erratic antibody response to immunization with buffy coat leucocytes given intravenously [11]. In his experience, one to two injections of leucocytes derived from 10–20 ml of blood given intradermally and followed 7 days later with a similar schedule of injections intravenously elicits leucocyte agglutinins in all subjects. It seems desirable to avoid using an intravenous route of immunization with the possible dangers of transfusion reaction. Such a risk may be negligible, but if repeated intradermal and subcutaneous injections can elicit an adequate response there is no reason for preferring the intravenous route. At present no careful study on the safest and most effective method of isoimmunization with leucocytes has been published.

Isoantigenic differences, though usually detected by isoimmune sera, may in some cases also be picked up with antisera produced by immunization across a species gap. The extent to which sera of this type are useful has not been fully explored. There is no doubt that frequently such antisera only contain species antibodies and are unable to discriminate between individuals of the same species [12], but this is not always the case. Gorer [13, 14] used rabbit anti-mouse sera for his early studies on H-2 antigens, and Metzgar *et al* [15] have observed that some chimpanzee anti-human leucocyte sera are capable of discriminating between the leucocytes of different humans.

* Except for antigens of the ABO system.

It is reasonable to suppose that if the immunogenetic gap is minimized by appropriate choice of the species to be immunized, one is more likely to obtain an antiserum capable of distinguishing intraspecies differences.

Absorption of antisera

Immunization with incompatible tissues usually produces a multiple antibody response since donor and host in most circumstances differ by a large number of antigens. Sera containing multiple antibodies obviously cannot be used for analytical purposes since subjects giving positive reactions may do so on account of different antibodies in the same serum. Failure to work with monospecific reagents has undoubtedly hampered the earliest attempts to serotype human tissues. For proper analysis of any H system, 'monospecific' reagents are needed. To obtain such reagents, absorption of unwanted antibodies in the serum is carried out.

The optimum proportions of serum and tissue for absorption differ according to the system being tested, and preliminary experiments to determine these are usually necessary. Absorption of H-2 antibodies *in vitro* may be carried out as follows. The liver and spleen are removed from an exsanguinated mouse of the pertinent genotype. After being homogenized in saline, the macerated tissue is washed three to four times in more saline, and firmly packed at the last centrifugation. Equal volumes of antiserum (diluted 1:4 or 1:8 if the haemagglutinin titre exceeds 1:1000) and homogenate are mixed and incubated for 1 hour at 37° C. It is usually necessary to repeat the absorption a second time for complete removal of all haemagglutinins.

Quantitative absorptions can be performed with counted numbers of live cells, or with weighed amounts of lyophilized tissue. The Möllers [16] mixed 15–60 million lymph node or tumour cells with 0·05 ml of serum diluted 1:4 or 0·1 ml diluted 1:8. The tubes were kept at bench temperature with frequent shaking for half an hour.

Non-specific absorption of antibody may sometimes be a troublesome feature. It may occur with strong antisera if successive absorptions are performed with liver tissue. But when working with weak antisera great care must be taken in performing absorption analyses to avoid non-specific absorption. An example of the necessity of absorbing with known small numbers of cells is shown in Table 30.2. The human isoantiserum, produced by immunizing JRB with a series of skin grafts from GP, was absorbed with increasing numbers of leucocytes from JRB and tested for cytotoxic activity on a positive reactor, RT. It can be seen in Table 30.2 that although of course JRB cells are not susceptible to the cytotoxic action of JRB anti-GP serum, absorption of aliquots of 0·1 ml of undiluted serum with more than 5·6 million JRB leucocytes significantly reduces the titre of antibody. It has therefore been our practice to perform absorptions of human isoantisera with not more than

5–6 million leucocytes per 0·1 ml of antiserum. In all except for one case this has been enough for the cells of known positive reactors to remove virtually all cytotoxic antibody which reacted with them. On the other hand non-specific absorption of antibody has been slight or absent when these proportions have been used.

In genetic experiments upon H antigens, the direct reactions of cells from an individual animal to antibody may sometimes be equivocal, and doubt as

TABLE 30.2

The cytotoxic activity of JRB anti-GP serum on RT lymphocytes, before and after absorption with JRB lymphocytes

Serum	Undiluted	Serum dilution 1 : 2	1 : 4	1 : 8	Serum control	Complement control
Unabsorbed	44%	20%	19%	9%	9%	2%
0·1 ml absorbed with 5·6 million JRB white cells	36%	15%	8%	4%	—	4%
0·1 ml absorbed with 11·1 million JRB white cells	15%	11%	12%	9%	—	—
0·1 ml absorbed with 14·9 million JRB white cells	15%	15%	14%	7%	—	—

Results are espressed as the percentage of non-viable cells present in each tube. Complement is omitted from the serum control tube, and antiserum from the complement control. Undiluted JRB anti-GP serum gives a value of 5 per cent non-viable cells when tested on JRB lymphocytes.

to the genotype will exist. One method for resolving this is to see whether antibody is absorbed by tissues of the animal in question. If the animal is to be preserved for a mating programme, absorption may be performed *in vivo* [17]. The technique has been of considerable value in work upon the genetics of mouse H antigens, but there is no reason why it cannot be applied in other experimental animals. In mouse work a convenient serum dose is 0·1 ml given intraperitoneally. If the animal possesses the antigens corresponding to the antiserum injected, absorption occurs rapidly, and no antibody is detected in its serum after approximately half an hour. Even if 0·5 ml of H-2 antiserum is injected, all haemagglutinins are absorbed within 2 hours. However, if the animal under examination lacks the pertinent antigen(s), antibody will persist in the serum for several days. The extracellular fluid pool into which the injected antibody passes has a volume of approximately 2 ml in an adult 25 g mouse. If 0·1 ml of an antiserum with a haemagglutinin titre of 1:4000 is injected, the expected titre after equilibration *in vivo* will be approximately one-twentieth of 1:4000 or 1:200.

Haemagglutination tests

The principle, of course, is that isoantibodies combine with H antigens present on the test red cells, causing them to agglutinate. The advantages of the technique are simplicity, reliability and sensitivity. The chief disadvantage is that not all H antigens can be detected by the test, either because they are completely absent from erythrocytes, or present in too small amounts. Haemagglutination tests were first used for the detection of H antigens in mice [14, 18]. Later it was found that mouse isohaemagglutinins were usually 'incomplete' and required special diluents if reliable results were to be obtained. Gorer & Mikulska [19] eventually developed a satisfactory method. In essence their method was to suspend the test red cells in human serum (or plasma) and to dilute the mouse isoantisera with a dextran solution. The details are as follows:

Human serum or, if convenient, plasma from outdated bank blood is obtained. This is heated to 56° C for half an hour to inactivate complement, and then absorbed with mouse red cells to remove natural anti-mouse hae-magglutinins present in human sera. Equal volumes of human serum/plasma and packed washed mouse red cells are incubated at 37° C for 1 hour. The absorption is repeated a second time, and the serum stored at −20° C until required. Washed mouse red cells for titrations are made up as a 2–5 per cent suspension in a solution of absorbed human plasma diluted with an equal volume of normal saline. In order to conserve absorbed human plasma, it is wise to calculate the volume of red cell suspension needed, and avoid making up much excess. Isoantiserum dilutions are made up in a solution of dextran. Intradex (Glaxo Ltd, Greenford, Middlesex), a 2 per cent solution of dextran (mol. wt. 100,000), in either 5 per cent glucose or normal saline, can be used. Not all other types of dextran have been satisfactory, and if used should be checked for suitability. Equal volumes (e.g. 0·025 ml) of the 2–5 per cent red cell suspension and isoantiserum dilutions are incubated in precipitin tubes for 1½ hours at 37° C. Controls consisting of one volume of dextran solution mixed with one volume of the red cell suspension should be included in each test. Known positive and negative antiserum controls may be advisable in certain circumstances. For reading, the contents of the tubes are taken up in a Pasteur pipette and streaked on to a broad glass slide. The slide is gently rocked three to four times so that antibody-induced red cell aggregates remain, but rouleaux formations due to the dextran are dispersed. The amount of rocking necessary can be gauged by the disappearance of rouleaux from the controls. A simple grading system of agglutination is:

+ + + strong agglutination, macroscopically visible, none or few unagglutinated cells in between clumps;

+ + macroscopically visible agglutinates, but numerous unagglutinated cells visible between clumps;

+ weak agglutination, just visible macroscopically;

± marginal agglutination, requiring microscopic confirmation.

Red cells of different mouse strains show variation in the ease with which they agglutinate. For example, strain A red cells are particularly reactive and useful for testing weak sera.

Stimpfling [20] has recommended a modification of the test so as to avoid using absorbed human serum. Instead, the red cell suspension is made up in a solution of polyvinylpyrrolidone (PVP) and the antiserum is diluted with normal saline. A 45 per cent aqueous solution of PVP* (mol. wt. 160,000) is diluted to 1·5 per cent with phosphate buffer (76·5 g NaCl, 7·25 g Na_2HPO_4, 2·12 g KH_2PO_4 in 10 litres of water). Two volumes of serum dilution are incubated with one volume of a 2 per cent red cell suspension, incubated for 2 hours, and read. Before reading, the tubes are centrifuged at 1000 g for 30 seconds. Ten volumes of saline are then added to each tube, and the red cells gently flushed from the bottom of the tube with a pasteur pipette. Agglutination is assessed macroscopically. The method is dependable and somewhat more simple than the dextran/human serum test.

If haemagglutination tests are performed in other species about which there is no previous information it is advisable to carry out titrations in the presence of 'developing agents' such as PVP or dextran before concluding that an antibody is absent.

Cytotoxic assays

Cytotoxic tests consist essentially of testing the permeability of cells after their incubation with antibody and complement. If cytotoxic antibody combines with the target cells, complement is fixed and cell permeability increases. It is usual to assess cell permeability by adding a solution of trypan blue or eosin which penetrates into dead cells, but leaves viable cells unstained.

Amongst the advantages of the technique are its relative simplicity, the fact that a wide range of nucleated cell types may be tested, and that it is capable of detecting certain H antigens present on white cells, but not on red cells. It is therefore a more widely applicable test than haemagglutination. However, it is rather less sensitive and more laborious to perform. H-2 antisera which give haemagglutination titres of, say, 1/8000–16,000 may show

* Antara Chemicals, 435 Hudson Street, New York 14, N.Y., U.S.A.

titres of 1/256 in a cytotoxic test performed on a suspension of lymph node cells. When reading the results of a haemagglutination test, scores are allotted after macroscopic inspection of tube contents with an occasional microscopic check, whereas for cytotoxic tests it is necessary to examine microscopically a sample from each tube, and count the number of stained cells present in fifty to one hundred cells.

The original cytotoxic test was devised by Gorer & O'Gorman [21]. Several refinements have now been introduced, but of course some of these will be unnecessary in a strongly reactive system. As in complement-fixation tests, the design of test chosen will depend upon how much sensitivity is needed. All tests require the use of monodiscrete cell suspensions with a high percentage of viable cells. It is preferable to avoid using suspensions with more than 15 per cent of non-viable cells. Not only do high background counts of non-viable cells cause doubt as to the significance of any particular test result, but non-viable cells can absorb antibody and complement, reducing the amounts available for reacting with viable cells. Suspensions of lymphoid or myeloid cells may be obtained by teasing the appropriate tissue (e.g. lymph nodes, spleen, thymus or bone marrow) in a balanced salt solution. If red cells are present in the suspension, they are easily recognized and may be excluded from counting.

Peripheral blood is a convenient source of lymphocytes for cytotoxic tests, particularly in the case of man. There are a number of methods for preparing lymphocyte suspensions from crude blood. The following one, developed by Dr D.B.Amos, has proved to be a satisfactory technique. Heparinized blood is filtered through a column of brushed nylon. Polymorphs adhere to the fibre, but lymphocytes and red cells pass through the column. The white cells are then separated from erythrocytes by sedimentation. To obtain approximately 1 ml of a suspension containing 3–4 million lymphocytes per ml, 7–10 ml of blood is withdrawn in a heparinized syringe. The nylon filter through which the blood is passed consists of a Pasteur pipette packed tightly with 0·8 g of washed nylon. The nylon (stable fibre type A, medium crimp-normal, semi-dull; obtainable from British Nylon Spinners, ICI Fibres Ltd, Pontypool, Monmouthshire, Wales) should be previously washed in detergent, and rinsed very thoroughly before drying. 0·8 g of washed nylon is combed over a stiff hair brush to separate the fibres and produce a uniform fluffy filter material. It is very firmly packed into a Pasteur pipette with the barrel of a tuberculin syringe. The broad-diameter end of the pipette is closed with a tight rubber or polythene cap which can be pierced by a syringe needle when filtration is carried out. Before the filter is used, 2 ml of saline should be forced through it to wet the fibres. Heparinized blood is then pressed out of the collecting syringe and through the filter so that it emerges from the Pasteur pipette at the rate of 20–30 drops per minute.

The filtered blood is mixed with 2·5 ml of 5 per cent dextran (mol. wt. 200,000, obtainable from Poviet Products N.V., Mauritskade 14, Amsterdam) to sediment the red cells rapidly. 0·5 ml of isotonic citrate solution is also added as an additional precaution against clotting. After approximately 45 minutes, the lymphocyte-rich supernate is removed, and the cells collected by gentle centrifugation. The lymphocytes and remaining erythrocytes are resuspended in approximately 1 ml of the supernatant dextran/plasma and a second sedimentation performed. After this, the lymphocytes and red cells remaining in suspension are removed, centrifuged down and resuspended in complement-fixation test buffer.

Suspensions of cells from solid tissues may be obtained by trypsinization. Boyse [22] has described a very successful method for producing high-quality suspensions. In this method tissue fragments are washed in saline and subjected to enzyme treatment in a small continuous circulation system. The circulation system consists of an inverted T-shaped glass reservoir with the two horizontal limbs of the T connected by a silicone rubber tube. The system is loaded with tissue fragments and trypsin solution (0·25 per cent in '199' medium) through the vertical limb of the glass reservoir. Circulation is maintained by a finger pump which squeezes the contents of the rubber tubing forward. The enzyme treatment causes exfoliation of cells from the tissue fragments, and with the use of 0·02 per cent desoxyribonuclease (DNase), a monodiscrete cell suspension can be harvested. The DNase prevents nucleoprotein liberated from disrupted cells from forming a viscous mass which entraps most of the live cells. Without its use, the yield is drastically reduced. The use of the finger pump ensures that a gentle but efficient circulatory force is applied. Magnetic stirrers have been employed, but the author has no personal experience of the quality of the cell suspensions produced by them.

Although good-quality cell suspensions may be obtained by this method of trypsinization, there is no doubt that the cells are more vulnerable to mechanical injury. Care should be taken during pipetting and centrifugation, and once a satisfactory suspension has been obtained it should be used without undue delay. Trypsinization does not appear to damage H-2 antigens since untreated and enzyme-treated cells of an ascites tumour have been found to be equally susceptible to the cytotoxic action of isoantibody. The possibility that other H antigens, including those of other species, are trypsin sensitive has not yet been tested. It is also possible that enzyme treatment may reveal further antigens.

The ease with which different tissues disintegrate varies considerably. Chemically induced murine sarcomas usually dissociate readily to produce a good suspension. Mouse mammary tumours require longer periods of trypsinization probably because of their fibrous stroma. The author has trypsinized a few human tumours by the same method and obtained monodiscrete suspensions of similar quality to those obtained from mouse tumours.

After having obtained a suitable cell suspension, the cytotoxic test is performed as follows. One volume of suspension is mixed with an equal volume of isoantibody dilution and one volume of complement added. Volumes of 0·025 ml are convenient and economical. After mixing, the reagents are incubated at 37° C for 30 minutes, the supernatant is removed, and a solution of dye is added to the cells in each tube. The tube contents are then examined microscopically.

Diluent

Although saline, 199 medium, or Ringer's solution may be used, veronal buffered saline with added optimal amounts of calcium and magnesium is preferable for maximum sensitivity (C.F.T. diluent tablets, obtainable from Oxoid Division, Oxo Ltd, London, S.E.1).

Cell concentration

Sensitivity is increased if the ratio of antibody to target cells is high. Suspensions of 2–3 millions per ml are easy to read and permit considerable sensitivity. If the test suspension contains less than 1 million cells per ml reading of the test is facilitated by using a Fuchs-Rosenthal haemocytometer which has a counting chamber depth of 0·2 mm. After incubation, the supernate should be removed before trypan blue or an alternative dye is added. This maintains the cell concentration at a maximum for reading of the test.

Complement

The source of complement requires consideration. In tests upon mouse H-2 antigens, fresh guinea-pig serum is usually a satisfactory source. Titration for activity should be carried out on each new batch of guinea-pig serum. In most cases it can be diluted to 1:2 for cytotoxic tests with mouse reactants. The majority of mouse tissues are unaffected by normal guinea-pig serum in the absence of specific isoantibody. However, thymic lymphocytes and some lymphomas are highly sensitive to guinea-pig serum *in vitro*. It appears that these cells share an antigen which reacts with a naturally occurring antibody present in all guinea-pig sera. It is possible to remove this antibody by absorption of guinea-pig serum for 30 minutes at 20–25° C with an equal volume of packed mouse thymic tissue. This procedure does not destroy all complementing activity judged either by a conventional sheep cell haemolytic system or a mouse H-2 isoantibody/lymphocyte system (Wakefield, unpublished).

Guinea-pig serum is a satisfactory source of complement for the investigation of dog H antigens [23]. In work upon chicken systems, no additional complement to that present in the isoantisera is necessary [24]. Fresh rat serum complements mouse isoantisera reacting with H-2 antigens, but it is less active than guinea-pig serum in this respect. Bogden & Aptekman [25] have used fresh rat serum to complement rat isoantisera combining with rat tumour cells. Rabbit serum is toxic for most mouse nucleated cells. However, it appears to be a highly active source of complement for human isoantibody systems. This discovery [26] has been of great importance for the study of human H antigens. One or two volumes of undiluted fresh rabbit serum provide good complement activity in cytotoxic tests upon human isoimmune systems. Other normal sera, including those of guinea-pig and humans, show much less complementing activity for human isoimmune systems.

Normal rabbit serum contains naturally occurring haemolysins for human erythrocytes, but no detectable antibodies with a cytotoxic effect upon human lymphocytes. Hence, in cytotoxic tests upon human cells, red cells which contaminate lymphocyte suspensions are lysed, whereas the lymphocytes remain unaffected unless specific isoantibody has been added to the tube. This increases the ease of reading a test greatly.

In all cytotoxic tests care must be taken to ensure that the system is adequately complemented. Mouse isoimmune sera have strong inhibitory effects upon guinea-pig complement and may cause prozones of incomplete cytotoxic activity in a titration. There are some reasons to suspect that this effect is due to competitive inhibition of C'_1 of guinea-pig complement by mouse C'_1 [27]. Heating of the mouse serum to 56° C for 10 minutes rapidly destroys the inhibitory activity. Alternatively the cytotoxic test may be set up merely as a mixture of antiserum and cells. After 30 minutes' incubation, the supernatant is removed and complement is added to the cells. Incubation is continued for a further 20 minutes before the test is read.

Strong anticomplementary effects in cytotoxic tests with human isoantisera are rare. However, if there is excessive red cell contamination of the lymphocyte suspension, much of the complement present in the rabbit serum may be consumed in lysis of the red cells. Hence a false negative result may be obtained.

All cytotoxic tests should be set up with proper controls to ensure that the antiserum or complement is not toxic *per se*. The complement control tubes should contain cell suspension, complement, and one volume of C.F.T. diluent substituted for isoantiserum. In the antiserum control, C.F.T. diluent is added in the place of complement.

Test reading
Trypan blue is the dye most commonly used for reading cytotoxic tests. Eosin has also been employed, but the author has no personal experience

with it. Cell viability may also be assessed by phase contrast microscopy. Trypan blue is made up as a 1 per cent stock solution in distilled water. When required the stock solution is diluted 1/8–1/10 with isotonic saline. It is advisable to test new supplies of trypan blue for toxicity.

In the interval between test incubation and reading all tubes should be held at 4° C, to prevent the reaction from proceeding further. Trypan blue solution should be added to the individual tubes 1–2 minutes before they are examined. Before adding trypan blue, the supernatant fluid should be removed from the tube, and two to three volumes of dye added. A sample is inspected in a microscope counting chamber, and the proportion of stained cells in a survey of fifty to one hundred cells is noted. Strong antisera produced unequivocal staining, but with weak reagents staining is frequently slight and the most obvious effect is a distortion of cell morphology. The cells may appear ballooned due to swelling of the nucleus or cytoplasm.

Results of a test are most clearly expressed as the percentage of non-viable cells in the population. Conversion of the results into a cytotoxic index conceals the actual values of the control tubes, and is therefore less informative.

Interpretation of results and analysis of H systems

So far the only H systems which have been extensively investigated by haemagglutination or cytotoxic methods are the H-2 of mouse, and the B locus of chickens. Preliminary studies have begun on rats, dogs and man, but only limited information is at present available upon these species. It is necessary, therefore, to rely heavily upon experience derived from studies on the H-2 and B systems in discussing the interpretation of tests, and how to set about the serological analysis of an H system. It must be appreciated, however, that these two systems may possess characteristics, e.g. of antigen distribution, which are not shared by the major H systems of other species, and generalizations should be treated with some caution. It must also be remembered that both of these systems are merely one amongst many present in the respective two species. Other systems, as yet uninvestigated, in mice and chickens may possess some different features.

Investigation of the H-2 system during the past two decades has shown that it consists of a complex of closely linked loci which determine the expression of a large number of antigens [see 28 for references]. H-2 antigens are known to be present on red cells and nucleated cells. The amount of antigen present varies according to the particular tissue. Lymphoid cells are rich, various parenchymatous cells such as liver and kidney less so; H-2 antigens appear to be absent from brain tissue. The concentration of H-2 antigens in neoplasms tends to resemble the tissue from which the malignant cells were derived. However, antigenic loss may occur.

Although a large number of H-2 antigens have been identified, it is most probable that many unidentified ones exist, particularly in random bred populations and the less commonly used inbred strains. Originally the various antigens were identified by letters, but since it is evident that more than twenty-six exist, the terminology has been revised and the antigens are now denoted by numbers. Table 30.3, taken from Snell *et al* [29], shows the antigens that have been identified so far by both haemagglutination and cytotoxic tests. Certain of the antigens are strong in the sense that they elicit good antibody titres; others are weak. The reasons for this variation are unknown. But it is of practical value when analysing the genotype of a mouse to begin by looking for the stronger antigens, such as antigen 4 (D) and 11 (K).

It can be seen from Table 30.3 that many mouse strains share individual H-2 antigens. The overall antigenic variability of the system is due not only to the large number of antigens, but also to the different combinations of antigens which may be present. To make a full serological analysis it is necessary to prepare antisera by immunizing each strain with tissues of all other strains. The antisera are then tested on each strain in turn. Since each serum is likely to contain a number of antibodies it is necessary to 'dissect' it at this stage so that an estimate of the number of antibodies present can be made. Analysis of each serum is conducted by absorbing it in turn with each positively reacting tissue and then retesting the absorbed serum on the other positively reacting tissues. Usually it will be necessary to perform sequential absorptions. The necessary analysis has not yet been conducted on the B system of chickens, but there is little reason to doubt that the B system, like the H-2 is compound. Immunization between lines of chickens known to differ at the B locus elicits sera which cross-react with several other strains. This can only mean that some antigens are shared by several strains. Evidence from dogs [30], and man [31] makes it plain that here also antigens may be shared by many members of the same species. Therefore, in any unknown situation a primary objective will be to discover how many antibodies a given isoantiserum contains, and until monospecific reagents have been obtained, further immunogenetic studies may be impossible to interpret accurately.

It should be noted that although in the H-2 system the majority of antigens are present on erythrocytes, this is not always the case. For example, antigens 32 (D^k) and 33 (K^b) cannot be detected by haemagglutination. Therefore, one cannot rely solely on haemagglutination tests for a complete analysis of an H system. It may be that haemagglutination tests will prove as useful for analysing H systems in other species as they have been in mice and chickens, and that most antigens of the major systems will turn out to be haemagglutinogens. It is already known that some important H antigens in rats are haemagglutinogens [32, 33, 7], and since incompatible skin grafts in dogs [8]

TABLE 30.3

The known alleles and alloantigenic specificities of the H-2 system and the inbred strains that carry them

H-2 alleles	A	D^b	C	D	E	F	G	H	I	J	K	M	N	P	Q	S	V	Y	A^1	B^1	C^1	D^1	E^d	D^k	K^b	Inbred strains
a	1	–	3	4	5	6	–	8	–	10	11	13	14	–	–	–	–	25	27	28	29	–	–	–	–	A, AKR.K, B10.A
b	–	2	–	–	5	6	–	–	–	–	–	–	14	–	–	–	22	–	27	28	29	–	–	–	33	A.BY, C3H.SW, C57BL/6, C57BL/10, C57L, CC57BR, CC57W, D1.LP, LP/J, ST/a, 129
c	*	–	3	4	?	*	–	8	–	*	–	13	*	–	–	–	*	*	27	28	29	–	*	*	*	D1.C
d	–	–	3	4	–	6	–	8	–	10	–	13	14	–	–	–	–	–	27	28	29	–	31	–	–	BALB/c, C57BL/Ks, B10.D2, DBA/2, ST.T6, WH, YBL/Rr, YBR/Wi
e	–	–	3	–	5	6	–	–	–	–	–	13	*	*	*	–	*	25	27	28	29	30	*	*	*	STOLI
f	*	–	–	–	–	?	7	8	9	*	–	–	*	*	*	–	*	–	27	–	–	–	*	*	*	A.CA, B10.M, RFM/Un
g	–	2	–	–	–	6	*	8	*	*	11	–	14	*	–	–	22	*	*	*	*	*	31	–	–	H-2G
h	1	–	3	4	5	6	*	8	*	*	11	–	?	*	–	–	–	*	*	*	*	*	–	–	–	H-2H, B10.A(2R)
i	*	–	3	–	5	6	*	*	*	*	–	13	*	*	–	–	22	*	*	*	*	*	–	–	33	H-21, B10.A(5R)
j	1	–	–	–	–	6	?	–	–	–	–	–	–	–	–	–	22	?	?	–	–	–	–	32	–	JK/St
k	1	–	3	–	5	–	–	8	–	–	11	–	–	–	–	–	–	25	–	–	–	–	–	32	–	AKR, B10.BR, CBA, CE, CHI, C3H, C57BR/a, C57BR/cd, C58, D1.ST, MA/J, RF/J, ST/bJ, 101
l	–	–	–	–	5	6	?	–	*	10	–	–	–	*	–	–	22	–	?	28	*	*	*	*	*	I/St, N/St(?)
m	*	–	3	–	5	?	?	8	*	*	11	13	*	*	–	–	*	*	27	28	29	30	*	*	*	AKR.M
n	1	–	–	–	5	6	*	8	*	10	–	–	14	*	–	–	–	*	?	?	*	*	*	*	*	F/St
o	1	*	3	–	5	*	*	8	*	*	–	–	*	*	*	*	–	*	*	*	*	*	31	*	*	H-20/Sf
p	*	–	?	–	5	?	*	–	–	*	–	–	*	16	*	*	–	*	–	–	–	–	*	*	*	P/Sn, C3H.NB
q	–	–	3	–	5	6	–	–	–	–	11	13	–	–	17	–	22	*	27	28	29	30	*	*	*	DBA/1, B10.Y(?), C/St, BUB
r	*	–	3	–	5	–	–	8	–	*	11	–	*	–	–	–	*	25	–	–	–	–	*	*	*	RIII/J, RIII/Wy, LP.RIII
s	*	*	3	–	5	6	7	–	–	*	–	–	*	*	–	19	*	*	*	28	–	–	–	*	*	A.SW, SJL

[a] An asterisk (*) indicates that no test has been made for the particular component; a negative (–) symbol denotes absence of the component; a question mark (?) indicates that the presence or absence of the component is uncertain.

and rabbits [34] provoke the formation of haemagglutinins, it is probable that in these species also a number of strong H antigens are borne by red cells. However, we must be prepared to find that in some species the majority of strong H antigens may not be haemagglutinogens. Preliminary studies on the antibody response to incompatible skin grafts in man (Batchelor, unpublished) indicate that haemagglutinins are not formed although lymphocytotoxic and leucoagglutinating antibodies have been detected. It is too early to conclude definitely that none of the strong human H antigens are haemagglutinogens, but clearly the analysis of H systems in man cannot be pursued merely by haemagglutination tests.

The second point to be emphasized is that not all haemagglutinating antibodies found in murine isoantisera are directed against H-2 antigens [35]. Identification of the antigen against which an unknown haemagglutinin reacts can be a difficult and laborious task. In some species a number of red cell antigens are known which do not appear to influence the compatibility of tissues other than red cells. For example, matching of red cell groups in man, except for the ABO system, does not materially affect the results of grafting allogenic kidneys.* The same can be said of the C and D antigens of rat erythrocytes and the survival of rat skin grafts. If foreign tissues provoke a haemagglutinin response, two questions must be answered. Is the haemagglutinin in question directed against an H antigen? If so, with which H antigen does it react?

In attempting to discover whether a particular haemagglutinogen is an H antigen, the ideal is to use a test population which is genetically uniform except with respect to the locus controlling the particular antigen under examination. If any tissue incompatibility exists between members of such a population, it can only be due to the antigen in question. Obviously it is not often possible to attain these ideal genetic conditions. However, an absolutely uniform genetic background is not essential. It is only necessary to use a population from which variation due to H antigens of equal or greater strength than the test antigen has been eliminated. Thus partially inbred animal lines may be satisfactory. If the test antigen is indeed an H antigen, grafts from antigen-positive donors to antigen-negative recipients will survive for significantly shorter periods than grafts made between subjects both of whom lack or possess the antigen.

The classical method of demonstrating that an antigen found in an inbred population is an H antigen is illustrated by one of Gorer's early experiments [14]. Strain A mice, which possessed antigen II on their erythrocytes and nucleated cells, were mated to C57BL partners which lacked the antigen. The hybrid offspring were either intermated giving rise to F_2 progeny, or they were mated to other C57BL mice to produce backcross mice. Both F_2 and

* Recent evidence suggests that compatibility is affected by the P system.

backcross mice were typed for the presence of antigen II and then challenged with an A strain tumour graft. It was observed that the tumour, which of course bore antigen II, was able to grow progressively only in those hosts which were antigen II positive. All antigen II-negative hosts rapidly rejected their tumour grafts. This kind of experiment may be performed using other types of graft, but the advantage of using tumour grafts, at least in mice, is that this type of tissue is relatively unaffected by antigenic differences of weak H systems. Hence the data obtained reflects chiefly the effects of strong H antigens. If more sensitive tissues, e.g. skin grafts, are used for testing histocompatibility, graft rejection due to weaker H system antigens complicates the results.

The difficulties of proving that an antigen found in a random bred population influences tissue compatibility are considerable. Survival of tissue grafts such as skin is affected by numerous antigens, and therefore the relationship of a particular antigenic difference to graft survival is in most cases obscure. If grafts between a large number of individuals are made, a significant number of prolonged survivals may be observed which indicates chance tissue compatibility between donor and recipient. In the cases when prolonged graft survival occurs there should be no examples of a donor possessing an antigen which is absent from the tissues of the recipient if the antigen in question is a strong H antigen. Obviously the validity of this type of evidence depends upon the numbers of prolonged graft survivals observed. Therefore, it is an advantage to work with as closely related a population as is feasible. In this way the numbers of prolonged graft survivals should be maximum. In humans, it is likely that this kind of study will have to be performed on families.

Another approach to the problem is by using a graft-versus-host reaction. So far these reactions have been employed for this purpose only infrequently. Brent & Medawar [36] devised the following method. When lymphocytes of one guinea-pig are injected intradermally into a genetically dissimilar partner, a skin reaction occurs which is believed to be a localized graft-versus-host reaction. Brent and Medawar have shown that the intensity of this reaction correlates with the survival time of skin transplanted from the host animal to the lymphocyte donor. Thus the skin reaction is a measure of the degree of histocompatibility. The possibility that this test may be of value in typing humans is being investigated at several laboratories. Simonsen [37] has pointed out that by using suitably low cell doses of lymphocytes, it should be possible to detect only the major incompatibilities. If the theoretical basis for these reactions put forward by Brent and Medawar proves to be correct, it may later be possible to correlate serologically defined antigenic differences with intradermal graft-versus-host reactions.

Once it has been established that an antigen influences tissue compatibility, the question arises as to which H system it belongs. It is only in inbred mice that studies have progressed to the point where several different systems have been delineated. However, with more widespread use of inbred rats it seems probable that data on linkage groups in rats will accumulate rapidly and that different H systems will prove convenient genetic markers. If compound H systems are the rule in other species besides mice and chickens, searches for linkage between different H antigens will be of great importance. It is beyond the scope of this chapter to describe methods of testing for linkage in random bred populations, and interested readers should consult appropriate text-books of genetics.

The question as to which H system an antigen detected in an inbred mouse strain belongs is answered by demonstrating that its inheritance is closely linked to that of a known H system. The principle is the same as that used for showing that an antigen influences compatibility. A convenient genetic marker for the known H system is chosen. This may be a visible physical feature, e.g. coat colour, provided that it is determined by another closely linked locus, or another antigen that has already been established as part of the known H system. Matings are set up between strains of animals possessing both the unknown antigen and the marker with members of a strain possessing neither. The F_1 hybrid offspring of the cross are either intermated to produce the F_2 generation, or are mated with animals of the parent strain lacking the test antigen and marker. The F_2 and backcross animals are classified for the presence of the test antigen and the marker. If inheritance of the test antigen is closely linked to the marker, the mice will tend to fall into two groups—i.e. those possessing both characters or those lacking both. If no linkage exists there will be four classes—animals bearing the marker with and without the test antigen, animals without the marker, again with and without the test antigen. If close linkage is found to be present, it may be inferred that the test antigen belongs to the known H system.

In the preceding discussion in which the evidence required to establish an antigen as an H antigen was considered, the significance of the capacity of an antigen to provoke the formation of cytotoxic antibodies was not mentioned. It is often tacitly assumed that only H antigens are capable of eliciting such antibodies. It is possible that this may prove to be true, but as yet it remains an assumption. It is already known that cytotoxic isoantibodies are not always directed against normal H antigens. It has been shown that many oncogenic viruses provoke the appearance of new antigens which are not present in the corresponding normal tissues of the same genetic origin [38]. Cytotoxic antibodies may be elicited by such antigens. The nature of such antigens is still obscure, but they are clearly not normal H antigens.

There is very little information from which we can judge how widespread this phenomenon is. Presumably it may occur as a result of infection with non-oncogenic viruses. It has been shown that HEp-2 cells infected with herpes simplex virus acquire a new antigenic specificity not present on uninfected cells or in infected cells before virus replication has taken place [39]. Incubation of infected cells with rabbit antibody directed specifically against the newly acquired antigen, plus complement, prevented the virus-containing cells from giving rise to plaques when seeded on to monolayers of uninfected HEp-2 cells. Other interpretations are possible but Roane and Roizman considered that the infected cells were killed by antibody. It is of course true that these experiments were pursued with a heterospecific rather than an isoantibody. Nevertheless, it does raise the possibility that non-oncogenic virus parasitization may induce the formation of new antigens, and that such antigens might elicit cytotoxic isoantibodies.

Somewhat similar is the 'antigenic conversion' of tumour cells by an oncogenic virus described by Stück, Old & Boyse [40]. In their system, infection of mice bearing transplanted lymphomas with Rauscher virus led to the tumours acquiring a new antigen, which had previously been found only in tumours induced by Rauscher or related viruses. The new antigen persisted through at least six serial transfers of the tumour. Presence of the antigen was detected by means of a direct cytotoxic test.

Old, Boyse and their colleagues [41] have also discovered a series of antigens which they have named TL^{1-3}. These antigens are present on normal thymuses of some mouse strains, and also certain thymic leukaemias. TL antigens elicit specifically reactive cytotoxic antibodies. The significance of the antigens is not understood, but they do not appear to be normal H antigens. There is some evidence to indicate that TL^1 does not affect tissue compatibility. Leukaemias bearing this antigen may arise in TL^1-negative hosts: furthermore, their growth in TL^1-negative hosts of the strain of tumour origin is unaffected even if such hosts are pre-immunized against TL^1-positive tissue and a cytotoxic antibody is present. Nevertheless, although exceptions exist, the demonstration that an antigen can elicit a cytotoxic antibody suggests that it is a normal histocompatibility antigen, particularly if the antigen is shown to be present on a variety of normal tissues including skin.

Acknowledgments

I am grateful to The Williams & Wilkins Co., Baltimore, Maryland, U.S.A., and to the authors, Drs Snell, Hoecker, Amos and Stimpfling for permission to reproduce Table 30.3. Dr Snell has kindly suggested some corrections which have been inserted.

References

[1] STETSON C.A. & JENSEN E. (1960) Humoral aspects of the immune response to homografts. *Ann. N.Y. Acad. Sci.* **87,** 249

[2] KALISS N. (1958) Immunological enhancement of tumour homografts in mice (A review). *Cancer Res.* **18,** 992

[3] BATCHELOR J.R. (1963) The mechanisms and significance of immunological enhancement. *Guy's Hospital Reports* **112,** 345

[4] GORER P.A. & AMOS D.B. (1956) Passive immunity in mice against C57BL leukosis E.L.4 by means of isoimmune serum. *Cancer Res.* **16,** 338

[5] MÖLLER G. (1961) Demonstration of mouse isoantigens at the cellular level by the fluorescent antibody technique. *J. exp. Med.,* **114,** 415

[6] BATCHELOR J.R. & HOWARD J.G. (1965) Synergic and antagonistic effects of isoantibody upon graft versus host disease. *Transplantation* **3,** 161

[7] PALM J. (1964) Serological detection of histocompatibility antigens in two strains of rats. *Transplantation* **2,** 603

[8] PUZA A., RUBINSTEIN P., KASAKURA S., VLAHOVIC S. & FERREBEE J.W. (1964) The production of isoantibodies in the dog by immunization with homologous tissue. *Transplantation* **2,** 722

[9] WALFORD R.L., GALLAGHER R. & TROUP G.M. (1965) Human lymphocyte typing with isologous antisera; technical considerations and a preliminary study of the cytotoxic reaction system. *Transplantation* **3,** 387

[10] FRIEDMAN E.A., RETAN J.W., MARSHALL D.C., HENRY L. & MERRILL J.P. (1961) Accelerated skin graft rejection in humans preimmunized with homologous peripheral leukocytes. *J. clin. Invest.* **40,** 2162

[11] ROOD J.J. VAN (1965) Discussion in *Histocompatibility Testing.* Publication 1229, National Academy of Sciences—National Research Council, Washington, D.C. p. 56

[12] SHULMAN N.R. (1965) Platelet and leukocyte isoantigens. In *Histocompatibility Testing.* Publication 1229, National Academy of Sciences—National Research Council, Washington, D.C., pp. 7–16

[13] GORER P.A. (1936) The detection of antigenic differences in mouse erythrocytes by the employment of immune sera. *Brit. J. exp. Path.* **17,** 42

[14] GORER P.A. (1937) The genetic and antigenic basis of tumour transplantation. *J. Path. Bact.* **44,** 691

[15] METZGAR R.S., ZMIJEWSKI C.M. & AMOS D.B. (1965) Serological activity of human and chimpanzee antisera to human leucocyte isoantigens. In *Histocompatibility Testing.* Publication 1229, National Academy of Sciences—National Research Council, Washington, D.C., pp. 45–56

[16] MÖLLER E. & MÖLLER G. (1962) Quantitative studies of the sensitivity of normal and neoplastic mouse cells to the cytotoxic action of isoantibodies. *J. exp. Med.* **115,** 527

[17] Amos D.B. (1955) The persistence of mouse isoantibodies *in vivo. Brit. J. Cancer* **9,** 216

[18] GORER P.A. (1938) The antigenic basis of tumour transplantation. *J. Path. Bact.* **47,** 231

[19] GORER P.A. & MIKULSKA Z.B. (1954) The antibody response to tumour inoculation. Improved methods of antibody detection. *Cancer Res.* **14,** 651

[20] STIMPFLING J. (1961) The use of PVP as a developing agent in mouse haemagglutination tests. *Transplantation Bull.* **27,** 109

[21] GORER P.A. & O'GORMAN P. (1956) The cytotoxic activity of isoantibodies in mice. *Transplantation Bull.* **3**, 142

[22] BOYSE E.A. (1960) A method for the production of viable cell suspensions from solid tumors. *Transplantation Bull.* **7**, 100

[23] ALTMAN B. & SIMONSEN M. (1964) Cytotoxic antibody and hemagglutinin in canine homotransplantation. *Ann. N.Y. Acad. Sci.* **120**, 28

[24] TERASAKI P., CANNON J.A., LONGMIRE W.P. & CHAMBERLAIN C.C. (1960) Antibody response to homografts: V. Cytotoxic effects upon lymphocytes as measured by time-lapse cinematography. *Ann. N.Y. Acad. Sci.* **87**, 258

[25] BOGDEN A.E. & APTEKMAN P.M. (1962) Histocompatibility antigens and haemagglutinogens in the rat. *Ann. N.Y. Acad. Sci.* **97**, 43

[26] WALFORD R.A., GALLAGHER R. & SJAARDA J.R. (1964) Serologic typing of human lymphocytes with immune serum obtained after homografting. *Science* **144**, 868

[27] WINN H.J. (1965) Effects of complement on sensitized nucleated cells. In *Ciba Found. Symposium on Complement*, eds. WOLSTENHOLME G.E.W. & KNIGHT J. Churchill, London, p. 133

[28] BATCHELOR J.R. (1965) Histocompatibility systems. *Brit. med. Bull.* **21**, 100

[29] SNELL G.D., HOECKER G., AMOS D.B. & STIMPFLING J. (1964) A revised nomenclature for the histocompatibility-2 locus of the mouse. *Transplantation* **2**, 777

[30] RUBINSTEIN P. & FERREBEE J.W. (1964) Efforts to differentiate leucocytotoxins in the dog. *Transplantation* **2**, 734

[31] *Histocompatibility Testing* (1965) Publication 1229, National Academy of Sciences—National Research Council, Washington D.C.

[32] BOGDEN A.E. & APTEKMAN P.M. (1960). The R-1 factor, a histocompatibility antigen in the rat. *Cancer Res.* **20**, 1237

[33] PALM J. (1962) Current status of blood groups in rats. *Ann. N.Y. Acad. Sci.* **97**, 57

[34] ZOTIKOV E.A. (1958) Humoral factors of immunity in tissue incompatibility of skin homografts in rabbits. *Transplantation Bull.* **5**, 67

[35] AMOS D.B., ZUMPFT M. & ARMSTRONG P. (1963) H-5A and H-6A, two mouse isoantigens on red cells and tissues detected serologically. *Transplantation* **1**, 270

[36] BRENT L. & MEDAWAR P.B. (1963) Tissue transplantation: A new approach to the 'typing' problem. *Brit. med. J.* **2**, 269

[37] SIMONSEN M. (1965) Strong transplantation antigens in man. *Lancet* i, 415

[38] OLD L.J. & BOYSE E.A. (1964) Immunology of experimental tumours. *Annu. Rev. Med.* **15**, 167

[39] ROANE P.R. & ROIZMAN B. (1964) Studies of the determinant antigens of viable cells. *Virology* **22**, 1

[40] STÜCK B., OLD L.J. & BOYSE E.A. (1964) Antigenic conversion of established leukaemias by an unrelated leukaemogenic virus. *Nature, Lond.* **202**, 1016

[41] BOYSE E.A., OLD L.J. & STOCKERT E. (1965) The TL (thymus leukaemia) antigen: A review. *Immunopathology, IVth International Symposium*, eds. GRABAR P. & MIESCHER P.A., SCHWABE, Basel, p. 23

CHAPTER 31

The Isolation of Lymphocytes and Macrophages

B.M.GESNER & J.G.HOWARD

Lymphocytes

General considerations

The preparation of suspensions of lymphocytes for experimental purposes presents certain conceptual as well as technical difficulties. The conceptual difficulties arise because of problems in deciding which cells shall be called lymphocytes. For many years, lymphocytes were defined primarily or solely on the basis of morphological appearance under the light microscope. It is now clear that it is inadequate to use gross morphological criteria alone to define lymphocytes since, for example, mononuclear cells which have similar appearance under the light microscope may belong to different cell lines [1, 2]. It is generally acknowledged that the mononuclear cells, 5–8 microns in diameter, which possess a dense nucleus surrounded by a narrow rim of cytoplasm containing few organelles and no well-developed endoplasmic reticulum, and which are the predominant cell type in mammalian lymph, are 'small lymphocytes'. These cells also exhibit certain behaviour in the living state which helps to distinguish them from other cells. They do not phagocytose bacteria [3]. They do not adhere to glass as firmly as other leucocytes [3]. They move in a characteristic fashion [4, 5, 6]. They do not respond to chemotactic stimuli to which other leucocytes react [3]. They do not ordinarily incorporate tritiated thymidine when incubated *in vitro* with this isotope [7, 8]. Recently it has been reported that under certain experimental conditions small lymphocytes, unlike macrophages, do not bind cytophilic antibody [9, 10]. When transfused intravenously, a large proportion of small lymphocytes 'home' to lymphoid tissues of the recipient and subsequently recirculate to the lymph [8, 11, 12, 13, 14, 15]. Thus far, the only specialized bodily function that has been established for small lymphocytes is that they participate in the immune response [for review, see 16, 17]. Cells which possess these morphological *and* behavioural characteristics are widely distributed in the animal. They are concentrated in the lymph and lymphoid tissues, and they also occur in the blood and in connective-tissue spaces. In all of these sites, small lymphocytes are interspersed amongst other cells.

Small lymphocytes, unlike erythrocytes, are not the end cell of their line.

Some small lymphocytes may survive as small lymphocytes in the body for at least 90 days [18]. However, it is now known that under appropriate conditions small lymphocytes can differentiate into a larger cell which possesses prominent nucleoli and abundant pyroninophilic cytoplasm [19, 20, 21, 22, 23, 24, 25]. There is evidence that these large cells may subsequently assume the appearance of the 'large lymphocyte' which then may divide to form typical small lymphocytes [26]. Thus, small lymphocytes can act as a source of more small lymphocytes. Presumably, different cells, i.e. a 'primary lymphocyte precursor', can also give rise to small lymphocytes. This line of production of small lymphocytes remains to be clarified. It should be emphasized that the demonstration that small lymphocytes can differentiate into another cell type cannot in itself be taken to substantiate the claims that small lymphocytes can 'transform' into fibroblasts, plasma cells, macrophages or multipotential stem cells (for review, see [16]). There is strong evidence that small lymphocytes cannot differentiate into multipotential stem cells [27, 28, 29]. The possibilities that lymphocytes may, under certain circumstances, differentiate into plasma cells or macrophages remain open, but these require further clarification.

From what has been said, it is apparent that morphological and behavioural differences will be encountered amongst cells in the lymphocyte series. A major difficulty, however, is that not all the cells which comprise the lymphocyte series are known. It would seem that clarification of the lymphocyte lineage and other advances in our knowledge of these cells would be served by confining the application of the term 'small lymphocyte' to those cells which have the *behavioural* as well as the morphological characteristics of the predominant small round cells in mammalian lymph. Further, if it is accepted that only such cells are 'small lymphocytes', then, in the strictest sense, it would be permissible to consider only those cells which have been demonstrated to be developmentally related to them to be members of the lymphocyte series.

Sources of lymphocytes for experimental use

The wide distribution of lymphocytes in the body makes it possible to choose a variety of sites for obtaining these cells. The source one selects will depend on the purpose of the experiment. To obtain suspensions of cells which contain lymphocytes, it is usually most convenient to use lymphoid tissue or blood as the source. However, for a number of reasons which will be made apparent below, it is often desirable to obtain cells from thoracic duct lymph.

Thoracic duct lymph

Thoracic duct lymph contain a physiologically selected and unique cell population. Erythrocytes, granulocytes and phagocytic mononuclear cells are largely excluded. The cell population is composed almost entirely of mononuclear cells which vary in size from about 5 to 20 microns in diameter. About 90 per cent of these are less than 8 microns and these, by definition, are small lymphocytes. Although this segment of the lymph cell population appears homogeneous in many respects there is little doubt that functional heterogeneity (e.g. with respect to immunological capacities) exists amongst its members [see 17]. The larger mononuclear cells in lymph have been called 'medium' and 'large lymphocytes' but the developmental relationships between all of the larger cells and typical small lymphocytes are incompletely understood. For example, some of the larger mononuclear cells in lymph contain a well-developed endoplasmic reticulum [e.g. 30, 31] and their relationship to small lymphocytes is not known. However, it is known that some of the larger mononuclear cells divide, *in vitro* [11, 32] and *in vivo* [8], to form small lymphocytes. Also, the larger cells exhibit the same behaviour with respect to phagocytosis of bacteria, adherence to glass, mode of loco-motion, and response to chemotactic stimuli as the small lymphocytes [3]. The common physiological selection of the larger mononuclear cells and small lymphocytes in the lymph, their similarities in behaviour and gross morphology, the information that *is* available concerning their developmental relationships, and a great deal of circumstantial evidence are all consistent with the view that the small and larger mononuclear cells in lymph are members of the same cell line. It must be emphasized, however, that this remains to be demonstrated for several of the cell forms which occur in lymph.

Cannulation of the main lymphatic duct and determinations of the outputs of lymphocytes have been achieved for most mammalian species commonly used for experimental purposes including man [e.g. 33], monkey [see 34], calf [35], dog [36; see also 37], cat [38, 39], rabbit [e.g. 38], guinea-pig [40], rat [11, 41], and mouse [42, 43, 44]; [for review, see also 34, 37]. The rat has been used most frequently. It is noteworthy that many workers have found it particularly difficult to cannulate the main lymphatic duct in guinea-pigs and maintain continuous drainage.

Mastering the technique of surgery which is described in various references cited above is only the first obstacle that must be overcome in order to obtain good lymphocyte preparations. Careful attention must be given to post-operative care of the experimental subject. In small laboratory animals the method of restraining the animal after cannulation is an important aspect of the procedure. Different methods have been described for different species, e.g. rat [45], mouse [43]. Once the animal (e.g. the rat) is cannulated, restrained and awake, it should be kept warm, comfortable, clean and as free of external stimuli as possible. The animal should have easy access to food and should be induced to drink if it does not do so spontaneously. If the animal does not drink, lymph flow is likely to be slow and clotting may continuously occur

KK

in the cannula. The animal may be induced to drink by leading its mouth to the drinking spout with a wet-cotton applicator stick and/or by adding glucose to the drinking water; rats and mice seem to find this palatable. Addition of salt to the drinking water increases the flow of lymph [46] and, therefore, reduces the risk of clotting. Getting the animal to drink may sometimes be enough of a problem to elect to do a gastrostomy with a continuous saline drip to ensure adequate lymph flow. Intravenous transfusion of heparin (1–2 units/ml) in physiological salt solutions also reduces the risk of clotting in the cannula. Clots are best removed from the cannula after they have retracted by twirling them around a thin wire or a hair. Occasionally bleeding into the cannula occurs after a day or two of drainage. This may be due to hypoprothombinaemia and if so, is correctable with injections of vitamin K [47]. These relatively mundane details of post-operative care are mentioned because they are easily neglected and frequently make the difference between success and failure of accomplishing an experiment.

The lymph which is obtained during the first few hours after cannulation is almost invariably contaminated with blood. J. Medawar [48] has shown that, in rabbits, the lymph obtained immediately after puncture of the thoracic duct contains phagocytic mononuclear cells. For these reasons it is often desirable to begin collection of thoracic duct cells about 6–10 hours after operation when bleeding has subsided, clots have been withdrawn from the cannula and free flow has been established.

The lymph may be collected in flasks containing heparin (20 units/ml) and antibiotics (e.g. streptomycin and penicillin, 200 μg/ml of each) in a physiological salt solution (e.g. Krebs–Ringer's). It is usually advisable to avoid having separate collection periods exceed 14–16 hours because the percentage of viable cells decreases with standing. However, holding the collection flasks at room temperature during 12-hour collection periods provides cell populations of greater than 95 per cent viability [e.g. 11].

The number of cells obtained depends, for example, on the species used. In general, species of smaller animals put out more cells per kilogram per hour than species of larger animals, but, the larger the animal, the greater is the total daily output [see 34, 37]. Thus, during the first 24 hours after cannulation, 25 g mice put out about 250×10^6 cells/kg/hr as calculated from a measured total output of about 150×10^6 cells [43], whereas 10 kg dogs put out about 20×10^6 cells/kg/hr with a total first day output of about 5×10^9 cells [see 37].

In all species tested, the daily output of cells falls as thoracic duct drainage continues. For example, in the rat, during the first day the average output per hour is about 35×10^6 cells; the second day, about 20×10^6 cells/hr; the third day, about 15×10^6 cells/hr; and the fourth day about 10×10^6 cells/ hr [12, 46]. Since there is a large-scale recirculation of small lymphocytes from the blood back to lymph via lymphoid tissue, tapping the thoracic duct and continuing drainage depletes small lymphocytes from all the reservoirs connected with the recirculating pool. Thus, after prolonged drainage, in the rat, there is a marked depletion of small lymphocytes in all the lymph nodes, the white pulp of the spleen, and in Peyer's patches [49]. These and other findings make it apparent that the small lymphocytes obtained during prolonged thoracic duct drainage are derived not only from the lymph nodes immediately drained by the duct but from all the lymph nodes in the body. The depletion of the recirculating pool of small lymphocytes is reflected in the drastic reduction in the numbers of small lymphocytes emanating from the duct after prolonged drainage. Many of the larger mononuclear cells found in lymph do not follow the same pattern of circulation as small lymphocytes [8, 20]. It has been found in rats [19] and mice [29] that the percentage of the larger cells increases as drainage continues. For example in the rat, lymph collected during the first 24 hours contains about 5 per cent large mononuclear cells whereas during the fifth to seventh day of drainage the large cells comprise about 30 per cent of the cell population [19]. Advantage of this phenomenon has been taken in experiments where lymph cell populations containing a relatively greater proportion of large cells was desired [e.g. 19].

Recently a method has been described for eliminating most of the larger mononuclear cells from the lymph cell population. The method depends upon the fact that when lymph cells are incubated *in vitro*, some of the larger cells divide to form small lymphocytes and the remainder of them die sooner than the small lymphocytes. Thus, when freshly collected rat lymph cells are suspended in 'medium 199' 20 per cent (v/v) isotonic phosphate buffer pH 7·4, 0·5 per cent (v/v) glucose and 1 per cent (v/v) rat serum in a concentration of 100×10^6 cells/ml, the flask then incubated and gently shaken at 37° C for 24 hours, populations consisting of greater than 99 per cent small lymphocytes may be obtained in which 70–80 per cent are viable [20].

For certain studies it is necessary to label lymphocytes in order to follow their fate. Two methods are generally used: (1) labelling with radioisotopes, (2) chromosome analysis. Lymphocytes have been labelled *in vitro* using several isotopes including ^{32}P [e.g. 14], ^{51}Cr [e.g. 14], ^{14}C [e.g. 19], and ^3H [e.g. 7, 8, 19]. An ^3H-containing compound is usually selected for radioautographic studies where identification of single cells is desired. When lymph cells are incubated *in vitro* with isotopes which are not incorporated exclusively into DNA, the small *and* the larger cells become labelled. For example, ^3H-adenosine, which is incorporated into RNA, is taken up *in vitro* both by small lymphocytes and by the larger mononuclear cells in lymph [e.g. 8]. However, when lymph cells are incubated *in vitro* with H^3-thymidine, which is incorporated into DNA, a great many (e.g. about 60–80 per cent) of the larger cells become labelled but the vast majority (e.g. about 99·5 per cent) of small lymphocytes do not [7, 8].

Lymph cells can also be labelled by injecting the isotope into the animal before cannulation of the thoracic duct. ^{32}P has been frequently used in this way [e.g. 11, 14]. When ^{3}H-thymidine is injected, only those cells which are synthesizing DNA become labelled [50, 51, 52]. A single injection of this isotope labels a high percentage of the larger cells (about 90 per cent), but only a very low percentage of the small lymphocytes (e.g. about 1 per cent) in lymph and in other sites of the body become labelled [7, 8, 53]. When ^{3}H-thymidine is transfused continuously, about 50 per cent of the small lymphocytes in the blood become labelled at the end of a month, and about 90 per cent at 80 days [18]. Such information has provided strong evidence for the long life-span of some small lymphocytes [see also 54]. The general advantages of using isotopes for labelling lymphocytes are apparent. The disadvantages of using isotopes which label protein and RNA are that they are turned over rather rapidly in lymphocytes, thus limiting the time that the labelled cell can be followed to a few days. With ^{3}H-adenosine, for example, the label remains well associated with donor small lymphocytes for 24 hours after they are injected into recipients [19]. However, after 2–3 days a large portion of the label is diluted out from the donor cells. ^{3}H-thymidine, which is incorporated exclusively into DNA, stays associated with donor lymphocytes for much longer periods of time. This isotopic compound remains largely undiluted in donor lymphocytes until the cells either die or divide and is, therefore, an excellent label for following the fate of these cells. Its chief disadvantage is that repeated injections of the isotope over long periods of time are required to label a high percentage of the small lymphocyte population in the body. In using any radioisotope to follow the fate of cells one must consider the possibility that the isotope has leaked from labelled cells and was reincorporated into others.

Chromosome analysis has also been used to advantage for following the fate of lymphocytes. For example, an unusual chromosome occurring within a species, such as the T6 chromosome in mice, has been used to distinguish cells with this chromosome marker from cells of other mice which do not possess it [e.g. 55]. Cells from animals of different species (e.g. rats and mice) can be told apart by their differences in karyotype [e.g. 20]. And cells of males can be distinguished from cells of females by the sex chromosomes [e.g. 22]. The advantage of using chromosomes to identify cells is that, unlike radioisotopes, there is virtually no risk of exchange of the marker between cells. The disadvantage is that cells can be identified by this method only when they are undergoing mitosis. Combined use of radioactive labelling and identification by chromosome analysis has proved very useful in elucidating the fate of lymphocytes [e.g. 20, 56]

Blood

The cellular contents of lymph are delivered to the blood stream and consequently the blood serves as a most convenient source of cell suspensions containing lymphocytes. The obvious disadvantage of blood as a source of lymphocytes is that it contains many types of cells in addition to those contributed to it via the lymph. A great variety of methods have been described for separating lymphocytes from other cell types in blood. Though many methods have been reported to be successful, there is no established procedure of choice and the technique selected has depended on the purposes of the experiment and the taste of the investigator. In general, the procedures used may be viewed to consist of (1) methods for separating erythrocytes from leucocytes, (2) methods for disassociating lymphocytes from other leucocytes.

Erythrocytes are usually separated from leucocytes by differential centrifugation and/or sedimentation in suspensions containing dextran or fibrinogen or PVP or another high molecular weight substance [for review see 57]. Agglutination of red cells (e.g. by phytohaemagglutination [25]) combined with differential centrifugation has also been used. These techniques do not remove all the red cells. If desired, elimination of most of the remaining erythrocytes can be achieved by lysing them in hypotonic saline [58] or in water [59]—suspending the leucocyte-rich suspension in hypotonic saline or water for about 3 seconds and then restoring isotonicity lyses red cells and leaves most of the leucocytes intact.

The methods used for separating lymphocytes from other leucocytes have utilized differences in the phagocytic [e.g. 60, 61, 62, 63] and adhesive properties of the cells. The most commonly used techniques have depended on the phenomenon that lymphocytes do not adhere to glass and other surfaces as firmly as other leucocytes. Thus, the heterogeneous cell suspension is incubated at 37° C in glass bottles, or with glass beads and/or glass wool, and the lymphocytes are subsequently washed off leaving other leucocytes attached to the glass [e.g. 64, 65, 66, 67, 68]. Other surfaces such as cotton wool [24, 69], nylon wool [70], and recently even ladies' nylon stockings have been used for this purpose [71, 72]. Separating leucocytes has become so popular that columns of nylon wool ('Leucopak'; Fenwall) for this purpose are available commercially.

The procedures for separating blood cells may begin by removing erythrocytes from anticoagulated blood followed by separation of leucocytes. Or, since lymphocytes and erythrocytes share the properties of adhering poorly to glass and being non-phagocytic, these two cell types may first be separated from other leucocytes, e.g. by defibrinating blood with glass beads [63, 73] followed by separation of red cells from lymphocytes. Regardless of the order chosen, the same general principles for separating lymphocytes from red cells and from other leucocytes are applied.

Using the various approaches outlined above, it has been reported that cell suspensions have been obtained containing 75–100 per cent small lymphocytes, with up to 98 per cent viability and with recoveries of 30–95 per cent of the original number of lymphocytes. Several points should be considered in regard to the techniques used and the assessment of the cell populations obtained: (1) All of the separation procedures involve risk of damage to lymphocytes. (2) Variations in procedure can result in substantial differences in the population of cells obtained. For example, the adherence of granulocytes and monocytes to glass is dependent on temperature and ions [e.g. 68]. (3) Methods which have been reported to be successful using blood of one species are not necessarily as satisfactory with blood of other species and modifications in procedure may be required. For example, Hildemann *et al* [74] have noted that procedures reported to be successful for separation of cells using human blood and those for chicken blood [75] had to be modified in order to get adequate separation using mouse blood. (4) In evaluating the percentage viability of the cells obtained, many workers have used resistance to staining with certain dyes (e.g. trypan blue, nigrosin, eosin Y) as the sole criterion of viability. It has been pointed out [e.g. 75] that inaccuracies may occur in judging viability by this means alone, since cells which lack other characteristics of viability may exclude these dyes. Other criteria, such as motility of the cells, morphological integrity or oxygen consumption should be used in addition to studying the uptake of vital dye in order to obtain a more meaningful assessment of cell viability. (5) The evaluation of the purity of the lymphocyte suspensions obtained by these techniques has rested largely upon the assumption that all mononuclear cells in blood which do not adhere to glass under the conditions of the procedure are small lymphocytes. It should be noted that the origins and developmental relationships of the mononuclear cells selected from blood by such techniques have not been fully described, and it remains possible that they are not all of the same lineage. Some investigators have attempted to further characterize the cell populations obtained by these methods by testing the cells for ability to phagocytose bacteria or other particles [e.g. 24, 68]. Such studies have revealed that a high percentage of the cells are non-phagocytic and this could be taken as another point in favour of the view that they are lymphocytes.

Lymph nodes

In laboratory animals, lymph nodes serve as a convenient source of lymphocytes. A substantial amount of nodal tissue containing great numbers of lymphocytes can be obtained with ease immediately after sacrificing the animal. In living rabbits and guinea-pigs the popliteal nodes are easily accessible. In rats, the mesenteric chain which lies alongside the ascending colon provides a large mass of nodes at one site. In mice, the cervical, axillary, inguinal and brachial nodes, as well as the mesenteric chain are easily accessible and are frequently pooled in order to obtain large numbers of cells. A simple procedure for obtaining the cells is to dissect out the nodes free of fat, place them in a Petri dish containing a physiological salt solution which may contain an anticoagulant such as heparin, and tease them each apart gently with forceps or needles. The tissue debris is removed by allowing it to settle out and/or by passing the suspension through a thin layer of glass wool. The cell suspension obtained in this manner is heterogeneous, containing small lymphocytes, some red cells, and various cells of the tissue including, presumably, other cell forms of the lymphocyte line. Cells with the general morphological features of small lymphocytes comprise about 70–90 per cent of the population, of which about 85–95 per cent are viable. No macrophages, as judged by vital staining with neutral red, are present in suspensions filtered through a 2 cm glass wool column [104]. Further purification of the cell population can be achieved by applying the methods of separation previously outlined. One problem encountered with concentrated lymph node cell suspensions is that they sometimes cause fatal emboli when injected intravenously into laboratory animals. Such mishaps are extremely rare using concentrated suspensions of thoracic duct cells.

Spleen
Lymphocytes are concentrated in the white pulp of the spleen, and, because of the relatively large size of this organ, a great number of lymphocytes may be obtained from it. However, lymphocytes comprise a small percentage of the total cell population in the spleen. The procedures that have been described for obtaining lymph node cell suspensions can be applied to obtain suspensions of spleen cells. Another commonly used technique is to press fragments of spleen on a wire mesh and collect the cells which pass through [77]. Two precautions should be observed with spleen cells to be used for intravenous transfusion. First, the cells must be washed to get rid of free cytoplasmic particles which are usually toxic. Second, suspensions should stand for 3–4 minutes to allow large aggregates of cells (which are difficult to dissociate) to settle out. The cell populations obtained have not been well characterized. The cellular constituents of blood, a variety of tissue cells in addition to small lymphocytes and cells related to them are obtained. Presumably, some separation of the cell population can be achieved by using procedures previously described.

Thymus
Suspensions of thymus cells can easily be prepared by dissociating the tissue with forceps or by pressing tissue fragments on a steel mesh. There can be

little doubt that the predominant cell types obtained are members of the lymphocyte line. However, it should be realized that thymus cell populations differ in some respects from other lymphoid cell populations. For example, there is evidence that differences occur in the distribution of thymus cells after intravenous transfusion as compared with that of thoracic duct cells and lymph node cells [78, 79]. Also, certain differences in the immunologic capabilities of thymus cells as compared with thoracic duct cells and lymph node cells have been reported [e.g. 80]. These points are made to emphasize that suspensions of thymocytes cannot be considered to be entirely equivalent to suspensions of non-thymic lymphoid cells.

Bone marrow

Bone marrow cells are usually obtained from small laboratory animals by means of flushing out the cavity of the femurs with a physiological salt solution. The cell populations obtained are, of course, heterogeneous. It is difficult to assess what percentage of the cells are lymphocytes from the information that is presently available since published estimates are based primarily on morphological criteria. It is now clear that there are mononuclear cells in bone marrow which resemble small lymphocytes but whose 'life history' and functions differ from that of the predominant cells in lymph. It, therefore, should be re-emphasized that it is inadequate to use gross anatomical features alone to characterize and identify mononuclear cells.

Macrophages

General considerations

The mononuclear cells comprising the macrophage (or reticuloendothelial) system are characterized by their highly developed capacity to phagocytose foreign particulate and colloidal materials. Since the ability to phagocytose these materials is the sole common behavioural characteristic used to designate members of this group, it is understandable that cells which differ in other functional capacities as well as in morphological appearance will be included in this heterogeneous system. The term 'macrophage' itself is now used fairly generally as a group designation for these various cells. Foreign particles can occasionally be found within the cytoplasm of lymphocytes [e.g. 81], but the extent of this is minimal when compared with the rapid and gross uptake by macrophages.

Although some macrophages might play a role in the initiation phase of an immune response, they are not 'immunologically competent' in the sense described for lymphocytes. Other major features which serve to differentiate macrophages from lymphocytes are:

1. Macrophages adhere very readily and firmly to glass surfaces or fibres—a property which can be exploited in separating these cells from mixed populations.

2. Lysosomes are prominent in macrophages and are responsible for the strong acid phosphatase reaction given in cytochemical preparations. Although lymphocytes are negative in this regard, Hirschhorn *et al* [82] have found that lymphocytes altered by phytohaemagglutinin contain cytochemically demonstrable lysosomal materials.

3. Macrophages in suspensions or monolayers are rapidly stained (within minutes) by a vital dye such as neutral red (2 ml 0·1 per cent neutral red added per 100 ml balanced salt solution), and can thereby be clearly distinguished from unstained lymphocytes present in a mixed preparation.

4. The surface membrane of macrophages possesses a well-developed receptor for free cytophilic antibodies (7S γ2) which is absent from lymphocytes and other cell types so far examined [9, 10].

5. Macrophages in suitably fixed preparations show a strong affinity for silver and other heavy metals [83]. This property correlates fairly well with the phagocytic potentiality of the living cell and can therefore be of value in identifying such cells in tissue sections.

Dissimilarities are known to occur between macrophages isolated from different parts of the body. The following points should be considered in selecting a suitable source of cells. First, peritoneal macrophages depend solely upon anaerobic glycolysis as an energy source for phagocytosis, whereas alveolar macrophages and Kupffer cells utilize oxidative phosphorylation as well [84, 85]. Second, the content of enzymes such as lysozyme, acid phosphatase and β-glucuronidase is up to ten times greater in alveolar macrophages than it is in peritoneal cells [86, 87, 88], although, rather surprisingly, this greater enzymatic activity is correlated *inversely* with the ability of these two cell types to kill phagocytosed bacteria [87]. Third, there appear to be differences in the phagocytic discrimination exhibited by Kupffer cells and spleen macrophages. For example, Salmonellae injected intravenously into colostrum-deprived newborn pigs (deficient in natural antibodies) are taken up mainly by the spleen, whereas colloidal carbon accumulates largely in the liver as it does in adult animals [89]. Again, ^{51}Cr-labelled human erythrocytes treated with strong agglutinating antibody or complement-binding incomplete antibody are phagocytosed quickly by the liver, whereas incomplete antibodies not binding complement promote a slower uptake by spleen macrophages with relatively few cells going to the liver [90, 91]. Finally, it seems that whereas antigens are rapidly rendered non-immunogenic when phagocytosed by Kupffer cells, they retain their antibody-stimulating capacity for a much longer period within spleen macrophages [92, 93].

Macrophages become 'activated' following the ingestion of particles or

KK*

endotoxin or by exposure to antigen in sensitized animals. The cells become larger, 'stickier', hyperphagocytic and show increased cytoplasmic vacuolation [see 94]. These changes are accompanied by an increase in the enzyme content of such cells [e.g. 95]. The ultrastructure of 'activated' macrophages taken from mice sensitized to *Listeria* differs from that of normal macrophages and is typical of differentiating cells [96].

The aforementioned variations in properties of macrophages should be considered in selecting both a suitable source of cells and a method for isolating them.

Compared with lymphocytes, our present knowledge of the origin, life history and interrelationships of the various macrophage groups is very incomplete and frequently controversial. Volkman & Gowans [1, 2] have recently shown decisively in rats that macrophages in foci of sterile acute inflammation are derived from a rapidly dividing cell line in the bone marrow. Peritoneal macrophages in radiation chimaeras are also derived from bone marrow [97, 98]. The macrophage (histiocyte) accumulations in various hypersensitivity reactions have also been shown to be derived from a rapidly dividing haematogenous precursor [99, 100]. Whether or not this represents a similar sequence to that of Volkman and Gowans remains to be determined. Macrophages in *in vitro* cultures of blood leucocytes are derived from monocytes and not from lymphocytes [101]. By a combination of ^{3}H-thymidine and particle labelling, Kelly *et al* [102] found that oestrogen stimulation of Kupffer cells was accompanied by division of pre-existing phagocytic cells. On the other hand, by means of the T6 marker chromosome, Howard *et al* [103, 104] found that a large percentage of liver macrophages was derived from thoracic duct cells during the graft-versus-host reaction and in radiation chimaeras stimulated with *Corynebacterium parvum*. In both these latter situations, however, macrophage proliferation is of far greater intensity than that induced by oestrogen.

The long persistence of heavy carbon labelling in peritoneal macrophages [94] and their ability to survive for months *in vitro* with little or no mitosis (see later) suggests that these cells can have a relatively slow turnover. This is supported by their low rate of mitosis *in vivo*. Only 1–3 per cent of peritoneal macrophages and 3·7 per cent of Kupffer cells took up ^{3}H-thymidine from a single pulse in normal mice [94, 105]. After a dose of colchicine, 0·1 per cent of normal Kupffer cells were found to be in mitosis [103].

Little is known of the circulation of macrophages in the body. Intensely stimulated Kupffer cells become detached and migrate to the lungs [e.g. 106], but to what extent this happens normally has not been determined so far. When peritoneal macrophages labelled with ^{198}Au are injected intravenously, the cells settle in the liver sinusoids and red pulp of the spleen after transient lodgement in the lungs [107].

Sources of macrophages for experimental use

1. *Peritoneal cells*

The serous cavities of normal animals contain a heterogeneous population of cells consisting of a variable percentage of macrophages and lymphocytes, together with some polymorphonuclear leucocytes and eosinophils. Because of its greater size and simplicity of washing out, the peritoneal cavity has been utilized far more frequently than have the pleural or pericardial cavities.

The suitability of peritoneal fluid as a source of non-activated macrophages varies greatly amongst the common laboratory mammals, because of wide differences in the cell yield per unit body weight. The number of cells which can be obtained from the rabbit is usually too low to be of much general use. Approximately $2-6 \times 10^7$ cells, of which 50–70 per cent are macrophages, can be obtained from a guinea-pig [108], although in some animals lymphocytes appear to be numerically predominant, whilst in others eosinophils are occasionally much in evidence [109]. A similar total cell yield from rats (2×10^7) contains somewhat fewer macrophages, with eosinophils usually comprising some 30 per cent [110]. The mouse has been used more frequently than other species as a source of normal peritoneal macrophages. According to the strain used, between 10^6 and 5×10^6 total cells can be obtained, of which, however, only 20–40 per cent are macrophages and 50–75 per cent are cells with lymphocyte morphology [e.g. 97, 98]. Balner found that only mouse peritoneal cells with a diameter greater than 10 μ were actively phagocytic towards carbon, whereas the smaller cells (taken to be lymphocyte forms) were not.

In general, considerably larger yields can be obtained from sterile peritoneal exudates induced by the intraperitoneal injection of various irritants 3–5 days earlier. The gain is greatest in species such as the rabbit where the normal cell content of the peritoneum is low, and least in the mouse which possesses a more cellular peritoneal fluid. In all animals, however, the macrophage becomes the predominant cell type in exudate cell populations. Consideration should be given, however, to whether or not the use of the more 'activated' type of macrophage found in these exudates is suitable. Sterile paraffin (mineral) oil is the most favoured material for this purpose in rabbits and guinea-pigs. For the former animal, 50 ml of a preparation such as Bayol F (many different proprietary oils have been adopted) warmed to 37° C should be injected 5 days before peritoneal lavage. As it is not uncommon for the bowel to be accidentally perforated in rabbits by the large needle (gauge 17) required, it is a wise precaution to first inject 5 ml saline and then to draw back so as to be sure that correct siting has been obtained. The cell yield in rabbits obtained by this method is usually $1-4 \times 10^8$, of which more than 90 per cent are macrophages [e.g. 86, 111, 112]. Oil droplets are present in 20–30 per cent of these cells. Glycogen may be used as an alternative inducer in a dose of 200 mg intraperitoneally per rabbit, but the cell yield is smaller. This is, however, the method of choice for obtaining very pure polymorphonuclear leucocytes, as they appear in large numbers before the stage of macrophage exudation. If the peritoneum is washed out only 4 hours after injection of glycogen, approximately 10^9 cells should be obtained which may be up to 99 per cent polymorphs. The best results are obtained with animals which are used repeatedly for this procedure at 1–3 week intervals [113].

For obtaining macrophage exudates in rats, Fishman [112] has favoured the use of 5 ml of beef heart infusion broth reinforced with 10 per cent proteose-peptone which gives average yields of 5×10^7 cells some 2–3 days later, although 'lymphocytes' are usually present at 20 per cent or so concentration. Franzl [93] has found that the best yield of macrophages in peritoneal exudates in mice were obtained by the injection of 1 ml 12 per cent sodium caseinate (Difco). (This material is prepared for use by adding slowly to saline at 80° C with vigorous stirring and is sterilized by autoclaving.) Exudates examined 3 days later contained 50 per cent macrophages, but as many as 45 per cent cells with lymphocyte morphology.

The peritoneal cavity should be washed out with a balanced salt solution (such as Hank's or Tyrode's) containing 5–20 units of heparin per ml. The volume used is at least 2 ml per mouse, 10 ml per rat, 20 ml per guinea-pig and 200 ml per rabbit. Gentle massage should be applied before attempting to withdraw the fluid. It is generally preferable to strip the abdominal skin before harvesting cells from the peritoneum. Fluid may be aspirated with a syringe and needle (multiple holes in the latter are an advantage) or in the case of small animals with a Pasteur pipette inserted through a small incision. A cannula sheathed by a perforated well tube [111] is a useful method for avoiding occlusion by the abdominal viscera. Multiple drainage tubes attached to large-bore needles are frequently useful for rabbits, especially when lavage with a large volume is being applied. This procedure (or a repeat wash through) is recommended when maximum yields are required. Cell suspensions can be centrifuged at 250–300 *g* for 5 minutes, and washed or resuspended as required. The speed of centrifugation should not exceed 350 *g* as cells then begin to show pronounced loss of phagocytic ability [68]. If oil has been used, the suspension should be first filtered through a wire mesh or gauze filter to remove particulate material. The free oil will form an upper layer after centrifugation.

2. *Lung (alveolar) macrophages*

Macrophages can be obtained with a greater degree of purity than those in peritoneal exudates by washing out the lungs via the trachea. As previously indicated, these cells differ from peritoneal macrophages, not only in their ability to utilize oxidative phosphorylation as well as glycolysis, but also in their greater content of enzymes such as lysozyme and acid phosphatase.

The yield from normal rabbits is usually $1-2 \times 10^7$ cells, of which at least 95 per cent are macrophages [86, 114]. A similar number of cells (2×10^7) can be obtained from the lungs of guinea-pigs, with a purity of 90–95 per cent [115]. Larger numbers of cells may be obtained by the establishment of granulomatous lesions in the lungs before washing out [86, 116, 117]. This can be done either by the intravenous injection of complete Freund's adjuvant (for example, 0·2 ml containing 0·5 mg *Myco. tuberculosis* per guinea-pig) or by two intravenous injections on successive days of lyophilized BCG (20 mg in 1 ml 0·01 per cent Tween 80 per rabbit). Cells should be harvested about 3 weeks later. The increment in cellular yield is greater in rabbits than it is in guinea-pigs. The former-treated animals usually give $1-3 \times 10^9$ cells with 85 per cent macrophages, and the remainder comprising lymphocytes and a few polymorphs. Freund's adjuvant will produce a five-fold increase in cell yield in guinea-pigs (10^8 cells) with a similar differential count to that described for rabbits. It should be noted that alveolar macrophages isolated from granulomatous lungs are far more 'activated' (with respect to their content of enzymes) than are normal alveolar macrophages [86].

The technique of washing out is as follows: The animal is best killed with an overdose of veterinary nembutal injected intraperitoneally and the skin reflected away from a midline ventral incision extending from the mandible to the lower abdomen. The upper end of the trachea is clamped off with a fine pair of artery forceps and divided immediately above. The entire trachea, lungs and heart are then dissected out *en bloc*, taking care to avoid puncturing the lungs. The excised thoracic organs are washed free from blood in a balanced salt solution and wrapped in moistened gauze. With the aid of an appropriately sized polythene cannula, a balanced salt solution is injected via the trachea into the lungs (20 ml for a guinea-pig, 50 ml for a rabbit). The point of insertion of the cannula into the trachea should be held firmly to avoid leakage. The fluid is then allowed to run out of the lungs (without squeezing) into a receptacle and the process is repeated once or twice more. The cells may then be centrifuged, washed and resuspended as described for peritoneal cells. There should be little or no contamination with blood—specimens which are clearly 'bloody' should be discarded. Pavillard [87] found that the yield of alveolar macrophages obtained from rats could be increased fivefold by including 0·2 per cent versene (EDTA) in the perfusion fluid.

3. *Blood monocytes*
These cells are the most readily accessible and frequently used type of RE cell both in birds and in man. Monolayers are readily prepared from buffy

coat cells as they stick firmly to glass surfaces and are difficult to dislodge with either trypsin or versene. Other blood leucocytes are washed off and in any case do not survive long on culturing. Both chicken and human monocytes on first isolation are smaller than typical macrophages, but rapidly enlarge after 2–3 days on glass surfaces [111, 118].

Terasaki [75] has described a useful technique for preparing suspensions of chicken monocytes from buffy coat cells cultured on plasma clots. The cells are grown in Ringer–bicarbonate containing 10–30 per cent chicken plasma for 9–10 days in Carrell flasks. Polymorphs rapidly disappear and lymphocytes are no longer viable after 5–7 days. The plasma clot is rinsed three times with Ringer–phosphate and digested for 10–20 minutes at room temperature or 37° C with 2–4 ml of 0·5 per cent 1:250 trypsin (Difco). The flasks are rinsed out with three volumes of Ringer–phosphate and the cells centrifuged, washed and resuspended. This procedure provides a fairly pure suspension of macrophages which stain vitally with neutral red and will proliferate. They have been used for the induction of transplantation tolerance.

Many workers have obtained human macrophages by applying a similar approach to buffy coat cells. Another recent method is to pass the mixed white cells through a glass bead column and to subsequently elute the adherent monocytes with EDTA [68]. First, the red cells are sedimented with 5 per cent dextran in Hank's solution (1 ml per 5 ml blood). The white cells are centrifuged and resuspended at 4× concentration in the original plasma. A maximum volume of 75 ml is loaded into a 40×2·5 cm column packed with glass beads and incubated at 37° C for 30 minutes. The column is then washed through at 37° C with 100 ml neat plasma and 500 ml 20 per cent plasma in Hank's solution, which removes lymphocytes and platelets respectively. This is followed by continued washing with 0·2 per cent EDTA in Ca and Mg-free buffered saline. The effluents are collected in fractions and examined microscopically. The first shower of cells to be released is predominantly polymorphs and is succeeded by another peak of monocytes. The yield of monocytes is only about 10 per cent of their starting value and contamination with polymorphs is about 25 per cent. The latter is greatly reduced by rerunning the cells through a smaller column. The isolated monocytes will develop into typical macrophages after 6–7 days' culture.

4. *Kupffer cells*

These cells are difficult to dislodge from the liver sinusoids by perfusion at raised pressure unless they have recently phagocytosed large amounts of colloidal material. (Stimulation by oestrogen also appears to facilitate their release *in vivo* [106].) The liver is perfused through the portal vein and the washings collected from the vena cava. When the blood has been cleared from the liver, the perfusion pressure should be raised, the outflow closed and the liver massaged gently. The swollen liver is then allowed to empty and the procedure repeated several times. Rous & Beard [119], working with rabbits and dogs, purified Kupffer cells from these washings by using magnetic iron oxide as their injected colloid and separating those cells containing it with the aid of a magnetic field. The cell yields from such methods are small, however, and St George *et al* [120] improved upon this by applying the iron oxide technique to whole rat livers which had been reduced to their constituent cells by passage through a garlic press. Nevertheless, these methods of extraction have been of limited usefulness and will not be described in detail here.

The undesirable preliminary of stuffing the cells with excess particles may be avoided by using Garvey's [121] technique of collagenase and trypsin digestion of liver fragments, which permits extraction of viable phagocytic cells in reasonable yield and tolerable purity. The technique which we have used extensively in mice is basically that described by Garvey [121] for the isolation of Kupffer cells from rabbit liver, but with a few modifications which we found advantageous in these experiments [103]. Mice are injected with 250 i.u. heparin intravenously and killed 5 minutes later. The inferior vena cava is severed whilst 2 ml GKN solution (Garvey) is perfused through the portal vein. The liver is then excised and cut up into small fragments (not more than 2 mm thick). These are transferred to 0·1 per cent collagenase (Sigma) in GKN solution (2 ml per liver) and incubated at 10° C with constant stirring for 3 hours. (We have found this concentration of collagenase gives better digestion of liver fragments and less parenchymal cell contamination than the 0·01 per cent recommended by Garvey, although this may only reflect differences in the specific activity of batches of enzyme.) The cells are centrifuged at 330 g and then incubated in 0·3 per cent trypsin (2 × crystallized, Light & Co.) at 37° C with mechanical stirring for 30 minutes. Gross debris is removed by filtration through a fine-mesh wire sieve, and the cells centrifuged and washed three to four times. Yields of cells should fall within the range 10–20 million from one normal liver, or 20–40 million from animals undergoing RE stimulation by graft-versus-host reaction or *Corynebacterium parvum*, for example.

The cell suspensions obtained are usually 85–90 per cent macrophage types, less than 7 per cent 'lymphocytes' and 1 per cent parenchymal cells together with an assortment of other cells in very small numbers. At least 80 per cent of the total cells show vital staining with neutral red and positive acid phosphatase reactions. The technique has been suitable in providing cells for chromosomal analysis in chimaeras [103]. Garvey [121] describes a technique for short-term tissue culture experiments with these cells. The method will require further refinement if the cells are to be used for intravenous injection, as the suspensions contain much debris which, furthermore, tends to aggregate during centrifugation carrying down with it an appreciable number of cells. It does offer at present, however, the best starting-point available for the isolation of functionally intact Kupffer cells in reasonable numbers.

5. *Spleen macrophages*

Little attention has so far been given to the extraction of macrophages from suspensions of spleen cells. Most studies on these cells have been restricted to the examination of monolayers which migrate from cultured spleen fragments. Initially, the halo of cells consists largely of polymorphonuclear leucocytes and lymphocytes, but by 4 days the further extension of the zone is predominantly due to macrophages [see 122]. Recently Bennett [130] has described a technique for obtaining virtually pure macrophage monolayers from mouse spleen cell suspensions whose content of erythrocytes had been reduced by prior organ perfusion. As lymphoid cells rapidly die off during cultivation, pure macrophages are generally obtained by 7 days.

In vitro **cultivation of macrophages**

Macrophages can be kept alive for much longer periods *in vitro* than can pure suspensions of lymphocytes. A careful study of the conditions necessary for the long-term cultivation of mouse peritoneal macrophages has been made by Chang [123]. The duration of his cultures, which were satisfactory on termination, was 172·5 days with a maximum of 220 days. Active phagocytosis was observable even after prolonged culturing. It is essential to adhere to the many minor details of technique found to be advantageous by Chang, if such prolonged survival is required. The main points to be observed are: (1) The peritoneal cells should be washed out with NCTC medium 109 and *not* centrifuged. (2) The best culture medium was found to be 50 per cent NCTC 109, 40 per cent horse serum and 10 per cent 1/5 beef embryo extract with penicillin (100 u/ml) and streptomycin (100 μg/ml). (3) Cultures are best maintained in a 5 per cent CO_2 : 95 per cent air mixture at $37°$ C and the medium changed twice a week. As the cells form adherent monolayers, a variety of culture vessels may be used including Leighton tubes (with flying cover slips) and Carrell flasks. Disposable polystyrene Petri dishes (36 mm diameter are economical) and Cooper dishes of similar material allow excellent microscopical observation of the monolayers.

Although it is frequently reported that macrophages do not normally divide *in vitro*, they will do so at a very low rate under suitable cultural conditions. Less than 1 per cent of mouse peritoneal macrophages became labelled when they were incubated with tritiated thymidine *in vitro* [124, 125]. The number of mitotic divisions observed by Chang [123] during the first few days of culturing mouse peritoneal macrophages was less than 0·05 per cent. Occasional mitotic figures were also noticed by Garvey [121] in her Kupffer cell cultures.

The rate of DNA synthesis in macrophage suspensions can be greatly enhanced by the subcutaneous injection of endotoxin 2 days before isolation [126] or of antigen 1 day previously to cells obtained from sensitized animals [125]. DNA synthesis is stimulated likewise by the *in vitro* addition of antigen to 'sensitized' macrophages [127].

A sudden and dramatic increase in the rate of mitosis frequently observed in long-term cultures of blood monocytes represents a fibroblastic conversion which rapidly overgrows the phagocytic cells [128, 129].

Labelled macrophages

Two methods are most frequently used for following the fate of macrophages or for determining the origin of these cells in chimaeric suspensions:

1. Labelling with phagocytosed particles which may be tagged with radioisotopes.
2. Chromosome analysis.

It is most convenient to allow macrophages to ingest particles before removing them from the animal, although this can be carried out *in vitro*. Peritoneal macrophages or Kupffer cells may be labelled with colloidal carbon (C11/1431a, Gunther Wagner, Hanover) or with colloidal ^{198}Au [107]. The latter isotope is, like ^{51}Cr (which has a longer half life) a useful marker for macrophages as it is not metabolised and remains fixed within the cells. With these techniques, the possibility must be considered that the marker material will be rephagocytosed by other cells on the death of the labelled macrophage. It is difficult to label more than a very small percentage of normal macrophages with ^{3}H-thymidine.

The mouse translocation chromosome (T6) incorporated in the CBA strain has been used for identifying the origin of Kupffer cell suspensions isolated from animals undergoing graft-versus-host reactions (C57BL or CBA→C57BL × CBA/T6) and from radiation chimaeras (CBA/T6→CBA). Use is made in these experiments of the histocompatibility of the strains CBA and CBA/T6. Colcemid (0·01 ml of 0·04 per cent solution per g body weight) should be injected 2 hours before beginning Kupffer cell extraction as described previously. The number of mitoses obtained from 'GVH' livers is adequate for analysis, but a previous injection of an RE stimulant (such as *Myco. tuberculosis* BCG or *Corynebacterium parvum*) is necessary for syngeneic radiation chimaeras. The fate of injected T6-labelled macrophages has not yet been investigated.

Balner [97] has described the use of a cytotoxic antibody assay for determining the origin of peritoneal macrophages in mouse radiation chimaeras.

References

[1] VOLKMAN A. & GOWANS J.L. (1965) The production of macrophages in the rat. *Brit. J. exp. Path.* **46,** 50

[2] VOLKMAN A. & GOWANS J.L. (1965) The origin of macrophages from bone marrow in the rat. *Brit. J. exp. Path.* **46,** 62

[3] HARRIS H. (1953) The movement of lymphocytes. *Brit. J. exp. Path.* **34,** 599

[4] LEWIS W.H. (1931) Locomotion of lymphocytes. *Johns Hopkins Hosp. Bull.* **49,** 29

[5] LEWIS W.H. (1933) Locomotion of rat lymphocytes in tissue cultures. *Johns Hopkins Hosp. Bull.* **53,** 147

[6] CLARK E.R., CLARK E.L. & REX R.O. (1936) Observations on polymorphonuclear leukocytes in the living animal. *Am. J. Anat.,* **59,** 123

[7] SCHOOLEY J.C., BRYANT B.J. & KELLEY L.S. (1959) Preliminary autoradiographic observations of cellular proliferation in lymphoid tissues, using tritiated thymidine. In *The Kinetics of Cellular Proliferation,* pp. 208–217, ed. STOHLMAN, FREDRICK JR. New York: Grune & Stratton

[8] GOWANS J.L. & KNIGHT E.J. (1964) The route of re-circulation of lymphocytes in the rat. *Proc. Roy. Soc.* (B) **159,** 257

[9] BOYDEN S.V. (1964) Cytophilic antibody in guinea pigs with delayed-type hypersensitivity. *Immunology* **7,** 474

[10] HOWARD J.G. & BENACERRAF B. (1966) Properties of macrophage receptors for cytophilic antibodies. *Brit. J. exp. Path.* **47,** 193

[11] GOWANS J.L. (1957) The effect of the continuous re-infusion of lymph and lymphocytes on the output of lymphocytes from the thoracic duct of unanaesthetized rats. *Brit. J. exp. Path.* **38,** 67

[12] GOWANS J.L. (1959) The recirculation of lymphocytes from blood to lymph in the rat. *J. Physiol.* **146,** 54

[13] GOWANS J.L. (1959) The transfusion of lymphocytes in experimental animals. In *The Kinetics of Cellular Proliferation,* pp. 64–68, ed. STOHLMAN, FREDRICK JR. New York: Grune & Stratton

[14] SHORTER R.G. & BOLLMAN J.L. (1960) Experimental transfusion of lymphocytes. *Amer. J. Physiol.* **198,** 1014

[15] EVERETT N.B., CAFFREY R.W. & RIEKE W.O. (1964) Recirculation of lymphocytes. *Ann. N.Y. Acad. Sci.* **113,** 887

[16] GESNER B.M. (1965) The 'life-history' and functions of lymphocytes. In *The Inflammatory Process,* pp. 281–322, ed. ZWEIFACH B., GRANT L. & McKLUSKEY R.T. New York: Academic Press

[17] GOWANS J.L. & McGREGOR D.D. (1965) The immunological activities of lymphocytes. *Progr. Allergy* **9,** 1–78. Basel and New York: Karger

[18] LITTLE J.R., BRECHER G., BRADLEY T.R. & ROSE S. (1962) Determination of lymphocyte turnover by continuous infusion of H^3 thymidine. *Blood* **19,** 236

[19] GOWANS J.L., GESNER B.M. & McGREGOR D.D. (1961) The immunological activity of lymphocytes. In Ciba Foundation Symposium No. 10, *Biological Activity of the Leucocyte,* pp. 32–44, ed. WOLSTENHOLME G.E.W. & O'CONNOR M. London: Churchill

[20] GOWANS J.L. (1962) The fate of parental strain small lymphocytes in F_1 hybrid rats. *Ann. N.Y. Acad. Sci.* **99,** 432

[21] PORTER K.A. & COOPER E.H. (1962) Transformation of adult allogeneic small lymphocytes after transfusion into newborn rats. *J. exp. Med.* **115,** 997

[22] PORTER K.A., CHAPIUS G. & FREEMAN M.K. (1962) Responsibility of small lymphocytes for the killing effect of blood-marrow mixtures on irradiated rabbits. *Ann. N.Y. Acad. Sci.* **99**, 456

[23] MACKINNEY A.A., STOHLMAN F. & BRECHER G. (1962) The kinetics of cell proliferation in cultures of human peripheral blood. *Blood* **19**, 349

[24] COOPER H.L. & RUBIN A.D. (1965) RNA metabolism in lymphocytes stimulated by phytohemagglutinin: Initial responses to phytohemagglutinin. *Blood* **25**, 1014

[25] MARSHALL W.H. & ROBERTS K.B. (1963) The growth and mitosis of human small lymphocytes with a phytohaemagglutinin. *Quart. J. Physiol.* **48**, 146

[26] GOWANS J.L., MCGREGOR D.D., COWEN D.M. & FORD C.E. (1962) Initiation of immune responses by small lymphocytes. *Nature, Lond.* **196**, 651

[27] VAN BEKKUM D.W. & VOS O. (1957) Immunological aspects of homo- and heterologous bone marrow transplantation in irradiated animals. *J. Cellular Comp. Physiol.* **50, Suppl. 1,** 139

[28] ANDERSON D.O. & WHITELAW D.M. (1960) Transfer of homologous thoracic duct lymphocytes to irradiated rats. *Amer. J. Physiol.* **199**, 824

[29] GESNER B.M. & GOWANS J.L. (1962) The fate of lethally irradiated mice given isologous and heterologous thoracic duct lymphocytes. *Brit. J. exp. Path.* **43**, 431

[30] MARCHESI V.T. & GOWANS J.L. (1964) The migration of lymphocytes through the endothelium of venules in lymph nodes: An electron microscope study. *Proc. Roy. Soc.* (B) **159**, 283

[31] ZUCKER-FRANKLIN D. (1963) The ultrastructure of cells in human thoracic duct lymph. *Ultrastructure Research* **9**, 325

[32] HALL J.W. & FURTH J. (1938) Cultural studies on the relationship of lymphocytes to monocytes and fibroblasts. *Arch. Path.* **25**, 46

[33] BIERMAN H.R., BYRON R.L., KELLEY K.H., GILFILLAN R.S., WHITE L.P. FREEMAN N.E. & PETRAKIS N.L. (1953) The characteristics of thoracic duct lymph in man. *J. clin. Invest.* **32**, 637

[34] REINHARDT W.O. (1964) Some factors influencing the thoracic duct output of lymphocytes. *Ann. N.Y. Acad. Sci.* **113**, 844

[35] CRONKITE E.P., JANSEN C.R., COTTIER H., RAI K. & SIPE C.R. (1964) Lymphocyte production measured by extracorporeal irradiation, cannulation, and labelling techniques. *Ann. N.Y. Acad. Sci.* **113**, 566

[36] GRINDLAY J.H., CAIN J.C., BOLLMAN J.L. & MANN F.L. (1950) Lymph fistulas in trained dogs. An experimental technique. *Surgery* **27**, 152

[37] YOFFEY J.M. & COURTICE F.C. (1956) *Lymphatics, Lymph and Lymphoid Tissue*, pp. 323–390. Mass.: Harvard University Press

[38] SANDERS A.G., FLOREY H. & BARNES J.M. (1940) The output of lymphocytes from the thoracic duct in cats and rabbits. *Brit. J. exp. Path.*, **21**, 254

[39] ADAMS W.S., SAUNDERS R.H. & LAWRENCE J.S. (1945) Output of lymphocytes in cats including studies on thoracic duct lymph and peripheral blood. *Amer. J. Physiol.* **144**, 297

[40] REINHARDT W.O. & YOFFEY J.M. (1957) Lymphocyte content of lymph from the thoracic duct and cervical ducts in the guinea pig. *J. Physiol.* **136**, 227

[41] BOLLMAN J.L., CAIN J.C. & GRINDLEY J.H. (1948) Techniques for the collection of lymph from the liver, small intestine or thoracic duct of the rat. *J. lab. clin. Med.* **33**, 1349

[42] SHREWSBURY M.M. (1959) Thoracic duct lymph in unanaesthetized mouse: Method of collection, rate of flow and cell count. *Proc. Soc. exp. Biol. Med.* **99**, 53

[43] GESNER B.M. & GOWANS J.L. (1962) The output of lymphocytes from the thoracic duct of unanaesthetized mice. *Brit. J. exp. Path.* **43**, 424

[44] BOAK J.L. & WOODRUFF M.F.A. (1965) Modified technique for collecting mouse thoracic duct lymph. *Nature, Lond.* **205**, 396

[45] BOLLMAN J.L. (1948) A cage which limits the activity of rats. *J. lab. clin. Med.* **33**, 1348

[46] MANN J.D. & HIGGINS G.M. (1950) Lymphocytes in thoracic duct, intestinal and hepatic lymph. *Blood* **5**, 177

[47] MANN J.D., MANN F.D. & BOLLMAN J.L. (1949) Hypoprothrombinemia due to loss of intestinal lymph. *Amer. J. Physiol.* **158**, 311

[48] MEDAWAR J. (1940) Observations on lymphocytes in tissue culture. *Brit. J. exp. Path.* **21**, 205

[49] McGREGOR D.D. & GOWANS J.L. (1963) The antibody response of rats depleted of lymphocytes by chronic drainage from the thoracic duct. *J. exp. Med.* **117**, 303

[50] HUGHES W.L., BOND V.P., BRECHER G., CRONKITE E.P., PAINTER R.B., QUASTLER H. & SHERMAN F.G. (1958) Cellular proliferation in the mouse as revealed by auto-radiography with tritiated thymidine. *Proc. nat. Acad. Sci. (Wash.)* **44**, 476

[51] AMANO M., MESSIER B. & LEBLOND C.P. (1959) Specificity of labelled thymidine as a deoxyribonucleic acid precursor in radioautography. *J. Histochem. Cytochem.* **7**, 153

[52] LEBLOND C.P., MESSIER B. & KAPRIWA B. (1959) Thymidine-H^3 as a tool for the investigation of the renewal of cell populations. *Lab. Invest.* **8**, 296

[53] YOFFEY J.M., EVERETT N.B. & REINHARDT W.O. (1958) Labeling of cells in thoracic duct lymph of guinea pigs after tritiated thymidine. *Nature, Lond.* **182**, 1608

[54] ROBINSON S.H., BRECHER G., LOURIE I. & HALEY J.E. (1965) Leukocyte labeling in rats during and after continuous infusion of tritiated thymidine: Implications for lymphocyte longevity and DNA reutilization. *Blood* **26**, 281

[55] FORD C.E., HAMERTON J.L., BARNES D.W.H. & LOUTIT J.F. (1956) Cytological identification of radiation chimeras. *Nature, Lond.* **177**, 452

[56] PORTER K.A. & COOPER E.H. (1962) Recognition of transformed small lymphocytes by combined chromosomal and isotopic labels. *Lancet*, **ii**, 317

[57] WALFORD R.L. (1960) *Leukocyte Antigens and Antibodies*, pp. 1–45. New York: Grune & Stratton

[58] FALLON H.J., FREI E., III, DAVIDSON J.D., TRIER J.S. & BURK D. (1962) Leukocyte preparations from human blood: Evaluation of their morphologic and metabolic state. *J. lab. clin. Med.* **59**, 779

[59] WALFORD R.L., PETERSON E.T. & DOYLE P. (1957) Leukocyte antibodies in human sera and in immune rabbit sera. *Blood*, **12**, 953

[60] LEVINE S. (1956) Magnetic techniques for *in vitro* isolation of leukocytes. *Science* **123**, 185

[61] CASSEN B., HITT J. & HAYS E.F. (1958) The efficient separation of lymphocytes from normal human blood. *J. lab. clin. Med.* **52**, 778

[62] HASTINGS J., FREEDMAN S., RENDON O., COOPER H.L. & HIRSCHHORN K. (1961) Culture of human white cells using differential leukocyte separation. *Nature, Lond.* **192**, 1214

[63] GRAY J.G. & RUSSELL P.S. (1965) Preparation of viable human lymphocytes. In *Histocompatibility Testing*, pp. 175–176. Washington: Nat. Res. Council

[64] WILDY P. & RIDLEY M. (1958) Separation of human leukocytes from blood. *Nature, Lond.* **182**, 1801

[65] JOHNSON T.M. & GARVIN J.E. (1959) Separation of lymphocytes in human blood by means of glass wool column. *Proc. Soc. exp. Biol. Med.* **102,** 333

[66] GARVIN J.E. (1961) Factors affecting the adhesiveness of human leukocytes and platelets *in vitro. J. exp. Med.* **114,** 51

[67] BRANDT L., BORJESON J., NORDEN A. & OLSSON I. (1962) Separation of lymphocytes from peripheral blood by means of a glass wool column. A method for *in vitro* culture of lymphocytes. *Acta med. scand.* **172,** 459

[68] RABINOWITZ Y. (1964) Separation of lymphocytes, polymorphonuclear leukocytes and monocytes on glass columns, including tissue culture observations. *Blood* **23,** 811

[69] FICHTELIUS K.E. (1950–1951) A simple method to separate lymphocytes from the blood. *Acta Soc. Med. Upsalien.* **56,** 27

[70] GREENWALT T.J., GAJEWSKI M. & McKENNA J.L. (1962) A new method for preparing buffy coat-poor blood. *Transfusion* **2,** 221

[71] HAMMOND D. & REISZ M. (1965) Manuscript in preparation

[72] HIRSCHHORN R. (1965) Personal communication

[73] CARPENTER C.B., GLASSOCK R.J. & MERRILL J.P. (1965) Normal lymphocyte transfer (NLT) test in humans. In *Histocompatibility Testing*, pp. 173–174. Washington: Nat. Res. Council

[74] HILDEMANN W.H., LINSCOTT W.D. & MARLINO M.J. (1962) Immunological competence of small lymphocytes in the graft-versus-host reaction in mice. In *Ciba Foundation Symposium on Transplantation*, pp. 236–263, ed. WOLSTENHOLME G.E.W. & CAMERON M.P. London: Churchill

[75] TERASAKI P.I. (1959) Identification of the type of blood cell responsible for the graft-versus-host reaction in chicks. *J. Embryol. exp. Morph.* **7,** 394

[76] TULLIS J.L. (1953) Preservation of leukocytes. *Blood* **8,** 563

[77] BILLINGHAM R.E. (1961) The induction of tolerance of homologous tissue grafts. In *Transplantation of Tissues and Cells*, pp. 87–106, ed. BILLINGHAM R.E. & SILVERS W.K. Philadelphia: The Wistar Institute Press

[78] GOWANS J.L. (1964) In *The Thymus in Immunobiology*, p. 287, ed. GOOD R.A. & GABRIELSEN A.E. New York: Harper & Row

[79] FICHTELIUS K.E. (1958) A difference between lymph nodal and thymic lymphocytes shown by transfusion of labelled cells. *Acta Anat.* **32,** 114

[80] BILLINGHAM R.E., DEFENDI V., SILVERS W.K. & STEINMULLER D. (1962) Quantitative studies on the induction of tolerance and on runt disease in neonatal rats. *J. nat. Cancer Inst.* **28,** 365

[81] ZUCKER-FRANKLIN D., DAVIDSON M., GESNER B. & THOMAS L. (1965) Phagocytosis of PPLO by mononuclear cells. (Abst.). *J. clin. Invest.* **44,** 1115

[82] HIRSCHHORN R., KAPLAN J.M., GOLDBERG A.F., HIRSCHHORN K. & WEISSMANN G. (1965) Acid phosphatase-rich granules: Appearance in human lymphocytes before mitosis induced by phytohaemagglutinin. *Science* **147,** 55

[83] MARSHALL A.H.E. (1956) Chapter 1 in *An Outline of the Cytology and Pathology of the Reticular Tissue*. Edinburgh: Oliver & Boyd

[84] OREN R., FARNHAM A.E., KAZUHISA S., MILOFSKY E. & KARNOVSKY M.L. (1963) Metabolic patterns in three types of phagocytizing cells. *J. cell. Biol.* **17,** 487

[85] ASIDDAO C.B., FILKINS J.P. & SMITH J.J. (1964) Metabolic and surface factors governing phagocytosis in the perfused rat liver. *J. Reticuloendothelial Soc.,* **1,** 393

[86] COHN Z.A. & WIENER E. (1963) The particulate hydrolases of macrophages. 1. Comparative enzymology, isolation and properties. *J. exp. Med.* **118,** 991

[87] PAVILLARD E.R. (1963) *In vitro* phagocytic and bactericidal ability of alveolar and peritoneal macrophages of normal rats. *Austral. J. exp. Biol.* **41,** 265

[88] LEAKE E.S., GONZALEZ-OJEDA D. & MYRVIK Q.N. (1964) Enzymatic differences between normal alveolar macrophages and oil-induced peritoneal macrophages obtained from rabbits. *Exp. Cell Res.* **33**, 553

[89] MOUTON D., BOUTHILLIER Y., BIOZZI G. & STIFFEL C. (1963) Phagocytosis of *Salmonellae* by reticulo-endothelial cells of new born piglets lacking natural antibody. *Nature, Lond.*, **197**, 706

[90] JANDL J.H., JONES A.R. & CASTLE W.J. (1957) The destruction of red cells by antibodies in man. 1. Observations on the sequestration and lysis of red cells altered by immune mechanisms. *J. clin. Invest.* **36**, 1428

[91] CUTBUSH M. & MOLLISON P.L. (1958) Relation between characteristics of bloodgroup antibodies *in vitro* and associated patterns of red cell destruction *in vivo*. *Brit. J. Haemat.* **4**, 115

[92] FRANZL R.E. (1962) Immunogenic sub-cellular particles obtained from spleens of antigen-injected mice. *Nature, Lond.* **195**, 457

[93] FRANZL R.E. Personal communication

[94] MIMS C.A. (1964) The peritoneal macrophages of mice. *Brit. J. exp. Path.* **45**, 37

[95] DANNENBERG A.M., WALTER P.C. & KAPRAL F.A. (1963) Histochemical study of phagocytic and enzymatic functions of rabbit mononuclear and polymorphonuclear exudate cells and alveolar macrophages. 2. The effect of particle ingestion on enzyme activity; two phases of *in vitro* activation. *J. Immunol.* **90**, 448

[96] NORTH R.J. & MACKANESS G.B. (1963) Electronmicroscopical observations on the peritoneal macrophages of normal mice and mice immunized with *Listeria monocytogenes*. II. Structure of macrophages from immune mice and early cytoplasmic response to the presence of ingested bacteria. *Brit. J. exp. Path.* **44**, 608

[97] BALNER H. (1963) Identification of peritoneal macrophages in mouse radiation chimaeras. *Transplantation* **1**, 217

[98] GOODMAN J.W. (1964) On the origin of peritoneal fluid cells. *Blood* **23**, 18

[99] KOSUNEN T.U., WAKSMAN B.H., FLAX M.H. & TIHEN W.S. (1963) Radioautographic study of cellular mechanisms in delayed hypersensitivity. I. Delayed reactions to tuberculin and purified proteins in the rat and guinea pig. *Immunology* **6**, 276

[100] KOSUNEN T.U., WAKSMAN B.H. & SAMUELSSON I.K. (1963) Radioautographic study of cellular mechanisms in delayed hypersensitivity. 2. Experimental allergic encephalomyelitis in the rat. *J. Neuropath.* **22**, 367

[101] RABINOWITZ Y. & SCHREK R. (1962) Studies of cell source of macrophages from human blood in slide chambers. *Proc. Soc. exp. Biol. N.Y.*, **110**, 429

[102] KELLY L.S., BROWN B.A. & DOBSON E.L. (1962) Cell divisions and phagocytic activity in liver reticuloendothelial cells. *Proc. Soc. exp. Biol. N.Y.* **110**, 555

[103] HOWARD J.G., BOAK J.L., CHRISTIE G.H. & EVANS-ANFOM E. (1965) Evidence for the conversion of lymphocytes into liver macrophages during graft-versus-host reaction pp 95–102. In *La Greffe des Cellules Hematopoietiques allogeniques*. Paris: C.N.R.S.

[104] HOWARD J.G., BOAK J.L. & CHRISTIE G.H. (1966) Further studies on the transformation of thoracic duct cells into liver macrophages. *Ann. N.Y. Acad. Sci.* **129**, 327–339

[105] EDWARDS J.L. & KLEIN R.E. (1961) Cell renewal in adult mouse tissues. *Amer. J. Path.* **38**, 437

[106] NICOL T. & BILBEY D.L.J. (1958) Elimination of macrophage cells of the reticuloendothelial system by way of the bronchial tree. *Nature, Lond.* **182**, 192

[107] ROSER B. (1965) The distribution of intravenously injected peritoneal macrophages in the mouse. *Austral. J. exp. Biol. Med. Sci.* **43**, 553

[108] VAUGHAN R.B. (1965) Interactions of macrophages and erythrocytes; Some further experiments. *Immunology* **8**, 245

[109] GARDNER L.V. (1929) Differential cell count of the peritoneal fluid from the normal guinea pig. *Proc. Soc. exp. Biol. Med.* **26,** 690

[110] PADAWER J. & GORDON A.S. (1956) Cellular elements in the peritoneal fluid of some mammals. *Anat. Rec.* **124,** 209

[111] MACKANESS G.B. (1952) The action of drugs on intracellular tubercle bacilli. *J. Path. Bact.* **64,** 429

[112] FISHMAN M. (1961) Antibody formation *in vitro. J. exp. Med.* **114,** 837

[113] COHN Z.A. & MORSE S.I. (1959) Interactions between rabbit polymorphonuclear leucocytes and staphylococci. *J. exp. Med.* **110,** 419

[114] MYRVIK Q.N., LEAKE E.S. & FARISS B. (1961) Studies on pulmonary alveolar macrophages from the normal rabbit: A technique to procure them in a high state of purity. *J. Immunol.* **86,** 128

[115] BERKEN A. & BENACERRAF B. Personal communication

[116] MYRVIK Q.N., LEAKE E.S. & OSHIMA S. (1962) A study of macrophages and epithelioid cells from granulomatous (BCG-induced) lungs of rabbits. *J. Immunol.* **89,** 745

[117] BERKEN A. & BENACERRAF B. (1966) *J. exp. Med.* **123,** 119

[118] WEISS L.P. & FAWCETT D.W. (1953) Cytochemical observations on chicken monocytes, macrophages and giant cells in tissue culture. *J. Histochem. Cytochem.* **1,** 47

[119] ROUS P. & BEARD J.W. (1934) Selection with the magnet and cultivation of reticuloendothelial cells (Kupffer cells). *J. exp. Med.* **59,** 577

[120] ST GEORGE S. FRIEDMAN M. & BYERS S.O. (1954) Mass separation of reticuloendothelial and parenchymal cells of rat's liver. *Science* **120,** 463

[121] GARVEY J.S. (1961) Separation and *in vitro* culture of cells from liver tissue. *Nature, Lond.* **191,** 972

[122] HEILMAN D.H. (1965) The selective toxicity of endotoxin for phagocytic cells of the reticuloendothelial system. *Intern. Arch. Allerg. Appl. Immunol.* **26,** 63

[123] CHANG Y.T. (1964) Long-term cultivation of mouse peritoneal macrophages. *J. nat. Cancer Inst.* **32,** 19

[124] SPEIRS R.S., WENCK Y. & JANSEN V. (1961) DNA synthesis in inflammatory cells of immunized and non-immunized mice. *Proc. Soc. exp. Biol. N.Y.* **106,** 251

[125] FORBES I.J. & MACKANESS G.B. (1963) Mitosis in macrophages. *Lancet* **2,** 1203

[126] FORBES I.J. (1965) Induction of mitosis in macrophages by endotoxin. *J. Immunol.* **94,** 37

[127] ROWLEY D. & LEUCHTENBERGER C. (1964) Antigen-stimulated desoxyribonucleic-acid synthesis *in vitro* by sensitized mouse macrophages. *Lancet* **2,** 734

[128] CARREL A. & EBELING A. (1922) Pure cultures of large mononuclear leucocytes. *J. exp. Med.* **36,** 365

[129] PAUL J. (1958) Establishment of permanent cell strains from human adult peripheral blood. *Nature, Lond.* **182,** 808

[130] BENNETT B. (1966) Isolation and cultivation *in vitro* of macrophages from various sources in the mouse. *Amer. J. Path.* **48,** 165

CHAPTER 32

Techniques for the Study of Phagocytes

A.E.STUART

Introduction

The techniques described in this section are based largely on routine methods used in the author's laboratory. References to alternative procedures are given at the end of the chapter.

Phagocytes *in vitro*

Animal peritoneal cells are composed of lymphocytes, macrophages and serosal cells. The phagocytic cells are readily cultured and the method described here, based on the work of Whitby & Rowley [1], is applicable to the mouse, rat, guinea-pig and rabbit. A better yield can be obtained with larger animals like the sheep if nutrient broth is injected into the pleural cavity 2 or 3 days before rinsing out the sac.

Material and methods

The mice should be 4–8 weeks old and free from infection. Cells from outbred mice give better cultures than those from highly inbred strains. Mice which are old or have splenomegaly or granulomata of the liver must not be used. The peritoneal cells from mice with chronic infection are often very rich in mast cells. The essential material required is shown in Fig. 32.1.

    1. Tissue culture medium 199 (Glaxo).

    2. Heparin.

    3. Sterile 10 ml graduated cylinder.

    4. One pair sharp pointed scissors.

    5. Sterile 5 ml or 2 ml syringe and needle.

    6. Cotton wool and methylated spirit.

    7. Three mice will yield sufficient cells to seed six to twelve tubes.

    8. Pyrex rimless tubes (16 × 125 mm) and rubber stoppers obtainable from Esco Rubber Ltd.

    9. No. 1 coverslips 19 × 6 mm.

Technique

Kill the mice by rapid dislocation of the neck and damp the fur with alcohol.

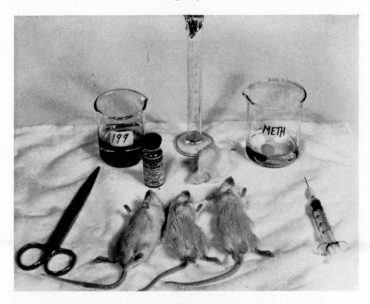

FIG. 32.1. Material required for tissue culture of macrophages.

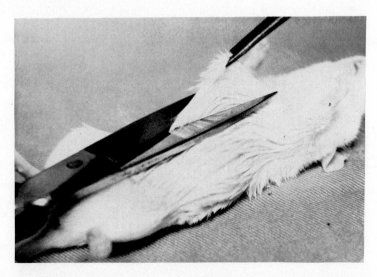

FIG. 32.2. Lifting the skin upwards with forceps to make a longitudinal incision $\frac{1}{2}$ in. long.

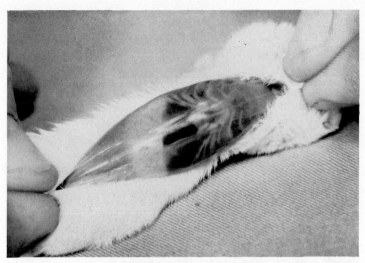

Fig. 32.3. Stripping back the fur with thumb and forefinger.

Lift the skin upwards from the abdominal wall (Fig. 32.2) with forceps and make a longitudinal incision $\frac{1}{2}$ in. long. Then strip back the fur with thumb and forefinger (Fig. 32.3.) and avoid touching the exposed abdominal wall. Inject 1·5–2·0 ml of medium 199 containing 5 units of heparin/ml. (If necessary heparin can be omitted.) The injection is made along the mid anterior line (Fig. 32.4) taking care to avoid puncture of the gut. Circulate the injected

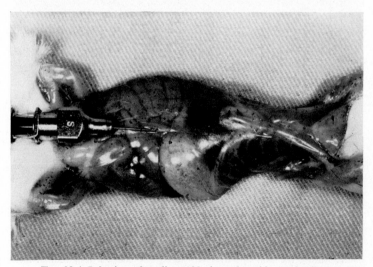

Fig. 32.4. Injection of medium 199 along the mid anterior line.

fluid by shaking or prodding. Remove the peritoneal fluid as follows: insert needle into flank (Fig. 32.5) and pull sideways so as to form a pocket of fluid. This prevents blockage of the needle with fat or intestine. Aspirate gently and transfer fluid to a sterile cylinder. The fluid may be pooled with other samples if large numbers of culture tubes are required. Mix the cell suspensions and remove a drop with a sterile Pasteur pipette. Count in a haemocytometer chamber using white cell diluting fluid and a white cell pipette at a dilution of 1/10. The nucleated cell count is usually between 1×10^6 and 3×10^6

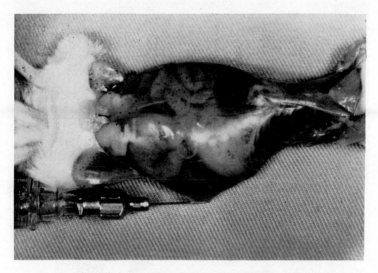

FIG. 32.5. Needle inserted into flank so as to form a pocket of fluid.

cells/ml. Add sterile calf serum (Burroughs Wellcome No. 1) to a final concentration of 10 per cent. Add 1·5 ml containing $1·5 \times 10^6$ cells to the tubes and incubate at 37° C. Change the medium 24 hours later and use the cells within 48–72 hours. When tubes quickly become bright yellow, then infection is probably present.

Examples of practical work with monolayers. Erythrophagocytosis
The monolayers should be 24 hours old. It is most important in studies on phagocytosis to use standard monolayers of the same age, and old cultures are unsuitable for macrophage red cell interactions. Tissue culture macrophages will ingest erythrocytes only if the latter are old or have been injured. Red cells coated with globulin are readily ingested. It is of interest that human red cells can be used for some experiments with animal macrophages although for some experimental work on immune isoantibodies it is of importance to use cells from inbred strains of mouse.

Technique

1. Obtain 24 hour cultures on coverslips of mouse macrophages grown in human AB serum.

2. Prepare a 10 per cent saline suspension of human red cells and incubate with an equal volume of diluted and heat inactivated haemolysin prepared in the rabbit against human erythrocytes.

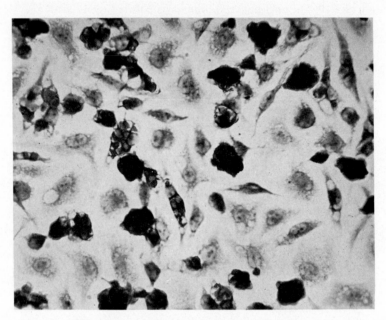

FIG. 32.6. Macrophage culture showing erythrophagocytosis.

3. After a 2–4 hour incubation at 37° C the cells may be used immediately or stored overnight at 4° C in 100 per cent serum.

4. Add 0·2 ml of the sensitized suspension to a monolayer containing 1 ml of culture medium and incubate at 37° C for 1 hour and also for 3 hours. Non-sensitized cells are used as controls. Even dispersal of the suspension is helped by using a Gallenkamp oscillating table, which gives a gentle lateral movement. It may be necessary to tap the cultures with the fingers at intervals of 30 minutes. Rotary shakers are not suitable and for class work one can manage without mechanical aids for dispersal.

5. After incubation the cultures must be rinsed thoroughly with two washes in physiological saline, dried by brief (2 minutes) exposure to methanol and stained by Leishman's method (Fig. 32.6).

Demonstration of erythrophagocytosis of old red cells

Time-expired blood transfusion samples are a useful source of red cells.

1. Samples of fresh cells (obtained by venepuncture) are used as controls and stored cells 4–8 weeks old as test examples. They are washed three times in physiological saline and made to a 5 per cent suspension. Add 0·2 ml to coverslip monolayers and incubate for approximately 1 hour before removing and staining.

Technical difficulties

1. Infection in the monolayer or of the sample added will give anomalous results. On most occasions chemically clean glassware is suitable, but sterile precautions are advisable for critical work. When this is necessary always keep at hand a blood agar bacteriological plate for direct culture of materials under investigation.

2. Adherence of red cells to macrophages may simulate phagocytosis. The outline of the cells in adherence is irregular and resembles a bunch of grapes. In phagocytosis the irregular masses of red cells are contained within a relatively smooth boundary. The characteristic feature of pronounced phagocytosis is the presence of large, round, clearly defined dark masses under the lower power of the microscope.

3. Avoid glassware cleaned with detergents. 'Lux' soap flakes are suitable.

4. Variables which influence the degree of phagocytosis are the age of the culture, the age of the red cell, the duration of sensitization and the concentration of the fluid suspension. For preliminary work use 24-hour-old cultures. As the culture ages the phagocytic properties become less. The red cells should preferably be fresh and stored in 100 per cent serum. The suspensions are used at a concentration of between 5 and 10 per cent.

Bacterial phagocytosis

The methods developed by Whitby & Rowley [1], Rowley [2] and Jenkin & Palmer [3] have probably been the most successful for the examination of the phagocytic and intracellular bactericidal properties of macrophages [4, 5, 6]. Cooper & West [7] studied the stimulatory effects of glyceryl trioleate on the peritoneal macrophage and their methods are used here as a guide in technique.

Example

Organisms

In the majority of experiments a Paracolobactrum strain with a low virulence for mice was used. The organisms are inoculated into 10 ml volumes of Hartley's tryptic broth and incubated for 2 hours at 37° C on a horizontal shaker after which they are centrifuged at 3000 rev/min for 20 minutes and finally resuspended in Tyrode's solution at a concentration of 4×10^5 organisms per ml by comparison with Brown's opacity tubes (Burroughs Wellcome and Co.). Opsonization of Gram-negative organisms is important for phagocytosis and the organisms are now incubated with an equal volume of normal animal serum for 15 minutes at 37° C and finally diluted 1/2000 in Tyrode's solution.

Preparation of peritoneal cells. This is done as before except that penicillin and streptomycin are omitted from the tissue culture medium. The cells are centrifuged once and suspended in Tyrode's solution or Glaxomedium 199. It is advisable in addition that the medium contains a 5 per cent concentration of serum; alternatively, 5 per cent of bovine serum albumin can be tried.

Determination of macrophage activity. Samples of 1 ml cell suspension containing 2×10^6 cells are distributed in 1 oz screw-capped bottles containing round No. 1 coverslips at the bottom. The bottles are incubated at 37° C for 1 hour. The coverslips are then removed, washed gently in medium and transferred to the diluted suspension (1 ml) of organisms in screw-capped bottles, the ratio of viable organisms to cells being approximately 100 : 1. They are then incubated at 37° C for 60 minutes. The coverslips are then removed, washed, transferred to 1 ml volumes of distilled water and the cells rinsed off. Bacterial counts are done on both the fragmented cells and the original supernatant [8]. Bottles containing macrophages heated to 100° C for 15 minutes are used as controls for bacterial growth during the incubation period. It is now possible to assess the extent of phagocytosis by the cells and the survival of organisms within the cells by the following calculations:

If N_1 = number of organisms in supernatant of heated cell bottles (controls)
N_2 = number of organisms in supernatant of experimental bottles
C = number of organisms in cells from the experimental bottles

then $\dfrac{N_1 - N_2}{N_1} \times 100$ = percentage of organisms phagocytosed by the cells.

and $\dfrac{C}{N_1 - N_2} \times 100$ = percentage of ingested organisms surviving within the cells.

Isolation and culture of human macrophages from the living and dead

Cadaveric macrophages
The subject should not be more than 2 hours dead and free from abdominal disease: the young or middle aged are more suitable than the elderly. Clean the skin over the left iliac fossa with 70 per cent ethyl alcohol. Insert a large-bore needle or small Trocar and avoid the bladder and bowel. Connect the trocar with plastic tubing to a 6 litre reservoir of physiological saline situated 10 to 12 ft above the body. Introduce 3-5 litres of saline into the peritoneal

sac. Repeatedly press the abdomen up and down whilst the saline is running. This takes 15–20 minutes. Then make an incision 1 in. long in the right iliac fossa and a hole $\frac{1}{4}$ in. in diameter in the peritoneum. Push $\frac{1}{2}$ in. plastic tubing through the hole for a distance of 6–9 in. The terminal 5 in. of this tube contains multiple perforations $\frac{1}{5}$ in. in diameter. Aspirate the abdominal fluid into flasks. When the holes of the intraperitoneal part of the tube are blocked by fat, close the vacuum and rotate the tube. Blood-stained fluids should not be used.

Macrophages from peritoneal dialysis
The fluid from patients treated by peritoneal dialysis for renal failure is a convenient and reliable source of macrophages. The fluid should be clear and straw coloured. A tinge of pink is acceptable but heavily blood-stained fluid is not recommended. All apparatus must be sterile.

Centrifuge the peritoneal fluid at 800 rev/min in 250 ml containers for 15 minutes at 10° C. Discard the supernatant and pool the deposits in Glaxo tissue culture medium 199 containing both penicillin and streptomycin. Centrifuge gently once more and resuspend in tissue culture medium containing 10 per cent human serum of any blood group. The nucleated cell count should be between $1\frac{1}{2}$ and 2 million cells per ml. The optimal volume for seeding coverslips in test tubes is 1·5 ml, for hexagonal Pyrex baby feeding bottles 10 ml and 50 ml for large Roux flasks. Incubate the cultures at 37° C for 48 hours when adherent red cells are detached by very gently flicking the tube with the forefinger and rinsing with medium 199. Replenish with fresh medium containing 10 per cent serum. Starch granules [9] give excellent results for phagocytosis but should be used in a high concentration from a suspension containing 1 mg/ml of starch.

Results
Most of the cells have adhered to coverslips within 48–72 hours and their cytoplasm has spread out on the glass (Fig. 32.7). Their shape is variable; many have numerous and short processes, some are round and others spindle-shaped. In all cases the nucleus is oval or indented, the nuclear membrane is clearly defined and nucleoli are absent. These cells avidly phagocytose starch granules (Fig. 32.8). There is a much smaller population of cells, between 5 and 10 per cent of the total, which do not phagocytose. They are often large and elongated although pleomorphic and triangular forms may be found. Their cytoplasm is deep blue with Leishman's stain and contains minute fenestrations. Longitudinal striae are present in the thicker parts of the cytoplasm. These cells never contain leucocytic granules. The processes are often long and tenuous. The nucleus is very large and characteristic. It is round or oval, finely granular and never indented or lobed. The nuclear

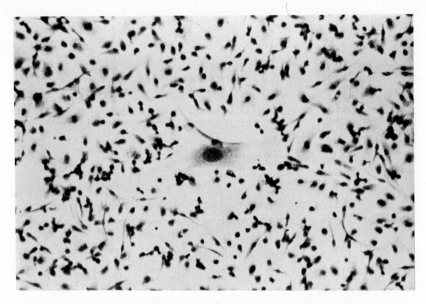

FIG. 32.7. Human peritoneal cells in culture. Note central large serosal cell.

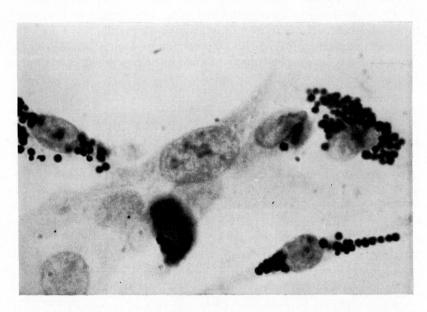

FIG. 32.8. Human peritoneal cells in culture showing phagocytosis of starch granules.

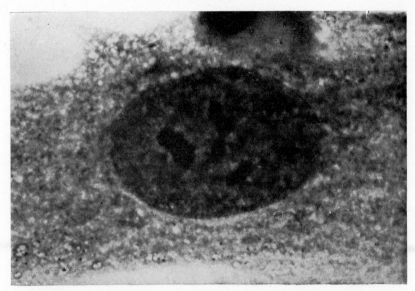

FIG. 32.9 Nuclear structure of human serosal cell showing intranuclear chromatin.

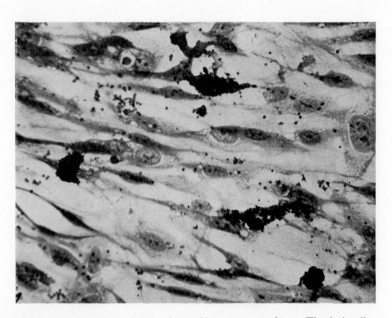

FIG. 32.10. Spindle cells in 10 day culture of human macrophages. The dark cells are filled with starch granules.

LL

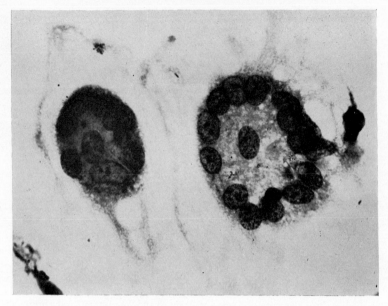

FIG. 32.11. Giant cells.

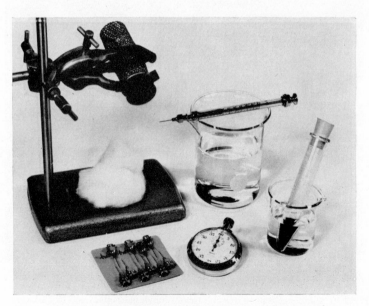

FIG. 32.12. Materials required for carbon clearance test.

membrane is rather irregular and poorly defined. The nucleus is very much less basophilic than the surrounding cytoplasm although the intranuclear chromatin is intensely basophilic. These chromatin bodies are distinctive, variable in shape but often round or Y-shaped (Fig. 32.9). Their borders are irregular and they number from two to five.

Between the fifth and tenth day of culture the cells visibly increase in number and the macrophages are relatively fewer. Mitotic figures are sometimes seen. Between the fifteenth and thirtieth day of culture the large non-phagocytic cells predominate. Fig. 32.10 shows a spindle cell culture containing only a few phagocytic cells which are filled with darkly staining starch granules. Fig. 32.11 shows a Touton giant cell.

The carbon clearance test for *in vivo* phagocytosis
This is based on the work of Biozzi, Halpern, Stiffel & Benacerraf [10]. These authors obtained a preparation of colloidal carbon which was stable in the bloodstream and, unlike Indian ink, did not cause thrombosis in the lungs. The carbon particles are uniform in size and measure 250 Å in diameter. When this preparation is injected intravenously the carbon is removed by the sessile intravascular phagocytes in the liver and spleen. The Kupffer cells of the liver take up approximately 90 per cent and the splenic macrophages 10 per cent. Provided the dose is standardized, the rate of removal from the bloodstream is a measure of reticulo-endothelial phagocytic activity. Very small doses of colloid are a measure of hepatic blood flow rather than phagocytic function. Massive doses result in some absorption of carbon by the parenchymatous cells of the liver. Other useful methods include the use of lipid emulsions [11], fluorescent particles [12], chromium phosphate [13] and albumin labelled with iodine [14, 15, 16]. It is useful to remember that most particles require opsonins for phagocytosis and depletion of opsonins may therefore inhibit phagocytosis.

Materials
The materials are shown in Figs. 32.12 and 32.18.
   1. A glass and metal tuberculin syringe. This is preferable to the all-glass kind. Slight pressure on the metal plunger enables the graduation marks to be easily seen despite the presence of carbon.
   2. A beaker of warm water and cotton wool for heating the tail of the mouse.
   3. A suspension of carbon in a stoppered tube at 37° C. The carbon is obtained from Gunther Wagner, Pelikan Werke, Hanover, Germany, and is stored in a stock solution of 64 mg/ml with a small amount of gelatin. The stock solution is melted in boiling water, thoroughly shaken and diluted to a concentration of either 8 mg/ml or 16 mg/ml.

If the reticulo-endothelial system (RES) is very active then the higher concentration is preferable.

4. A stop watch.

5. Stand with heavy base and wire cage with cork containing V-shaped slit at periphery for tail of animal.

6. Rack with six rimless tubes 70 × 11 mm each containing 2·0 ml distilled water.

7. 0·025 ml pipette for withdrawal of blood samples.

8. Grease pencil.

The pipette must have a sharp but relatively stout end; they are most easily prepared from old or broken 1 ml graduated pipettes.

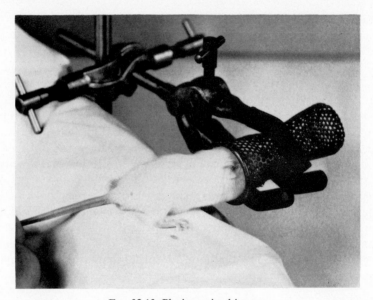

FIG. 32.13. Placing animal in cage.

Method

1. Weigh the mouse. The dose of carbon for a 21 g animal is 0·21 ml, for a 16 g animal 0·16 ml. Divide the weight by 100 to obtain the amount in millilitres for injection.

2. Place mouse on coat sleeve with head facing cage and exert gentle traction on tail (Fig. 32.13). Nearly always the animal will enter the cage. Insert stopper with V-shaped slit and warm the tail with water and cotton wool.

3. The upper and undersurfaces of the tail both contain a large vein which is suitable for intravenous injection. Avoid the lateral veins which are rather

difficult to enter. Always start injections at the extremity and if unsuccessful move further upwards. Hold the tail between finger and thumb (Fig. 32.14) at an angle of 45° and inject tangentially. The syringe should be completely free from air bubbles.

4. Remove serial samples of 0·025 ml from the retro-orbital venous plexus at intervals of approximately 3, 6, 9, 12, 15 minutes. The mouse must be held gently but firmly by the scruff of the neck with the thumb over the flank. The sharp end of the pipette is inserted rapidly and not too far (Fig. 32.15) and the blood allowed to run slightly above the 0·025 ml mark. Expel any

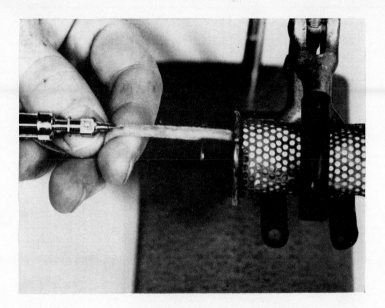

Fig. 32.14. Injecting the carbon.

excess by touching the lip of the pipette with blotting paper and transfer content to a tube containing distilled water. Rinse the pipette once in saline and once in heparin before taking the next sample. At the end of the experiment the mouse (Fig. 32.16) should be in good condition and completely free from any signs of distress, although the nose, paws and ears will have a black colour. Beginners are recommended to try the technique in the first instance by using fully anaesthetized animals.

5. The relative amounts of carbon are now estimated in an EEL photoelectric colorimeter using a 1 ml adaptor for the blood samples and a red filter. The density readings are converted to a logarithmic scale and plotted against time. The slope of the line is called the phagocytic coefficient K.

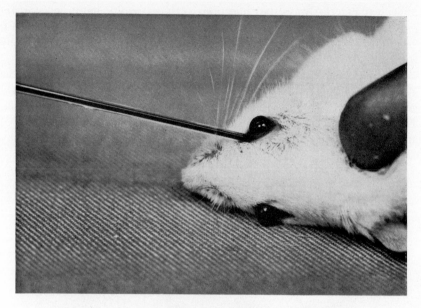

FIG. 32.15. Removal of blood samples from retro-orbital plexus.

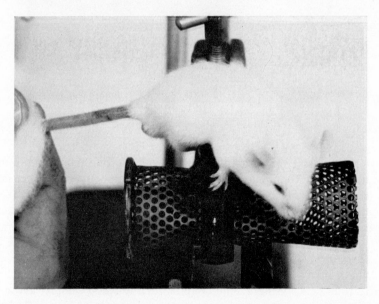

FIG. 32.16. After injection the nose, paws and ears are slightly blackened; the animal is in good condition.

6. The mouse is killed and the liver and spleen removed and weighed individually. Spleen weight should be constant. Mice with large spleens or livers commonly give elevated K values which are misleading. If the strain of animal used shows marked variation in spleen weight then it is quite unsuitable for measurement of RES function.

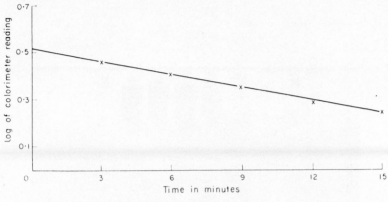

FIG. 32.17

Example

Example of carbon clearance using carbon at 16 mg/ml

Mouse weight	(w)	20	g
Spleen weight		0·09	g
Liver weight		1·07	g
Combined weight of liver and spleen (wls)		1·16	g

Ratio of body weight (w) to combined weight of liver and spleen (wls)

$$\equiv \frac{w}{wls} = \frac{20}{1 \cdot 16} = 17 \cdot 2$$

Time	Colorimeter reading	Log of colorimeter reading
3	2·87	0·46
6	2·53	0·40
9	2·51	0·39
12	1·91	0·28
15	1·74	0·24

From Fig. 32.17

Phagocytic index $K_{16} = \dfrac{0 \cdot 51 - 0 \cdot 33}{10} = 0 \cdot 018.$

Because a carbon dose of 8 mg/100 g mouse weight is commonly used it is convenient to reduce all results of K_8 as follows:

$K_8 = \cdot036$ $\sqrt[3]{K_8} = 0\cdot330$.

The corrected phagocytic index α is a measure of phagocytic activity per unit weight of tissue and is given by the formula

$$\alpha = \frac{w}{wls} \times \sqrt[3]{K_8}$$

$$\alpha = 17\cdot2 \times 0\cdot330 = 5\cdot7.$$

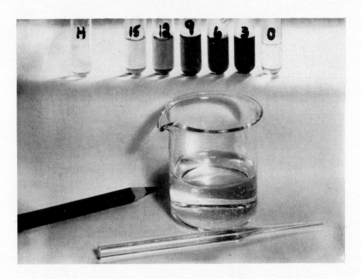

FIG. 32.18. Showing pipette for removal of blood samples, beaker of water and tube H containing heparin for rinsing pipette. Grease pencil for marking tubes with time of removal of blood samples, e.g. 0, 3, 6, 9, 12, 15 minutes.

Stimulation of the reticulo-endothelial system

Small doses of inert colloids produce a mild and transitory stimulation of phagocytic function. Repeated doses of colloid result in cellular hyperplasia and a more pronounced degree of activity. Bacterial infections also stimulate the RES as in experimental typhoid infection and the injection of BCG. The RES-stimulating material commonly used are bacterial extracts [17], yeast extracts [18, 19], simple lipids [20] and hormones [21]. Bacterial and yeast extracts cause granulomatous lesions in the recipient whereas hormones and simple lipids do not.

Examples

Bacterial extracts. The anaerobic strain 936B of *Corynebacterium parvum* causes widespread lympho-reticular hyperplasia. The organisms are heat killed, formalized and kept at 4° C. The mice are given 0·1 ml IV or IP, i.e. 255 µg dry weight of bacteria. The RES stimulation lasts for 8–10 days.

Hormones. Diethyl stilboestrol in a dose of 0·5 mg in 0·1 ml arachnis oil is injected into mice subcutaneously once daily for 6 days. The phagocytic index K is raised to approximately five times that of normal on the eighth day. The increased RES activity lasts for a week. The reticulo-endothelial phagocytes continue to respond to stimulation during repeated courses with diethyl stilboestrol and large doses cause the animals to lose weight. In adult rats a dose of 0·2 mg ethinyl oestradiol/day is recommended. The doses of oestrogens required to activate the RES is much is excess of the calculated physiologically available hormone.

Endotoxin. 'Difco' Escherichia coli O111 : B4 lipopolysaccharide is made as a solution in 0·9 per cent sodium chloride containing 200 µg per ml. 0·1 ml volumes (20 µg) are given intravenously to each mouse. The phagocytic index K is elevated at 24 hours, reaches a peak within 2–3 days and returns to normal within 4–5 days.

Triglycerides. The most useful are glyceryl trioleate and glyceryl tricaprate. The lipid is made into a suspension and injected intravenously. This is followed by a prompt elevation of K values which is sustained for about 4–5 days. Repeated doses can be given. In the doses used here a large amount of the injected suspension is trapped in the lung but does not cause infarction or a foreign body reaction. Improved methods for the preparation of more uniform suspensions have been described in the literature but are not discussed here because relatively little is known about their effects on the RES.

Preparation of triolein suspensions
Triolein (glycerol trioleate, British Drug Houses) is prepared as a 20 per cent v/v suspension immediately before injection. 1 ml of triolein is added to 4 ml of 5 per cent dextrose water (Evans Medical) containing 0·04 ml Tween 20 (L. Light & Co.). The mixture is stirred rapidly in an M.S.E. homogenizer for 3–5 minutes and 0·05 ml volumes (11·5 mg triolein) are injected into the tail veins of mice.

Depression of the reticulo-endothelial system
This is readily accomplished by saturation with inert particulate matter such as carbon or thorotrast, injection of cortisone or administration of the alkyl esters of fatty acids such as ethyl oleate, ethyl stearate, ethyl palmitate and methyl palmitate. The intravenous administration of particulate matter suppresses phagocytic activity in the liver and spleen but does not affect lymph nodes.

LL*

Technique and dosage for the depression of RES phagocytic function with ethyl palmitate

Preparation of ethyl palmitate suspension. 15 ml of ethyl palmitate is mixed with 2·5 ml of ethyl alcohol and the mixture kept at 45° C. This is slowly added by pipette to 32·5 ml of 1 per cent of Tween 20 dissolved in 5 per cent dextrose water, the mixture being homogenized for 4 or 5 minutes in an M.S.E. homogenizer surrounded by a water jacket at 45–50° C. The suspension is then transferred to Visking cellophane tubing and the ends carefully tied without leaving an air space. The material is dialysed overnight against excess 5 per cent dextrose water buffered with phosphate to pH 7·2 at 37° C. The addition of alcohol reduces the size of the particles.

Dosage: 0·1–0·2 ml per 10 g body weight is injected intravenously.

It is important to use BDH technical grade ester since the highly purified Pfluka preparations are toxic (personal communication from Professor K. Flemming, Freiburg). However, purified methyl palmitate has been used successfully [22] when prepared by ultrasonic disintegration. Although no direct comparison has been made of the depressant effect of ethyl palmitate prepared as above and the ultrasonicated methyl ester, the particle size of the latter preparation seems more suitable for intravenous injection.

References

[1] WHITBY J.L. & ROWLEY D. (1959) The role of the macrophage in the elimination of bacteria from the mouse peritoneum. *Brit. J. exp. Path.* **40,** 357

[2] ROWLEY D. (1960) The role of osponins in non-specific immunity. *J. exp. Med.* **111,** 137

[3] JENKIN C. & PALMER D.L. (1960) Changes in the titre of serum opsonins and phagocytic properties of mouse peritoneal macrophages following injection of endotoxin. *J. exp. Med.* **112,** 419

[4] JENKIN C., ROWLEY D. & AUZINS I. (1964) The basis for immunity to mouse typhoid. *Aust. J. Exp. Biol. and Med. Sci.* **42,** 215

[5] JENKIN C. and BENACERRAF B. (1960) *In vitro* studies on the interaction between mouse peritoneal macrophages and strains of Salmonella and Escherichia coli. *J. exp. Med.* **112,** 403

[6] MACMASTERS M.M., BAIRD P.D., HOLZAPFEL M.M. & RIST C.E. (1955) Preparation of starch from *Amaranthus cruentus* seed. *Economic Botany* **9,** 300

[7] COOPER G.N. & WEST D. (1962) Effect of simple lipids on the phagocytic properties of peritoneal macrophages. 1. Stimulating effects of glyceryl trioleate. *Aust. J. Exp. Biol. and Med. Sci.* **40,** 485

[8] MILES A.A., MISRA S.S. & IRWIN J.D. (1938) The estimation of the bacterial power of the blood. *J. Hyg. Camb.* **38,** 732

[9] THORPE, BERT D. & MARCUS, STANLEY (1964) Comparison of two techniques to study *in vitro* uptake and fate of *Pasteurella tularensis. Journal of the Reticulo-endothelial Society* **1,** 418

[10] BIOZZI G., BENACERRAF B., STIFFEL C. & HALPERN B.N. (1954) Étude Quantitative du l'activité granulopexique du système réticuloendothélial chez la souris. *C.R. Soc. Biol., Paris* **148,** 431

[11] DI LUZIO N.R. & RIGGI S.J. (1964) The development of a lipid emulsion for the measurement of R.E.S. function. *Journal of the Reticulo-endothelial Society* **1,** 136

[12] JUHLIN L. (1960) Effect of starvation on the reticulo-endothelial system as evaluated by means of a new fluorescent particle technique. In *Reticulo-endothelial Structure and Function*, ed. HELLER J.H. New York: The Ronald Press Co.

[13] SNELL J.F. (1960) Relationship of chromium phosphate clearance rates to resistance: Effects of some cortico-steroids on blood clearance rates in mice. In *Reticulo-endothelial Structure and Function*, ed. HELLER J.H. New York: The Ronald Press Co.

[14] BENACERRAF B., BIOZZI G., HALPERN B.N., STIFFEL C. & MOUTON D. (1957) Phagocytosis of heat denatured serum albumin labelled with I^{131} and its use as a means of investigating liver blood flow. *Brit. J. exp. Path.* **38,** 35

[15] BIOZZI G., BENACERRAF B., HALPERN B.N., STIFFEL C. & HILLEMAND B. (1958) Exploration of the phagocytic function of the recticulo-endothelial system with heat denatured serum albumin labelled with I^{131} and application to liver blood flow in normal man and in some pathologic conditions. *J. lab. clin. Med.* **51,** 230

[16] BASES R.E. & KRAKOFF I.H. (1965) Enhanced reticulo-endothelial phagocytic activity in myeloproliferative diseases. Colloidal heat denatured albumen labelled I^{131} was used to investigate phagocytic activity in human beings. *Journal of the Reticulo-endothelial Society* **2,** 1

[17] HALPERN B.N., PRÉVOT A-R., BIOZZI G., STIFFEL C., MOUTON D., MORARD J.C., BOUTHILLIER Y. & DECREUSEFOND C. (1964) Stimulation de l'activité phagocytaire du système réticuloendothélial provoquée par Corynebacterium parvum. *Journal of the Reticulo-endothelial Society* **1,** 77

[18] HELLER J.H. (1960) The effect of zymosan on the R.E.S. In *Reticulo-endothelial Structure and Function*, ed. HELLER J.H. New York: The Ronald Press Co.

[19] FITZPATRICK F.W., HAYNES L.J., SILVER N.J. & DICARLO F.J. (1964) Effect of glucan derivatives upon phagocytosis by mice. *Journal of the Reticulo-endothelial Society* **1,** 423

[20] COOPER G.N. (1964) Functional modification of reticulo-endothelial cells by simple triglycerides. *Journal of the Reticulo-endothelial Society* **1,** 50

[21] BILBEY D.L.J. & NICOL T. (1962) The molecular basis of drug effect on R.E.S. activity. *Colloq. Int. duc C.N.R.S.* No. 115, p. 109

[22] BLICKENS D.A. & DI LUZIO N.R. (1965) Metabolism of methyl palmitate, a phagocytic and immunologic depressant, and its influence on tissue lipids. *Journal of the Reticulo-endothelial Society* **2,** 60

CHAPTER 33

Localized Haemolysis in Gel

D.W.DRESSER & H.H.WORTIS*

Prior to the development of the localized haemolysis in gel (LHG) assay, antibody produced by single cells had been detected by immunofluorescence and microdroplet assays. In the former technique, developed by Coons and his co-workers [4], the antibody is detected specifically in sections or smears by means of antigen labelled with a fluorescent dye; in the microdroplet assays the fluid of a drop containing a single cell is assayed for anti-bacteriophage antibody [1] or the specific inhibition of bacterial movement by antibody to the flagellae of *Salmonellae* [17]. Both these elegant and sensitive techniques are difficult and time consuming, so that the development of the easier LHG assay by Jerne, Nordin & Henry [12] and Ingraham & Bussard [11] has considerably speeded the study of cellular events of interest to the immunologist.

Principle
The LHG assay is similar in principle to the plaque or colony techniques of the microbiologist. It is essentially a situation in which a visible plaque is formed round those cells producing antibody. In this way a population of lymphoid cells can be screened for plaque-forming cells (PFC) (antibody producers). For example, a suspension of spleen cells from a mouse immunized against sheep red blood cells (SRBC) is mixed with SRBC in a semisolid medium which is made to form a thin film. The plates are incubated for a few hours and then complement (fresh guinea-pig serum) is added before the plates are reincubated for a further 40–50 minutes. Complement-dependent lysis occurs around those lymphoid cells which have produced specific haemolysing antibody. With suitable illumination these plaques are clearly visible to the naked eye and with slight magnification can be counted with great precision and rapidity. The LGH techniques, as originally described by Jerne *et al* [12], detected only those lymphoid cells producing antibody capable of lysing erythrocytes (mostly γM (19S) antibody) but not other classes of antibody which could agglutinate or bind to erythrocytes but not fix complement (γG, γA (7S) antibodies). Other workers have shown that these other classes of antibody will fix complement and form plaques if an anti-globulin-developing serum is used [6, 23].

* USPHS Special Research Fellow, No, 2F3AM 29,299–02.

1054

The following description of the technique is based on our [27, 28] further modifications of the original method of Jerne *et al* [12]. Before a decision was reached as to what we thought was the best procedure to adopt, the following points were considered:

(a) Conditions necessary for obtaining the maximum PFC from a given population of lymphoid cells.

(b) Economy of materials.

(c) Efficiency of the laboratory operation in terms of the number of plates that can be used and lymphoid cell suspensions studied in a day.

Reagents and equipment

9 cm disposable polystyrene Petri dishes, grease-free, no irregular edges.
46° C water-bath fitted with racks for 12 × 90 mm test tubes. 50 – 55° C hot plate (magnetic stirrer).
Level platform—sheet of plate glass and three lumps of plasticine.
Automatic pipetting devices for 7·5 ml, 2 ml, 1 ml and 0·1 ml.
Agarose—L'Industrie Biologique, Gennevilliers, Seine—stating in the order that the agarose must be free of anti-complementarity.
Concentrated PBS solution A(× 10)
Concentrated Gey's solution A (× 10) } see page 1068
Dulbecco's PBS solutions B and C and Gey's solutions B and C

For each separate pool of lymphoid cells:

A very loose, all-glass or PTFE/glass, homogenizer, with 1 mm clearance.
10 ml conical graduated centrifuge tube (or graduated cylinder).
A 60 hole/cm stainless steel mesh sieve (shaped to fit on top of centrifuge tube).
Test tubes, racks and ice water-bath.
5 ml, 1 ml, 0·2 ml graduated blow-out pipettes.
Balances to measure organ and animal weights.
A water-jacketed incubator set at 37° C, with a humid atmosphere of 96 per cent air and 4 per cent carbon dioxide.
As a source of complement, 1 ml of 10 per cent fresh guinea-pig serum in Gey's for each plate. (Freshly reconstituted freeze-dried guinea-pig serum—commercially available—is a satisfactory, if expensive, substitute.)

Procedure
Bottom layer
Two layers of gel are required; the bottom layer is to provide a smooth non-toxic level surface for the top layer which contains the lymphoid cells and the indicator RBC. The bottom layer also prevents the top layer forming a meniscus with a significant proportion of its volume. The bottom layer is

made from 7·5 ml of 1·2 per cent (w/v) agarose in Dulbecco's phosphate buffered saline (PBS).

If the total volume of bottom layer for an experiment is x ml then the required amount of agarose is 0·012 x g, and this is suspended in 0·4 x ml distilled water by stirring vigorously. The agarose is then dissolved by bringing the mixture to the boil while shaking vigorously. After the agarose is dissolved a further 0·5 x ml of cool distilled water is added to lower the temperature. When the temperature is 60° C or slightly less, 0·08 x ml of concentrated (X10) PBS solution A is added, followed by 0·01 x ml of solution B and 0·01 x ml of C. The solution is maintained at 50–55° C with continual stirring. Using a prewarmed automatic pipette (or a graduated pipette), 7·5 ml is added to each Petri dish, spread and allowed to set on the level platform. These prepared plates can be used at once or stored for up to 48 hours, but NOT longer, at 4° C. Plates stored in the cold should be warmed (20–30° C) immediately before addition of the top layer.

Top layer

Each top layer for a 9 cm plate requires 2 ml of solution, which is 0·6 per cent agarose in Gey's solution. Sufficient agarose to make a 0·6 per cent solution is put into a flask with 0·8 y ml distilled water (where y ml is the required volume of top layer solution), and fully dispersed before being brought to the boil. 0·1 y ml concentrated Gey's A is now added, followed by 0·05 y ml of B and then 0·05 y ml of C. The solution is then filtered through a medium grade (No. 3) scintered glass filter which has been preheated to about 60° C. Two millilitre aliquots of the top solution are now dispensed into 12 × 90 mm tubes, set in racks in a water-bath at 46–48° C. A prewarmed automatic pipetting device can be used here.

If developing sera (see later) are to be used, they should be added now. A considerable speeding up of the operation can be achieved by having space in the racks for all the tubes necessary for any one day's experiment.

Preparation of lymphoid cell suspensions

Lymphoid cells are prepared from various organs, for instance spleens, by gentle homogenization in a very loose-fitting homogenizer. We use Jencon's '15 ml' PTFE pestles cut down with a fine screw thread finish to give a 1 mm clearance in MSE 15 ml round-bottom glass centrifuge tubes. The organ is gently squeezed in 1–2 ml Gey's solution until the lymphoid cells are released. When it is anticipated that the number of PFC per organ is very low, high numbers of lymphoid cells are added to each plate—in these circumstances the lymphoid cell suspension is 'washed' by addition of 8–10 ml Gey's solution, centrifugation at 600 **g** for 5 minutes, removal of supernatant and making up the volume to that required (say 3 ml). This suspension is then passed through a stainless-steel sieve. Lymphoid cell suspensions which are expected to have higher numbers of PFC are used relatively more dilute, do not need to be washed and are sieved immediately after homogenization. *After rinsing the sieve, the final volume of the lymphoid cell suspension is noted. The number of 'live' lymphoid cells in a suspension is measured with small samples removed immediatey after sieving and after the cells have been shaken into suspension and the lumps allowed to settle for 1 minute. At the same time 1–2 ml of the suspension is carefully removed to a second tube for dilution or to be used without further dilution, for addition to the assay plates.

When using peripheral leucocytes in the LHG assay we have found it necessary to remove platelets. This can be done by defibrination of the blood, followed by taking the buffy coat and washing the leucocytes.

Cells are counted either by (a) haemocytometer, using dye exclusion (0·1 per cent eosin freshly made in Gey's solution from a stock 1 per cent in 0·9 per cent saline kept at 4° C) to give 'live' and 'dead' counts; or (b) particle counter, e.g. Coulter or Celloscope, to give total cell counts and to estimate the number of 'live' cells by means of a viability constant (e.g. mean 'live' cells from 4-month-old CBA male spleens is 77·2 per cent when prepared by these techniques).

Lymphoid cell suspensions are made up so that the number of cells required on each plate is contained in 0·1 ml, or occasionally 0·2 ml.

Homogenization should be carried out within minutes of the organ's removal from the freshly killed animal. From this point onwards, except during centrifugation, and until addition to the agarose top layer solution, the lymphoid cells MUST BE KEPT IN AN ICE WATER-BATH.

Red blood cells
Bleed sheep (or other animal) into sterile Alsever's solution or buy as a sterile suspension in Alsever's solution (commercially available). Use 5–21 days after bleeding. Use 0·1 ml of a 20 per cent suspension (packed cell volume—1750 *g* for 5 min) for each plate. The SRBC suspension is washed twice in citrate-saline (or Alsever's solution) and twice in Gey's, and is finally made up as a 20 per cent suspension in Gey's solution. The buffy coat should be removed after the first centrifugation. We have noted that clumps of lymphoid cells of any origin can form non-specific fresh serum-dependent plaques.

Preparation of the assay plates
This operation is most easily carried out by three operators. The first operator selects a tube containing top layer from the 46° C water-bath, removes it,

*To prevent competition of non-specific mouse γ-globulin with specific mouse antibody for the developing antiserum, we now 'wash' all cell suspensions.

quickly dries the outside and adds 0·1 ml of the RBC suspension (indicator erythrocyte). The tube is handed to the second operator who, having ensured that the lymphoid cells are evenly in suspension, pipettes 0·1 ml of this lymphoid cell suspension into the top layer tube, gently shaking the tube to mix the red cells and lymphoid cells before handing the tube to the third operator who pours the contents into a prepared Petri dish containing a bottom layer, shaking out as much of the solution from the tube as possible

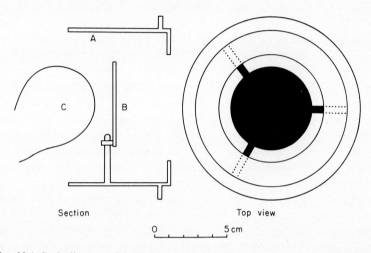

Section   Top view

0 _____ 5 cm

Fig. 33.1. Scale diagram of dark ground adaptor for colony counter. Made in brass. Surface A is polished metal; surface B is painted matt black; C is a 15 or 25 watt bulb which is shown at an angle to the adaptor because the front of the colony counter is at about 35° from the horizontal. The electrode which makes permanent contact with the gel medium should have a flexible wire to facilitate movement of the plate whilst counting.

before gently swirling the top layer over the surface of the bottom layer and then placing the plate on to the level platform while the agarose sets. At this stage, plates have been kept for up to 45 minutes at room temperature before incubation without causing any detectable effect.

Incubation and complement addition

The plates are incubated at 37° C in a humid atmosphere of 96 per cent air and 4 per cent carbon dioxide for 2 hours, after which 1 ml of the freshly diluted complement is added to each plate and spread evenly over the surface by gentle shaking. The plates are then incubated at 37° C for a further 40–50 minutes.

Counting the plaques

We count the plaques under slight magnification using a 'conductivity' type of colony counter (Scientifica Ltd—Model 1) which has been modified so that we can use dark ground illumination (Fig. 33.1). Plates may be stored at 4° C for 24 hours without any detectable change. Plates stored at room temperature may develop colonies of haemolytic bacteria within 24 hours.

Plates can be stained by pouring off the complement solution and then flooding with a freshly prepared mixture of 10 ml of a 2 per cent benzidine solution in glacial acetic acid, plus 10 ml of 5 per cent H_2O_2, plus 80 ml distilled water. This is NOT RECOMMENDED as a routine procedure as the benzidine is highly carcinogenic.

TABLE 33.1
An example of a calculation of mean PFC per spleen from plaque counts
Experiment STR-1; group 1.
Mice A strain males 4 months old; dose 4×10^5 SRBC ip; day 4 after immunization.

Animal No.	Live cells $\times 10^6$ per ml.	Dead cells $\times 10^6$ per ml.	Suspension total	vol. ml. per plate	Direct (γM) plaques	Developed plaques	Mean* direct plaques/ plate	Mean* total plaques on treated plate
1.	35	13	4·0	0·1	3, 2,	3, 6,	2·00	4·24
2.	37	18	4·0	0·1	3, 12,	15, 13,	6·21	13·97
3.	38	17	4·0	0·1	23, 18,	34, 24,	20·35	28·58

	Mean*	mean (log (x+1))	S^2 (log (x+1))
Direct (γM) PFC per spleen	253·4	2·4056	0·2514
Direct PFC per million live cells	3·8	0·6796	0·1373
Developed (non-γM) PFC per spleen	316·7	2·5019	0·1096
Developed PFC per million cells	2·3	0·5164	0·0399

Developing serum, polyspecific; KI = 0·93; KD = 1·38 (see Figs. 33.2 and 33.3)

*Mean $= \text{antilog} \dfrac{\log (x+1)}{n} - 1$; where x is either the number of plaques on a plate, the calculated number of developed PFC per spleen (mouse) or the number of direct (γM) PFC per spleen. n is the number of plates or mice.

Plates can be fixed unstained by washing out protein overnight with Gey's solution (4° C) and after pouring off the Gey's solution, adding 2 per cent formalin in PBS.

Statistics

A frequency distribution made of the number of plaques found on each of a large number of plates containing cells from a single population is not normal. Furthermore, the standard deviation of plaque counts per plate increases linearly with the mean of the plaque count (unpublished observations). In these circumstances it is necessary to calculate geometric means on transformed data. We use $\log(x+1)$ although other transformations may be used [20]. For similar reasons, the same transformation is used for calculating the mean number of PFC per organ or PFC per million live lymphoid cells. A sample calculation is presented in Table 33.1.

When the main consideration of the experiment is the measurement of the immune response in terms of PFC per organ or million lymphoid cells, the chief source of variation is between the different cell suspensions (animals) and not between samples taken from any one suspension. In this instance we sample 4–10 animals per 'point' but only do duplicate plates. If the main interest is an *in vitro* treatment (say a KI or KD titration as below) using a common pool of lymphoid cells for all the experimental groups, it is necessary to use more plates: the actual number depending on the magnitude of difference which must be detected.

Developing and inhibiting sera

The LHG assay relies on antibody-mediated complement-dependent lysis. Where a single γM molecule on an erythrocyte can fix complement and cause lysis, several thousand γG_2 antibody molecules are required for the same effect, and γG_1 and γA molecules have never been shown to fix complement at all, but an antiserum specific for these immunoglobulin molecules can form γ globulin complexes which do fix complement and cause lysis. Inhibition of γM plaques by anti-γM sera (which may be due to decreased diffusion or to steric hindrance of binding to antigen or complement) will be discussed below.

Developing or inhibiting sera should be diluted with PBS so that 0·1 ml added to the top layer solution results in the desired concentration of serum. The sera should be added to the 2 ml aliquots of top layer in the 46° C waterbath shortly before the assays are carried out.

Production of antisera

Antisera which are intended to react with one class of immunoglobulin must not contain cross-reacting or contaminating antibodies directed against other immunoglobulins because (a) plaques round mouse γM producing cells are strongly inhibited by antisera specific for μ chain or for Fab piece, but are not inhibited by anti-γ or anti-α chain sera; (b) the relative numbers of cells producing different classes of antibody molecules depend on the dose of antigen and time of immunization. 'Specificity' of the developing antisera is therefore essential if valid comparisons are to be made between experiments (unpublished data). This specificity can be obtained by immunizing with pure antigens, by standard absorption procedures, or a combination of both.

Myeloma proteins prepared from serum of mice carrying the tumour or directly from the tumour itself can be prepared by standard methods. Rabbits can be injected twice intramuscularly with 200–1000 μg protein in complete Freunds adjuvant, the first injection into the left thigh, followed 1 week later by the second into the right thigh. After 4–5 weeks the rabbits should be test bled and the sera run on immunoelectrophoresis and immuno-diffusion plates. If necessary the rabbits can be given further injections of antigen, either by twenty to forty simultaneous small subcutaneous injections totalling 200 μg protein in complete Freunds, spread as widely as possible over the body, or by an intraperitoneal injection of 200–500 μg of the protein after alum precipitation. Microsomes prepared from solid myeloma tumours can be successfully substituted for protein, but with the added complication that antisera prepared in this way have always contained a great deal of anti-α globulin.

Anti-allotype sera can also be used as developing sera [24, 26]. Anti-allotype sera can be prepared by the method of Dubiski [7]. We have found that in mice *H. pertussis* is more satisfactory than *B. proteus*. For instance, CBA mice are immunized two or three times at 10–20 day intervals with 2×10^9 pertussis organisms, and they are bled a few weeks later. Pertussis organisms are incubated at 20–22° C with some of the CBA anti-pertussis serum and then centrifuged out of suspension and either (a) washed twice with PBS, or (b) injected without washing. 1–2 $\times 10^9$ of the pertussis organisms coated with CBA immunoglobulin are now injected into C57BL/6 mice (repeated two or three times) which subsequently show anti-γ globulin anti-bodies which react with γ globulin from CBA and a few other strains of mice. With alternative (a) the antiserum will be against Ig-1^a (the locus and allele name) which is on the γG$_{2a}$class of molecules, and alternative (b) would also show antibodies against Ig-3 (on γG$_{2b}$ molecules). The difference is presumably because the γG$_{2b}$ binds to the pertussis organisms less strongly than γG$_{2a}$ and is washed off in procedure (a). A large number of other specificities can be prepared in this way. (See Herzenberg [9] for details of the allotype loci in mice.) Repeated injections of small amounts of myeloma protein in complete Freunds adjuvant into appropriate mice can also lead to the production of antisera with allotypic specificity [19].

Titration of sera: constants
All sera should have their complement destroyed by being heated to 56° C for 30 minutes, and anti-SRBC antibodies should be absorbed out by adding 1/8 volume of packed SRBC, incubating half-hour and then centrifuging; this should be done twice.

The inhibitory effect of sera on mouse γM plaques can be measured by adding serial dilutions of the serum to the top layer, and using spleen cells from mice injected intraperitoneally with 4×10^7 SRBC 2 days before. In CBA mice the great majority of PFC at this time are producing γM antibody, and it can be shown that relatively high concentrations of anti-mouse Fab piece or μ chain will inhibit them (unpublished data). Figure 33.2 shows a typical experiment to measure an inhibition constant (KI). If the experiment is repeated, but using spleen cells taken 9–12 days after immunization, then

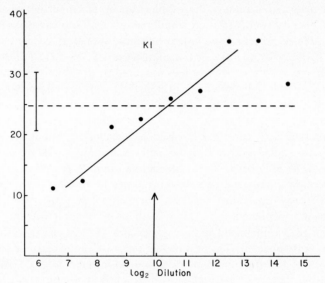

FIG. 33.2. Plot of a KI titration, using spleen cells from CBA males injected i.p. 2 days before with 4×10^7 SRBC. The abscissa is the $\log_2$ concentration of the developing serum in the top layer solution. The ordinate is the mean number of PFC per plate. The dashed line indicates the mean number of PFC on twelve untreated plates, with one standard deviation indicated. The vertical arrow indicates 0·1 per cent serum, the concentration of developing serum it was decided to use in subsequent experiments (see Table 33.1). KI is calculated as follows:

$$KI_{0.1} \text{ per cent} = \frac{\text{Mean PFC with serum}}{\text{Mean PFC without serum}} = \frac{23.0}{24.8} = 0.93.$$

the developing effect on non-γM PFC can be measured after allowance has been made for the inhibitory effect on γM PFC. Figure 33.3 shows a typical experiment from which a development constant (KD) for a given concentration of developing serum can be calculated. Ideally the KI and KD of a developing serum should be 1·0 if the serum does not react with γM and if used at optimal concentration. In view of the way the calculation is carried out, it is better that KI should equal 1·0 even if the KD is large. The basis of the calculation of γM (direct) PFC and, say, γG_1 (developed) PFC per spleen for each animal, is as follows:

'Developed' PFC = [Total PFC on treated plate—KI (PFC on untreated plate)] KD.

Geometric mean PFC/spleen for a group of animals is calculated on the basis of each of the derived numbers.

Variations of the method

As described, the technique is not carried out under sterile conditions. However, this method can be adapted for this purpose although this is appreciably more tedious. The agarose can be simultaneously dissolved and sterilized by autoclaving at 10 lb/sq. in. for 10 minutes.

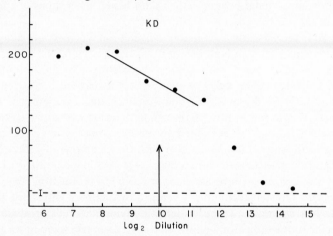

Fig. 33.3. Plot of KD titration, using cells 9 days after immunization. Similar to Fig. 2. KD is calculated as follows:

$$KD_{0 \cdot 1} \text{ per cent} = \frac{\text{Maximum PFC/plate obtained} - (\gamma M \times KI \text{ at that concentration})}{\text{PFC/plate at } 0 \cdot 1 \text{ per cent} - (\gamma M \times KI \text{ at } 0 \cdot 1 \text{ per cent})}$$

$$= \frac{210 - (20 \times 0 \cdot 6)}{162 - (20 \times 0 \cdot 93)} = \frac{198}{143} = 1 \cdot 38.$$

Agarose can be replaced by less expensive agar (Difco Noble Agar) to which has been added 0·5 mg/ml of DEAE-dextran (Pharmacia Ltd). This substitute is more difficult to handle and, in our experience, decreases the number and size of plaques.

In the preparation of bottom and top layers, the concentrated A solutions (PBS and Gey's) can readily be replaced by concentrated salt solutions of standard tissue culture media such as Parker's 199 or Eagle's.

The basic method described here has been evolved to enable us to obtain the maximum daily 'output' with three or four persons. Using machine data processing and graph plotting we can regularly examine twenty to forty mice (spleen cell suspensions) and use from 200–350 plates every day. By reducing the size of experiments it is possible for two persons to carry out LHG experiments using up to 200 plates per day, especially if the help of a third person can be obtained for the short time necessary to complete and add the top layers to the plates.

(Other plaque assays)

Ingraham & Bassard [11] developed a similar LHG assay which used a gum of carboxymethyl cellulose which is prepared by mechanical dispersion of the cellulose in a nutritive medium. Advantages of this method may be that it is possible to carry out microscopic procedures or micromanipulation and, furthermore, being a gum rather than a gel, macrophages and other motile cells may be free to move about.

Two LHG assays using small-scale cultures on microscope slides, both of which may possibly be adaptable for use in autoradiographic and immunofluorescence studies, have been developed recently [23, 26]. Cunningham [5] has developed an LHG assay of great sensitivity carried out with a monolayer of indicator SRBC in a thin chamber on a microscope slide. Plaques due to the lysis of as few as fifty SRBC can be detected microscopically.

Individual PFC can be examined by electron microscopy [10], and the LHG assay can be used in conjunction with the technique of Till & McCullough [25] in which there are colonies (clones) of cells in recolonized irradiated spleens. These colonies can be assayed for antibody production [18, 13, 3].

The 'rosette' (cluster) technique developed by Zaalberg [29] is not an LHG assay, but it is a simple method of detecting lymphoid cells producing antibody specific to the indicator cell, which can be an erythrocyte or an erythrocyte coated with some other antigen. The indicator cells stick to and cluster round those cells releasing the antibody and can be seen microscopically. Zaalberg [30] has compared the LHG and 'rosette' assays.

Non-erythrocyte antigens

Several workers [8, 14, 16] have shown that sheep erythrocytes can be coated with various lipopolysaccharides of bacterial origin and that these coated RBC can be used in the LHG assay as indicator cells to detect cells producing anti-polysaccharide antibodies. Merchant & Hraba [15] have further extended this approach by being able to detect anti-arsenilic acid antibodies, using hapten/sheep RBC as the indicator system in the LHG assay.

In unpublished preliminary experiments we have shown that the LHG assay can be used to detect cells producing anti-protein antibody: (a) Sheep RBC were coated with human or bovine serum albumin (HSA and BSA) by the tanned RBC method [22] (see Chapter 21). The lymphoid cells were prepared from the popliteal lymph nodes of adult CBA male mice injected in the foot pads once with 200 μg of alum-precipitated protein mixed with 2×10^9 pertussis. A polyspecific (anti-mouse 7S globulin) developing serum was used. Table 33.2 presents these results. In other experiments specific anti-BSA plaques were obtained in suspensions of lymphoid cells from popliteal lymph nodes of CBA mice 2 weeks after the last of three injections made at weekly intervals. Each injection consisted of 400 μg alum precipitated BSA plus 1×10^9 pertussis organisms. (b) Similar experiments were carried out with bovine γG globulins (DEAE-cellulose cut) coupled to sheep RBC by means of

TABLE 33.2

Results of a test of specificity of the LHG technique
using protein-coated tanned sheep RBC

Protein used for immunization	Mouse number	Protein coated on sheep RBC Plaque count	
		HSA	BSA
HSA	1	89 156*	0 0
	2	144 251	0 1
BSA	1	0 0	44 46
	2	0 1	20 29

* Number of plaques per 10^6 popliteal lymph node cells as counted on duplicate plates. A developing serum which reacted with all mouse '7S' immunoglobulins was used at optimal concentration on all the plates. The plaques were counted by someone with no knowledge of the experimental protocol.

bis-diazo-benzidine (BDB) [21] (see Chapter 21). Specific anti-protein plaques were detected when CBA male mice were immunized in the foot pads with 200 μg alum precipitated bovine γ globulin plus 1×10^9 pertussis organisms and the popliteal lymph nodes used as a source of lymphoid cells for the LHG assay.

No specific anti-protein plaques were obtained with other lymphoid organs nor with other routes of immunization. In this experiment, as with the anti-BSA experiment, a polyspecific developing serum was used. However, in this case it was found necessary to absorb the developing serum (rabbit anti-mouse 7S γ globulins) with bovine γ globulin (Armour & Co.—BGG). The BGG used for absorption was cross-linked and thereby insolubilized by BDB [2].

We have found that using BDB to couple proteins on to sheep RBC makes them more liable to spontaneous lysis. For this reason it is necessary to use fresh sheep RBC, to carry out the whole coupling procedure and centrifugations at 0° C to keep the prepared RBC in 1 per cent normal rabbit serum (complement destroyed and absorbed with sheep RBC) in veronal saline buffer and to use the prepared RBC in the LHG assay within 18 hours of preparation.

References

[1] ATTARDI G., COHN M., HORIBATA K. & LENNOX E.S. (1959) Symposium on the biology of cells modified by viruses or antigens. II. On the analysis of antibody synthesis at the cellular level. *Bact. Rev.* **23,** 213

[2] BERNIER G.M. & CEBRA J.J. (1965) Frequency distribution of α, γ, κ and λ polypeptide chains in human lymphoid tissues. *J. Immunol.* **95,** 246

[3] CELADA F. & WIGZELL H. (1966) Immune responses in spleen colonies. I. Clonal distribution of haemolytic plaque-forming cells. *Immunology* **10,** 231

[4] COONS A.H. (1958) Fluorescent antibody methods. In *General Cytochemical Methods*, ed. DANIELLI J.F. **1,** 400

[5] CUNNINGHAM A.J. (1965) A method of increased sensitivity for detecting single antibody-forming cells. *Nature Lond.* **207,** 1106

[6] DRESSER D.W. & WORTIS H.H. (1965) Use of an antiglobulin serum to detect cells producing antibody with low haemolytic efficiency. *Nature Lond.* **208,** 859

[7] DUBISKI S. (1958) Studies on antigenicity of immune globulins. I. Immune globulins as iso-antigens and auto-antigens. *Folia biol., Krakow* **6,** 47

[8] HALLIDAY W.J. & WEBB M. (1965) A plaque technique for counting cells which produce antibacterial antibody. *Aust. J. exp. Biol.* **43,** 163

[9] HERZENBERG L.A. (1964) A chromosome region for gamma$_{2a}$ and beta$_{2a}$ globulin H chain isoantigens in the mouse. *Cold Spring Harbour Symposia on Quantitative Biology* **29,** 455

[10] HUMMELER K., HARRIS T.N., TOMASSINI N., HECHTEL M. & FARBER M.B. (1966) Electron microscopic observations on antibody-producing cells in lymph and blood. *J. exp. Med.* **124,** 255

[11] INGRAHAM J.S. & BUSSARD A. (1964) Application of a localized hemolysin reaction for specific detection of individual antibody-forming cells. *J. exp. Med.* **119,** 667

[12] JERNE N.K., NORDIN A.A. & HENRY C. (1963) The agar plaque technique for recognizing antibody producing cells. In *'Cell-bound antibodies'*, p. 109. Philadelphia: Wistar Institute Press.

[13] KENNEDY J.C., SIMINOVITCH L., TILL J.E. & McCULLOCH E.A. (1965) A transplantation assay for mouse cells responsive to antigenic stimulation by sheep erythrocytes. *Proc. Soc. exp. Biol. N.Y.*, **120,** 868

[14] LANDY M., SANDERSON R.P. & JACKSON A.L. (1965) Humoral and cellular aspects of the immune response to the somatic antigen of *Salmonella enteritidis. J. exp. Med.* **122,** 483

[15] MERCHANT B. & HRABA T. (1966) Lymphoid cells producing antibody against simple haptens; detection and enumeration. *Science* **152,** 1378

[16] MÖLLER G. (1965) 19S antibody production against soluble lipo-polysaccharide antigens by individual lymphoid cells *in vitro. Nature Lond.* **207,** 1166

[17] NOSSAL G.J.V. (1962) Cellular genetics of immune responses. *Adv. Immunol.* **2,** 163

[18] PLAYFAIR J.H.L., PAPERMASTER B.W. & COLE L.J. (1965) Focal antibody production by transferred spleen cells in irradiated mice. *Science* **149,** 998

[19] POTTER M., LIEBERMAN R. & DRAY S. (1966) Isoantibodies specific for myeloma γG and γH immunoglobulins of BALB/C mice. *J. mol. Biol.* **16,** 334

[20] QUENOUILLE M.H. (1950) *Introductory Statistics.* Chapter 8. Transformations and non-normal distributions. London: Butterworth-Springer

[21] RANGEL H. & REPKA D. (1965) The use of passive haemolysis in the quantitative estimation of anti-protein antibodies. *Immunology* **8,** 618

[22] STAVITSKY A.B. & ARQUILLA E.R. (1958) Studies of proteins and antibodies by specific hemagglutination and hemolysis of protein-conjugated erythrocytes. *Int. Arch. Allergy* **13,** 1

[23] STERZL J. & RIHA I. (1965) Detection of cells producing 7S antibodies by the plaque technique. *Nature Lond.* **208,** 857

[24] TAYLOR R.B., WORTIS H.H. & DRESSER D.W. (1966) Production of class-specific immunoglobulin and antibody by thymectomized-irradiated mice bearing syngeneic and allogeneic thymus grafts. Chapter 27 in *Society for Developmental Biology Symposium on Lymphocytes in Immunology and Haemophoesis,* ed. YOFFEY J.M.

[25] TILL J.E. & McCULLOCH E.A. (1961) A direct measurement of the radiation sensitivity of normal mouse bone marrow cells. *Radiation Res.* **14,** 213

[26] WEILER E., MELLETZ E.W. & BREUNINGER-PECK E. (1965) Facilitation of immune hemolysis by an interaction between red cell-sensitizing antibody and γ-globulin allotype antibody. *Proc. nat. Acad. Sci. (Wash.)* **54,** 1310

[27] WORTIS H.H., TAYLOR R.B. & DRESSER D.W. (1966) Antibody production studied by means of the LHG assay. I. The splenic response of CBA mice to sheep erythrocytes. *Immunology* **11,** 603

[28] WORTIS H.H., TAYLOR R.B. & DRESSER D.W. (1967) Antibody production studied by means of the LHG assay. II. Assay procedure. *Immunology* (in press)

[29] ZAALBERG O.B. (1964) Simple method for detecting single antibody-forming cells. *Nature Lond.* **202,** 1231

[30] ZAALBERG O.B. (1966) Antibody production by single spleen cells: A comparative study of the cluster and agar-plaque formation. *Nature Lond.* **210,** 544

Solutions for LHG

Dulbecco's PBS

Solution A (conc. × 10)
NaCl 8·09 g
KCl 0·29 g
KH_2PO_4 0·290 g
Na_2HPO_4 1·159 g
Water up to 80 ml

Solution B (*not* concentrated)
$CaCl_2$ 0·19 g
Water up to 100 ml

Solution C (*not* concentrated)
$MgCl_2 \cdot 6H_2O$ 0·19 g
Water up to 100 ml

Sterilize all solutions by autoclaving 10 minutes at 10 lb/sq. in. 80 ml A + 900 ml dist. water + 10 ml B and 10 ml C gives 1 litre PBS

Gey's solution

Solution A (conc. × 10)
NaCl 70·0 g
KCl 3·7 g
$Na_2HPO_4 \cdot 12 H_2O$ 3·01 g
KH_2PO_4 0·237 g
Glucose 10·0 g
Phenol red 0·1 g
Water to 1 litre

Solution B (*not* concentrated)
$MgCl_2 \cdot 6H_2O$ 0·42 g
$MgSO_4 \cdot 7H_2O$ 0·14 g
$CaCl_2$ 0·34 g
Dist. water to 100 ml.

Solution C (*not* concentrated)
$NaHCO_3$ 2·25 g
Dist. water to 100 ml.

Sterilize all solutions by autoclaving 10 minutes at 10 lb/sq. in. 10 ml A + 80 ml dist. water + 5 ml B and 5 ml C gives 100 ml Gey's solution: the pH of this solution can be adjusted by the addition of CO_2 to the bottle.

At a pH of 7·2 the colour should be orange.

Methods for the Study of Allergic Reactions

CHAPTER 34

Notes on Problems Associated with *in vitro* Sensitization and Antigen–Antibody Reactions

W.E.BROCKLEHURST

Hartley showed in 1939 that tissue could become sensitized to a given antigen by the simple process of being soaked in serum containing the appropriate antibody [1]. Dale realized the need to get thorough penetration of the tissue and to maintain it in reasonable physiological condition, and he sought to do this by perfusion, in the cold [2]. The principles of this early work form the basis of present methods of sensitization *in vitro*.

The early workers detected hypersensitivity by an anaphylactic contraction of some smooth muscle such as gut or uterus, that is by the Schultz-Dale reaction. In recent studies, most workers assess the level of sensitization by the amount of a specific biologically active substance, e.g. histamine, set free from the tissue, thus minimizing biological variation by reducing the number of steps between the actual challenge and the observed response. An added advantage is that many non-contractile tissues can be studied without difficulty. Lytic reactions and agglutination phenomena are sometimes used, but their specificity and their relation to allergic reactions must always be in doubt and necessitate supplementary studies. Damage to mast cells in the tissue is not 'all or none', and histamine release occurs in mild antigen–antibody reactions without obvious damage to mast cells.

Tissues which have been employed include chopped or sliced lung, whole gut or uterus from small animals, thin strips of smooth muscle (e.g. gut or uterus), sheets of mesentery, leucocytes. The choice depends very largely upon the purpose of the study, but properties which make tissue satisfactory in use include:

(a) The ability to remain in a substantially normal metabolic condition during long periods in simple physiological media.

(b) The presence of relatively few different types of cell, all freely accessible to large molecules present in the bathing fluid.

(c) The availability of a reasonable amount of the tissue in one animal and the production of a measurable product or change which is quantitatively related to the severity of the antigen–antibody reaction.

When studying the quantity of antibody attached to cell surfaces there are obvious advantages in using uniform intact cells, such as erythrocytes, basophils or small lymphocytes. The difficulty of maintaining the histamine content of basophils suggests that even when no damage is observed the cells may be quite unrepresentative of those *in vivo*. The use of pieces of mesentery similarly permits a reasonable assessment of the surface area of the tissue and avoids errors due to dead or badly damaged tissue. However, there is much mesenteric epithelium with only a small number of cells embedded in it, and one may reasonably assume that much of the antibody taken up is attached to non-reactive sites.

There can be no justification for the use of any tissue which is too thick to receive adequate oxygenation and exchange of nutrition and waste. The limit of acceptable thickness will depend on the experiment, but will usually be less than 1 mm, especially if the tissue is sheathed in intact membranes. In pharmacological experiments using rat diaphragm, better responses are obtained with muscle from 100 g rats (about 0·5 mm thick) than from larger animals, indicating that thicker tissue does not permit adequate diffusion of the nutritional requirements of a moderately active tissue. The innermost cells of thick pieces of tissue will certainly not have physiological integrity and may even be dead, with serious repercussions on adjacent cells.

When tissue is being sensitized by soaking in antibody, even under favourable conditions, there is a delay of at least an hour before the deepest tissue has become exposed to a concentration of γ globulin comparable to that in the bathing fluid. Brocklehurst & Colquhoun [3] found that for chopped lung in rods of nominal dimensions 0·4 × 0·4 mm it took at least 2 hours for the deep antibody concentration to approximate to equilibrium, and about the same time for maximum sensitization to occur, when low concentrations of purified homologous antibody were used.

The difficulties of diffusion are overcome to large measure if the tissue can be perfused, i.e. the sensitizing and challenging substances gaining intimate access to the whole organ via the blood vessels. For qualitative studies this procedure has much to recommend it since the whole organ, or at least a large intact segment of it, is used, and the tissue is never subjected to physical trauma, since the only operative procedure is the insertion of a cannula into the arterial supply. Provided that such an artery is present and can be dissected out, and that the use of an anticoagulant pending the establishment of perfusion is acceptable, perfusion is practicable. The main drawbacks are:

(a) The experiment must be fairly short as the tissue tends to become 'waterlogged' and perfusion is then inadequate or patchy.

(b) It cannot be assumed that *all* the tissue is being adequately perfused or that it is receiving adequate oxygenation (unless blood is used—which is not usually practicable or desirable), indeed it is so often clear that perfusion is uneven in spite of a very high rate of flow of perfusate through the tissue.

(c) Replicates are not possible, and rather large numbers of animals and amounts of substances (e.g. antigen and antibody) will be needed.

(d) Unless the rate of flow through the tissue is greatly diminished or, alternatively, unless the perfusate is recycled, the concentration of any substance released will be low, and the volume of solution to be processed will be large.

The application of perfusion techniques is dealt with in a critical review by Kellaway [4].

The optimum conditions for sensitization of isolated tissue have usually to take second place to the conditions necessary to keep the tissue in good condition.

Isolated rat mast cells must be kept cold and in a solution containing albumin. Even so their useful life *in vitro* is under 2 hours according to Keller [5], who also considers that 'reactivity' should be checked by release of histamine with 'Compound 48/40' from a few cells, at the same time as anaphylactic release of histamine is expected. 48/80 releases histamine by the activation of cellular enzymes in a manner comparable with the antigen–antibody reaction [6].

In contrast, well-washed uterus, gut and lung (sliced or in rods) are surprisingly robust and will remain usable in Tyrode or Krebs solution for 5 or 6 hours at room temperature, or up to 36 hours at $4°$ C with only one or two changes of solution and moderate oxygenation. It is, however, important to keep the tissue in a fairly large volume of solution and to cool it, preferably to about $10°$ C, as early as possible. Human lung keeps satisfactorily for 24 hours either chopped or in whole segments provided it remains cold at all times and is placed in pre-oxygenated solution shortly after excision. Tyrode solution is satisfactory for chopped-tissue experiments, but Krebs solution is better for isolated bronchial muscle. Solutions should be pre-oxygenated by bubbling O_2 containing 5 per cent CO_2 through a sintered glass disk, and if tissue is to be stored without rocking for more than 5 hours a large vessel should be chosen so that there is plenty of space above the solution which can be flushed out with O_2/CO_2 and then closed. If oxygen has to be bubbled through a solution containing tissue for more than a few minutes, it must be saturated with water and the rate of oxygenation kept low to minimize change of pH. Gases may be cleaned and saturated with water by passing them through a column of water as very small bubbles, e.g. via a sintered glass disk. When tissue is in small vessels in shallow pools of solution and gently rocked there is usually no need for oxygenation. The vessels should simply be lightly covered, and the experiment limited to about 3 hours. If practicable the bathing solution should be changed for fresh warm pre-oxygenated solution at intervals of 1 hour.

In sensitizing human tissue, the balance of advantage seems to rest with a long exposure to antibody at a temperature of 10–15° C, standing in an oxygen-rich atmosphere and very gently agitated. It is suggested that in this case minimal amounts of sensitizing antibody are available, and that exchange with antibody already on the tissue will be slow, especially in the face of competition from the other antibody present in the sensitizing antiserum.

The time for antigen to reach and 'challenge' cells below the surface of the piece of tissue must be considerable and will depend on the dimensions of the antigen molecule in solution. With molecules as large as haemocyamin and pneumococcal polysaccharide, challenge may well be so retarded as to result in a greatly diminished reaction. The work of Mongar & Schild [7] shows that for chopped lung it is necessary to strike a balance between having tissue pieces large enough to contain predominantly viable cells—i.e. not lose their histamine stores—and having pieces small enough to permit rapid entry of antigen. These workers found that when antigen had to penetrate more than 0·2 mm into lung tissue there was a diminished reaction.

It follows that the concentration of antigen must influence the rate of the reaction and thus the total response. Too high concentrations are, however, inhibitory [8] and concentrations of 10^{-4} or 10^{-5} g antigen/ml are commonly used for substances of molecular weight less than 100,000. Since an adequate concentration will depend on the number of molecules and the molecular size (which may not be known for all antigens), preliminary trials may be necessary.

It is important to avoid errors due to inhomogeneity of tissue samples. Pieces of tissue taken from two sites only a few inches apart in the same ileum may vary in their responsiveness to histamine, and therefore in their response to otherwise equal anaphylactic reactions. Variations will be minimized by mixing the samples of tissue so that each 'replicate' sample for comparison is composed of many small pieces of tissue taken at random from the total tissue available. If this cannot be done—e.g. where the contraction of larger pieces of tissue forms part of the study—it is necessary to greatly increase the number of tests in order to overcome error due to biological variations. The closest approach to true tissue replicates is achieved by chopping the tissue into uniform slices or rods, which are thoroughly mixed and washed in one lot, then subdivided into equal amounts, each of which contains as many as fifty individual pieces. This method was introduced by Mongar & Schild [7] who used guinea-pig lung. When lungs from larger animals are used, the pleura may be too tough to permit regular chopping and may comprise only a small part of the total tissue although it contains a larger proportion of the histamine. There is plenty of releasable histamine in the parenchmyal tissue of the lung, and if possible this should be cut away from the pleura and from all obvious vessels and bronchioles to exclude these from the test tissue. Human lung is best treated in this way. It must be emphasized that uniformly chopped and sliced tissue is essential if undue scatter in results is to be avoided.

At least three replicates of each test are usually necessary to give a sufficiently reliable result. As there may be a difference in the size of samples (which must be distributed quickly whilst quite moist), it is advisable to assay the total histamine content of each sample and to calculate the amount released by the anaphylactic reaction as a percentage of the total. Total release from small fragments is achieved by boiling the tissue in Tyrode solution (5 ml) for 5 minutes, the sample must then stand in the cold for at least 30 minutes to allow diffusion into the solution. The tube is then shaken to mix thoroughly and allowed to stand for a few minutes for the tissue to settle before assaying the supernatant. Histamine is released in the tissue by the antigen–antibody reaction in the first few minutes after challenge, but continues to diffuse out slowly to reach a maximum in the supernatant solution in about 10 minutes. It is therefore usual to remove the supernatant at 15 or 20 minutes after challenge [9]. Longer periods of incubation result in loss of histamine—presumably by enzymic processes—and are therefore not advisable unless the tissue is rather thick. After removal through a cotton-wool 'brush', the supernatant is at once boiled for 2 or 3 minutes and then stored in ice. After boiling, solutions may be kept frozen ($-15°$ C) for up to a week whilst awaiting assay.

References

[1] HARTLEY P. (1938) Anaphylaxis: Passive sensitization *in vitro. Proc. 3rd Int. Congr. Microbiol.* p, 763

[2] DALE H.H. (1912) The anaphylactic reaction of plain muscle in the guineapig. *J. Pharmac. exp. Therap.* **4,** 167

[3] BROCKLEHURST W.E. & COLQUHOUN D. (1965) Adsorption and diffusion of γ-globulin during passive sensitization of chopped guineapig lung. *J. Physiol.* **181,** 760

[4] KELLAWAY C.H. (1947) The perfusion experiment in the study of tissue injury. *Edinb. med. J.* **54,** 333

[5] KELLER R. (1965) *Mast Cells in Immune Reactions.* Basel: Karger

[6] CHAKRAVARTY N., HOGBERG B. & UVNAS B. (1959) Mechanism of the release by compound 48/80 of histamine and of a lipid-soluble smooth-muscle stimulating principle ('SRS'). *Acta physiol. scand.* **45,** 255

[7] MONGAR J.L. & SCHILD H.O. (1956) Effect of antigen and organic bases on intracellular histamine in guineapig lung. *J. Physiol.* **131,** 207

[8] BROCKLEHURST W.E., HUMPHREY J.H. & PERRY W.L.M. (1961) The *in vitro* uptake of rabbit antibody by chopped guineapig lung and its relationship to anaphylactic sensitization. *Immunology* **4,** 67

[9] AUSTEN K.F. & BROCKLEHURST W.E. (1961) Anaphylaxis in chopped guineapig lung. I. Effect of peptidase substrates and inhibitors. *J. exp. Med.* **113,** 521

CHAPTER 35

Demonstration of Reagins in the Serum of Allergic Subjects

ROSA AUGUSTIN

Introduction

Reagins occur characteristically in the blood and other tissues of hay fever and asthma sufferers and their existence was clearly demonstrated for the first time in 1921 [1], nearly 50 years after Blackley [2] had shown that the skin and mucous membranes of hay fever sufferers react specifically and in a violent manner to the introduction of a small quantity of the offending pollen. Prausnitz & Kuestner [1] demonstrated that the factor responsible for producing the histamine-like skin reactions with the allergen resides in the serum of the afflicted subject and can be transferred to a localized area of normal non-reactive skin by the intradermal injection of a small quantity of the serum of the hay fever sufferer. The injected area then exhibits the specific skin reactivity of the serum donor.

Although the test had been ingeniously devised in a deliberate attempt to produce local anaphylaxis in man by means of serum antibodies of hay fever sufferers, contemporaries remained unconvinced of the antibody nature of the serum transferable activity and named it therefore, non-committally, a 'reagin' [3]. Indeed, the antibody nature of reagins has remained unconvincing in various respects until quite recently; for not only has it consistently proved impossible to sensitize guinea-pigs anaphylactically with reaginic serum [1, 4–7]—unless these sera contained antibodies other than reagins for the allergens [7, 8]—but strict evidence to show that 'reagins had appeared as the result of immunological stimulation' [3] was not forthcoming until quite recently [9–11]. Furthermore, reagins fail to give any of the traditional tests for antibodies (precipitation, agglutination, complement fixation), either because they are intrinsically incapable of doing so or because their concentration in serum is too low to give these tests. In addition, it has proved impossible to isolate reagins by methods established for the isolation of other antibodies; the physico-chemical properties of reagins do, in fact, differ from those of other known antibodies; and not until 1959/1960 were reagins prepared essentially free from serum proteins other than medium-fast 7S γ globulins [12–14]; and it was not until 1960 [16, 17] that reagins

1076

were finally proved to belong after all, at least immunochemically, to the family of immunoglobulins—like other antibodies. This was done by precipitation with rabbit antiserum 'R92', prepared by immunization with what we now call pure γG globulin [15] (eluted from DEAE-cellulose with 0·01 M phosphate at pH 7·4 [12–14]); i.e. on immunoelectrophoresis the eighteen bleedings of this rabbit (immunization over 12 months) never gave more than the one characteristic single γG globulin line against whole human serum [12–14] and had, incidentally, no antibodies specific for γA globulin (although γA was precipitated by cross-reactivity of the light chains common to γG and γA globulins). Since then, much evidence has accrued that appeared to show that reagins belong, in fact, to the subgroup of γA globulins [7, 14, 18–21] although there have also been dissentive voices [22–25]. Currently, this aspect is once more under investigation in this and other laboratories, but need not concern us here. Suffice it to say that most of the published work suffers as yet from lack of quantitation. Often there seems to have been lack of a proper appreciation that the lability of highly dilute protein solutions affects their activity and that losses are incurred during fractionation and sterilization (sometimes by Seitz filtration!) together with the dangers of using an exquisitely sensitive test (like the Prausnitz-Kuestener = PK test) without quantitation in relation to comparatively insensitive (qualitative) analyses for γA by immunoelectrophoresis, etc. [25].

The problem of assaying reagins thus poses great difficulties; for not only are the usual methods for assaying antibodies not applicable and not only is the chemical nature of reaginic antibodies still under investigation, but enough is known to make it certain that the concentration of these antibodies in serum must be very low indeed [24]. That is, not only have special methods to be devised, but these methods must also be exceptionally sensitive. Nevertheless, a number of such tests are beginning to be available now, nearly 50 years after the discovery of the PK test and nearly 100 years after Blackley's discovery of the special skin reactivity of hay fever sufferers for their allergen.

Yet, whatever the chemical nature of reagins, they have certain biological properties which distinguish them from other antibodies and it is these which have been pressed into use for the demonstration of reagins. That is, all tests for reagins have so far involved the use of live tissues, even when done *in vitro*.

The most important biological properties that distinguish reagins from other human antibodies is their high affinity for skin and other human (and primate) tissues and the special nature of this attachment which causes release of histamine and other pharmacologically active substances as a consequence of interaction of the specific antigen with the tissue-fixed antibodies. Indeed, it has been known for a long time that passively sensitized human skin sites may remain reactive for many weeks and dilatation of small blood vessels with extravasation of fluid (oedema in skin and lungs, nasal congestion, lachrymation) and contraction of smooth muscles (bronchial spasms) are well-known features of human asthma and hay fever. In other words, reagins appear to have the properties characteristic of Dale's anaphylactic antibodies [26, 27] and we have called reagins 'anaphylactic antibodies par excellence' [7] because of their exceptionally high affinity for tissues. As long as all animal antibodies were thought to have this special affinity for tissues and thus all to be able to act as anaphylactic antibodies [28], there was much hesitation about accepting reagins as man's anaphylactic antibodies (as opposed to γG antibodies, etc.). The idea that reagins alone of all human antibodies have anaphylactic properties and that these are lacking in other types of human antibodies may become more acceptable now that it is known that not only human but also guinea-pig [29, 30], rat [31] and rabbit antibodies [32, 33] may be divided into anaphylactic and non-anaphylactic antibodies. Antigen-induced release of histamine and other pharmacologically active substances as well as antigen-induced smooth muscle contraction due to interaction with tissue-fixed reagins and the demonstration of tissue fixation itself thus have all become legitimate measures of reaginic activity—always provided correlation with PK tests and clinical history can be demonstrated and provided these reactions are indeed not given by antibodies other than reagins.

Most proponents of new tests for reagins have so far usually been content to demonstrate that the tests are given by reaginic sera although such sera contain many other types of antibodies in addition to reagins. As we have now been concerned for a long time with the separation of reaginic from non-reaginic antibodies [12–14, 7], we have paid special attention to this aspect; and in confirmation and extension of our previous work we have invariably found that only reagins are capable of anaphylactically sensitizing primate tissues while what are now [15] called (human) γG antibodies (at least those failing to be retained on DEAE-cellulose at pH 7·4) cannot do this although they are capable of anaphylactically sensitizing guinea-pig tissues (see later).

Antigen-induced histamine release from human leucocytes and antigen-induced leucocyte damage as a measure of reaginic activity has been under investigation for some 25 years [34–47], but has only quite recently with the evolvement of a highly sensitive fluorimetric test for estimating histamine [48, 49] become acceptable as a test for reagins (not described here). Originally, these tests measured antigen-induced histamine release from leucocytes of allergic subjects, i.e. from *in vivo* sensitized leucocytes [50]; however, the *in vitro* sensitization of normal leucocytes with reaginic serum is also being elaborated and with this the demonstration of *serum* reagins [51]. Similarly, antigen-induced *in vitro* histamine release from human asthmatic lung has been demonstrated some 15 years ago [52] while antigen-induced histamine release from *in vitro* sensitized normal human lung tissue has only quite recently been attempted by us [53, 54] and is here proposed as a further test for reaginic activity. Anaphylactic *in vitro* sensitization of smooth guinea-pig muscle preparations was already achieved by Dale [26] and was subsequently confirmed and extended by Hartley [55], Kulka [56] and Halpern *et al* [57]. Arbesman *et al* [58] found that some reaginic sera are also capable of anaphylactically sensitizing guinea-pig ileum although this has not proved possible in our hands and may have been due to antibodies other than reagins (see later). However, Arbesman *et al* [58] as well as ourselves have been able to sensitize monkey ileum *in vitro* with reaginic sera and subsequent antigen-induced contraction is here described as yet another test for demonstrating reagins in human serum. A further test developed in the author's laboratory uses antigen-induced contraction of reagin-sensitized human bronchi and is also given here. Attempts have also been made to sensitize strips of human appendix and human uterus with reagins [59], but the sensitivity of these tissues turned out to be of a very low order.

Lastly, the so-called DLLA test is described which exploits solely the cytophilic nature of reagins [54] and is not concerned with any further cell-damaging sequence of the anaphylactic reaction such as histamine release.

MATERIALS

Antigens

Pollen extracts
The free-flowing pollen (throughout this work cocksfoot grass pollen—*Dactylis glomerata**—was used) is first quickly extracted with distilled water to remove impurities [60] and then with buffered saline to prepare the antigen solution used in our tests. Ten millilitres distilled water is used per gramme of pollen to make a suspension which is thoroughly shaken for exactly 45 seconds and quickly filtered over a thin pad of supercel (Hyflo-Supercel, Johns Manville Co., California) on a Buchner funnel furnished with a No. 54 Whatman filter paper; the whole operation (from suspending the pollen to obtaining a compact filter cake) must not take more than 1 minute as otherwise too much activity is lost with the impurities in this first extract which is discarded. The pollen filter cake is then suspended in 50 ml of Coca's solution [61], omitting the phenol (5 g NaCl and 2·75 g Na_2HCO_3 per 1000

* Obtained from the Wright-Fleming Pollen Farm, Weybridge, Surrey, through the courtesy of Dr A.W.Frankland of the Wright-Fleming Institute, St Mary's Hospital Medical School, London.

ml distilled water, pH = 8·2), and put for half an hour on a mechanical shaker (for quantities of 1–5 g of pollen a pipette shaker may be used). If necessary, the pH is then readjusted to 8·2–8·5 and the extraction allowed to continue overnight in the coldroom. A second or third shaking period (with pH adjustments) follows. After 48 hours the extract is filtered once more over a filter pad, sterilized by passing through a Swinney filter (Millipore Filter Corp., V.A.Howe & Co. Ltd, London) and stored at 4° C. Extracts thus prepared have been shown [60] to contain at least 100,000 Noon units/ml. Suitable dilutions are prepared in saline or Tyrode, etc., as required for the test in hand.

Thyroglobulin (TG)
Freeze-dried human thyroglobulin was kindly supplied by Dr D. Doniach and Dr I.M.Roitt of the Middlesex Hospital, London.

Horse serum
The sterile serum was purchased from Evans Medical Ltd, Speke, Liverpool.

Egg albumin (Ea)
This was obtained in crystalline form from Armour Pharmaceutical Co. Ltd, Eastbourne.

Aspergillus fumigatus *antigen*
Freeze-dried culture extracts were obtained from Bencard Ltd, Beecham Research Labs, Surrey, and had to be dialysed to removed substances interfering with our tests; these mostly relaxed guinea-pig and monkey ileum. 'Antigens No. 1 and No. 2' as provided by Bencard Ltd, were used for gel diffusion as well as for the anaphylactic tests.

Antibodies

Human sera
Pollen reaginic sera from treated and untreated grass pollen-sensitive highly skin reactive subjects were available as well as sera from normal subjects hyperimmunized with *Dactylis glomerata* [62]. The latter as well as the post-treatment sera contained γG antibodies as demonstrated by the bis-diazotized benzidine (BDB) method [63] (see Chapter 21). All but the sera from the hyperimmunized normal subjects contained reagins for grass pollens.

In addition to these we had at our disposal sera from subjects sensitive to *Aspergillus fumigatus* (containing reagins and/or precipitins for the mould), serum sickness sera (with precipitating as well as reaginic antibodies for horse serum proteins) and Hashimoto sera (with precipitating non-complement-fixing γG antibodies for TG).

Rabbit antisera
These were prepared by multiple depot injections [64] with egg albumin and grass pollen extracts.

Purified antibody preparations
Sera containing γG antibodies as well as reagins were fractionated on DEAE-cellulose with and without preceding salt fractionations to prepare γG antibodies free from reagins and reagins essentially free from γG antibodies. Slight modifications of our previously described methods [12–14] were used.

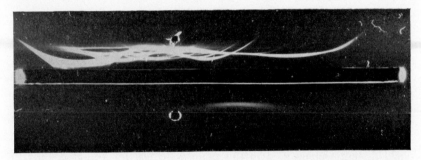

FIG. 35.1. Immunoelectrophoresis of a PK-reactive γA globulin fraction (lower well) isolated from a pollen hay fever serum and of the unfractionated serum (upper well). The central trough contained rabbit antiserum for whole human serum.

Essentially, the γ globulins were precipitated at Na_2SO_4 concentrations of 24 per cent (i.e. at a slightly higher concentration than had previously [14] been found to precipitate practically all the γA globulins). After further purification by salt fractionation this was followed by ion-exchange chromatography. As before, the pH 7·4 eluate (0·01 M Na phosphate) proved to be pure γG globulin ($<0·01$ per cent of γA by immuno-diffusion). After removal of residual γG globulin (at the cost of some γA globulin as well as siderophilin, etc.) essentially γG-free γA globulin (Fig. 35.1) was eluted at pH 6·0 (0·04 M phosphate). All our γG fractions thus prepared, whatever their source, proved to be free from reaginic activity, in confirmation of previous work [7, 12–14] while all the essentially γG-free γA fractions contained the serum reagins.

We had thus at our disposal reagin-free human γG antibodies for thyroglobulin, pollen antigen and horse serum components as well as essentially γG-free reagins for *Dactylis glomerata*, horse serum proteins and *Aspergillus fumigatus*.

Regardless of whether reagins are indeed γA globulins or are contained in our γA fractions as an impurity, these fractionations enabled us to contrast sensitization due to reaginic antibodies with sensitization due to pure γG antibodies.

Table 35.1 summarizes data of representative sera and some of their non-reaginic γG and reaginic γA fractions which have been used in the following tests.

Test subjects

Volunteers for PK tests
All tests reported here were done on one non-allergic subject (R.A.) whose skin tests to pollen extracts (up to 1,000,000 Noon units/ml) were negative and whose serum has always given negative results in passive haemagglutination tests [63] for pollen as well as in PCA tests in monkeys and guinea-pigs; i.e. this subject does not possess any demonstrable reaginic or indeed other types of antibodies for grass pollen antigens. The reaginic sera used in the PK tests were derived from donors personally known to the author and had as far as could be ascertained never suffered from serum jaundice or in any way been in contact with serum jaundice cases.

It should perhaps be added that in view of the risk of serum jaundice we usually do not feel justified in this country to ask for volunteers for PK tests.

Monkeys
Rhesus monkeys were used throughout and were mostly post-malarial subjects (fully recovered from experimental malarial infections) kindly put at our disposal by the staff of the Liverpool School of Tropical Medicine. These monkeys weighed 8–16 lb and proved entirely satisfactory for PCA tests.

Guinea-pigs
Albino guinea-pigs weighing 250–300 g purchased from Tuck & Son Ltd, Rayleigh, were used for PCA tests and also for most of the tests requiring guinea-pig tissues.

Tissues

Human lung and bronchi
Pieces removed during operation (mostly from operations for lung cancer, normal tissues only being selected) were collected directly from the operating

table, and put immediately in excess oxygenated Tyrode (room temperature or lower). The tissue was transferred within the hour to the laboratory where it was worked up either immediately or after storage in the coldroom (4–8° C). Continuous rocking in a large excess of oxygenated Tyrode appeared, if anything, to improve subsequent antibody uptake, probably by washing out residual blood. Lung tissue kept under these conditions could some-times still be satisfactorily sensitized even after 4 days (when antibiotics were added as preservative) and was usually quite satisfactory after 24–48 hours. Pieces containing bronchi were kept in Krebs-Henseleit solution saturated with a mixture of 95 per cent O_2 and 5 per cent CO_2. Tetracyclidine* at a concentration of 0·01 mg/ml was added as a preservative for storage above 24 hours.

Monkey ileum and colon
For preference rhesus monkeys weighing 5–10 lb are chosen. Dying malarial monkeys have proved quite suitable. Just before death the monkeys were anaesthetized, bled out and the organs immediately removed to oxygenated Tyrode. The ileum from Patas monkeys similarly removed through the courtesy of Glaxo Laboratories Ltd (Stoke Poges, Bucks) and transferred by air to Liverpool in an insulated container filled with Tyrode (4° C) was found to be some one hundred times less sensitive.

Guinea-pig lung, trachea and bronchi
After the animals were killed by a blow on the back of the head, ileum, colon and heart-lung-trachea preparations were immediately removed to warm Tyrode (37° C) solutions in which they were dissected and/or cleaned as required. The tissues were mostly used immediately after killing, but could usually still be used after several days in the coldroom (as described for human tissues). To obtain maximally reactive ileum and colon the animals had to be starved for at least 24 hours before killing.

METHODS

A. *In vivo*

I. Cutaneous transfer methods

(a) The PK test in man
For over 40 years the PK transfer test has been the only means of demonstrat-ing and measuring reagins; it remains the basis of comparison for any new

* = Achromycin, kindly donated by Lederle Laboratories, Cyanamid Division, London.

MM*

TABLE 35.1

Some representative sera used in ensuing experiments. PK, BDB and tanned cell titres given as reciprocals of dilution end point. +: positive result. −: negative result. N.D.: not done

Type of serum	Data relevant to serum donor		PK titre	Gel diffusion	γG antibodies			Complement fixation
	Antigen injections	Skin test to antigen			BDB	Tanned cells	mg/Ab/ml	
Pollen reaginic:								
Flah	No	+	1000	−	−	N.D.	N.D.	N.D.
Wes	No	+	300	−	−	N.D.	N.D.	N.D.
Leo	Yes	+	100	−	4,000	N.D.	N.D.	N.D.
Lee	No	+	128	−	−	−	N.D.	N.D.
Gill (normal)	Hyperimmunized to pollen [62]	−	−	+	20,000	N.D.	N.D.	N.D.
Gill γG fraction			−	+	10,000	N.D.	N.D.	N.D.
Gill 'γA' fraction			−	−	256	N.D.	N.D.	N.D.
Aspergillus antisera:								
Taylor	Yes	+	N.D.	+	N.D.	N.D.	0·1	N.D.
Taylor γG fraction			−	+	N.D.	N.D.	N.D.	N.D.
Taylor 'γA' fraction			+	−	N.D.	N.D.	N.D.	N.D.
LA	(Farmer's lung)	−	N.D.	+	N.D.	N.D.	N.D.	N.D.

TABLE 35.1 (*continued*)

| Type of serum | Data relevant to serum donor | | | Gel diffusion | γG antibodies | | | |
	Antigen injections	Skin test to antigen	PK titre		BDB	Tanned cells	mg/Ab/ml	Complement fixation
Hashimoto sera:								
GY	None	N.D.	—	+	400,000	>80,000,000	N.D.	—
GY γG fraction		N.D.	—	+	200,000	N.D.	N.D.	N.D.
GY 'γA' fraction		N.D.	+	—	100	N.D.	N.D.	N.D.
Fish		N.D.	N.D.	+	N.D.	>80,000,000	N.D.	—
Heath		N.D.	N.D.	+	100,000	N.D.	N.D.	256
Serum sickness serum:								
Dodgs.	horse anti-tetanus	+ (urticaria)	N.D.	+	N.D.	N.D.	N.D.	N.D.
Dodgs γG fraction		N.D.	N.D.	+	N.D.	N.D.	N.D.	N.D.
Dodgs 'γA' fraction		N.D.	N.D.	—	N.D.	N.D.	N.D.	N.D.
Rabbit sera:								
Anti-egg albumin	Yes acc. to [64]	N.D.	—	+	N.D.	N.D.	0·5	N.D.
Anti-pollen	Yes	N.D.	—	+	50,000	N.D.	0·1	N.D.

test that may be devised. It is therefore essential to have a proper understanding of all the factors influencing the test and its accuracy. There is the danger of transferring serum jaundice and the inconvenience of having to use man as a test subject, but apart from this the PK test, as such, remains one of the more easily performed as well as one of the most sensitive tests for reagins.

The test is still usually done in the classical manner, i.e. the intradermal injection of the reaginic serum is followed about 24 hours later by an intradermal injection of the corresponding antigen, the allergen responsible for the clinical symptoms of the serum donor. These intradermal injections necessarily produce non-specific wheal and flare injection wheals. Yet while it is possible to wait for the reagin injection wheal to subside before challenging with allergen, the non-specific wheal and flare reaction produced by the intradermal injection of the allergen interferes with the reading 20 minutes later of the ensuing histamine wheal. To overcome this difficulty, various authors have injected the allergen not in the reagin-sensitized site, but some distance away from it. Wherever the antigen was introduced, the ensuing reaction occurred always at the antibody site, i.e. the allergen always travelled to the site where the other reactant, the reagin, appeared to be truly 'fixed'. In particular, the contralateral challenging procedure of Gay & Chant [65] may be mentioned where the reaginic serum is injected in one arm and the allergen solution in the other. This way of challenging requires, however, very concentrated allergen solutions, the reactions take at least 30 minutes to appear and are different from the classical PK reactions. At first white papules are formed taking a crescent shape in another 15 minutes. The complete wheal takes 1 hour to form, has a depression in the centre and persists for 5–24 hours. Payling Wright & Hopkins [66] have done reverse type of PK reactions with horse reaginic sera and obtained much larger reactions than with the direct PK test, but here maximum reaction was not achieved until about 12 hours after challenge although the reactions started within 30 minutes. One wonders what exactly is the relationship of these modified tests to the PK test proper, and with horse serum as the antigen a possibility of mixed PK–Arthus type reactions cannot be excluded since serum sickness type sera (= horse reaginic sera) are known to contain precipitins as well as reagins for horse serum.

However, difficulties of non-specific whealing due to intradermal injections in the direct skin test in allergic subjects have been overcome by pricking through a drop of the allergen extract instead of injecting it [67]. This causes no irritation whatever and Squire [68] has shown that a superficial prick (done so as not to draw blood) introduces the equivalent of an intradermally injected dose of 3×10^{-6} ml. Prick tests have been used in all our work on allergens [69, 70] and as a logical development also for PK tests [14]. Challenging by prick has also been used by Stanworth & Kuhns [71]. Squire [68] has evaluated the accuracy of skin testing by measuring the size of wheals produced by pricking through known concentrations of histamine and found a coefficient of variation for a single direct prick through a solution of histamine to be of the order of 16 per cent. In the hands of Stanworth & Kuhns [71] coefficients of variations of the same order—or only slightly higher (20 per cent, and occasionally 30 per cent) were obtained for wheals > 50 mm^2 and 50 per cent for wheals < 50 mm^2. Stanworth and Kuhns thus used wheal size as a quantitative indicator of potency rather than a dilution end-point type of reaction although the latter is done by most other workers. The accuracy of the dilution end-point method has not been assessed statistically, but seems to be of the same order as the method using wheal size as the indicator (see later). In practice, we have found it convenient to employ a combination of the two methods, i.e. by comparing the wheal sizes of several dilutions which include the dilution end-point.

A further quantitative modification of the PK test is the neutralization method [72]. Here increasing amounts of allergen mixed with constant amounts of reagin are injected intradermally. Above a threshold concentration of antigen and antibody, wheals of increasing size are formed until a concentration ratio of allergen to reagin is reached which is sufficiently large for all the reagin to react and thus to be 'used up'. In practice, this neutralization point is found by challenging the sites with allergen 48 hours after injecting the allergen–reagin mixtures; only sites containing excess ('unreacted') reagin can give a wheal at this time, i.e. only sites up to an antigen concentration insufficient to have neutralized—reacted with—the available reagin; thus, the first site NOT to give a wheal on challenging at 48 hours may be regarded as the neutralization point and may be expressed in terms of the amount of allergen contained in this injection. All subsequent sites— containing still larger amounts of allergen—will of course also fail to react to the 48 hour challenge.

The accuracy of the test must depend on the minimum amount of (residual) reagin capable of giving a PK reaction to the 48 hour challenge and has not been assessed; it may be expected to be of the same order as the amount of reagin reactive in the dilution end-point of the dilution method and the sensitivity of the two methods may be of the same order. The attraction of the test is that it makes it possible to express reaginic potency in absolute terms (of allergen) which may become of great practical value once we have available recognized pure allergen standards. However, we do not know whether this potency would be the same in different test subjects. Also, this is one of the more tedious forms of the PK test and requires a rather larger number of injections than others. Nevertheless, replacement of the intradermal challenge by prick and a quantitative assessment of the method may well prove very much worth while.

Although many statements can be found in the literature regarding the long persistence of reagins in human skin, this must vary with the original concentration of the reagin; no quantitative assessment seems to have been made of this, nor indeed is there much knowledge about the speed of fixation of reagins. There is an early investigation by Loveless [73] who found that after a blood transfusion with reaginic serum, reagins disappeared from the blood-stream of the normal recipient in less than 24 hours while cutaneous sensitivity could be discovered $1\frac{1}{4}$ hours after transfusion, conjunctival and nasal responses appearing somewhat later and disappearing earlier than the cutaneous responses. Skin sensitization was at a maximum from 1–5 days and stayed at this level for 24 days. However, these conditions are not exactly comparable with what happens following an intradermal introduction of reagin. Stanworth & Kuhns [71] claim to have obtained some indication that maximal sensitization may not occur until 50 hours after the injection of the reagins, but they also state that time intervals (2–168 hours) between transfer and challenge have, on the whole, little effect on wheal size.

As all these factors influence the PK test, attempts have been made by us to find out more about the rate of fixation of reagin, the permissible distance between PK sites and the effect of excess allergen or excess reagin at any site on the reactions at neighbouring PK sites. In addition, the half-life of persistence of reagins in skin has been determined. The quantitative conclusions reached by Stanworth & Kuhns [71] have been largely confirmed.

Procedure

Reasonably unblemished skin sites are selected, preferably on the back of a non-allergic subject although upper arms and thighs also offer sufficiently large areas for many tests under similar conditions. The future injection sites are lightly marked with a ballpoint pen. They are spaced at least 3–4 cm apart and the same distance is maintained between consecutive rows of tests. Parallel rows of sites are arranged so that each site is placed midway between two sites in the rows above and below. 0·05 ml amounts of the sterile reaginic serum (or a dilution of it) are then injected intradermally in the indicated positions, using for preference a disposable 1 ml tuberculin syringe (available in sterile packs ready supplied with 28 gauge needles: 'Plastipak', Becton, Dickinson & Co. Ltd., Drogheda, Ireland). Care is taken to inject as far as possible always to the same depth of skin. The resulting injection wheals are then carefully outlined with a black or blue 'Platignum' felt pen or otherwise marked so as not to rub off easily. Twenty-four hours later—or as soon after this as all non-specific irritation due to the injection has completely subsided—the sites are challenged by pricking the epidermis through a drop of the allergen solution centrally placed over the outlined injection wheal. The pricking must never be deep enough to draw blood and may be done in a variety of ways. Haagedorn, syringe, and even sewing needles are all suitable, provided the pricking is always done in the same manner. After 10–15 seconds the allergen solution is gently wiped off with soft absorbent tissue or cotton wool. At a reactive site itching usually starts within 3 minutes of challenging, whealing begins soon afterwards and reaches a maximum at about 20 minutes when itching has ceased.* The reaction wheals are outlined with a ballpoint or felt pen and a suitable piece of 'Sellotape' stuck over them; on pulling it off, the injection wheals as well as the reaction wheals will be found outlined on the 'Sellotape' (and are therefore best drawn in contrasting colours) which are then stuck on graph paper. This gives a permanent record and makes it easy to count the outlined square millimetres of the reaction area.

As controls, prick tests are made through a drop of the allergen solution on unsensitized skin and through a drop of physiological saline on sensitized skin. Both must be entirely negative. In addition, histamine prick tests may be done to test possible variability of skin reactivity at different sites.

Whenever possible, reagin solutions of low protein content are used in the tests. The higher the protein content, the more non-specific reactions occur and the longer it takes for them to subside. High molecular weight proteins, e.g. α_2M and γM globulins, are particularly obnoxious in this respect. It is absolutely essential to wait until the injected skin is once more completely smooth and even, before challenging. Reagin solutions may be sterilized by filtration through Swinney filters (Millipore (U.K.) Ltd, London) and dilutions are made in physiological saline (0·15 M NaCl) or phosphate–saline buffer (0·01 M phosphate pH 7·5). All high dilutions are made just before testing since low-protein reagin solutions deteriorate on storage. Deterioration may be reduced by adding serum albumin or normal serum [14, 71].

Influence of site of reagin injection on wheal size
Skin reactivity to histamine—and thus direct skin tests in allergic subjects as well as PK tests (in normal subjects)—vary with the site of injection. It is well known that size of wheal formation decreases as the forearm is descended and when passing from the ulnar to the radial side [74]. Parallel conditions apply to the thighs. There is usually much less variability—if any—at the back [71] and some subjects show very little variability on the upper parts of the forearms and even less on the frontal parts of the thighs.

Do reagins spread outside the outlined injection areas?
A normal skin site was sensitized with a 1/50 dilution of a pollen reaginic

* The reaction wheals can be seen best by pressing a glass slide over them. This can be particularly important when judging dilution end-points.

serum (Wes) of dilution end-point 1/300. Twenty-four hours later the site was challenged by migration, i.e. by pricking in the allergen at a distance of 1 cm from the periphery of the reagin site. Within 10–15 minutes a very small wheal formed at the allergen site—i.e. some reagin had indeed spread 1 cm away from the periphery. The wheal increased a little in size up to 15 minutes and by 20–25 minutes a very small wheal also formed in the centre of the reagin-injected area. We may conclude that a small quantity of reagin had moved 1 cm outwards from the injected area, possibly before 'fixation' could occur and that this was the reagin which after fixation outside the original injection area produced the first small wheal, 1 cm from the periphery of the reagin site. The second (central) wheal may have been caused by excess allergen moving to the site of highest reagin concentration; the remaining area presumably did not contain sufficient reagin to produce even a threshold reaction.

To test this theory further, another reagin site was challenged by pricking with allergen in many places at 1 cm distant from the periphery. Within 15 minutes an erythema formed around the reagin site together with a little whealing here and there within the 1 cm ring around the reagin site (Fig. 35.2). Simultaneously, a big wheal formed at 15 minutes at that side of the reagin injection site into which the needle of the reagin-filled syringe had pointed towards during the injection, i.e. presumably at the site of the highest reagin concentration. Within another 10 minutes four big wheals spreading from the outside to the centre of the reagin site filled the reagin site while another similar reagin site, injected centrally with but one-twentieth of the total amount used around the periphery of the first reagin site, produced within 15 minutes a large wheal spreading similarly, but evenly outside the reagin area. A further two sites, sensitized with one-tenth of the amount of reagin used to sensitize the first two sites, produced on challenge a small central wheal which failed to fill the sensitized area—i.e. a wheal was once more only produced at the site of the highest reagin concentration. The fourth site was challenged as before by migration at a distance of 1 cm from the periphery of the original reagin injection area; this once more produced first a small wheal at the allergen injection site which soon disappeared and was followed by another small wheal just inside the outlined reagin injection area.

The reagin site challenged by multiple peripheral pricking at a distance of 1 cm (1 hour after challenge), eventually produced a large, uneven and diffuse wheal, with the swelling persisting for longer than 5 hours and still present to a slight extent next morning. Direct central pricking of a similar reagin site produced a much more transient wheal and the reaction had subsided in less than 1 hour. Presumably, the more intense migratory reaction may have been caused by a much larger than usual amount of allergen gradually reaching the reagin site. At no time was there again any whealing in the peripheral 1 cm ring produced by the allergen pricking around the reagin area, i.e. any reagin 'fixed' after spreading outside the original reagin injection area must have been 'silently' discharged by the allergen diffusing in. By implication, only very little reagin can have spread to this outer ring and 'silent' discharge appears to occur mainly where there is not quite enough reagin to give a visible reaction.

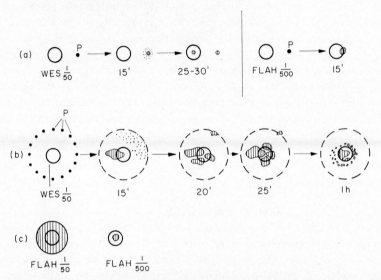

FIG. 35.2. Fixation of reagin and relative movements of reagin and allergen in human skin. Tracings of reagin injection wheals are indicated by solid lines and the prick sites of the allergen (P) by heavy dots. Wheals forming after challenge (challenging 24 hours after sensitization with reagin) at the indicated times (minutes after challenging) are drawn as solid black areas and erythema is indicated by faint stippling. A: challenge by a single prick 1 cm distant from the periphery of the reagin site. B: challenge by multiple pricking all around the reagin injection site at a distance of 1 cm from the periphery. C: direct central challenge by single prick (routine method). The challenging solution (*Dactylis glomerata*) contained 500,000 Noon units/ml and the reaginic serum was diluted 50-fold.

That 'silent' neutralization of reagin-sensitized sites is possible has already been shown by Spies *et al* [75] who found that it can be produced by allergen migration from a distance of 5 cm by sixteen to one hundred times the amount of allergen that would neutralize when injected centrally into the reagin site. As much as a thousand times the normal amount of allergen was required to produce the usual wheal reaction when the allergen was injected at a distance of 5 cm instead of centrally, while in the above experiments only about twenty times as much was required when injected at a distance of 1 cm. These figures can be seen to be of a comparable order when it is considered that the injected allergen presumably spreads roughly in a hemisphere or circle, with the allergen injection site as the centre; i.e. the amounts of allergen reaching the reagin site at a given time will vary with the square of the radius. This would necessitate a 500-fold dose (not too different from the 1000-fold dose found by Spies *et al*) at a distance of 5 cm instead of the 20-fold dose found by us at a distance of 1 cm. The smaller amount required by us may, in part, be due to our using multiple divided doses strategically placed, rather than the single dose placed to one side of the reagin site by Spies *et al* [75].

In conclusion, reagin does not appear to move far or in large amounts from the actual injection sites—another proof of very quick 'fixation'. This contrasts greatly with the very fast spread of the allergen. This statement in no way contradicts Stanworth & Kuhns [71] who found—as indeed is also shown here—that there is a gradient from the centre of injection and that a slight spread of reagin outside the reagin injection wheal can be demonstrated. We find that antigen-induced histamine whealing outside the original injection wheal only occurs above a certain reagin concentration—as if only a limited amount of reagin could be fixed in a given area, the rest 'fixing' in immediately adjacent areas.

Minimum distance permissible between adjacent PK sites
Adjacent PK reactions may interfere with each other (a) quasimechanically by confluence of excessively large histamine wheals at sites containing excessively large amounts of reagin; i.e. where, for instance, only some of the injected reagin could be contained and 'fixed' within the actual injection sites (as shown in the previous experiment); in other words, there is a danger that individual reagin sites are much larger than can be judged from the actual injection areas. (b) Interference may also be possible by excess allergen migrating out from low-reagin sites where only a small part may become neutralized and 'fixed' by the reagin. This can be seen to be a lesser evil than excess reagin at a site, when it is considered that even if all the injected allergen were capable of spreading almost instantaneously (contralateral challenging has been shown [65] to induce wheal formation in reagin sites within 30 minutes), the allergen will necessarily be distributed over an ever-increasing area; i.e. at 1 cm distance $\frac{1}{2r^2\pi}$ or 1/600 of the original amount will reach each square-millimetre—and 1/600 of the usual allergen challenge (of 3 Noon units) has already been shown to have very little whealing effect at a distance of 1 cm. However, a danger of 'silent' discharge remains and was put to the test as set out in Fig. 35.3.

A minimal reactive dose of reagin (reaginic serum Flah, 1/500) was injected in one site and ten times as high doses at distances of 1 and 2 cm from it, followed by two further doses of 1/50 dilutions of Flah at 2 cm distances. The minimal reactive dose was challenged first, 24 hours after sensitization. This caused, as expected, a very small reaction, yet nevertheless no allergen appeared to reach the 1/50 sites; at least, there was no visible reaction at either adjacent site; i.e. some allergen was obviously used up at site 2, since the same amount of allergen placed similarly in a non-sensitized site at 1 cm from the reagin site did produce a reaction (Fig. 35.2). Thirty minutes later site 4 was pricked with allergen (Fig. 35.3). This caused the expected wheal formation in site 4, but was without effect on either sites 3 or 5 at 10 minutes, with possibly some very slight effect at site 5 at 20 minutes after challenge. Two and a half hours later, site 4 still exhibited some slight swelling. At this time site 2 was challenged a second time, producing once more a very slight reaction—with once more a chance of excess of allergen spreading to sites 1 and 3. However, there was again no visible reaction or itching at either sites 1 or 3 and sites 1 and 5 were challenged; both the latter

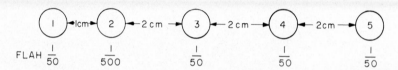

FIG. 35.3. Schematic representation of placing of reagin injection wheals in relation to the challenging (prick) sites to find the minimum distance permissible between PK wheals. Sites were sensitized throughout with Flah 1/50 except in site 2 (sensitized with Flah 1/500) and challenged by prick as indicated in the text. Reagin injection wheals outlined by solid lines and prick sites given as heavy dots as in Fig. 35.2.

sites reacted maximally, i.e. had not been visibly affected by the allergen injections in either sites 2 or 4. At this stage the last available site, 3, was challenged and reacted strongly, although certainly not maximally; i.e. this site may have been affected by the earlier challenge and/or reaction at site 4. We may conclude that a 2 cm distance between PK sites is insufficient.

This possibility was tested in a further experiment (Fig. 35.4) which was set out to test the effect of challenges 1, 2, 3 and 4 cm distant from reaginic sites. Site 8 (Fig. 35.4) was pricked with allergen once and sites 7, 9 and 10 three times in quick succession, all of them 24 hours after sensitization of sites 6, 7A, 8, 9A and 10A with reagin (1/50 dilution of 'Flah'). Ten minutes after challenging, site 8 reacted strongly, as expected, with a maximum reaction at 20 minutes. There was a tiny reaction at site 10A—confirming once more that there is some effect at a distance of 1 cm, with no visible reactions at sites 7A or 9A (distances of 2 and 3 cm). Forty-five minutes later sites 6, 7A, 9A and 10A were challenged; all reacted maximally, i.e. once more, there had not been any noticeable 'silent' discharge.

We may conclude that PK sites producing, on challenge, wheal areas of about 1 cm^2 may safely be situated within 3–4 cm of each other, but that 2 cm is too small a distance.

Rate of fixation of reagin

Reagin sites (1/50 dilutions of 'Flah') were spaced 4 cm apart from each other. Three sites were challenged centrally, 2, 5 and 24 hours after sensitization and another three sites after the same time-intervals, by migration from

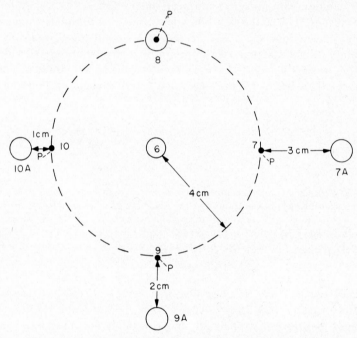

FIG. 35.4. Schematic representation of a further series of reagin injection wheals and their challenging sites. Sensitization throughout with Flah 1/50. Conventions as in Fig. 35.3.

1 cm outside the injection wheal periphery. At this relatively high serum dilution, the non-specific injection wheals had completely subsided 2 hours after the injection.

The central allergen pricks produced, 2 hours after sensitization, a large ill-defined, not very compact wheal which spread well outside the original sensitization area and continued to grow quickly for 30 minutes and even after that. A large swelling persisted well over 4 hours. The impression was gained that the reagin was not properly 'fixed' and continued to spread over an ever-increasing area, only gradually 'fixing' and thus producing a long-drawn-out, ill-defined reaction. This impression was borne out by the fact that no reaction whatever was produced by the 1 cm distant 2 hour challenge, presumably because too little reagin was 'fixed' either centrally or at the 1 cm distant site to be affected from a distance of 1 cm or at the 1 cm distant site itself to give a reaction there.

At 5 hours the central prick produced a compact, well-defined wheal reaching its maximum at 20 minutes, in every way very much resembling a routine 24 hour reaction. However, the 1 cm 5 hour reaction was very different from the corresponding 24 hour 1 cm distant reaction; there was much itching and a transient big wheal formed at the allergen injection site with ensuing double wheal formation which covered both the allergen and reagin sites. The wheals subsided in less than 30 minutes. The 5 hour 1 cm distant reaction thus indicated that there was, at that time, quite a lot of presumably 'unfixed' or 'lightly fixed' reagin 1 cm distant from the reagin injection area. This reactive reagin must have arrived there in the period between the 2 and 5 hour challenges.

The 24 hour central challenge produced the routine compact raised wheal reaching a maximum at 20 minutes and exhibiting a large erythema. The 1 cm distant challenge produced a very small, transient, wheal at the allergen injection site—i.e. by 24 hours little reagin was available outside the actual reagin injection site.

We may conclude that the fixation of reaginic antibodies—like that of other anaphylactic antibodies—requires time although some of the injected reagin is indeed probably fixed almost immediately. Yet some of the injected reagin appears to get away from the injected site before it can become fixed— and reacts well outside the actual reagin injection area 2 hours after sensitization. Proportionately more reagin can be expected to escape when higher concentrations of reagin are injected and this may be one reason for the flattening out of the dose-response curves at the higher reagin concentrations (see later).

Half-life of persistence of reagins in human skin
Several rows of doubling dilutions of a reaginic serum of dilution end-point 1/128 were injected intradermally. At suitable time intervals the dilution end-points were determined by challenging sets of dilutions with allergen (prick method, 100,000 Noon units/ml). As the period between sensitization and challenge increased, fewer and fewer sites reacted until, finally, even the sites injected with undiluted serum no longer gave a response. The experiment lasted for 90 days and during this long period great care had to be taken to preserve the markings, which had to be retraced at frequent intervals.

In Fig. 35.5 reciprocals of dilution end-points have been plotted against time (in days) elapsed since sensitization by the intradermal injections of reagin. An exponential-type curve was obtained from which it can already be seen that it always took about 15 days for the activity to drop to half its value.

In Fig. 35.6 the logs of the dilution end-points have been plotted against

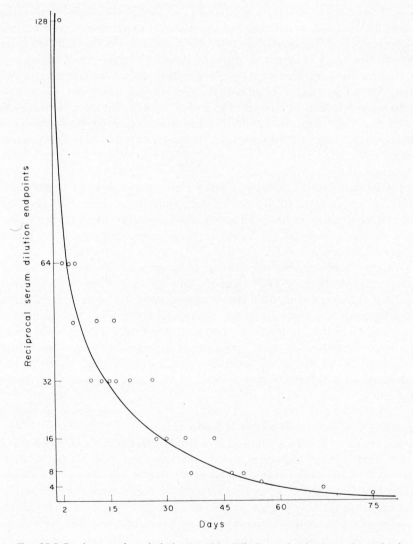

FIG. 35.5. Persistence of reagin in human skin. Dilution end-points were determined at varying times after sensitization with reaginic serum Lee. Plots of reciprocals of dilution end-points against time intervals between sensitization and challenge (in days),

time elapsed since the reagin injection; a straight-line relationship was obtained from which the half-life of persistence of reagins in human skin could be calculated with the help of the general equation:

$$n_1 = n_0 e^{-\lambda t} \tag{1}$$

where n_1 = the number of molecules persisting at a given site after time t since sensitization. n_0 = original number of molecules at the site and λ = what is usually called the decay constant and refers here to the disappearance

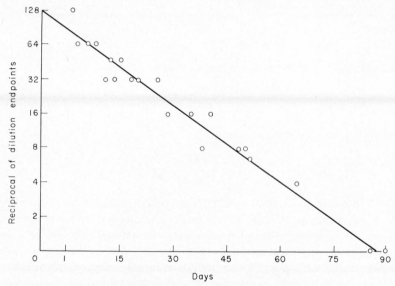

FIG. 35.6. Persistence of reagin in human skin. Logs of reciprocals of dilution end-points plotted against time elapsed between sensitization and challenge.

of reagin molecules from a given site. For two sites injected with different amounts of reagin $(n_1)_0$ and $(n_2)_0$, dilution end-points (which, by definition must contain identical numbers of reagin molecules, i.e. $n_1 = n_2$) will be reached at different times t_1 and t_2.

$$\ln \frac{n_1}{(n_1)_0} = -\lambda t_1 \tag{2}$$

$$\ln \frac{n_2}{(n_2)_0} = -\lambda t_2 \tag{3}$$

Hence
$$n \frac{(n_1)_0}{n_1} - \ln \frac{(n_2)_0}{n_2} = \lambda (t_1 - t_2) \tag{4}$$

At dilution end-point, $n_1 = n_2$, thus

$$\ln \frac{(n_1)_0}{(n_2)_0} = \lambda (t_1 - t_2) \tag{5}$$

From Fig. 35.6, reciprocal dilution end-points dropped from 32 to 2 between 74 and 21 days, thus

$$2\cdot 3 \times \log_{10} \frac{32}{2} = \lambda (74\text{–}21)$$

hence

$$\lambda = \frac{2\cdot 3 \times \log_{10} 16}{53} \tag{6}$$

From (1) $\dfrac{n_0}{n_1} = 2$ at the half-life period τ, and therefore

$$\tau = \frac{\ln 2}{\lambda} \tag{7}$$

Substituting for λ from (6) we obtain

$$\tau = \frac{\ln 2 \times 53}{2\cdot 3 \times \log_{10} 16} = 13\cdot 3$$

The half-life of persistence of reagins in human skin is thus of the order of 13 days. Although this figure may be expected to vary to some extent in different subjects, this order of persistence of an antibody protein at a skin site is certainly quite exceptionally high. In the absence of any absolute measure of reaginic activity, Kuhns [76] some time ago ingeniously sought to determine the half-life of persistence of what he thought to be reaginic anti-diphtheria toxin, from the neutralization of a given quantity of toxin. Although it has since been shown that the allergen responsible for the immediate-type skin reactions to diphtheria toxoid in sensitized atopic subjects is not due to the toxin itself, but to a contaminant [77], Kuhns's experiments remain important and can be used to deduce the half-life of persistence of non-reaginic human γG antibodies which can be calculated to be 12 hours. This compares with 8 hours for rabbit antibodies in guinea-pig skin [78].

The half-life of persistence of about 13 days deduced here for reagins is, on the whole, in agreement with experiments of Stanworth & Kuhns [71] who could find no significant reduction in response on testing for 7 days the persistence of reaginic activity in the serum of a subject sensitive to horse dander which was injected at a dilution of 1/1·5 and had a dilution end-point of about 50–100; and, indeed, with a half-life of about 13 days and a coefficient of variation of the PK test of around 20 per cent, a reduction of activity by about 25 per cent in 7 days would not be recognized as significant.

Quantitative considerations

Figure 35.7 gives a log (dose)-response curve, where the logarithms of serum dilutions are plotted against the wheal responses in square millimetres. Two curves are shown, one composed of area readings obtained 12 minutes after challenging and the other taken after the usual 20 minutes. The 12 minute curve is considerably lower, but parallel to, the 20 minutes' curve and

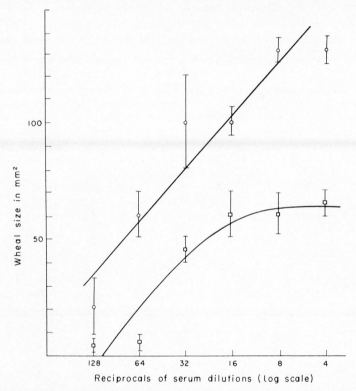

Fig. 35.7. Dose-response relationship in PK testing. Lower curve: readings taken 12 minutes after challenge. Upper curve: readings taken 20 minutes after challenge (when wheals were fully developed).

flattens out sooner, due to the wheals not being fully developed 12 minutes after challenge. In confirmation of Stanworth & Kuhns [71], wheals read 20 minutes after challenge gave a roughly straight line relationship up to a wheal area of about 120 mm². Above this size, the response curve flattens out, as shown by our experiments described earlier, presumably because the maximum amount of reagin that can be held in that area has been exceeded and has, in part, diffused away. Again in confirmation of Stanworth & Kuhns [71], coefficients of variation were found to be of the order of 10–30 per cent

Allergic Reactions

for wheal sizes $> 50 < 100$ mm^2 and it can be seen that, in this range of wheal sizes, a tenfold increase in dose produces but a twofold increase in response. There is a fourfold increase in wheal size for a tenfold increase in dose over the lower wheal area range (20–80 mm^2), but here the error of estimation is higher, i.e. frequently coefficients of variations as high as 50 per cent have been found by statistical analysis [71].

The latter high coefficient of variation obviously applies also to the dilution end-point. However, as here also a steeper dose/response relationship applies, the accuracy of the dilution method may be of the same order as

TABLE 35.2

Dilution end-point method. Limiting wheal: +, 1–3 mm diameter; wheals of increasing size indicated by increasing numbers of + signs; ± trace wheal; ± ? no wheal, but slight erythema and itching. Results of doubling dilutions and closer tests on Flah and Wes. Wheals elicited 24 hours after sensitization; challenging solution 500,000 Noon units/ml. N.D. = not done.

Serum	Serum dilutions							
	1/100	1/200	1/400	1/800	1/1600	1/800	1/1000	1/1300
Flah	+ + + +	+ + +	+	+	±	+	+	—
	+ + + +	+ + +	+	+	—	+	±	±
	+ + + +	+ + +	+	+	±	+	+	±
	+ + + +	+ + +	+	+	—	+	+	—
	+ + + +	+ + +	+	+	—	+	+	—
						1/200	1/300	1/400
Wes	+ + +	+	± ?	—	N.D.	+	+	±
	+ + +	+	±	—	N.D.	+	+	+
	+ + +	+	—	—	N.D.	+	±	—
	+ +	+	+	—	N.D.	+	+	—
	+ + +	+	—	—	N.D.	N.D.	N.D.	N.D.

that of the wheal area method. In practice, coefficients of variation of the order of 30 per cent were obtained. In other words, doubling dilutions are always clearly distinguished from each other by the dilution end-point method (as also borne out by incidental figures given by Stanworth and Kuhns) and it is generally possible to distinguish dilutions differing by 30 per cent (Table 35.2). Below this percentage difference, dilution end-points become less and less distinguishable from each other.

As already pointed out, we generally attempt to inject a small range of dilutions covering areas from 50–100 mm^2 which is made to include the dilution end-point.

In conclusion, reagins are shown to possess for human skin, to an exceptionally high degree, the most fundamental characteristic of anaphylactic antibodies, namely, affinity for tissue, in such a way that histamine (and other substances) is specifically released on interaction with the corresponding antigen. Despite the low concentration of reagins, this fixation is shown to start immediately on injection, to be complete within a few hours and to have the extraordinarily long half-life of persistence of 13 days. Combination of this with the fact that human skin is a particularly sensitive indicator of histamine, gives the PK test its great sensitivity. It is also confirmed that the PK test is a reasonably accurate biological test (coefficient of variation 20–30 per cent). The test is easily performed and when challenging by prick instead of by intradermal injection, controls are invariably negative. All this, together with its insensitivity in respect to variations in time of challenge, must surely make it an almost ideal biological test—if it were not for the risks involved in using man himself as the experimental animal.

(b) PCA in monkeys

It has been known for some time that a type of PK reaction can also be produced by reaginic sera in monkeys. Caulfield *et al* [79] and Strauss [80] obtained whealing of reagin-sensitized sites following intravenously injected antigen and Walzer *et al* [81] succeeded in sensitizing with reagins rhesus monkey intestine and other abdominal organs. Unfortunately, PK wheals produced in the monkey are rather flat and diffuse and lack the surrounding erythema that is produced in man; i.e. the monkey PK test is an altogether much less well-defined reaction than in man and high concentrations of reagin and allergen are required to produce it. It was therefore a finding of great importance when Layton *et al* [82, 83] showed that a PCA reaction could be produced in monkeys with the sera of allergic subjects in exactly the same manner as PCA is produced in guinea-pigs with rabbit antisera [84], i.e. by challenging intradermally sensitized sites with intravenously injected antigen plus dye. Well-defined blue areas appear indicating the sites of antigen-induced extravasation of fluid due to interaction with tissue-fixed antibody (see Brocklehurst, Chapter 22). There was, however, the possibility that the reactions were produced by antibodies other than reagins in the allergic sera, particularly as non-reaginic antibodies do occur in allergic sera in addition to the reagins and reagins have consistently been shown not to give PCA reactions in guinea-pigs [1, 4–6] although they are given by non-reaginic human γG antibodies. However, Augustin *et al* [7, 110] found that reagin-free pure human γG precipitins for horse serum gave negative PCA reactions in monkeys, while the reaginic γA fractions isolated from the same serum, as well as from pollen-reaginic sera, were positive. Similar results have since been obtained by Buckley & Metzgar [85] with the reaginic γA fractions of ragweed reaginic serum, i.e. PCA reactions in monkeys may indeed be regarded as a true equivalent of the PK reactions in man.

Procedure

Apart from a few minor alterations the technique of Layton *et al* [86] was employed.

Five to nine pound rhesus monkeys were injected with 'Sernylan' (Parke, Davis & Co., Hounslow, Middlesex) rather than with nembutal. Intramuscular injections of 4 mg usually tranquillized satisfactorily a 7–9 lb monkey within 10–20 minutes. Under these conditions, the eyes remain open while the animal can be handled with ease for the next hour or so. Also, there is no need to gag or strap it as was found necessary by Layton and colleagues [82]. A second injection can be given if necessary. Usually, the abdomen only is used, but tests can also be done satisfactorily on the back, thighs, arms, neck and cheeks. Where necessary, hair is removed by means of electric clippers. Intradermal injections (disposable tuberculin syringes furnished with 28 gauge needles) of 0·1 ml serum, or dilutions of it, are then positioned according to a premarked grid (outlined in red indelible dye) and the ensuing raised injection blebs are marked similarly. Twenty-four hours later the femoral vein is used for injecting the dye plus antigen. We generally use 'Coomassie blue' (Medical, ICI Ltd, Cheshire), a dye specifically developed for use in human heart disease because of its very low toxicity and quick excretion—a particularly important consideration for us as the monkeys had to be used later for other experiments. In man the half-life of persistence of 'Coomassie blue' in plasma was found to be 15–30 minutes [87] and appears to be similar in monkeys; at least, blue-coloured urine was at times excreted 10 minutes after an intravenous injection. The dye is supplied in sterile ampoules (2 per cent w/v) and we usually injected 3–5 ml. This amount does not tint the skin while giving well-defined, strongly blue spots after challenge with antigen. The exact amount of dye to be injected is readily and accurately judged by watching for the first blue hue tinting gums and tongue of the monkey. This can usually readily be seen, as the animals tend to yawn a lot due to 'Sernylan'. As soon as a blue tint appears, the injection of dye is stopped, leaving the syringe *in situ*. The skin is then quickly examined and a note made of any non-specific blueing due to trauma or scratching, etc. Leaving the needle *in situ*, the dye-filled syringe is replaced 5 minutes later by the antigen-filled syringe and the antigen solution injected. For challenging grass pollen reaginic sites, we usually injected 1–5 ml of concentrated pollen extract (1,000,000 Noon units/ml, prepared by adding freeze-dried purified pollen protein to the usual 100,000 Noon units/ml extracts). To locate serum sickness reagins, as much as 5 ml of horse serum may be injected and for milk antibodies up to 5 ml of cow's milk. It is possible to challenge with more than one antigen when it may be convenient to allow a short interval between injections to record the first set of results before producing the second set (reaginic sera often contain reagins to a number of substances).

All the intravenous injections are done very slowly and stopped at the first indication of specific blueing. This occurs within 3–5 minutes after starting the antigen injections.

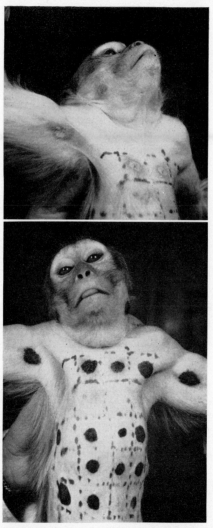

FIG. 35.8. PCA testing in rhesus monkey. Upper photograph taken 3 minutes after challenging—reaction areas can be seen to develop from the periphery. Lower photograph: fully developed reaction sites.

Allergic Reactions

As many as fifty and more tests can be done on the abdomen of a single animal with the help of the painted-on grid system. The slight blueish, somewhat patchy, natural skin coloration of many rhesus monkeys can be safely ignored, since it is never confused with the well-defined blue antigen–antibody reaction spots. The reactions are fully developed 10–15 minutes after challenging and are recorded and/or photographed (Fig. 35.8).

Persistence of human reagins in monkey skin

Ag-chall. hours after sensit.	Neat	$\frac{1}{2}$	$\frac{1}{4}$	$\frac{1}{8}$	$\frac{1}{16}$	$\frac{1}{32}$	$\frac{1}{64}$	$\frac{1}{128}$
196	++++++	N.D.	++	+	Nil	Nil	N.D.	N.D.
101	++++	+++	+++	+	Nil	Nil	N.D.	N.D.
53	++.++++	N.D.	+++++	++++	+++	? tr	Nil	Nil
30	N.D.	N.D.	++++	++++	++++	++	+	Nil
7	+++++	N.D.	++++	++++	+++	+++	tr	Nil
2·5	+++	N.D.	+++	(+)	? tr	Nil	Nil	N.D

FIG. 35.9. Persistence of human reagins in monkey skin. Schematic lay-out of the reagin injection sites on the chest and abdomen of the monkey and the reaction results when challenged at the indicated times after sensitization. Number of + signs indicate strength of reaction, tr = trace, ?tr = trace reaction of questionable significance, Nil = no reaction, N.D. = site not tested.

Rate of fixation and persistence of human reagins in monkey skin

This was determined similarly as described for human skin. Rows of doubling serum dilutions were injected at intervals and challenged all together 10 days later. Figure 35.9 gives schematically the lay-out of the experiment and in Fig. 35.10 the logarithms of the reciprocals of the resulting serum dilution end-points have been plotted against time elapsed since sensitization. As for man, a roughly straight-line relationship resulted, from which a half-life of persistence of about 55 hours can be deduced. As the injected serum had a dilution end-point of 1/64 in the monkey we used, some of the undiluted serum would be expected to persist demonstrably for six half-lives, i.e. for 13–14 days. This is roughly in agreement with Buckley & Metzgar [85] who stated that passive sensitization with sera of dilution end-points 1/32 to 1/64 could be demonstrated for at least 2 weeks.

Figures 35.9 and 35.10 pinpoint another important feature. It can be seen that the dilution end-point determined $2\frac{1}{2}$ hours after sensitization was scarcely 1/8 and that maximum sensitization was probably reached soon

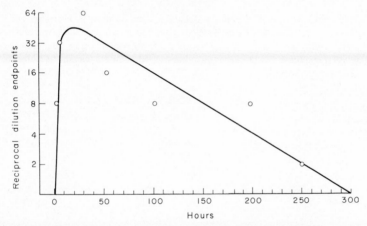

FIG. 35.10. Persistence of human reagins in monkey skin. Plot of log of reciprocals of serum dilutions against time elapsed between sensitization and challenge.

after 7 hours. The experiment records a sensitization peak at 30 hours after sensitization which was already well passed 53 hours after sensitization. This means that—unlike in man—challenging in the monkey must not be delayed much above 24 hours after sensitization, but that it would probably be permissible to challenge 12 hours after sensitization. This would be quite possible in monkeys, where usually very little trauma due to the serum injections is seen.

PCA reactions in monkeys thus occupy an intermediate position between PK reactions in man and PCA reactions in guinea-pigs, in that human reagins take longer to become 'fixed' to monkey skin than to human skin and persist considerably less long in monkey skin than in human skin, although longer than rabbit antibodies in guinea-pig skin—8 hours according to Ovary *et al* [78]. An attempt was therefore made to examine more closely the affinity of rabbit and human γG antibodies for monkey skin.

Affinity of rabbit and human γG antibodies for monkey skin

A serum sickness serum (i.e. the serum of a person sensitized with horse serum antigens—e.g. through injection with anti-tetanus preparations— and possessing reaginic as well as γG precipitating antibodies for horse serum antigens) and the pure γG precipitin fraction isolated from it as well as a pollen reaginic serum from a subject also slightly sensitive to horse serum (Wes) and a rabbit antiserum for cocksfoot were all injected intra- dermally at the back of a monkey, 30 hours and $2\frac{1}{2}$ hours before challenging first with horse serum (plus dye) and then with pollen extract (plus dye). The ensuing reactions are given in Table 35.3. At the $2\frac{1}{2}$ hour sites, strongly

TABLE 35.3

PCA reactions in monkey skin after challenging consecutively with grass pol- len extract (C) and horse serum (Ho), $2\frac{1}{2}$ and 30 hours after the intradermal serum injections. Dodgs: serum sickness serum containing reagins as well as γG precipitins (= Dodgs I) for horse serum: Wes: serum of subject strongly sensitive to C and weakly to H; R-a-C: rabbit antiserum for C; +, + +, + + +, + + + +: positive reactions of increasing size.

| Sensitizing sera and serum fractions | Antigen-induced reactions | | | |
| | At $2\frac{1}{2}$ hours | | At 30 hours | |
	With Ho	With C	With Ho	With C
Dodgs I (= γG)	+ + +	Nil	Nil	Nil
Dodgs	+ + + +	Nil	+ + + +	Nil
Wes	+	+ + + +	+	+ + + +
R-a-C	Nil	Diffuse, weak	Nil	Nil

marked, compact blueing reactions appeared at both the serum sickness sites and a weak reaction at the Wes site after challenge with horse serum, while only the latter (+) and the unfractionated serum sickness site (+ + + +) reacted at the 30 hour sites; in confirmation of our earlier work [110], the isolated γG precipitins from the horse serum sickness serum gave no reaction 30 hours after sensitization. The rabbit antiserum for pollen (rabbit anti- cocksfoot) gave, as expected, no reaction on challenge with horse serum, either $2\frac{1}{2}$ hours or 30 hours after sensitization, demonstrating the specificity of the reactions. The subsequent intravenous injections of pollen extract produced, as expected, from our previous experiments strongly positive reac- tions in the $2\frac{1}{2}$ hour as well as the 30 hour sites sensitized with pollen reaginic serum Wes; there was an unexpected, diffuse, weak, blueing reaction at the $2\frac{1}{2}$ hour rabbit serum site.

We may conclude that human γG antibodies also have, after all, some—

albeit short-lived—affinity for monkey skin and that there is even some very slight affinity for rabbit antibodies. In monkeys it is therefore important not to challenge too soon after sensitization, as this could lead to interference by non-reaginic antibodies.

Site variability

Claims have been made that eyelids and cheeks are more reactive sites than chest and abdomen, but in our hands all these sites gave roughly equal reactions, at least when sensitized with slightly diluted reaginic serum (1/4), while somewhat larger reactions were given at the insides of the upper arms and upper thighs.

Repeated testing on the same animal

Although 'Coomassie blue' is quickly excreted [87] and the animal soon appears to be normal once more, we found it inadvisable to do PCA tests more than once on the same animal, although this is recommended by Rose *et al* [88]. However, these workers also report that the skin of animals that have been used several times becomes less reactive. The latter has been also our experience; indeed almost complete refractoriness was sometimes experienced even at intervals of 2–3 weeks between tests.

This could be due to the formation of blocking antibodies to the intravenously injected antigen, a danger pointed out by other workers. However, we had definite proof that there is an even greater likelihood of sufficient antigen remaining in the circulation for sufficiently long periods to discharge reagin-sensitized test sites as soon as the injections are made; in consequence, challenge with antigen (plus dye) the next day fails to produce a reaction. A case in point was a monkey that had been used twice before for PCA tests with pollen reaginic sera. Excellent reactions had been obtained the first time, but there were unexplained, irregular results and low end-points the second time. Three weeks later the animal was sensitized intradermally with one exceptionally potent pollen reaginic serum (Flah), neat and at a dilution 1/10, and with three less potent sera at the same two dilutions. There were no visible reactions. Next day, we injected, as usual the dye before the antigen, when immediately, large blue areas formed in both the Flah sites as well as one weakly positive reaction with one of the other undiluted sera. These reactions must have been due to pollen antigen remaining in circulation from the previous tests, since the subsequent injection of the antigen produced no further blueing at any of the sensitized sites; one is therefore forced to conclude that most of the sites had already been discharged 'silently' the previous day in absence of the dye indicator, but that the reaction was still going on in the most active reaginic sites 24 hours later, as was seen on injecting the dye (without the antigen).

NN

There is also a danger of producing anaphylaxis and/or a type of serum sickness on using animals more than once, as has been shown by Feinberg *et al* for guinea-pigs that had been used several times for PCA tests [89]. The monkey described above was challenged once more intravenously with pollen extract after injecting dye. The injection was stopped after the administration of 1 ml of dye because the animal began to moan and there was heavy breathing. And suddenly the face, hands, feet, ears and genitals 'blushed' dark blue. Gradually, the body skin also became a mottled blue, although the face remained most strongly coloured. Repetition of a similar procedure 4 weeks later also produced increases in basophil and eosinophil counts similar to those described by Feinberg *et al* in guinea-pigs [89].

However, the anaphylactic reactions produced in the monkey were presumably due to reagin formation to the injected pollen antigens, while the reactions described by Feinberg *et al* appear to have occurred in response to the intradermally injected heterologous serum.

Reliability and sensitivity of the test

Nine normal, non-reaginic sera and sixteen sera from pollen-allergic subjects were tested blind, undiluted and diluted 1/10, by PCA in a monkey, challenging, as usual, with cocksfoot pollen extract as the antigen. All the non-reaginic sera gave negative reactions, while fourteen out of the sixteen hay fever sera gave positive results at both the serum concentrations. One of the 'false' negatives turned out to come from the serum of a patient who, on further examination, was found to give negative skin reactions for cocksfoot and timothy pollen extracts although giving positive reactions to other grass pollen extracts. Not surprisingly, therefore, our tests with cocksfoot pollen extract were negative. There was no opportunity of pursuing the other apparently 'false' negative. Eight of the reaginic sera came from untreated and eight from treated (depot injections) hay fever subjects [54]. The former had passive haemagglutination titres [63] not exceeding 1/40, while those of the latter ranged from about 1/600–1/5000 which did not, however, appear to interfere with the PCA reactions. However, a special study of the effect of γG antibodies—presumably including blocking antibodies—on the PCA reaction in monkeys has not yet been made.

Monkey PCA titres, for sera giving PK titres of around 1/100–1/300, ranged from 1/10 to 1/64, while one serum of PK titre 1/1000 gave a PCA titre in monkey skin of 1/100. In our hands, PCA in monkeys is thus a less sensitive test than the PK test in man. This agrees with the findings of Buckley & Metzgar [85] although Rose *et al* [88] claim comparable sensitivity for the two tests.

So far no statistical assessment of the accuracy of the test is available.

PCA tests for reagins in primates other than rhesus monkeys and in lower animal orders

Layton *et al* [86, 82, 83] have made an intensive study of reagin transfer to a number of higher primates as well as to prosimii, the primate-like tree shrew and representatives of lower orders of animals [90]. Only primates proper were found to be successfully sensitized and the reaction was most intense in the higher primates (monkeys and apes).

In conclusion, although the affinity of human reaginic antibodies is shown to be not nearly as high for monkeys as for human skin, it is still much higher than that of human γG antibodies for either monkey or human skin and very much higher than that of rabbit antibodies for primate skin. Under the proper conditions, PCA in monkeys is given by human reagins and NOT by human γG antibodies or by rabbit antibodies. PCA in monkeys is therefore a valuable equivalent of the PK test in man for demonstrating reagins, even though it is a somewhat less sensitive reaction. Certain precautions are necessary; e.g. time of challenge is more critical than in the PK test and should be done within 16–30 hours of sensitization; although challenging by intradermal injection of the antigen is possible [88], this is less reliable than intravenous challenge and the latter naturally requires much larger amounts of allergen than are needed for the PK test. There remains the fact that monkeys are expensive animals and can be used reliably only once for PCA tests. There is further, the hazard of transmitting B virus through bites during the handling of the animals. The latter is, however, greatly minimized by quarantining animals for at least 6 weeks after arrival and 'Sernylan'-treated animals are very easy to handle. Fifty and more samples can be injected in about 1 hour, with the challenging the next day taking only minutes. PCA in monkeys is thus a relatively quick and easy method for demonstrating reagins.

B. *In vitro*

I. Test based on antigen-induced histamine release from *in vitro*-sensitized human lung

Fifteen years ago, Schild and colleagues [52] showed that perfused, human, asthmatic lung could be made to release histamine *in vitro* when perfused with the antigen to which the lung donor was sensitive. This clearly demonstrated that reagins were anaphylactically 'fixed' to this asthmatic lung. And nearly 10 years ago Mongar & Schild [91, 92] and more recently, others [93–95] showed that normal chopped guinea-pig lung can take up rabbit antibodies *in vitro* in such a way that added antigen releases histamine. Unfortunately, we found that guinea-pig lung cannot be similarly sensitized with human reagins. This was not unexpected in view of our inability to anaphylactically sensitize other guinea-pig tissue, e.g. guinea-pig skin, with human reagins. We therefore took the obvious next step and proceeded to sensitize normal chopped human lung with reagins. This proved successful and has been developed into an assay method for reagins.

A homogeneous tissue suspension was prepared from human lung essentially as described by Mongar & Schild [96] and Brocklehurst *et al* [93] for guinea-pig lung, except that mechanical aids could not be used because of the much greater toughness of the human compared with the animal material; cutting with a McIlwain chopper proved unsatisfactory with our material and no attempt was made to remove the tough pleura since this is said to contain the majority of the lung mast cells [97] which appear to be the cells involved in anaphylactic histamine release [98, 99]. Tissue aliquots were then sensitized by incubation with reaginic serum and subsequently challenged with the appropriate allergen. This caused release of histamine (and SRS-A, etc.) which was measured in the conventional manner on the atropinized guinea-pig ileum; and we have also successfully used guinea-pig colon for the same purpose. Figure 35.11 shows part of the tracings obtained in a typical experiment.

Procedure

Preparation of chopped lung

Pieces of lung weighing about 20 g were usually worked up to yield twenty-five to fifty, homogeneous, washed, chopped tissue samples of 100–120 mg each.

The 20 g piece is placed in a 100 ml beaker containing at least 40 ml of Tyrode (37° C), to ensure that all the tissue remains covered during the ensuing chopping. This is done by snipping repeatedly slantwise in quick succession into the tissue, using pointed, thin-bladed, surgical scissors. Two 5 minute sessions of snipping reduces the tissue to fairly even sized pieces, about 2 mm in length. In the process, cells are disrupted and the liquid becomes murky with blood, mucous and often also with soot. Disposable surgical gloves ('Dispos-a-glove', Ethicon Ltd) and a face mask are worn for protection. The murky suspension is then filtered by gentle suction over a Buchner funnel furnished with surgical gauze between two layers of filter paper (Whatman No. 54). The tissue is washed once on the filter with warm Tyrode (37° C), taking care not to let it drain dry. The gauze is then lifted off, with the top filter paper on it holding the chopped tissue. With the help of curved 'dental' forceps (no teeth, to avoid injuring the tissue) the tissue is transferred to a 50 ml beaker containing 20 ml Tyrode (37° C) for yet a further cutting with scissors (5 minutes) which reduces the particle size to pieces about 0·5 mm long. The washing on the Buchner funnel is then repeated and the drained tissue quickly divided into uniform samples of

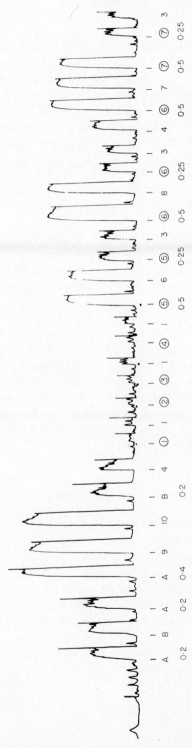

Fig. 35.11. Antigen-induced histamine release from reagin-sensitized human lung; part of a typical experiment. Tracings obtained from the contraction of guinea-pig ileum challenged with histamine (unringed figures indicate amounts in 10^{-9} g per ml tissue bath) and with supernatants of the antigen-challenged reagin-sensitized chopped lung samples (ringed sample numbers). ①, ②, ③ and ④ are negative controls where antigen and antibody have in turn been replaced by Tyrode solution; one antibody solution is replaced by normal serum and usually the effect of several antigen concentrations is tested in the absence of reagin. ⑤ is a positive control where a standard reaginic serum was used. Unless otherwise indicated, 0.5 ml aliquots of the supernatants were added to the 10 ml tissue bath. Samples A and B were derived from lung tissue where the total histamine had been released in a boiling water-bath.

100–120 mg by pushing the pieces tightly into even-sized holes in a perspex tray as described by Mongar & Schild [96], any excess liquid being removed with the help of a home-made nylon suction brush described by Brocklehurst *et al* [93].

Meanwhile, a polystyrene rack containing fifty flat-bottomed polystyrene tubes (6 × 1·3 cm, S42–141 capped specimen tubes type No. 10, Griffin & George Ltd, Manchester), each supplied with 2 ml warm Tyrode (37° C), has been placed in a water-bath (37° C) and connected to a motor to enable rocking from side to side through an angle of 60° every second or so as described by Mongar & Schild [96].

The tissue cylinders are pushed one by one into the prepared polystyrene tubes, great care being taken to ensure even suspension in the fluid. Preparation of twenty-four such samples from the original piece of lung takes about 45 minutes.

The tissue samples may then be washed once more with 1 ml quantities of Tyrode (37° C) which is then removed as completely as possible with the nylon suction brush and replaced with 0·5 ml of Tyrode (37° C). The sample tubes are then rocked in the 37° C bath for 5–10 minutes to ensure adequate equilibration.

Sensitization with antibody
0·5 ml antibody solutions (or Tyrode in the 'control' tubes) are added, the tubes swirled round and capped. Incubation in the rocking bath (37° C) is allowed to proceed for 3 hours. The sera are then removed with the nylon suction brush and the tissue pieces washed with 2 ml Tyrode solution (37° C). As before, the liquids are then removed as completely as possible with the nylon brush and 1 ml Tyrode (37° C) added to each sample, followed by 10 minutes' rocking at 37° C for equilibration.

Antigen challenge
One millilitre of antigen in Tyrode (37° C) is then added to each of the antibody-sensitized tissue samples and allowed to remain in contact for 20 minutes (37° C, rocking bath). The tubes are then plunged into ice water and the supernatants quickly separated from the tissues by means of capillary-tipped pipettes loosely plugged with non-absorbent, teased cotton wool [96], transferred to Pyrex tubes and heated for 2–3 minutes in a boiling water-bath [96]. The released histamine is then assayed on either the guinea-pig ileum or the guinea-pig colon, either immediately or after storage in the frozen state (−15° C) within the next 2–3 days (see Brocklehurst, Chapter 36).

Influence of time of incubation with antibody on histamine release
From similar work with guinea-pig lung and guinea-pig ileum it is known

that the time required for sensitization of tissues varies with the antibody concentration, periods of only a few minutes being required with highly potent rabbit antibody preparations where 50 per cent of the proteins consist of antibody [93].

Halpern *et al* [57] found, similarly, that full sensitization of guinea-pig gut was achieved with antibody protein concentrations of 7 μg/ml during 1 hour at 37° C. However, as the concentration of reaginic antibody in human serum is known to be very low, optimum incubation times had to be carefully determined. Figure 35.12 shows that histamine release could be detected after

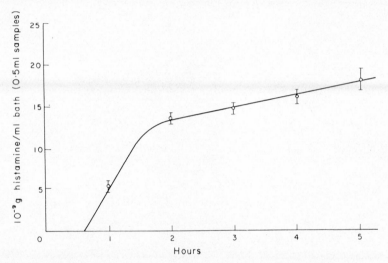

Fig. 35.12. Pollen antigen-induced histamine release from reagin-sensitized human lung. Influence of time of incubation (hours) of chopped lung with antibody on histamine release. Vertical bars show the standard deviations of the means.

a 1 hour contact with reagin at 37° C and that the tissues were almost fully sensitized after incubation times of 3 hours. Further incubation (up to 5 hours was tested) brought little further improvement in the subsequent antigen-induced histamine release and an incubation time of 3 hours was therefore chosen in all later experiments. It is interesting to remember that a minimum period of 3 hours was also required for the sensitization of human leucocytes with reagins [54].

Influence of time of contact with antigen on histamine release
Brocklehurst *et al* [93] found a 3 minute contact with antigen sufficient for maximum release of histamine from *in vivo* sensitized guinea-pig lung (perfused free from blood) and with *in vitro* sensitized guinea-pig lung Colquhoun

& Brocklehurst [95] found incubation periods of 15 minutes with antigen sufficient to cause histamine release. Figure 35.13 shows the course of antigen-induced histamine release for reagin-sensitized human lung; from this it can

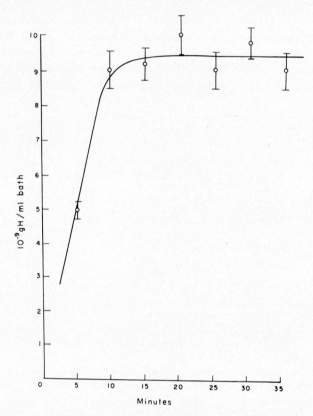

FIG. 35.13. Pollen antigen-induced histamine release from reagin-sensitized human lung. Influence of time of contact (minutes) of chopped lung with antigen on histamine release. Vertical bars show the standard deviations of the means.

be seen that the curve is only just about entering its flat part at 15 minutes and contact for 20 rather than 15 minutes was therefore chosen for our experiments.

Influence of antigen concentration on histamine release
Figure 35.14 shows little significant variation in histamine release over a 1000-fold range of pollen antigen concentration (100–100,000 Noon units/ml), but there was a distinct decrease of histamine release below 100 Noon units/ml. As high concentrations of antigen sometimes cause non-specific release of

histamine and/or contraction of guinea-pig ileum, the antigen concentrations were kept as low as was compatible with efficiency. We chose a concentration of 100 Noon units/ml.

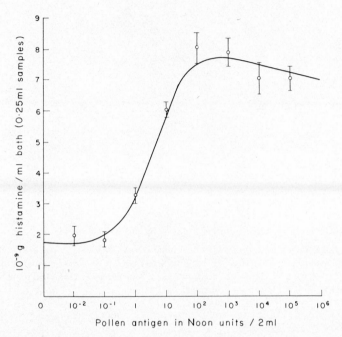

Fig. 35.14. Pollen antigen-induced histamine release from reagin-sensitized human lung. Influence of antigen concentration on histamine release from chopped lung. Vertical bars show the standard deviations of the means.

Histamine release in relation to antibody concentration—dose response curves
One to three per cent of the total histamine content of human lung tissue is spontaneously released during the 3 hour incubation with antibody (control value) while incubation with reaginic serum, followed by antigen challenge, releases 15–50 per cent of the total histamine content, depending on antibody concentration. Figure 35.15 shows that histamine release falls off sharply with decrease in antibody concentration; indeed, control release values are reached at 32-fold dilutions of even our most potent reaginic sera where maximum histamine release is achieved at fourfold dilutions of the sera. We have never obtained histamine releases of more than 50 per cent with any of our reaginic sera. It can be seen that the dose/response curves are reasonably parallel. The quick fall-off of histamine release may be taken as a reflection of the low reagin content of reaginic sera.

NN*

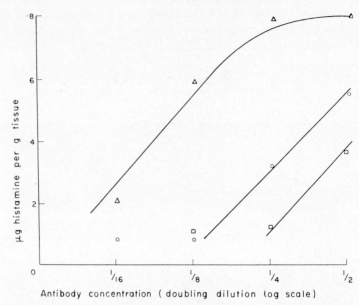

FIG. 35.15. Pollen antigen-induced histamine release from reagin-sensitized human lung. Dose/response curves with reaginic sera Flah. (-△-), Wes (-○-) and Stopford (-□-) which gave 47, 35 and 22 per cent release, respectively, of total histamine when diluted 1 : 2. Total histamine content 17 μg/g tissue.

Specificity of the reaction

Table 35.4 shows that only pollen antigen was capable of releasing histamine from lung sensitized with pollen reaginic serum and not BSA nor Ea nor thyroglobulin nor *Aspergillus fumigatus* antigen; and solely the latter was

TABLE 35.4

Specificity of antigen-induced histamine release from reagin-sensitized human lung. Flah, pollen reaginic; Tay, *aspergillus* sensitive.

| Antigen | Per cent histamine release from human lung sensitized with | |
	Flah 1/2	Tay
Dactylis glomerata	50	1–3
Egg albumin (Ea)	1–3	1–3
Thyroglobulin	1–3	1–3
Aspergillus fumigatus	1–3	20
BSA	1–3	1–3

capable of releasing histamine from lung sensitized with the serum of a subject sensitive to *A. fumigatus.*

Antigen-induced release of slow reacting substance (SRS-A) in addition to histamine

Figure 35.16 shows that the presence of 10^{-6} M mepyramine in the tissue bath containing the guinea-pig ileum almost completely inhibited the response to added histamine and altered the histamine-type response usually given by the eluates of the antigen-challenged reagin-sensitized lung tissue to one characteristic of SRS-A [100].

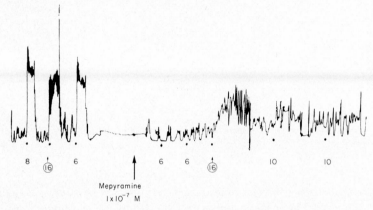

Mepyramine
1×10^{-7} M

Fig. 35.16. Pollen antigen-induced release of substances (ringed 16) from reagin-sensitized human lung tested on guinea-pig ileum before and after addition of mepyramine maleate (10^{-7} M). Additions of histamine indicated in plain figures as ng/ml bath.

Are antibodies other than reagins capable of anaphylactically sensitizing human lung?

The γG globulin fraction of a human antipollen serum prepared by immunizing a non-atopic subject with large quantities of pollen extract [62], that of a serum sickness serum and of a high-titre Hashimoto serum were all found to contain the bulk of the precipitating antibodies of the unfractionated sera (as demonstrated by gel diffusion and/or passive haemagglutination tests) and to be free from reaginic activity (as demonstrated by PK transfer and PCA in monkeys). These γG antibody preparations were used to sensitize human lung exactly as described for reagins and this was followed by 20 minutes' incubation with the corresponding antigens. Yet no histamine release could be discovered; nor did similarly used precipitating rabbit antisera for cocksfoot pollen induce anaphylactic sensitization. Yet these four sera were capable of anaphylactically sensitizing chopped guinea-pig lung.

Destruction of sensitizing capacity of reagins by heating at 56° C
Figure 35.17 shows for two sera that heating at 56° C destroys 50 per cent of the sensitizing capacity of reaginic serum for lung within ½–1½ hours and that no demonstrable reaginic activity may be left after heating for 2 hours.

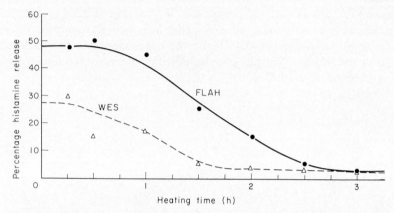

FIG. 35.17. Destruction of sensitizing capacity of reaginic serum for human lung by heating at 56° C. Histamine release from human lung sensitized with Flah (-●-) and Wes (--△--).

Sensitizing activity remaining in the serum after optimally sensitizing lung tissue
After the usual 3 hour incubation with human lung, the antibody layers were transferred to 100 mg quantities of fresh, chopped, human lung and proved capable of anaphylactically sensitizing this too (Table 35.5). The degree of sensitization of the second piece of lung was similar to that given by the original serum when similarly diluted. Very little antibody can therefore have been 'used up' in the sensitization process.

Reaginic and non-reaginic sera assayed blind on human lung
Coded sera were tested blind. All the nine normal human sera failed to sensitize for histamine release by pollen antigen, while the sixteen reaginic sera (from treated as well as untreated hay fever subjects) all did.

The results were in good agreement with the clinical history of the patients as well as with the PCA tests in monkey and the DLLA tests they gave [53, 54]. There appeared to be some interference by high titres of γG antibodies, which would be expected to include blocking antibodies, and this point warrants further investigation.

In conclusion, it emerges clearly that only reagins and not human γG antibodies or rabbit antibodies are capable of anaphylactically sensitizing chopped human lung. SRS-A as well as histamine is shown to be released in the process, as has been shown previously for perfused, whole human, asthmatic lung [100] and for *in vitro* sensitized, chopped, guinea-pig lung [101, 102]. The antibody/response relation is reasonably steep and a fourfold increase in antibody dose more than doubles the amount of histamine released (Fig. 35.14); this is a much more satisfactory relationship than obtains with the PK test where a tenfold increase in antibody dose is required to give a two- to fourfold increase in response (cf. p. 1099 and Fig. 35.7).

The method has also the advantage that a large amount of relatively homogeneous tissue is available, i.e. many duplicate estimations can readily be made on a serum and so statistically significant results obtained. Furthermore, sufficient histamine is released per sample (100–800 ng in 2 ml) to

TABLE 35.5

Sensitizing activity remaining after sensitization of one piece of lung

	Reaginic serum added	Per cent antigen-induced histamine release
Lung I + 1 ml Tyrode	1 ml neat	50
Lung II + 1 ml Tyrode	1 ml 1/2	22
Lung II + Nil	2 ml supernatant from Lung I after 3 hours' incubation	20

allow ten to fifty histamine analyses to be made on each when using a 1 ml bath together with the automatic biological assay apparatus devised by Boura *et al* [103]. Results of reasonable and known accuracy can thus be obtained.

Allergen-induced histamine release from human lung is, however, not the most sensitive test for reagins. Histamine is released over a rather small range of dilutions of reaginic serum—a reflection, no doubt, of the low concentration of reagin in these sera. With blank (control) values (where antigen and antibody respectively are replaced by Tyrode during the various incubations) of 1–3 per cent of the total histamine available in the tissue, we arbitrarily demand a release of at least 10 per cent for the demonstration of reaginic activity. Most reaginic sera drop to this value already at four to eightfold dilutions. With one single serum (PK titre 1/1000) a significant histamine release was still given at a 30-fold dilution.

Histamine release from human lung is therefore a relatively accurate and reliable, but not very sensitive, measure of reaginic antibodies.

II. Tests based on antigen-induced contraction of *in vitro*-sensitized primate tissues

(a) Using monkey ileum and monkey colon

That guinea-pig ileum can be passively sensitized *in vitro* was discovered by Dale [26] in his early experiments on anaphylaxis. It was confirmed by Hartley [55] and Kulka [56] and has more recently been examined in detail by Halpern *et al* [57]. However, the serological system used seems to have been almost invariably Ea with rabbit anti-Ea and our attempts to sensitize guinea-pig ileum with human reaginic antibodies failed—as with other guinea-pig tissue. As human ileum is not easy to come by, the obvious solution was to use monkey ileum and Arbesman *et al* [58] and we ourselves found that monkey ileum is very readily anaphylactically sensitized by reaginic sera, even at high dilutions. However, Arbesman *et al* [58] were also able to sensitize guinea-pig ileum with reaginic serum and monkey ileum with rabbit antiserum. In view of our own negative results with guinea-pig ileum, we felt that an investigation of the various types of antibodies involved in these reactions was urgently required.

Procedure

For preference rhesus monkeys weighing 8–10 lb are chosen. Dying malarial monkeys have proved quite suitable. The animals are injected intravenously (back of leg) with 'Sernylan' (Parke, Davis & Co., 0·2 ml per 8 lb monkey) to which they succumb almost instantaneously. They are then canulated and bled out via the vena cava. The abdomen is then quickly opened and the caecal end of the ileum immediately transferred gently without stretching (the mesentery rather than the ileum itself is handled) to oxygenated Tyrode.

Pieces 1·5-2·0 cm in length are cut, starting at the caecal end. Keeping to the natural sequence, each piece is placed in one of a consecutive row of Petri dishes filled with warm Tyrode. Each piece is then gently washed as free as possible from faecal matter by allowing Tyrode from a 10 ml pipette to flow gently—under gravity only—through the lumen of the piece of ileum (no stretching). The washed pieces (suitably trimmed from excess mesentery) are then put in sequence in consecutively numbered 'Universal containers', each equipped with about 10 ml of oxygenated Tyrode, the piece nearest the caecal end being labelled No. 1. It is convenient to keep this order since the pieces nearest the caecal end usually exhibit greatest sensitivity.

The pieces of gut are best used immediately, but can be kept in the cold (4° C) for several days in oxygenated Tyrode. Pieces stored thus have remained active at times for 5 days although time required to revive responsiveness increases with length of storage.

Each piece of monkey ileum can then be sensitized with human serum in exactly the same manner in which guinea-pig ileum is sensitized with rabbit or guinea-pig serum [26, 55–57]. We found incubation for 1 hour at 37° C most convenient, a method also used by Arbesman *et al* [58]. This incubation can be undertaken in small, stoppered tubes in a shaker in a water-bath; whenever possible we prefer, however, to suspend the piece of ileum in a 10 ml Schultz-Dale type tissue bath, in the usual manner, to allow it to be buffeted by oxygen. One end of the gut is fixed to the bottom of the bath and the other end attached to a lever which records the contractions on a drum. In place of the drum arrangements, transducer equipment may be used. Response to histamine is then tested and incubation with serum is started once a reasonably good histamine response has been established. After incubation, the gut is washed several times with warm Tyrode (37° C) and again tested for response to histamine. Fresh guts tend to respond immediately, but stored guts may sometimes require many histamine additions before the original histamine response is established once more. A suitable amount of antigen is then added to the bath liquid and allowed to remain in contact with the gut for 2–5 minutes. Highly sensitized guts contract immediately, while lightly sensitized guts may exhibit a short lag period. The gut is then washed as before and the antigen response checked for its histamine equivalent. Antigen is then added again, when a second and with further antigen, even third and fourth series of contractions may be obtained with highly sensitized specimens of ileum. Eventually, however, the ileum appears to be desensitized to the antigen on further challenge; it is important to check that sensitivity to histamine has been retained, while specificity of the reaction is checked by challenge with unrelated antigens which must not give a response. Non-reactivity of the chosen antigen concentration must be ensured on a non-sensitized piece of the same ileum. Only one antibody concentration can be tested on each piece of ileum. With two tissue baths, four to possibly six samples may be tested by one worker in a day, depending on the ease with which different specimens of ileum can be made to respond.

Although some pieces of monkey ileum are as sensitive to histamine as guinea-pig ileum, the majority are less sensitive. While guinea-pig ileum can almost always be made to respond to 1–2 ng/ml bath liquid, some specimens of monkey ileum do not respond to less than 5 ng histamine/ml bath liquid.

Great care must be taken to ensure that all the sera and antigens used are free from substances giving non-specific contractions (or relaxations) of the monkey ileum. This is usually achieved by working with sterile solutions free from preservative and often dialysis successfully removes interfering substances.

Monkey ileum sensitized with reaginic serum and failure of sensitization with other antibodies

Figure 35.18 gives a typical tracing showing the antigen contractions obtained before and after incubation with the reaginic serum in relation to the responses to added histamine. Although this ileum typically only barely responded to 5 ng of histamine/ml bath, a very good response was obtained on challenging with antigen. It can also be seen that three additions of antigen were required for desensitization. Additions of unrelated antigens (Ea, horse serum and BSA) failed to give a response (not shown). Moreover, this same, admittedly highly potent reaginic serum (Flah) still sensitized monkey ileum when

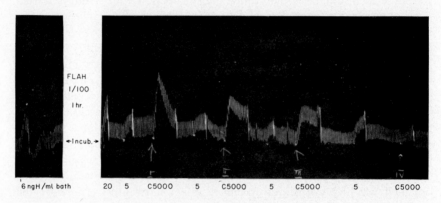

FIG. 35.18. Monkey ileum: pollen antigen-(5000 Noon units/ml bath)-induced contractions after incubation with a 1/100 dilution of pollen reaginic serum (Flah). Note, desensitization required four antigen additions. In between pollen challenges additions of histamine in ng/ml bath.

diluted 10,000-fold when desensitization was complete after a single addition of pollen antigen. Other reaginic sera sensitized down to 100- and 1000-fold dilutions and so did the reaginic γA fractions of horse serum sickness serum.

All our attempts to sensitize monkey ileum with human γG antibodies free from reagins failed—as did our attempts to sensitize with rabbit anti-pollen and rabbit anti-Ea serum.

Monkey colon sensitized with reaginic serum

Monkey colon responds much more slowly and ponderously than monkey ileum. Nevertheless, the sensitivity of the colon to histamine is often of the same order as that of the ileum and this tissue too can be successfully sensitized with reaginic serum. Figure 35.19 shows a typical result. The antigen-induced contractions—although quite distinct—are smaller than can be obtained with the ileum. Nevertheless, it can be seen that here, too, three additions of

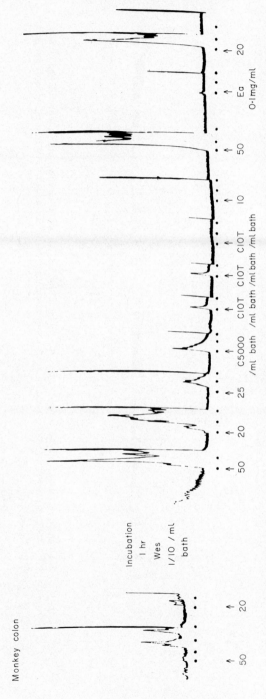

Fig. 35.19. Monkey colon: pollen antigen–(5000 and 10,000 Noon units/ml bath)–induced contractions after incubation with a 1/10 dilution of pollen reaginic serum. Note, desensitization required four antigen additions. Figures not preceded by C indicate added histamine in ng/ml bath. Reaction to C specific—no reaction with Ea. 0·1 mg/ml. Dots indicate minutes.

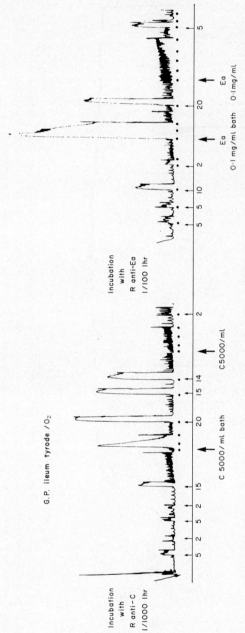

FIG. 35.20. Guinea-pig ileum: sensitized consecutively with rabbit antipollen (C) serum (1/1000) and rabbit anti-egg albumin serum (1/100). Challenge with antigen indicated by arrows and amounts of histamine added to bath in ng/ml bath indicated by plain figures.

antigen were required for desensitization. However, there was usually little response after incubation with 100-fold dilutions of reaginic sera. Challenging with unrelated antigen, e.g. Ea, can be seen not to give a response.

Guinea-pig ileum sensitized with rabbit antisera and human γG antibodies; failure to sensitize with reagins

Figure 35.20 gives a typical tracing obtained after sensitization with rabbit anti-pollen (rabbit anti-cocksfoot). It can be seen that the response to the same amount of antigen that was used with the reagin-sensitized monkey ileum (Fig. 35.18) gives here a rather smaller response and that a single addition of antigen was sufficient to desensitize. Figure 35.20 also shows that it is possible to sensitize the same ileum successfully with more than one antiserum.

Figure 35.21 gives the results of the sensitization with one of the same human γG antibody preparations that failed to sensitize monkey ileum. Good responses were nevertheless obtained with guinea-pig ileum and three additions of horse serum antigen were required for desensitization (not shown). The reaction was specific and neither Ea nor C produced responses.

In no instance have we been able to sensitize guinea-pig ileum with a reaginic serum, not even with Flah.

In conclusion, antigen-induced contraction of monkey ileum is a highly sensitive test for reaginic antibodies, surpassing even the sensitivity of PK tests. Antigen as well as antibody specificity has been demonstrated for human γG antibody preparations, which were highly active with guinea-pig ileum, failed to produce any reaction with monkey ileum and the opposite held true with reaginic serum. We may therefore conclude that the sensitization of guinea-pig ileum obtained by Arbesman *et al* with reaginic serum was due to human γG and not to the reaginic antibodies in these sera. Their sensitization of monkey ileum with rabbit antiserum is not supported by our experiments.

(b) Using human bronchi

Bronchial smooth muscle strips or chains from animals and man have been prepared in a number of ways and have been shown to react to the addition of histamine, SRS-A, bradykinin, etc., mostly to give a contraction like other smooth muscle preparations [104–108]. Moreover, several workers have shown [105, 52, 106] that when such preparations are derived from asthmatic subjects, they contract upon addition of the allergen to which the patient is sensitive. We therefore attempted to sensitize normal human bronchi *in vitro* with reaginic serum in the hope of obtaining allergen-specific contractions similar to those obtained with monkey ileum. However, although isolated human bronchial muscle strips had been found to be roughly

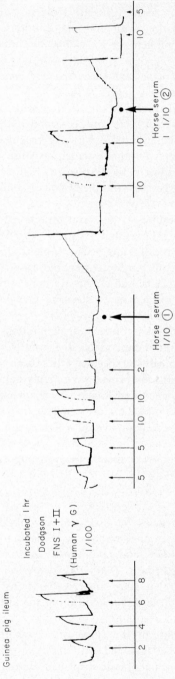

FIG. 35.21. Guinea-pig ileum: response to horse serum antigen after sensitization (1 hour incubation) with γG antibody isolated from human serum sickness serum.

as sensitive to SRS-A as is guinea-pig ileum, it was already known that they are much less sensitive to histamine than is guinea-pig ileum [108, 109]. Therefore, although sensitivity to histamine is not necessarily a guide to anaphylactic sensitivity, we did not expect the same high degree of sensitivity which we had found with monkey ileum which was unfortunately borne out by our experiments.

Preparation and type of response given by broncho-tracheal tissues
Rosa & McDowall [105] and Schild *et al* [52] fastened human bronchial rings together with cotton thread to make a contractile chain while Rosa & McDowall [105] also made spiral cuts from human bronchi and Bhoola *et al* [107] prepared strips by opening bronchial tubes longitudinally and making transverse cuts successively from alternate sides, so that they overlap one another without transepting the preparation.

We had little success with preparations made according to Bhoola *et al* [107], but did succeed with spiral cuts and chains of tracheo-bronchial rings. These were made from human quaternary bronchi (dissected out from suitable pieces of lung obtained from operations and, as before, immediately removed to oxygenated isotonic saline buffer to keep the tissues alive) as well as from guinea-pig trachea. Spiral cuts of the human bronchi were made by inserting an orange stick or narrow metal rod (of a diameter slightly smaller than that of the bronchial tube), etc., into the bronchus to serve as a guide and support during the dissection, which greatly facilitated the procedure. Guinea-pig trachea can readily be dissected without such a support. Later we found, however, that bronchial rings knotted together with cotton thread give possibly more reliable reactive preparations which may be slightly more sensitive. However, sensitivity varied considerably in all instances.

Krebs-Henseleit buffer rather than Tyrode solution was used for the tracheal and bronchial preparations as recommended by others [105–108]. The bronchial (or tracheal) muscle strips or chains were suspended in a 10 ml tissue bath as described for the ileum pieces. A mixture of 95 per cent O_2 and 5 per cent CO_2 was bubbled through in place of the pure O_2 used with the ileum.

In confirmation and extension of previous work [105, 107, 108] the sensitivity of the bronchial strips and chains to histamine was found to be fifty to five hundred times less than that of the ileum preparations; microgramme rather than nanogramme concentrations of histamine were required to obtain contractions and there was little difference between the responses given by the human and guinea-pig preparations. The contractions were, moreover, very much slower than ileum contractions and periods of a minimum of 10 minutes (guinea-pig) to 30 minutes (human) had to elapse between additions of histamine, etc., to enable the writing pointer of the lever to return to the

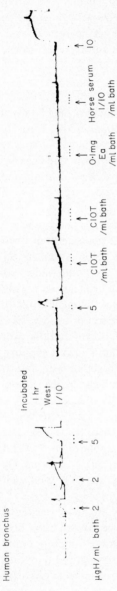

Human bronchus

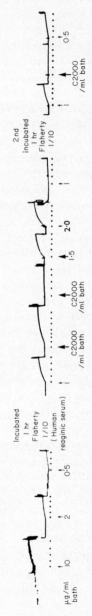

Human bronchus (rings)
(K—H medium O₂)

Fig. 35.22. Human bronchus (spiral cut). Response to pollen antigen (C, 10,000 Noon units/ml bath) after sensitization (1 hour incubation) with human pollen reaginic serum (Wes) 1/10. Plain figures indicate histamine responses in μg/ml bath. Added substances left in bath in contact with tissue for 5 minutes (minutes indicated by dots). Drum speed 1 mm per second. Note, no response to challenge with unrelated antigens (Ea and horse serum).

Fig. 35.23. Human bronchus (ring preparation). Sensitization with Flah 1/10. Responses after challenging with pollen antigen (C, 2000 Noon units/ml bath)—desensitization after one addition of the pollen antigen. A second sensitization with Flah 1/10 failed in spite of the tissue still fully reacting to histamine (0·5 μg histamine per ml bath).

base line. Also, to reach maximum response, the histamine had to be left in the bath for 5 minutes instead of the 30 seconds with guinea-pig ileum. It is possible that the relative insensitivity of the tissues is, in part, due to injury incurred during dissection. Yet, despite the relative insensitivity of these muscle preparations to *added* histamine, the *in vitro* sensitization with suitable antibody solutions, followed by challenge with the corresponding antigen, gave quite unequivocal specific contractions (Figs. 35.22–35.24).

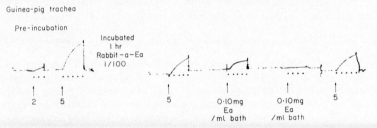

FIG. 35.24. Guinea-pig trachea: response to Ea after incubation with rabbit anti-Ea 1/100. Plain figures indicate histamine responses in $\mu g/ml$ bath. Added substances left in bath in contact with tissue for 5 minutes (minutes indicated by dots).

Procedure
The bronchial (or tracheal) strips or chains suspended like ileum in a tissue bath are first tested with histamine; only after sufficiently large responses have been obtained (>1 cm for 1–5 μg histamine/ml bath liquid), is the washed tissue incubated with the antibody solution in the tissue bath (37° C, CO_2 plus O_2). Serum dilutions of 1/10 and even 1/100 were effective. After 1 hour the antibody-containing serum is removed by washing three or more times and the response to histamine tested once more until a response at least equal to that registered before incubation is obtained. At this stage antigen is added and left in the bath for 5 minutes. Contractions usually start almost immediately. Table 35.6 shows that they were antigen-specific.

TABLE 35.6

Specificity of antigen-induced contraction of reagin-sensitized human bronchus. +, positive reaction; −, no contraction; (+) contraction of secondary importance.

| | Challenging antigen | | |
Serum	Horse serum	Cocksfoot	Egg albumin
Dodgs	+	−	−
Flah	−	+	−
Wes	(+)	+	−

The tissue was usually specifically desensitized to the antigen after a single addition of the antigen while continuing to react to histamine as before (Figs. 35.23, 35.24).

Results

Table 35.7 shows, once more, that only the human tissues could be sensitized with reaginic antibodies which failed to sensitize guinea-pig trachea, while the rabbit antibodies sensitized guinea-pig trachea and failed to sensitize human bronchus. Human γG antibodies not only failed to sensitize human

TABLE 35.7

Antigen-induced contractions of human and guinea-pig bronchial muscle preparations sensitized *in vitro* with various types of antibody. Each muscle strip was challenged with four antigens: pollen extract 10,000 Noon units/ml, Horse serum 1/10, egg albumin (Ea) 0·1 mg/ml, thyroglobulin (TG) 0·1 mg/ml. +, contractions on challenging with antigen; −, failure to contract on challenging with antigen; ±, very faint contraction.

| | Challenging antigen for | | | | | | | |
| | Human bronchus | | | | Guinea-pig trachea | | | |
Sensitizing serum	Pollen	Horse serum	Ea	TG	Pollen	Horse serum	Ea	TG
Pollen reaginic 1/10	+	−	−	−	−	−	−	−
Hodg reaginic fraction for horse serum 1/10	−	+	−	−	−	−	−	−
Hodg γG antibodies for horse serum 1/10	−	−	−	−	−	±	−	−
Hashimoto serum GY* 1/10	+	−	−	−	−	−	−	±
Hashimoto serum Heath 1/10	−	−	−	+	−	−	−	−
Rabbit anti-Ea 1/10	−	−	−	−	−	−	+	−

* This serum contained reagins for grass pollens as well as precipitins for TG.

bronchus, but also gave only very weak sensitization of guinea-pig trachea—a not altogether unexpected result in view of the rather low sensitivity of excised guinea-pig trachea, not only to histamine but also to SRS-A [108, 109]. In view of this, it is in fact remarkable that rabbit anti-Ea serum diluted 100-fold nevertheless still sensitized guinea-pig trachea sufficiently to cause definite contractions on addition of the corresponding antigen (Fig. 35.24). The human γG antibodies—which have a lesser affinity for guinea-pig tissues than rabbit antibodies—barely sensitized guinea-pig trachea at a dilution of 1/10 although sensitization of guinea-pig ileum was possible at 1/100 (cf. Fig. 35.21).

Figures 35.22 and 35.23 give similar tracings obtained with reagin-sensitized human bronchi. Figure 35.22 shows this to be antigen-specific and Fig. 35.23 shows that an attempt at a second sensitization with the same reaginic serum failed.

Ten-fold dilutions of six pollen reaginic sera all gave antigen-specific positive results with some human bronchial preparations, but other such preparations failed to become sensitized, although responding similarly to added histamine. Normal non-reaginic sera were consistently negative.

In conclusion, it is shown that human bronchi—like other primate tissues—can be specifically sensitized with reaginic antibodies and that reagins fail to sensitize guinea-pig trachea. The latter tissue is, as expected, sensitized by rabbit antibodies and only—very feebly—by human γG antibodies. Human bronchial muscle preparations are thus an additional tissue that can be used for the specific *in vitro* demonstration of reagins, but in view of the low sensitivity it is perhaps of greater theoretical than practical significance.

We are told by Dr H.O.J. Collier (of Parke, Davis & Co., Hounslow) that he also has been able to sensitize guinea-pig trachea with rabbit antibodies, but that his attempts with human bronchi have been too erratic to be convincing, especially as the best contractions were obtained with rabbit antisera and no attempt was made to distinguish between different types of antibodies.

III. The DLLA test—based on the cytophilic properties of reagins

During 1962 it was found that washed human leucocytes are capable of adsorbing, *in vitro*, reagins from grass pollen reaginic sera [110]. This has been made the basis of a test for reagins [54] the principle of which is set out schematically in Fig. 35.25.

Washed leucocytes are sensitized with reagins and then reacted with the corresponding antigen, e.g. grass pollen allergen. This does not cause agglutination, presumably because of steric hindrance, but specific antigen attachment is demonstrated by the subsequent addition of precipitating indicator serum for the antigen which does produce agglutination. Agglutination fails to occur when either the reaginic or the indicator serum is replaced by the corresponding normal serum or when the specific antigen is replaced by some unrelated antigen.

Preparation of washed leucocytes
Twenty millilitres of freshly taken blood is heparinized (500 units of heparin), mixed at 37° C with 2 ml of dextran (a commercial 6 per cent w/v solution of dextran in physiological saline—ex Benger's Laboratories, Holmes

Chapel, Cheshire) and slanted in test tubes (15×1.5 cm) at an angle of
$45°$ in a water-bath ($37°$ C). After about 20 minutes, a leucocyte layer of
altogether 7 ml can be recovered from the top of the tubes. This supernatant
is then centrifuged in capillary-tipped tubes for 10 minutes at 400 *g* (Martin
Christ Junior centrifuge II, Harz, Germany, 1700 rev/min) and the supernatant (LY layer) discarded. The deposit consists mostly of neutrophils (with
basophils and eosinophils in roughly the usual proportions), lymphocytes

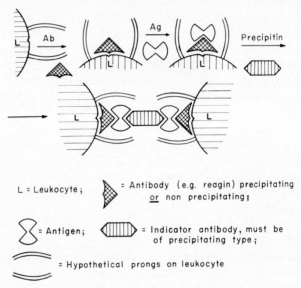

L = Leucocyte; = Antibody (e.g. reagin) precipitating
                  or non precipitating;

 = Antigen; = Indicator antibody, must be
              of precipitating type;

 = Hypothetical prongs on leukocyte

FIG. 35.25. Double-layer leucocyte agglutination. Diagrammatic representation of the
method.

and about equal numbers of erythrocytes. The cells are resuspended in about
5 ml of Tyrode buffer, followed by sedimentation for 5 minutes at 400 *g*.
This washing is repeated twice more. The cells are then evenly resuspended
in the buffer and divided into four to five equal portions.

Procedure
The washed leucocytes are gently suspended in 0.20 ml of the various sera
under test. This is followed by incubation for 3 hours, the leucocytes being
resuspended from time to time as they sediment. Lesser times proved
insufficient for sensitization and longer periods are inadvisable as leucocytes then tend to agglutinate non-specifically. The cells are then sedimented as before and washed five times in Tyrode (0.2 ml). After this, the
serum-treated cells are suspended in pollen extract (0.20 ml; 3300 Noon
units/ml) and incubated for 25 minutes. This is followed by eight 5 minute

washings (500 *g*) to remove every trace of non-specifically absorbed pollen antigen and the sedimented cells are then incubated for 25 minutes in 0·25 ml of the indicator serum (a precipitating antiserum for the antigen, e.g. rabbit antiserum for pollen antigen). Finally, each washed cell sample is resuspended in about 0·2 ml of Tyrode solution, depending on the number of cells still available. One drop of the suspension is then mixed in a small tube with 2 drops of Tuerk's diluting fluid. An appropriate portion is immediately transferred to a Neubauer counting chamber, the cell density being arranged such that the total number of cells in the large central square lies between 150 and 400, i.e. a density of 1500 to 4000 cells per mm^3 is aimed at.

During the whole of this procedure a temperature of 37° C (water-bath) is maintained.

Cell counting
At least sixteen of the twenty-five squares in the large central square are counted according to the usual conventions. No distinction is made between polymorphs and lymphocytes (although the latter do not take part in the agglutination reaction, see later). Agglutinates of two to eight cells are counted as 'clumps' and distinguished from single cells. Occasional large clumps are ignored as non-specific, those few preparations which contained many such clumps being discarded. The total number of cells in the (small) clumps is divided by the sum of single cells plus the cells in the clumps and is reported as 'percentage agglutination'. At least three independent counts are averaged for each test.

Controls, non-specific agglutination and optimum number of cells per test
Each series of tests done with a particular leucocyte preparation should include two known negative and one known positive controls. In the positive controls a known reaginic serum is used, while in the two negative controls the reaginic and indicator sera are replaced, respectively, by normal human and normal rabbit serum. While very little non-specific agglutination occurs on replacing the indicator serum with normal rabbit serum, a permissible base-line agglutination of up to 19 per cent had to be allowed for normal non-reaginic sera (Fig. 35.26); in fact, when taking single counts and working at room temperature, there was some overlap between reaginic and non-reaginic sera in the region of 18-22 per cent agglutination. This overlap was considerably reduced by working at 37° C and taking the average of three counts per test sample. It was further found that apparently positive results (about 19 per cent agglutination) were often due to overcrowding and could be largely avoided by keeping the total number of cells per square milli-metre below 400.

Types of cells involved in the reaction

Figure 35.27 gives a microphotograph of the type of agglutination seen before staining with Tuerk's fluid, i.e. before removing the residual red cells; the clumps can already be seen to contain mostly large polymorphs, with some red cells also caught up in the clumps. There are free red cells, some single polymorphs and free smaller lymphocyte-like cells. Dissolution of the red cells with Tuerk's fluid leaves the clumped, lightly stained, polymorphs (Fig. 35.28B) a number of single polymorphs and a few single lymphocyte-like cells. Figures 35.28C and D show the corresponding controls.

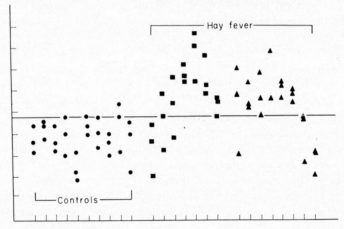

FIG. 35.26. Double-layer leucocyte agglutination. Percentage agglutination obtained in individual single estimates. Note overlap at the 19 per cent level. ● Normal controls, ■ treated hay fever subjects, ▲ untreated hay fever subjects.

To evaluate the role—if any—of red cells in the agglutination reaction, leucocyte-free red cells were incubated with reaginic serum, followed by allergen and indicator serum as in the usual test. However, there was no clumping. Participation of lymphocytes could be similarly excluded by repeating the reagin-allergen-indicator serum incubations with the almost polymorph-free lymphocyte suspensions. The latter were prepared by brief sedimentation (400 *g*) of the lymphocyte-rich layer 'LY' which is normally discarded when preparing the leucocytes for the test (see under 'Preparation of washed leucocytes'). The lymphocytes were not agglutinated, presumably because they had not taken up any antibodies.

Romanovsky staining showed an occasional inclusion of basophilic and/or eosinophilic cells in the clumps, but the former were mostly found degranulated already after the first few washings of the leucocytes. Obviously, from the large numbers of polymorphs alone which can be seen to be involved in clump formation, the polymorphs had to be largely neutrophils.

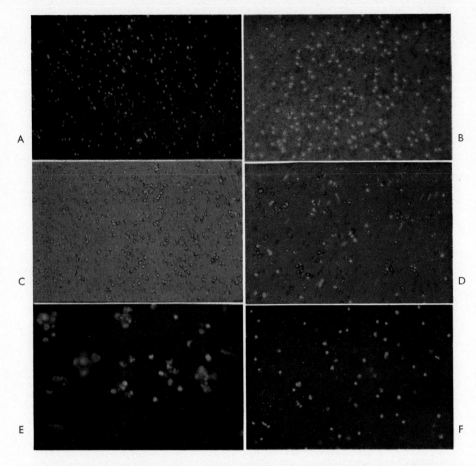

FIG. 35.28. Double-layer leucocyte agglutination. Micro-photographs after staining with acridine orange. A and B: negative controls (B enlarged); C, D and E: positive controls (D and E enlarged). F gives an example of the highly homogeneous preparations of lymphocytes that can be obtained from the LY layer.

(*Facing page* 1135)

Further confirmation that the agglutinates consisted of polymorphs was obtained by fluorescent staining with acridine orange, a dye giving apple-green fluorescent staining with DNA and brown to bright orange-red fluorescence with RNA [111, 112]. Therefore, lymphocytes—with their large nuclei

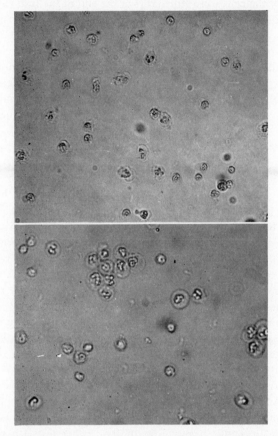

FIG. 35.27. Double-layer leucocyte agglutination. Micro-photographs of agglutination after treatment with Tuerk's fluid; top: negative control—cells are unagglutinated; bottom: positive results—agglutination of cells.

—show up as small green disks (with just a trace of peripheral orange) while polymorphs—which possess fairly large amounts of cytoplasmic RNA—show characteristic bright orange circular fluorescent patches (Fig. 35.28). When a drop of acridine orange solution is mixed with a drop of the agglutinated leucocyte preparation, it can readily be seen that the clumps all consist of comparatively large cells which contain brilliantly fluorescent (orange) patches (besides the green nuclei) and do not include small (green) lymphocytes, although the latter can be seen in the surrounding medium; red cells show up hardly at all and can only be seen with difficulty as black disks since the haemoglobin quenches fluorescence.

Dye exclusion experiments, according to Schrek, [113] indicated that 90–100 per cent of the cells were still viable at the end of the tests, i.e. just before adding the indicator serum to the antigen-treated antibody-sensitized cells.

Antibody type involved in the test

When originally working at room temperature [114], we found that human γG-antibodies as well as reagins were taken up although to a lesser extent, but there was little, if any, uptake of γG antibodies at 37° C. Similarly, rabbit antibodies also do not appear to become attached to human leucocytes.

Blind test of the method

Sera from untreated and treated (injections of pollen extract) grass pollen hay fever subjects, as well as from non-allergic subjects with negative skin tests to grass pollen extracts, were coded and tested blind, the coding key remaining in the possession of the physician responsible for collecting the bloods who had no further contact with the laboratory where the tests were done. The results were summarized in Table 35.8 which contains, in addition, results of passive haemagglutination tests ('BDB') which measure the γG antibodies for the pollen antigens, of monkey PCA tests and of antigen-induced histamine release in human lung as well as results of the skin tests done on the serum donors.

It can be seen that all but one of the normal nine control sera gave negative results by the DLLA method, as long as it was done at 37° C, but that there was a considerable amount of non-specific agglutination (in five out of nine sera) at room temperature. No false positives were obtained by the other two tests for reagins. The DLLA test scored as positive six out of the possible eight sera from untreated hay fever subjects and five out of the possible eight post-treatment sera. However, R14, one of the negatively scoring post-treatment sera, was also negative by the two other tests for reagins (PCA in monkeys and antigen-induced histamine release from reagin-treated human lung). A second DLLA-negative post-treatment serum (R35) gave equivocal results by the two other reagin tests and had an exceptionally high BDB titre (? blocking antibody titre). The BDB titre for the third DLLA-negative post-treatment serum was also fairly high, but no higher than for four other DLLA-positive post-treatment sera.

The patient giving negative results for reagins by all three tests with pollen antigens from *Dactylis glomerata* was recalled. The fact that his serum gave a BDB titre of 640 proved that no mix-up with a normal serum had occurred inadvertently and he was found to be only very slightly

TABLE 35.8

Comparison of blind DLLA results (at 37° C and at room temperature) with blind results obtained with two other tests for reagins (antigen-mediated histamine release from *in vitro* sensitized human lung and passive cutaneous anaphylaxis in monkeys) in relation to clinical status, skin tests and BDB titres.

Serial No. of patients	Clinical status	DLLA 37°C	RT	Histamine release from human lung (μg/g)	PCA (monkey) intradermal serum Neat	1/10	BDB test reciprocal titre	Skin tests
	Normal							
R07	control	—	—	—	—	—	10	—
R20	,,	—	+	—	—	—	20	—
R27	,,	—	—	—	—	—	20	—
R46	,,	—	+	—	—	—	20	—
R50	,,	—	+	—	—	—	20	—
R57	,,	?+	—	—	—	—	10	—
R61	,,	—	?−	—	—	—	10	—
R71	,,	—	?+	—	—	—	20	—
R81	,,	—	+	—	—	—	20	—
	Untreated							
R36	hay fever	—	+	+	+	+	20	++
R38	,,	+	+	+	+	+	20	++
R47	,,	+	?+	+	+	+	10	+++
R54	,,	+	+	+	+	+	20	++
R64	,,	+	?+	+	+	+	20	++
R68	,,	—	?+	+	+	+	40	++
R82	,,	+	—	+	+	+	20	+
R96	,,	+	—	+	—	—	20	+
	Treated hay fever*							Before After treatment
R14**		—	—	—	—	—	640	++** ++**
R26	,,	+	+	+	±	+	1280	++ ++
R35	,,	—	?+	+	±	+	5120	++ ++
R42	,,	+	—	+	—	+	1280	++ ++
R56	,,	—	?+	+	+	+	640	++ +
R62	,,	+	+	+	+	+	1280	+++ ++
R66	,,	+	?−	+	+	+	20	++ ++
R86	,,	+	+	+	+	+	640	++ +

DLLA results are given as average scores of triplicate tests. —, negative results, +, positive results. Widely discrepant or near-border line results being preceded by ?. RT = room temperature. BDB (bis-diazotized benzidine) agglutination results in triplicate, but single results for histamine release and PCA.

Skin tests are recorded as +, ++ and +++ according to size of reaction.

* All these patients had been treated during the current year with mixed grass pollen emulsion vaccine (Bencard Ltd) with the exception of R66 who had had an incomplete course of aqueous pollen injection treatment.

** This patient proved subsequently to have very weak skin tests for *Dactylis glomerata* (the antigen used in all the laboratory tests), but large skin responses for meadow (*Poa sp.* and wild oat (*Avena fatua*) grass pollens, and weak reactions for *Phleum pratense*.

skin-sensitive to our test antigen 'C' (cocksfoot—*Dactylis glomerata*) while giving good skin responses to pollen extracts of *Poa* sp. and *Avena fatua*.

Correct results were thus scored for twenty (eight plus six plus six) out of twenty-five sera by the DLLA method when done at 37° C, i.e. in 80 per cent of the cases. Table 35.8 shows that this compares with 100 per cent correct results for histamine release from human lung and 96 per cent correct results for PCA in monkeys.

In conclusion, the DLLA test is shown to be capable of demonstrating reagins in the great majority of cases. The main difficulty to be guarded against

TABLE 35.9
Eight tests for reagins summarized and compared

Test	Sensitivity Dilution end-point of serum	Challenging dose of allergen in Noon units	Accuracy	Total histamine per g test tissue (μg)	Sensitivity of test tissue to H in 10^{-9} g
PK	Usual:1/100 Occ: 1/1000 and higher	1–3 (as i.d. dose)	±20–30%	4–8 (human skin)	About 0·1 (i.d., no dye)
PCA (monkey)	Usual:1/10–1/60 Occ.: 1/100 and higher	100,000 i.v.	N.D., but likely as for PK	Similar to human skin	About 0·1 (i.d. with dye indic.)
Histamine release from human lung	Usual:1/10–1/20 Occ.: up to 1/30	10–10,000	Depends on number of tests done ±5–10%	Usual: 17 Range: 12–35	1–2 (guinea-pig ileum)
Contraction of monkey ileum	Usual:1/100–1/1000 Occ.: 1/10,000	1000–5000	Not known, but low	About 10	1–5 (colon: 5)
Contraction of human bronchi	1/10	1000–5000	Not known, but low	About 8	50–500
DLLA	1/10	3000	Not known, but low	Not relevant	Not relevant
Histamine release from human leucocytes	about 1/10	About 20	Not known, preliminary results only	About 0·15 per $1·3 \times 10^7$ leucocytes	Not relevant
Basophil degranulation (indirect test)	Not known	Variable, so as to give negative controls	Not known	10 per 10^7 cells	Not relevant

is non-specific agglutination of the leucocytes which could not be entirely suppressed. It has also to be admitted that the test, in its present form, is somewhat exacting, as well as a little tedious, as all the stages have to be done on the same day, since it is not possible to preserve leucocytes in a viable un-agglutinated state overnight. In a blind study, the test has nevertheless proved to correlate well with clinical results and with the results of two other tests for reagins in twenty-one out of the twenty-five cases investigated.

DISCUSSION

Together with antigen-induced histamine release from reagin-sensitized human leucocytes—and leaving aside Shelley's basophil degranulation test

[47] (which most probably measures antibodies other than reagins unless human basophils are used)—there are now, in addition to the PK transfer test, six further tests available for measuring reagins. Five of these as well as the PK test itself are described here. All the tests are based on the anaphylactic properties of reagins and it has to be admitted that none of the tests can be regarded as easy and convenient; they are either laborious (histamine release from leucocytes, DLLA) or hazardous (PK, PCA in monkeys) or expensive (monkey PCA and contraction of monkey ileum) or involve materials which are not commercially available (human lung, bronchi and

TABLE 35.9 (*continued*)

Time of incubation		No. of samples which can be done in 1 day	Second day required	Type of antibody involved in reaction			Cost of materials
With Ab (hours)	With Ag (minutes)			Reagin	γG	Rabbit	
24–140	20	50 and more on one volunteer	Yes, for challenging	Yes	No	No	Expl. animal = man Hazardous (serum jaundice)
16–30	10	50 and more per monkey in 1 hour	Yes, for challenging	Yes	No	No	Cost of monkey (plus 6 weeks' quarantine)
3	20	50 in afternoon or morning	Yes, for convenience, but can be finished 1st day	Yes	No	No	None—operational waste
1		3–4	No	Yes	No	Usually No	1 monkey for 8–12 tests (over 3 days)
	5	3–4	No	Yes	No	No	None—operational waste, but difficult to come by
3	25		No	Yes	±	No	Panel of leucocyte donors required
2–4	30	About 10	Yes, for convenience	Yes	Not known		Panel of leucocyte donors required
A few minutes (various modifications of test)	Many	Yes, for convenience (cell counts of stained slides)		Not known (probably NOT reagins unless human cells used)			Negligible

leucocytes—and man himself). The difficulty of assaying reagins arises, in essence, from the fact that all the tests (even those done *in vitro*) require live primate tissues; for in every case investigated, reagins, the anaphylactic antibodies of man, had no demonstrable anaphylactic affinity for species other than primates, either because they really intrinsically lack such an affinity or because their concentration in human serum is below the sensitivity of anaphylactic reactions in non-primates (see later). The sudden evolvement of so many alternatives to the PK test is nevertheless of considerable practical as well as theoretical importance.

Comparison of the tests
In Table 35.9 the sensitivity, accuracy and other details relevant to eight tests claimed to measure reagins are compiled.

Most of the tests depend on the measurement of histamine released during interaction of allergen with tissue-fixed reagin. This released histamine is either measured in a separate test (see Brocklehurst, Chapter 36) biologically, by the guinea-pig ileum test for histamine or chemically, by a fluorimetric method [48, 49]—or the challenged tissue is used as its own indicator; e.g. the wheal size in the PK test and the size of blue area in the PCA test are indicators of the amount of histamine released and therefore of reaginic potency; so is the antigen-induced contraction of reagin-sensitized smooth muscle preparations. Other things being equal, the 'self indicator' systems are the much more sensitive measures of reaginic activity, for all the released active substances are able to react directly on the target tissue in the concentration in which they are released, without being diluted out by the surrounding fluid; also, it has been suggested [27] that smooth muscle contraction may, to some extent, be a direct consequence of antigen–antibody interaction, and may not necessarily be mediated by histamine and other contractile substances released during the reaction. It is therefore not surprising that the most sensitive tests are the two self-indicatory *in vivo* tests (PK and monkey PCA) and the *in vitro* monkey ileum test—the latter being the most sensitive test of all. Although the bronchial test also is a self-indicatory method, this tissue can be seen to be much less sensitive to (added) histamine than monkey ileum; yet it must be emphasized that sensitivity to external histamine is not necessarily an indicator of the size of response produced by challenging the sensitized tissue with antigen; for the latter releases much more than just histamine and there may be other factors.

As we are concerned with measuring antibodies, sensitivity refers here to the amount of antibody capable of anaphylactically sensitizing a tissue, although anaphylactic sensitivity has also been described in terms of the amount of antigen capable of producing an anaphylactic response with antibody-sensitized tissue [115]. These two definitions of anaphylactic sensitivity are not necessarily identical as can be seen from the table.

Table 35.9 shows that only very few of the tests have, as yet, been explored quantitatively and that the lung test is the most accurate although not the most sensitive test. This is not unexpected since this method has the advantage of using aliquots of a reasonably homogeneous tissue preparation where each sample releases sufficient histamine for many duplicate estimations. The sensitivity of the test is limited by the fact that there is a spontaneous base-line release of histamine (the 1–3 per cent reported here for human lung is similar to the 1–2 per cent released from chopped guinea-pig lung reported by Mongar & Schild [116]) and the sensitivity of the test would not be improved by using still more sensitive methods of estimating histamine. For the same reason, accuracy, but not sensitivity, would be improved by using larger samples of chopped lung; a similar situation arises in histamine release from leucocytes, with a spontaneous histamine release of a similar order [50]. We have arbitrarily postulated a histamine release above 10 per cent as significant of reaginic activity in the lung test. The highest releases obtained by us were about 50 per cent of total histamine. The dose/response curves are reasonably steep (Fig. 35.15) and are similar to those shown by Colquhoun & Brocklehurst [95] for histamine release from chopped guinea-pig lung. Unfortunately, the measuring range is short, the curves flattening out (for guinea-pig as well as for human lung) once a histamine release of 50 per cent is reached; presumably a similar range will apply to antigen-induced histamine release from passively sensitized leucocytes. In this latter test accuracy could be improved as in the lung test by doing many duplicates with a reasonably homogeneous tissue. In practice, the number of samples that can be done is limited by leucocyte supply, as well as by the fact that the test is very time-consuming.

The lung test is more laborious than the *in vivo* methods, but not excessively so. PCA tests in monkeys are somewhat more sensitive than the lung test and are particularly easy and quick tests to do—as indeed is the PK test. All the other tests are rather inaccurate and no more sensitive than the lung test. Choice of test must obviously depend on what type of primate tissue is available and whether accuracy or sensitivity is the primary consideration in a particular situation. Although most of these tests are eminently suitable for distinguishing reaginic from non-reaginic sera and for determining reaginic specificity and although the tests were found to correlate well with clinical history and skin tests of the serum donors, they are none of them particularly suited to follow fractionations of reaginic sera; unless large quantities of serum are available, the PK test may still be the method of choice, since it enables one to assay with a fair degree of accuracy, highly diluted samples, and so entails little loss during fractionation. No very great dilution is possible with the lung test and samples containing 10 per cent of the starting activity may escape discovery unless highly potent sera are employed; and the highly sensitive monkey ileum test is very inaccurate. However, a combination of different tests may solve the problem without recourse to the PK test.

Reagins as anaphylactic antibodies par excellence *and their absolute amounts in human serum*
With a half-life of persistence of 13 days for reagins in human skin, compared with 8 hours for rabbit antibody in guinea-pig skin, one of the characteristics of anaphylactic antibodies—affinity for tissues—can be seen to be exceptionally highly developed in human reagins; also, exceptionally minute quantities suffice to produce anaphylactic sensitization. Ishizaka & Ishizaka [24] have recently deduced that as little as 10^{-5} μg reagin N may be sufficient to give a positive PK reaction, while the limiting sensitivity of PCA reactions given by

rabbit and guinea-pig antibodies in guinea-pig skin is said to be 0·003–0·01 μg N [84]; i.e. the anaphylactic response of (human) skin may be a hundred to a thousand times as strong for (human) reagins as for other antibodies. Whichever way it is considered, reagins emerge as particularly powerful anaphylactic antibodies—a fact well known to clinicians who know that mere traces of allergen can kill, with quantities very much smaller than those capable of killing anaphylactically sensitized guinea-pigs [60].

The above figure of 10^{-5} μg reagin N for a PK test can be used to arrive at some estimate of the amount of reagin in human serum. Assuming a PK titre of 1000, this gives about 0·01 μg reagin N/ml reaginic serum.

Antibodies involved in reaginic reactions and the question of species specificity
Table 35.10 summarizes our attempts to sensitize primate tissues with human γG and rabbit antibodies and non-primate tissues with human γG antibodies and reagins. From this, reagins appear to sensitize only homologous primate tissue, while the (for man) non-anaphylactic human γG antibodies appear to have affinity (and anaphylactic sensitizing power) for non-primate tissue—albeit to a lesser degree than the non-primate anaphylactic antibodies, that is, non-anaphylactic antibodies appear to be able to cross species barriers while anaphylactic-type antibodies do not. However, closer investigation shows that this generalization may not be justified. For while it is an experimental fact that reaginic sera do not sensitize guinea-pig tissues, this may have nothing to do with an intrinsic inability, but could be due to the low concentration of reagins; e.g. 0·01 μg reagin N/ml serum is within the lower limits of sensitivity (0·003–0·01 μg N) for rabbit antibody for the PCA reaction in guinea-pigs. And not only is this sensitivity known to be reduced in the presence of undiluted serum, but human antibodies are known to have about ten times less affinity for guinea-pig skin than rabbit antibodies (threshold values of 0·10–0·15 μg N [117]) that is, even 0·01 μg N of human γG antibody/ml serum would be too small an amount to sensitize guinea-pig skin.

The failure of human γG antibodies and rabbit antibodies to sensitize primate tissues stands on much firmer ground since high antibody concentrations could be employed. It is interesting to note that human γG antibodies, which have no anaphylactic affinity whatever for human skin, did have at least some such affinity for monkey skin, while rabbit antibodies have none. Arbesman's claim [58] that rabbit antibodies sensitize monkey ileum has not been supported here, but sera may vary; e.g. Sherman [118] found that certain specially prepared rabbit antisera gave positive PK tests in man.

Although it is, at this stage, on the whole correct to say that the anaphylactic antibodies of one species will not anaphylactically sensitize another species, while the non-anaphylactic antibodies of one species may have (fortuitous) anaphylactic affinity for other species (not always—ungulate antibodies were

TABLE 35.10

Demonstration of *in vitro* anaphylaxis in different tissues of two primate and one non-primate species after passive *in vitro* sensitization with different types of human and animal antibodies. Reactions after challenge with antigen corresponding to the sensitizing antibody: +, ±, positive responses (histamine release, contraction etc.); tr, trace; −, negative response; N.D., not done in this or other laboratories. All results obtained in this laboratory except for the following: *[59], **[50, 51], ***[95].

Antigen-induced reactions of the following sensitized tissues

Sensitizing antibody	Guinea-pig				Monkey				Man					
	Skin (PCA)	Lung	Ileum	Trachea	Skin (PCA)	Lung	Ileum	Trachea	Skin (PK)	Lung	Ileum*	Bronchi	Leucocytes**	DLLA
Human reaginic:														
Pollen reaginic serum	−	N.D.	−	−	+	N.D.	+	N.D.	+	+	+	+	+	+
Horse reaginic γG-free fraction	N.D.	N.D.	−	−	+	N.D.	+	N.D.	+	+	N.D.	+	N.D.	+
Human γG antibody														
Against horse serum	+	N.D.	+	−	−	N.D.	−	N.D.	−	−	N.D.	−	N.D.	N.D.
Against thyroglobulin	+	N.D.	±	±	N.D.	N.D.	−	N.D.	−	−	N.D.	−	N.D.	±
Against *Aspergillus fumigatus*	+	N.D.	N.D.	N.D.	N.D.	N.D.	N.D.	N.D.	N.D.	−	N.D.	N.D.	N.D.	N.D.
Rabbit antibody:														
Against egg albumin	+	+	+	+	−	N.D.	−	N.D.	−	−	N.D.	−	N.D.	−
Against pollen	+	+	+	+	−	N.D.	−	N.D.	−	−	N.D.	N.D.	N.D.	−
Guinea-pig antibody:*														
γ1 (guinea-pig 'reagin')	+	+	N.D.	N.D.	N.D.	N.D.	N.D.	N.D.	N.D.	N.D.	N.D.	N.D.	N.D.	N.D.
γ2 (guinea-pig 'γ-G')	tr	tr	N.D.	N.D.	N.D.	N.D.	N.D.	N.D.	N.D.	N.D.	N.D.	N.D.	N.D.	N.D.

found incapable of sensitizing guinea-pig skin), more quantitative studies may show this to be more apparent than real.

Further outlook

Despite the recent spate of tests capable of measuring reagins, there is obviously still room for the evolvement of a reasonably simple, accurate and sensitive *in vitro* test, particularly one that does not involve the use of primate tissue. Although it might be possible to attach reagins to globulins (or globulin fragments) with affinity for, say, guinea-pig tissues, this would be unlikely to bring success in view of the—compared with man—very low sensitivity of anaphylactic reactions in guinea-pigs. In other words, the problem of measuring reaginic antibodies now clearly emerges mainly as a sensitivity problem—there are now no intrinsic difficulties.

Summary

Six (two *in vivo* and four *in vitro*) tests for the assay of reagins are described in detail and a further two *in vitro* tests (not described) are included in the discussions. Sensitivities and difficulties involved in the tests are given in detail and it is shown that for practical purposes neither human γG nor rabbit antibodies have anaphylactic affinity for human tissues, although they do have anaphylactic affinity for guinea-pig tissues.

The half-life of persistence of reagins in human and monkey skin has been determined and it is shown that the anaphylactic properties of reagins for human tissues greatly surpass those of guinea-pig and rabbit antibodies for guinea-pig tissues. In view of this and the low concentrations of reagins in human serum, it is concluded that the sensitivity of tests for reagins has to be much higher than for any other antibodies. Failure to measure reagins by conventional tests may merely be a reflection of this and more concentrated solutions of reagins—if and when available—may well be measurable in the conventional manner.

ACKNOWLEDGMENTS

The author wishes to acknowledge closest collaboration from her colleagues with the experimental work reported here; Mr S.A.O'Sullivan, Mrs P.J.Frank and Mr C.R.West have shared in the lung and gut experiments, Mr R.A. Muirhead has been responsible for the protein fractionations, Miss M.E. Fitzpatrick for many of the DLLA tests and Mr R.C.Connolly has done agglutination and gel-diffusion tests. Lungs were obtained from Aintree Hospital, Liverpool, through the courtesy of Mr J.K.B.Waddington, Consultant Thoracic Surgeon, and staff, and latterly also from Broadgreen Hospital, Liverpool, through the courtesy of Mr F.R.Edwards, Consultant Thoracic Surgeon, and staff, to all of whom grateful thanks are expressed. Drs D.B.Macaulay (Consultant Allergist, Liverpool Allergy Clinic) and M.B.Macaulay (David Lewis Northern Hospital, Liverpool) have most kindly collected for us many hay fever as well as normal human sera and I also wish to thank the secretarial staff of the United Liverpool Hospital Board of Rodney Street, Liverpool, and numerous colleagues and friends who have allowed us to take blood from them. I also thank Dr R.E.C.Altuonyan of Benger's Ltd, Holmes Chapel, Cheshire, for hay fever sera. Hashimoto sera were obtained through the kindness of Drs D.Doniach and I.M.Roitt of the Middlesex Hospital, London, and Dr W.H.Cook and Mr P.Hawe of the David Lewis Northern Hospital, Liverpool. Dr A.W.Frankland of the Wright-Fleming Institute, London, very kindly supplied us with grass pollen. I further wish to thank Professor A.Wilson of this University for advice and hospitality in his laboratory with Schultz-Dale experiments. I am especially grateful to Dr W.E.Brocklehurst of Edinburgh University who most kindly came to initiate us into chopped-lung experiments at our own laboratory. Grateful thanks are further due to Professor B.G.Maegraith and Dr K.A. Fletcher of the Liverpool School of Tropical Medicine for allowing us to do PCA tests on their post-malarial monkeys and for tissues from moribund malarial monkeys. Dr K.A.Fletcher, Mr F.Swain and Dr Panata Migasena of the School of Tropical Medicine have also been most helpful with advice about the handling of these animals and with injections which have been greatly appreciated. I further wish to thank Dr A.C.Laursen of Glaxo Laboratories, Stoke Poges, who has sent us a number of ileums from Patas monkeys. Thanks are also due to Miss P.Franklin of the author's laboratories and Mr J.Brady of the Liverpool School of Tropical Medicine who have been responsible for the photographs.

The author further wishes to acknowledge financial assistance from the North West Cancer Research Fund, the Asthma Research Council and the United and Regional Liverpool Hospital Boards.

Finally, thanks are due to the Editors of *Immunology* for permission to reproduce material from papers published or submitted by me for publication to this journal.

Referencee

[1] PRAUSNITZ C. & KUESTNER H. (1921) Studien ueber die Ueberempfindlichkeit. *Zbl. Bakt., Abt. I. (Orig)* **86,** 160
[2] BLACKLEY C.H. (1873) *Experimental Researches on Hay Fever.* Balliere, Tindall & Cox; reprinted 1959, London: Dawson's of Pall Mall

[3] COCA A.F. & GROVE E.F. (1925) Studies in hypersensitivity. XIII. A study of the atopic reagins. *J. Immun.* **10,** 445

[4] AUGUSTIN R. (1955) Chemical, biochemical and immunological advances in allergy, with special reference to pollens and their standardization. *Quart. Rev. Allergy* **9,** 504

[5] FISHER J.P., MIDDLETON E. JR. & MENZEL A.E.O. (1956) Studies on passive cutaneous anaphylaxis with serum of allergic patients. *J. Allergy* **27,** 256

[6] FISHER J.P. & COOKE R.A. (1957) Passive cutaneous anaphylaxis in the guinea pig. An immunological and pathological study. *J. Allergy* **28,** 151

[7] AUGUSTIN R., CONNOLLY R.C. & LLOYD G.M. (1964) Atopic reagins as a prototype of cytophilic antibodies. *Proc. 11th Colloquium Protides Biol. Fluids, Bruges 1963,* pp. 56–66. Amsterdam: Elsevier Publ. Co., 1964

[8] FISHER J.P. & CONNELL J.T. (1962) Passive cutaneous anaphylaxis in the guinea pig with serum of allergic patients treated with ragweed extract emulsions. *J. Allergy* **33,** 59

[9] FINE A.J. & ABRAM L.E. (1960) The period of sensitization in immigrant hay fever patients. *J. Allergy* **31,** 375

[10] HUGHES R.F. (1959) Incidence of hay fever in recent immigrants to Canada. *Canad. M.A.J.* **80,** 651

[11] SHILKRET H.H. & LAZAROWITZ L.C. (1953) Hay fever in immigrants. *Ann. Allergy* **11,** 194

[12] AUGUSTIN R. & HAYWARD B.J. (1960) Grass pollen and mould antigens and their antibodies, including reagins. *Proc. 7th Colloquium Protides Biol. Fluids, Bruges 1959,* pp. 314–322. Amsterdam: Elsevier Publ. Co., 1960

[13] AUGUSTIN R. (1960) On the nature of the antibody response to allergens. *Proc. Symposium 'Mechanisms of antibody formation', 1959,* pp. 94–104. Prague: Publ. House Czech. Acad. Sci.

[14] AUGUSTIN R. & HAYWARD B.J. (1960) Human reagins to grass pollens and moulds: Their purification and physico-chemical characterization. *Immunology* **3,** 45–73

[15] World Health Organization meeting on 'Nomenclature of human immunoglobulins' (1964). *Bull. Wld Hlth Org.* **30,** 447

[16] AUGUSTIN R. (1960) Immunological aspects of diagnosis and treatment in allergy. *Proc. Europ. Acad. Allergy, Barcelona* 1960, pp. 19–26. Leiden: H.E.Stenfert Kroese N.V.

[17] AUGUSTIN R. (1961) Precipitins, reagins and blocking antibodies. *Acta Allergol.* **16,** 473

[18] HEREMANS J.F. & VAERMAN J.P. (1962) β_2A-globulin as a possible carrier of allergic reaginic activity. *Nature, Lond.* **193,** 1091

[19] FIREMAN P., VANNIER W.E. & GOODMAN H.C. (1963) The association of skin-sensitizing antibody with the β_2A-globulins in sera from ragweed-sensitive patients. *J. exp. Med.* **117,** 603

[20] ISHIZAKA K., ISHIZAKA T. & HORNBROOK M.M. (1963) Blocking of Prausnitz-Kustner sensitization with reagin by normal human β_2A-globulin. *J. Allergy* **34,** 395

[21] VAERMAN J.P., EPSTEIN W., FUDENBERG H. & ISHIZAKA K. (1964) Direct demonstration of reagin activity in purified γ_1A-globulin. *Nature, Lond.* **203,** 1046

[22] LOVELESS M.H. (1964) Reagin production in a healthy male who forms no detectable β_2A immunoglobulins. *Fed. Proc.* **23,** 403

[23] ROCKEY J.H., HANSON L.A., HEREMANS J.F. & KUNKEL H.G. (1964) β_2A aglobulinemia in two healthy men. *J. lab. clin. Med.* **63,** 205

[24] ISHIZAKA K. & ISHIZAKA T. (1966) Physico-chemical properties of reaginic antibody. 1. Association of reaginic activity with an immunoglobulin other than γA– or γG–globulin. *J. Allergy* **37,** 169

[25] REID R.T., MINDEN P. & FARR R.S. (1966) Reaginic activity associated with IgG immunoglobulin. *J. exp. Med.* **123,** 845

[26] DALE H.H. (1913) The anaphylactic reaction of plain muscle in the guinea pig. *J. Pharmacol. exptl. Therap.* **4,** 167, 517

[27] DALE H.H. (1952) The mechanism of anaphylaxis. *Acta Allergol.* **5,** 191; (1958) Biochemical aspects of hypersensitivity. *Proc. III Int. Congr. Allergol.,* p. 337

[28] BENACERRAF B. & KABAT E.A. (1949) A quantitative study of passive anaphylaxis in the guinea pig. V. The latent period in passive anaphylaxis and its relation to the dose of rabbit anti-ovalbumin. *J. Immun.* **62,** 517

[29] OVARY Z., BENACERRAF B. & BLOCH K.J. (1963) Properties of guinea pig 7S antibodies. II. Identification of antibodies involved in passive cutaneous and systemic anaphylaxis. *J. exp. Med.* **117,** 951

[30] WHITE R.G., JENKINS G.C. & WILKINSON P.C. (1963) The production of skin-sensitizing antibody in the guinea pig. *Int. Arch. Allergy* **22,** 156

[31] MOTA I. (1963) Mast cells and anaphylaxis. *Ann. N.Y. Acad. Sci.* **103,** 264

[32] ONOUE K., YAGI Y. & PRESSMAN D. (1966) Isolation of rabbit IgA antihapten antibody and demonstration of skin-sensitizing activity in homologous skin. *J. exp. Med.* **123,** 173

[33] ZVAIFLER N.J. & BECKER E.L. (1966) Rabbit anaphylactic antibody. *J. exp. Med.* **123,** 935

[34] KATZ G. (1940) Histamine release from blood cells in anaphylaxis *in vitro. Science* **91,** 221

[35] KATZ G. & COHEN S. (1941) Experimental evidence of histamine release in allergy. *J. Am. Med. Assoc.* **117,** 1782

[36] SQUIRE T.L. & LEE H.J. (1947) Lysis *in vitro* of sensitized leukocytes by ragweed antigen. *J. Allergy* **18,** 156

[37] FAVOUR C.B. (1947) Lytic effect of bacterial products on lymphocytes of tuberculous animals. *Proc. Soc. exp. Biol. Med.* **65,** 269

[38] CHAMBERS V.V., HUDSON B.H. & GLASER J. (1958) A study of the reactions of human polymorphonuclear leukocytes to various allergens. *J. Allergy* **29,** 93

[39] SPAIN W.C., STRAUSS M.B. & NEUMANN E. (1950) *In vitro* release of histamine by hypersensitive (allergic) serum in contrast to immune (treated) allergic serum in antigen and normal rabbit blood mixtures. *J. Allergy* **21,** 318

[40] WAKSMAN B.H. & GAULITZ D. (1953) Specific white cell lysis production by combination of rabbit antiserum to purified protein (ovalbumin, bovine gamma globulin) with homologous antigen. *J. Immun.* **70,** 331

[41] HARTMAN J.D. & HOCH W.S. (1955) Changes in blood leucocytes resulting from an antigen-antibody reaction. *Amer. J. Physiol.* **183,** 214

[42] BLACK A.P. (1956) A new diagnostic method in allergic disease. *Pediatrics* **17,** 716

[43] MIDDLETON E., SHERMAN W.B., FLEMING W.J. & VAN ARSDEL P. (1960) Characteristics of allergic histamine release from leukocytes. *J. Allergy* **31,** 448

[44] PETTIT H., SULLIVAN H.E. & HART E.D. (1961) Leukocytolysis in presence of allergenic extracts. *J. Allergy* **32,** 30

[45] VAN ARSDEL P. & MIDDLETON E. (1961) The effect of hyposensitization on histamine release. *J. Allergy* **32,** 348

[46] FRANKLIN W. & LOWELL F.C. (1949) Failutre of ragweed pollen extract to destroy white cells from ragweed-sensitive patients. *J. Allergy* **20,** 375

OO*

[47] SHELLEY W.B. (1963) Indirect basophil degranulation test of allergy to penicillin and other drugs. *J. Am. Med. Assoc.* **184,** 171

[48] SHORE P.A., BURKHALTER A. & COHN V.H. JR. (1959) A method for the fluorimetric assay of histamine in tissues. *J. Pharmacol. and Exp. Therap.* **127,** 182

[49] KREMZNER L.T. & WILSON I.B. (1961) A procedure for the determination of histamine. *Biochem. biophys. Acta* **50,** 364

[50] LICHTENSTEIN L.M. & OSLER A.G. (1964) Studies on the mechanisms of hypersensitivity phenomena. IX. Histamine release from human leukocytes by ragweed pollen antigen. *J. exp. Med.* **120,** 507

[51] VAN ARSDEL P. & SELLS C.J. (1963) Antigenic histamine release from passively sensitized human leucocytes. *Science* **141,** 1190

[52] SCHILD H.O., HAWKINS D.F., MONGOR J.L. & HERXHEIMER H. (1951) Reactions of isolated human asthmatic lung and bronchial tissue to a specific antigen. *Lancet* **ii,** 376

[53] AUGUSTIN R., O'SULLIVAN S.A. & CONNOLLY R.C. (1966) Reagins as the anaphylactic antibodies of man. Feb. Meeting Brit. Allergy Soc. (*Acta allergol.* **31,** 430)

[54] FITZPATRICK M.E., CONNOLLY R.C., LEA D.J., O'SULLIVAN S.A., AUGUSTIN R. & MACAULAY M.B. (1967) *In vitro* detection of human reagins by double layer leukocyte agglutination method and controlled blind study. *Immunology* **12,** 1

[55] HARTLEY P. (1939) Passive sensitization *in vitro. Proc. III congr. intern. Microbiol., New York*, p. 343. Intern. Assoc. Microbiol.

[56] KULKA A.M. (1943) Studies on antibody–antigen mixtures. II. The effect on normal living excised tissue and its dependence on the presence of free antibody in the mixture. *J. Immun.* **46,** 235

[57] HALPERN B.N., LIACOPOULOS P., LIACOPOULOS-BRIOT N., BINAGHI L.R. & VAN NEER F. (1959) Patterns of *in vitro* sensitization of isolated smooth muscle tissues with antibody. *Immunology* **2,** 351

[58] ARBESMAN C.E., GIRARD P. & ROSE N.R. (1964) *In vitro* passive sensitization of monkey ileum with human sera. *J. Allergy* **35,** 535

[59] KOVACS C.B.A., GOODFRIEND L. & ROSE B. (1964) *In vitro* detection of reagins to ragweed. (Abstr. 2786) *Fed. Proc.* **24,** 633

[60] AUGUSTIN R. & HAYWARD B.J. (1962) Grass pollen allergens. IV. The isolation of some of the principal allergens of *Phleum pratense* and *Dactylis glomerata* and their sensitivity spectra in patients. *Immunology* **5,** 424

[61] COCA A.F. (1922) Studies in specific hypersensitiveness. V. The preparation of fluid extracts and solutions for use in the diagnosis and treatment of the allergies with notes on the collection of pollens. *J. Immun.* **7,** 163

[62] AUGUSTIN R., CONNOLLY R.C., LLOYD G.M. & RICKARDS J. (1966) Reaginic precipitins to grass pollens in allergic and non-allergic subjects (in preparation)

[63] STAVITSKY A.B. & ARQUILLA E.R. (1958) Studes of proteins and antibodies by specific hemagglutination and hemolysis of protein-conjugated erythrocytes. *Int. Arch. Allergy* **13,** 1

[64] HAYWARD B.J. & AUGUSTIN R. (1957) Quantitative gel diffusion methods for assay of antigens and antibodies. *Int. Arch. Allergy* **11,** 192

[65] GAY L.N. & CHANT E. (1927) Passive transfer of hypersensitivity. *Bull. Johns Hopkins Hosp.* **40,** 270

[66] PAYLING-WRIGHT G. & HOPKINS S.J. (1941) Reversed passive skin sensitization to horse serum in human beings. *J. Path. Bact.* **53,** 243

[67] HARLEY D. (1953) The prick method of skin testing. *Int. Arch. Allergy* **4,** 455

[68] SQUIRE J.R. (1950) The relationship between horse dandruff and horse serum antigens in asthma. *Clin. Sci.* **9**, 127

[69] AUGUSTIN R. (1959) Grass pollen allergens. I. Paper chromatography and membrane diffusion studies. *Immunology* **2**, 1

[70] FRANKLAND A.W. & AUGUSTIN R. (1962) Grass pollen antigens effective in treatment. *Clin. Sci.* **23**, 95

[71] STANWORTH D.R. & KUHNS W.J (1965) Quantitative studies on the assay of human skin sensitizing antibodies (reagins). I. An examination of factors affecting the accuracy of the Prausnitz-Kuestner (PK) test. *Immunology* **8**, 323

[72] LOVELESS M.H. (1940) Immunological studies of pollinosis. I. The presence of two antibodies related to the same pollen antigen in the serum of treated hay fever patients. *J. Immun.* **38**, 25

[73] LOVELESS M.H. (1941) Immunological studies of pollinosis. II. Passive sensitization of man through transfusion. *J. Immun.* **41**, 15

[74] BECKER E.L. & RAPPAPORT B.Z. (1948) Quantitative studies in skin testing. II. The form of the dose-response curve utilizing a quantitative response. *J. Allergy* **19**, 317

[75] SPIES J.R., BERNTON H.S. & CHAMBERS D.C. (1960) Migration of intracutaneously injected cottonseed allergen. *J. Allergy* **31**, 175

[76] KUHNS W.J. (1961) Disappearance of diphtheria antitoxin from skin. *Proc. Soc. exp. Biol.* **108**, 63

[77] HENOCQ E., RELYVELD E.H. & RAYNAUD M. (1962) La sensibilisation aux antigènes diphthériques. *Int. Arch. Allergy* **20**, 262

[78] OVARY Z. & BIER E.G. (1953) Quantitative studies on passive cutaneous anaphylaxis in the guinea pig and its relationship to the Arthus phenomenon. *J. Immun.* **71**, 6

[79] CAULFIELD A.H.W., BROWN N.H. & WATERS E.T. (1936) Suitability of the monkey (*Macacus rhesus*) as a recipient for the Prausnitz-Kustner reactions. *Proc. Soc. exp. Biol. Med.* **35**, 109

[80] STRAUSS H.W. (1937) Studies in experimental hypersensitiveness in the rhesus monkey II. Passive local cutaneous sensitization with human reaginic sera. *J. Immun.* **32**, 251

[81] WALZER M., GRAY I., STRAUSS H.W. & LIVINGSTONE S. (1938) Studies in experimental hypersensitiveness in the rhesus monkey. IV. The allergic reaction in passively locally sensitized abdominal organs (a preliminary report). *J. Immun.* **34**, 91

[82] LAYTON L.L., YAMANAKA E., LEE S. & GREEN T.W. (1962) Multiple allergies to the pollen and seed antigens of *Ricinus communis* (castor bean). *J. Allergy* **33**, 232–235, 257, 271

[83] LAYTON L.L., YAMANAKA E., GREENE F.C. & PERLMAN N.F. (1963) Atopic reagins to penicillin, pollens and seeds; thermolability, titer and persistence in the skin of passively sensitized Macaque monkeys. *Int. Arch. Allergy* **23**, 87, 94, 176

[84] OVARY Z. (1958) Immediate reactions in the skin of experimental animals provoked by antibody–antigen interaction. *Progress in Allergy* **5**, 459

[85] BUCKLEY R.H. & METZGAR R.S. (1965) The use of non-human primates for studies of reagins. *J. Allergy* **36**, 382

[86] LAYTON L.L., LEE S. & DE EDS F. (1961) Diagnosis of human allergy utilizing passive skin-sensitization in the monkey (*Macaca irus*). *Proc. Soc. exp. Biol. Med.* **108**, 623

[87] TAYLOR S.H. & THORP J.M. (1959) Properties and biological behaviour of Coomassie blue. *Brit. Heart J.* **21**, 492

[88] ROSE N.R., KENT J.H., REISMAN R.E. & ARBESMAN C.E. (1964) Passive sensitization of monkey with human sera. *J. Allergy* **35**, 520

[89] FEINBERG J.G., DEWDNEY J.M. & TEMPLE A. (1965) Serum sickness in guinea pigs. *Int. Arch. Allergy* **27**, 175

[90] LAYTON L.L. (1965) Passive transfer of human atopic allergies into primates. *J. Allergy* **36**, 523

[91] MONGAR J.L. & SCHILD H.O. (1957) Effect of temperature on the anaphylactic reaction. *J. Physiol. (London)* **135**, 320

[92] MONGAR J.L. & SCHILD H.O. (1958) The effect of calcium and pH on the anaphylactic reaction. *J. Physiol. (London)* **140**, 272

[93] BROCKLEHURST W.E., HUMPHREY J.H. & PERRY W.L.M. (1961) The *in vitro* uptake of rabbit antibody by chopped guinea pig lung and its relationship to anaphylactic sensitization. *Immunology* **4**, 67

[94] BAKER A.R., BLOCH K.J. & AUSTEN K.F. (1964) *In vitro* passive sensitization of chopped guinea pig lung by guinea pig 7S antibodies. *J. Immun.* **93**, 525

[95] COLQUHOUN D. & BROCKLEHURST W.E. (1965) Passive sensitization of skin and lung by guinea pig immunoglobulins. *Immunology* **9**, 591

[96] MONGAR J.L. & SCHILD H.O. (1953) Quantitative measurement of the histamine releasing activity of a series of mono-alkyl amines using minced guinea pig lung. *Brit. J. Pharmacol.* **8**, 103

[97] HOLCZABEK W. (1963) Die Mastzellen der Lunge des Menschen. *Dtsch. Ztschr. gesamt. gerichtl., Med.* **54**, 175

[98] MOTA I. (1959) Effect of antigen versus octylamine on mast cell and histamine content of sensitized guinea pig tissues. *J. Physiol. (Lond)* **147**, 425

[99] HUMPHREY J.H. & MOTA I. (1959) The mechanism of anaphylaxis: Specificity of antigen-induced mast cell damage in anaphylaxis in the guinea pig. *Immunology* **2**, 31

[100] BROCKLEHURST W.E. (1960) The release of histamine and formation of a slow reacting substance (SRS-A) during anaphylactic shock. *J. Physiol. (London)* **151**, 416

[101] CHAKRAVARTY, N. (1960) The occurrence of a lipid-soluble smooth muscle stimulating principle ('SRS') in anaphylactic reaction. *Acta physiol. Scand.* **48**, 167

[102] AUSTEN K.F. & BROCKLEHURST W.E. (1961) Anaphylaxis in chopped guinea pig lung. II. Enhancement of the anaphylactic release of histamine and slow-reacting substance by certain dibasic aliphatic acids and inhibition by monobasic fatty acids. *J. exp. Med.* **113**, 541

[103] BOURA A., MONGAR J.L. & SCHILD H.O. (1954) Improved automatic apparatus for pharmacological assays on isolated antigens. *Brit. J. Pharmacol.* **9**, 24

[104] CASTILLO J.C. & DE BEER E.J. (1947) The tracheal chain. I. A preparation for the study of antispasmodics with particular reference to bronchodilator drugs. *J. Pharmacol.* **90**, 104

[105] ROSA L.M. & McDOWALL R.J. (1951) The action of the local hormones on the isolated human bronchus. *Acta allergol.* **4**, 293

[106] HAWKINS D.F. & SCHILD H.O. (1951) The action of drugs on isolated human bronchial chains. *Brit. J. Pharmacol.* **6**, 82

[107] BHOOLA K.D., COLLIER H.O.J., SCHACHTER M. & SHORLEY P.G. (1962) Action of some peptides on bronchial muscle. *Brit. J. Pharmacol.* **19**, 190

[108] BERRY P.A. & COLLIER H.O.J. (1964) Broncho constrictor action and antagonism of a slow reacting substance from anaphylaxis of guinea pig isolated lung. *Brit. J. Pharmacol.* **23**, 201

[109] BROCKLEHURST W.E. (1962) Slow reacting substance and related compounds. *Progress in Allergy* **6**, 539

[110] Augustin R. (1963) Allergens and other antigens of grass pollens: Their isolation, characterization and standardization in relation to immune responses evoked in animals and man. *Fifth European Congr. Allergy, Basel* 1962, pp. 137–146. Selbstverlag Schweiz. Allergieges (Druck: Schwabe & Co. Basle 1963)

[111] Schiffer L.M. (1962) Fluorescence microscopy with acridine orange: A study of hemopoetic cells in fixed preparations. *Blood* **10**, 200

[112] Bertalanffy F.D. (1960) Fluorescence microscopy for the rapid diagnosis of malignant cells by exfoliative cytology. *Mikroskopie (Vienna)* **15**, 67

[113] Schrek R. (1936) A method for counting the viable cells in normal and malignant cell suspension. *Am. J. Cancer* **28**, 389

[114] Ridges A.P. & Augustin R. (1964) An *in vitro* test for atopic reagins by double layer leukocyte agglutination. *Nature, Lond.* **202**, 667

[115] Dale M.M. (1965) The applicability of anaphylactic tests in studies of antigen mixtures. I. The sensitivity of the tests, and II. The discriminatory capacity of the tests. *Immunology* **8**, 435–443, 444

[116] Mongar J.L. & Schild H.O. (1957) Inhibition of the anaphylactic reaction. *J. Physiol (London)* **135**, 301

[117] Ovary Z. & Biozzi G. (1954) Passive sensitization of the skin of the guinea pig with human antibody. *Int. Arch. Allergy* **5**, 241

[118] Sherman W.B. (1953) Experimental production of skin-sensitizing antibodies. In *The Nature and Significance of the Antibody Response*, pp. 126–144, ed. Pappenheimer A.M. Jr. New York: Columbia University Press

CHAPTER 36

The Assays of Mediators in Hypersensitivity Reactions

W.E.BROCKLEHURST

Introduction

The list of substances which may play an active part in the production of the complex pattern of allergic manifestations is considerable. Fortunately the evidence implicating most of them is indirect, so that the need, indeed the opportunity, for making a quantitative assessment does not arise.

If the mediator is extremely labile *in vivo*, or if the reaction is protracted, it may only be possible to infer that it was involved by showing an increase in a characteristic metabolite or the diminution of stores of the active substance itself or its precursors. The metabolites will generally not be susceptible to biological assay, but may be assayed chemically. The precursor may usually be activated ready for assay, but to do this quantitatively may be difficult because enzymes in the tissue or extract will often cause severe loss of biological activity. Where stores of active substance are present in a tissue loss by enzyme action may be minimized by cold, or avoided by dropping the tissue into boiling water or an appropriate solvent.

The substances which are known to be involved in allergic reactions are, in historical sequence, histamine, slow-reacting substance (of anaphylaxis), 5-hydroxytryptamine ('serotonin') and bradykinin (or closely related kinins). Acetylcholine has never been demonstrated, but the method and sensitivity of the biological assay may nevertheless be of interest. Each of these substances can be assayed at very low concentration on selected isolated tissues. In the case of histamine and 5-HT (5-hydroxytryptamine) there are also physicochemical procedures which permit evaluation of somewhat greater concentrations.

The choice of the method of assay

It is important to appreciate the less obvious disadvantages of the biological and chemical methods of estimation.

The machine, usually an expensive spectro-fluorimetric device, is unlikely to drift or fail half-way through the assay—the tissue often will, and on some days may not be sufficiently sensitive and stable for use. The machine cannot distinguish the active material from closely related molecules. These are often quite difficult to separate chemically and the process frequently involves serious loss. Purification adds to the labour, and manipulation affords chances of error—for very small samples it may be impractical. The solutions must be absolutely clear.

The biological method will often permit the use of crude samples and will record only active materials, but it is necessary (at least in initial experiments) to use antagonists to show that the contraction is due to the substance being evaluated. Satisfactorily specific antagonists of histamine and 5-HT are available. The assay of histamine is the simplest, and usually affords a reliable assessment of the intensity of antigen–antibody reactions of immediate type.

General considerations concerning biological assay

The tissues suggested for bioassay will cover all five substances and permit assays accurate to ± 10 per cent with comparatively little labour *once the assay has started*. This accuracy is possible because these tissues when properly used all show a steep dose-response relationship—i.e. there is a considerable increase in response for a moderate increase in dose. Bradykinin, SRS-A (slow reacting substance of anaphylaxis) and ACh (acetylcholine) can only be assayed biologically. In the case of bradykinin and SRS-A, characterization by inhibitors is not possible, and procedures such as parallel quantitative assay and destruction by enzyme action may be necessary in preliminary experiments to show that the assay is truly that of the supposed substance. 'Parallel quantitative assay' is the comparison of the substance under test and the authentic material with which it is supposed to be identical. Assay on at least three different kinds of test tissue should give the same assay value in each case.

In the course of routine assay, it is usual to compare the authentic and test samples at two different dose levels, and if the assay value at the different levels of comparison is not the same, the two substances cannot be identical. The difficulty may be resolved by preliminary purification or by the use of antagonists to exclude interference by other active substances including the presence of K^+ or other ions in excess. Comparison at two dose levels is called a $2+2$ assay, and if there is a sufficient number of tests, performed in a random sequence to offset interference between one dose and the next, the results can be treated mathematically and the accuracy of the assay established (Schild [1]).

Usually an assay value which is only approximate is all that is needed, and in many cases may be all that is practicable because the size of the sample is small. Then, a 2+1 assay is performed in which two slightly different doses of authentic substance are used alternately to give two slightly different levels of response, and the test sample is diluted until it gives a response which matches one of these, or falls between them so that interpolation is possible. It must be remembered that all dose-response lines are sigmoid, but may be converted to a linear form by plotting response upon the logarithm of the dose. The part of the sigmoid line between about 30 per cent and 70 per cent of the maximum response is regarded for purposes of interpolation as straight over short distances. This is also the steepest part of the line and therefore provides the most accurate assay. It is usual to begin an assay with the lower of the standard doses giving 30–40 per cent of the maximum contraction, because the response to a given dose usually increases as the assay proceeds.

General instructions for setting up isolated organs

The animal is killed instantaneously, usually by a blow on the head; there is no need to exsanguinate. The organ is dissected out quickly and cleanly, so that it may be washed in the physiological saline to be used in the organ bath, and is then ready for setting up without further handling. The tissue should be grasped with forceps only in parts which will not be used in the final preparation, and must not be exposed to gut contents or any other noxious substance. Care must be taken not to stretch it, and this includes distension whilst washing through the lumen. Plenty of the appropriate physiological saline, at room temperature (or a little warmer), should be available for washing. A triangular cutting needle as used for skin sutures is satisfactory for passing the threads through the tissue, because this makes a hole large enough for the wet thread to pass without undue resistance. If it is necessary to touch the tissue with the fingers, these must be clean and moistened with the physiological saline.

The apparatus must be quite ready to receive the tissue. All vessels must be clean and the whole apparatus must be thoroughly washed out with distilled water both at the end of the experiment and the start of the next. Red rubber tubing should be avoided, as filler and anti-oxidant substances are toxic to tissue. Unvulcanized latex, silicone rubber, or PVC intended for surgical or transfusion purposes are all satisfactory, but should be soaked in water and washed through for 24 hours before being used for the first time. Clips for closing tubes from the outside are more satisfactory than stopcocks. Fittings inside the bath, such as oxygen tube or tissue anchorage, are best of glass, but polythene can be used, and a very little stainless steel or silver is also permissible. Before receiving the tissue, the bath should be at the correct temperature, should have been flushed through with several changes of the bathing solution and have the oxygen supply turned on.

The tissue should be exposed to the air for only a few moments whilst being fixed in the bath, and should at once be washed with two changes of bathing solution and then left to settle down with the bath fluid being changed (automatically) about every 2 minutes. Standard (authentic drug) solutions should be made fresh and kept in ice during the experiment. Final dilutions of the solutions should not be left unused for more than 1 hour and, in the case of bradykinin and purified SRS-A, are best kept in polythene or silicone-treated vessels to avoid loss by adsorption.

Extensive literature on assay methods and apparatus can be traced by reference to the *Handbook of Experimental Pharmacology* [2]. The details given are those preferred by the author.

TABLE 36.1

Composition of physiological saline solutions (g/L)

	Locke (1901)	Tyrode (1910)	Krebs-Henseleit (1932)	De Jalon (1940)
NaCl	9·2	8·0	6·87	9·0
KCl	0·42	0·2	0·4	0·42
CaCl$_2$	0·24	0·2	0·28	0·06
MgCl$_2$	—	0·1	—	—
MgSO$_4$	—	—	0·14	—
NaH$_2$PO$_4$	—	0·05	0·14	—
NaHCO$_3$	—	1·0	2·1	0·5
Glucose	1·0	1·0	2·0	0·5

Only glass distilled water or good quality ion-exchange water and analytical grade reagents should be used; even so some samples of glucose are unsuitable.

Note. The CaCl$_2$ and MgCl$_2$ should be kept as concentrated solutions (e.g. 0·2 g/ml) made from the hydrated crystalline salts, and calculated to correct for water content. When all the salts have been dissolved and the solution made up almost to volume, the Ca and Mg solutions are mixed in. The bicarbonate may be added solid, but must be the *last* ingredient.

Assays of histamine and SRS-A

A guinea-pig of 300–500 g, which has had an adequate diet including fresh greens, is killed by a sharp blow on the head, or by dislocation of the neck.

(It is best, though not essential, to have given the animal no food for the preceding few hours.) The abdomen is opened widely in the midline, and the caecum located. Very near the ileo-caecal valve is a larger Peyer's patch, cut the ileum just above this and dissect the mesentery away cleanly as the ileum is lifted free. Do not stretch the ileum, or handle it, or let it come in contact with gut contents. Take about 9 in. and make a cut half-way through at the proximal end. Here insert the tip of a tube holding about 50 ml Tyrode solution and wash through the lumen of the gut thoroughly with the whole piece of tissue immersed in Tyrode solution. Cut two lengths (of about 2 in.) from the lower end of the ileum, for use, and store the whole in clean Tyrode solution at laboratory temperature.

There are several ways of attaching the tissue to the fixed support, and to the thread which leads to the lever or isotonic recording device. Sewing cotton is satisfactory, and separate threads are passed through one wall of the gut about 3 mm from each end, using a triangular cutting needle. The lower end of the ileum is fixed to the oxygenation tube, which acts as an anchor. (It is sometimes an advantage to split the tissue from the bottom nearly to the top along the line of attachment of the mesentery.) The lever should be truly isotonic and free-moving, and is loaded to exert a pull of 0·5 g on the ileum. If a kymograph* is used, the writing point must be 'frictionless' (e.g. fine rounded glass) and is usually mounted on a swinging arm, the moments about the pivot being arranged so that the pressure of the writing point on the kymograph is approximately constant for movements of the lever 10° either way from the horizontal position. A lever magnification of about 5:1 is suitable.

Make sure the organ bath is ready and at 37° C. Place the tissue in a Petri dish containing Tyrode solution, fix one end to the oxygen tube and leave a long thread at the other end for attachment to the lever. Carry the tissue on the oxygen tube during transfer to the organ bath. Fix the oxygen tube and adjust to give a gentle stream of bubbles. Attach the long thread from the tissue to the lever with a small piece of plasticine and check the tension exerted on the tissue. Replace the bath fluid, leave to relax for a few minutes, give a series of 10–20 small doses of histamine (e.g. 5 ng/ml) first, then raise the dose to 10 μg/ml if no satisfactory contraction has occurred. The doses actually used for assay will depend on the response of the tissue, but doses larger than 10 ng/ml should never be needed, and 5 ng/ml or less is desirable. The time-cycle suggested for histamine assay is:

Add drug and wait 20 seconds or until the maximum response has passed.
Drain and refill bath, stop kymograph.
Drain and refill bath.

* C.F.Palmer Ltd., Effra Road, London, S.W.2, supply suitable apparatus.

Rest 40–60 seconds.

Start kymograph.

The tissue will also respond to the following concentrations of other substances in the organ bath:

Acetylcholine	2 ng/ml
5-hydroxytryptamine	10 ng/ml
Bradykinin	20 ng/ml
KCl	300 μg/ml

(Doses of organic salts are quoted as the base.)

Too much spontaneous rhythm may be controlled by atropine 10^{-7} g/ml in *all* washing and bath fluid. This will raise the effective dose of ACh to about 1 μg/ml and of 5-HT to about 0·2 μg/ml.

A kymograph record of a $2+2$ assay may be found in the papers by Schild [1, 3], which also give a method of calculating the limits of error of the assay value.

The cycle for SRS-A will need longer for relaxation and it is advisable to wash at least three times between doses spaced at least 5 (and usually 10) minutes apart. The assay is performed in the presence of mepyramine 10^{-6} M (400 ng/ml) and atropine 5×10^{-7} M (100 ng/ml) which are added to all the Tyrode solution used. If an automatic assay machine* is used, it is convenient to set it for a 2 minute contact period, and a 4 minute rest including three washes, and to have Tyrode solution added instead of a dose of SRS-A, in every alternate cycle.

The tissue will give threshold responses to $<0·4$ units of activity/ml, and doses of 1–2 units/ml give responses suitable for assay purposes [4].

Mepyramine cannot easily be removed from glassware or tubing, and it is therefore an advantage to use separate organ baths and associated apparatus for histamine and SRS-A assays, and to mark all volumetric glassware used for strong solutions of potent inhibitor substances.

A critical review of the methods available for histamine assay, based on the experience of members of the 'Histamine Club', deals with both biological and spectro-fluorimetric methods [5]. The most recent work on fluorimetric assay by Kremsner & Pfeiffer [6] refers to the need to exclude spermidine from brain extracts, since this enhances the fluorescence and gives assay values which are too high. This refinement will seldom concern immunologists, who will find the articles by Shore [7] Carlini & Green [8] and Aures *et al* [9] useful.

It is easy to confirm that the substance being assayed is histamine, by

* Such a machine is described by Boura, Mongar and Schild [3] and is marketed by Vickers Instruments, London, S.W.1.

showing abolition of the contraction by a moderate concentration of an anti-histamine drug (e.g. mepyramine 0·1 μg/ml). The characterization of SRS-A is much more difficult, and for completeness demands the use of the rat uterus (to exclude plasma kinins) and the hamster colon (to exclude prostaglandins). It will frequently be adequate, however, to use only the guinea-pig ileum as above, and to show that the contraction is unaffected by the presence of BOL (bromolysergic acid diethylamide) 1 μg/ml and incubation of the active substance with crystalline trypsin 0·1 mg/ml at 37° C for 30 minutes, thus excluding 5-HT and kinins.

The chief metabolic end-product of released histamine is imidazole acetic acid (IAA), which is excreted in the urine, but in man N-methyl histamine and riboside derivatives are also formed [10]. Furthermore, the large but variable amounts of histamine in the diet and formed by bacterial action in the intestine are the principal source of the products of histamine found in urine. It is therefore evident that the study of IAA levels will not generally be applicable in studies of allergic reactions *in vivo*.

Biological assay of acetylcholine

The longitudinal muscle of the leech *Hirudo medicinalis* gives a rather slow contraction to ACh (base) 1 or 2×10^{-9} g/ml in the presence of eserine, and can therefore be used to detect the ACh released physiologically. Leeches are stored at about 4° C in ion-exchange water, in a large jar, half-filled and covered with muslin or a fine grid. The water is changed once a week. Every 2 months the creatures must be fed with liver or a bag of clotted blood, and then the water is changed daily.

Diluted Locke solution (five-seventh concentration) is used to bathe the tissue. Put the leech on a cork board, catch it through the mouth and tail suckers with pins and extend to about two-thirds stretched length, suckers upwards. With scissors, cut along the two pale lateral lines from the mouth nearly to the tail and take most of the internal organs out with the ventral body-wall at the second incision. Do NOT allow the external surface ever to touch exposed tissue. With the dorsal half of the leech still pinned to the board, carefully cut out all internal organs down to the mucilaginous connective tissue overlying the muscle. Pin out at either side and impale the selected length of muscle with cutting needles ready threaded. Split the muscle longitudinally with a scalpel, and set the preparation up in a bath about 5 cm long (3–5 ml) at room temperature with gentle aeration with air or O_2/CO_2. A low friction lever exerts a load of 2–2·5 g and records at × 10 magnification on a lightly smoked kymograph. Vibration of the lever improves the kymograph records. Either isometric or isotonic transducers can be used.

Wash every 15 minutes for *3 hours before* adding eserine (5×10^{-6} g/ml) to all bathing fluids. Start the assay 20 minutes later. Allow *exactly 2 minutes* contact with ACh, even if the contraction is not complete, wash well and allow 12–15 minutes for relaxation between doses. Relaxation may be assisted by vibrating but not by a greater load. A satisfactory 15 minute cycle of operations during assay is:

Start kymograph, 1 cm/min ($\frac{1}{2}$ min).
Drain bath and *at once* refill with test solution in leech–Locke.
After 2 minutes contact, stop drum, drain and refill with leech–Locke.
Wash tissue after further intervals of 1 minute and 2 minutes, using leech–Locke.
Five minutes before next cycle, drain and refill with leech–Locke + eserine.

Steady responses are reached after only three doses, and the assay can then start, but a fixed time of contact and cycle is important. It is practicable to run four preparations concurrently (from two leeches).

Assays of 5-hydroxytryptamine and plasma kinins

The rat uterus preparation is essentially similar to the guinea-pig ileum. A virgin rat of 200 to 300 g is brought into full oestrus with stilboestrol 0·1 mg/kg (i.e. 10–15 μg/rat, as 20 μg/ml solution in 25 per cent ethanol) given subcutaneously 18–20 hours beforehand. It is killed by a blow on the head. One horn of the uterus is cut at the bifurcation and the cut end lifted with blunt forceps whilst the mesentery and fat are cut cleanly away with sharp scissors. The horn is then cut off near the ovary, and placed in cold de Jalon's solution. It is often useful to split the organ longitudinally along the side furthest from the mesentery (and two preparations can be made by splitting along the line of the mesentery also).

Set up the piece of tissue in de Jalon's solution (low Ca^{++}) at 30–32° C, with an isotonic lever giving tension of 0·3–0·5 g, and magnification of 4:1. The bath fluid should be changed at intervals of 10 minutes or less whilst the tissue is allowed to settle during at least 30 minutes. A suitable cycle of operations is as follows:

Add active substance* and wait 2 minutes or until contraction has passed maximum (for 5-HT this may be only 20 seconds).
Wash by overflow,† wait 1 minute.
Wash, wait 3 minutes.
Wash, wait 1 minute (optional).

* Add (in about one-twentieth bath volume) *quickly* from a syringe, through a fine needle inserted deep into the bath to ensure rapid mixing.
† Rat uterus will usually contract spontaneously when exposed to the air or when not

This preparation is unresponsive to histamine in small amounts, but high concentrations are inhibitory. If the tissue is stretched during setting up, it is liable to give troublesome spontaneous rhythm which is not controlled by atropine.

The preparation should respond to the following concentrations of drugs (salts expressed as base):

ACh	2–10 ng/ml
Carbachol	0·2–0·5 μg/ml
5-HT	5–10 ng
Bradykinin	0·2 ng/ml

Too large doses or too short rest periods lead to loss of sensitivity or the onset of spontaneous contractions. The dose-response relationship for this tissue is extremely steep, and a $2+1$ assay can often be performed with standard doses as close as 0·2 ng/ml and 0·22 ng/ml bradykinin. This makes matching tedious, but provides a very accurate assay.

The rat uterus preparation is readily stimulated to contract by many substances other than the plasma kinins, and it is necessary to characterize the substance by other means before accepting the assay as indicating that a certain amount of bradykinin is actually present.

The easiest test is to show that the active material is a polypeptide which is rapidly destroyed by chymotrypsin. If a sample of authentic bradykinin is incubated with crystalline chymotrypsin (0·25 mg/ml) at pH 7·4 for 30 minutes, little if any of the activity will survive. The authentic bradykinin and the crude sample, roughly matched for biological activity, are incubated in parallel using silicone-coated or polythene tubes. The loss of biological activity should be very high (>90 per cent) and comparable in each tube. If the crude sample contains a large amount of protein this may protect peptides present and should therefore be removed [11]. When this is not possible, some allowance must be made, such as extra enzyme or longer incubation. If the biological activity is clearly due to a polypeptide, the characterization may be further narrowed by showing that it will cause relaxation of the rat duodenum [12], which occurs only with bradykinin and closely related substances, whereas substance P, angiotensin and other peptides cause this tissue to contact.

A long strip cut from the fundus of the stomach of the rat is satisfactory for the assay of 5-HT, but not for bradykinin [13, 14]. It needs a somewhat

---

supported by the bathing fluid. It is therefore usual to change the bath fluid by allowing about $1\frac{1}{2}$ times the bath volume to enter at the bottom and displace the used solution which is sucked off from the top of the bath, or simply allowed to flow over the edge.

larger bath than the uterus, it must be stretched after each contraction, by temporarily increasing the load, and it does not give a level baseline. The advantages are that it rarely gives troublesome spontaneous movements, that its threshold for a contractile response is low (0·1–0·2 ng/ml) and that doses up to at least twenty times threshold seldom cause aberrant behaviour. The preparation contracts in response to many substances, including histamine and vasopressin, but is comparatively unreactive to bradykinin.

5-HT is most commonly assayed by spectrofluorimetric methods, although these do not always correlate very well with biological assay. When the assay of the metabolites is necessary, there is no alternative to the spectrofluorimetric method. The principal metabolite of 5-HT is 5-hydroxyindoleacetic acid (5-HIAA), and the inactivation of 5-HT *in vivo* is so rapid that unless its release is both sudden and very great, no active 5-HT will be detectable, and the role of 5-HT may only be inferred from changes in the output of 5-HIAA in the urine. The release of 5-HT *in vitro* may be studied directly provided that the substance is quickly stabilized by acidification to pH 4 or 5, usually with HCl. Measurement of 5-HT in plasma is complicated by the large amount of the substance in the platelets, where it is bound to ATP. It is released as soon as clotting begins or the platelets start to age, and this must be avoided by immediately treating the blood with heparin or versene (EDTA) and then centrifuging it at once in the cold at high g to ensure sedimentation of the platelets.

Fluorimetric methods should not be employed unless the dangers of error due to related indole compounds have been correctly assessed and are acceptable. These hazards will vary with different types of experiment and will usually necessitate some preliminary checks, such as showing that the assay value remains unchanged in spite of deliberately adding to the starting material the substance(s) suspected of introducing error. Reference to a detailed treatise on fluorimetric methods and apparatus (e.g. Udenfriend [15] or Maickel & Weissbach [16]) is strongly advised. Qualitative chromatographic methods for the separation and identification of indole compounds and their metabolites in biological material [17] may afford further evidence for the purity of samples used in spectrofluorimetry as well as better understanding of the normal pattern of metabolism, and the detection of major changes. Certain items of diet contain large amounts of tryptamine or 5-hydroxyindole substances which may distort the pattern of metabolites found in the urine, and will certainly alter the output of 5-HIAA. These foods include fruits such as bananas, tomatoes and pineapples [18, 19] and mature cheeses. In the absence of fluctuations due to diet, the 24 hour excretion of 5-HT is comparatively constant for a given person, although individual values differ widely, even within apparently similar groups of people.

References

[1] SCHILD H.O. (1942) A method of conducting a biological assay on a preparation giving repeated graded responses illustrated by the estimation of histamine. *J. Physiol.* **101,** 115

[2] *Handbook of Experimental Pharmacology, Histamine,* Vol. 18 (1966); *5-Hydroxytryptamine,* Vol. 19 (1966). Berlin: Springer

[3] BOURA A., MONGAR J.L. & SCHILD H.O. (1954) Improved automatic apparatus for pharmacological assays on isolated preparations. *Br. J. Pharmac. Chemother.* **9,** 24

[4] BROCKLEHURST W.E. (1962) SRS-A and related substances. *Prog. Allergy.* **6,** 540

[5] Les méthodes employées pour l'étude du métabolism et de la liberation de l'histamine. *J. de Physiol. (Paris)* **53,** 847

[6] KREMSNER L.T. & PFEIFFER C.C. (1966) Identification of substances interfering with the fluorimetric determination of brain histamine. *Biochem Pharmac.* **15,** 197

[7] SHORE P.A. (1964) Fluorimetric measurement of histamine. *Meth. med. Res.* **10,** 173

[8] CARLINI E.A. & GREEN J.P. (1963) The subcellular distribution of histamine, slow-reacting substance, and 5-hydroxytryptamine in the brain of the rat. *Br. J. Pharmac. Chemother.* **20,** 264

[9] AURES D., WINQUIST G. & HANSSON E. (1965) Histamine formation in the blood and bone marrow of the guineapig. *Am. J. Physiol.* **208,** 186

[10] SCHAYER R.W. (1963) Histamine metabolism in the mammal. *Henry Ford Hospital Symposium,* p. 227. London: Churchill

[11] ZEITLIN I.J. & BROCKLEHURST W.E. (1966) The measurement of normal values of kininogen and plasma kinins in human plasma by a method suitable for use under clinical conditions. In preparation

[12] GADDUM J.H. & HORTON E.W. (1959) The extraction of human urinary kinin (substance Z) and its relation to the plasma kinins. *Br. J. Pharmac. Chemother.* **14,** 117

[13] VANE J.R. (1957) A sensitive method for the assay of 5-hydroxytryptamine. *Br. J. Pharmac. Chemother.* **12,** 344

[14] VANE J.R. (1959) The relative activities of some tryptamine analogues on the isolated rat stomach strip preparation. *Br. J. Pharmac. Chemother.* **14,** 87

[15] UDENFRIEND S. (1965) *Fluorescence Assay in Biology and Medicine.* New York: Academic Press

[16] MAICKEL R.P. & WEISSBACH H. (1962) Recent developments in chemical and biochemical assay techniques applicable in pharmacology. *A. Rev. Pharmac.* **2,** 399

[17] CRAWFORD T.B.B., ASHCROFT G.W., ECCLESTON D. & SMITH A.N. (1965) Some observations on the metabolism of indoles in two patients with the carcinoid syndrome. *Gastroenterology* **48,** 745

[18] WEST G.B. (1958) Tryptamine in edible fruits. *J. Pharm. Pharmac.* **10,** 589

[19] WEST G.B. (1960) Carcinoid tumours and pineapples. *J. Pharm. Pharmac.* **12,** 768

Statistical Methods as Applied to Immunological Data

W.LUTZ

Introduction

In recent years several excellent books have appeared dealing specifically with the application of statistics to biology and an even larger number of publications has devoted one or more chapters to the subject. To attempt again, in condensed form, what others have done so well, did not appeal to us.

Co-operation between biologist and statistician has fortunately become quite common and this has certainly been to the benefit of the statistician. The bulk of the advice and assistance a statistician is called upon to give relates to some of the more standard tests and techniques which many biologists use both routinely and competently. Yet we have been struck by the surprising frequency with which certain queries relating to those standard methods and their application are raised. We felt, therefore, that a discussion of some of these points might be of more interest than a systematic resumé of basic statistical techniques.

Contingency tables

The observations of an experiment are usually expressed either as measurements of some characteristics or recorded as the number of occasions the subjects belonged to a specific class. The data in Table A1.1 on cholera-vaccinated rabbits, subsequently challenged, provides an example:*

The basic requirements for statistical analysis of classificatory data are:

1. The number of classes are exhaustive. No subject at the end of the experiment falls into an unspecified category.

2. Every subject falls into one, but *only* one, group or class.

3. The subjects are statistically independent, i.e. the response of subject A in no way influences the response of any of the other subjects in the experiment.

* Data from 'Studies in Experimental Cholera', Ph.D. thesis, 1965, by Dr H.K.Gosh, Dept. of Bacteriology, Edinburgh University.

Classificatory results (or counts) such as those of Table A1.1 are best analysed by using the χ^2 test (chi-square test). This is a very satisfactory approximate method, easily applied, but, like all tests, it is inappropriate under some conditions.

The method proceeds as follows:

Corresponding to each observed 'cell' count, compute the 'expected' frequency on the assumption that all the treatments have the same effect.

TABLE A1.1

	Died	Survived	Total	Deaths (%)
Live vacc. 834, 2 doses	4	13	17	23·5
Live vacc. 834, 4 doses	3	6	9	33·3
Formalized 834, 4 doses	3	7	10	30·0
O antigen 834, 4 doses	4	6	10	40·0
Total	14	32	46	

This is done by dividing the product of the row and column totals of the cell under consideration by the grand total. Thus, in cell one, four deaths were observed, the corresponding expected frequency is

$$\frac{14 \times 17}{46} = 5\cdot174 \text{ or } 5\cdot2 \text{ approximately.}$$

A convenient layout for the computations is illustrated in Table A1.2

TABLE A1.2

O (observed frequency)	E (expected frequency)	$D = (O-E) \pm \frac{1}{2}$	D^2/E
4	= 5·2	−0·7	0·094
13	= 11·8	0·7	0·042
3	2·7	−0·2	0·015
6	6·3	0·2	0·006
3	3·0	0·0	0·000
7	7·0	0·0	0·000
4	3·0	0·5	0·083
6	7·0	−0·5	0·036
46	46·0		0·276 = χ^2 : totals

To obtain column D subtract E from the corresponding observed value O. Add $\frac{1}{2}$ to this difference if negative, otherwise subtract $\frac{1}{2}$ unless the difference is zero. (If zero, do not correct by either adding or subtracting $\frac{1}{2}$.) This is known as Yates's correction. Its use is recommended as a routine, although not really necessary when all the E values are large.

The total of the last column yields the computed χ^2 value with $(r-1)(c-1)$ degrees of freedom (d.f.). Here r, c denote the number of rows and columns in the 'contingency' table as Table A1.1 is often called. In this example r = 4, c = 2 and d.f. = 3, with $\chi^2 = 0\cdot276$. From χ^2 tables [3, p. 36], the probability that $\chi^2 \leqslant 7\cdot815$ is given as:

$P(\chi^2 < 7\cdot815;\ 3\ \text{d.f}) = 0\cdot95$, so that the result of $\chi^2 = 0\cdot276$ (being less than 7·815) is not statistically significant. There is no reason, as far as this data goes, for rejecting the proposition that the percentage of deaths is the same for all four vaccination treatments.

TABLE A1.3

Antibody

Liver histology	Present	Absent	Total	Percent with antibody
Damage present	12	7	19	63·2
Normal	1	11	12	8·3
Total	13	18	31	

The term 'significantly different' when applied to the comparison of two or more treatments requires clarification. A statistician's use of the term is rather different from that of most biologists. When comparing two or more treatment results, the statistician assumes the null hypothesis to hold. This hypothesis asserts that the various treatments all exert the same effect and that any differences observed in the experimental results are explicable in terms of random fluctuations and error only. On the basis of this assumption, the probability of obtaining the observed experimental outcome is computed. When this probability is small, say 0·05 or 0·01, the null hypothesis which formed the basis of our calculations is rejected as unreasonable.

Rejecting, or at any rate seriously questioning the validity of, the null hypothesis is equivalent to accepting that the treatments do not all have the same effect. In other words, the observed differences in the experimental results cannot reasonably be explained as random experimental error or variation. It should be noted that the term 'significantly different' as used in the above sense does not depend on any consideration whether the treatment differences are of any biological interest or importance.

An m × 2 contingency table (m rows, 2 columns) or a 2 × m table (2 rows, m columns) can be interpreted as a set of percentages or proportions relating to m different treatments or situations. Testing such contingency tables for a significant difference is equivalent to testing for a significant difference in the m percentages.

Frequently only two percentages are to be compared. Such comparisons may be set out as a 2 × 2 contingency (fourfold) table. Table 3 relates to the data of Weir on liver auto-antibodies [10].

Proceeding as before:

O	E	D	D^2/E
12	8·0	3·5	1·53
7	11·0	−3·5	1·11
1	5·0	−3·5	2·45
11	7·0	3·5	1·75
31	31·0		$\chi^2 = 6\cdot84$, with $(2-1)(2-1) = 1$ d.f.

From χ^2 tables in *Documenta Geigy Scientific Tables*, p. 36 [3] we find

$$P(\chi^2 < 6\cdot635; \text{d.f} = 1) = 0\cdot99$$

Thus as a random value of χ^2 (1 d.f) will exceed the value 6·635 only once in 100 trials, we conclude that the observed χ^2 value of 6·84 is rather unlikely to occur randomly. The null hypothesis of no treatment (liver damage) effect on which the computation is based seems unreasonable. The data, therefore, suggests rather strongly that liver damage affects the percentage of subjects with antibody present.

As already indicated, the χ^2 test for contingency tables is an approximate method. This approximation tends to become unsatisfactory when the expected frequency for any cell is small, say less than five. If the grand total exceeds forty and the number of cells is not less than six, say, we might still accept the method for one of the E's as small as three. In Table A1.2 the method was accepted although an E = 2·7 occurred. For a large grand total (70 or more, say) and no fewer than six cells, a single E as small as two might still pass. Nevertheless, this is stretching the applicability of the χ^2 test as applied to contingency tables about as far as it will go. When these conditions do not apply, the exact (but very long and tedious) method for analysing contingency tables can be used (see Maxwell [5]).

For 2×2 tables, tables giving the results of the exact method can be used when the χ^2 method fails as a result of one or more of the E's being too small (*Documenta Geigy*, p. 109 [3]). To use the *Documenta Geigy* tables, arrange the 2×2 contingency table in the form:

	Column 1	Column 2	Total
Row 1	x_1	$N_1 - x_1$	N_1
Row 2	x_2	$N_2 - x_2$	N_2
Total	$X = x_1 + x_2$	$N_1 + N_2 - x_1 - x_2$	$N = N_1 + N_2$

where care is taken to ensure

(a) $N_1 \leqslant N_2$

(b) $x_1 \leqslant N_1 - x_1$.

The *Documenta Geigy* tables are then entered with the values N, N_1 and x_1. As an illustration, consider Table A1.4 relating to data on liver auto-antibodies [10].

TABLE A1.4

Antibody

Liver histology	Present	Absent	Total	Per cent with antibody
Normal	1	4	5	20·0
Damage present	12	3	15	80·0
Total	13	7	20	

Here $N_1 = 5 \leqslant N_2 = 15$

$x_1 = 1 \leqslant N_1 - x_1 = 4$.

The *Documenta Geigy* tables are entered with $N = 20$, $N_1 = 5$, $x_1 = 1$. The tables give the limits within which $X = x_1 + x_2$ must lie for the results of the table to be non-significant. At the 5 per cent level, X in this example must lie within $0 \leqslant X \leqslant 14$. Since the observed $X = 13$ does lie within this range, the observed percentages of 80 per cent and 20 per cent antibody present are not significantly different. This example emphasizes that quite striking percentage differences in small samples can still be reasonably accounted for by random fluctuation and random experimental errors.

TABLE A1.5

	Survived	Died	Total	Deaths (%)
Control	0	7	7	100·0
Immunized	6	1	7	14·3
Total	6	8	14	

The above exact method can be applied just as easily to a 2×2 table when all the subjects on one trial fall into the same class. Unpublished data kindly supplied by Dr W.J.Herbert* furnishes an example on reaction of mice to a trypanosome challenge. In this example $N = 14$, $N_1 = 7$, $x_1 = 0$ and $X = 6$. The relevant tables show that at the 5 per cent level X should lie between 0 and 5, whilst at the 2 per cent level X should not exceed 6. Hence the probability of observing the above table of results on the null hypothesis (that immunization has no effect) lies between 0·05 and 0·02. This is clearly unreasonable and we conclude that the results are significantly different.

The χ^2 test is an extremely versatile and powerful statistical method, particularly for large samples. For an excellent account of its varied applications with worked examples see Maxwell [5].

The normal distribution and tests of significance
Most of the well-known statistical tests require that the measurements be sampled from a 'normal distribution'.† The normal curve is, of course, a mathematical abstraction which no set of data completely satisfies. Fortunately most of the elementary tests are robust with respect to normality, i.e. moderate departures of the data from the normal distribution do not materially affect the results or the validity of the tests.

Table A1.6 Fig. A1.1 gives the observed distribution of height of seventy-one boys at non-fee paying schools in Edinburgh.‡

The distribution of biological measurements does not often fit the normal curve so well. A rather more typical example of biological data is given in

* Dr W.J.Herbert, Dept. of Animal Health, Edinburgh University.
† For simple tests not requiring assumptions of normality see [8].
‡ Data from 'Edinburgh Dental Survey 1952' kindly made available by Mr S.A.Sklaroff, Dept. of Social Medicine, Edinburgh University.

TABLE A1.6

Height (in.)	Observed frequency	Fitted normal frequency
< 57	4	4·92
57 < 59	7	7·95
59 < 61	17	13·17
61 < 63	15	15·91
63 < 65	14	13·99
65 < 67	8	8·88
67 < 69	3	4·27
69 +	3	1·90
Total	71	70·99

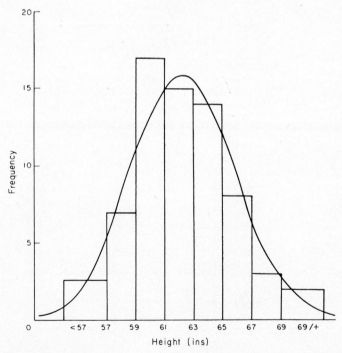

FIG. A1.1. Frequency distribution of the height of seventy-one boys at non-fee paying schools in Edinburgh.

TABLE A1.7A

Area of weal (mm²)	Observed frequency
35– 44	1
45– 54	4
55– 64	5
65– 74	8
75– 84	7
85– 94	6
95–104	4
105–114	1
Total	36

TABLE A1.7B

Distribution of haemoglobin levels
303 patients

$6 \cdot 5 < 7 \cdot 0$	4
$7 \cdot 0 < 7 \cdot 5$	3
$7 \cdot 5 < 8 \cdot 0$	10
$8 \cdot 0 < 8 \cdot 5$	5
$8 \cdot 5 < 9 \cdot 0$	4
$9 \cdot 0 < 9 \cdot 5$	8
$9 \cdot 5 < 10 \cdot 0$	4
$10 \cdot 0 < 10 \cdot 5$	6
$10 \cdot 5 < 11 \cdot 0$	14
$11 \cdot 0 < 11 \cdot 5$	19
$11 \cdot 5 < 12 \cdot 0$	9
$12 \cdot 0 < 12 \cdot 5$	23
$12 \cdot 5 < 13 \cdot 0$	37
$13 \cdot 0 < 13 \cdot 5$	21
$13 \cdot 5 < 14 \cdot 0$	27
$14 \cdot 0 < 14 \cdot 5$	23
$14 \cdot 5 < 15 \cdot 0$	29
$15 \cdot 0 < 15 \cdot 5$	14
$15 \cdot 5 < 16 \cdot 0$	17
$16 \cdot 0 < 16 \cdot 5$	10
$16 \cdot 5 < 17 \cdot 0$	6
$17 \cdot 0 < 17 \cdot 5$	3
$17 \cdot 5 < 18 \cdot 0$	5
$18 \cdot 0 < 18 \cdot 5$	2
	303

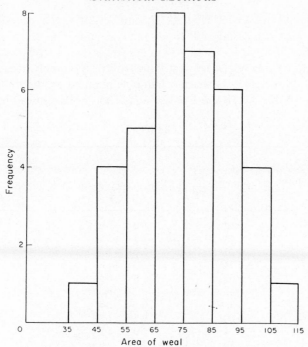

Fɪɢ. A1.2A. Distribution of weal size using a P-K test.

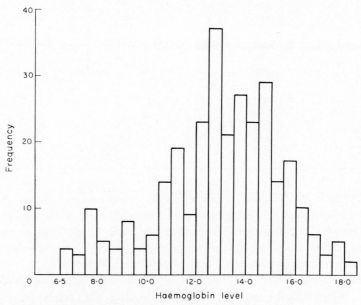

Fɪɢ. A1.2B. Frequency distribution of the haemoglobin level of 300 patients.

Table A1.7A [9] and A1.7B* (Figs. A1.2A and A1.2B) which records the distribution of weal size using a P-K test and haemoglobin levels in patients respectively.

The data in Table A1.7A are distributed a little too evenly over the central values and do not have as sharp a hump as required by the normal curve. The data of Table A1.7B are likewise a little too evenly spread between the

TABLE A1.8A

x ovulation response (estimated number of eggs)	$\tanh^{-1}\left(\dfrac{x+1}{1700}-1\right)$	Frequency distribution of $\tanh^{-1}\left(\dfrac{x+1}{1700}-1\right)$	
2717	0·69	$-4\cdot0 < -3\cdot5$	1
3214	1·43	$-2\cdot5 < -2\cdot0$	3
2386	0·43	$-2\cdot0 < -1\cdot5$	—
584	−0·78	$-1\cdot5 < -1\cdot0$	—
702	−0·67	$-1\cdot0 < -0\cdot5$	3
2449	0·47	$-0\cdot5 < 0$	6
2319	0·38	$0 < 0\cdot5$	5
2614	0·60	$0\cdot5 < 1\cdot0$	3
1464	−0·14	$1\cdot0 < 1\cdot5$	2
17	−2·50	$1\cdot5 < 2\cdot0$	—
1627	−0·04	$2\cdot0 < 2\cdot5$	1
3043	1·07		
1475	−0·13		
803	−0·59		
1127	−0·35		
2289	0·36		
3551	2·10		
2567	0·56		
1115	−0·36		
1838	−0·08		
35	−2·30		
38	−2·20		
1208	−0·29		
0	−4·00		

values 12 to 15 and are clearly skew with a disproportional number of smaller values. Nevertheless, we would not hesitate to apply most of the tests requiring 'normality' to such data. The pronounced central hump and absence of extreme values are a rough and ready rule quite good enough for most practical purposes, particularly if the sample exceeds fifteen or so.

Unfortunately examples abound of biological data departing markedly

* Dr S.H.Davies, Dept. of Haematology, Royal Infirmary, Edinburgh.

and in important respects from normality. Tables A1.8A and A1.8B Fig. A1.3 give the ovulation response of *Xenopus laevis* to hormone treatment.*

As the above ovulation figures show no noticeable central hump and the range of values is extreme, it would be hazardous to rely on the validity of tests requiring normal data if applied mechanically to such readings.

TABLE A1.8B

No. of eggs laid	Observed frequency
0 < 500	4
500 < 1000	3
1000 < 1500	5
1500 < 2000	2
2000 < 2500	4
2500 < 3000	3
3000 < 3500	3
	24

The arithmetic mean and variance

'Raw' experimental data in general convey little clear information. The need is soon felt for one or two constants which in some sense are typical and convey the essential features of the measurements. The sheer variability of most results requires that any 'descriptive' or 'representative' constants computed from the observations be more stable than the individual readings.

The mean (arithmetic) and variance are more stable than the individual measurements in the sense that means and variances computed from samples of replicated experiments are demonstrably less variable than the readings themselves. (The standard deviation is, of course, computed as well and is simply obtained by finding the square root of the variance which is computed first.) Calculating the mean and variance from a set of data is a simple enough process, an illustration of which is given below using the data in Table A1.9.†

The standard deviation (as well as the variance) is a 'measure' of the spread or variability of the data. The reason for introducing both the standard deviation and the variance is that the latter has pleasing mathematical and

---

* Unpublished data supplied by Dr A.Barr, Pregnancy Diagnosis Laboratory, Edinburgh University.
† H.K.Ghosh, ibid.

statistical properties whereas the former appears in expressions of the form $\mu \pm K\sigma$ relating the mean (μ) and the standard deviation (σ) to the area under the normal curve for some given constant K.

The geometric mean

On occasion the geometric mean (GM) is used instead of the arithmetic mean (AM). The geometric mean is found by computing the product of the

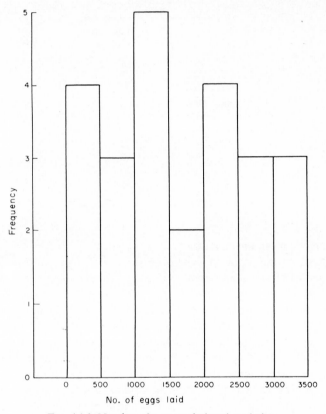

FIG. A1.3. Number of eggs per induced ovulation.

n sample results and then taking the nth root of this product. As an example the AM of a sample of three readings 2, 3 and 3 is

$$AM = \frac{2+3+3}{3} = 2{\cdot}667.$$

The GM of the same readings is: $GM = \sqrt[3]{2 \times 3 \times 3} = 2{\cdot}621$.

The GM will never exceed the AM value. Thus for very positively skew data, i.e. data which contain a fairly high proportion of very large values, the GM value is nearer the median than is the AM. (The median is defined as that particular value of a set of observations such that half the readings are less than or equal to the median value.) Under these circumstances the GM appears to our commonsense as being a more 'typical' value.

TABLE A1.9

Survival in hours of rabbits after cholera challenge

Vaccinated group (x)		Control group (ly)			
29	30	24	34	24	24
56	32	34	20	24	
48	32	28	22	28	
32		22	28	20	
		32	34	28	
		28	24	20	
		28	28	24	

$N_x = 7$

Sum (x) = Σx = 259

Sum (x²) = Σx^2 = 10253.

Sample mean (x) = x = $\dfrac{259}{7}$ = 37·0.

Sample variance (x) = S_x^2

$= \dfrac{1}{(N_x-1)}\left(\Sigma x^2 - \dfrac{(\Sigma x)^2}{N_x}\right)$

$= \dfrac{1}{6}\left(10253 - \dfrac{(259)^2}{7}\right)$

= 111·7.

Standard deviation (x) = S_x

$\qquad = \sqrt{111\cdot7}$

$\qquad = 10\cdot6.$

$N_y = 22$

Sum (y) = Σy = 578.

Sum (y²) = Σy^2 = 15604.

Sample mean (y) = $\bar{y}$ = $\dfrac{578}{22}$ = 26·3

Sample variance (y) = S_y^2

$= \dfrac{1}{(N_y-1)}\left(\Sigma y^2 - \dfrac{(\Sigma y)^2}{N_y}\right)$

$= \dfrac{1}{21}\left(15604 - \dfrac{(578)^2}{22}\right)$

= 19·92.

Standard deviation (y) = S_y

$\qquad = \sqrt{19\cdot92}$

$\qquad = 4\cdot46.$

One advantage of the GM is that if the readings are such that their logarithm is normally distributed, then log (GM) = arithmetic mean of the logarithm of the individual readings. Using the above three values for illustration:

$$\log (GM) = \log (2\cdot621) = 0\cdot4185.$$

$$\text{AM of log (titre)} = \frac{\log 2 + \log(3) + \log(3)}{3} = 0\cdot4184.$$

There are, however, disadvantages attached to the general use of the GM. In the first instance it is less easily computed than the AM. The result that

GM < AM is only desirable if the data is positively skew. If the data has a high proportion of very low values, the use of the AM might be more justifiable. For an extreme example consider the set of readings

$$1, 2, 100, 100, 100, 100, 100, 150, 200, 200.$$

AM = 105·3

GM = $\sqrt[10]{12 \times 10^{16}}$ = 51·04, an 'unreasonably' low value.

A great deal is known about the statistical properties of an arithmetic mean. Our knowledge concerning the GM is not so complete. Furthermore, use of the GM is severely restricted in that it can be applied only to positive (non-zero) values. No such restriction applies to the AM.

The use of GM is usually advocated where the recorded readings are proportional to some applied effect. But for such readings the logarithm of the reading has, as often as not, more desirable statistical properties than the initial readings themselves. When dealing with the logarithms of the readings, one should use the AM. In the final process of converting back to the actual readings, the anti-log of the AM of the log (readings) will, of course, be the GM.

My own preference, in general, is not to use the GM. Should the data be very skew, some mathematical transformation, such as taking the logs or the square root of the readings, may be desirable. The transformed variables are likely to have an almost symmetrical histogram, in which case the AM should be used.

The F-test

The aim of most experiments is to record the effect of a change in method or treatment. This effect often expresses itself as a shift in the percentage reacting, a change in the average or in the variability of the readings. Of course, even the basic distribution form of the data could be affected, but such radical change following an alteration in treatment is comparitively rare.

There is no way of knowing before the completion of the experiments whether the average or the variance (i.e. variability) or both will be affected significantly by a change in method or treatment. Yet it never ceases to surprise how frequently only the average is affected to any extent, whilst the variance is unaltered for all practical purposes. Consider, for instance, some data on bacterial colony counts obtained by two methods.*

Σx = 4090	Σy = 4423
Σx^2 = 1,674,290	Σy^2 = 1,959,387
sample mean (x) = $\bar{x}$ = 409·0	sample mean (y) = $\bar{y}$ = 442·3
sample variance (x) = S_x^2 = 164·4	sample variance (y) = S_y^2 = 343·8.

* H.K.Ghosh, ibid, reading altered for illustrative purposes.

The F-test (also known as the variance ratio test or Fisher's test) can be applied to test whether S_x^2 and S_y^2 are significantly different. The assumptions made by this test are:

1. Readings and samples must be independent.
2. Readings are 'normally' distributed.

On such small samples a formal test of normality is not really practicable. But the absence of extreme values and possibly a 'feeling' about how such data is generated would, we feel, justify accepting the data as normal. The independence is 'obvious' from the experimental procedure.

$$F = \frac{\text{larger sample variance}}{\text{smaller sample variance}} = \frac{343 \cdot 8}{164 \cdot 4} = 2 \cdot 09,$$

with degrees of freedom ($v_1 = 9$; $v_2 = 9$).

The d.f. are given by sample size less one $= 10 - 1 = 9$ for both the above samples. (It is important to put $v_1 = n_L - 1$, where n_L is the sample size of the larger variance; $v_1 \neq v_2$ when the two samples are not of equal size.)

TABLE A1.10

Spread plate method x		Pour plate method y	
396	412	406	446
410	397	443	454
403	437	423	444
420	413	426	462
395	407	461	458

From the F-tables [3, p. 40], $P(F > 3 \cdot 18; v_1 = 9, v_2 = 9) = 0 \cdot 05$. Since $F = 2 \cdot 09 < 3 \cdot 18$ these sample variances are not significantly different.

The use of a single pooled estimate of the variance would now be justified if required. It is computed by the formula:

$$S^2 = \frac{(N_x - 1) S_x^2 + (N_y - 1) S_y^2}{N_x + N_y - 2}$$

$$= \frac{9 (164 \cdot 4) + 9 (343 \cdot 8)}{18} = 254 \cdot 1.$$

Table A1.9 provides an example of a situation where a change in treatment apparently affects the variability of the data.

$$F = \frac{111 \cdot 7}{19 \cdot 92} = 5 \cdot 61 \text{ with d.f. } (v_1 = 6; v_2 = 21).$$

Tables for F give:

$$P(F \geqslant 2 \cdot 57; v_1 = 6, \quad v_2 = 21) = 0 \cdot 05$$

and $$P(F \geqslant 3 \cdot 81; v_1 = 6, \quad v_2 = 21) = 0 \cdot 01,$$

so that the sample variances are significantly different at the 1 per cent level.

When more than two treatments are being studied, at least as many samples as there are treatments are obtained. Although it is possible to compare the sample variances, two at a time, running through all possible comparison, this procedure is not recommended. It leads eventually to the minimum and maximum observed variances being contrasted and this comparison will have an unnaturally enhanced probability of being significant. In such cases a single multiple comparison is possible using Bartlett's test (*Documenta Geigy* [3], see worked example, p. 172).

Students' distribution

The classical experimental pattern is to perform an experiment under certain fixed conditions, possibly repeating it several times under the same conditions. One or more aspects of the treatment or method are then changed and the experiment is performed under the altered conditions. A fairly typical example is given by the data on bacterial counts in Table A1.10. The question posed is whether the change in method causes the bacterial counts to differ materially. Some difference due to random errors is, in any case, to be expected even if the methods exert no effect. A test is thus required for deciding whether the observed difference is significant in the statistical sense.

The t-test (Students' distribution) is usually the first test thought of in this connection. It is a rather limited test but powerful, provided the following conditions are satisfied:

(a) The individual observations as well as the two samples are independent.
(b) The data are normally distributed.
(c) The sample variances of the two samples are not significantly different.

This last condition is equivalent to asserting that the t-test can be applied when a change of treatment may affect the average value but does not affect the variance: in other words the variance is independent of the mean. This condition, at first sight very restrictive, is satisfied in many situations. Occasions on which a change of treatment radically alters the variance are comparatively rare, but by no means unknown. In passing, it should be mentioned that the t-test is 'robust' with respect to both conditions (b) and (c) and will not be greatly affected by moderate departures of the data from either of these requirements.

The first step in applying the t-test is to ascertain whether the requirements of the test are reasonably met. The bacterial count data, consisting of repeated counts on separate plates, can be assumed to be independent. The assumption of normality can, on such small samples, be taken on trust but the absence of any large outlying results, i.e. no values that are several times as small or as large as the average, does lend some support to it. The equality of variance can be tested for, using the F-test, as has already been done in the previous section.

Given that the F-test accepts the sample variances as not differing significantly, the next stop is to compute the pooled variance, which for the data of Table A1.10 was found to be $S^2 = 254 \cdot 1$.

$$t = \frac{\bar{x} - \bar{y}}{S \sqrt{\dfrac{1}{N_x} + \dfrac{1}{N_y}}}, \text{ with d.f.} = N_x + N_y - 2,$$

$(N_x, N_y$ are the two sample sizes)

$$= -4 \cdot 43 \text{ with d.f.} = 18 \text{ for the data of Table A1.10.}$$

The t-tables (*Documenta Geigy* [3], p. 32) at the 5 per cent level and d.f. = 18 give the value $2 \cdot 1009$. This implies that if the computed t-value lies within the interval $-2 \cdot 1009$ to $+2 \cdot 1009$ the result is not significant. Actually, since $P(-3 \cdot 922 < t < 3 \cdot 922) = 0 \cdot 999$, the observed result of $t = -4 \cdot 43$ is significant at the $0 \cdot 001$ level. There seems to be little room for doubt that the spread plate method yields a bacterial count different from that of the pour plate method, possibly owing to liquid adhering to the glass rod.

The data of Table A1.9 are an example of an experiment in which treatment apparently affects both means and variance. The F-test on the sample variances was found to be significant, hence the t-test cannot be applied. Of the various methods of dealing with this problem the most reliable is probably Behrens distribution. For details of the computations required see Fisher & Yates [2, Table V_1] and Finney [1].

The stringent condition that the samples must be independent can be relaxed in the case of some 'follow-up' studies. The observations within each sample must, however, be absolutely independent. In a 'follow-up' study each subject has a measurement or response recorded on at least two occasions, possibly with a change of treatment intervening between the readings. An example is provided by Table A1.11* which records the glucose level of pregnant women at 36 weeks, 38 weeks and during delivery.

The average of the column of differences (x) is tested against the hypothesis

* Unpublished data from Professor J.O.Forfar, Dept. of Child Life and Health, University of Edinburgh.

PP*

TABLE A1.11

I 36 weeks	Glucose level II 38 weeks	III Delivery	x = Difference I − II	A = Average I & II	y = Difference A − III
92	94	110	−2	93·0	−17·0
106	79	81	27	92·5	11·5
80	87	91	−7	83·5	−7·5
86	84	128	2	85·0	−43·0
89	91	129	−2	90·0	−39·0
74	85	120	−11	79·5	−40·5
85	73	120	12	79·0	−41·0
75	101	124	−26	88·0	−36·0
102	97	119	5	99·5	−19·5
89	92	80	−3	90·5	10·5
91	78	99	13	84·5	−14·5
100	94	125	6	97·0	−28·0
−	88	99	—	88·0	−11·0
108	73	92	35	90·5	−1·5
92	90	112	2	91·0	−21·0
93	102	97	−9	97·5	0·5
96	—	128	—	96·0	32·0
91	96	100	−5	93·5	−6·5
132	93	135	39	112·5	−22·5
117	—	150	—	117·0	−33·0
104	110	121	−6	107·0	−14·0
95	84	75	11	89·5	14·5
90	84	100	6	87·0	−13·0

$$n = 20 \quad n = 23$$
$$\Sigma x = 87 \quad \Sigma y = -403·5$$
$$\Sigma x^2 = 5019 \quad \Sigma y^2 = 13750·75$$
$$S_x^2 = 244·24 \quad S_y^2 = 303·27$$
$$\bar{x} = 4·35 \quad \bar{y} = -17·54$$

that if there is no shift in glucose level between 36 and 38 weeks, this column ought to have a theoretical mean of zero.

$$t = \frac{\bar{x} - 0}{\sqrt{\frac{S^2}{N}}} \text{ with } (N-1) \text{ d.f., where } N = \text{number of differences}$$

$$= \frac{4·35}{\sqrt{\frac{244·24}{20}}} = 1·24, \text{ d.f.} = 19.$$

Since this result clearly permits us to assume that no change in glucose level has taken place, the average level of 36 and 38 weeks is next computed and the difference found between this value and the level at delivery (column y). Performing the same computation but this time with 23 paired differences, we find

$$t = \frac{-17 \cdot 54}{\sqrt{\dfrac{303 \cdot 27}{23}}} = -4 \cdot 83, \text{ d.f.} = 22.$$

Since $P(-3 \cdot 792 < t < 3 \cdot 792) = 0 \cdot 999$ this result is highly significant.

The conclusion that the glucose level for most women rises during delivery seems well established by these results. One point should be noted. This method of taking the difference between two consecutive readings overcomes the difficulty that the consecutive results are not, in general, independent. The statistical price we pay is that the number of d.f. is reduced to half of what it would have been had the two samples been independent.

Statistical independence
An essential requirement for both the F- and the t-test is that the samples, are well as the individual observations within each sample, be independent. Mathematically this independence is simple enough to define. In specific applications it is not always obvious whether or not the data are independent.

Consider two events A and B with the probability of each occurring on its own, without reference to the other, being p(A) and p(B) respectively. If the probability of both occurring is p(A.B) then the events A and B are said to be statistically or stochastically independent if it is true to say that: $p(A.B) = p(A) \cdot p(B)$. In other words if the value of the probability of both A and B occurring together equals the product of the probabilities of A and B occurring without reference to each other, then A and B are independent. Dice-throwing provides the simplest example. From considerations of symmetry it follows that the probability of throwing two consective two's is $\frac{1}{36}$. The probability of throwing a two on any occasion is $\frac{1}{6}$. Since $\frac{1}{36} = \frac{1}{6} \cdot \frac{1}{6}$, the product of throwing a 'two' on two consecutive occasions, we can state that the throws are stochastically independent.

The following statement is a rough guide: If knowing the value of the present observation throws no light on the value of any subsequent readings and in particular does not restrict the range of the subsequent observations, then the readings can be assumed to be independent. A simple case is that of a newborn infant weighing 9 lb. To predict the exact weight of this child 1 week later is not possible, but it is almost bound to be 9 ± 1 lb, i.e. between 8 and 10 lb. Had we, however, chosen at random some other 1-week-old child the possible range of its weight could have been anything between about 4 lb and 11 lb, possibly even wider. In the first case a knowledge of the weight at birth imposes restrictions on the variation or range of the weight at 1 week. Not so in the second case, where the weight of the first child at birth cannot give any information regarding the weight of the randomly chosen 1-week-old. Hence the latter two results are independent whilst the former are dependent. The repeated readings on the same child separated by a 1-week interval is a typical case of a 'follow-up' study and such studies frequently lead to highly interdependent data. For this reason growth and development curves, whether relating to weight or the trend in antibody response, give rise to a series of dependent readings if the observations relate to the same subject or even to the same sample of subjects. Table A1.12* gives an example of the development of antibody response to ovalbumin in water-in-oil emulsion in a sample of ten mice observed over a period of 365 days. This data is shown graphically in Fig. A1.4.

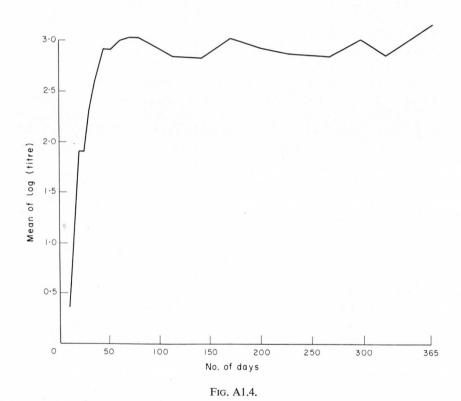

FIG. A1.4.

* Dr W.J.Herbert, ibid,

TABLE A1.12

Days after inoculation	Average log (titre)	Days after inoculation	Average log (titre)
10	0·3643	80	3·0187
15	1·0602	114	2·8301
20	1·9031	142	2·7949
25	1·9031	170	2·9857
30	2·3206	198	2·8903
37	2·5893	226	2·8426
45	2·8755	266	2·7949
51	2·8755	296	2·9674
61	2·9710	320	2·8105
71	3·0187	365	3·0869

An example where dependence is not so obvious is given by Table A1.13.* The data relates to a sequence of amplitude of rectum contractions. These contractions were recorded for 5 minutes, gastrin was then injected, and the contractions recorded for a further 5 minutes.

It is well known that contractions follow a cycle, i.e. the amplitude readings increase until a maximum is reached, then decrease to a minimum. This cycle repeats itself more or less evenly unless disturbed by some activity or treatment. Hence, given that the cycle is known, even roughly, the value of a reading will in some degree depend on the position on the cycle at which it was taken. To this extent the reading depends on the preceding values. As a result of this dependence in the above readings, it would not be advisable to test for a difference in average amplitude value before and after gastrin injection by means of the t-test. The results do not constitute two samples of size four and six, each consisting of independent measurements.

TABLE A1.13

Amplitude

Before gastrin injection	After gastrin injection
10·2, 10·2, 12·5, 14·5,	10·2, 11·6, 12·8, 14·8, 15·5, 16·8

In general, data taken over time on the same subjects present difficulties to the statistician. The mathematical difficulty with dependent data is that it cannot be adequately analysed until the type of dependence between an observation and those preceding it is known. Unfortunately the kind of dependence, whether expressed mathematically or not, is usually not even approximately known to us. Even if the dependence is assumed to be of a

* Unpublished data collected by Dr A.N.Smith, Dept. of Clinical Surgery, University of Edinburgh.

very simple type, the resulting mathematical and statistical problems are considerable. Perhaps the easiest way to ensure independence is to take only one reading per randomly chosen subject. This, however, is not always feasible and sometimes not even desirable.

Non-normal data

The assumption that our readings are normally distributed, or at least approximately so, forms the theoretical basis of the F- and t-tests. Statistical tests applied in regression analysis as well as in the analysis of variance also assume the data to have a normal distribution. Unfortunately, biological data are often non-normal in the extreme.

A simple mathematical transformation such as taking the logarithm or the square root of the readings will often result in a 'transformed variable' which is very nearly normally distributed. No simple rule is known to us for deciding whether a particular transformation will be satisfactory. For large samples of thirty or more, various transformations can be tried, the histogram drawn of the transformed variables and the most 'normal' one finally chosen to work with.

For small samples, experience or some theoretical assumption concerning the nature of the measurements has to act as a guide in choosing a particular transformation. Occasionally large samples of a similar type of measurement are available, for which a particular transformation has been found useful. The same transformation could then be accepted for the small sample.

Table A1.14* illustrates the application of the log transformation to white blood cell counts of 101 patients. The frequency distribution A, Table A.14, records the actual white blood cell counts and B gives the distribution of the logarithm of the same readings. The distribution in A is most definitely non-normal whereas the distribution in B must be very close to normal (see Figs. A1.5 and A1.6).

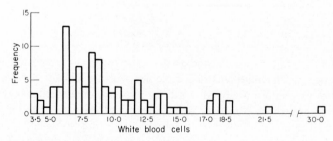

FIG. A1.5. Distribution of the white blood cell count in 101 patients.

* Dr S.H.Davies, ibid.

TABLE A1.14

White blood cell count Distribution of 101 Patients		White blood cell count (logarithms) Distribution of same 101 patients Log No.	Frequency
3·5 < 4·0	3	0·5000 < 0·6000	3
4·0 < 4·5	2	0·6000 < 0·7000	4
4·5 < 5·0	1	0·7000 < 0·8000	14
5·0 < 5·5	4	0·8000 < 0·9000	22
5·5 < 6·0	4	0·9000 < 1·000	24
6·0 < 6·5	13	1·0000 < 1·1000	15
6·5 < 7·0	5	1·1000 < 1·2000	10
7·0 < 7·5	7	1·2000 < 1·3000	7
7·5 < 8·0	4	1·3000 < 1·4000	1
8·0 < 8·5	9	1·4000 < 1·5000	1
8·5 < 9·0	8		
9·0 < 9·5	4		
9·5 < 10·0	3		
10·0 < 10·5	4		
10·5 < 11·0	2		
11·0 < 11·5	2		
11·5 < 12·0	5		
12·0 < 12·5	2		
12·5 < 13·0	1		
13·0 < 13·5	3		
13·5 < 14·0	3		
14·0 < 14·5	1		
14·5 < 15·0	1		
15·0 < 15·5	1		
15·5 < 16·0	0		
16·0 < 16·5	0		
16·5 < 17·0	0		
17·0 < 17·5	2		
17·5 < 18·0	3		
18·0 < 18·5	0		
18·5 < 19·0	2		
21·5 < 22·0	1		
30·0 < 30·5	1		
Total	101	Total	101

Any single transformation, such as taking logs, will not in all circumstances produce a transformed variable with normal properties. A case in point is given by the ovulation data (Table A1.8A). Here both the log or the square root transformation are inappropriate. However, the $\tanh^{-1}$ transformation,

Appendixes

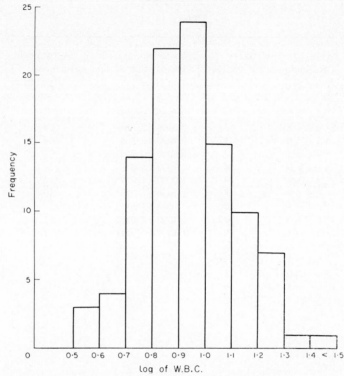

Fig. A1.6. Distribution of the logarithm of the white blood cell count in 101 patients.

TABLE A1.15 A, B and C

Titres of mouse sera collected on the ninety-fourth day after S/C inoculation of 2 mg of ovalbumin in a water-in-oil emulsion (twenty-seven mice)

A		B		C	
		Dilution counts (titre			
Titre		10 taken		Log	
values	Frequency	as 1)	Frequency	(titre)	Frequency
40	1	3	1	1·6021	1
80	1	4	1	1·9031	1
160	3	5	3	2·2041	3
320	4	6	4	2·5051	4
640	10	7	10	2·8062	10
1280	6	8	6	3·1072	6
2560	1	9	1	3·4082	1
5120	1	10	1	3·7093	1
	Total 27		Total 27		Total 27

i.e. the inverse hyperbolic tangent, will do. We have assumed the ovulation range to be 0 to 3400 and have worked with

$$\left(\frac{x+1-1700}{1700}\right) = \left(\frac{x+1}{1700} - 1\right),$$

where x is the observed number of eggs laid (1700 represents both the theoretical mean and the mid-range of the data). x + 1, instead of x, was used to avoid 1−occurring in the expression when no ovulation took place. See Fig. A1.7.

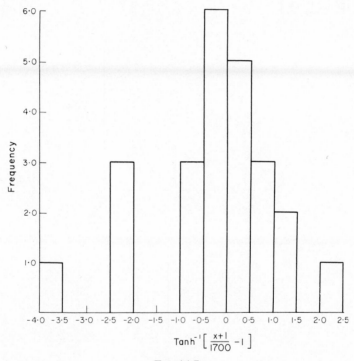

$$\mathrm{Tanh}^{-1}\left[\frac{x+1}{1700} - 1\right]$$

Fɪɢ. A1.7

Analysing titre results

Titre readings usually have an extremely skew distribution. Table A1.15A* records the frequency distribution of the antibody titres of the sera of twenty-seven mice collected on the ninety-fourth day after inoculation with 2 mg of ovalbumin S/C in a water-in-oil emulsion. These sera were tested in doubling dilution series starting at a dilution of 1:10. Figure A1.8 A, B and C

* Dr W.J.Herbert, ibid.

displays the corresponding three bar diagrams; the original data are clearly 'non-normal'. Apart from a change of scale, Tables A1.15B and A1.15C are identical as is borne out by their bar diagrams.

There exists a simple mathematical relationship between the titre value T

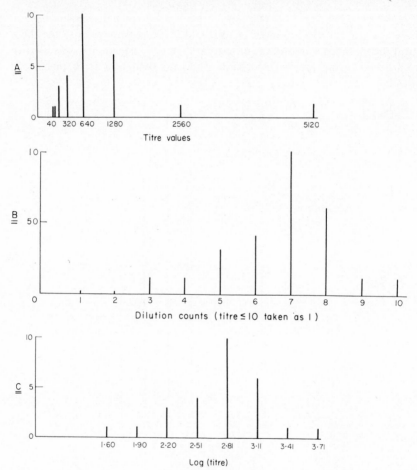

FIG. A1.8. A, B and C

and the 'titre count' c. If 'a' is the original dilution of the sera (1:10 in Table A1.15) and 'b' the dilution factor (b = 2 in the above example since a doubling dilution series was used) then:

$$T = a.b^{(c-1)} \qquad (1)$$

Hence log (T) = log (a)+(c−1) log (b)

$$= \log (a/b)+c \log (b) \qquad (2)$$

In general c can be expected to have more pleasing statistical properties than the titre value T itself, if only because it has a smaller range. It follows from equation 2 above that log (T) will then be easier to work with than T.

There is no mathematical reason why the dilution factor b should remain constant throughout the titre determination. When the dilution is close to the final titration value, a finer dilution factor such as 4:5 or 9:10 instead of 1:2, say, might in many instances reveal c to have an almost normal distribution.

Certainly the final titre values would not then increase with such huge leaps, which are statistically a little disturbing.

The use of the log transformation rather than the dilution counts enables a change on the dilution factor at any stage of the titre determination to be effected. A change of dilution factor midway would, of course, invalidate the use of the dilution count as an indicator of antibody concentration.

Table A1.16 provides us with a fairly typical example of titre results.

TABLE A1.16

| | Group A Titre value | | | Group B Titre value | |
Weight	21st day	35th day	Weight	21st day	35th day
30	20	20	31	<10	20
22	40	160	25	40	40
31	160	160	31	20	20
26	40	160	28	20	20
31	20	160	25	20	80
26	40	80	25	40	40

$\Sigma W = 166$
$\Sigma W^2 = 4658$

$\Sigma W = 165$
$\Sigma W^2 = 4581$

The data records the haemagglutination inhibition titres against influenza virus A_2/Singapore/57 of mice immunized with an influenza virus vaccine prepared either as a water-in-oil emulsion or as a multiple emulsion. The same quantity of antigen was given to the mice in each group. The initial dilution was 1:10 with subsequent doubling.

Dr Herbert has raised the following questions concerning this data:
1. Are the groups too small?
2. Is the variation in weights unacceptable?
3. Is the difference in mean titres between the two groups significant on either day?
4. How does one deal with a reading of <10 (first titre result of group B at 21 days)?

There was no reaction in the 1:10 dilution but there might have been one at a dilution of 1:5 or 2:5.

To deal with (2) first: computing the sum and the sum of squares of the mice weights gave:

A: $\Sigma x_A = 166$; $\Sigma x_A^2 = 4658$; $N_A = 6$.

B: $\Sigma x_B = 165$; $\Sigma x_B^2 = 4581$; $N_B = 6$.

As these totals are exceedingly close, there really is no need for a formal t- and F-test to show that the weight can be taken as evenly distributed between the two groups.

To deal with question (4) next: there is no satisfactory way of coping with a situation where only the upper (or lower) bound of a value is known. Further titrations done at 1:5 or 2:5 dilution provides the only secure means of removing doubt about this titre value. Statistically there remains the possibility of examining the effect on the t-value of using 'likely' values of the missing titre value such as 1:10, 1:5 and 2:5.

Working with log (titre) we tried all three of these 'likely' values for the first titre with the following results:

| | Group A | Group B | | |
| | | Dilution of the missing titre | | |
	1:10	1:10	1:5	2:5
Sum	9·6125	8·1072	7·8062	7·5051
Sum of squares	15·9439	11·2113	10·6999	10·3696
Mean	1·6021	1·3512	1·3010	1·2509
Mean square	0·1088	0·0514	0·1088	0·1964

Comparing the 'extreme' mean squares:

$$F = \frac{0·1088}{0·0514} = 2·1167; \text{ d.f. } (5,5).$$

Since this F-value is clearly not significant, the t-test on the log (titre) values is in order.

The largest of the differences between the means in groups A and B arose when the missing titre result for B was assumed to be 2·5:

$$t = \frac{1·6021 - 1·2509}{0·3906\sqrt{1/6 + 1/6}} = 1·5574; \text{ d.f. } = 10.$$

Since this, the largest of the differences in the means, is not significant, none of the other differences will be significant. There is thus no strong evidence to suggest that a real difference exists in the haemagglutination titre results at 21 days between groups A and B.

Similar computations at 35 days likewise gave a non-significant F-value. At 35 days we found

$$t = 2.79; \text{ d.f.} = 10.$$

Since $P(-2.764 < t < 2.764) = 0.98$, this value of t is significant, i.e. at 35 days the two types of emulsion do 'cause' a difference in titre values. Whether two groups of six mice are a sufficiently large sample is not easily decided. Clearly at 35 days the difference in the sample means is sufficiently large to be detected by the two groups of six subjects. On the other hand, if there is a real difference at 21 days, it is clearly smaller and will need a larger sample to detect it.

In general it is possible to determine the sample size required to detect with a given probability a stated difference in the averages due to various treatments. Unless one has knowledge of the variances involved, either from previous or from similar work, some assumptions concerning the magnitude of the variances will have to be made. Unfortunately, a discussion of how to determine the required sample size would lead us rather far afield.

More than two samples
That it is unwise to use the F-test repeatedly when more than two samples are available has been stressed. The reason is that pairwise comparisons eventually lead to testing the highest and the lowest sample variances. This results in an artificially high probability of obtaining a 'significant' result.

A similar objection holds for comparing more than two sample averages. It is inadvisable to make all possible pairwise comparisons using the t-test. For more than two independent samples the method of analysis for comparing the averages depends upon the experimental design.

Experimental design is almost a separate branch of statistics. Properly designed experiments permit simultaneous comparison between a multiplicity of factors and treatments as well as their possible interactions, often using only a comparatively small number of subjects. In the simplest design as illustrated in Table A1.17* one factor or treatment varies. Table A1.17 records the titre values of anti-ovalbumin antibodies in the sera of mice, all immunized 31 days previously. Four different doses of ovalbumin were applied in a water-in-oil emulsion.

The main questions raised by this experiment are:

(a) The same dose was administered to all mice on the same treatment irrespective of weight. Is there evidence that the distribution of weight is different for any of the groups?

* Dr W.J.Herbert, ibid.

TABLE A1.17

Group A 1333 μg each			Group B 200 μg each			Group C 20 μg each			Group D 2 μg each		
Weight	Titre	Log (titre)	Weight	Titre	Log (titre)	Weight	Titre	Log (titre)	Weight	Titre	Log (titre)
36·5	320	2·5051	33·3	5120	3·7093	29	1280	3·1072	33·2	40	1·6021
33·0	160	2·2041	33·0	2560	3·4082	34·4	2560	3·4082	29·2	1280	3·1072
30·5	1280	3·1072	37·0	640	2·8062	34·0	1280	3·1072	29·2	10	1·0000
29·0	160	2·2041	34·0	2560	3·4082	35·8	20	1·3010	33·2	20	1·3010
34·0	640	2·8062	29·6	5120	3·7092	32·9	1280	3·1072	32·2	80	1·9031
36·0	1280	3·1072	31·4	5120	3·7092	32·0	1280	3·1072	33·6	160	2·2041
37·2	2560	3·4082	31·4	5120	3·7092	31·0	320	2·5051	34·0	Died	—
34·5	2560	3·4082	30·5	2560	3·4082	34·0	160	2·2041	33·5	Died	—
30·0	2560	3·4082	32·8	Died	—	35·9	1280	3·1072	38·0	1280	3·1072
360	640	2·8062	35·5	Died	—	30·0	320	2·5051	29·2	80	1·9031
336·7		28·9647	328·5		27·8680	329·0		27·4595	325·3		16·1278

(b) Is the antibody level affected by a change in ovalbumin dosage? Since antibody level is measured by its titre value, this is equivalent to asking whether the average titre values are different for the four groups.

The analysis of variance is based on the simple algebraic result that a sum of squares about the general mean of several treatments can be partitioned into several separate (and statistically independent) sums of squares about the various group and treatment means. For instance, for the one-way analysis of variance as applied to Table A1.17,

$$\sum_{i=1}^{k} \sum_{j=1}^{n_i} (x_{ij} - \bar{x})^2 = \sum_{i=1}^{k} \sum_{j=1}^{n_i} (x_{ij} - \bar{x}_i)^2 + \sum_{i=1}^{k} n_i (\bar{x}_i - \bar{x})^2$$

where (1) x_{ij} denotes the jth reading in the ith group, there being k distinct and independent groups.

(2) $\bar{x}$ is the general mean of all groups combined.

(3) $\bar{x}_i$ is the mean of the ith group only.

The first term on the right,

$$\sum_{i=1}^{k} \sum_{j=1}^{n_i} (x_{ij} - \bar{x}_i)^2$$

is a measure of the variability of the observations within each group about the group means $\bar{x}_i$. The second term is a measure of the variability of the group or treatment averages $\bar{x}_i$ about the general mean $\bar{x}$. The division of each of these terms by their respective degrees of freedom yields the two 'mean squares' which are independent estimates of the population variance if the treatments exert no effect. The d.f. are given by $n - k$ and $k - 1$ respectively, where n is the total number of observations and k is the number of different treatments tried; n_i equals the number of subjects on the ith treatment.

The 'treatment' mean square,

$$\frac{1}{(k-1)} \sum_{i=1}^{k} n_i (\bar{x}_i - \bar{x})^2,$$

will be increased if the treatments are exerting an effect on the measurements. Compared with the 'error' mean square,

$$\frac{1}{(n-k)} \sum_{i=1}^{k} \sum_{j=1}^{n_i} (x_{ij} - \bar{x}_i)^2,$$

the treatment mean square will tend to be much larger if the treatments are exerting an effect, but not otherwise.

The calculations are straightforward. For each group (i.e. treatment) compute the sum and the sum of squares, recording these sums. Next total both the treatment sums and the treatment sums of squares. A worked example follows using the weights of mice on the four treatments as given in Table A1.17.

Weights	A	B	C	D	Total
Sample size	$10 = n_1$	$10 = n_2$	$10 = n_3$	$10 = n_4$	$40 = n$
Sum	$336.7 = T_1$	$328.5 = T_2$	$329.0 = T_3$	$325.3 = T_4$	$1319.5 = T$
Group average	33.7	32.9	32.9	32.5	
Sum of squares	11414.59	10837.31	10874.22	10650.45	43776.57

Then the left-hand expression $\Sigma\Sigma(x_{ij}-\bar{x})^2 = \Sigma\Sigma x_{ij}{}^2 - \dfrac{T^2}{n}$

$$= 43776.57 - \frac{(1319.5)^2}{40}$$

$$= 249.56.$$

The second right-hand term, $\displaystyle\sum_{i=1}^{k} n_i(\bar{x}_i - \bar{x})^2$

$$= \sum_{i=1}^{k} \frac{T_i{}^2}{n_i} - \frac{T^2}{n}$$

$$= \frac{(336.7)^2}{10} + \frac{(328.5)^2}{10} + \frac{(329.0)^2}{10} + \frac{(325.3)^2}{10} = \frac{(1319.5)^2}{40}$$

$$= 7.02.$$

The difference between these two values (subject to no arithmetical errors) equals the first right-hand term, $\Sigma\Sigma(x_{ij}-\bar{x}_i)^2$

$$= 249.56 - 7.02 = 242.54.$$

Finally we set up the following table:

Source of variation	d.f.	Sums of squares about means	Mean square	
Treatment	3	7.02	$\dfrac{7.02}{3} = 2.34$	$F = \dfrac{6.74}{2.34} = 2.88$
Error	36	242.54	$\dfrac{242.54}{36} = 6.74$	
Total	39	249.56		

F has d.f. (36;3), so that $F = 2\cdot88$ is not significant. This confirms the impression that the four groups of mice are comparable with regard to their weight. In this example the treatment mean square is less than the error mean square which is rather unusual. On theoretical grounds the expected value of the treatment mean square should either equal or exceed the error mean square. Had the treatment mean square been significantly less than the error mean square we would question the assumption of randomness in the experiment. In fact we might then have suspected that the mice had been carefully selected for group allocation in such a way as to ensure a similar average weight for each group. To analyse the titre values, we carried out a similar analysis as for the weights, using log (titre) instead of the actual titre results. The arithmetical results are given below:

Log (titre)	A	B	C	D	Total
Sample size	$10 = n_1$	$8 = n_2$	$10 = n_3$	$8 = n_4$	$n = 36$
Sum	$28\cdot9647 = T_1$	$27\cdot8677 = T_2$	$27\cdot4595 = T_3$	$16\cdot1278 = T_4$	$100\cdot4197 = T$
Group average	$2\cdot90$	$3\cdot48$	$2\cdot75$	$2\cdot02$	
Sum of squares	$85\cdot8980$	$97\cdot7556$	$78\cdot9910$	$36\cdot6703$	$299\cdot3149$

$$\sum_{i=1}^{k} \sum_{j=1}^{n_i} (y_{ij} - \bar{y})^2 = \Sigma\Sigma y_{ij}^2 - \frac{T^2}{n} = 299\cdot3149 - \frac{(100\cdot4197)^2}{36} = 19\cdot2006.$$

$$\sum_{i=1}^{k} n_i (\bar{y}_i - \bar{y})^2 = \sum_{i=1}^{k} \frac{T_i^2}{n_i} - \frac{T^2}{n}$$

$$= \frac{(28\cdot9647)^2}{10} + \frac{(27\cdot8680)^2}{8} + \frac{(27\cdot4595)^2}{10} + \frac{(16\cdot1278)^2}{8} - \frac{(100\cdot4197)^2}{36} = 8\cdot7727.$$

Finally:

Source of variation	d.f.	Sum of squares about means	Mean squares	
Treatment	3	$8\cdot7727$	$\dfrac{8\cdot7727}{3} = 2\cdot9244$	$F = \dfrac{2\cdot9242}{0\cdot3258} = 8\cdot975$
Error	32	$10\cdot4279$	$\dfrac{10\cdot4279}{32} = 0\cdot3258$	
Total	35	$19\cdot2006$		

With d.f. (3;32) an F-value of $8\cdot975$ is significant at the $0\cdot1$ per cent level, in fact $P(F > 6\cdot94) = 0\cdot001$. The average of $3\cdot48$ for group B exceeds the means of the other treatments although it is not the highest dose group. It was observed that all mice in this group developed an abscess at the site of injection, suggesting contamination of the ovalbumin. It is conjectured that the unexpectedly high 'mean of log (titre)' for this group is due both to dose strength and to a 'contamination' effect.

The high mean value for group B raises the further question whether dose differences on their own can change the average log (titre) value, i.e. do groups A, C and D differ significantly. To answer this question we repeated the analysis on groups A, C and D, omitting group B.

Log (titre)	A	C	D	Total
Sample size	10	10	8	28
Sum	28·9647	27·4595	16·1278	72·5520
Sum of square	85·8980	78·9910	36·6703	201·5593

$$\sum_{i=1}^{k} \sum_{j=1}^{n_i} (y_{ij} - \bar{y})^2 = 201\ 5593 - \frac{(72\cdot5520)^2}{28} = 13\cdot5667$$

$$\sum_{i=1}^{k} n_i (\bar{y}_i - \bar{y})^2 = \frac{(28\cdot9647)^2}{10} + \frac{(27\cdot4595)^2}{10} + \frac{(16\cdot1278)^2}{8} - \frac{(72\cdot5520)^2}{28}$$

$$= 3\cdot8184.$$

Source of variation	d.f.	Sum of squares about means	Means squares	
Treatments	2	3·8184	$\dfrac{3\cdot8184}{2} = 1\cdot9092$	$F = \dfrac{1\cdot9092}{0\cdot3900} = 4\cdot895$
Error	25	9·7483	$\dfrac{9\cdot7483}{25} = 0\cdot3900$	
Total	27	13·5667		

From the F-tables, for d.f. (2;25):

$$P(F \geqslant 4\cdot29) = 0\cdot025; \quad P(F \geqslant 5\cdot57) = 0\cdot01$$

The result, $F = 4\cdot895$, is therefore significant at the $2\frac{1}{2}$ per cent level. Various doses of ovalbumin do appear to exert a differential effect on the titre values. (If the log (titre) results are significantly different for the groups A, C and D, so too are the actual titre results.)

The above method of analysis is often referred to as the one-way analysis of variance. Like any statistical technique it requires that certain conditions are met before it can be validly applied. These are the same as for the t-test, and the comments made in that section are equally pertinent here. There are, as before, three conditions:

(a) All observations and samples are independent.
(b) The readings in each sample are normally distributed, but need not have the same mean.
(c) The variances of the observations from each sample are equal.

This last condition is equivalent to assuming that if the various treatments exert an effect, this expresses itself by raising or lowering the value of the readings, i.e. it affects the average but leaves the variance unaffected.

One final condition should be stressed as it is frequently required both in such simple experimental designs as the above and in more complicated designs, i.e. the subjects must be randomly allocated to their treatments. Matching or other procedures to ensure maximum comparability of subjects on the various treatments is considered for this purpose as part of the experimental method. However, sets of comparable subjects having been selected, the allocation of these subjects to the various treatments must be done randomly. Considering the ease with which randomization can be ensured in most laboratory situations, it is rather surprising to find this aspect of the experiment frequently neglected. All too often it is considered adequate to remove from the nearest cage the first animal unable to escape our grasp.

Regression analysis
Frequently both a change in treatment and reactions to the change can be expressed numerically. For instance, if the only change from experiment to experiment is a change of concentration or dose, then these changes are expressed numerically. If the corresponding response or reaction to these treatment changes can also be measured and expressed numerically, then the results of each trial can be plotted on a graph. The 'curve' traced out by changes in response value as the treatment alters is of considerable interest. Estimates of the mathematical equation representing this curve can sometimes be found, particularly if the number of different treatment levels is large and the response curve is of a simple mathematical type, e.g. a straight line, an exponential curve, a quadratic etc. Even if the response can be expressed only as a percentage, e.g. percentage of flies surviving a given concentration of DDT, it is quite in order, and usually very helpful, to plot these percentages against treatment level to show the change in percentage in relation to changes in treatment value.

The response curve as shown in Fig. A1.9 is sigmoidal and is probably difficult to fit in its entirety. But such a curve can readily be approximated by a straight line for the carrageenin dose range 0·45 to 1·3 μg. This fitted straight line (fitted admittedly over only a section of the response curve) can be used by means of 'probit analysis' to determine fairly accurately the carrageenin dose at which the per cent lysis is 50 per cent (or some other required per cent lysis between about 25 and 75 per cent). For details of this method see Finney [1].

If the same subject, or sample of subjects, is exposed to the various levels of treatment on different occasions, the resulting response curve passes through points which may, or may not, be independent. If, however, each subject is treated once only the results are sure to be independent. In the latter method the evaluation of the results is statistically simpler and the

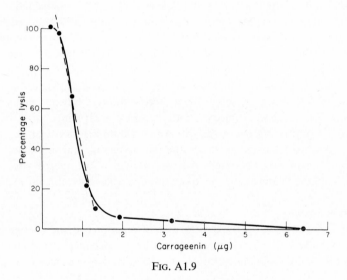

FIG. A1.9

procedures more firmly established. The most straightforward case occurs when the response curve is linear, or can be made so by a suitable transformation, and passes through stochastically independent observations.

An example of a linear regression line passing through independent observations is given in Table A.18*. This data relates the X-ray 'opaqueness' as measured in radiodens (radio-density)† to the ash content of the X-rayed bone. The experiment arose out of an attempt to measure the calcium content to detect possible calcium changes in the bone by utilizing the patient's

* Unpublished data by Dr J.Chalmers, Dept. of Orthopaedic Surgery, University of Edinburgh.

† Radio-density—using a wedge containing a 100 per cent weight by volume solution of dipotassium hydrogen phosphate as a standard, the radio-density unit quoted is the thickness of that wedge which produces blackening on a wrist X-ray equal to that at the lower end of the radius.

radioden value. In this experiment, the wrist bone of twenty-one cadavers was X-rayed under water and the ash content subsequently determined chemically.

TABLE A.1.18

X radiodens (cm)	Y ash (g)
4·3	0·64
5·9	0·76
3·3	0·45
4·4	0·69
5·6	0·75
4·3	0·60
2·6	0·45
5·2	0·77
5·4	0·82
4·1	0·63
4·4	0·60
4·3	0·54
2·5	0·38
4·7	0·54
3·1	0·49
5·5	0·83
3·8	0·66
6·0	0·82
4·7	0·74
2·6	0·53
4·7	0·76

The computations are fairly straightforward.

Compute: $\Sigma X = 91\cdot4$; $\quad\quad \Sigma Y = 13\cdot45$

$\quad\quad\quad\quad \Sigma X^2 = 420\cdot60$; $\quad \Sigma Y^2 = 8\cdot9837$.

Mean $X = \bar{X} = 4\cdot35$

Mean $Y = \bar{Y} = 0\cdot640$.

We also require the 'sum of cross-products', i.e. the product of the radioden value and the corresponding ash content for each subject. It was found to be:

$$\Sigma XY = 61\cdot112.$$

Since a knowledge of the variances involved and of the correlation coefficient between radioden and ash content is useful, these quantities might just as well be computed first and then used to fit the line to the data.

Appendixes

$$S^2(x) = \frac{1}{N-1}\left(\Sigma X^2 - \frac{(\Sigma X)^2}{N}\right) = 1 \cdot 140$$

$$S^2(y) = \frac{1}{N-1}\left(\Sigma Y^2 - \frac{(\Sigma Y)^2}{N}\right) = 0 \cdot 1847.$$

$$\text{Covariance }(X, Y) = \frac{1}{N-1}\left(\Sigma XY - \frac{(\Sigma X)(\Sigma Y)}{N}\right) = 0 \cdot 1286.$$

The correlation coefficient =

$$r = \frac{\text{Covariance}(XY)}{S(x) \cdot S(y)} = 0 \cdot 886,$$

where $S(x) = \sqrt{S(x)^2}$ and similarly for $S(y)$.

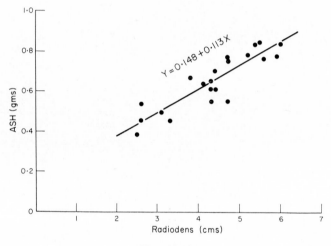

FIG. A1.10

This is rather a high value for a correlation since r is restricted mathematically to lie within the range -1 to $+1$.

The equation of the 'regression line' as shown in the 'scatter diagram', Fig. A.10, is:

$$Y = A + BX$$

$$\text{where } B = \frac{\text{Covariance }(X, Y)}{S^2(x)} = \frac{0 \cdot 1286}{1 \cdot 140} = 0 \cdot 113$$

$$\text{and } A = \overline{Y} - B\overline{X} = 0 \cdot 148.$$

Thus the estimated equation 'best' fitting the experimental points as given in Fig. A.10 is:

$$Y = 0{\cdot}148 + 0{\cdot}113X.$$

Two points ought to be emphasized:

(a) Despite the strong positive correlation indicating that a high radioden value is associated in general with a high ash content, the prediction of ash content when the radioden value is known cannot be very precise. This is clearly indicated in the scatter diagram, Fig. A1.10, showing how wide is the spread of points about the line.

(b) In the fitting of a regression line, the value to be predicted must be denoted by Y and the 'known' or directly measured quantity by X. In the above examples the line would be used to predict ash or Ca content (Y) for patients whose radioden (X) value was known from an X-ray reading.

The estimated slope B of the line is subject to random sampling fluctuations as is any other constant computed from sample results. If the line were really horizontal, i.e. had zero slope, then the response would be insensitive to treatment changes. The estimated variance of the computed sample slope B is given by the expression

$$\frac{S^2(y)(1-r^2)}{S^2(x)(n-2)} = \frac{0{\cdot}1847(1-0{\cdot}886^2)}{1{\cdot}140(19)} = 0{\cdot}001833 = S_B^2.$$

To test whether the computed sample slope B is significantly different from zero, we calculate:

$$t = \frac{B}{S_B}, \text{ with } (n-2) \text{ degrees of freedom}$$

$$= \frac{0{\cdot}113}{\sqrt{0{\cdot}001833}} = 2{\cdot}579.$$

The t-tables with 19 d.f. at the 2 per cent level give the critical value: 2·539. As the slope of the regression line appears not to be zero, a genuine relationship between radioden and ash content is indicated.

To return to the ovalbumin injection experiment, Table A1.17—it is easy to be wise after the event, but the result of the experiment shows that a more decisive result would probably have been obtained if the experiment had been planned with regression analysis in mind. The following is one of many possible designs that could have been used.

Having chosen eight levels, randomly allocate five subjects to each level, thus using the same numbers of subjects as previously. Since there is a chance that the relationship between log (titre) and log (dose) is a simple one, possibly even linear as a first approximation over the range of dose levels considered, there is some arithmetical advantage in taking the dose levels a geometric progression. This is so since the logarithms of the term of a geometric progression are equally spaced from each other. If approximately the range previously used is kept, suitable values to use are: 10, 20, 40, ..., 1280, μg, eight in all.

The computations are illustrated by fitting a straight line to the data of Table A1.17, but it must be emphasized that fitting any curve, even a straight line, to only four points is not a very securely based procedure. Moreover, the unexplained high antibody level for group B raises doubts as to the linearity of the relationship. For the sake of computational illustration, these difficulties are ignored. A 'typical' regression computation lay-out is given below:

Group	x = log (dose)	n = sample size	y = total of log (titre)	nx	nx²	xy
A	3·124	10	28·96	31·24	97·59	90·47
B	2·301	8	27·87	18·41	42·36	64·06
C	1·301	10	27·46	13·01	16·93	35·78
D	0·301	8	16·13	2·41	0·72	4·86
		36	100·42	65·07	157·60	195·17

$$\bar{x} = \frac{65·07}{36} = 1·81; \quad \Sigma x = 65·07$$

$$\Sigma y = 100·42$$

$$\bar{y} = \frac{100·42}{36} = 2·79; \quad \Sigma xy = 195·17$$

$$\Sigma x^2 = 157·60.$$

We assume the regression equation is of the form $Y = A + BX$, where

$$X = \log (\text{dose})$$
$$Y = \log (\text{titre}).$$

A and B are of course constants whose value is to be estimated from the sample results by means of the calculations given above.

$$B = \frac{\Sigma xy - \bar{x}\Sigma y}{\Sigma x^2 - \bar{x}\Sigma x} = \frac{195·17 - 1·81 (100·42)}{157·60 - 1·81 (65·07)} = 0·342$$

and
$$A = \bar{y} - B\bar{x} = 2·17.$$

Hence the estimated regression line of Y on X is: $Y = 2·17 + 0·342X$.

The regression line is shown in Fig. A1.11.

We would emphasize again that the high value of group B throws some doubts on the assumption that the relationship between log (titre) and log (dose) as assumed in the regression analysis, is linear. Had more dose levels and fewer subjects per level been employed, this point would undoubtedly have been clarified.

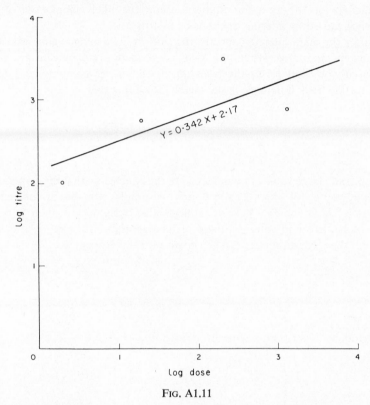

FIG. A1.11

Confidence limits

Tests of significance perform an invaluable service in that they enable us to judge when the observed disagreement of results can no longer be attributed solely to random errors. They serve as an alert to show when the biologist is almost certainly on to some genuine effect or response brought about by changed conditions or by an experiment.

Yet in another sense, a significance test begs the question: If the observed difference cannot reasonably be explained by random fluctuations, how large is this difference? The observed difference, whether in the means, the variances or some other statistic, is derived from sample results. These observed differences will vary with each repetition of the experiment. Hence, no single observed difference can be taken as a true or reliable measure of the shift in value brought about by a change of method or treatment. On this and related questions, the formal tests of significance give no direct answers. Fortunately, a little extra arithmetic, using the computational results of the significance test, enables us to say a fair amount about the likely magnitude of the difference caused by altering methods or treatments.

Usually the main interest concerns the shift in the average value following a change in conditions. When only two independent sample means are being compared, the t-test forms the basis on which we can compute confidence limits for the 'real' difference in the means. Recalling that

$$t = \frac{\bar{x}_1 - \bar{x}_2}{S\sqrt{\dfrac{1}{n_1} + \dfrac{1}{n_2}}}; \quad \text{d.f.} = n_1 + n_2 - 2,$$

a significantly large value of t would lead to the conclusion that the population means μ_1 and μ_2, of which $\bar{x}_1$ and $\bar{x}_2$ are the sample estimates, are not equal. Let $\mu_1 - \mu_2 = D$ and $\bar{x}_1 - \bar{x}_2 = d$. If the t-value is significant, then D is unlikely to be zero and some estimate of its magnitude is therefore desirable.

Under these conditions, it can be shown that the expression

$$\frac{D - d}{S\sqrt{\dfrac{1}{n_1} + \dfrac{1}{n_2}}}$$

has a students' distribution with d.f. equal to $n_1 + n_2 - 2$.

Hence
$$P\left\{ -t_{(0\cdot95)} \leqslant \frac{D - d}{S\sqrt{\dfrac{1}{n_1} + \dfrac{1}{n_2}}} \leqslant t_{(0\cdot95)} \right\} = 0\cdot95$$

and
$$P\left\{ -t_{(0\cdot99)} \leqslant \frac{D - d}{S\sqrt{\dfrac{1}{n_1} + \dfrac{1}{n_2}}} \leqslant t_{(0\cdot99)} \right\} = 0\cdot99.$$

A little algebra shows that:

$$d - t_{(0\cdot95)}\, S\sqrt{\frac{1}{n_1} + \frac{1}{n_2}} \leqslant D \leqslant d + t_{(0\cdot95)}\, S\sqrt{\frac{1}{n_1} + \frac{1}{n_2}}$$

with a probability equal to 0·95. A similar result holds if we use $t_{(0·99)}$ or any other convenient $t_{(\alpha)}$ value.

The lower limit,

$$d - t_{(0·95)} \cdot S \sqrt{\frac{1}{n_1} + \frac{1}{n_2}}$$

and the upper limit,

$$d + t_{(0·95)} \cdot S \sqrt{\frac{1}{n_1} + \frac{1}{n_2}}$$

define the '95 per cent confidence interval' for the real difference D. Such an interval can always be computed whenever the t-test is applicable. D is of course considered as a population constant, but the values of the upper and lower limits as computed from the samples are subject to random fluctuations. On average in only one in twenty cases do we expect the computed '95 per cent confidence interval' not to cover or overlap D. If the '99 per cent confidence interval' were computed instead, the interval would be large but our confidence that this interval overlaps the unknown D would be increased to 0·99, i.e. there is a probability of 0·01 that the computed interval is so far out as not to cover the unknown D. Even when the t-test turns out to be non-significant, it may be useful to compute the upper and lower 'confidence limits' of D. In this case, the lower value will be negative and the upper value positive, thus enclosing the origin or zero point. These limits serve to remind us that μ_1 and μ_2 might not really be identical despite the non-significant t-value. Moreover, these limits give a good indication of the magnitude of the difference should $D = \mu_1 - \mu_2$ not be zero.

To refer to the data in Table A.10, the mean difference in bacterial count between the spread plate and pour plate methods was found to be significant. An estimate of the magnitude of the 'underestimate' given by the spread plate method can be found using the above formula.

$$d = 409·0 - 442·3 = -33·3; \quad S = \sqrt{254·1} \text{ (see page 1177).}$$

Hence
$$S\sqrt{\tfrac{1}{10} + \tfrac{1}{10}} = 7·13$$

$$t_{(0·95)} = 2·1009; \quad \text{d.f.} = 18.$$

Hence
$$d - t_{(0·95)} S\sqrt{\tfrac{1}{10} + \tfrac{1}{10}} = -48·3$$

$$d + t_{(0·95)} S\sqrt{\tfrac{1}{10} + \tfrac{1}{10}} = -18·3.$$

The claim that $-48·3 \leqslant D \leqslant -18·3$ can be made with '95 per cent confidence', i.e. the probability of this computed range not overlapping the true difference in the mean values of these two bacterial count methods is only

0·05. Had we used $t_{(0·99)}$ instead of $t_{(0·95)}$ the range would have been: $-58·3$ to $-12·8$.

This is, of course, longer than the previous 95 per cent confidence interval, but our 'confidence' that $\mu_1 - \mu_2 = D$ does not have a value lying outside the above range has increased. The probability of D having a value not covered by $-58·3$ to $-12·8$ is reduced to 0·01. It should be noted how wide are both the 95 per cent and the 99 per cent confidence limits. The two samples, each of size ten, were quite adequate to decide that the spread plate method 'underestimates' the bacterial count and cannot be considered an 'equivalent method' to the pour plate method. Yet the samples are too small to enable the average difference in these two counting procedures to be estimated with any precision.

A slightly different problem arises when the analysis of variance leads to a 'significant' result. Clearly one or more of the averages are not in agreement with the rest.

Often the set of sample means is not sufficiently heterogeneous to allow groups of similar means to be picked out with any confidence from the whole set.

The Tukey or the Scheffe 'Method for Multiple Comparisons' can be used to test whether any subgroup of means is significantly different from the remaining averages of the set. Readers interested in following up these two useful techniques are referred to Geunther [4].

Finally, we append a list of texts written for the non-statistician, none of which are very mathematical. It is hoped that these may be of assistance to biologists working without the aid of a statistician.

References

[1] FINNEY D.J. (1964) *Statistical Method in Biological Assay*, 2nd edition. Charles Griffis & Co. Ltd
[2] FISHER & YATES *Statistical Tables for Biological, Agricultural and Medical Research.* Oliver & Boyd
[3] *Scientific Tables—Documenta Geigy*, 6th edition (1962). Manchester: Geigy Pharmaceutical Co. Ltd
[4] GEUNTHER, WILLIAM C. (1964) *Analysis of Variance.* New York: Prentice Hall
[5] MAXWELL A.E. (1961) *Analysing Qualitative Data.* Methuen & Co.
[6] SIMPSON G.G., ROE A. & LAVENTIN R.C. (1960) *Qualitative Zoology.* New York: Harcourt, Bruce & Co.
[7] SNEDECAR, GEORGE W. (1965) *Statistical Methods*, Seventh Printing, 5th edition. The Iowa State University Press
[8] SEGEL S. (1956) *Non-parametric Statistics.* McGraw-Hill Book Co.
[9] STANWORTH D.R. & KULRO W.J. (1965) *Immunology* **8**, 323
[10] WEIR D.M. (1963) Liver autoantibodies in the rat. *Immunology* **6**, 581
[11] WILLIAMS E.J. (1959) *Regression Analysis.* New York: John Wiley & Sons.

Methods for the Preparation of Water-in-oil, and Multiple, Emulsions for Use as Antigen Adjuvants; and Notes on their Use in Immunization Procedures.

W.J.HERBERT

Introduction

The researches of the late Jules Freund rekindled the interest of immunologists in emulsions of water in mineral-oil and showed that they act as most efficient adjuvants to an antigen incorporated in the dispersed (water) phase. A single injection of a vaccine prepared in this way stimulates a high and remarkably long-lasting antibody response [1, 2, 3]. Antigen has been detected in the emulsion depot up to 544 days after inoculation and the adjuvant activity appears to be due to slow release of the antigen, for which emulsions of this type are ideally suited [3, 4]. If dead mycobacteria are added to the continuous (oil) phase, guinea-pigs produce an additional type of antibody [5] and the development of the hypersensitive state is potentiated [6, 7].

To achieve a stable mixture of water and mineral oil in the form of a water-in-oil emulsion, it is necessary to have a stabilizer present which is capable of promoting an emulsion of this type. Emulsifiers such as lanolin [8], the ointment bases 'Aquaphor' [9] and 'Falba' [10] have been used but, since the investigations of Salk, Laurent & Bailey [11], it is now usual to employ one of the sorbitan emulsifiers. A highly purified and non-toxic one of these is known as 'Arlacel A', an emulsifier which has been used safely in vaccines given to man [2, 12].

Water-in-oil emulsions are highly viscous and consequently are difficult to manipulate and inject. It has, however, been found possible to overcome this difficulty by re-emulsifying water-in-oil emulsions in a further water phase, thus producing multiple (or double) emulsions [13]. These are free-flowing, milk-like liquids which have an adjuvant action equivalent to that of the classical water-in-oil emulsions. Additionally they are very stable, remaining in good condition for much longer periods than the water-in-oil emulsions from which they are made, and being less prone to break-down when subjected to repeated temperature changes.

Emulsions, particularly those of the water-in-oil type, are notoriously difficult to prepare. The earliest adjuvant emulsions were prepared by mixing the materials in a mortar [8, 14], but recycling through a syringe [15] or a vibratory shaker can also be used [16], and a system employing two syringes coupled with a double-hubbed needle has been described [17]. If available, mechanical emulsifiers of the Silverson rotary type* [18, 19] are very convenient to use, and models can be obtained which are suitable for volumes of a few millilitres, or for several litres. Powerful machines of the piston type† [20] are very efficient, but these are most suitable for use with large quantities of material, say over 100 ml.

In many immunological experimental procedures, the supply of antigen may be limited, and only a small quantity of the adjuvant emulsion is required. A method is described here which is suitable for the preparation of small (2–5 ml) volumes of emulsified vaccine. This method may also be used as the first stage of a process suitable for the preparation of larger quantities of vaccine with the aid of a cheap and readily available emulsifying machine.

Methods

Water-in-oil emulsions

Light liquid paraffin (Manchester Refinery (Sales) Ltd, London) or Drakeol 6VR (Pennsylvania Refining Co., Butler, Pennsylvania) is mixed with Arlacel A (Atlas Chemical Industries, Wilmington, Delaware; Honeywill & Stein, Carshalton, Surrey) in the ratio 9 parts of oil to 1 part of emulsifier. The mixture can be made up either by weight or volume; Arlacel A is a very viscous liquid and it is usually more convenient to weigh it out rather than to use a pipette. The two liquids are well mixed and then sterilized by Seitz filtration. They should not be autoclaved as heating may cause them to become toxic. The sterile mixture may safely be stored frozen at $-20°$ C for a year or more, but if it is kept at room temperature it should be used within a few weeks of preparation, for its emulsifying capacity deteriorates with time. The use of mixtures made up in a ratio other than 9 to 1 has not been found to be advantageous, even with materials found difficult to emulsify properly.

The antigen to be used is dissolved in physiological saline or in distilled water, concentrations of protein antigens up to 100 mg per ml usually producing stable emulsions. Materials such as whole serum may have to be diluted to at least 1 in 64 with physiological saline before a stable emulsion can be obtained, due to their high electrolyte content.

Equal volumes of the oil-emulsifier mixture and of the antigen solution are put in two immunologically clean, dry, sterile, wide-mouthed, screw-capped,

---

* Silverson Machines Ltd, London.

† T. Giusti & Son Ltd, London; Omerod Engineers Ltd, Rochdale, England.

glass bottles of suitable size. 'Universal' containers are suitable for volumes of finished vaccine up to 20 ml; 5 ml 'Bijou' bottles may be used for smaller quantities [21].

Using a disposable 2 ml or 5 ml syringe and a fine-bore (0·5 mm) needle, a small volume of the antigen solution is taken up and, with the point of the needle held below the surface of the oil, injected *vigorously* into it. The quantity injected is such that the whole volume of the antigen solution is added to the oil in five to ten stages. Between each addition the bottle is capped and shaken. This should result in the production of a coarse water-in-oil emulsion. On standing for a few minutes no accumulation of the water phase should be seen at the bottom of the bottle. If any does appear, it may be taken up with the syringe and reinjected into the oily layer. Disposable syringes are used for this process in preference to glass ones as it is difficult to remove all traces of oil from the latter after use. Disposable syringes may, however, have been lubricated with silicone oils and detergents which could be inimical to the preparation of stable emulsions [22].

The stability and the duration of immunological activity of an emulsion prepared in this way is greatly improved by breaking up the water phase into very small droplets under 1 μ in diameter. If only a small volume of vaccine is to be prepared, the dispersion of the water phase may be increased by repeatedly taking the emulsion up in the syringe, either without a needle, or using one of large bore, and then ejecting it through a smaller-bore needle. As the dispersion increases, the emulsion becomes much more viscous so that relatively large needles may have to be used. Otherwise an excessive force may have to be applied to the syringe which may cause it to fracture. Recycling the emulsion through a syringe in this way is hard work, syringes sometimes collapse, it is difficult to maintain sterility, and the product is unevenly emulsified.

The use of a more powerful mechanical emulsifier is to be preferred, but as the use of this may involve the loss of up to 5 ml of emulsion, which irretrievably coats the surfaces of the machine, it is only suitable where rather larger volumes of vaccine are being prepared. The ordinary 'Bel' kitchen cream-maker (Royston (Bel) Sales, Erith, Kent) can readily be modified, as shown in Fig. A2.1, to handle sterile material. Three of the four holes at the bottom of the barrel are closed off with screwed plugs and soldered. A brass or copper 'funnel' is then attached to the side of the cylinder to envelope the remaining hole so that fluid can be drawn into the cylinder without coming in contact with the plastic bowl which cannot conveniently be sterilized. The 'funnel' is extended upwards, as shown, to encircle the top of the barrel; in this way any emulsion which leaks past the piston is not lost but is returned to the barrel. Finally, the mixing or stirring ring (not shown in Fig. A2.1), which is found attached to the piston lever, is removed. All parts of the machine which come into contact with the emulsion can now readily be dismantled and sterilized in an autoclave.

Assembly of the sterile emulsifier must be accomplished without contaminating the parts which will come in contact with the emulsion. The plastic cup is held in a stand by a clamp round the base. The barrel is fitted into it and the nut which holds it is tightened by hand. The emulsifying valve

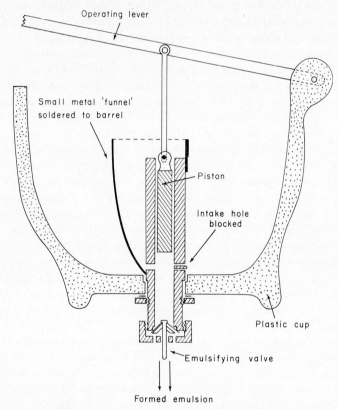

FIG. A2.1. Diagrammatic cross-section though modified 'Bel' emulsifier used to prepare water-in-oil and multiple emulsions.

is assembled with sterile forceps and placed in position, being tightened and adjusted with forceps, a protected hand, or sterile spanner. Experience with the machine is necessary to judge the correct tightness of the valve but usually it requires to be screwed up firmly. Emulsion which has already been prepared by the syringe method is then poured into the funnel and forced through the valve into a sterile bottle below by working the piston lever.

A single pass is usually sufficient to produce a good emulsion of medium viscosity.

After preparation, by syringe alone, or with the aid of the machine, all water-in-oil emulsions should be checked by allowing a few drops to fall into a beaker of cold water. The first drop often spreads over the surface, but subsequent ones should remain as discrete white drops below the surface, indicating that the water phase containing the antigen is entirely enclosed within the oil. If, on the other hand, the emulsion forms a cloud of tiny particles when dropped into the water it is an oil-in-water emulsion. Emulsions of this type are ineffective as adjuvants [23].

Multiple (double) emulsions
A multiple emulsion is prepared from a water-in-oil emulsion, preferably one with a well dispersed water phase made with the aid of an emulsifying machine. An equal volume of a sterile 2 per cent solution of Tween 80 (Atlas Chemical Industries, Wilmington, Delaware; Honeywill & Stein, Carshalton, Surrey) in physiological saline is added to the emulsion and the whole well shaken by hand. The mixture is then fed into the modified 'Bel' emulsifier, the valve of which has been slackened slightly. If this machine has been used to prepare the original water-in-oil emulsion there is no need to clean it of remaining emulsion before the second emulsification, though allowance should be made for the volume of emulsion still adherent to its parts. If the valve has been correctly set, a single pass through the machine is usually sufficient to produce a multiple emulsion whose primary disperse phase droplets are 5–10 μ in diameter. In some cases, however, it may be necessary to pass the emulsion through the machine a second time. Before use, the emulsion is checked under the oil-immersion objective of a microscope to ensure that it is of the correct form, i.e. tiny water droplets within larger oil drops as shown in Fig. A2.2. It is necessary to dilute the emulsion by running a little water in at the edge of the cover-slip before making this observation.

Notes on immunization

The antibody response following a single subcutaneous inoculation of antigen in a water-in-oil emulsion adjuvant does not reach a peak until about the sixtieth day. Thereafter the response may remain at a constant 'plateau' level for a year or more [3, 23]. During this period a subcutaneous second inoculation of soluble protein antigen in physiological saline alone will stimulate a strong secondary response [24]. A good secondary response to the antigens of bacteria such as the Enterobacteriacae may, however, only be obtained if the second dose is given intravenously [23].

QQ*

Precipitating sera for use in double-diffusion tests, etc., should be collected from immunized animals 5–7 days after a booster inoculation (without adjuvant) has been given at the peak of the antibody response 2 months after the initial inoculation. Booster doses given during the first 20 days may be ineffective in increasing the antibody titre [24]. Those given thereafter, but before the peak titre is reached, do increase the antibody response, but not so effectively as those given later. After boosting and collection of serum, the animal may usually be kept for an extended period of time, being similarly inoculated whenever a further supply of serum is required. It is prudent to have adrenalin or antihistamine available to combat shock when this is done. Arthus reactions may also occur and require local treatment.

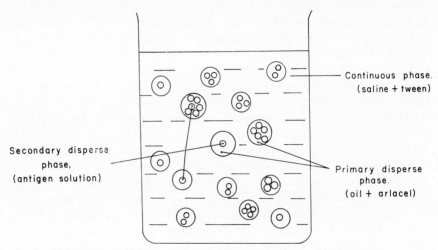

Fig. A2.2. Diagrammatic representation of a multiple emulsion [13].

It is doubtful whether distribution of the original water-in-oil emulsion inoculum, in small quantities, to many sites over the body is advantageous. Injection into the foot-pads is also to be discouraged, especially if myco-bacteria are included in the oil, because of the painful reactions produced. The effectiveness of water-in-oil emulsion adjuvants depends on their ability continually to release the antigen which is locked up by the oil phase. The antigen released must, however, be undegraded and fully antigenic even though it has been kept in saline at body temperature for an extended period of time within the emulsion. In many cases the antigen will not be stable under these conditions, which can be duplicated in an incubator as a check. If the antigen is very labile, immunization may be accomplished by mimicking the action of the emulsion [4]. The antigen is prepared as one batch which is divided into aliquots containing a few microgrammes each and preserved by freezing. One of the aliquots is then inoculated subcutaneously each day into the animal to be immunized for 2 months [25] before a larger secondary inoculation is given and serum collected.

The intramuscular inoculation of water-in-oil emulsions may produce a more rapid, less persistent response. Multiple emulsions can safely be given intravenously to the larger experimental animals, but in mice, administration by this route may be dangerous unless the primary dispersed phase particles are small. The antibody response is very rapid after immunization by the intravenous route and sera should be collected after the first week. Thereafter the titre falls quickly, so that simultaneous inoculation by the subcutaneous and intravenous routes may be useful in some cases to obtain both an early and a persistent response.

References

[1] TALMAGE D.W. & DIXON F.J. (1953) The influence of adjuvants on the elimination of soluble protein antigens and the associated antibody responses. *J. infect. Dis.* **93,** 176–180

[2] HERBERT W.J., SELWYN S. & PHILP J.R. (1965) Field trials of adjuvant and saline influenza vaccines. *Br. J. prev. soc. Med.* **19,** 97–100

[3] HERBERT W.J. (in press) Some investigations into the mode of action of the water-in-mineral-oil emulsion antigen adjuvants. *Progr. immunobiol. Standard.* Basel: Karger

[4] HERBERT W.J. (1966) Antigenicity of soluble protein in the presence of high levels of antibody: A possible mode of action of the antigen adjuvants. *Nature, Lond.* **210,** 747–748

[5] WHITE R.G., JENKINS G.C. & WILKINSON P.C. (1963) The production of skin-sensitizing antibody in the guinea-pig. *Int. Arch. Allergy* **22,** 156

[6] FREUND J., THOMPSON K.J., HOUGH H.B., SOMMER H.E. & PISANI T.M. (1948) Antibody formation and sensitization with the aid of adjuvants. *J. Immunol.* **60,** 383–398

[7] WHITE R.G., COONS A.H. & CONNOLLY J.M. (1955) Studies on antibody production. IV. The role of wax fraction of *Mycobacterium tuberculosis* in adjuvant emulsions on the production of antibody to egg albumin. *J. exp. Med.* **102,** 83–103

[8] LE MOIGNIC & PINOY E. (1916) Les vaccines en emulsion dans le corps gras ou 'lipovaccine'. *C.R. Soc. Biol., Paris* **79,** 201

[9] KABAT E.A., WOLF A. & BEZER A.E. (1947) The rapid production of acute disseminated encephalomyelitis in rhesus monkeys by injection of heterologous and homologous brain tissue with adjuvants. *J. exp. Med.* **85,** 117–129

[10] HALBERT S.P., SMOLENS J. & MUDD S. (1945) Reduced acute toxicity of antigens in saline-in-mineral oil emulsions. *J. Immunol.* **51,** 39–43

[11] SALK J.E., LAURENT A.A.M. & BAILEY M.L. (1951) Direction of research on vaccination against influenza. New studies with immunologic adjuvants. *Amer. J. pub. Health* **41,** 669–677

[12] DAVENPORT F.M. (1961) Applied immunology of mineral oil adjuvants. *J. Allergy* **32,** 177–189

[13] HERBERT W.J. (1965) Multiple emulsions; a new form of mineral-oil antigen adjuvant. *Lancet* **2,** 771

[14] FREUND J. & MCDERMOTT K. (1942) Sensitization to horse serum by means of adjuvants. *Proc. Soc. exp. Biol., N.Y.* **49**, 548–553

[15] FREUND J. & THOMPSON K.J. (1945) A simple rapid technique of preparing water-in-oil emulsions of penicillin, drugs and biologics. *Science* **101**, 468

[16] RAFFEL S. Personal communication

[17] BERLIN B.S. & MCKINNEY R.W. (1958) A simple device for making emulsified vaccines. *J. Lab. clin. Med.* **52**, 657–658

[18] WIBBERLEY K. Personal communication

[19] GANGULI P. Personal communication

[20] HIMMELWEIT F. (1960) Serological responses and clinical reactions to influenza virus vaccines. *Brit. med. J.* **2**, 1690–1694

[21] CRUICKSHANK R. (1965) *Medical Microbiology*, 11th ed., p. 723. Edinburgh: Livingstone

[22] DOWD J.M., EDWARDS E.A., MARTIN C.E., MILLER C.H. & PIERCE W.E. (1965) Large scale trial of adjuvant and aqueous polyvalent influenza vaccines: Short-term side effects and antibody response in a young adult population. *U.S. Naval Medical Research Unit* **4**, 1–29

[23] FREUND J. (1947) Some aspects of active immunization. *Ann. Rev. Microbiol.* **1**, 291–308

[24] HERBERT W.J. (in press) Observations of practical interest in the use of water-in-mineral-oil emulsion antigen adjuvants. *Progr. immunobiol. Standard.* Basel: Karger

[25] Adam K.M.G. Personal communication

Index

1215